Don't Go TO THE Cosmetics Counter Without Me

7th Edition

A unique guide to thousands of skin-care and cosmetic products, plus the latest research on keeping skin beautiful at every age

PAULA BEGOUN

with Bryan Barron

Contributing Author: Bryan Barron
Editors: Sigrid Asmus, John Hopper, Stephanie Parsons, Jill Irwin
Art Direction, Cover Design, and Typography: Erin Smith Bloom, Beginning Press
Printing: RR Donnelley
Research Director: Tama Bruton
Research Assistant: Raizel Druxman

Publisher: Beginning Press
1030 SW 34th Street, Suite A
Renton, Washington 98057

Seventh Edition Printing: January 2008

ISBN-13: 978-1-877988-32-5
ISBN-10: 1-877988-32-4
10 9 8 7 6 5 4 3 2 1

This book is distributed to the United States book trade by:

Publishers Group West
1700 Fourth Street
Berkeley, California 94710
(800) 788-3123

And to the Canadian book trade by:

Raincoast Books Limited
9050 Shaughnessy Street
Vancouver, British Columbia, V6P 6E5 CANADA
(604) 633-5714

And in Australia and New Zealand by:

Peribo Pty Limited
58 Beaumont Road
Mount Kuring-gai NSW 2080 AUSTRALIA
Tel: (02) 9457 0011

BE BETTER INFORMED THAN EVER BEFORE!
WWW.BEAUTYPEDIA.COM

www.Beautypedia.com
Thousands of precise, accurate, and controversial reviews – all online in an easily searchable product database!

Subscribe Today
Subscribers will have exclusive access to over 35,000 product reviews, full ingredient lists of every skin care product reviewed, plus analytical evaluation of cosmetic formulations.

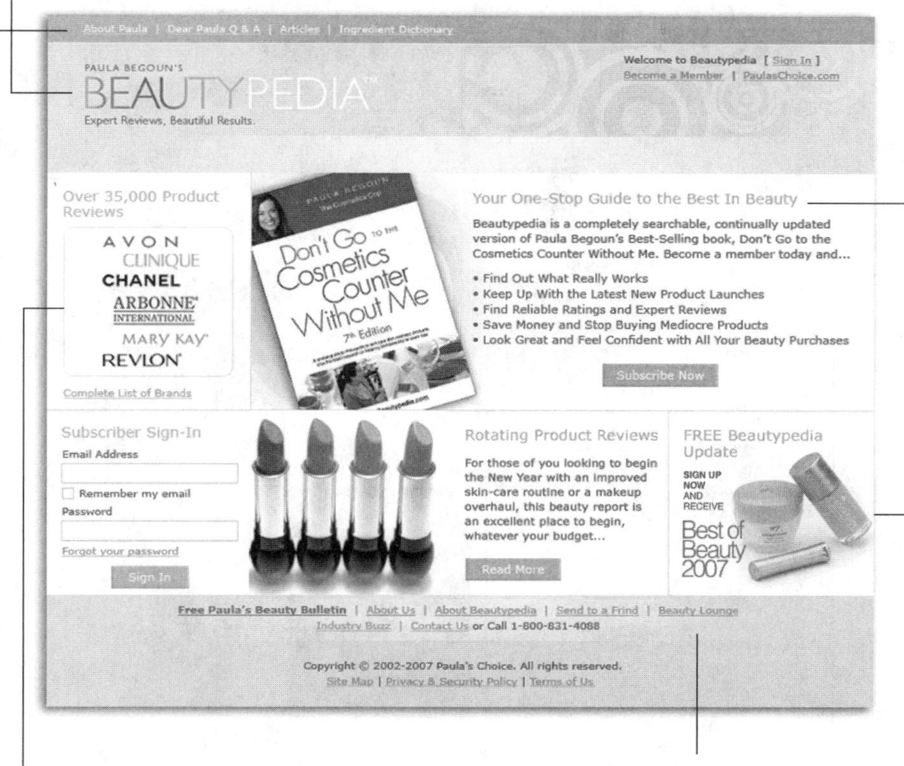

Real Time Updates
New product reviews will be added daily in real time. You will be better informed than ever before!

Community Forum
Subscribers have exclusive access to our "Beauty Lounge" community forum, where you can become part of a growing global network of cosmetics cops!

Free Content
Read Paula's latest articles on skin care, new ingredients, industry controversies, and answers to readers' questions.

Free Email Updates
Want to know what's new on Beautypedia.com? Get the inside scoop by signing up for Paula's free Beautypedia Update.

Stay Updated with Paula's Web Site
www.CosmeticsCop.com

Live Chat
Need help? Our Customer Service Specialists are only a click away. Live Chat is now available 7 days a week. We look forward to chatting with you soon!

FREE email Beauty Bulletins
Sign up for Paula's Beauty Bulletins and stay informed about what's happening in the cosmetics industry. Free product reviews, intriguing special reports, "Dear Paula" Q&As, and more.

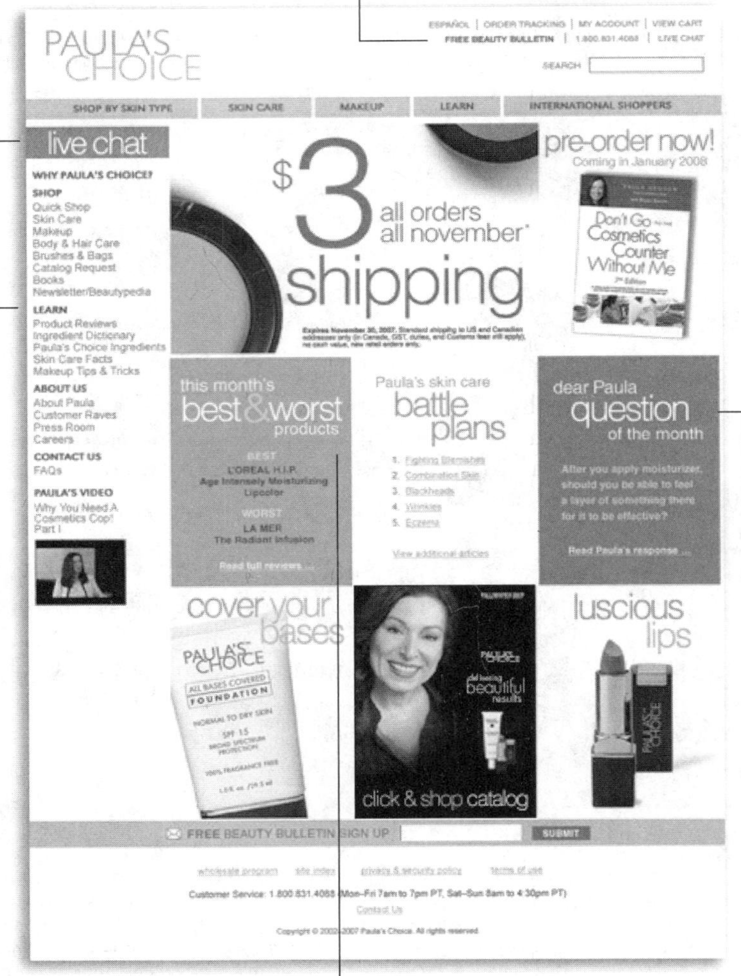

Learn
Find extensive information on how to determine and manage your skin type, sensible battle plans for everything from wrinkles to blemish-fighting, and ingredient updates! Read all about beauty facts and fiction, and pick up expert tips on how to apply makeup to your advantage!

Best & Worst Products
Every month, Paula reviews new products and awards a "best" and "worst" product. Find out if your favorite products meet the Cosmetic Cop's strict criteria!

Dear Paula
Check out the current "Dear Paula" Question of the Month for the latest pressing skin care questions and beauty concerns. Better yet, submit your beauty questions and concerns to Paula today!

FROM THE PUBLISHER

Paula Begoun is the best-selling author of *Don't Go to the Cosmetics Counter Without Me*, *The Beauty Bible*, *Don't Go Shopping for Hair Care Products Without Me*, and *Blue Eyeshadow Should Be Illegal.* She has sold millions of books, educating women about the facts and secrets the beauty industry doesn't want them to know.

Paula is nationally recognized as a consumer advocate, covering the cosmetics and hair-care industries. She is called upon regularly by reporters and producers from television, newspapers, magazines, and radio as a cosmetics industry expert. She has appeared on hundreds of talk shows over the years, including *The View, Dateline NBC, Good Morning America, 20/20, Today, Later Today, CBS Morning News, Hard Copy, Canada AM*, and National Public Radio, and has made more than a dozen appearances on *The Oprah Winfrey Show*. Today, with the success of Paula's web site, www.CosmeticsCop.com, women all over the world consider Paula the most reliable source for straightforward information about all their beauty questions.

In 1996 Ms. Begoun launched her own line of skin-care products, called Paula's Choice. This distinctive line of products, available online at www.paulaschoice.com, is renowned for its effectiveness and affordability. While Paula is proud of her line, she realizes that there are vast numbers of product options for women to consider. As a result, she continues to provide her readers with substantiated and documented studies and analysis about skin-care and makeup products from other lines based on her extensive research and years of experience. The ratings in this edition show as many "happy faces" as "unhappy" and "neutral" ones. In her reviews and critiques, it is clear that Paula continues to maintain her evenhanded approach to offering readers an unprecedented assortment of choices for their cosmetic purchases.

PUBLISHER'S DISCLAIMER

The intent of this book is to present the author's ideas and perceptions about the marketing, selling, and use of cosmetics. The author's sole purpose is to present consumer information and advice regarding the purchase of makeup and skin-care products. The information and recommendations presented strictly reflect the author's opinions, perceptions, and knowledge about the subject and products mentioned. Some women may find success with a particular product that is not recommended or even mentioned in this book, or they may be partial to a skin-care routine Paula has reviewed negatively. It is everyone's unalienable right to judge products by their own criteria and to disagree with the author.

More important, because everyone's skin can, and probably will, react to an external stimulus at some time, any product can cause a negative reaction on skin at one time or another. If you develop skin sensitivity to a cosmetic, stop using it immediately and consult your physician. If you need medical advice about your skin, it is best to consult a dermatologist.

ACKNOWLEDGMENTS

There are no words that can adequately express the challenge and commitment required for writing a book of this scope and nature. The energy and resourcefulness needed to research, compile, review, write, and edit a 1000+ page book is an almost endless undertaking. If it were not for Tama Bruton and Bryan Barron, this book would not have been possible. Their perseverance and devotion to completing the project go beyond anything I could have hoped for. Not only did they meet deadline after deadline, they did it with an accuracy and exactness that exceeded my every expectation. Tama and Bryan bring new meaning to the concepts of proficiency and integrity. I am blessed to have these two people in my life. Without their feedback, patience, and contributions, this book would have been a very good idea but an absolutely unconquerable task.

DEDICATION

This book is dedicated to the Bryan Barron. Bryan has been my research assistant and co-writer for over seven years. His writing style is flawless and his voice seamlessly echoes mine. We are soul-mates residing on some astral plane where writers must dwell. Bryan has also been my right hand, my alter ego, and a steadfast colleague on whom I can rely without hesitation. There is no question that my success is a direct result of his talent, wit, skill, and tenacity. Through it all, Bryan's sense of humor and flexibility has gotten us past many perilous deadlines and cosmetic industry encounters. I can't imagine life without him and it is my deepest prayer I will never have to face that possibility.

CHAPTER ONE

Knowledge Is Beautiful

NEVER SAY NEVER

When I wrote the 6th Edition of this book, I said in the opening chapter that it would be the last one. It was truly my intent to never write another edition of *Don't Go to the Cosmetics Counter Without Me*. As I stated then, after 22 years of writing books about the marvels and chicanery of the cosmetics industry, it felt like I could never possibly write another book. It is still true that I have a love/hate relationship with what I do. The physical burden, time, organization, and research involved in putting together this kind of tome is overwhelming. On the one hand, it is a fascinating experience to create a book that page after page uncovers and reveals the web of secrets, missteps, and duplicity the cosmetics industry spins out of thin air and puts on exhibit for unsuspecting but captivated consumers.

On the other hand, I know that speaking up for reality and honesty in this business is an endless battle that even after thousands of pages, I know I can never win. It's true that I have seen significant changes in the industry, and I honestly believe what I've done is at least partially responsible for some of them, but there are still countless bogus claims being made, substandard products being created, ads fashioned with misleading pictures or empty bravado, and unethical "scientific" research espoused and presented as valid when it is anything but. Perhaps the worst part, though, is knowing that millions and millions of women are seduced by all of it, wasting billions of dollars on hopes and dreams that can never be achieved—at least not the way the industry suggests they can.

It is a struggle to deal with this insanity day in and day out. The frustration sometimes leaves me ranting in my office, my staff listening compassionately and offering their commiseration, and reminding me that my work isn't all for naught. Yet at the end of every book, I never want to see another moisturizer, toner, mascara, cleanser, or lipstick again for as long as I live!

Why did I change my mind? I'm not sure what to say, except that I couldn't help myself. The questions from consumers continue, thousands each month, and my passion for revealing what I know to be true hasn't altered one iota. I also have one of the best research staffs available and their efforts are unrelenting and exacting. Their desire for accuracy and truthfulness is wonderful to be a part of. So I am still the Cosmetics Cop, sharing with you the information you need to make wise decisions about the beauty products you buy.

BEAUTYPEDIA.COM

Don't Go to the Cosmetics Counter Without Me is now online at www.Beautypedia.com (this site can also be accessed from www.cosmeticscop.com). The online version is a subscribable database of this book that will be updated weekly. We will continually be adding new reviews, changing reviews as new research comes to light, updating the ingredient dictionary, and adding articles to let you know what is going on in the world of skin care, dermatology, plastic surgery, and makeup. Beautypedia will be the living version of *Don't Go to the Cosmetics Counter Without Me*, so you won't have to wait for another edition to get current information or lug my book around when shopping for makeup (I know, you're right, it is a really big book!). You can now have a direct, readily available link that you can visit to access the information you need with just a few clicks on your computer!

HOW I BECAME A COSMETICS COP

I often marvel at how I happened into this unusual occupation. It's not as if you can answer an ad for this kind of job, and clearly the cosmetics industry and beauty magazines aren't interested in hiring someone to do what I do. Yet, from the beginning, it was clear that there was a demand from consumers for this kind of information. With over 2 million books sold, I'm certainly glad I gave up my day job working at cosmetics counters, and eventually began writing my books.

From a very young age I struggled with debilitating, painful eczema over most of my body. Then at puberty I developed acne that lingers even now. I spent a good deal of my childhood and teen years in dermatologists' offices and at cosmetics counters or drugstores, trying every possible treatment or product that promised to give me normal skin. It never happened.

Struggling with my own skin has been a lifelong quest. Then, in 1977, I took my first job at a department-store makeup counter to supplement my income as a freelance makeup artist (I always had a knack for doing makeup). As a young makeup artist in Washington, DC, where I was living at the time, I had built up a list of political and celebrity clients and was doing quite well, both financially and professionally. I found the artistry of creating beautiful makeup styles for women intriguing, and the world of fashion and glamour thoroughly exciting. At the age of 24, I was thrilled with my career. My clients wanted only me, and they were some of the most powerful and formidable women in Washington. But, as with any business, it had its ups and downs. A store at a mall in Silver Spring, Maryland, had an opening for a cosmetics salesperson. They hired me on the spot because, as I was told, I looked the part, wearing nice makeup and dressing well. Amazingly (to me anyway) they weren't interested in my makeup experience; I had to be retrained to sell products, especially skin-care products.

Even back then, I knew something was awry with a lot of the cosmetics and the advertising for them, particularly in the skin-care arena. Having struggled for years with oily skin and blemishes, I knew from personal experience that astringents didn't close pores, products claiming not to cause breakouts made me break out, and most products that promised to clear up acne only made my skin more red and irritated. I didn't yet know all the technical details of why skin-care products failed abysmally at what they claimed they could do, but it was blatantly obvious that plenty of mascaras with claims of being flakeproof weren't, that foundations claiming to keep oil at bay didn't, and on and on. More often than not, the claims made about what the products would do rarely matched their performance. However, while it seemed certain to me that much of the cosmetics industry was grossly misrepresenting its products, at the time I had no way to confirm my suspicions.

But back to 1977 when I started at the department-store cosmetics counter. On my first day, I was assigned to work behind the Calvin Klein counter (Klein had a makeup line then that lasted only a brief period; it was resurrected in 1999 and then again in 2007; perhaps the third time will be the charm) and the Elizabeth Arden counter. With no previous training or information about these lines, I was told to sell the products. I did the best I could. Unfortunately, my notion of how to help customers was completely different from that of the other salespeople and, more important, different from that of the line manager. My first mistake was telling several customers not to bother using an astringent because alcohol-based products wouldn't stop oil production and would only create more skin problems, causing skin to become dry, red, flaky, and irritated. By the end of the second day, the woman working next to me was mortified. She called in the line representative, who made it clear that I should keep my personal opinions to myself and just sell the products. I said I would do my best. This was only my second day! Things had to get better, I thought. They didn't.

After I complained that the two lines I was assigned to didn't always have the best makeup colors or skin-care products for every woman I talked to, the cosmetics manager told me, "All the customer wants to know is what you tell her; the customers never ask questions, because they trust our products." Several disagreements later, I was out of a job.

Shortly after my brief stint in the department store, I read *The Great American Skin Game* by Toni Stabille. It changed my life. This landmark book conveyed in clear, concise terms the processes and techniques the cosmetics industry uses to sell hope to gullible and uninformed consumers. In fact, Stabille was largely responsible for proposing many present-day Food and Drug Administration (FDA) regulations, including advertising guidelines, safety regulations, and mandatory ingredient lists. Her work confirmed what I had already reasoned must be true, and significantly changed the way I approached cosmetics.

Although it sounds a bit melodramatic, I couldn't continue selling something I knew to be a waste of money or just plain bad for the skin. Consumers (including myself) deserved better. I wasn't anti-makeup—just the opposite—but I was (and am) anti-hype and against misleading information. Thus I took my first steps on a long career path—longer and more consistent in some ways than I could ever have imagined—that went from owning my own cosmetics stores in 1980 to working as a TV news reporter at a local Seattle TV station, to owning my own publishing company in 1985, and back to creating and owning my own skin-care and makeup company in 1995, Paula's Choice.

With every step, my goal has been to do whatever it takes to find out and expose the truth behind the ads and the literally unbelievable claims thrown about by the cosmetics world. After all, one good sales pitch about an "exclusive formula" or a revolutionary new ingredient, and your pocketbook could easily be lighter—by $100 to $500—for a 1-ounce jar of standard cosmetic ingredients, or for ingredients that can't possibly live up to the claims made for them.

I know that I can't stop the cosmetics industry from force-feeding consumers an endless stream of expensive products and misleading or erroneous claims and information, but I also know there are enough women who are interested in seeing the other side of the picture to motivate me to continue to do what I do. Knowing the "rest of the story" can only help you feel and look more beautiful in the long run.

WHY YOU NEED A COSMETICS COP!

The answer to that question is: Because the cosmetics industry is a jungle and you need someone to help you get through it. As was true for all previous editions of this book, this one covers many of the new lines that have appeared, while many of the previously included lines have been entirely re-reviewed, critiqued, and balanced against current studies to make sure that the analysis reflects the most current research about ingredient efficacy, performance, and product integrity.

Do you need this book? If you've ever felt uncertain about a product, or too short of time or energy to figure out for yourself which foundations are too pink or too orange, which eyeshadows are too shiny or too difficult to use, which powders go on too chalky, which cleansers are too greasy, which toners are too harsh, what makes one moisturizer different from another, or how wrinkle creams differ, then, yes, you need (and will benefit from) this book. As you read the various skin-care and makeup reviews, you will start to get a better understanding of how the cosmetics industry really works. I've also included a summary chapter of best finds and best buys, but don't jump to that one first. It is important to read the individual product assessments and criteria so you understand *exactly* what standards were used to evaluate each particular category.

Skin-care products were evaluated almost entirely by analyzing the ingredient list and comparing the ingredients listed to the claims made about the product. If a toner asserts that it is designed for sensitive skin, it should not contain ingredients that irritate skin. If a moisturizer claims it can hydrate the skin, it should contain ingredients that can do just that. In addition, I make a point of challenging the inflated claims made about myriad ingredients. I also explain why seemingly impressive-sounding ingredients might indeed benefit the skin or might hurt the skin, and I often elaborate on the validity or usefulness of a specific ingredient or combination of ingredients. In short, the skin-care reviews separate the state-of-the-art products from the so-so and "oh, no!" products found in line after line after line.

For the makeup reviews, each product is described in terms of its reliability, value, texture, application, and effect. Within every category of product—foundations, mascaras, blushes, eyeshadows, concealers, powders, lipsticks, brushes, and pencils—I established specific criteria, and I evaluate the products based on those criteria. For example, according to my criteria, a foundation meant for someone with oily skin should be matte, contain minimal to no greasy or emollient ingredients, blend easily, leave a smooth, even finish, and have no blatant breakout-triggering ingredients. All foundations must match skin tones exactly; they should not be any noticeable shade of orange, peach, rose, pink, or ash, because people are not orange, peach, rose, pink, or ash. I established similar criteria for mascaras, blushes, eyeshadows, concealers, pressed powders, lipsticks, and pencils. I relied on my more than 20 years as a professional makeup artist to help establish guidelines for the quality of a product and its application, and I compared and contrasted hundreds of similar makeup products from different lines throughout the review process.

HOW DO THEY GET AWAY WITH IT?

I'm sure you've heard the remark that if you repeat a lie often enough it can become fact for many people, and that is how it is in the cosmetics industry. The need for an eye cream is ludicrous (I will explain why later in this book), but these products are accepted as standard by most women. Many women believe a skin-care product can work better than Botox (after all, that's what the ads say), but nothing could be further from the truth.

I am often asked, "How do they get away with it?" How do cosmetics companies get away with what is either misleading information or out-and-out lying to the public? Because for these companies, getting around cosmetics regulations worldwide has become an art that has left the consumer between a rock and a hard place.

By the time regulatory boards get around to challenging cosmetics advertising claims the ads have long since been replaced with a new product launch. My favorite example is the case of StriVectin, which used the slogan "Better Than Botox!" to take a $1 million dollar annual revenue product to a $150 million dollar gold mine. Then, as a result of FDA pressure and legal threats from Allergan, when StriVectin couldn't prove its claim that it was Better Than Botox!, their ads went from Better Than Botox! (a declarative statement) to Better Than Botox? (a question). That little change of punctuation satisfied the FDA and "truth" in advertising (Source: www.fda.gov). I'm sure the change was lost (as it was intended to be) on many a consumer.

The only part of the cosmetics industry that is strictly regulated for the consumer's protection is the ingredient list, but even there I see lots of problems. Since 1978, cosmetics companies have been required to divulge all the contents in their products, and to list them in the order of concentration from most to least. Unfortunately, the vast majority of consumers don't know how to read a cosmetic's ingredient list because it is phenomenally technical and vast (there are thousands and thousands of cosmetic ingredients). That complexity means that most of us can only rely on the unregulated claims and assertions the marketing copy boasts about. Yet taking the time to decipher the ingredient lists is the only way to make a rational decision when it comes time to purchase skin-care products. But then again, that's my job security!

CLAIM SUBSTANTIATION

How many times in skin-care advertising have you seen the claim "our studies show"? Aside from how often this claim is made, it may surprise you that, even though we call every company whose products we review and ask them to share their research with us, I can count on one hand the actual number of studies we've received. We get plenty of press releases, but we never get the actual studies.

Why is it so important to get the actual study, if it really exists? And when it does exist, why am I often very skeptical about what such studies report? Because in the world of skin care, there is an entire business known as claim substantiation. Laboratories, including those at some respected universities and colleges, are expert at setting up a study so that the results will back up whatever the label or advertisements say a product can do. One important thing that many consumers and physicians aren't aware of, and this includes lots of physicians who are involved in these bogus studies, is the question, "Under what conditions were the studies performed?" Maybe it takes some experience even to ask. For example, in a skin-care study, the subjects participating often begin by washing their face and then stripping it clear with alcohol. Then the "before" photos are taken and measurements (wrinkle depth, skin tone, and water loss, among other parameters) are recorded. With that starting point, it's hardly surprising that the "before" situation is so much worse than the "after" results. What would the results have been if the woman had started by using a gentle cleanser, a good moisturizer, and sunscreen (for example, effective ones different from those being tested)? There are lots of ways to use pseudo-science to create proof for a claim that, in reality, has very little to do with science and everything to do with marketing. Following are a few of my favorite examples from the "Our Studies Show" file.

A favorite of mine is the study used to "prove" that Clarisonic, a $195 battery-driven facial cleansing brush is something you must have. This is a hand-held device that is supposed to work like SoniCare (the battery-driven toothbrush), which isn't surprising considering that the same engineers who created SoniCare make the Clarisonic. The technical selling point is that the bristles of the face brush are designed to traverse facial dermatoglyphics (the scientific study of fingerprints—which for some marketing reason is being used to sound impressive for this product—just to be clear, wrinkles are not related to fingerprints in any way), pores, and scars. The sonic motion of the brush also aids in dislodging facial debris, much like the sonic surgical-instrument cleansers that are used to clean liposuction cannulas and reusable injection needles.

But again, upon closer examination, the study itself is far less convincing. In a "split-forehead" randomized study using six subjects (not exactly an extensive sample population), equal amounts of fluorescent makeup were placed on the forehead of each subject. Photographs of the forehead were then taken using a digital camera with a UV flash. An aesthetician then cleansed half of the forehead with the Clarisonic brush and the other half by hand. Both sides of the forehead were then rinsed with equal amounts of water and left to air dry. After drying, the subject's forehead was again photographed. The higher the level of glowing makeup, the less effective the cleansing was considered to be for dirty skin (less glow would mean cleaner skin). As you might suspect, the side of the face cleansed with the brush was cleaner than the side washed by hand. That might lead you to run out and buy the Clarisonic, but more careful scrutiny might save you $195. What this study didn't compare was what would have happened if the types of cleansing were more equal. Suppose one side of the face had been cleansed with the Clarisonic and the other half with a washcloth and gentle cleanser? Or what if a makeup remover had been applied, and the skin then washed with a gentle cleanser and washcloth? It is also possible that the aesthetician was not as zealous cleansing one side of the face as much as the other (after all this person was part of the study proving the value of the Clarisonic). Either way, the study does not in any way indicate or establish the value of this rotating brush for cleansing the face.

Just as an aside: Because SoniCare and Clarisonic are related, it's interesting to realize that research published in the *Journal of the International Academy of Periodontology*, July 2006, pages 83–88, revealed that SoniCare was no more effective than just using a toothbrush.

SO WHY CAN'T "ANTI-WRINKLE" CREAMS WORK BETTER THAN BOTOX?

Or dermal fillers? Or laser resurfacing? Or chemical peels? Or endoscopic facelifts? Or plastic surgery? Because they simply cannot address the complex physiological processes that cause wrinkles. Here are some of the factors we face:

- **Sun damage!** Caused by pervasive, recurring, cumulative, unprotected, or inadequate sun protection (Sources: *Archives of Dermatological Research*, January 2006, pages

294–302; *British Journal of Dermatology*, December 2005, Supplemental, pages 37–46; *Journal of Dermatology*, August 2004, pages 603–609; and *Journal of Investigative Dermatology*, September 2003, pages 578–586).

- **Fat depletion and movement in the face.** The fat pads of the cheek, forehead, and jaw move down and in on the face as the skin becomes less supple and firm (Sources: *Journal of Drugs in Dermatology*, November–December 2006, pages 959–964; *Dermatologic Surgery*, August 2006, pages 1058–1069; *Annals of Plastic Surgery*, March 2004, pages 234–239; and *Dermatologic Surgery*, October 2003, pages 1019–1026).
- **Loss of estrogen due to menopause or illness.** Hormone levels and the stress of illness add more factors (Sources: *Climacteric Journal of the International Menopause Society*, August 2007, pages 289–297; and *Experimental Dermatology*, February 2005, page 156).
- **Genetics.** This speaks for itself. The genes you inherit may hinder or help a great deal, but they too are only part of the picture given environmental influences and the other factors listed here (Sources: *Current Problems in Dermatology*, 2007, volume 35, pages 28–38; and *Journal of Investigative Dermatology*, February 2006, pages 277–282).
- **Bone loss.** As the skeletal support structure of the face loses density and bulk, it provides less architectural support for skin (Sources: *Facial Plastic Surgery Clinics of North America*, May 2007, pages 221–228; *Skin Therapy Letter*, April 2006, pages 1–3; and *Journal of the American Academy of Dermatology*, February 1998, pages 248–255).
- **Cell senescence.** This takes place in skin cells as they eventually lose the capacity to divide and re-create themselves. The result is thin, inelastic, dry skin and generally impaired skin function. This process is known as the "Hayflick phenomenon," named after Dr. Leonard Hayflick, who identified the condition in 1965; it has also been called genetically programmed cell death (Sources: *Dermatology*, August 2007, pages 352–360; *Molecular Biology Reports*, September 2006, pages 181–186; and *Cell Cycle*, September 2004, pages 1127–1129).

No cosmetic or skin-care product can address all of these physiological issues and problems. A combination of products and medical treatments can achieve some success against these elements, but to imagine that a single miracle cream can do this all by itself is just not realistic.

BUZZWORDS

The following are a few of the more popular terms you may have seen or heard in marketing jargon for cosmetic products that get hyped and overhyped by the cosmetics industry. Although you might have heard them, you may not be aware that they have little to no meaning when it comes to what you will actually be putting on your skin or what is effective or a waste of your money. Here's what's behind the buzz.

All Natural: This term is used to convey the idea that the ingredients in a given product or product line were derived from plants or other organic material, as opposed to being produced synthetically. While this implication of "natural" ingredients resonates with consumers, it doesn't assure you that you are getting an accurate picture of safety or effectiveness, much less reliable facts. Natural ingredient claims are not regulated by the FDA. Although the FDA has tried to establish official definitions and guidelines for the use of terms such as "natural," its regulation proposals were overturned in court. Therefore, cosmetics companies can use the "all natural" term on ingredient lists to mean anything they want, and almost always it means nothing at all.

Many companies even claim their products are all natural when in fact they contain a preponderance of unnatural ingredients. Further, there is no convincing research showing that "natural ingredients" are better for skin than synthetic versions. In fact, there are lots of natural ingredients that show up in skin-care products that are either toxic (Source: *Toxicology In Vitro*, June 2006, pages 480–489), carcinogenic, or irritating to skin—and irritation causes all kinds of havoc for skin (Sources: *Skin Research and Technology*, August 2004, pages 144–148). And finally, when a plant product is added to a cosmetic, and is preserved, stabilized, and mixed with other ingredients, it loses most, if not all, of its natural orientation (Source: *FDA Consumer* magazine, May–June 1998; revised May 1998 and August 2000).

Organic Cosmetics: Since October 2002, according to the U.S. Department of Agriculture (USDA), national regulations have been on the books that specify exact standards for determining what precisely is meant when food is labeled "organic," whether it is grown in the United States or imported from other countries. As is stated on the USDA Web site, "Organic food is produced by farmers who emphasize the use of renewable resources and the conservation of soil and water to enhance environmental quality for future generations. Organic meat, poultry, eggs, and dairy products come from animals that are given no antibiotics or growth hormones. Organic food is produced without using most conventional pesticides, fertilizers made with synthetic ingredients or sewage sludge, bioengineering, or ionizing radiation. Before a product can be labeled 'organic,' a government-approved certifier inspects the farm where the food is grown to make sure the farmer is following all the rules necessary to meet USDA organic standards. Companies that handle or process organic food before it gets to your local supermarket or restaurant must be certified, too."

What does any of this have to do with cosmetics? Many consumers are already attracted to any cosmetic that claims to be natural, no matter how bogus the claim. To make their products stand out from the rest, cosmetics companies are starting to use the term "organic" on their product labels. But as *Consumer Reports* (August 2003, page 61) stated, "With no hearings or public discussion, the USDA extended its rules on organic labeling to cosmetics. There are now shampoos and body lotions labeled 70% organic based on the fact that their main ingredient is … water in which something organic, such as an organic lavender leaf, has been soaked."

It takes only a quick look at the ingredients list on a cosmetic to notice that there are a lot of words that are completely unrelated to anything resembling a plant, much less a plant that can be labeled "organic." Plenty of synthetic ingredients are found in products of cosmetics lines that boast about their all "natural" and now "organic" content. Yet the hope and desire for healthier products will be an emotional pull for lots of women. The situation becomes even more confusing when you consider that most "natural" cosmetics lines are sold at supermarkets that showcase organic produce and food products. When specialty grocery stores sell products that have strictly regulated organic labeling, many customers will never notice that the products in the other half of the store, where the cosmetics are sold, are backed by no such regulation, despite the similar labeling.

For more detailed information on the USDA organic standards, visit their Web site at www.ams.usda.gov/nop or call the National Organic Program at (202) 720-3252.

Hypoallergenic or Good for Sensitive Skin: These terms suggest to the consumer that the product is less likely to cause allergic reactions or skin sensitivities. However, there are no standard testing restrictions or regulations for determining whether a product qualifies as meeting this claim. A company can label their product as "hypoallergenic" or "good for sensitive skin" without providing any substantiation for the claim. This is also true for terms such as "dermatologist-tested," "sensitivity tested," "allergy tested," or "nonirritating." None of these terms are required to be backed up by any proof that they are better for your skin than products without these claims, because there are no standardized guidelines (Source: www.fda.gov). You will also be surprised at the number of products in this edition that get rated with an unhappy face because the product is labeled for sensitive skin, but contains a preponderance of irritating or sensitizing ingredients.

Alcohol-Free: This generally means that a product does not contain denatured alcohol, ethyl alcohol, methanol, benzyl alcohol, isopropyl (rubbing) alcohol, or sd alcohol, all of which are akin to grain alcohol, which is very drying and irritating for skin (Source: *Contact Dermatitis*, February 2005, pages 82–87, and *The Lancet*, April 2002, pages 1489–1490). However, many cosmetics may contain other "alcohol" compounds, such as cetyl alcohol, stearyl alcohol, cetearyl alcohol, or lanolin alcohol, also known as fatty alcohols, and you should know that what these do is completely unrelated to the effect of grain alcohol on the skin. As is true for any skin irritant, the higher up on the ingredient list the alcohol is, the greater the risk of irritation. Grain-type alcohols that appear after or just before the list of preservatives rarely pose an irritation problem for skin.

Fragrance-Free: This is supposed to indicate to the consumer that a product contains no perfume or fragrant ingredients, but it ends up having little meaning. Despite this labeling, many products use fragrant plant extracts that can cause skin irritation, allergic reactions, or a phototoxic response on skin (meaning they enhance the negative effects of the sun on your skin). Fragrances, natural or otherwise, are not benign ingredients (Source: *Acta Dermato-Venereology*, July 2007, pages 312–316).

It is important to know that fragrant ingredients (including fragrant plant oils and extracts) may be added to a "fragrance-free" cosmetic to mask any offensive odor originating from the raw materials used, but in such a small amount that they may not impart a noticeable scent. So, "fragrance-free" can mean that a product does not exude a noticeable aroma, although it can still contain those types of ingredients. Either way, because "fragrance-free" is not a term regulated by the FDA, it ends up being useless information on a product's label unless you know what to watch out for on the ingredient list (Source: www.fda.gov).

Noncomedogenic and Nonacnegenic: These terms are not regulated by the FDA or any other regulatory board anywhere in the world, and as such have no legal meaning. Again, any product can spotlight these terms. In real life, the search for products that won't cause breakouts remains a struggle. Wouldn't it be nice if a product could live up to this claim? But given that almost all cosmetic ingredients can trigger breakouts for some people, and that the problem is not so much with a single ingredient as with combinations of ingredients, and given there are millions of permutations of ingredients, there is no way to determine exactly which combination is a problem. We've all bought products labeled "noncomedogenic" that have made us break out. The fact is, these terms are not only bogus, they can never really be true (Source: www.fda.gov).

Dermatologist Tested: No matter how impressive this wording sounds, and as long as there are no reliable published data stating otherwise, this term can mean simply that a doctor applied the product to his or her skin or watched someone else do that and then said they liked the product. It doesn't tell you anything about efficacy or how one product compares to any other product. A similar empty phrase that's often seen is "dermatologist approved" (Source: www.fda.gov).

Laboratory Tested: A laboratory sounds so scientific—but any place a study is done can be referred to as a "laboratory" setting. Once you get past the scientific impression the term may give you, you realize that the testing issues are rarely logical, and that the tests are often engineered in advance to give the company precisely the results they paid for.

Patented Secrets or Patented Ingredients: There is no such thing as a patented secret. The very concept is an oxymoron. The only way to *obtain* a patent is to *divulge* the complete contents of the product and its intended use! There are also no patents that deal with proof of efficacy. All a patent can legally do is attribute to an ingredient or formulation the capability to be used for a specific purpose (such as wrinkles, acne, exfoliation, or skin-lightening). That has nothing to do with whether or not those ingredients can do anything at all. Patents also do not indicate or validate the quality, reliability, or usefulness of a product, nor does a patent mean that certain established ingredients can't be used by other companies for other purposes (Source: United States Patent and Trademark Office, www.uspto.gov).

Essential Oils: There is nothing essential about essential oils. It is a term attributed to fragrant oils to bestow an aura of effective skin care upon them, where, in almost every case, none exists. Hundreds of cosmetics companies market products that contain essential oils and assert that these oils are good for skin and are suitable for even the most sensitive skin. If there is any consistent lie that won't go away in the cosmetics industry (aside from undoing wrinkles), it is this one. It is well established in scientific and dermatological journals that fragrance, whether natural or synthetic, is problematic for skin (Sources: *Acta Dermato-Venereology*, 2007; volume 87, issue 4, pages 312–316); *Dermatology*, 2002, volume 205, number 1, pages 98–102; *Contact Dermatitis*, December 2001, pages 333–340; and *Toxicology and Applied Pharmacology*, May 2001, pages 172–178). For any company to suggest that products containing volatile ingredients such as rose, orange oil, pine oil, and musk are gentle, helpful, or hypoallergenic is not just misleading—it's harmful for skin.

COSMECEUTICAL

Cosmeceutical is a buzzword that deserves its own section. The products in this group are loosely (and I mean really loosely) defined as products combining the benefits of a cosmetic and a pharmaceutical. The term is used by many skin-care companies, especially for products sold or endorsed by dermatologists, to give the impression that the products have more effective or more biologically active ingredients than just ordinary cosmetics. As more and more doctors get into selling or endorsing skin-care products, you will hear more and more about cosmeceuticals. Dr. Tina Alster is the spokesperson for Lancome; Dr. Karyn Grossman is the spokesperson for Prescriptives; Dr. Patricia Wexler has her namesake products, Patricia Wexler M.D. Dermatology; Skin Effects by Dr. Jeffrey Dover is at CVS; Dr. Sheldon Pinnell's SkinCeuticals line has been purchased by L'Oreal; and, of course, there's N.V. Perricone, M.D. Upping the ante in this group is Dr. Howard Sobel, who has some of the most expensive skin-care products being sold today.

Despite all these medical pedigrees, the term "cosmeceutical" is not in any way regulated or controlled, and anyone can slap that label on their products to promote them as being more "medical." Cosmeceutical is nothing more than a marketing term with illusions of grandeur. Even the FDA says cosmeceuticals don't exist, and considers these products to be merely cosmetics with clever marketing language attached.

Do cosmeceuticals really differ from any other cosmetics? The answer is a resounding no, because no matter how a product is labeled and marketed, as a cosmeceutical or otherwise, many skin-care treatments contain ingredients that affect the biological function of skin. The biologically active ingredients to look for include antioxidants (most of which have anti-inflammatory properties), cell-communicating ingredients, exfoliants, skin-lightening ingredients, and intercellular substances (ingredients that mimic skin structure).

I will talk about all these types of ingredients throughout this book, but suffice it to say that "cosmeceutical" is nothing more than a marketing term, it doesn't prove anything about the effectiveness of the formulation in comparison to any other product.

(Sources for the above information: *Archives of Dermatological Research*, April 2005, pages 473–481; *American Journal of Clinical Dermatology*, March–April 2000, pages 81–88, and September-October 2000, pages 261–268; *Biofactors*, January–February 2002, pages 29–43; *Biological & Pharmaceutical Bulletin*, April 2004, pages 510–514; *Bioorganic and Medicinal Chemistry*, December 2003, pages 5345–5352; *British Journal of Dermatology*, November 1995, pages 679–685, and September 2000, pages 524–531; *Business Week Online, An Ugly Truth About Cosmetics*, November 30, 2004; *Contact Dermatitis*, June 2002, pages 331–338; *Cutis*, February 2004, pages 3–13 Supplemental; *Clinical and Geriatric Medicine*, February 2002, pages 103–120; *Dermatology*, February 2002, pages 153–158, April 2002, pages 281–286, and 2005, 210 Supplemental 1, pages 6–13; www.emedicine.com/derm/topic509.htm; *Experimental Dermatology*, 2003, 12 Supplemental 2, pages 57–63, and 2004, 13 Supplemental 4, pages 16–21; *Facial Plastic Surgery Clinics of North America*, August 2004, pages 363–372; *Free Radical Research*, April 2002, pages 471–477; *Journal of Cosmetic Science*, September–October 2002, pages 269–282; *Journal of the European Academy of Dermatology & Venereology*, November 2002, pages 587–594; *Mutation Research*, April 2005, pages 153–173; *Nutrition and Cancer*, February 2003, pages 181–187; *Photochemistry and Photobiology*, January–February 2005, pages 38–45; *Plastic and Reconstructive Surgery*, February 2005, pages 515–528, and April 2005, pages 1156–1162; *Progress in Lipid Research*, January 2003, pages 1–36; *Skin Pharmacology and Applied Physiology*, September–October 2004, pages 207–213; *Skin Therapy Letter*, June–July 2004, pages 1–3; and *Toxicological Sciences*, September 2004, pages 43–49.)

I could go on and on, and I will throughout the next thousand-plus pages as I describe and cite sources that explain what works and what doesn't when it comes to skin-care products. The information I provide just restates everything the cosmetics industry already knows to be true (it's their information directly from their sources). I simply add what they won't tell you: what you absolutely need to know to make sensible, cost-effective decisions about what you put on your skin.

Take This to the Bank: Expensive Doesn't Mean Better

The amount of money you spend on skin-care products has nothing to do with how your skin looks. In other words, spending more money does not affect the status of your skin. What does affect the status of your skin are the products you use. An expensive soap by Erno Laszlo is no better for your skin than an inexpensive bar soap such as Dove (though I suggest that both are potentially too irritating and drying for all skin types). On the other hand, an irritant-free toner by Neutrogena can be just as good as, or maybe even better than, an irritant-free toner by Orlane or La Prairie (depending on the formulation), and *any* irritant-free toner is infinitely better than a toner that contains alcohol, peppermint, menthol, essential oils, eucalyptus, lemon, or other irritants, no matter how natural-sounding the ingredients are and regardless of the price or claim. Spending less doesn't hurt your skin, and spending more doesn't necessarily help it. Simple, but true!

Ingredients

To make it easier for you to become familiar with what you'll find on ingredient lists, I have completely revised and updated Chapter Seven, *Cosmetic Ingredient Dictionary*. Please refer to it when you don't know what an ingredient is or does, or when you hear a claim that a particular ingredient has some miraculous properties for skin. You will be amazed at how legitimate research rarely matches what a cosmetics company wants you to believe.

CHAPTER TWO

Healthy Skin: Rules to Live By

CAN YOU HAVE GREAT SKIN?

You can obtain the best skin possible for your skin type, but there are no cures or absolutes. We are all going to grow up, and skin-care products can't stop that. *Don't Go to the Cosmetics Counter Without Me* is primarily a product review guide. It is meant as a source that tells you specifically what products live up to their claims, what products don't, and what products waste your money.

Over the past several years, the amount of documented and peer-reviewed research on skin-care and cosmetic ingredients has grown tremendously. Serious investigation has increased exponentially on all fronts—from antioxidants, anti-irritants, skin-identical ingredients, and cell-communicating ingredients, to how skin ages, why skin wrinkles, how skin heals, what the effects of hormones are on skin function, and how to treat blackheads and acne, not to mention giving us a better understanding of how sun and oxygen destroy skin and why irritation is harmful for skin. Cosmetic dermatology and plastic surgery procedures have greatly improved, but the array of options has become more extensive and the risks more difficult to easily quantify and evaluate.

It is amazing how far the cosmetics world has advanced in understanding how skin behaves and reacts to environmental factors, to the passing of time, and to the products we put on it. Yet for all this progress, I am still shocked at how much has remained the same when it comes to misleading claims, poor formulations, products that contain ingredients that can hurt skin, and products that are priced with nothing more in mind than seducing women who are tempted by high prices because they are forever convinced that expensive means better. Once you have some basic information, you can use this book to decide what products best meet your needs and budget.

THE BASIC FACTS

The questions I have been asked repeatedly over the years are these: If the cosmetics industry's promises and claims are often disingenuous, if many companies operate under shared ownership, and if you can't rely on what the ads or products describe, then what is real? What is and isn't possible when it comes to treating your skin and skin-care needs? Although following the premises laid out in this book can prevent you from wasting money on overpriced or ineffective skin-care products, or perhaps stop you from being persuaded the next time you hear a sales pitch for a miraculous (or even semi-miraculous) sounding skin-care product or routine, you still need to know how to evaluate what to use and know what to avoid for your own specific personal needs.

The following is an overview to give you some insight into how to begin making decisions to create a skin-care routine that can help you achieve optimum benefits and results. Keeping these "rules" in mind and diligently following them will not only help you keep the craziness of the cosmetics industry in perspective, but also result in healthy skin—and that's the truth. But first it is important to grasp the universal, overly glorified world of moisturizers.

WHAT IS A STATE-OF-THE-ART MOISTURIZER?

Moisturizer is a ubiquitous term that has lost meaning over the years. With all the anti-aging, anti-wrinkling, lifting, firming, nourishing, organic, works-like-Botox, eye cream, neck cream, and throat cream products touting their miracle formulations, it's hard to know where moisturizers fit into the picture. In actuality, regardless of the name or claim, "moisturizers," or whatever the industry calls them in terms of their anti-wrinkle benefit, whether they are in cream, lotion, serum, or even liquid form, must supply the skin with ingredients that maintain its structure, reduce free-radical damage (environmental assaults on the skin from sun, pollution, and air), and help cells function more normally. When moisturizers contain the well-researched, effective groups of ingredients that can do these things, they are as close to "anti-aging," or "anti-wrinkling," or "repairing" as any skin-care product can get.

Contrary to what the cosmetics industry at large would like you to believe, a state-of-the-art moisturizer does not rely on one "star" ingredient to enhance skin's appearance or function or to improve the appearance of wrinkles. Month after month, consumers are faced with new ingredients, each claiming superiority over any number of earlier stars, although the majority have no substantiated, non-company–funded research to prove these assertions. This constant yet ever-changing list of "best" ingredients may keep things interesting for cosmetics marketing departments, but it rarely helps the consumer determine what is needed to maintain healthy, radiant skin.

All skin types will benefit from daily, topical application of cell-communicating antioxidants, anti-irritants, skin-identical ingredients, and water-binding agents that together work to improve and re-create the structure and function of healthy skin. Those are the ingredients that make the most difference and have the most impact on the function of the skin (and the research, as you'll see, is abundant and overflowing on this topic).

The brilliance of cosmetics chemists and advanced ingredient technology allows for the creation of all types of moisturizers (with and without sunscreen) that have elegant textures, silky applications, and superb finishes. The days of plain water-and-wax moisturizers are over (though many lines still sell such formulations to unwary customers). Using these antiquated formulations would be like using a computer made in the 1980s. It would also be cheating your skin by not giving it the best that's out there to help it (dare I say it) "look younger."

SHOULD YOU USE A LOTION, CREAM, GEL, SERUM, LIQUID, MOUSSE, OR BALM?

Aside from the actual antioxidants, cell-communicating ingredients, and ingredients that mimic skin structure, the question women are most confused by is: What should the consistency of their moisturizer or anti-wrinkle product be? The answer is: It doesn't matter. This is all about personal preference. State-of-the-art ingredients are the necessary substances in any "moisturizer" or "specialty product," but the base—the ingredients that make the product a gel, cream, lotion, serum, liquid, or mousse—are inconsequential. Think of it like a chocolate dessert. You might prefer a torte, pudding, bonbon, cake, ice cream, or some other form, but the chocolate is what counts; the other ingredients are there simply to carry the important taste of chocolate to your mouth.

As a general rule, those with oily or combination skin will prefer lighter-weight lotions, gels, serums, or liquids (think of really well-formulated toners without irritants, and with lots of state-of-the-art ingredients). Those with dry skin usually prefer creams or more emollient formulations to make up for what their oil glands don't provide. And those with blemish-prone skin generally do better with moisturizers that have a thinner consistency.

DAYTIME VS. NIGHTTIME MOISTURIZERS

Putting aside the claims, hype, and misleading information you may have heard, the only real difference between a daytime and nighttime moisturizer is that the daytime version should contain a well-formulated sunscreen. For daytime wear, unless your foundation contains an effective sunscreen, it is essential that your moisturizer feature a well-formulated, broad-spectrum sunscreen rated SPF 15 or higher. Well-formulated means that it contains UVA-protecting ingredients, specifically titanium dioxide, zinc oxide, avobenzone (also called butyl methoxydibenzoylmethane or Parsol 1789), Tinosorb, or Mexoryl SX (ecamsule). Regardless of the time of day, your skin needs all the current state-of-the-art ingredients I describe in the following paragraphs. Your skin doesn't do special healing at night, despite what you might have heard from a cosmetics salesperson.

SKIN-IDENTICAL INGREDIENTS

Ingredients that mimic skin structure are referred to in different ways. They are often called skin-identical ingredients or intercellular matrix substances, but they can also be termed natural moisturizing factors (NMF), and I have often referred to them in my books as water-binding agents. By any name these are brilliant ingredients for all skin types because they improve the function of skin and provide the barrier protection that is critical to having and maintaining healthy skin.

The term "skin-identical ingredients" refers to the substances between skin cells that keep skin cells connected and help maintain skin's fundamental external structure. Many ingredients have these functions. Humectants, of which glycerin is a classic example, draw water to skin and are one vital component of a moisturizer. But what good is attracting water to the skin if the structure isn't there to keep the water from leaving?

It turns out that skin cells usually have plenty of water if they don't become damaged, and the water content of healthy skin typically ranges from 10–30%. Once skin is irritated, overcleansed, exposed to the sun, or dehydrated by air conditioning or indoor heaters, its integrity is compromised and water loss ensues. This occurs when the substances that keep the skin cells bound together to create the surface structure we see as skin (the intercellular matrix) are depleted.

This intercellular structure is made up of many different components, ranging from ceramides to lecithin, glycerin, polysaccharides, hyaluronic acid, sodium hyaluronate, sodium PCA, collagen, elastin, proteins, amino acids, cholesterol, glucose, sucrose, fructose, glycogen, phospholipids, glycosphingolipids, glycosaminoglycans, and many more. All of these give the skin what it needs to keep its cells intact. Just adding water is meaningless if the intercellular matrix is damaged. When a moisturizer does contain a combination of these, it can help reinforce the skin's natural ability to function normally, improve skin's texture, and—with continual use of products containing the ingredients mentioned above—can eliminate dry skin.

ANTIOXIDANTS

Antioxidants are essential elements of a state-of-the-art moisturizer. A growing body of research continues to show that antioxidants are a potential panacea for skin's ills, and to ignore this benefit while you're shopping for moisturizers is shortchanging your skin. One thing that makes antioxidants so intriguing is that they seem to have the ability to reduce or prevent some amount of the oxidative damage that destroys and depletes the skin's function and structure, while also preventing some amount of the degeneration of skin and its support structure caused by sunlight. Another good thing is that there are hundreds of antioxidants (Sources: *Journal of Medicinal Food*, June 2007, pages 337–344; *Cellular and Molecular Biology*, April 2007, pages 1–2; *Cosmetic Dermatology*, December 2001, pages 37–40; *Current Opinion of Investigational Drugs*, May 2007, pages 390–400; *Dermatologic Surgery*, "The Antioxidant Network of the Stratum Corneum," July 31, 2005, pages 814–817; and *Journal of Pharmaceutical and Biomedical Analysis*, February 23, 2005, pages 287–295).

A key point to keep in mind when considering a moisturizer with antioxidants is packaging. Although antioxidants have great ability to intercept and mitigate free-radical damage, it's ironic that their main drawback in a cosmetic is that they deteriorate when repeatedly exposed to air (oxygen) and sunlight. Therefore, an antioxidant-laden moisturizer packaged in a jar or clear (instead of opaque) container will likely lose its antioxidant benefit within weeks (or days, depending on the formula) of being opened. Look for moisturizers with antioxidants that are packaged in opaque tubes or bottles, and be sure the opening that dispenses the product is small so as to minimize exposing the product to air.

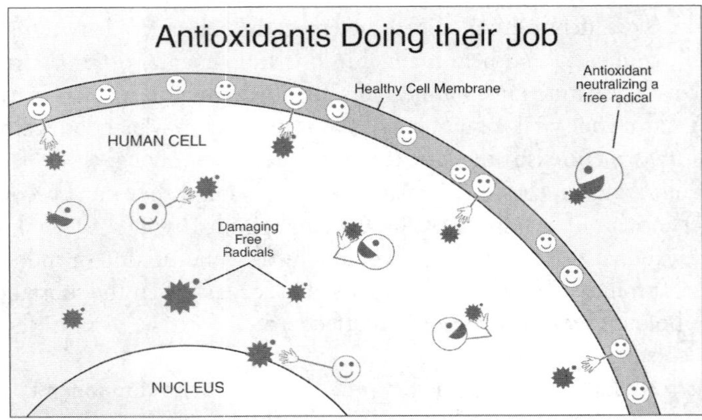

CELL-COMMUNICATING INGREDIENTS

The ingredients in the group known as cell-communicating ingredients are getting attention for their role in helping skin function more normally. Medical journals refer to these as "cell-signaling" substances—but I think "cell-communicating" is more descriptive of what they do in relation to skin care.

Whereas the antioxidants described above work by intervening in a chain-reaction process called free-radical damage ("grabbing" the loose-cannon molecule that causes free-radical damage to nullify it), cell-communicating ingredients, theoretically, have other valuable effects. These include the ability to tell a skin cell to look, act, and behave better, more like a normal healthy skin cell would, and also to stop other substances from telling the cell to behave badly or abnormally. This is exciting news, because on their own antioxidants lack the ability to "tell" a damaged skin cell to behave more normally. Years of unprotected or poorly protected sun exposure cause abnormal skin cells to be produced. Usually the skin regenerates itself with normal, round, even, and completely intact skin cells, but when damaged cells reproduce, the new cells are uneven, flat, and lack structural integrity. As a result of these deformities, they behave poorly. This is where cell-communicating ingredients (examples are niacinamide and adenosine triphosphate) have the potential to help.

Every cell has a vast series of receptor sites for different substances. These receptor sites are the cell's communication hookup. When the right ingredient for a specific site shows up, it has the ability to attach itself to the cell and transmit information. In the case of skin, this means telling the cell to start doing the things a healthy skin cell should be doing. If the cell accepts the message, it then shares the same healthy message with other nearby cells in a continuing process.

As long as there is an open receptor site and the appropriate, healthy signaling substance is present, a lot of beneficial communication takes place. But a cell's communication network is more complex than any worldwide telephone system ever made. The array of receptor sites and the substances that can make connections to them comprise a huge, complex, and varied group, with incredible limitations and convoluted pathways that we are still finding out about. And as far as skin care is concerned, it's an area of research that's in its infancy. No doubt you will be hearing more and more about cell-communicating or cell-signaling ingredients being used in skin-care products, despite the lack of solid research. The good news is that, theoretically, this new horizon in skin care is incredibly exciting (Sources: *Microscopy Research and Technique*, January 2003, pages 107–114; *Nature Medicine*, February 2003, pages 225–229; *Journal of Investigative Dermatology*, March 2002, pages 402–408; *International Journal of Biochemistry and Cell Biology*, July 2004, pages 1141–1146; *Experimental Cell Research*, March 2002, pages 130–137; *Skin Pharmacology and Applied Skin Physiology*, September–October 2002, pages 316–320; and www.signaling-gateway.org).

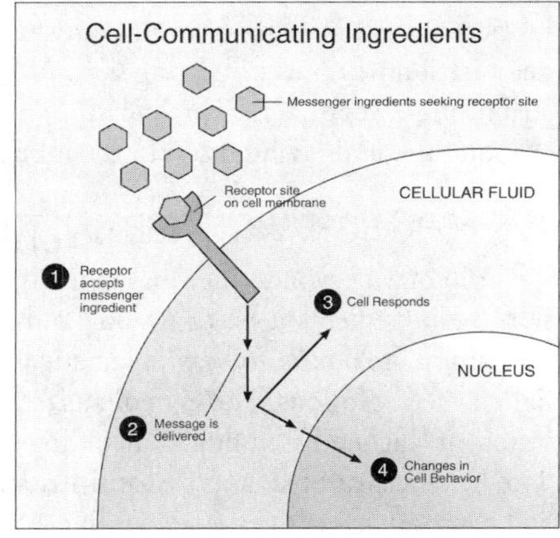

ANTI-IRRITANTS

Anti-irritants are another element vital for good skin-care formulations. Regardless of the source, irritation is a problem for all skin types, yet it is almost impossible to avoid. Whether it is from the sun or is oxidative damage from pollution, the environment, or from the skin-care products a person uses, irritation can be a constant assault on the skin. Ironically, even such necessary ingredients as sunscreen agents, preservatives, exfoliants, and cleansing agents can cause irritation. Other ingredients, such as fragrance, menthol, and sensitizing plant extracts, are primary irritants and are typically void of genuine benefits for skin, so their use in skin-care products is not a positive thing, at least if you're serious about creating and maintaining healthy skin.

Anti-irritants are incredibly helpful because they allow skin extra healing time and can reduce the problems caused by oxidative and other sources of external damage. Anti-irritants include substances such as allantoin, aloe, bisabolol, burdock root, chamomile extract, glycyrrhetinic acid, grape extract, green tea, licorice root, vitamin C, white willow, willow bark, willowherb, and many, many more. Their benefit for skin should be strongly considered because they are that rare thing—a case where too much of a good thing is better!

EMOLLIENTS

For those with truly dry skin—that is, where the dryness is not caused by irritating or drying skin-care products—emollients provide lubricating ingredients that are critical for making skin feel hydrated. Emollients provide dry skin with the one thing it's missing—moisture—in the form of substances that resemble those the skin should produce for itself. Emollients are ingredients like plant oils, mineral oil, shea butter, cocoa butter, petrolatum, fatty alcohols, and animal oils (including emu, mink, and lanolin, the latter probably the one ingredient that is most like our own skin's oil). All of these are exceptionally beneficial for all cases of dry skin, and are easily recognizable on an ingredient list.

More technical-sounding emollient ingredients like triglycerides, benzoates, myristates, palmitates, and stearates are generally waxy in texture and appearance, but they are what provide most moisturizers with their elegant texture and feel. Overall, emollients create the fundamental base and texture of a moisturizer and impart a creamy, smooth feel on the skin. Silicones (listed on labels in terms ending in "siloxane") are another interesting group of lubricants for skin. They have an exquisite, silky texture and an incredible ability to prevent dehydration without suffocating skin. All of these ingredients spread over the skin to create a thin, imperceptible layer, re-creating the benefits of our own oil production, preventing evaporation, and giving dry skin the lubrication it is missing.

FOR THOSE WITH NORMAL TO OILY SKIN OR MINIMAL DRYNESS

You may be wondering what to use if you don't have dryness, but still want to give your skin the ingredients it needs to look and feel better. Moisturizers in cream, balm, or ointment form are bound to be problematic if you have any degree of oiliness, and so are many lighter-weight lotions. The ingredients to look for that will work more effectively for you are water- or silicone-based fluids (including well-formulated toners) or serums that are loaded with beneficial antioxidants and anti-irritants. Look for ingredients that mimic the structure and function of healthy skin, including water-binding agents such as glycerin or lecithin and cell-communicating ingredients such as niacinamide or adenosine triphosphate. Using such products will give your skin what it needs without layering on emollients, thickeners, or other heavier ingredients that, although elemental for dealing with dry skin, are often troublesome for combination or oily skin. If you have combination skin but also have some very dry areas, you may have no choice but to address the dryness with a more emollient moisturizer. The key is to apply it only to the dry areas and make sure it doesn't migrate to oily zones.

(Other sources for this article: *Current Molecular Medicine*, March 2005, pages 171–177; *Applied Spectroscopy*, July 1998, pages 1001–1007; *Skin Research and Technology*, November 2003, pages 306–311; *Journal of the American Academy of Dermatology*, March 2003, pages 352–358; *Skin Pharmacology and Applied Skin Physiology*, November–December 1999, pages 344–351; and *Dermatology*, February 2005, pages 128–134.)

Essential Point: All of the elements above are prime factors that contribute to making what I (and many cosmetic ingredient researchers and chemists) consider a state-of-the-art moisturizer. It is important to know that there is no single "best" moisturizer available. Instead, there are many brilliant formulations, and informed consumers can find truly elegant products for their specific skin type, be it a serum-type moisturizer for use on combination or oily skin or an emollient-rich product to help remedy dry skin.

YOU DON'T NEED EYE CREAMS!

Most women believe that eye creams are specially formulated for the skin around the eye area. Although the eye area does tend to be more prone to allergic or sensitizing reactions, and often shows wrinkles before other areas of the face, it turns out that product formulations for eye creams don't differ from those for face products. There is no evidence, research, or documentation to validate the claim that eye creams have special formulations that set them apart from or make them superior to other facial moisturizers. I have never found a dermatologist or cosmetics chemist who can tell me what special ingredients the eye area needs that the face doesn't—or vice versa. It only takes a quick look at the ingredient labels of any moisturizer or eye moisturizer to see that they don't differ except for the price and the tiny containers the eye creams come in. Eye creams are a whim of the cosmetics industry designed to evoke the sale of two products when only one is needed.

The only time you might want to use a different product around the eyes is if the skin there happens to indeed be different from the skin on the rest of your face. For example, if your face is normal to oily and doesn't require a moisturizer except occasionally on the cheeks or around the eyes, then an emollient, well-formulated moisturizer of any kind will work beautifully.

Ironically, one of the real drawbacks of many so-called eye creams is that they rarely contain sunscreen. For daytime, that makes most eye creams a serious problem for the health of skin. You could believe that you were doing something special for your eyes, but you would actually be putting them at risk of sun damage and wrinkling by using an eye cream without sunscreen. This is another example of the way cosmetics marketing and misleading information can waste your money and hurt your skin.

WHY IRRITATION IS SO BAD FOR SKIN

Throughout this book you will repeatedly read cautions and warnings encouraging you to avoid products or skin-care routines that can cause irritation and inflammation. I cannot stress enough (as you undoubtedly will be able to tell after reading only a few paragraphs of this book) how bad it is to irritate or inflame skin—I mean really, really bad. The research about this issue is overwhelming, yet on an ongoing basis we subject our skin to those elements that can cause a long list of unwanted problems.

Irritation and inflammation, whether it is from unprotected sun exposure, free-radical damage from the very air we breathe, eating unhealthy foods, smoking, or pollution is a terrible problem. Yet equally as problematic are skin-care products that contain irritating ingredients, using very hot water, or over-scrubbing skin. Our skin can barely keep up with the assault; in the long run it doesn't, and it suffers irreparable damage.

There is a litany of negative effects that occur when skin is irritated or inflamed, but fundamentally this results in the skin's immune system becoming impaired, collagen breaking down, and the skin being stripped of its outer protective barrier. What is perhaps most shocking is that all of these damaging responses can be taking place underneath the skin and you wouldn't even notice it on the surface, not until many years later. The clearest example of this is the significant and carcinogenic effect of the sun's silent UVA rays. You don't feel the penetration of these mutagenic rays, but they are taking a toll on the skin nonetheless.

For the overall health of your skin, anything you can do to treat it gently is a good thing. Treating skin gently encourages normal collagen production, helps skin fight infection, maintains a smooth and radiant surface, and helps skin protect itself from environmental stressors.

With the goal being to eliminate anything that unnecessarily irritates and inflames skin, the following is a list of typical skin-care culprits that are not helpful in the least and that are potentially damaging to your skin. The skin can react negatively to all of the following products, procedures, and ingredients.

IRRITATING SKIN-CARE STEPS AND PRODUCTS TO AVOID

- Overly abrasive scrubs (such as those that contain aluminum oxide crystals, walnut shells, or pumice)
- Astringents containing irritating ingredients (alcohol and menthol being the prime offenders)
- Toners containing irritating ingredients (alcohol and menthol being the prime offenders)
- Scrub mitts
- Cold or hot water
- Steaming or icing the skin
- Facial masks containing irritating ingredients (watch out for fragrant essential oils, alcohol, and menthol)
- Loofahs
- Bar soaps and bar cleansers

(Sources: *International Journal of Dermatology*, August 2002, pages 494–499; *Skin Research and Technology*, May 2001, pages 98–104; and *Dermatology*, March 1997, pages 258–262.)

IRRITATING INGREDIENTS TO AVOID

Keep in mind that all of these ingredients are of greater concern when they appear near the top of the ingredient list, although because women often use numerous products, the repeated aggravation to skin means it is best to avoid these regardless of concentration.

Alcohol or sd alcohol deserves a bit more explanation than the other substances listed below. Not all "alcohols" are problematic. These exceptions include, among others, cetyl alcohol and stearyl alcohol, which are standard, benign, waxlike cosmetic thickening agents that are completely nonirritating and safe to use; sd alcohols are not considered problematic when they are used in minute amounts, as is the case with some ingredient mixtures.

Ammonia
Arnica
Balm mint
Balsam
Bentonite
Benzalkonium chloride
Benzyl alcohol
Bergamot
Camphor
Cinnamon
Citrus juices and oils
Clove
Clover blossom
Coriander
Cornstarch
Essential oils
Eucalyptus
Eugenol
Fennel
Fennel oil
Fir needle
Fragrance
Geranium
Grapefruit
Horsetail
Lavender
Lemon
Lemongrass
Lime
Linalool
Marjoram
Melissa (lemon balm)
Menthol
Menthyl acetate
Mint
Oak bark
Orange
Papaya
Peppermint
Phenol
Sandalwood oil
Sodium C14-16 olefin sulfate
Sodium lauryl sulfate
TEA-lauryl sulfate
Thyme
Wintergreen
Witch hazel
Ylang ylang

Many of the ingredients in this list are extremely common, showing up in skin-care products for all skin types. And because many of these are recognizable, "natural/botanical" names, consumers often perceive them as "good" ingredients when in fact they are anything but.

(Sources for the information in this section on irritation include *Journal of Cosmetic Dermatology*, March 2006, pages 30–38; *International Journal of Toxicology*, May–June 2006, pages 183–193; *Skin Research and Technology*; November 2001, pages 227–237; *Dermatologic Therapy*, January 2004, pages 16–25; *American Journal of Clinical Dermatology*, May 2004, pages 327–337; *Journal of the European Academy of Dermatology and Venereology*, November 2003, pages 663–669; *Drugs*, 2003, volume 63, issue 15, pages 1579–1596; *Clinical and Experimental Dermatology*, March 2002, pages 138–146; *Cosmetics & Toiletries*, November 2003, page 63; *Global Cosmetics*, February 2000, pages 46–49; and *Contact Dermatitis*, February 1995, pages 83–87.)

IRRITANTS AND COUNTER-IRRITANTS

For those of you who are familiar with my reviews, you may notice that I am now much more cautious about products that contain almost any amount of irritating ingredients, particularly those containing any form of grain alcohol (ethyl, ethanol, methanol, benzyl, or sd alcohol). This also goes for irritants like lemon, grapefruit, mint, peppermint, menthol, camphor, eucalyptus, ivy, fragrant oils, and overly drying or irritating detergent cleansing agents. My more exacting criteria in this area reflect the growing body of research indicating that irritation damages skin and disrupts the skin's healing process (Sources: *Skin Research and Technology*, November 2001, pages 227–237; and *Microscopy Research and Technique*, volume 37, issue 3, pages 193–199). In the midst of our daily battle against sun damage, wrinkles, and breakouts, there is never a reason to unnecessarily irritate the skin with ingredients like these, which provide no benefit whatsoever for the face or body and can prevent the skin from healing.

It turns out that much of what we know about skin aging, wrinkles, and skin healing involves a better understanding of the skin's inflammatory reaction to sun exposure (UV radiation), pollution, and cigarette smoke. These elements trigger an inflammatory process that leads to the accumulation of damage in the skin, in turn resulting in deterioration of collagen and elastin, depletion of disease-fighting cells, and free-radical damage (Sources: *Biogerontology*, 2001, volume 2, number 4, pages 219–229; *Ageing Research Reviews*, June 2002, pages 367–380; and *Journal of the International Union of Biochemistry and Molecular Biology*, October–November 2000, pages 279–289). Therefore, it never makes sense to use irritating ingredients on skin when they have no additional beneficial purpose (as topical disinfectants or certain exfoliants do). These ingredients can only hurt the skin and contribute to complications that make matters far worse for skin, not better.

What about counter-irritants? There is a misperception among many in the cosmetics industry, as well as among consumers, that ingredients considered to be counter-irritants, such as menthol, peppermint, camphor, eucalyptus, and mint, have anti-inflammatory or anti-irritant properties, but that is absolutely not true (Sources: *Archives of Dermatological Research*, May 1996, pages 245–248; and *Code of Federal Regulations*, Title 21—Food and Drugs, revised April 1, 2001, at 21CFR310.545, www.fda.gov). In fact, counter-irritants induce local inflammation as a way to relieve inflammation in deeper or adjacent tissues. In other words, they substitute one kind of inflammation for another. That is never good for skin. Both irritation and inflammation, no matter what causes them or how it happens, impair the skin's immune and healing response (Source: *Skin Pharmacology and Applied Skin Physiology*, November–December 2000, pages 358–371). Although your skin may not show it, or may not react in an irritated fashion, if you apply irritants to your skin the damage is still taking place, and the effects are ongoing and add up over time (Source: *Skin Research and Technology*, November 2001, pages 227–237).

What Makes Skin Happy—and What Doesn't

GENTLY CLEAN YOUR SKIN. Research proving that you should clean the skin gently is now well established. This is the basic first step for all skin types, from normal to oily, dry, blemish-prone, or sun-damaged. Nevertheless, no matter what your skin type, it is impossible and unhealthy to "deep-clean" skin. You can't get inside a pore and clean it out like a dentist with a drill. Even if you could get inside a pore and clean it out, the damage you would do to the skin would negate any benefit of deep cleaning. (I know a blackhead looks like it's dirty, but dirt isn't what's making it look black!)

Expensive water-soluble cleansers will not make your face any cleaner, nor are they necessarily any gentler than the less expensive water-soluble cleansers. In fact, the handful of standard cleansing agents used in cleansers is the same all across the cosmetics spectrum, regardless of price.

One more point: The wrong cleanser can cause headaches for your skin. For example, a cleanser that is too greasy can create blemishes and make skin feel greasy or oily. A cleanser that is too drying can create combination skin, because drying up skin doesn't stop or change the amount of oil your oil glands produce.

(Sources: *International Journal of Dermatology*, August 2002, pages 494–499; *Cosmetic Dermatology*, August 2000, pages 58–62; *Cutis*, December 2001, volume 68, number 5, Supplemental; *Skin Research and Technology*, February 2001, pages 49–55; *Dermatology*, 1997, volume 195, number 3, pages 258–262; and *Journal of the American Medical Association*, April 1980, pages 1640–1643.)

Thankfully, overly drying cleansing agents are being used less and less. Yet there are still products that include them, especially bar soaps and bar cleansers, which are typically far more drying than water-soluble cleansers that use gentle cleansing agents.

Essential Point: Use a gentle, water-soluble cleanser that doesn't dry out the skin or leave it feeling greasy, and that can remove most types of eye makeup without irritating the eyes.

USE EYE-MAKEUP REMOVER. Removing all of your eye makeup is more important than you may think. I was asked to be part of a medical advisory group attended by some of the most prominent dermatologists in the field. Of the topics discussed, the most fascinating were discussions about anti-wrinkle products, the validity (or lack thereof) of how effective they are, and the ways the cosmetics industry and the medical community have collaborated to create studies that prove a product is beneficial when in truth the study proves nothing at all (but makes for great marketing copy). What a great meeting!

On a seemingly far more mundane level there was a also brief dialogue about makeup removal. I mentioned that a basic remedy for puffy, irritated, crepey skin around the eyes was being sure to remove every last trace of eye makeup before you go to bed. One of the dermatologists echoed that and voiced a concern, mentioning that when she looks at her patients' skin under a magnifying glass, she is always surprised to see how much makeup is crusted into the lines around the eyes. Not a pretty picture.

That got me thinking about the need for makeup remover. In the past, I would have recommended using only a gentle, water-soluble cleanser for cleaning your face and removing makeup, and for some women who wear minimal makeup that works great. But for those who apply foundation, concealer, eyeshadows, eye pencils, and mascara, it takes more diligence to get these off the skin (because leaving them on overnight causes problems). In those cases, a dedicated makeup remover needs to be part of your nightly routine. I still feel it is important to begin by washing your face with a gentle, water-soluble cleanser and removing as much makeup as you can that way. Gently massaging a cleanser over the face and eyes prevents tugging and pulling, which is far better for skin. Then you can remove the last traces of makeup with a gentle makeup remover and soft pad of cotton (pulling and tugging as little as possible).

EVEN MINIMAL UNPROTECTED SUN EXPOSURE IS DAMAGING TO THE SKIN. Consumers clamor for the latest anti-wrinkle cream or serum, but all of that is meaningless if you aren't using an effective sunscreen every day of your life. Whether you tan or not (though tanning is particularly damning for skin), the damaging rays of the sun are taking a toll that begins the moment your skin sees daylight.

If you are exposed to the sun, even for as little as a few minutes every day—and that includes walking to your car, walking to the bus, or sitting next to a window during the day (the sun's damaging UVA rays come through window glass)—regardless of the season, that exposure adds up over the years, and it will wrinkle your skin, cause skin discolorations, and potentially result in skin cancer. If exposure that minimal can wrinkle the skin, imagine how much worse the impact of being in the sun for a long period of time can be and how ultimately detrimental sunbathing can be. No skin-care product except a sunscreen with an SPF of 15 or greater that includes the appropriate UVA-protecting ingredients of titanium dioxide, zinc oxide, avobenzone (butyl methoxydibenzylmethane), Mexoryl SX (ecamsule), or Tinosorb can help prevent that excessive and relentless damage from taking place.

And you must apply sunscreen liberally! That means that using an expensive sunscreen can be dangerous if it discourages you from applying it generously. For more specifics about sun protection, including SPF ratings and UVA versus UVB protection, refer to Chapter Seven, *Cosmetic Ingredient Dictionary*.

Bottom Line: There is no such thing as a safe tan, either from the sun or from tanning beds (in fact, tanning beds are far more dangerous than the sun) (Source: *Cancer Epidemiology, Biomarkers, and Prevention*, March 2005, pages 562–566). Any amount of skin turning color from the sun means that your skin is being seriously damaged.

Essential Point: Sunscreen and being smart about exposing your skin to the sun is the most important part of any skin-care routine.

MANY SKIN-CARE PROBLEMS ARE CAUSED BY THE SKIN-CARE PRODUCTS SOLD TO PREVENT THEM. Most consumers would be shocked to learn that many of the products they buy to treat a specific skin condition can actually make matters worse. Overly emollient and too-thick moisturizers can clog pores, even if those products claim to be noncomedogenic or nonacnegenic. Products designed to control oily skin often contain ingredients that can make skin oilier. For example, oil-free products often contain potential pore-clogging, emollient ingredients that don't sound like they would be a problem—yet nevertheless they are. And then there are the many products that contain irritants that can cause a range of skin problems. Countless skin-care products, even from the most expensive lines, contain such irritating ingredients as fragrance, alcohol, peppermint, lemon, camphor, menthol, horsetail, arnica, and on and on. All these ingredients can contribute to the very skin problems you are trying to eliminate from your face and your life. I would estimate that most combination skin problems are caused by using products that are poorly formulated or wrong for the individual's skin type.

Essential Point: Allergic, sensitizing, or irritating skin reactions are often caused by skin-care products that contain problematic ingredients such as irritating plant extracts. Some of the ones to watch out for are camphor, menthol, lemon, lime, eucalyptus, peppermint, fragrant oils, and grain alcohol. In addition, products that are too emollient can make oily or blemish-prone skin as well as dry skin worse, and products that are too drying can also make both skin types worse, just for different reasons.

DRY SKIN DOESN'T WRINKLE ANY MORE OR LESS THAN OILY SKIN—AND ALL THE MOISTURIZERS IN THE WORLD WON'T STOP WRINKLING. Oily skin may *look* less wrinkled, but that is only because oily skin has its own built-in moisturizer, namely the oil produced by the skin's oil glands. Wrinkles, sagging, and skin discolorations are caused by a combination of events, and the primary culprits are sun exposure, genetic inheritance, sagging muscles (not from lack of exercise, but from the stretching and laxity that occur with use), loss of subcutaneous fat, thinning of skin due to cell senescence, menopause (estrogen depletion), and normal aging. But dry skin does not cause wrinkles.

That's not to say moisturizers (in their varying forms) can't do amazing things for skin, because they can, and more and more research is showing this to be the case. Moisturizers with significant amounts of skin-identical ingredients, water-binding agents, state-of-the-art antioxidants, and anti-irritants can temporarily make skin look smoother, help skin function better, reduce the effects of sun damage, help improve texture, and much, much more. However, the notion that even reliable use of a good moisturizer will somehow substitute for the work of a plastic surgeon or be enough to defend skin from further signs of aging is sheer fantasy.

Essential Point: What causes wrinkles to appear is *not* related to how dry or oily the skin may be. Wrinkles are caused by a number of factors, chiefly years of unprotected sun exposure and a person's own genetics.

EXFOLIATE REGULARLY. Exfoliation is the natural process all skin goes through in which the outermost layers of skin are sloughed off and replaced by the new cells that move to the surface. This endless inside-out rotation is the hallmark of healthy skin. For many reasons this healthy cell turnover may get impaired, causing problems for many skin types. An excess of surface skin cells that don't shed normally can be the result of sun damage (sun damage causes the surface layer of skin to become thick and scaly, while it thins and depletes the support structures in the layers below the surface). However, it can also be caused by oily skin preventing natural exfoliation because the excess oil makes skin cells stick to the surface. Overly emollient skin-care products that basically hold skin cells down can do the same thing. For some skin disorders and as a result of sun damage, abnormally generated skin cells adhere unevenly and tenaciously to the surface of skin, another problem that slows down healthy exfoliation.

Exfoliation is very important for many skin types. For dry skin, removing the excess layers of skin can help the skin better absorb moisturizers, stimulate collagen production, improve cell turnover and skin texture, and reduce the appearance of skin discolorations. Those with oily skin will find that regular exfoliation can prevent clogged pores, can keep skin clear and even-toned, and can improve cell turnover.

Perhaps the only skin type that cannot benefit from some form of exfoliation is extremely sensitive skin or skin that has become thin due to the cell senescence that begins to occur when a woman is in her 70s. Yet even very sensitive skin may be able to tolerate (and will benefit from) occasional, extra-gentle exfoliation.

Among the most effective methods of exfoliation are topical scrubs, which can be as simple as using a washcloth, or a cosmetic cleanser that contains an abrasive material. However, research has established that salicylic acid (BHA), for normal to oily or blemish-prone skin, and alpha hydroxy acid (AHA) or polyhydroxy acid (PHA), for normal to dry skin, are not only effective exfoliants but also increase collagen production, improve the overall health of the skin, increase cell turnover, and reduce the appearance of skin discolorations. Therefore, those types of exfoliants are preferred to scrubs because they deliver greater results.

(Sources for the above information: *Cutis*, August 2001, pages 135–142; *Journal of the European Academy of Dermatology and Venereology*, July 2000, pages 280–284; *American Journal of Clinical Dermatology*, March–April 2000, pages 81–88; *Skin Pharmacology and Applied Skin Physiology*, May–June 1999, pages 111–119; *Dermatologic Surgery*, August 1997, pages 689–694, and May 2001, pages 1–5; *Journal of Cell Physiology*, October 1999, pages 14–23; and *British Journal of Dermatology*, December 1996, pages 867–875.)

Essential Point: Regular exfoliation is beneficial for almost all skin types, particularly oily skin and dry skin.

DO NOT AUTOMATICALLY BUY SKIN-CARE PRODUCTS BASED ON THE NOTION OF AGE. Many products on the market are supposedly designed specifically for women who are in their 30s, 40s, or 50 or older. Before you buy into these arbitrary divisions, ask yourself why the over-50 group is always lumped together. Isn't it odd that women between the ages of 20 and 49 have skin that requires three or four categories, but those women over the age of 50 (often referred to as "mature skin") need only one? There are a lot of years between 50 and 90! According to this logic, someone who is 40 to 49 shouldn't be using the same products as someone who is 50 or 51, but someone who is 80 should be using the same products as someone who is 50. Skin has different needs based on how dry, sun-damaged, oily, sensitive, thin, blemished, or normal it is, all of which have little to do with age. Plenty of young women have severely dry skin, and plenty of older women have oily skin and breakouts (particularly those women experiencing perimenopausal or menopausal hormone fluctuations). Turning 40 or 50 does not mean a woman should assume that her skin is drying up and that she must begin using overly emollient moisturizers or skin creams. And it definitely does not mean that the battle with blemishes is over.

Essential Point: Categorizing skin-care products by age groups is nothing more than a marketing device designed to sell products; it does not correlate at all with age-specific benefits to the skin.

DO NOT AUTOMATICALLY BUY SKIN-CARE PRODUCTS BASED ON YOUR SKIN TYPE. I know that statement sounds strange, but there are several reasons for this rule. It's not that skin type isn't important, but more often than not your skin type is not what you think it is. It's even possible that your skin type has been created by the products you are already using. Soap can severely dry the skin, overly emollient moisturizers can clog pores and cause blemishes, and alcohol-based toners can irritate the skin and cause dryness while doing nothing to change oil production (a situation that can create classic combination skin). To know what your skin type really is, you must start from square one with healthy gentle basics that won't alter or adversely affect your skin. That means using a gentle, water-soluble cleanser along with an irritant-free toner (or a disinfectant if you tend to break out) that contains effective water-binding agents, skin-identical ingredients, antioxidants, anti-irritants, or gentle detergent cleansing agents. You will also want an effective exfoliator (such as an AHA product if you have sun-damaged skin and/or a BHA product for breakouts), a sunscreen for daytime (this can be included in your moisturizer or foundation), and a well-formulated moisturizer, serum, or toner at night.

For those with oily, combination, or blemish-prone skin, using a moisturizer, even if it's one of those that claims to be oil-free or specially formulated for oily skin, can cause more problems for you than it can possibly solve. If you still want the benefits of all the new skin-identical ingredients, antioxidants, water-binding agents, and anti-irritants, they can be obtained from a well-formulated toner or gel/serum-type product, products that typically don't contain the thickening agents (ingredients that create lotion or cream textures) that can cause problems for oily or blemish-prone skin.

Essential Point: The intense cosmetics hype insisting that everyone needs a moisturizer is absolutely not true. But all skin types need antioxidants, cell-communicating ingredients, water-binding agents, and skin-identical ingredients to have and maintain healthy skin.

TREAT THE SKIN YOU HAVE TODAY, NOT THE SKIN YOU HAD LAST MONTH, LAST WEEK, OR YESTERDAY. Your skin type can and will fluctuate. Skin-care routines based on a specific skin type don't take into consideration the fact that your skin changes with the season, your emotions, the climate (humidity, dryness, cold, and heat all affect your skin), and your menstrual cycle. Pay attention to what your skin tells you it needs at any given time. This month you might need an extra-moisturizing sunscreen during the day, and a more emollient nighttime moisturizer. Next month you may only need a lightweight sunscreen or a foundation with sunscreen during the day and no moisturizer at night. The same is true for oily skin and breakouts. In fact, those dealing with breakouts may find that alternating their routine (such as using a disinfectant one evening and a BHA product the next) is necessary to balance the benefits with the potential side effects. But all of that doesn't mean you need new products every month—it just means you may need to use less of one item or more of another, adapting your routine flexibly according to your skin's current needs.

Essential Point: Don't hold fast to the idea that your skin fits squarely into and remains only one type—it changes, and so should your skin-care routine.

TEENAGERS ARE NOT THE ONLY ONES WHO HAVE ACNE. One of the biggest skin-care myths ever is that women over the age of 20 are not supposed to break out, and that when they do, it is the exception to the rule. What a mistaken belief that is! Women in their 30s, 40s, and 50s can have acne just like teenagers, and the treatment principles remain the same.

Essential Point: Not everyone who has acne as a teenager will grow out of it, and even if you had clear skin as a teenager, that's no guarantee that you won't get acne later in life. You can blame this often-maddening inconsistency on hormones!

BATTLING BLEMISHES OR ACNE IS NOT A MYSTERY, BUT IT DOES REQUIRE SPECIFIC TYPES OF PRODUCTS AND INGREDIENTS. Unfortunately, many cosmetics companies don't use those specific ingredients in their products for blemish-prone skin. As I wrote the reviews for this edition, I was flabbergasted that so few product lines contain truly effective products for dealing with blemishes. This is one category of products where needless irritation is not the exception, but rather the unfortunate norm. The following is a very brief overview of how to win the battle against blemishes.

The goals of effective blemish treatment are to reduce excess oil production, to eliminate skin-cell buildup on the surface of the skin and in the pore, and to kill the bacteria (*Propionibacterium acnes*) that cause the inflammation in the first place. This is best accomplished using a gentle, water-soluble cleanser, exfoliating on the surface and in the pore lining with a pH-correct BHA product, and using a topical disinfectant (benzoyl peroxide is considered the most effective over-the-counter topical disinfectant. One study in the December 2004 issue of the British medical journal *Lancet*, pages 2188–2195, showed benzoyl peroxide to be as effective and more stable than oral antibiotics). You can also improve new skin-cell production with topical prescription products such as Retin-A, Renova, Tazorac, or Differin, which also help restructure the pore to allow for it to function normally.

Essential Point: Battling blemishes requires experimenting to find the right combination of products, although a gentle cleanser, exfoliant, and topical disinfectant are the basics.

SKIN LIGHTENING

Regardless of your ethnic background or skin color, eventually most of us will struggle with some kind of brown or ashen pigmentation problem. Skin will either appear lighter or darker than normal in concentrated areas, or you may notice blotchy, uneven patches of brown to gray discoloration or freckling. Skin pigmentation disorders occur because the body produces either too much or too little of the pigment melanin. Melanin is produced by specific cells (melanocytes). Melanocytes are triggered by an enzyme called tyrosinase, which creates the color of our skin, eyes, and hair. (Melanin actually has two major forms that combine to create varying skin tones. Eumelanin produces a range of brown skin and hair color, while pheomelanin imparts a yellow to reddish hue.)

As far as skin is concerned, melanin, depending on how much is present, does provide some amount of protection from the sun by absorbing the sun's UV light. This explains why darker skin is less susceptible to sunburn as well as to the overall effects of sun damage. However, less susceptible does not mean immune to problems.

Increased or unwanted melanin production—also known as hyperpigmentation—is often referred to as melasma, chloasma, or solar lentigenes. Melasma is a general term describing darkening of the skin. Chloasma is typically used to describe skin discolorations caused by hormones. These hormonal changes are usually the result of pregnancy, use of birth control pills, or estrogen replacement therapy. Solar lentigenes is the technical term for darkened spots on the skin caused by the sun (solar refers to sunlight, and lentigene describes a darkened area of skin). These spots are quite common in adults with a long history of unprotected sun exposure.

By far, for all skin colors, the most typical cause of darkened areas of skin, brown spots, or areas of discoloration is unprotected sun exposure. Once incorrectly referred to as liver spots, these pigment problems have nothing whatsoever to do with the liver. In fact, these discolorations wouldn't have appeared in the first place if the skin had been diligently protected from the sun over the years.

On lighter to medium skin tones, solar lentigenes emerge as small- to medium-sized brown patches of freckling that can grow and accumulate over time on areas of the body that receive the most unprotected sun exposure, such as the back of the hands, forearms, chest, and face. For those with darker skin colors, these discolorations can appear as patches or areas of ashen-gray skin. Regardless of how or why these benign discolorations occur, the response to them is the same worldwide: this is something women want to get rid of and prevent from recurring, or to prevent in the first place.

COMBINATION TREATMENT

Melanin production is stimulated by a complex process that is partially controlled by the enzyme tyrosinase. Most skin-lightening treatments are aimed at inhibiting this enzyme, which can reduce or block some amount of melanin production. There are many options to consider when searching for a solution. The most successful treatments use a combination of topical lotions or gels containing melanin-inhibiting ingredients, a well-formulated sunscreen, and a prescription retinoid (such as Renova, TriLuma, or generic versions containing tretinoin, a type of retinoid). Depending on how the skin responds to these treatments, exfoliants—either in the form of topical cosmetic or chemical peels—as well as lasers are also able to further affect pigment and can definitely enhance results (Sources: *Journal of the American Academy of Dermatology*, May 2006, Supplemental, pages 272–281; *Dermatologic Surgery*, March 2006, pages 365–371; *Journal of Drugs in Dermatology*, September–October 2004, Supplemental, pages 27–34; *International Journal of Dermatology*, December 2003, pages 966–972; and *Archives of Dermatology*, December 2002, pages 1578–1582).

SUNSCREEN

Without question, the first line of defense is smart sun behavior. That means avoiding sunlight, and welcoming sunscreen. The key is daily use (365 days a year) and liberal application (and, when needed, reapplication) of a well-formulated sunscreen. Diligent use of a sunscreen alone allows some repair as well as protection from further sun damage, which is what created the problem to begin with (Sources: *Journal of the American Academy of Dermatology*, May 2005, pages 786–792; *American Journal of Epidemiology*, April 2005, pages 620–627; and *The British Journal of Dermatology*, December 1996, pages 867–875). No other aspect of controlling or reducing skin discolorations is as important as being careful about exposing your skin to the sun and the regular use of sunscreen, SPF 15 or greater (and greater is usually better). And make sure that the sunscreen includes the UVA-protecting ingredients of titanium dioxide, zinc oxide, avobenzone, Tinosorb, or Mexoryl SX. Using skin-lightening products, exfoliants, peels, or laser treatments without also using a sunscreen will prove to be a waste of time and money.

HYDROQUINONE

Topical hydroquinone is the next step in reducing or eliminating skin discolorations. In fact, topical application of hydroquinone is considered by many dermatologists to be a safe option. It is as effective (if not more so) as laser or deep peel treatments, and far less expensive. Topical hydroquinone is available at a 2% concentration in cosmetic products and up to a 4% concentration that is available only from a physician or by prescription. Whether it is used alone or in combination with tretinoin 0.05% to 0.1%, it has an impressive track record. Research has repeatedly shown that hydroquinone and tretinoin are powerful tools against sun- or hormone-induced melasma (Source: *Dermatologic Surgery*, March 2006, pages 365–371).

Some concerns about hydroquinone's safety on skin have been expressed, but when it comes to topical application, the research indicates that negative reactions are minor or a result of using extremely high concentrations—or are caused by adulterated products in some countries that use glucocorticoids or mercury iodine. This is particularly true in Africa, where tainted skin-lightening products are commonplace (Sources: *British Journal of Dermatology*, March 2003, pages 493–500; *Critical Reviews in Toxicology*, May 1999, pages 283–330; and *Journal of Toxicology and Environmental Health*, September 1998, pages 301–317).

Despite hydroquinone's impressive track record and efficacy, in September 2006 the Food and Drug Administration (FDA) recommended that products containing hydroquinone be sold only with a prescription due to their opinion that it posed certain health risks. The FDA asserts there are animal studies that show it may be a possible carcinogen, and studies from Africa showed its use was linked with a risk of a skin disorder called ochronosis (Source: www.fda.gov/ohrms/dockets/98fr/E6-14263.htm).

However, there is abundant research from reputable sources that shows hydroquinone to be safe and extremely effective (Sources: *Cutis*, August 2006, Supplemental, pages 6–19; *Journal of Cosmetic Laser Therapy*, September 2006, pages 121–127; *American Journal of Clinical Dermatology*, July 2006, pages 223–230; and *Journal of the American Academy of Dermatology*, May 2006, Supplemental, pages 272–281). Surprisingly, there is even research showing that workers who handle pure hydroquinone actually have lower incidences of cancer than the population as a whole (Source: *Critical Reviews in Toxicology*, May 1999, pages 283–330).

Hydroquinone can be an unstable ingredient in cosmetic formulations. When exposed to air or sunlight it can turn a strange shade of brown. Therefore, when you are considering a hydroquinone product, it is essential to make sure it is packaged in a non-transparent container that doesn't let light in and that minimizes air exposure. Hydroquinone products packaged in jars are not recommended because the jars will allow the product to become ineffective shortly after opening.

AZELAIC ACID, KOJIC ACID, AND GLYCOLIC ACID

Some research has shown that topical azelaic acid in 15% to 20% concentrations is as efficacious as hydroquinone, and with a decreased risk of irritation, but this is minor in comparison to the research about hydroquinone. Kojic acid, alone or in combination with glycolic acid or hydroquinone, also has shown good results, thanks to its inhibitory action on tyrosinase. But kojic acid has also had its share of problems in terms of stability and potential negative effects on the skin, and is rarely used nowadays, at least by itself. Several plant extracts and vitamin C also have some research showing them to be effective for inhibiting melanin production (Sources: *Journal of the American Academy of Dermatology*, May 2006, pages S272–S281; *International Journal of Dermatology*, August 2004, pages 604–607; *The American Journal of Clinical Dermatology*, September–October 2000, pages 261–268; and *Archives of Pharmacal Research*, August 2001, pages 307–311).

Glycolic acid, kojic acid, or glycolic acid with hydroquinone are all effective in reducing the pigment in melasma patients (Source: *Dermatological Surgery*, May 1996, pages 443–447). So why aren't there more products available containing kojic acid? Because it is an extremely unstable ingredient in cosmetic formulations. On exposure to air or sunlight it turns a strange shade of brown and loses its efficacy. Many cosmetics companies use kojic dipalmitate as an alternative because it is far more stable in formulations. However, there is no research showing kojic dipalmitate to be as effective as kojic acid, although it is a good antioxidant. Further, some controversial research has shown kojic acid to have some carcinogenic properties (Sources: *Mutation Research, Genetic Toxicology and Environmental Mutagenesis*, June 2005, pages 133–1450; and *Toxicological Sciences*, September 2004, pages 43–49).

OTHER ALTERNATIVES

Although hydroquinone has the highest efficacy and a long history of safe use behind it, there are other alternatives that have shown promise for lightening skin. However, these have been far less researched, and their effectiveness often pales in comparison to that of hydroquinone. It is interesting to point out that some of these alternative ingredients are, perhaps not surprisingly, derivatives of hydroquinone. They include *Mitracarpus scaber* extract, *Uva ursi* (bearberry) extract, *Morus bombycis* (mulberry), *Morus alba* (white mulberry), and *Broussonetia papyrifera* (paper mulberry), all of which contain arbutin. Technically known as hydroquinone-beta-D-glucoside, arbutin can inhibit melanin production. Pure forms of arbutin, such as alpha-arbutin, beta-arbutin, and deoxy-arbutin, are considered more potent for skin lightening. Other options with some amount of research about their potential skin-lightening abilities are licorice extract (specifically glabridin), azelaic acid, and stabilized vitamin C (L-ascorbic acid, ascorbic acid, and magnesium ascorbyl phosphate). What has not been conclusively established for most of these hydroquinone alternatives is how much is needed in a cosmetic lotion or cream to obtain an effect.

There is also a small amount of research showing that oral supplements of pomegranate extract, ellagic acid, vitamin E, and ferulic acid can inhibit melanin production. All of these options are worth considering and experimenting with. However, compared with the extensive research on hydroquinone's effect on inhibiting melanin production, these alternatives may very well disappoint, although their natural allure is hard for consumers to ignore.

(Sources: *Experimental Dermatology*, August 2005, pages 601–608; *Bioscience, Biotechnology, and Biochemistry*, December 2005, pages 2368–2373; *International Journal of Dermatology*, August 2004, pages 604–607; *Journal of Drugs in Dermatology*, July–August 2004, pages 377–381; *Facial and Plastic Surgery*, February 2004, pages 3–9; *Dermatologic Surgery*, March 2004, pages 385–388; *Journal of Bioscience and Bioengineering*, March 2005, pages 272–276; *Journal of Biological Chemistry*, November 7, 2003, pages 44320–44325; *Journal of Agriculture and Food Chemistry*, February 2003, pages 1201–1207; *International Journal of Cosmetic Science*, August 2000, pages 291–303; and *Anti-Cancer Research*, September–October 1999, pages 3769–3774.)

ARBUTIN

A bit more information on arbutin is warranted. As mentioned above, arbutin contains a form of hydroquinone derived from the leaves of bearberry, cranberry, mulberry, or blueberry shrubs, and also is present in most types of pears. Because of arbutin's hydroquinone content it can have melanin-inhibiting properties (Source: *The Journal of Pharmacology and Experimental Therapeutics*, February 1996, pages 765–769). Although the research describing arbutin's effectiveness is persuasive (even if most of the research was done in vitro), concentration protocols have not been established. That means we don't know how much arbutin it takes to lighten skin when it is added to a cosmetic formulation. Moreover, most cosmetics companies don't use arbutin because of its cost. To get around this problem, many cosmetics companies use plant extracts that contain arbutin. Unfortunately, there is little to no research to show that the plant-extract sources of arbutin have any impact on skin, especially not in the tiny amounts present in cosmetics.

Arbutin is the most intriguing alternative to hydroquinone, but even so, it is arbutin's hydroquinone content that gives it its melanin-inhibiting properties (Sources: *Analytical Biochemistry*, June 2002, pages 260–268, and June 1999, pages 207–219; *Pigment Cell Research*, August 1998, pages 206–212; and *Journal of Pharmacology and Experimental Therapeutics*, February 1996, pages 765–769).

Mulberry extract, which contains arbutin, has one study showing that it does have minimal effectiveness, although almost none when compared with the effectiveness of hydroquinone (Source: *Cosmetics & Toiletries*, 1997, volume 112, pages 59–62); plus, the study used a pure concentration of mulberry extract, not the minimal amounts that are present in cosmetics.

TRETINOIN

A great deal of research has shown that the use of tretinoin (also known as all-trans retinoic acid, as found in the prescription medications Renova and Retin-A) can be effective in treating skin discolorations (Sources: *Tissue & Cell*, April 2004, pages 95–105; *Dermatologic Surgery*, March 2006, pages 365–371; *Journal of Dermatologic Science*, August 2001, Supplemental, pages S68-S75; *Acta Dermato-Venereology*, July 1999, pages 305–310; *International Journal of Dermatology*, April 1998, pages 286–292; and *Journal of the American Academy of Dermatology*, March 1997, pages S27–S36). However, when tretinoin is used in combination with hydroquinone, skin discolorations can show a far more noticeable and impressive improvement. Because of this, tretinoin is generally not recommended as the only topical option for melasma, but is best used to reduce darkened areas of skin in combination with other effective topicals, particularly sunscreen and hydroquinone (Source: *eMedicine Journal*, www.emedicine.com, November 15, 2001).

ALPHA HYDROXY ACIDS

Alpha hydroxy acids (AHA), primarily in the form of lactic acid and glycolic acid, are the most researched forms of substances for skin lightening because they have a molecular size that allows them to effectively penetrate into the top layers of skin. It is generally assumed that, in and of themselves, AHAs at concentrations of 4% to 15% are not effective for inhibiting melanin production. Yet because they improve the appearance and function of skin's outer layer, skin tone and color can show overall improvement. AHAs help cell turnover rates and remove unhealthy or abnormal layers of superficial skin cells (exfoliation) where hyperpigmented cells can accumulate, and this can create a marked improvement. There is also other research that has shown that lactic and glycolic acids can indeed inhibit melanin production apart from their actions as exfoliants on skin (Source: *Experimental Dermatology*, January 2003, Supplemental, pages 43–50).

Either way, there is a good amount of evidence that in combination with other treatments—such as hydroquinone, azelaic acid, laser resurfacing, and, of course, an effective sunscreen—AHAs can be very effective for improving the overall appearance of sun-damaged skin and possibly helping other ingredients better penetrate skin. While there is no comparative research in regard to salicylic acid (BHA) and its effect on melasma, it makes sense to assume that because salicylic acid exerts an action on skin that is similar to that of AHAs, it will have similar results for improving skin color.

Much like laser treatments, AHA peels (using 50% concentrations or greater) have shown impressive results for removing skin discolorations (Sources: *Dermatologic Surgery*, February 2005, pages 149–154; *Journal of Cutaneous Medicine and Surgery*, April 2004, pages 97–102; *Cutis*, February 2004, Supplemental, pages 18–24; *Dermatologic Therapy*, June 2004, pages 196–205; and *Dermatological Surgery*, June 1999, pages 450–454). Only a physician should perform facial peels using these high concentrations of AHAs.

VITAMIN C

Magnesium ascorbyl phosphate, L-ascorbic acid, ascorbyl glucosamine, and ascorbic acid are the various forms of vitamin C considered stable and effective antioxidants for skin. Very few studies show them to have benefit for inhibiting melanin production, but what little there is has been positive. The problem is that in these studies, researchers used high concentrations (more than 5%) of these ingredients, an amount rarely used in cosmetic formulations. However, in combination with other treatments, vitamin C is an extra step that can help reduce skin discolorations (Sources: *International Journal of Dermatology*, August 2004, page 604; *Dermatology*, April 2003, pages 316–320; and *Journal of the American Academy of Dermatology*, January 1996, pages 29–33).

LASER TREATMENTS

Both ablative and nonablative lasers can have a profound effect on melasma. However, the results are not always consistent, and problems can occur (such as hypo- or hyperpigmentation). Moreover, laser treatments of this kind are often a problem for those with darker skin tones due to the manner in which they affect skin color. Nonetheless, when laser treatments work they make a marked difference in the skin's appearance, especially when used in combination with the topical treatments previously mentioned. The results can be startling, and although they are expensive, lasers are absolutely worth a try for stubborn discolorations. There are many types of lasers that can be successful for this purpose. Which one is optimal for you is best determined by a skilled dermatologist who has a practice that incorporates a variety of different lasers (Sources: *Journal of the American Academy of Dermatology*, May 2006, Supplemental, pages 262–271; *Dermatologic Therapy*, January 2001, page 46; *Journal of Cosmetic and Laser Therapy*, March 2005, pages 39–43; Journal of Cutaneous Medicine and Surgery, April 2004, pages 97–102; *Journal of Drugs in Dermatology*, November–December 2005, pages 770–774; *Dermatologic Surgery*, October 2005, page 1263; and *Lasers in Surgery and Medicine*, April 2000, pages 376–379).

Regardless of which skin-lightening ingredient or product you decide to try, a well-formulated sunscreen used diligently, 365 days a year over exposed parts of the body, is absolutely the most effective way to prevent and reduce skin discolorations. Also, an effective AHA product (meaning one with a 4% to 10% concentration of AHA and with a pH of 3 to 4) can help encourage cell turnover, and that has been shown to improve skin discolorations, too.

Essential Point: When it comes to choosing the best ingredient for lightening sun-caused or hormone-induced skin discolorations, hydroquinone is the star of the show. No other skin-lightening ingredient has a more substantiated, successful track record.

BATTLE PLANS FOR BLEMISHES

There is very little mystery about how a pimple is created. It essentially starts with hormones causing excess oil production in the pore. For some reason, the oil cannot get out in an even flow, possibly as a result of an abnormally shaped pore. This backed-up oil, along with a buildup of dead skin cells in the pore lining, forms a blockage—and eventually a clogged pore. A specific type of bacteria (*Propionibacterium acnes*) in the pore thrives on the oil and dead skin cells, flourishes, and as a result causes the skin to become inflamed. The inflammation and proliferation of bacteria result in a pimple (Sources: *Drugs*, 2003, volume 63, issue 15, pages 1579–1596; and *Advances in Dermatology*, January 2003, pages 1–10).

A limited number of studies have looked at the role diet plays in causing and/or treating acne. For some individuals an allergic reaction to certain foods such as nuts, salmon, or dairy products can trigger inflammation in the pore, resulting in blemishes. Research indicates that dietary supplements, such as zinc or vitamin A, are most likely not effective in the treatment of acne, and these supplements may very well be unhealthy if too much is taken (Sources: *Journal of Pediatric Hematology and Oncology*, October 2002, pages 582–584; *Journal of the American Academy of Dermatology*, August 2002, pages 231–240; and *European Journal of Dermatology*, June 2000, pages 269–273).

For optimal results when fighting blemishes and acne:

- Reduce oil to eliminate the environment in which acne-causing bacteria thrive.
- Exfoliate the skin's surface and within the pore to improve the shape and function of the pore.
- Disinfect the skin to eliminate acne-causing bacteria.

Over-the-counter and prescription options abound for fighting blemishes, and that makes it a confusing battle to fight. It's confusing because there isn't one routine or medication (or combination of therapies) that works for everyone. Finding the combination that works for you is the goal, and that requires experimentation.

FIGHTING BLEMISHES, STEP BY STEP

Cleansing the Face: Use a gentle, water-soluble cleanser. One of the most common myths in skin care is that a cooling or tingling sensation means that a product is "working," which couldn't be further from the truth. That feeling is actually just your skin responding to irritation, and products that produce that sensation can actually damage the skin's healing process, make scarring worse, and encourage the bacteria that cause pimples. Using cleansers that contain pore-clogging ingredients (like soaps or bar cleansers) can also make matters worse (Source: *Dermatologic Therapy*, February 2004, Supplement, pages 16–25 and 26–34). The essential first step is to find a gentle, water-soluble cleanser.

If you are removing stubborn or waterproof makeup, you may need to use a washcloth to be sure you really remove all of your makeup. To prevent bacterial growth on that washcloth, use a clean one every time you wash your face.

Exfoliating: Use a 1% to 2% beta hydroxy acid (BHA) product or an 8% alpha hydroxy acid (AHA) product to exfoliate the skin. As a general rule, for all forms of breakouts, including blackheads, BHA is preferred over AHA because BHA is better at cutting through the oil inside the pore (Source: *Cosmetic Dermatology*, October 2001, pages 65–72). Penetrating the pore is necessary to exfoliate the pore lining. However, some people (including those allergic to aspirin) can't use BHA, so an AHA is the next option to consider.

A topical scrub or a washcloth can be used as a mechanical exfoliant. To remove dead skin cells, this can be helpful for some people—but it does not in any way take the place of an effective BHA, AHA, or topical prescription treatment. Be careful never to overscrub when using a mechanical scrub—too much abrasion can disrupt the skin's ability to heal.

Topical Disinfecting: Benzoyl peroxide is considered the most effective over-the-counter choice for a topical disinfectant to fight blemishes (Source: *Skin Pharmacology and Applied Skin Physiology*, September–October 2000, pages 292–296). The amount of research demonstrating the effectiveness of benzoyl peroxide is exhaustive and conclusive (Sources: *American Journal of Clinical Dermatology*, April 2004, pages 261–265; and *Journal of the American Academy of Dermatology*, November 1999, pages 710–716). Among benzoyl peroxide's attributes is its ability to penetrate into the hair follicle to reach the problem-causing bacteria and kill them—with a low risk of irritation. Furthermore, it doesn't pose the problem of bacterial resistance that occurs with some prescription topical antibacterials (antibiotics) (Source: *Dermatology*, 1998, volume 196, issue 1, pages 119–125).

There aren't many other options for disinfecting the skin. Alcohol and sulfur are good disinfectants, but they are also too drying and irritating, and they can make matters worse for skin by damaging the skin's ability to heal (Sources: *American Journal of Clinical Dermatology*, April 2004, pages 217–223; *Cosmetics & Toiletries Magazine*, March 2004, page 6; and *Infection*, March–April 1995, pages 89–93).

Tea tree oil has some interesting research showing it to be an effective disinfectant. The *Medical Journal of Australia* (October 1990, pages 455–458) compared the efficacy of 5% tea tree oil with that of 5% benzoyl peroxide for the treatment of acne. The conclusion was that "both treatments were effective in reducing the number of inflamed lesions throughout the trial, with a significantly better result for benzoyl peroxide when compared to the tea tree oil. Skin oiliness was lessened significantly in the benzoyl peroxide group versus the tea tree oil group." Unfortunately, most products on the market contain little more than a 1% concentration of tea tree oil, not the 5% strength used in the study.

For some people, a topical disinfectant may be enough, but that is generally the exception. Using a topical antibacterial along with an exfoliant gives you a powerful combination in winning the battle against blemishes. That is, cleaning the skin by exfoliating alone or by disinfecting alone can give fairly good results, but used together they are a formidable defense against blemishes.

Note: Benzoyl peroxide negates the effectiveness of most retinoids (such as Retin-A and Tazorac) and, therefore, these two products cannot be used at the same time. To get the benefits of both, you can use benzoyl peroxide in the morning and the retinoid in the evening. However, Differin (adapalene) has been shown to remain stable and effective when used with benzoyl peroxide (Source: *British Journal of Dermatology*, October 1998, page 139).

Absorbing Excess Oil: This is perhaps one of the most difficult skin-care problems to control. Because oil production is triggered only by hormones, there is nothing you can apply topically to stop your skin's oil glands from making more oil. What you can do to make sure you don't make matters worse is avoid products that contain oils or emollient ingredients.

To absorb surface oil, forms of clay masks can help a lot, although avoid masks that contain irritating ingredients. As strange as it sounds, Phillip's Milk of Magnesia can be used as a facial mask. It is nothing more than liquid magnesium hydroxide, which does a very good job of absorbing oil. How often to use a mask depends on your skin type; some people use it every day, others once a week. This type of mask may be used after cleansing, left on for 10–15 minutes, then rinsed with tepid water.

MEDICAL OPTIONS

Retinoids: Aside from exfoliation, prescription options for improving the shape of the pore include Retin-A (tretinoin), Differin (adapalene), and Tazorac (tazarotene). There is an immense amount of research showing these to be effective in treating acne (Source: *Journal of the American Medical Association*, August 11, 2004, pages 726–735). Depending on your skin type, you can use them up to twice a day. You also can try using them only at night, and then use a BHA or AHA during the day. As an alternative, some dermatologists recommend applying the BHA or AHA first, then applying Retin-A, Differin, or Tazorac. The thought is that the BHA or AHA boosts the effectiveness of the prescription products by helping them penetrate the skin better. Again, talk to your doctor and experiment to see which frequency, combination, and sequence of application works best for your skin.

Oral Antibiotics: If none of the nonprescription options previously discussed (i.e., gentle cleansing, exfoliants, and antibacterial agents) work for you and if prescription retinoids also fail to give you satisfactory results, an oral antibiotic prescribed by a doctor is another option. Several studies have shown that oral antibiotics, used in conjunction with topical tretinoins or topical exfoliants, can control and greatly reduce breakouts (Sources: *Cutis*, June 2004, pages 6–10; and *International Journal of Dermatology*, January 2000, pages 45–50).

However, as effective as oral antibiotics can be, they should be considered carefully. A serious, problematic side effect is that acne-causing bacteria can become immune to the antibiotic after a short period of time, causing the acne to return (Sources: *Dermatology*, January 2003, pages 54–56; *American Journal of Clinical Dermatology*, April 2003, pages 813–831, and March 2001, pages 135–141; and *The General Meeting of the American Society for Microbiology*, May 2001). Whatever course of action you take should be discussed at length with your dermatologist, who, like you, should also be carefully monitoring you for any side effects.

Photodynamic Therapy: This treatment, also called Light Therapy, has been shown to effectively treat acne (Source: *Journal of Cosmetic Laser Therapy*, June 2004, pages 91–95). This medical treatment uses a topical medication called aminolevulinic acid (a drug used for treatment of precancerous skin conditions) in conjunction with non-skin–damaging lasers or a light source called blue light (Source: American Academy of Dermatology, www.aad.org). After the topical medication is applied, the patient sits in front of the light source for 15 to 30 minutes. It is often necessary to have three to five sessions over a period of time before lasting improvement is seen.

WHEN ALL ELSE FAILS

If your breakouts persist after you've tried the options I've described, it may be necessary to consider more serious treatment, such as hormone blockers or birth control pills designed to reduce breakouts.

Accutane is one of the last options to consider in this lineup of last resorts because of its very serious potential side effects, especially if a woman becomes pregnant while using it, which is why its use must be discussed with your physician. However, Accutane is the **only** option that can potentially cure breakouts; all of the other methods merely keep the problem reduced or at bay. More than 50% of the people who take Accutane for one round never break out again, and it eliminates oily skin altogether. Those odds are increased significantly for people who take it a second time (Sources: *Skin Therapy Letter*, March 2004, pages 1–4; *Expert Opinion on Drug Safety*, February 2004, pages 119–129; and *Journal of the American Medical Association*, August 2004, pages 726–735).

BATTLE PLANS FOR WRINKLES

The plan below is designed to improve the overall appearance of your skin by supplying it with gentle, effective, and protective ingredients that have a proven track record for helping wrinkled skin look and feel better. Providing such benefits to skin on a daily basis will enhance its health and appearance, encourage collagen production, and help generate normalized skin cells, which altogether means wrinkles can be greatly reduced! Notice that I did *not* write that wrinkles can be "eliminated"! Regrettably, there is no magic potion or combination of products in any price range that can make wrinkles truly disappear. The wrinkles you see and agonize over (not to be confused with fine lines caused by dryness, which are easily remedied with a good moisturizer) are the result of cumulative sun damage and the inevitable breakdown of the skin's natural support structure. Skin-care ingredients, no matter who is selling them or what claims they assert, cannot replace what plastic surgeons or cosmetic dermatologists can do.

With that in mind, the basic place to start is by following a step-by-step plan that provides what the skin needs to repair itself and function optimally.

A state-of-the-art sunscreen whose formula goes beyond basic (and critical) sun protection. The first and foremost best defense against wrinkles is the daily use of an effective, well-formulated sunscreen rated SPF 15 or higher. Daily application of a sunscreen (be it in your moisturizer or foundation, which must be applied all over your face) is critical to preventing new wrinkles and keeping existing lines from deepening each year. Ignoring this fundamental principle and focusing instead on anti-aging claims (which, if they don't involve sunscreen, don't require proof of efficacy) is an open invitation for more wrinkles, skin discolorations, and, potentially, skin cancer. The basics to look for are a product rated SPF 15 or higher, and make sure it has one of the following ingredients listed as active to ensure adequate protection from UVA rays: avobenzone (also known as Parsol 1789 or butyl methoxydibenzoylmethane), titanium dioxide, zinc oxide, Mexoryl SX (ecamsule), or Tinosorb. These are all effective UVA-protecting ingredients.

Beyond that, it is extremely beneficial if the sunscreen you choose is also loaded with antioxidants, anti-irritants, cell-communicating ingredients, and ingredients that mimic the structure and function of healthy skin. An abundant and ever-expanding amount of scientific research is proving how antioxidants not only boost a sunscreen's efficacy but also play a role in mitigating sun damage by reducing the free radicals and skin inflammation that sun exposure generates. A state-of-the-art sunscreen contains not only effective UVA-protecting ingredients but also antioxidants and other ingredients that help skin look and feel better. In short, for optimal benefit and healing, your sunscreen needs to go beyond just deflecting UV rays; it must also work on a cellular level to prevent damage (Sources: *Journal of the American Academy of Dermatology*, June 2005, pages 937–958; *Photodermatology, Photoimmunology, and Photomedicine*, August 2004, pages 200–204; and *Cutis*, September 2003, pages 11–15).

Retin-A, Renova, Avita (drug name tretinoin), **and Tazorac** (drug name tazarotene), prescribed by your doctor or dermatologist, are still the gold standards among topical prescription products for improving the appearance of sun-damaged (wrinkled and discolored) skin. Tretinoin has the ability to return abnormal skin-cell production back to some level of normalcy—think of it as the guru of cell-communicating ingredients. The result in most cases is an improvement in skin's collagen production, which makes skin smoother and offers a modest (but noticeable) decrease in the depth and appearance of wrinkles. Tazarotene is believed to work similarly to tretinoin (Sources: *Cutis*, February 2005, pages 10–13; *Mechanisms of Ageing and Development*, July 2004, pages 465–473; and *Dermatologic Surgery*, June 2004, pages 864–866).

An effective AHA or BHA product. One significant consequence of sun damage is that the outer layer of skin becomes thickened, discolored, rough, and uneven. The best way to help skin shed abnormally built-up layers of dead, unhealthy skin is to use a well-formulated AHA or BHA product. Such exfoliation will not just even out skin tone, it will also produce a significant improvement in the texture of skin. Another benefit is that exfoliating accumulated layers of dead skin cells helps other products you use, particularly moisturizers, penetrate your skin and be far more effective. The most researched forms of AHAs are glycolic or lactic acids. Salicylic acid is the sole BHA option. For AHAs, look for products that contain at least 5% AHA, but preferably 8% to 10%. If the percentage isn't listed on the label, then the ingredient should be at the top of the ingredient list. For BHA products, 0.5% to 2% concentrations are available.

The difference in concentrations between the AHAs and BHA is not a qualitative one. AHAs are not more effective or better than BHA just because AHAs have higher concentrations. Rather, it's just that leave-on, daily-use AHAs are effective at 5% to 10% and BHA is effective at 1% to 2% (Sources: *Women's Health in Primary Care*, July 2003, pages 333–339; *Journal of Dermatological Treatment*, April 2004, pages 88–93; *Dermatology*, January 1999, pages 50–53; and *Journal of the American Academy of Dermatology*, April 1997, pages 589–593). There are many such examples in skin care (and in cooking and baking for that matter) where a higher percentage or concentration of an ingredient doesn't necessarily correlate with superior performance.

If you are battling wrinkles and stubborn blemishes or blackheads, BHA is the better choice because salicylic acid can also improve the shape of the pore. Whether you choose an AHA or BHA product, it is essential that the product itself have a pH between 3 and 4. This range is necessary for either ingredient to exfoliate skin. You can find products with a pH lower than 3, but these tend to be too irritating for all skin types, which negates their benefits. (When I rate skin-care products with AHA or BHA, I always test the pH to be sure that it does indeed allow the acid to exfoliate skin.) (Sources: *Plastic and Reconstructive Surgery*, April 2005, pages 1156–1162; *Dermatologic Surgery*, February 2005, pages 149–154; and *Experimental Dermatology*, December 2003, pages 57–63.)

Be gentle! Don't forget that gentle cleansers and products that don't contain irritating ingredients play an important part in helping your skin look better. Using a gentle, water-soluble cleanser further minimizes skin irritation, prevents moisture loss, and won't leave a skin-dulling residue. No cleanser will change a wrinkle, but cleansing skin gently and reducing irritation and inflammation helps the healing process that results from such products as sunscreens and tretinoin.

A well-formulated, state-of-the-art moisturizer is basic. Choose a serum or liquid texture if you have normal to oily or blemish-prone skin, and a cream or emollient lotion for dry skin. A good moisturizer can go a long way toward improving skin's texture, enhancing its radiance, and creating a smoother, more supple surface. A gel, cream, serum, or lotion that is loaded with antioxidants, ingredients that mimic the structure of skin, cell-communicating ingredients, and anti-irritants can generate new collagen, create normalized skin cells, and lessen further damage. Make sure the packaging will keep the beneficial ingredients inside stable once the product is opened. That means, look for opaque tubes or bottles with pump applicators or small openings, and avoid clear packaging and jars of any kind. For more details, see the section in this chapter entitled "What Is a State-of-the-Art Moisturizer?"

Cosmetics companies (and the cosmetics industry at large) are acutely aware of the consumer's desire to forestall aging and stop wrinkles in their tracks. That's why, at every retail venue you visit, you will repeatedly encounter products promising to lift, firm, and tone the skin, along with decreasing (or dramatically reducing) wrinkles via this week's miracle ingredient or complex. Don't fall for it! And especially not at the expense of not using an effective sunscreen, or using the proven options described above for improving the appearance of sun-damaged (wrinkled) skin. Almost without exception, if an expensive (often very expensive) anti-wrinkle claim sounds too good to be true, it probably is. That doesn't mean the product in question isn't worth considering, just that it isn't the fountain of youth so many of us are perpetually seeking.

BATTLE PLANS FOR DRY SKIN

Before you begin creating a battle plan for dry skin anywhere on your body, it is essential to have a fundamental understanding of what dry skin is all about. Ironically, dry skin is not as simple as being about a lack of moisture. The studies that have compared the water content of dry skin to that of normal or oily skin show that there doesn't appear to be a statistically significant difference. And adding more moisture to the skin is not necessarily a good thing—if anything, too much moisture, like soaking in a bathtub, is bad for skin because it disrupts the skin's intracellular matrix by breaking down the substances that keep skin cells functioning normally and in good shape (Source: *Journal of Investigative Dermatology*, February 2003, pages 275–284).

What is thought to be taking place when dry skin occurs is that the intracellular matrix (the substances between skin cells that keep them intact, smooth, and healthy) has become depleted or damaged, bringing about water loss. To prevent dry skin, the primary goal is to reduce the damage to, as well as preserve and enhance, the intracellular matrix so that the skin can maintain its natural moisture homeostasis. (For example, think about kids who rarely have dry skin because their skin hasn't yet suffered damage from the sun or other factors that prevent the skin from taking care of itself.)

To reduce damage to the skin's matrix, never use drying skin-care products such as soaps, harsh cleansers, or products with irritating ingredients. These problematic products can disrupt the outer layer of the skin, destroying the intracellular matrix and eventually causing flakiness and roughness.

Constant exposure to arid environments and cold weather, as well as to dry, low-humidity air blasting from heaters or air conditioners, are all problematic because they destroy the skin's matrix. Adding a humidifier to your home can make a world of difference!

Believe it or not, sun damage plays a major role in skin becoming dry at any time of the year. Unprotected sun exposure creates a damaged outer layer of skin where skin cells adhere poorly to each other. The result is that the surface of new skin being formed just below it is continually unhealthy and impaired. Sun damage also disrupts and destroys the skin's intra-cellular matrix. Every day of the year, so long as there is daylight, the skin is subject to sun damage. Keep in mind that the sun's damaging rays come through office and car windows, too. Daily sun protection is vital to the health of skin.

Improving cell turnover is another important consideration in getting rid of dry skin and improving its appearance. Dry skin does not shed as it should, and those built-up layers of dead skin cells can feel rough and cause skin to look flaky and dull. A well-formulated, pH-correct exfoliant such as an AHA (glycolic or lactic acid) or BHA (salicylic acid) can handle this problem beautifully.

Genetically, age also is a cause of dryness because as a woman's levels of estrogen drop the skin becomes thinner and the fat deposits under the skin (part of the skin's protective barrier) also become thinner or depleted altogether. Regrettably, there is little that can be done about this other than using various types of hormone replacement therapy or plant-based hormone replacement (phytoestrogens), which you can get by consuming soy-based food or drinks.

By the way, while drinking eight glasses of water a day is great for your body, it won't work to improve or reduce dry skin. If all it took to get rid of dry skin was drinking more water, then no one would have dry skin and moisturizers would stop being sold. Keeping your liquid intake up is fine, but the causes of and treatments for dry skin are far more complicated than that. Following are some great options for winning the dry skin battle:

- **Wear sunscreen:** Daylight, even dim, obscure daylight, causes skin damage, which means your skin slowly becomes less and less able to hold moisture or feel smooth.
- **Use state-of-the-art moisturizers:** Moisturizers should be filled to the brim with antioxidants, water-binding agents, and anti-inflammatory ingredients. If you have persistent or exceptionally dry skin, the moisturizers you use should also contain various forms of lipids such as lecithin, cholesterol, glycerol, glycerides, and plant oils. Anything less leaves your skin incapable of warding off the environmental causes of dry skin. To ensure stability of the light- and air-sensitive ingredients, make sure whatever moisturizer you choose does not come in clear or jar packaging.
- **Apply and reapply moisturizer:** If you have dry skin, you really can't use too much. So whenever your skin starts feeling dry, put more on. It is also important to be diligent about reapplying moisturizer every time you wash your hands. Don't forget tokeep a moisturizer in your purse, at your desk, and in every bathroom in your home.
- **Avoid soap—use only gentle, nondrying cleansers:** This cannot be stressed enough. Never use a cleanser that leaves a dry feeling on your skin, and that includes skin from the neck down. Do not overscrub skin—you can't scour away dryness.

- **Avoid soaking in the bathtub or Jacuzzi or taking long showers:** As wonderful as a leisurely bath or shower feels, too much water is bad for skin because it breaks down the skin's intracellular matrix, destroying the substances that keep skin cells intact. Keep showers or baths as short as possible.
- **Get a humidifier:** Low humidity is the cause of most weather-related dry skin, regardless of a person being in a winter or a desert environment. Humidifiers are relatively inexpensive, last a long time, and work for the whole family. If you have a large or multilevel home, you may need two or three humidifiers to gain benefit.
- **Avoid bath oils in the bath:** It does not make much sense to pour bath oils into the bathwater because most of the oil ends up going down the drain, not to mention that it makes the bathtub slippery and dangerous. Bath oils also encourage you to soak in the tub for longer periods of time and that isn't good for skin. There is also research showing that oil can trap cleansing ingredients on skin, causing irritation and dryness. Oils are best applied when you get out of the bath or shower, after you are well rinsed off and gently towel dried.
- **Exfoliate:** Skin cell turnover (exfoliation) is a function of healthy skin, but due to sun damage, skin more often than not needs help with this process. A well-formulated AHA or BHA can help skin cells turn over in a more natural, youthful manner by removing the buildup of old skin cells and allowing them to be replaced by newer, smoother ones.
- **Use a pure plant oil, such as olive oil, after your moisturizer over dry areas:** At night, after you've applied your moisturizer, massage a few drops of plant oil over stubborn dry areas. Pure olive oil is a great option because it is rich in antioxidants.
- **Don't forget your lips:** The skin on lips is the least capable of staying smooth and soft when the air becomes dry. Your lips lack the lipids and cell structure the rest of the face has and, as a result, they are far more vulnerable to the effects of dry air. During the day apply and reapply an emollient lipstick or gloss. At night be sure to do the same. Do not go to sleep without protecting your lips. An emollient lip balm worn throughout the night can prevent dry lips all year round. Be sure it doesn't contain any irritating ingredients; peppermint and menthol (often found in lip balms) can cause irritation and that won't help dry lips.
- **Never use products that contain drying or irritating ingredients:** But you already knew that one, right?

(Additional sources: *Dermatologic Therapy*, 2004, volume 17, issue 1, Supplemental, pages 43-48; *American Journal of Clinical Dermatology*, April 2003, pages 771–788; *Journal of the American Academy of Dermatology*, March 2003, pages 352–358; *Skin Research and Technology*, November 2003, pages 306–311; *American Journal of Clinical Dermatology*, April 2003, pages 771–788.)

Please note: For other skin disorders, such as rosacea, psoriasis, severe dry skin, or wound and scar treatments, and more details about all skin-care concerns and options, refer to my Web site at www.cosmeticscop.com.

CHAPTER THREE

Explanation of Reviews

HOW PRODUCTS ARE RATED

Rating a wide variety of cosmetic products is a rigorous, complex process. Establishing criteria that will let someone distinguish and differentiate a terrible product from a great one, or a good product from one that's just mediocre, requires exact and consistently applied guidelines, and, moreover, guidelines that must be substantiated with published research that used clear criteria and rigorous scientific methods. These are exactly the criteria I've created for each product type that I review in this book.

First—and above all—you need to know that I do not base any rating decision on my own personal experience with a product. In other words, just because I like the way a cleanser or a moisturizer feels on my skin, I know it doesn't mean that thousands of others will feel the same way about it. Personal feelings won't help you evaluate whether a product may hurt your skin or live up to any part of the claims showcased on the label. There are lots of online beauty chat rooms and bulletin boards, fashion magazines, and friends who love to share their personal experiences about the products they use (some even publish online reviews). That might be interesting and entertaining, but it's important to recognize that lots of people also like things that aren't good for them. Some people may like suntanning, others may use products that contain irritating ingredients because they believe the tingling feeling means it's "working." Most people have no idea what kinds of ingredients can damage skin.

Even more to the point, these friendly recommendations don't know that there are other products that perform equally as well if not better, and for a lot less money. If you're going to spend money on a product, why not find out first whether or not it can live up to its claims, based on formulary or comparison performance issues, and then see how you can expect it to perform on you? That is what you will find out from the reviews in this book.

All the ratings for the skin-care products in this book are based primarily on formulation of the individual product. I have consulted countless published, peer-reviewed studies about the ingredients in the product, and have considered the possible resulting interactions, with each other and with your skin. I also evaluate these formulas based on published cosmetics chemistry data about ingredient performance and consistency. From that I can assess a product's potential for irritation, dryness, breakouts, sensitivities, greasiness, and other issues of texture and performance.

Makeup products are evaluated more subjectively than skin-care products with regard to their application, color selection, texture, and how they compare to similar products from myriad other lines. Formulation is also a consideration for makeup products, but predominantly for claims made in regard to skin care and for any makeup product that includes an SPF rating.

This rating process is more challenging than I can describe, because even if I think a company is absurdly overcharging for its products or is exceedingly dishonest in its claims and advertising, and no matter how unethical it seems to me, it does not prevent me from saying that a product of theirs is good for a particular skin type. Though I do often say, "This is a good product but what a shame the price has to be so absurd and the claims so ridiculous!"

Overall, the evaluation process for this 7th Edition of *Don't Go to the Cosmetics Counter Without Me* is the same as for previous editions. However, you will find one major difference that has had a direct impact on the product ratings: In this edition, I use a far more stringent standard for excellence for every category of product. Happy faces are no longer awarded to ordinary, perfunctory products with mediocre, standard, or even decent formulations. For example, if a product makes claims about containing antioxidants or anti-irritants, then it better contain a convincing amount of these ingredients. What you will notice is that many more products receive neutral ratings in this edition than in previous editions (many because of inadequate packaging).

Each cosmetics line is reviewed on the basis of several different elements. The first consideration is overall presentation and how user-friendly the displays or company literature are. For lines available at retail locations, I consider it an asset if their display units are set up with convenient color groups, such as colors divided into warm (yellow) and cool (blue) tones, and are easily accessible. Skin-care and makeup products that are convenient to sample without the help of a salesperson are also rated high. For drugstore lines, colors must be easy to see, and samples or tester units are considered a (rare) bonus.

For infomercial and in-home shopping channel companies, my major criterion is the organization and logic of their skin-care routines. Generally, ordering products from these sources means you are buying a set of products, not picking and selecting from what is being offered. If these prefabricated kits do not include an adequate sunscreen, or if the kit for someone with breakouts is only minimally different from the kit for someone with dry skin, then the overall rating goes down dramatically. (Skin-care products with ingredients that are good for someone with dry skin are rarely suited for someone with oily, acne-prone skin.)

I am also leery of any company that claims to be the best or to have state-of-the-art formulations when they don't include a sunscreen of SPF 15 or greater that is formulated with UVA-protecting ingredients (avobenzone, titanium dioxide, zinc oxide, Mexoryl SX, or Tinosorb) as part of their daily skin-care regimen. Any company purporting to have worthwhile products or well-researched formulations could not possibly be telling the truth if they are not even aware of the well-known and easily accessible information on sunscreen ingredients (Sources: Food and Drug Administration at www.fda.gov; American Academy of Dermatology at www.aad.org).

In this book, I make the final and fundamental determination for each individual product rating based on specific criteria established for each product category. For every category, from lipsticks, blushes, mascaras, and eyeshadows to concealers, foundations, cleansers, toners, scrubs, moisturizers, facial masks, AHA products, wrinkle creams, and brushes, I've created specific standards that the products must meet to garner a happy, unhappy, or neutral (meaning unimpressive but not bad) face.

Makeup products are assessed primarily on texture and application using professional tools (brushes). Was it silky-smooth or grainy and hard? But also important is color (was a wide range of colors available, and was there an adequate selection for women of color?), ease of use (was the container poorly designed, were colors placed too close together in an eyeshadow set, was foundation put in a pump container that squirted too much product or didn't reach to the bottom of the jar?), and, finally, price. More specific criteria for each makeup category is discussed further in this chapter.

Skin-care products are evaluated almost exclusively on the basis of content versus claim. For example, if a product claims to be good for sensitive skin, it cannot contain irritants, skin sensitizers, drying ingredients, and so on.

I also asked the following questions to see if a product can measure up to its claims, based on established and published research:

1. Given the ingredient list, and based on published research—not just on what the cosmetics company wants you to believe—can the product really do what it promises?
2. How does the product differ from similar types of products?
3. If a special ingredient (or ingredients) are showcased, how much of it is actually in the product, and is there independent research verifying the claims for it?
4. Does the product contain problematic fragrances (including volatile fragrance components), plants, topical irritants, or other questionable ingredients that could cause problems for skin?
5. How farfetched are the product's claims?
6. Based on what's known about the ingredients it contains, is the product safe? Are there risks such as allergic reactions, increased sun sensitivity, insufficient sunscreen formulations, or potentially toxic ingredients?

I wish I had the space to challenge and explain every single exaggerated claim and lofty explanation that accompanies the products listed in this book, but there is just not enough room (or time) to tackle that prodigious task. I cover most of the distortions and some of the hyperbole about products and ingredients in the reviews and in Chapter Seven, *Cosmetic Ingredient Dictionary*. Also I provide extensive information on my Web site (www.cosmeticscop.com) explaining everything you need to know about taking care of oily skin, dry skin, wrinkles, and other special skin-care needs, as well as a description of hundreds of skin-care ingredients and much more!

EVALUATING SKIN-CARE PRODUCTS

My reviews of skin-care products in each line are, with some exceptions, organized in the following categories: cleansers, eye-makeup removers, scrubs, toners, alpha hydroxy acid or beta hydroxy acid exfoliants, moisturizers (all kinds, regardless of the claim or type, such as eye or neck creams), specialty products, sunscreens, acne products, and facial masks. The criteria I used to evaluate the quality of the products in each of the different categories of skin-care products are explained below.

CLEANSERS: In reviewing facial cleansers, the primary criteria were how genuinely water-soluble they were, and how gentle. Facial cleansers should rinse off easily, with or without the aid of a washcloth, and remove all traces of makeup, including eye makeup. Once a water-soluble cleanser is rinsed off, it should not leave the skin feeling dry, greasy, or filmy. And it should never burn the eyes, irritate the skin, or taste bad.

Removing makeup with cold cream–style, rinseable cleansers in lotion or cream form is an option for some women with extremely dry skin. In the past, I have been hesitant to recommend these because they do not remove makeup very well and they require heavy wiping and pulling of the skin to remove the makeup. However, for someone with dry skin, these might be the only good, soothing, nondrying products to clean their skin, when used along with a soft washcloth.

I do not recommend cleansers just because they contain alpha hydroxy acids (AHA) or beta hydroxy acid (BHA) or topical disinfectants such as benzoyl peroxide or triclosan. These ingredients are quite helpful in other skin-care products, but in a cleanser they are rinsed off your face and down the drain before they have a chance to have any effect on your skin. Another concern is that these ingredients can inadvertently get into your eye when rinsing the cleanser off your face. (I should also mention, just in case someone might think that if they leave the cleanser on their face, then the AHA or BHA could exfoliate, and that I have never found a cleanser that includes enough AHA or BHA or that has a base with an appropriate pH to allow exfoliation. In other words, an AHA or BHA is useless in a cleanser, although I'm sure some consumers are misled into believing they could have an effect on skin.)

EYE-MAKEUP REMOVERS: As I mentioned in the section on eye-makeup removers in Chapter Two, I have changed my position on using a separate eye-makeup remover as an extra step. When you aren't wearing much makeup, an effective but gentle, water-soluble cleanser should take off all your makeup, including your eye makeup, without irritating the eyes. But for those who are wearing lots of eye makeup, a water-soluble cleanser won't be adequate because it will leave makeup behind, which can cause swelling, puffiness, irritation, redness, and exaggerated wrinkling. The problem with wiping off makeup is simply that you have to wipe and pull at your skin to get the stuff off. That repetitive pulling and wiping is not good for skin, particularly in the eye area, so be as gentle as possible. It is also a good idea to wash your face first with a water-soluble cleanser and then gently go over the eye area with the eye-makeup remover to be sure you remove all of your eye makeup.

It is important to note that the vast majority of eye-makeup removers contain many of the exact same ingredients found in water-soluble cleansers! In other words, more often than not eye-makeup removers contain a lightweight surfactant (detergent cleansing agent). In those instances, sticking with the water-soluble cleanser makes more sense. Other eye-makeup removers use either oils (plant or mineral) or silicones. These can help remove makeup without causing dryness, and for some skin types or personal preferences that can be beneficial.

Eye-makeup removers are one of the categories in which the products are nearly indistinguishable from one another. They are formulated so similarly that there are no surprises or real cautions needed. Eye makeup removers rated as Paula's Picks were assigned that distinction because of their exceptionally gentle, fragrance-free formulas that remain effective for their intended purpose.

SCRUBS: With the advent of alpha hydroxy acids (AHA) and the increased use of beta hydroxy acid (BHA; technical name, salicylic acid), there is less reason than ever before to use a mechanical exfoliant on the skin. Mechanical exfoliant is just a fancy name for scrubs, brushes, or washcloths that remove skin cells as you massage them over the skin. Even when a scrub's particles are small and uniform in size, this procedure can still abrade the skin and be harsher than necessary, causing damage and affecting the skin's healing process. That means that the major consideration for any topical scrub is that it must be gentle on the skin and not rough or overly abrasive. It is also important for it to rinse off easily without leaving any residue or greasy feel on the skin. Some women prefer the feeling of a scrub on their skin, but there aren't many scrubs that are any better than just a clean, soft washcloth with a gentle, water-soluble cleanser. Scrubs rated as Paula's Picks met the criteria above and had additional positive traits such as being fragrance-free or containing buffering agents that do not impede rinsing or hinder effectiveness.

ALPHA HYDROXY ACID (AHA) AND BETA HYDROXY ACID (BHA) PRODUCTS: Although AHAs and BHA can be effective as moisturizing ingredients, this is not what they do best for skin. Above all else, AHAs and BHA excel at exfoliating skin.

There is only one BHA (salicylic acid), but there are a variety of AHAs. The five major types of AHAs that show up in skin-care products are glycolic, lactic, malic, citric, and tartaric acids. Of these, the most commonly used AHAs are glycolic and lactic acids, because of their special ability to penetrate the skin and because they have the most accumulated research on their functionality for skin. A search of the published literature for glycolic and lactic acids lists over 200 studies, while there are only a handful for the other three AHAs combined, and that includes the infrequently used AHA alternative mandelic acid. A similar literature search for BHA reveals over 450 different published studies evaluating its effectiveness.

What glycolic, lactic, and salicylic acids can do is "unglue" the outer layer of dead skin cells. This helps to increase cell turnover by removing the built-up top layers of skin, allowing healthier cells to come to the surface. Removing layers of dead skin cells can improve skin texture and color, unclog pores, and allow moisturizers to be better absorbed by the skin. Both AHAs and BHA affect the top layers of skin, where they help to improve the appearance of sun-damaged skin, dry skin, and thickened skin caused by a variety of factors, including abnormal cell growth, smoking, and heavy moisturizers. A reminder: Sun damage in particular causes the top layer of skin to thicken, creating a dull, rough texture and appearance on the surface of skin; AHAs nicely remove this thickened layer, revealing the more normal-appearing skin cells underneath (Sources: *Archives of Dermatological Research*, June 1997, pages 404–409; and *Dermatologic Surgery*, May 1998, pages 573–577).

There is also a good deal of research showing that the use of glycolic acid (and most likely lactic acid) can improve the appearance of skin discolorations, increase collagen production, and reinforce the barrier function of skin (Sources: *Dermatologic Surgery*, May 2001, pages 429–433; and *American Journal of Clinical Dermatology*, March–April 2000, pages 81–88).

The fundamental difference between AHAs and BHA is that AHAs are water soluble, while BHA is lipid soluble (that is, oil soluble). This unique property of BHA allows it to penetrate the oil in the pores and exfoliate the built-up skin cells that are inside the pore lining (follicle). AHAs are not able to penetrate oil and so can't get through the fat content (sebum) of the skin and into the pores. Therefore, BHA is the best choice where blackheads and blemishes are the issue, and AHAs are more suitable for sun-damaged, thickened, or dry skin where breakouts are not a problem (Source: *Global Cosmetic Industry*, November 2000, pages 56–57).

I use very specific criteria to determine if an AHA or BHA product will be an effective exfoliant. I wish you could tell if it would be effective by reading the label, but that just isn't possible. With very few exceptions, there are no claims or promises on the product, or even on the ingredient label, that will tell you whether you are purchasing an effective AHA or BHA product.

When it comes to AHAs and BHA, the crucial information comes in two parts. One is the type of ingredient and its concentration in the product, and the other is the pH of the product. AHAs work best at concentrations of 5% to 8% in a base with a pH of 3 to 4 (this is more acid than neutral), and their effectiveness diminishes as the pH rises above 4.5. BHA works best at concentrations of between 1% and 2% at an optimal pH of 3, diminishing in effectiveness as the pH increases beyond 4. The effectiveness of both AHAs and BHA decreases as a product's pH increases and as the concentration of the ingredient decreases. This relationship is so central to the entire subject of exfoliation and cell turnover that it bears repeating: AHAs work best in a 5% to 8% concentration, in a product with a pH of 3 to 4; BHA works best in a 1% to 2% concentration, in a product with a pH of 3 to 4 (Source: *Cosmetic Dermatology*, October 2001, pages 15–18).

Salicylic acid (BHA), although it provides more penetrating exfoliation into the pore, is less irritating than AHAs because of its close chemical relation to aspirin. Salicylic acid is derived from acetylsalicylic acid, which is the technical name for aspirin, and aspirin has anti-inflammatory properties. When applied topically on the skin, the salicylic acid in BHA products retains many of these anti-inflammatory effects.

AHA and BHA products can definitely smooth the skin, improve texture, unclog pores, and give the appearance of plumper, firmer skin (because more healthy skin cells are now on the surface). But the change isn't permanent; when you stop using them the skin goes back to the condition it was in before you started.

Products that contain AHA sound-alikes, including sugarcane extract, mixed fruit acids, fruit extracts, milk extract, and citrus extract, or BHA sound-alikes, such as wintergreen extract or willow bark extract, cannot exfoliate skin, or do much of anything else (though willow bark has anti-inflammatory properties). Therefore, I rate products that contain these ingredients as not effective. You might think these are better because they appear to be a more natural form of AHA or BHA when you see these less technical, more familiar plant names on the label, but that perception is not reality.

As a general rule I do not recommend products that use both AHAs and BHA together because each has its specialized action, and that does not translate to all skin types. As mentioned previously, AHAs work on the surface of the skin and are best for sun-damaged skin that has developed a thickened outer layer, or for someone with dry skin who has a buildup of layers of skin that make the skin look dull and impede cell turnover. BHA can exfoliate on the surface of the skin much like AHAs can, but BHA can also cut through the lipid layer of skin and, therefore, works better in the pore, helping skin to shed cells and also loosening any plugs in the skin, improving the size and function of the pore. If you don't have breakouts, you don't need that kind of penetration; if you do have breakouts, AHAs may help to some extent, but the penetration from the BHA can be more effective. But for some skin types a combination can be preferred. This is an area that takes experimentation to see what works on your skin.

One word of caution: Anytime you use a well-formulated AHA product that contains more than 5% AHA, some stinging can occur, although this can diminish as the skin gets used to it. You should not let AHA or BHA products come in contact with the eyes, eyelids, or any mucous membranes. It is also possible that you may have an irritation reaction or sensitivity to AHAs or BHA. Slight stinging is expected, but continued stinging is not; if the stinging continues, stop using it. Ditto for persistent redness.

FACIAL MASKS: Many facial masks contain claylike ingredients that absorb oil and, to some degree, exfoliate the skin, which can be beneficial for someone with oily skin. The problem with many masks is that they often contain additional ingredients that are irritating or that can clog pores. Although your face may feel smooth when the mask is first rinsed off, after a short period of time you may experience problems created by the mask's drying effect. Even the few clay masks that contain emollients and moisturizing ingredients can still be too drying for dry skin yet can cause oily skin to break out. There is also a range of masks that contain plasticizing (hairspray-like) ingredients that you peel off the face like a layer of plastic. These take a layer of skin off when removed, and that can make skin feel temporarily smoother, but there is no long-term benefit to be gained.

The claims that clay from one part of the world or another, or from some part of the ocean or from a volcanic region is best for skin are backed up by no research of any kind showing that to be true. In essence, there isn't any research anywhere showing that clay can do anything beneficial for skin other than absorb oil, and there is not a shred of research showing that plasticizing masks have any benefit whatsoever. Moreover, any skin-care step used occasionally simply can't have as much value as a better routine used daily.

Another type of facial mask that shows up is the kind with strictly moisturizing ingredients. Basically these don't differ from other moisturizers except that they are thicker formulations. Calling the product a mask seems to make women feel like they are doing something special for their skin, when, with very few exceptions, they aren't. Despite all these shortcomings, which I point out in the individual reviews, there are masks in this book that did get happy face and Paula's Pick ratings, either because of their potential benefit for dry skin (if they contained reliable ingredients for this condition) or because of their absorbency for oily skin.

Masks are rated based on compatibility for each skin type and on whether or not they contain irritants. For dry skin the mask must have emollient properties and for oily skin it must have absorbent ingredients. Masks rated as Paula's Pick exceeded those criteria and went above and beyond by either offering fragrance-free formulas or unique extras with genuine benefit for skin.

TONERS: Toners, astringents, fresheners, tonics, and other liquids meant to refresh the skin or remove the last traces of makeup after a cleanser is rinsed off should not contain any irritants whatsoever. I evaluated these products primarily on this basis because, for the most part, that is all the industry has to offer—which is why so many of these products receive a neutral face rating. Toners tend to be ordinary, banal formulas with very little benefit for skin beyond the basics and, to their detriment, many in this category often contain irritants, making them unacceptable for any skin type.

Claims that toners can close pores or refine the skin are unachievable, so I ignore such language and look for toners that leave the face feeling smooth and soft, can remove the last traces of makeup, and do not irritate the skin. The best of this group are those that contain a good assortment of state-of-the-art ingredients (cell-communicating ingredients, water-binding agents, anti-irritants, antioxidants, and skin-identical ingredients). These are rated as being optimal for all skin types and get happy face and, occasionally, Paula's Pick ratings. Toners that add plant oils or emollients to those preferred ingredients are rated best for normal to dry skin. Toners that add mild detergent cleansing agents with no emollients, but that also include all the other state-of-the-art ingredients, are generally rated best for normal to oily skin.

For some skin types, a toner can be the only "moisturizer" the skin needs. Even for someone with dry skin, toners can be a great lightweight start to add an extra helping of brilliant, healthy ingredients to skin.

MOISTURIZERS: Despite all the fuss, assertions, and price differences among anti-wrinkle, firming, antiaging, and "renewing" supplements and treatments that claim to restore youth to skin, in truth these products are nothing more than moisturizers. A plethora of these products are being marketed to women, but I can tell you that not one plastic surgeon is going out of business because of them.

As a general category, "moisturizers" were quite easy to review because what constitutes a state-of-the-art product in this category is well established. They must contain ingredients that can smooth and soothe dry skin, keep water in the skin cell, help maintain or reinforce the skin's protective barrier, protect skin from free-radical damage, reduce inflammation or irritation, and contain cell-communicating ingredients to optimize healthy cell production, all in an elegant, silky base. Almost all other claims for this immense group of products are exaggerated and misleading, not to mention never-ending!

A recurring myth espoused at cosmetics counters and routinely in fashion magazines is that oily skin "needs" a moisturizer. In other words, you may be told that oily skin makes more oil because it is combating some form of underlying dryness. No part of that is true. Oil production is controlled and regulated by hormones (Sources: *Clinical and Experimental Dermatology*, October 2001, pages 600–607; and *Seminars in Cutaneous Medicine and Surgery*, September 2001, pages 144–153). If dry skin could induce oil production, then everyone with dry skin would be oozing oil, but they aren't, because physiologically that isn't how skin works (and the insanity of that hurts my brain). All skin types *need* healthy state-of-the-art ingredients, but they do not have to come in a lotion, balm, or cream form; gels, liquids, and serums serve that purpose perfectly.

While multitudes of ingredients are potentially helpful for skin, there are also a number that are a waste of time, or worse. These range from bee pollen to gold to animal extracts from thymus, spleen, and placenta, as well as plant extracts that can be potential skin irritants, and I point out as many of these as I can in my reviews. If there is no research showing any of these are helpful for skin, then they are there for marketing purposes only, and that doesn't help your skin. Those ingredients are explained in Chapter Seven, *Cosmetic Ingredient Dictionary*, of this book.

In addition, it is important to pay attention to the order in which the beneficial ingredients in moisturizers and serums are listed on the packaging. Just as with food labels, the ingredients present in the largest amounts are listed first. Often, the most interesting or the most extolled ingredients are so far down the list that the amount of them in the product means they are practically nonexistent. Just because an ingredient appears on an ingredient label doesn't mean there's enough of it to have any impact on skin or to make a difference of any kind.

There are also moisturizers that companies promote as being great for combination skin because they claim they can release moisturizing ingredients over dry areas and oil-absorbing ingredients over oily areas. This is categorically impossible. A product cannot hold certain ingredients back from the skin—where would they go? Imagine a lotion touching your skin and separating so the ingredients for the oily parts get up and run over here and the ones for the dry area get up and head over there. It just isn't feasible in any way, shape, or form. If you have combination skin (meaning slightly dry to dry areas accompanied by oily areas) you only need to apply a moisturizer over the dry parts of your face, including around the eyes, if applicable. If you have combination skin and wish to use something all over your face, shop for water- or silicone-based gel or serum-type moisturizers so as not to make oily areas worse.

MOISTURIZERS FOR OILY SKIN: Even when skin is oily, it can still (and does) benefit from the application of products that contain water-binding agents, antioxidants, anti-irritants, skin-identical ingredients, and cell-communicating ingredients.

When a product, particularly a moisturizer, claims to be oil-free, noncomedogenic, or non-acnegenic, it often misleads consumers into thinking they are buying a product that won't clog pores. But those terms are not regulated by the FDA and have no legal meaning. A cosmetics company can use any or all of those terms without any qualifying ingredient listing or substantiation. Bacon grease could be labeled non-comedogenic, as could any substance or product that may, in fact, clog pores.

The term "oil-free" is probably the most misleading, because there are plenty of ingredients that don't sound like oils but that will absolutely aggravate breakouts. Many cosmetics contain waxlike thickening agents that can clog pores. These ingredients are used in moisturizers because they duplicate the natural lipids (sebum or oil) in our skin, or prevent dehydration, and that's great. But if you have problems already with the oil being created in your pores, adding more of the same kind of substance will only make things worse. Despite the problems these ingredients can cause, they show up in lots and lots of so-called oil-free products.

While there is evidence that some specific ingredients can trigger breakouts, there are no absolutes. I wish there were, but there aren't.

There are no easy answers for this one, but you can understand that trying to research, categorize, classify, and make absolute conclusions about 50,000 ingredients with an infinite number of possible combinations is just not humanly possible.

However, here are a few ideas to at least point you in the right direction. Because a thicker formulation is more likely to contain problematic ingredients, just as a highly emollient product can, it is far better for normal to oily skin types to use gel- or serum-type products that leave out most, if not all, thickening agents. Moisturizers for oily skin are rated as being preferred for that skin type if they are lightweight and have minimal to no waxy or emollient ingredients of any kind listed near the beginning of the ingredient list (because emollients can theoretically clog pores).

DAY CREAMS VS. NIGHT CREAMS: There is no difference between what the skin needs during the day and what it needs at night, except for sunscreen. Other than that, there are no formulation variances that make one preferable over the other. Many moisturizing formulations now have great sun protection, and that is the only way you should differentiate a daytime product from a nighttime version. All other claims on the label are rhetoric you should ignore.

EYE, THROAT, CHEST, NECK, AND OTHER SPECIALTY CREAMS, SERUMS, OR GELS: Buying a separate product for a special area of the face or body, whether it is in the form of a cream, gel, lotion, or serum, is altogether unnecessary. Almost without exception, the ingredient lists and formulations for these products are identical to other creams, gels, lotions, or serums identified as being only for the face. That doesn't mean there aren't some great specialty products out there for different skin types, but why buy a second moisturizer for the eye area when the one you are already using on the rest of your face is virtually identical?

The cosmetics industry makes a lot of money selling women extra products they don't need by dividing the body into different parts, each with purportedly different skin-care needs. Because of the relentless advertising pushing this erroneous concept, women stay tied to the belief that the eye area, throat, chest, legs, and hands all have different skin-care needs. Even more bothersome is the fact that most cosmetics companies give you only a tiny amount of the so-called specialty product, and then charge you a lot more for that tiny tube of product than they do for a large tube of face cream, despite the similar formulations. Moreover, many eye products don't contain sunscreen. If your well-formulated face moisturizer contains sunscreen but your eye product doesn't, then you would actually be allowing damage to occur on the skin around your eye by not using your face moisturizer with sunscreen in this area.

SUNSCREENS: Valid scientific research abounds demonstrating that wrinkles, skin damage, many skin discolorations, and many skin cancers are primarily a result of unprotected sun exposure (Sources: *British Journal of Dermatology*, July 2007, pages 26–32; *Journal of Cutaneous Pathology*, May 2007, pages 376–380; *Radiation and Environmental Biophysics*, March 2007, pages 61–68; and *Mechanisms of Ageing and Development*, April 2002, pages 801–810). Clearly this subject has to do not only with cosmetics, but also with serious health issues. It is well established that the only true, first-line-of-defense anti-wrinkle product is a well-formulated and carefully applied sunscreen. My Web site, www.cosmeticscop.com, has extensive information on the wide variety of concerns, problems, and cautions regarding sunscreen formulations and application.

The main criterion for a well-formulated sunscreen is the SPF rating, with SPF 15 being the standard. SPF 15 or greater is considered the basic standard by the FDA, the American Academy of Dermatology, the American Academy of Pediatrics, and the National Cancer Institute. However, the SPF number only tells you how long you can stay in the sun without getting sunburned, which is caused by the sun's UVB rays. While that is helpful, it is only part of the protection you need. It is now known that most wrinkling, and possibly skin cancer, is a result of unprotected exposure to the sun's UVA rays. Because of the difference between UVA damage and UVB damage, and because there is still no UVA rating system, to ensure you are getting adequate UVA protection your sunscreen must contain one of the five UVA-protecting ingredients, and they must be listed as an active ingredient on the label. These active ingredients are avobenzone (also called Parsol 1789 or butyl methoxydibenzoylmethane), titanium dioxide, zinc oxide, Tinosorb, and Mexoryl SX (ecamsule) (Sources: *Free Radical Research*, April 2007, pages 461–468; *Mutation Research*, April 2007, pages 71–78; *International Journal of Radiation Biology*, November 2006, pages 781–792; *Photodermatology, Photoimmunology, & Photomedicine*, December 2000, pages 250–255; and *Photochemistry and Photobiology*, March 2000, pages 314–320).

No sunscreen receives a happy face rating unless one of those UVA-protecting ingredients is listed on the active ingredient part of the ingredient list and it has an SPF of 15 or greater.

Beauty Note: If you are using more than one product that contains sunscreen, such as an SPF 15 moisturizer and an SPF 8 foundation, it's the one with the higher SPF number that must contain the UVA-protecting ingredients. However, it's important to understand that if you are using two sunscreens, you *cannot* add the SPF numbers to figure out what kind of protection you're getting. In other words, using an SPF 6 sunscreen and an SPF 10 sunscreen does *not* mean that you're getting protection equivalent to an SPF 16. You would be getting some degree of increased protection, but there is no way to know what rating that increased protection would be. In addition, there is no way to know if the formulations are complementary or if the sunscreen ingredients are stable when combined. If you want to make sure you're getting an SPF 30's worth of protection, you should look for one product that has that SPF number.

Synthetic sunscreen ingredients (only titanium dioxide and zinc oxide are considered to be mineral or "natural" ingredients) can be irritating to skin no matter what the product's label says. You have to experiment to find the one that works best for you. The sunscreens that contain only mineral ingredients are considered almost completely nonirritating; however, they can still pose problems for someone with oily or acne-prone skin because their occlusive composition means they can clog pores and aggravate breakouts. This is not to say that someone with blemish-prone skin should avoid these active ingredients. It is not a given that they will make you break out, just something to be aware of as you're experimenting with various sunscreens.

One More Beauty Note: Proper and diligent sunscreen application is of vital importance to obtain protection from the sun. Protection is determined not only by the SPF number and the UVA-protecting ingredients the product contains, but also by how thickly and evenly the sunscreen is applied, and when, where, and how often it's reapplied. There is a mismatch between the expectation and the reality of actual use (Sources: *Journal of Photochemistry and Photobiology*, November 2001, pages 105–108; and *American Journal of Clinical Dermatology*, 2002, volume 3, issue 3, pages 185–191). Keep in mind that an everyday liberal application of sunscreen, applied 20 minutes before you step outside (not after you get in the car, or after you get to the beach, or after you do anything—but *before* you leave the house) is the key to getting the best protection possible. But in your skin-care routine, exactly when does sunscreen get applied? If you are applying several skin-care products, ranging from toners to acne medications to moisturizers, the rule is that the last item you apply should be your sunscreen. If you apply sunscreen and then apply, say, your moisturizer or an acne product over it, you could inadvertently be diluting or breaking down the effectiveness of the sunscreen you've just applied. If you are applying makeup (particularly foundation) over a daytime moisturizer with sunscreen, make sure you do so in a manner that does not rub off your sunscreen. Foundations with sunscreens can add an extra measure of protection, as can allowing your daytime moisturizer several minutes to absorb before proceeding to makeup.

Applying sunscreen liberally is indispensable for the health of skin, which means that all expensive sunscreens are potentially dangerous for skin, not because they don't provide the proper protection, but because their high cost might discourage you from applying it liberally. Think about it—how liberally would you apply a $50-for-1-ounce sunscreen to your face or body versus a product that costs only $20 for 2, 4, or 6 ounces?

SUNSCREENS FOR OILY OR COMBINATION SKIN: Sunscreens are a very tricky category for someone with oily or combination skin. It takes experimentation to find the one that will work best for you. The problem is that the ingredients used to suspend the active ingredients are not necessarily the best for oily skin. What I generally recommend is that someone with oily or combination skin select a foundation or pressed powder that contains well-formulated sunscreens. Pre-makeup with sunscreen, you can apply an appropriate lightweight moisturizer over dry areas or just use a well-formulated toner all over, which can be enough "moisturizing" for that skin type.

SUNSCREENS FOR SENSITIVE SKIN: The nonirritating nature of titanium dioxide and zinc oxide, when they are the only active(s) listed on the ingredient label, assures you that you are getting an optimal product for sensitive skin. Neither ingredient is known for causing an irritant response or a sensitizing reaction on skin (Sources: *Cosmetics & Toiletries*, October 2003, pages 73–78; and *Cutis*, September 2004, pages 13–16 and 32–34). But remember, mineral sunscreen ingredients are occlusive and may clog pores and aggravate breakouts. This is less of a concern when the amount of active ingredient used is lower (for example, an in-part oxide sunscreen with 4% of this active is less likely to clog pores than a pure zinc oxide sunscreen containing, say, 10% of this active ingredient).

WATER-RESISTANT SUNSCREENS: The FDA's December 2002 regulations regarding sunscreen require companies to eliminate the use of the word "waterproof" as a valid claim. In truth, no sunscreen can really be "waterproof" because it must be reapplied if you have been sweating or immersed in water for a period of time. The only terms approved for use on sunscreens are "water-resistant" and "very water-resistant." This FDA ruling reflects research data from studies that prove these products have only a limited ability to stay in place when people are in water or sweating. To determine a product's water resistance, the SPF value is measured directly after application and then again after a period of immersion in water. A "water-resistant" product means that its labeled SPF value measured directly after application and then again after 40 minutes of immersion is the same; that is, it maintains its SPF value over the entire 40 minutes of immersion. A "very water-resistant" product means that the SPF value on the label remained the same after 80 minutes of water immersion (Source: www.fda.gov).

If you are swimming or sweating, you absolutely should use a sunscreen that's labeled water-resistant or very water-resistant, and reapply it frequently. These sunscreens are formulated differently from regular sunscreens, using acrylate and silicone polymer technology in their formulations, which helps them hold up remarkably well under water. Acrylate-type ingredients are, like hairspray, holding agents. These plasticizing ingredients form a film over the skin and can take a great deal of wear and tear in contact with water and friction before the sunscreen protection is rinsed away.

SELF-TANNERS: All self-tanning products, whether you choose one made by Bain de Soleil, Clarins, Decleor Paris, or Estee Lauder, are created equal. The active ingredient in every one of these products is dihydroxyacetone, which is what turns the surface layer of skin brown. This ingredient acts on the skin cells and their amino acid content, causing a chemical reaction that temporarily gives the skin a darker color. These products are considered completely safe for skin (Source: *American Journal of Clinical Dermatology*, 2002, volume 3, number 5, pages 317–318).

Some self-tanners add a tint of color to help you see where you've applied the product, which helps you create a smoother, more even application. Additionally, some self-tanners contain dihydroxyacetone along with erythrulose, a chemical that acts similar to dihydroxyacetone but takes longer (usually 2 to 3 days) to show color.

Your personal preference as to how self-tanners make your skin appear actually has less to do with the product itself than with the nature of your own skin cells. The interaction between the active ingredient and your skin is controlled more by your body's chemistry than anything else. That's why your friend or sister may have brilliant results with a self-tanner that made your skin look rust-colored or unnaturally orange.

You may not like the smell of one product versus another, but that is merely a function of the fragrance added to the product to mask the smell of the dihydroxyacetone. A masking fragrance might be pleasant, but it doesn't change how the product functions, and the natural odor of the product is transient. Where self-tanners do differ is in the amount of dihydroxyacetone, although there is no surefire way to judge that from the ingredient list unless it is near the end. However, you can assume that those self-tanners rated as light, medium, and dark have the corresponding amount of dihydroxyacetone. You can also assume that self-tanners without any stated level have a low to moderate concentration of dihydroxyacetone.

For more specific critiques of self-tanning products, you'll find the Web site www.sunless.com incredibly helpful, and I strongly recommend a visit.

ACNE PRODUCTS: From all the research I've seen, particularly in dermatological journals and literature from the American Academy of Dermatology, acne products need to deliver four categories of performance to deal with breakouts: (1) gentle cleansing (to remove excess oil and reduce inflammation), (2) effective exfoliation to unblock pores and reshape the pore lining, (3) disinfection, and (4) absorption of excess oil (Source: *American Journal of Clinical Dermatology*, 2001, volume 2, number 3, pages 135–141). I base my reviews for these types of products according to how they measure up to these four important skin-care needs.

CLEANSERS FOR ACNE PRONE SKIN: Using a gentle, water-soluble cleanser is standard for any skin-care routine, and it is equally necessary for those with blemish-prone skin. Often skin-care routines aimed at those with oily skin or acne recommend cleansers that are exceptionally drying or irritating, which can increase inflammation. Yet, as I've mentioned several times throughout this introduction, inflammation damages the skin's healing process and that will make matters worse. Think about it this way: What color is acne? Red! So why use any product that makes skin redder? Inflammation can also increase the presence of acne-causing bacteria in the skin and increase the odds that you will be dealing with post-inflammatory hyperpigmentation once the acne lesion has subsided.

I also never recommend bar soap for acne or breakouts. Bar soaps of any kind are kept in their bar form by ingredients that can potentially clog pores. Research also shows that high-pH cleansers (soaps usually have a pH greater than 8) can increase the presence of bacteria in the skin (Source: *Cutis*, December 2001, Supplemental, pages 12–19). To that end, I rate gentle, water-soluble cleansers high if they do not contain irritating or excessively drying ingredients.

EXFOLIATING: See the section above on "Scrubs" and "Alpha Hydroxy Acid (AHA) and Beta Hydroxy Acid (BHA) Products."

DISINFECTING: To kill the bacteria in the skin that cause blemishes (*Propionibacterium acnes*), you need a reliable topical disinfectant (available over the counter) or topical antibiotic (available by prescription). There aren't many options when it comes to disinfecting the skin with over-the-counter products. The best over-the-counter topical disinfectant is either a 2.5%, 5%, or 10% benzoyl peroxide product—but only if no irritating ingredients are added. In fact, research has established benzoyl peroxide as one of the most effective treatments for mild to moderate acne (Sources: *Drugs in Dermatology*, June 2007, pages 616–622; *Cutis*, June 2007, Supplemental, pages 9–25; and *Lancet*, December 2004, pages 2188–2195). As a general rule, it is better to begin with a 2.5% strength benzoyl peroxide solution to see if it is effective, rather than starting with the more potent, and somewhat more irritating 5% or 10% concentrations. If those options don't work, the next step is to see a dermatologist to investigate the options of a topical antibiotic in association with a topical retinoid such as Retin-A, Differin, Tazorac, or Avita. For more information on using topical antibiotics and retinoids along with other treatments for acne, please refer to my Web site www.cosmeticscop.com.

ABSORBING EXCESS OIL: There are many types of skin-care and makeup products designed to create a matte finish or oil-absorbing layer of ingredients on the skin. Although these products often work well to absorb excess oil and keep shine under control, none of them can stop oil production because oil production is primarily a result of your hormones, and that cannot be affected from the outside with cosmetics.

I often point out my concern that oil-absorbing ingredients like rice starch, cornstarch, and other food products are typically considered problematic for those who have breakouts. Food substances can get into pores and encourage bacteria production (after all, bacteria thrive on organic substances), which is not the best when your goal is fighting off bacteria.

Clay masks are popular options for absorbing excess oil on the skin. While they can help, they often contain other ingredients that are skin irritants, can clog pores, or are too emollient for oily skin. I primarily rate clay masks and other masks on whether or not they contain irritating or emollient ingredients that would not be appropriate for blemish-prone skin.

PORE STRIPS: These are not to be used for blemishes. In all their varying incarnations, pore strips are only meant to remove blackheads, and they do this only superficially. You place a piece of cloth with a sticky substance on it over your face, as you might do with a Band-Aid, wait a bit for it to dry, and then rip it off. Along with some skin, blackheads are supposed to stick to it and come right out of your nose. There is nothing miraculous about these products, nor do they work all that well. The main ingredient on these strips is a hairspray-type product. If you follow the instructions closely you can see some benefit in removing the very surface of a blackhead. In fact, you may at first be very impressed with what comes off your nose. Unfortunately, that leaves the majority of the problem deep in the pore. What concerns me most about pore strips is that they are accompanied by a strong warning not to use them over any area other than the intended area (nose, chin, or forehead) and not to use them over pimples or inflamed, swollen, sunburned, or excessively dry skin. It also states that if the strip is too painful to remove, you should wet it and then carefully remove it. What a warning!

Also, despite the warning on the package, I suspect most women will try these strips wherever they see breakouts. If I didn't know better, I know I would. The way these strips adhere, they can absolutely injure or tear skin. They are especially unsafe if you've been using tretinoin, Differin, AHA, or BHA; are having facial peels or laser procedures; taking Accutane; or if you have naturally thin skin or any skin disorder such as rosacea, psoriasis, or seborrhea.

SKIN-LIGHTENING PRODUCTS: Regardless of whether they come in cream, lotion, gel, or liquid form, all skin-lightening products should contain at least 2% hydroquinone and/or an impressive amount of alternative ingredients (such as arbutin or magnesium ascorbyl phosphate) that have research demonstrating their ability to affect melanin production as a means of lightening sun- or hormone-induced skin discolorations. Although there are still no formulary protocols for alternative skin-lightening agents, the research that does exist examined higher concentrations. Therefore, a tiny amount of vitamin C in a skin-lightening product was considered ineffective (or, at best, minimally effective—and who wants that?). The other major considerations when reviewing skin-lightening products were packaging and the presence of needless irritants. All skin-lightening ingredients, and particularly hydroquinone, are light- and air-sensitive. Packaging for these ingredients must be opaque, as airtight as possible, and of a material that has good barrier properties to protect it from light and oxygen degradation. Skin-lightening products packaged in a jar were rated as being ineffective, regardless of the amount of active ingredient. Skin-lightening products in an alcohol base or those that contained other irritants such as peppermint or troublesome plant extracts are not recommended. The skin-lightening products that received a Paula's Pick rating met all of the criteria above and had additional bonuses, such as being fragrance-free or including anti-irritants.

ROSACEA PRODUCTS: Although rosacea is thought to afflict at least 30% of the Caucasian population, there are still only a handful of treatments for it, and they are all available by prescription only. These include the topical applications called MetroGel, MetroCream, MetroLotion, and Noritate. The active ingredient in each of these is metronidazole, which is considered the primary treatment for rosacea (Source: *Skin Therapy Letter*, January 2002, pages 1–6). Occasionally, azelaic acid and oral antibiotics are also a treatment option. Because you must experiment until you find what works best for your skin, all of these should be considered when developing your own battle plan for treating rosacea. One key point: When considering an oral antibiotic you must also consider the risk of the microbe adapting to the antibiotic after prolonged use. If that happens, that specific oral antibiotic won't be effective to help deal with other types of infections you may encounter.

Cosmetic skin-care products can help mitigate rosacea exacerbations, but there are no cosmetic products that can have an effect on the microbe that causes this skin disorder. Because redness, irritation, and skin sensitivities are part and parcel of rosacea itself, anything that makes these worse will cause more problems. In this regard, according to the National Rosacea Society (www.rosacea.org), gentle, nonirritating skin-care products are essential. Of course, I concur; and any skin-care products claiming to be helpful for rosacea must be completely irritant-free to receive a favorable rating.

WHAT WORKS VS. MARKETING CLAIMS

While I want to emphasize how extensive the misleading portrayals of skin-care products made by the cosmetics industry are, I also want to underscore that there are hundreds of great products for all skin types. When I describe my elation or enthusiasm about any product,

I am also always careful to let you know what can really be expected and, where applicable, how out-of-line the price often is for what you are getting. So just because I think a formula can be amazing for dry skin, that doesn't mean I concur with its claims about firming, lifting, undoing or preventing wrinkling, reducing lines, fighting stress, erasing cellulite, and on and on and on....

Every skin-care product is evaluated on the basis of the ingredients it contains because it is the ingredients (and their potential effects) that are the basis for whether a claim can be verified. Unlike my reviews in earlier editions of *Don't Go to the Cosmetics Counter Without Me*, I do not routinely summarize the ingredient list for every skin-care product in this edition. I wanted to review as many new lines as possible, and the repetitive "this product contains" list—and from your letters that was not everyone's cup of tea—took up an incredible amount of space. Unless I feel that this kind of information is needed to help understand a product's performance, I provide just a general summary of the product's ingredients and then describe what it can and can't do. When I do list a product's ingredients, it is always in the order in which they appear on the ingredient list. I often comment about how a product compares to similar or better versions that cost much less. Of course, you will have to test for yourself how a specific product feels on your skin and how you react to its fragrance or lack thereof.

When I list a product's ingredients in the product reviews, I frequently use the phrase "contains mostly," often followed by one or all of the following terms: thickener or thickening agent, slip agent, water-binding agent, film-forming agent, scrub agent, absorbent, detergent cleansing agent or standard detergent cleanser, disinfectant, preservative, fragrance, plant extract or plant oil, vitamin, antioxidant, and anti-irritant. It was easiest to summarize groups of ingredients using these general terms, but please read the following explanations of the terms before you read the reviews.

INGREDIENT HIGHLIGHTS

When reading ingredient lists, remember that the closer a specific ingredient is to a **preservative** (such as methylparaben, propylparaben, ethylparaben, imidazolidinyl urea, or quaternium-15) or a **fragrance** (listed as fragrance or often as an individual essential oil such as lavender or bergamot oil), or the closer it is to the end of the ingredient list, the less likely it is that there is a significant amount of it in the product. That means its impact, for better or worse, is negligible.

When I used the term **"thickeners"** to describe ingredients, I'm referring to those components that add texture, thickness, viscosity, spreadability, and stability to a product. Thickeners that function as emulsifiers are also vital for helping to keep other ingredients mixed together. **Thickening agents** often have a waxlike texture or a creamy, emollient feel, and can be great lubricants. There are literally thousands of ingredients in this category, and they are the staples of every skin-care product out there, regardless of the product's price or claims about "natural" ingredients.

Slip agents help other ingredients spread over or penetrate the skin and they also have humectant properties. Slip agents include propylene glycol, butylene glycol, and hexylene glycol, among many others. The misleading information you read about these being bad for skin is related only to the amount. At 100% concentrations they are definitely too strong and irritating; however, at a 100% concentration, lots of things are too strong and irritating.

Abrasive or **scrub** ingredients are found in cleansing scrubs or in some facial masks meant to remove dead skin cells. The most typical scrub particles are polyethylene, almond meal, cornmeal, ground apricot kernels, jojoba beads, and almond pits. Polyethylene is the most common form of plastic used in the world and the most popular scrub agent. It is flexible and has a smooth, waxy feel. When ground up, the small particles appear in scrubs as a fairly gentle abrasive. Seashells (listed as diatomaceous earth on the ingredient label) are also used as abrasives in scrubs, but they can be extremely rough on skin.

Aluminum oxide (also listed as alumina), the same substance used in microdermabrasion treatments, is also starting to show up in scrub products. This substance can be extremely gritty and irritating for skin and may be too harsh for regular use.

Absorbents in skin-care and makeup products are designed to create a matte finish or oil-absorbing film layer on the skin. These absorbent materials are typically talc, silicates (such as magnesium aluminum silicate), clays, dry-finish silicones or silicone polymers (usually cyclopentasiloxane or phenyl trimethicone), nylon-12, and film-forming agents (hairspray-like ingredients), and all of these can absorb oil effectively. Some have drier finishes than others, but that depends on the specific formulation and the amount of the ingredient. As I often point out, my concern about ingredients like rice starch, cornstarch, and other food products is that they are typically problematic for breakouts. Food substances can get into pores and encourage bacteria production, which is not the best when fighting off bacteria is the goal.

Film-forming agents are ingredients such as PVP (polyvinyl pyrrolidone), methylacrylate, and the polyglycerylacrylates currently being used in a vast number of moisturizers, wrinkle creams, and eye gels to help the skin look smoother. Film-forming agents are usually found in hairsprays and hairstyling products like gels and mousses because they place a thin, transparent, plastic-like layer over the hair (and skin). In the past, the kinds of film-forming agents used were problematic for some skin types; today, with the advent of new polymers, these ingredients do a good job of keeping moisture in the skin and are generally used in such tiny amounts that they are unlikely to be a problem for most skin types. They can also absorb oil in some formulations. When these film-forming agents are listed higher up on a product's ingredient list, they might be present at an amount that can leave a slightly tacky feeling on the skin.

Most skin cleansers include ingredients known as surfactants. Surfactant is a technical term that refers to a large number of ingredients that can cleanse as well as degrease. When cleansers contain surfactants as the primary cleansing agent, I use the phrases **detergent-based**, **detergent cleansing agent**, or **standard detergent cleanser**. Ingredients in this category include cocoamidopropyl betaine, sodium laureth sulfate, TEA-lauryl sulfate, cocamide DEA, ammonium laureth sulfate, and ammonium lauryl sulfate, to name a few (although these are the most common). Because sodium lauryl sulfate, TEA-lauryl sulfate, and sodium C14-16 olefin sulfate are very strong detergent cleansing agents and are known for their irritation potential (Sources: *British Journal of Dermatology*, May 2002, pages 792–800; and *Toxicology in Vitro*, August–October 2001, pages 597–600), I warn against using a product that contains them when they appear in the first part of the ingredient list.

A profusion of **plant extracts** are used in cosmetics, so many that it's impossible to list them all individually and explain their purpose or lack of purpose. As far as the world of cosmetics is concerned, if it grows, it can change skin for the better. However, there is no consensus on which plant (or plants) is the most amazing. According to the various cosmetics companies, the plants they use have the most astonishing merits. When plants are an issue in a skin-care product, I point out the known benefits of those plants, such as antioxidant, anti-irritant, or antibacterial properties. I also explain when plants are a problem in cosmetics due to their potential for causing irritation or a sensitizing reaction. There are occasions when a plant has irritation potential and antioxidant properties (a good example is horsetail extract). In these instances I generally cite the irritation potential because there are so many other plant extracts that have antioxidant properties without the irritation.

Nonfragrant plant oils or nonvolatile oils are almost always beneficial as emollients and lubricants. The debate about whether or not emu, mink, sunflower, olive, canola, or any of myriad other oils or blends of oils is superior is a marketing game to showcase a product. There also is research, especially over the past two years, showing that many plant oils have antioxidant properties of one kind or another.

I often list the exact name of a **vitamin** included in a product. Regardless of the individual vitamin—whether it is vitamin A, C, or E—vitamins in skin-care products can't feed the skin or provide nutrition from the outside in. However, many of them can work as antioxidants and that can benefit the skin.

Even plain **water** gets overhyped in skin-care products. Many products use an assortment of exclusive-sounding adjectives—deionized, declustered, purified, triple-purified, demineralized, fossilized—to describe what is nothing more than just plain water. These terms indicate that the water has gone through some kind of purification process or was taken from a specific water source, but that is standard for cosmetics. You will also find phrases such as "infusions of" or "aqueous extracts of" followed by the name of one or more plants. That means you're getting what I call "plant tea," essentially plant juice and water. Although descriptions like this indicate that you are getting mostly water and a hint of plant extract, they sound so pure and natural that they create the impression that they must be better for the skin. It turns out, as you might expect, that water is water. The kind of water used does not affect the skin or the final product. After the water is combined with other ingredients, its original status is unimportant.

Silicones are a remarkable, diverse, and ubiquitous group of ingredients that show up in over 80% of all cosmetic products being sold. Silicones may look, act, and have a feel reminiscent of oil, but these ingredients are not oils. Technically speaking, silicone as a chemical compound is related to fluid technology. Either way, regardless of the precise name, silicone is an elegant skin-care ingredient that has an exquisite, silky, somewhat slippery feel; it also has an affinity for skin and "dries" to an almost imperceptible finish. Its popularity in formulations reflects its versatility and the finish it gives products. For someone with oily or acne-prone skin, silicone is not necessarily a problem, because there are new silicone polymers that have oil-absorbing properties and can leave a soft matte finish on skin.

Antibacterial soaps and cleansers are those that contain **triclosan** or **triclocarban** (the most typical antibacterial agents used), but there is little to no independent scientific data published to suggest that these products prevent infection. In addition, and even more problematic, is a finding that triclosan-resistant bacteria have recently been identified (Source: *American Journal of Infection Control*, October 2001, pages 281–283). Similar concerns were discussed in *Emerging Infectious Diseases* (2001, volume 7, issue 3, Supplemental, pages

512–515). The article stated that "The recent entry of products containing antibacterial agents into healthy households has escalated from a few dozen products in the mid-1990s to more than 700 today. Antibacterial products were developed and have been successfully used to prevent transmission of disease-causing microorganisms among patients, particularly in hospitals. They are now being added to products used in healthy households, even though an added health benefit has not been demonstrated. Scientists are concerned that the antibacterial agents will select bacteria resistant to them and cross-resistant to antibiotics. Moreover, if they alter a person's microflora [the body's useful and functional bacteria], they may negatively affect the normal maturation of the T helper cell response of the immune system to commensal flora antigens; this change could lead to a greater chance of allergies in children." In other words, if we are too clean, we actually prevent our bodies from developing healthy and natural immunities to many "germs" in our environment.

The April 19, 1999, issue of the *Journal of Biological Chemistry* concluded that the ability of *E. coli* bacteria "to acquire genetic resistance to triclosan [the antibacterial agent found in many antibacterial hand creams and toothpastes] ... suggests that the widespread use of this drug will lead to the appearance of resistant organisms that will compromise the usefulness of triclosan."

Because of the limited research demonstrating the need for antibacterial products in daily skin care, these products are not recommended for their stated purpose.

PACKAGING MATTERS: AN AIRTIGHT ALIBI

Because many ingredients, particularly plant extracts, vitamins, antioxidants in general, and plant oils, break down and deteriorate in the presence of air and light, any packaging that isn't airtight means the product will not be recommended. This includes primarily jars, because they allow air penetration, and clear glass or plastic containers, because they allow light in. This kind of packaging means that the air- and light-sensitive ingredients will become ineffective within a short period of time after the container is opened. While a formula may indeed be brilliant, and contain all the necessary bells and whistles, if its packaging doesn't keep the ingredients stable the product will not receive a happy face rating; rather, it will receive a neutral rating.

EVALUATION OF MAKEUP PRODUCTS

For each product category, as I mentioned previously, I developed a list of specific criteria and guidelines that I use, along with other factors, to determine a product's performance, reliability, or value to skin. The following describes the criteria and guidelines I use to evaluate each category of makeup product.

FOUNDATIONS: My fundamental expectation for any foundation, regardless of type (liquid, pressed powder, loose powder, stick, or cream-to-powder), is that it not be any shade or tone of orange, peach, pink, rose, green, or ash—because there are no people with skin that color. Consistency, coverage, and feel are important. All foundations, regardless of texture, must go on smoothly and evenly, not separate or turn color, and be easy to blend. Foundations that claim to be matte must be truly matte, meaning no shine or dewy finish, and they must have the potential to last most of the day. Foundations that claim to moisturize must contain ingredients that can do that yet without being so slick that blending was difficult and coverage was spotty.

The very good news is that foundations continue to improve, in some cases dramatically so. More than ever, it is easier to find not only a broad selection of neutral shades encompassing many skin tones, but the textures are superb. That means today's best foundations work to make skin look beautifully smooth and even, rather than heavy or mask-like. I am consistently amazed at how many foundations today can make skin look incredible without seeming obvious. Even cream-to-powder foundations have come a long way and have some of the smoothest textures and most natural-looking results around.

FOUNDATIONS WITH SUNSCREENS: Foundations with sunscreens are held to the same standards as all other sunscreens, which means they must have at least an SPF 15 and must list a UVA-protecting ingredient as one of the active ingredients on the label. The only acceptable UVA-protecting ingredients are titanium dioxide, zinc oxide, avobenzone (also called Parsol 1789 or its technical name butyl methoxydibenzoylmethane), Tinosorb (technical name bis-ethylhexyloxyphenol methoxyphenyl triazine), and Mexoryl SX (technical name terephthalylidene dicamphor sulfonic acid; also known as ecamsule). In the reviews, you will notice that foundations with poor or inadequate sunscreens are criticized severely, and do not receive better than a neutral face rating. In some situations, the performance of the foundations was considered excellent, but the foundation could not be relied on for sun protection and would require a well-formulated sunscreen to be worn underneath. For more details, see the information on sunscreens presented in the "Evaluating Skin-Care Products" section.

Beauty Note: Color suggestions for makeup products are based primarily on products that were purchased, but some are based on tester units available at the cosmetics counter or on samples.The color, shade, or tone of a particular product can fluctuate for a number of reasons. If I refer to a particular foundation as being "too peach" and you find that it's just right, it may be that we simply disagree, or it may be that the product I tested or bought was different from the one you ended up buying. Whenever possible, every foundation has its entire shade range reviewed in person, with detailed notes for the good and poor shades.

CONCEALERS: Concealers should never be any shade of orange, peach, pink, rose, green, or ash, and they should not slip into the lines around the eye. I look for smooth textures that go on easily without pulling the skin, don't look dry and pasty, provide sufficient coverage, and, perhaps most important, do not crease into lines. I generally do not recommend using thick or creamy concealers over blemishes (liquid concealers with a matte finish are preferred), but there is rarely a problem with using such concealers on other parts of the face if they match the skin.

I don't recommend medicated concealers because they are rarely, if ever, "medicated" with ingredients or formulations that can affect breakouts. For medicated concealers to work, they would need to contain an effective exfoliant or an effective disinfectant, and I have yet to test one that meets those criteria and has a color that anyone would dare put on their face (though the colors have been getting better).

Despite claims that a product may make for oily skin versus dry skin, please keep in mind that companies can make these claims regardless of what ingredients the product contains. In general, the thicker and greasier the product, the more likely it is to be problematic for oily, acne-prone skin. However, anything you apply over skin can cause problems. Just because a product does or doesn't contain oil is no guarantee one way or the other that it won't cause problems. There are also lots of ingredients that don't sound like oil that can cause problems for skin. Generally, a matte-finish product is best for oily skin, but that still won't ensure a lack of breakouts.

COLOR CORRECTORS: I am not a fan of color correctors in any form. Color correctors are usually a group of concealers you apply before you apply your foundation color. They generally come in shades of yellow, mauve, pink, or mint green. Color correctors are marketed as a way to change skin color, so that if your skin has pink undertones, a yellow color corrector is supposed to even that out. The only thing these products do is give the skin a strange hue. Does anyone think the colored layer isn't noticeable? That yellow or mauve layer then mixes with your foundation, giving it a strange color. Another problem with this kind of product is that it adds another layer on the skin, and the buildup of cosmetic ingredients on the face can be pore-clogging. A well-chosen foundation color and blush can easily provide the color balance you are looking for without adding another layer of strange makeup colors to your skin.

FACE POWDERS: Face powders come in two basic forms: pressed and loose. I evaluate them on the basis of whether they go on sheer, shiny, chalky, or heavy, and whether they are too pink, peach, ash, or rose. I consistently give higher marks to powders that go on sheer and have a silky-soft texture and a natural beige, tan, or rich brown finish with no overtones of red, peach, orange, yellow, or green. It is getting more and more difficult to find a bad powder in any format. Thanks to improved milling processes and pigment technology, today's best powders are capable of making all skin types look polished while helping to set makeup and prolong its wear.

Talc is the most frequently used ingredient in powders in all price ranges, and it is one of the best for absorbing oil and giving a smooth finish to the face. Some companies make claims about their grade of talc being better than another company's. The issue of a grade difference cannot be proven and is irrelevant unless the product's feel and performance are affected.

Other minerals are used for the same purpose as talc, and though they may sound more exotic, they are not any better for the skin. Including cornstarch or rice starch in powders can help create a beautiful texture and these are interesting substitutes for talc, but they can also be a skin concern because there is evidence that they can clog pores and cause breakouts. I try to screen for these in that regard.

When it comes to bronzing powders, I generally suggest using them as a contour color and not as an all-over face color. Darkening the face almost always makes for an overdone look. After all, if a foundation is supposed to match the skin, how can you rationalize using a powder that darkens the skin? Using a bronzing powder will make your face a color decidedly different from your neck, and there will be a line of demarcation where the color starts and stops. Also, many bronzing powders are iridescent. Dusting a color over your face that is darker than your skin tone is bad enough, but why make it more obvious with particles of shine all over, particularly in daylight? The few bronzing powders without any hint of shine or those that produce a soft glow rather than apparent sparkles are rated highest.

Numerous shiny powders are being sold today in loose and pressed forms, and I rate these products on ease of use, how well they last, how much they flake, and how sheer and easy they are to blend. Shiny powder as an oil-absorbent is never deemed a good idea because if the intent is to powder down shine, then applying more shine doesn't make sense. These products are an option for those who want to add sparkle to their all-over makeup appearance.

Powders are often designated by the cosmetics companies as being specifically for dry skin or for oily skin. Those designations are often bogus, however, with little if any real difference between the formulations. I rate a face powder as being good for oily skin if it contains minimal waxy or oily ingredients and has good absorbency without being heavy or thick on the skin. Powders recommended for dry skin are those that contain moisturizing agents or that have a finish that is satin-like rather than blatantly matte. Powders for dry skin should also have an almost creamy texture, despite the absorbent nature of the main ingredients.

There is absolutely no reason to spend a lot of money on powders. Regardless of formulation, there is nothing about price that differentiates one from the other. Some of the best powders, including those with sun protection, are also available at the drugstore.

Beauty Note: Talc is often criticized as an awful cosmetic ingredient that should be avoided. The concern about talc is not about how it is used in makeup, but, rather, when it is used in pure, large concentrations in the form of talcum powder. Part of the story dates back to several studies published in the 1990s that found a significant increase in the risk of ovarian cancer from vaginal (perineal) application of talcum powder (Sources: *American Journal of Epidemiology*, March 1997, pages 459–465; *International Journal of Cancer*, May 1999, pages 351–356; *Seminars in Oncology*, June 1998, pages 255–264; and *Cancer*, June 1997, pages 2396–2401). However, subsequent and concurrent studies cast doubt on the way these studies were conducted and on the conclusions they reached (Sources: *Journal of the National Cancer Institute*, February 2000, pages 249–252; *American Journal of Obstetrics and Gynecology*, March 2000, pages 720–724; and *Obstetrics and Gynecology*, March 1999, pages 372–376).

While more research in this area is being carried out to clear up the confusion, none of the research about the use of talc is related to the way women use makeup. There is no indication anywhere that there is any risk for the face from using products that contain talc. That means you need not avoid using eyeshadows, blushes, or face powders that contain talc. But it does mean you should consider not using talcum powder on your children or on yourself vaginally. If you still would rather avoid talc in makeup, it is easy enough to do by just checking the ingredient list. I comment on whether or not any powder reviewed in this book contains talc, except for those few instances where, for whatever reason, the company did not make an ingredient list available to verify whether the powder was talc-based or not.

FACE POWDERS WITH SUNSCREEN: There are a few pressed powders available that have a reliable SPF 15 or greater and that contain UVA-protecting ingredients. That is great news. However, I am concerned about this because of the way women often use these products. While I don't doubt the validity of the SPF number, I worry that most women won't apply pressed powders with sunscreen liberally enough to get the amount of protection indicated on the label. If you lightly dust the powder over your skin, you will not be getting the SPF protection indicated on the label. You must be sure you apply the pressed powder in a manner that liberally, completely, and evenly covers your face. I feel that pressed powders with sunscreen are an iffy choice if they are the only product used for sun protection, although they are a great way to touch up your makeup during the day and reapply sunscreen at the same time.

BLUSHES: I consider it essential for blushes to have a smooth texture, to blend on easily, and to have a silky feel on the skin. Overall, I don't recommend obviously shiny blushes.

Although they don't make cheeks look as crepey or wrinkly as shiny eyeshadows do the eyes, sparkling cheeks look out of place during the day. There are many blushes whose finish casts an attractive, non-sparkly glow on skin. These were rated highly, provided other attributes remained strong. I also commented when a powder blush's pigmentation was strong, which means less is needed per application (and you may in fact prefer a sheer blush instead).

Cream blushes, cream-to-powder blushes, and liquid or gel blushes are rated on their blendability, whether they streak, how greasy or dry they feel, how fast they set, and how well they last. I also describe which cream blushes tend to work better over foundation and which ones perform better if applied directly on the skin. As a general rule, liquid blushes are best used on bare skin and are not recommended for anyone with large pores in the cheek area.

EYESHADOWS: It won't surprise most of you who have read any of my previous books or newsletters to find out that I don't recommend eyeshadows of any intense shade of blue, violet, green, or red, whether they shine or not. Intense hues may be a personal preference, but I don't encourage anyone to use them. Makeup that speaks louder than you do may be kicky and fun, but it doesn't help empower a woman or help her be taken seriously. But, if being taken seriously isn't your goal in life, then feel free to ignore my color and shine recommendations.

Regardless of color or shine, I evaluate all eyeshadows on the basis of texture and ease of application. I point out which colors have heavy or grainy textures because they can be hard to blend and can easily crease or flake. Eyeshadows that are too sheer or too powdery are also a problem because the color tends to fade as the day wears on; they can also be difficult to apply, flaking all over the place. I am also leery of eyeshadow sets that include difficult-to-use color combinations. Many lines offer duo, trio, and quad sets of eyeshadows with the most bizarre color combinations imaginable. Sets of colors must be usable as a set and coordinated in complementary colors; they should never paint a rainbow or kaleidoscope of color across the eye. However, if you are looking for a kaleidoscope effect, I've pointed them out; they just have an unhappy face rating next to them. Generally, it is best to buy eyeshadow colors singly, not in sets. That way you can be assured of liking all the colors you buy, not just two out of three or four. Powder eyeshadows are by far the most prevalent format, and as such the most attention was paid to this type of eyeshadow. Regarding shine, you will notice in this edition that I am a bit more lenient based on the fact that many of the best eyeshadows have a subtle shine that can light up the eye area without looking obvious. Such eyeshadows are still a tricky proposition for someone with pronounced wrinkles, but can still be used on the brow bone as a highlighter.

Specialty eyeshadow products such as liquids, creams, powdery or creamy pencils, and loose-powder eyeshadows are evaluated on ease of use, blendability, staying power, and how well they work over and with other products. My reviews indicate a clear bias toward matte eyeshadow powders as opposed to any other type of eyeshadow. I find liquids and creams hard to control, and even more difficult to blend with other colors, though there are some exceptions. Most of them also tend to crease easily, and they almost always lose intensity throughout the day. But again, some products in these formats surprised me, and the positive reviews indicate as much.

EYE AND BROW SHAPERS: Basically, all pencils, regardless of brand, have more similarities than differences. Most eye pencils, lip pencils, and eyebrow pencils are manufactured by the same companies (meaning the same manufacturing plants) and then sold to hundreds of different cosmetics lines. Whether they cost $30 from Chanel or $7 from Almay, they are likely to be exactly the same product. Some pencils are greasier or drier than others, but for the most part there are few marked differences among them. Eye pencils that smudge and smear and eyebrow pencils that go on like a crayon—meaning thick and greasy—are always rated ineffective, because they can get very messy as the day goes by. Keep in mind that whether an eye pencil smears along the lower eyelashes depends to a large extent on the number of lines around your eye, how much moisturizer you use around the eye area, the type of under-eye concealer you use, and how greasy the pencil is. The greasier the moisturizer or the under-eye concealer, the more likely any pencil will smear, and you can't blame that on the pencil.

Liquid eyeliners are rated on how easy they are to apply, the type of brush they have, how quickly they dry, and their potential to last all day. The way these types of liners last throughout the day is also a consideration because many liquid liners tend to flake and peel. Another bothersome issue with several liquid liners is that the color fades as you apply it along the lash line, meaning you need to do successive coats—and that increases the chance of smearing.

As a general rule, I do not recommend pencils for filling in the brow. Eyebrow pencil almost always looks harsh and artificial next to an eyebrow. I use only powder, and I encourage you to do the same. Any eyeshadow color that matches your eyebrow color as closely as possible can do the trick, applied with a tiny eyeliner or angle brush. The goal is to create a brow that is as natural looking as possible. Brow mascaras and eyeshadow or brow shadow work superbly together to fill in the brow. A handful of companies make a clear brow gel meant to keep eyebrows in place without adding color or thickness. This works well, but no better than hairspray on a toothbrush brushed through the brow. The only brow pencils I enthusiastically reviewed are those whose performance mimics that of filling in brows with a powder eyeshadow or brow powder.

LIPSTICKS, LIP GLOSS, AND LIP LINER: Every woman has her own needs and preferences when it comes to lipstick. Some women like sheer applications; others prefer glossy or matte finishes. Colors are also difficult to recommend because of the wide variation in taste. Given those limitations, I primarily review the range of colors and textures available, only commenting on texture rather than critiquing it, because personal preference is vital to a final decision. The general groupings are glossy or sheer, creamy, creamy with shine or iridescence, matte, and semi-matte. As a matter of preference, because of staying power and coverage, I give the highest marks to creamy or semi-matte lipsticks that go on evenly and aren't glossy, sticky, thick, or drying.

Lip paints replaced ultra-matte lipsticks, and, for the most part, are an improvement. Several companies offer their version of the 2-step process first introduced with Max Factor's Lipfinity. Step 1 involves painting the lips with color, waiting a couple of minutes for it to dry (which becomes increasingly uncomfortable because these paints are not moist in the least) and then finishing with a glossy top coat. The top coat provides moisture, a shiny finish, and doesn't disrupt the color coat applied beneath it. With few exceptions, the lip paints were rated highly, with some clear favorites emerging.

I evaluate lip pencils according to whether they go on smoothly without being greasy or dry and how well they stay in place once paired with a lipstick. I also comment on the shade range relative to the number of lipstick shades a company offers. You'd be surprised how many companies offer dozens of lipstick shades and only four or five color options for lip pencil.

Lip glosses were primarily evaluated based on their texture, application, finish (particularly level of stickiness) and longevity. Those that went on smoothly, provided a suitably glossy finish, and came in a beautiful range of colors of varying intensity were rated highest. When a lip gloss has greater pigmentation (some go on as intensely as a lipstick), this was mentioned in the review. I also screened for irritants such as peppermint, pepper extracts, and menthol. For sanitary reasons, lip glosses that come in a tube or wand rather than a pot were preferred.

MASCARAS: Mascaras should go on easily and quickly while building length and at least some thickness. Mascara brush shapes have improved phenomenally over the years, although there are those that can still be awkward to use because they are too big or too small. When applicable, I comment on a mascara's brush and how it helps or hinders application. Mascara should never smear or flake, regardless of price.

Whether or not mascaras smear is difficult to assess. No matter how well formulated it is, no mascara can hold up to a heavy layer of moisturizer around the eyes. If you wear an extremely emollient moisturizer around your eyes and a lot of it, your mascara will smear.

I don't recommend waterproof mascaras except for swimming and for special occasions that likely will involve tears. All the pulling and wiping that is necessary to get waterproof mascara off isn't good for the skin and tends to pull lashes out. There are hundreds of waterproof mascaras out there, but only a few capture the best traits of non-waterproof mascaras while still being waterproof. Keep in mind, however, that although waterproof mascaras might stay on better than water-soluble ones when in contact with water, they both break down just as easily when in contact with emollients from moisturizers, sunscreens, under-eye creams, foundations, creamy under-eye concealers, and other specialty products applied around the eye. Waterproof does not guarantee smudge-proof, all day wear.

In general, I tried to include information on how quickly a mascara produced great (or not so great) results, how well it wears, whether or not it made lashes feel soft and conditioned or brittle and dry, and how easy it was to remove with a water-soluble cleanser. When a separate makeup remover was needed, the review indicates that.

Beauty Note: I should mention that I have a personal preference for mascaras that produce long, thick lashes. I admit that my own preference in this regard can get in the way of my evaluations, so understand that I get particularly excited about mascaras, such as L'Oreal 3-D Lash Architect, that build thick, long lashes fast and easily without smearing or flaking, albeit with some clumping that must be combed through.

FACE AND BODY ILLUMINATING/SHIMMER PRODUCTS: This is a new category added to the makeup review section of this book. Given the ever-expanding number of choices for this group, it was time to separate them when a line offered such products (and clearly, many women want some element of shine to be part of their makeup wardrobe). Whether in liquid, cream, or powder format, shimmer products were rated on texture, application, finish (was it greasy or silky), level of shine, and the ability of the shine to cling to skin rather than flake off on you and your clothing. I also commented on shade ranges where applicable and mentioned when certain shimmer products would actually be better mixed with other makeup items, such as foundation. Special attention was paid to whether the amount of shine was a sophisticated, radiant glow or all-out Las Vegas glitter. The latter was not rated as highly because, almost without exception, performance and aesthetic issues existed.

BRUSHES: Brushes are essential for applying makeup correctly and beautifully. Blush and eyeshadow brushes are offered by some of the major cosmetics lines, and all of the makeup artistry lines offer at least the essentials for a complete makeup application. Brushes are rated on overall shape and function as well as on the softness and density of the bristles. Eyeshadow or blush brushes with scratchy, stiff, or loose bristles are not recommended. As a rule, be cautious about buying brush sets because many include brushes you don't need or can't use. Brush cases and other accessories were rated on their functionality, construction, ease of use, and, in some instances, portability. All closures were tested to ensure ease of use, and special care was taken to note the level of craftsmanship, especially for such items sold in department stores.

UNDERSTANDING THE RATING SYSTEM

The rating symbols I use to rate the products reviewed in this book are described below. These simple, but succinct (albeit cute), symbols denote approval or disapproval of a specific product and provide an at-a-glance comparison of expensive and inexpensive choices.

For those who are familiar with my reviews and ratings from previous editions of my books and newsletters, this edition has incorporated a major shift in what constitutes an expensive and reasonably priced product and what constitutes a product that is well-formulated and state-of-the-art. A significant change in this edition is that products containing antioxidants, plant extracts, vitamins, or any other light- or air-sensitive ingredients were evaluated based on their packaging as well as on their ingredients. A superior formula loaded with these kinds of ingredients is useless for your skin if it is packaged in a container that isn't airtight, or that allows light in, such as a jar or a clear container. Such packaging quickly renders antioxidants and other sensitive ingredients ineffective. Consequently, if its packaging is inappropriate and allows an unstable ingredient to break down, even a brilliantly formulated product is rated with only a neutral face.

✓☺ Excellent (Paula's Pick!) and ✓☺$$$ Excellent (Paula's Pick but overpriced). I use this rating to designate the products I found to be the best of the best. It is judiciously assigned whenever a product exceeds expectations, meets the criteria for a product in its category with minimal to no concerns (except for price, which is indicated by the dollar signs), and surpasses expectations of any comparable product. For this edition of *Don't Go to the Cosmetics Counter Without Me*, you will find that my "Best Products" list now includes only products that receive a Paula's Pick rating, divided by price. This reduces the number of best products in each category (which makes shopping easier) and assures my readers that they are getting what my experience and substantiated research indicates are truly state-of-the-art products, regardless of how much they choose to spend.

☺ **Very Good.** This smiling face designates a great product that meets and/or surpasses the criteria set for that category of product, and that I recommend highly because of its performance or its impressive formulary characteristics. The smiling face means the product is definitely worth checking into and potentially worth buying, especially considering that it is so reasonably priced. Products receiving this symbol have prices that are eminently more affordable on an ounce-per-ounce basis than other similar and equally well-formulated products.

☺ **$$$ Very Good (but overpriced).** This symbol designates a great product that meets and/or surpasses the criteria set for that category of product. However, just because the product is well-formulated doesn't mean it is worth the money. Almost without exception there are always reasonably priced versions of a product that meet or exceed the same standards as the more expensive versions. Whether or not a product received the "$$$" designation depends on a pricing versus size threshold my team and I set based on industry-wide averages per category. For example, if a cleanser costs more than $15 for 4 ounces or less of product, it is considered expensive and would receive the "$$$" symbol. Same thing for moisturizers priced mores than $30 for 1 ounce, and so on.

😐 **Average.** This neutral face indicates an OK, but unimpressive, product that can cause problems for certain skin types or a well-formulated product with packaging that compromises the effectiveness and stability of its ingredients. I often use this face to portray a dated or old-fashioned formulation. That doesn't mean it's a bad product, just that it isn't very interesting or is lacking some of the newer water-binding ingredients, antioxidants, anti-irritants, emollients, or nonirritating ingredients for its intended skin type. I also use the neutral face to reflect a makeup product that isn't really bad, but that is completely unnecessary or is unnecessarily overpriced for such an ordinary product that could easily be replaced with a far less expensive version from the drugstore. Depending on your personal preferences, products rated with the neutral face may be worth checking out, but they're nothing to get excited about and, in the case of skin-care items, should be avoided if the neutral face rating is due to poor packaging.

😐 **$$$ Average (but overpriced, so why bother?).** This symbol indicates an ordinary, boring product whose excessive price makes it ludicrous to consider, especially if it is an otherwise great formula with inappropriate packaging. For skin-care products, this rating may reflect a lack of unique or interesting water-binding agents, anti-irritants, emollients, antioxidants, effective exfoliants, gentle cleansing agents, or combinations of those in a given formulation. For makeup, it reflects a performance that pales in comparison to other far better formulations, but that still can look OK when applied, or an acceptable product for those who want a no-frills product for minimal accentuation.

☹ **Poor (don't buy!).** For many reasons, this frowning face reflects a product that is truly a poor choice for skin from almost every standpoint, including price, dated formulation, performance, application, and texture, as well as potential for irritation, skin reactions, and breakouts. Because any unhappy face rating is never a product I recommend, you will not find such products rated with the "$$$" designation. After all, who wants to pay extra for a truly inferior product destined to disappoint?

WHEN YOU AND I DISAGREE

Please be aware that you may not and need not agree with all my reviews to benefit from the information in this book. As you read my comments, you may very well find yourself disagreeing with me. That is perfectly understandable and as it should be, because the criteria you use to evaluate cosmetics may differ from mine. Or, for any one of a dozen reasons (personal preference, different expectations, actual usage such as once a week versus twice a day), a product I dislike may work well for you. Or just the opposite can be true: you may hate a product I rate highly. What I cannot account for is how millions of women will feel or react to a particular product. However, what you can learn here is whether your expectations about a product's efficacy are based on a worthwhile formulation or on nothing more than a placebo effect.

WHY REVIEWS CHANGE

Over the years, in each edition of my books, my reviews and comments change from those in previous editions. There are three major reasons why: (1) I have acquired new research that supports a different evaluation, (2) Other products in a category are significantly better and, therefore, the original evaluation of superior performance may be downgraded due to the comparison to superior formulations being sold now, and (3) The company changed the product since I last tested it.

CHAPTER FOUR

Product-by-Product Reviews

ALMAY

ALMAY AT-A-GLANCE

Strengths: Several very good sunscreens, moisturizers, and fragrance-free cleansers; an excellent assortment of foundations with sunscreen; very good powders, liquid eyeliner, lip pencil, and mascaras; inviting and well-organized in-store displays.

Weaknesses: A lack of effective products to address common concerns such as blemishes, hyperpigmentation, and uneven skin tone/texture; bar cleansers; despite their hypoallergenic claims they still included potentially irritating and sensitizing ingredients; mediocre blush and eyeshadows; lipsticks with sunscreen that do not provide sufficient UVA protection.

For more information about Almay, call (800) 992-5629 or visit www.almay.com or www.Beautypedia.com.

ALMAY SKIN CARE

ALMAY ANTI-AGING LINE

😐 **Anti-Aging Booster Serum** *($19.99 for 0.6 ounce)* is supposed to contain a special blend of moringa seed to heal and rejuvenate skin. There is still no research to support the use of the moringa plant in skin-care products, but components of this plant have demonstrated antifungal, antiviral, and antioxidant activity (Sources: *International Journal of Food Sciences and Nutrition*, June 2005, pages 287–291; and *Antiviral Research*, November 2003, pages 175–180), but that research is about eating the plant, not topical application. Antioxidants are good for skin, but moringa has no advantage over dozens of other options, including green tea or pomegranate. Exotic-sounding plant extracts tend to be a good hook for consumers who are looking for something new to address concerns about their skin, but up to this point no special plant (or any ingredient for that matter) has been proven to be the sole answer for wrinkles.

This water-based serum contains salicylic acid, but the pH of 4.2 means the exfoliating properties are weak (a pH of 3 to 3.5 would be better). A few vitamin-based antioxidants are included, too, and the opaque glass packaging will help keep them stable. All in all, this gel-like serum is a decent option for normal to dry skin, provided you keep your antiwrinkle expectations realistic. This product does contain a tiny amount of mica, which adds a soft glow to skin.

😐 **Anti-Aging Daily Cream SPF 15** *($19.99 for 1.6 ounces)* brags about the antioxidants it contains, but although they're present the amounts are scant, and the jar packaging won't keep them stable once the product is opened. The only reason to consider this product is for its value as an in-part avobenzone sunscreen for normal to slightly dry skin. However, you don't need to spend this much money for an effective daytime moisturizer with sunscreen, and I would encourage you to check out the non-jar-packaged options from Dove, Olay, or Paula's Choice before this one.

☺ **Anti-Aging Daily Lotion SPF 15** *($19.99 for 1.6 ounces)* has opaque, pump-bottle packaging and is an in-part avobenzone sunscreen (similar to the Anti-Aging Daily Cream SPF 15 above), although this version is a lightweight lotion suitable for normal to slightly oily skin. I wish the antioxidants were more plentiful, but there's a nice variety present, along with some good skin-identical ingredients, making this a well-formulated daytime moisturizer to consider.

😐 **Anti-Aging Eye Cream** *($19.99 for 0.5 ounce)* has a somewhat uninspired formula that is dated if you're looking for a state-of-the-art moisturizer—and you should be. There is nothing in this product that will restore firmness or reduce puffy eyes. Although some good antioxidants are included, the jar packaging will quickly reduce their effectiveness.

☺ **Anti-Aging Night Concentrate** *($19.99 for 1.7 ounces)* has a high concentration of silicones, which help make skin feel silky-smooth, but silicones don't have an impact on the skin's firmness or elasticity, they just make skin feel good. This serum works well as a lightweight moisturizer for all skin types, and it contains lots of antioxidants, although not in impressive proportions. Still, the packaging will keep them stable and there are several skin-identical ingredients to keep normal to slightly oily skin hydrated without feeling greasy.

ALMAY DRY SKIN LINE

☺ **Cleansing Lotion for Dry Skin with Cucumber** *($9.99 for 4 ounces)* is a gentle, water- and silicone-based cleanser that is suitable for dry or sensitive skin. It contains a mild detergent cleansing agent along with plant oil to help dissolve makeup, and it rinses well without leaving skin greasy. Although this does contain cucumber extract, with the claim that it can hydrate or replenish skin, it can't. It is great that this cleanser is fragrance-free.

☹ **Facial Soap for Dry Skin** *($3.69 for 3.5-ounce bar)* is a very standard bar soap with a few vitamins thrown in, more for show than effect. It is too drying for any skin type, but especially so for someone with dry skin. It is not recommended.

😐 **Toner for Dry Skin with Cucumber** *($8.79 for 5.1 ounces)* is a fairly basic, do-nothing toner that doesn't deserve consideration for two reasons: The amount of witch hazel is potentially drying, and the salicylic acid is wasted due to the product's pH level, which prevents it from working as an effective exfoliant. Does anyone really think cucumber is a great ingredient? What a dated gimmick.

☺ **Daily Moisturizer for Dry Skin with Cucumber SPF 15** *($11.99 for 4 ounces)* is actually a far better formula than Almay's Anti-Aging Daily Cream SPF 15 above, yet it costs less and you receive more product. The in-part avobenzone sunscreen provides UVA protection, while the opaque bottle packaging keeps the antioxidants stable. Someone with dry skin will likely find this not emollient enough, but it is recommended if you have normal to slightly dry skin, and it works well under makeup. This moisturizer with sunscreen is fragrance-free. It almost received a Paula's Pick rating, but isn't quite as impressive as similar options from Dove, Clinique, and Estee Lauder.

ALMAY NORMAL/COMBINATION SKIN LINE

☺ **Cleansing Lotion for Normal/Combo Skin with Grape Seed** *($9.99 for 4 ounces)* is a cleanser that is better for normal to dry skin due to the presence of thickeners and wax. This detergent-based cleansing lotion is fragrance-free and rinses relatively well, and it effectively removes all but the most tenacious makeup.

☹ **Facial Soap for Normal/Combo Skin** *($3.69 for 3.5-ounce bar)* is standard-issue bar soap and is not recommended for any skin type because it can be too drying and irritating.

😐 **Toner for Normal/Combo Skin with Grape Extract** *($8.79 for 5.1 ounces)* is similar to the Toner for Dry Skin with Cucumber above, only this replaces the cucumber with antioxidant grape extract. Otherwise the same review applies, and the clear packaging won't keep the grape extract potent for long.

✓☺ **Daily Moisturizer for Normal/Combo Skin with Grape Seed SPF 15** *($11.99 for 4 ounces)* is an excellent, in-part avobenzone sunscreen that is indeed appropriate for its designated skin type. The formula has a significant amount of antioxidants. Additionally, it comes in packaging that keeps these skin-beneficial ingredients stable. It's unfortunate that all of Almay's daily moisturizers with sunscreen didn't follow this protocol, but at least they got this one 100% right, and it's fragrance-free, too!

ALMAY OILY SKIN LINE

Almay included menthol in almost every product of their oily skin group of products. Yet there is nothing beneficial about menthol for any skin type. It doesn't reduce oil production, disinfect, or have any benefit for helping skin to function more normally. If anything, menthol is a skin irritant. Often it is mistakenly thought to be beneficial because of its use in anti-itch products, but it works in those kinds of products by causing irritation that distracts from the itch. That is not good for daily skin care.

☹ **Cleansing Lotion for Oily Skin with Meadowsweet** *($9.99 for 3.8 ounces)*. This water-soluble lotion would have been an option, but the menthol it contains will be a problem if it gets in the eye, and the same goes for the salicylic acid—plus menthol is a skin irritant.

☹ **Facial Soap for Oily Skin** *($3.69 for 3.5-ounce bar)* is similar to the other Almay facial soaps reviewed above, and the same review applies.

☹ **Toner for Oily Skin with Meadowsweet** *($8.79 for 5.1 ounces)* does contain salicylic acid, and has a pH that makes it effective for exfoliation, but this toner does not contain a significant amount of it. Plus the amount of menthol in this product is potentially irritating for all skin types, hence the unhappy rating.

☹ **Daily Moisturizer for Oily Skin with Meadowsweet SPF 15** *($11.99 for 4 ounces)* accomplishes the goal of providing skin with UVA protection, courtesy of avobenzone, but it remains a poor choice for any skin type due to the inclusion of menthol.

ALMAY SUN PROTECTION PRODUCTS

✓☺ **Sun Protector for Body SPF 30** *($8.99 for 4.2 ounces)* is a very good, in-part zinc-oxide sunscreen for normal to dry skin. Its smooth lotion texture isn't too thick or occlusive. As a skin-boosting bonus, it contains several antioxidants, and the opaque tube packaging helps keep them stable.

✓☺ **Sun Protector for Face SPF 30** *($8.99 for 4.2 ounces)* is identical in every respect to the Sun Protector for Body SPF 30 above, and either product can be used on the face or from the neck down. Of course, the same review applies.

☹ **Sun Protector Spray for Body SPF 30** *($8.99 for 4.2 ounces)* disappoints compared to the Sun Protector for Body SPF 30 above, but not because of its active ingredients, which include avobenzone. The problem is that the base formula is primarily alcohol, making this sunscreen too drying and irritating for all skin types.

☺ **Sunless Tanning Cream for Body SPF 15** *($9.99 for 4.2 ounces)* combines an in-part avobenzone sunscreen with dihydroxyacetone, the ingredient included in most self-tanners to create a tan-looking skin color. Although this might seem like a convenient two-in-one product, the drawback is that you don't need to apply a self-tanner with the same frequency as a sunscreen, and applying this liberally (as you should with sunscreen) may produce a tan that's too dark or blotchy, or waste perfectly good self-tanner that can be used more sparingly. If you're keen to experiment with such a product, this is one to try, but it is best alternated with a self-tanner that does not contain sunscreen—and sunscreen still needs to be applied daily, because the color you get from a self-tanning product does not provide any sun protection.

☺ **Sunless Tanning Cream for Face SPF 15** *($9.99 for 1.7 ounces)* is similar to the Sunless Tanning Cream for Body SPF 15 above, except this version has a higher concentration of dihydroxyacetone. That means deeper color, but also a greater chance of streaking or blotching if you treat this as a sunscreen, and you should, so apply it liberally. Otherwise, the same basic comments apply.

✓☺ **Sunless Tanning Gel for Body** *($9.99 for 4.2 ounces)* is a very good, antioxidant-enriched self-tanning gel that is also appropriate for use on your face. It contains dihydroxyacetone, the same ingredient used in almost every self-tanner being sold. This rises above many more basic formulas, and is appropriate for all skin types, including blemish-prone skin. Sunless Tanning Gel for Body is tinted to make application easier (you'll see any missed spots before the product dries).

✓☺ **Sunless Tanning Gel for Face** *($9.99 for 1.7 ounces)* is nearly identical to the Sunless Tanning Gel for Body above, which provides nearly three times as much product for the same price. It's up to you, but either product is suitable for facial application—you don't need a separate self-tanner for different parts of the body unless, for example, your face is oily and blemish-prone but you're dry from the neck down.

😐 **Sunless Tanning Mist** *($9.99 for 4.2 ounces)* is an aerosol self-tanner that contains enough alcohol to be a concern for irritation. However, in this mist form it evaporates quickly, allowing you to get dressed shortly after application. It's a tradeoff, and the misting is tricky to get right (you'll need practice). But if you're willing to experiment, this may be worth a shot. Oddly, all of the antioxidants included in the self-tanning options above are absent here.

😐 **Tan Prep Exfoliator** *($8.99 for 5.1 ounces)* is a lotion-like body scrub that contains walnut shells and almond-seed meal as the abrasive agents. Although these are natural substances and sound like they would be helpful for skin, they tend to be rougher on skin due to the irregular edges of the particles. There is no reason to consider this over a more gentle scrub, or better yet, a washcloth, a perfectly good option for manual exfoliation!

OTHER ALMAY PRODUCTS

☹ **15 Minute Facial** *($6.99 for 3.4 ounces)* combines the basic elements of a facial scrub and clay mask, and includes some antioxidants and salicylic acid for good measure. However, the pH is too high for the salicylic acid to exfoliate, and the menthol in this product subjects your skin to 15 minutes of irritation and beyond. That's probably not what you had in mind, and this isn't any more akin to a facial than asparagus is to ice cream.

☹ **Blemish Healer** *($7.19 for 0.5 ounce)* contains 1% salicylic acid and has a pH of 3.8. But before you get too excited, this anti-acne product contains enough alcohol and witch hazel to make matters worse for skin, and because of that it is absolutely not recommended.

😐 **Pore Minimizer** *($7.19 for 0.5 ounce)* contains mostly water, silicone, alcohol, film-forming agent, slip agent, absorbents, antioxidants, anti-irritant, more film-forming agents, and preservatives. This serum has a matte finish, but whether or not you see a change in the size of your pores is more wishful thinking than anything else. The alcohol has slight potential to cause irritation, which makes this an OK option, though it's not preferred to similar options from Clinique and Smashbox.

☺ **Makeup Remover Towelettes** *($8.69 for 30 towelettes)* is essentially a gentle, water-soluble cleanser in premoistened cloth form. This basic formula will remove a light makeup application but is not capable of removing mascara, long-wearing foundation, or lip color. It is best for normal to slightly dry or slightly oily skin.

☺ **Moisturizing Eye Makeup Remover Gel** *($5.19 for 1.5 ounces)* is a standard, mineral oil–based cleansing lotion that efficiently removes eye makeup, though not without leaving a greasy residue. The gentle, fragrance-free formula is best used prior to cleansing.

☺ **Moisturizing Eye Makeup Remover Liquid** *($5.99 for 4 ounces)* is nearly identical to the Moisturizing Eye Makeup Remover Gel above, save for its shorter ingredient list. Otherwise, the same review applies.

☺ **Moisturizing Eye Makeup Remover Pads** *($5.49 for 80 pads)* is nearly identical to the Moisturizing Eye Makeup Remover Gel above, except for the pad format, which some consumers may prefer.

☺ **Oil Free Eye Makeup Remover Gel** *($5.19 for 1.5 ounces)* is oil-free and gel-textured, and works well to remove most eye makeup. The lack of silicone or oils makes it a poor choice to remove waterproof mascara. This is also fragrance-free.

☺ **Oil Free Eye Makeup Remover Liquid** *($5.99 for 4 ounces)* is nearly identical to the Oil Free Eye Makeup Remover Gel above, and the same review applies.

☺ **Oil Free Eye Makeup Remover Pads** *($5.49 for 80 pads)* is nearly identical to the Oil Free Eye Makeup Remover Gel above, only in pad form, so the same review applies.

😐 **Moisture Stick** *($9.99 for 0.25 ounce)* claims to be infused with cucumber, and it is, but cucumber won't do the trick when it comes to hydrating skin; in fact, cucumber isn't even an impressive antioxidant or anything else for that matter when it come to skin. Rather, the emollients and oils in this twist-up stick moisturizer are what's working to protect skin and ease signs of dryness. Instead of the cucumber, this product would have benefited from the inclusion of a few state-of-the-art skin-friendly ingredients. This product is fragrance-free.

ALMAY MAKEUP

FOUNDATION: ✓☺ **Nearly Naked Liquid Makeup SPF 15** *($12.49)* was one of the new foundations Almay added in early 2006, and is easily their best liquid foundation. Its lightweight cream texture blends superbly, setting to a smooth matte finish that enhances skin without looking flat, fake, or the least bit unnatural. Well-suited for someone with normal to oily skin, it offers sheer to light coverage and excellent sun protection from its in-part titanium dioxide and zinc oxide sunscreen. More good news: The nine shades are beautifully neutral, with options for fair to tan skin tones. ✓☺ **Clear Complexion Liquid Makeup** *($12.49)* is a foundation that promises to "heal blemishes." It contains salicylic acid as the anti-acne active, but in an amount that's too low (0.6%) and at a pH that's too high (pH 6) to be helpful for skin. Even though the salicylic acid in this makeup won't help with blemishes, this still offers an enviably smooth, liquid texture that blends onto skin with ease, providing light to medium coverage and a natural matte finish. It is a great example of how beautiful a foundation can look on the skin. Eight shades are available, and almost all of them are exquisite. Only Warm and Honey should be viewed with caution; these may be too peach for some medium to tan skin tones. There are no options for very light or dark skin tones. One caution: Because of the salicylic acid, this product should not be used around the eyes or on the eyelids. This foundation is one to try if you have normal to very oily skin, though it would need to be paired with an effective sunscreen rated SPF 15 or higher for daytime use.

☺ **Line Smoothing Makeup SPF 15** *($13.99)* offers excellent UVA protection thanks to its titanium dioxide and zinc oxide sunscreen. It has a slightly thick, initially creamy texture that blends smoothly, provides light to medium coverage, and has a satin matte finish. I disagree with Almay's claim that this formula "hydrates all day" because it contains minimal ingredients with substantial moisturizing properties for skin. The nine shades are mostly neutral and include options for fair to tan skin. Beige and Warm suffer from a noticeable peach cast, and are the only shades to avoid. This foundation is best for normal to slightly dry skin and, contrary to its name, doesn't do much to smooth the appearance of lines.

☺ **Line Smoothing Compact Makeup SPF 15** *($14.99)* has a creamy texture that blends well and achieves a smooth texture with medium coverage, though it can be blended to have a sheer appearance if desired. It sets to a natural-looking finish that will only slip and fade if you have oily areas. Best for normal to dry skin, Line Smoothing Compact Makeup comes in eight shades, suitable for fair to medium skin, and all of them are outstanding.

☺ **Pure Blends Mineral Makeup SPF 15** *($12.49)* includes 20% zinc oxide, which not only provides excellent broad-spectrum sun protection but also lends an opacity and dry finish to this well-packaged loose powder makeup. The powder is housed in a central chamber and is shot onto an attached (and surprisingly soft) brush, allowing you to dust it over your face. The result is a sheer application whose initial light coverage can be built to medium with successive coats. However, adding more powder tends to make this look and feel too dry, not only because of the amount of zinc oxide but also because the other main ingredient is aluminum starch octenylsuccinate, which has an absorbent finish. Almay wisely recommends using this as secondary rather than primary sun protection because you'd have to pile this on to ensure your skin is sufficiently shielded. The finish feels very matte but tends to look a bit shiny on skin. That helps it not appear too dull, but it won't make someone with very oily skin happy, unless they don't want to downplay the shine. As is typical of Almay, all six shades (including options for fair to medium skin tones) are soft and neutral. This product is recommended as an adjunct to your sun protection, whether it's in addition to your foundation or daytime moisturizer. It doesn't have the best feel or performance when worn alone.

☺ **Smart Shade Makeup SPF 15** *($13.99)* is available in only three shades, and the logic from Almay is that this colorless makeup (I'll explain that in a moment) transforms to complement your skin tone, thus taking the guesswork out of choosing a foundation shade. If only it were that simple! Addressing the preliminaries, this liquid foundation has a titanium dioxide and zinc oxide sunscreen, which is great, and it also lends some opacity and coverage. Unfortunately, it also creates a somewhat flat finish. Coverage is sheer to medium (if you're up for layering), and for those with oily skin or oily areas, it does a great job of keeping shine to a minimum. As you dispense each shade, it appears grayish white. As you blend, it turns into a flesh tone and feels surprisingly light. Each shade blends well and does not streak or look "dotted" on skin, though its initial appearance is admittedly startling.

Almay has divided the shades by depth of skin color. The Light shade fares best because it is the most neutral, and is a versatile option for fair to light skin, but may be too yellow for some fair skin tones. Light/Medium is OK for medium skin tones, but is too peach for lighter skin, while Medium has a rosy tone that makes it unsuitable for most skin colors. Unlike Cover Girl's TruBlend or Max Factor's Colour Adapt foundations, you won't be able to wear more than one shade and have it look convincing. In fact, given the limitations of the shades Almay created, consumers may end up more frustrated than satisfied by this attempt to streamline foundation shade choices. If one of these shades works for you, this is an impressive, long-wearing foundation for normal to very oily skin. Note, however, that it will take more than a water-soluble cleanser to remove it. (I used a silicone-based makeup remover with a washcloth to get it off.)

☹ **Clear Complexion Compact Makeup** *($13.49)* is a pressed-powder foundation that contains 0.6% salicylic acid, but since you cannot establish a pH in a product without water, even a larger amount of this ingredient couldn't exfoliate skin. As a powder foundation the talc-based formula goes on sheer and has a drier-than-usual finish that looks chalky. The six shades appear very pink and peach in their compacts, but since each goes on sheer, it's not much of an issue. Still, there are many powder foundations (and standard pressed powders) that outperform this.

☺ **Touchpad Nearly Naked Makeup SPF 12** *($12.49)* is a sheer, nonaqueous, silicone-based foundation that has a foundation-soaked sponge firmly attached to the base of a compact. You touch the damp sponge and apply the makeup with your fingers. It's a bit inelegant but nevertheless is a method of application many women won't mind. The good news is double, because this has a titanium dioxide and zinc oxide sunscreen (even if SPF 12 is a bit disappointing, when SPF 15 is the standard set by all medical associations), and it also blends so well, drying to a natural satin-matte finish that feels smooth and weightless. Nearly Naked is aptly named, because this formula isn't much for coverage, though if you prefer sheer to light coverage this won't be an issue. The six shades (though ever-so-slightly peach) are all excellent, but because of the way this foundation is packaged, it is impossible to see the real color, which makes choosing the best shade a guessing game.

CONCEALER: ☺ **Clear Complexion Concealer** *($7.99)* contains, like all of Almay's Clear Complexion products, salicylic acid. It's present here at 1%, but the pH is over 4, so it won't exfoliate skin and can't help to reduce blemishes and blackheads. This is still a worthwhile liquid concealer that provides medium coverage and a soft, somewhat dry matte finish. It's an option for concealing blemishes or red spots, but be aware of the salicylic acid and keep it away from the eyelid area. All three shades are recommended.

☺ **Nearly Naked Cover-Up Stick** *($7.69)* pales in comparison to Almay's other concealers, but still has merit for someone with dry skin. The coverage this lipstick-style concealer provides is not "Nearly Naked" and it tends to crease into lines under the eye, though that can be reduced by setting it with powder. The wax content of this concealer makes it completely inappropriate for use over blemishes. Three shades are available, each suitably neutral. ☺ **Line Smoothing Concealer SPF 10** *($10.49)* works beautifully as an under-eye concealer thanks to its fluid, smooth application, just the right amount of slip, and soft matte finish. The sole sunscreen active is titanium dioxide, a gentle choice for a product meant to be used around the eyes, but it's disappointing the SPF rating is not 15. Three shades are available, all excellent.

POWDER: ✓ ☺ Line Smoothing Pressed Powder *($13.99)* feels silky, goes on sheer and exceptionally smooth, and makes normal to dry skin look polished, not powdered. The slight satin finish of this powder won't exaggerate wrinkles, but powders (this one included) don't do much to smooth their appearance, either. That doesn't mean this outstanding option isn't worth considering, and if you have light to medium skin, the three shades are geared for you.

✓ ☺ Nearly Naked Loose Powder *$12.49)* promises a "flawless, natural-looking finish" and delivers! This talc-based powder has an ultra-silky texture that feels weightless and sets makeup without looking flat or dry. All three shades are suitable for most skin tones since they are so translucent. Someone with very oily skin will likely want a more absorbent powder, but all other skin types will appreciate what this has to offer.

😐 Clear Complexion Pressed Powder *($12.49)* claims to clear blemishes with salicylic acid (present at 0.6%), but since a pH value cannot be obtained from a powder, it won't work for that purpose. The formula is talc-based and the texture is unusually dry, though it doesn't look chalky on skin. It contains cornstarch, not the best ingredient to use on blemish-prone skin, but it is absorbent. Three sheer shades are available, and all have merit. **😐 Powder Bronzer** *($10.29)* is pressed and has a dry texture; the two believable tan shades go on sheer, though each leaves sparkles on skin that tend to flake off and land where you don't want them.

BLUSH: 😐 Powder Blush *($10.29)* is a below-standard pressed-powder blush that comes in an attractive range of shades and has a reasonably smooth application. The problem is the sparkly particles woven into each shade. They don't do this blush any favors, are distracting in daylight, and tend to flake. Powder blush is one area where Almay never seems to pull ahead.

☺ Touchpad Blush *($10.29)* takes the concept of sheer blush almost all the way to invisible! An attached "touchpad" sponge is infused with liquid silicone blush and the result is a very soft wash of translucent color. Unfortunately, the slick nature of silicone makes this tricky to blend. It meshes well with skin, but controlling where the blush goes is difficult because of the product's slip. Still, for those willing to be patient and adapt to a unique application, this is a way to (barely) blush and leave skin with a subtle glow, courtesy of each shade's low level of shimmer. The available shades are so sheer, only those with porcelain to medium skin should use them. Darker or tan skin tones will be left wondering why no color is showing up after repeated applications!

☺ Smart Shade Blush *($8.99)* is said to be so smart, it blushes for you—thanks to shade-sensing "smart beads" that transform to your ideal blush color. Available in Pink, Berry, or Natural tone, each offers very soft, sheer color that requires several layers to really register as blush. The liquid texture is surprisingly easy to blend, and sets quickly to a soft matte finish. You may be wondering if this blush can really self-adjust to each individual's skin tone, and the simple answer is: it cannot. However, like any color cosmetic, the way it looks on your skin will be (to varying degrees) different from how the same shade looks on someone else's skin. Almay is taking the obvious and trying to make it sound customized, but all they've really created is a good liquid blush for normal to oily skin (Note to those with large pores: This does not magnify them or make them look "dotted with color"). **😐 Smart Shade Bronzer** *($8.99)* is nearly identical to the Smart Shade Blush above, except the color saturation is stronger, so you need less per application to produce noticeable results. The blending qualities and soft matte finish remain the same, as does the fact that this liquid bronzer is best for normal to oily skin. The main drawback is the color itself, which tends toward orange regardless of your skin tone. That limits the appeal and doesn't make this preferred to other bronzing options.

EYESHADOW: ☹ **Intense i-Color Powder Shadow** *($6.99)* presents a collection of four eyeshadow trios, each with shades meant to complement your eye color (a misguided notion, but I'll get to that in a moment). The texture of these shadows is smooth yet powdery, so unless you're careful some flaking is imminent and application can be messy. These go on quite soft, and every shade in each trio has an obvious shine that borders on overpowering the underlying color of the eyeshadow itself.

The trios for green eyes and blue eyes should be avoided because eyeshadow is not about matching your eye color, it's about shading and shaping the eye area. Even if your goal is to enhance your eye color, to do that effectively you would choose *contrasting*, not matching, shades. For example, if you want to make white look whiter, you don't put another shade of white next to it, you pair it with a dark shade, like slate or black. Applying blue eyeshadow (actually, don't apply it, ever, but just for example…) when you have blue eyes means that you're adding color that will visually compete with your eyes, whereas brown shades, or pale peach, caramel, or taupe colors will enhance them. It really is that simple. These trios from Almay are intended to make eyeshadow shopping easier but end up not helping in the least. They just point women back to a makeup theory that hasn't made it into the fashion magazines since the '70s. I'm sorry to report that according to the Almay representative I spoke with, these trios have been exceedingly popular.

☺ **Intense i-Color Eye Shadow Extension Play Up Trio** *($7.49)* has the same texture and application traits as the Intense i-Color Powder Shadow above, but most of the trios offer suitable, contrasting shadow shades that really do enhance one's eye color. For example, the Play Up Trio for Browns features a pale peach, medium brown, and muted plum shade, while the Play Up Trio for Hazels features pale pink and taupes, all of which work for, not against, those eye colors. Avoid the Play Up Trios for Green and Blue eyes because each contains at least one inappropriate color.

EYE AND BROW SHAPER: ✓☺ **Liquid Eyeliner** *($6.49)* remains one of the very best liquid liners at any price. It goes on smoothly and easily, creating a dramatic line—thin or thick—without flaking, chipping, or looking crinkled. Two shades (classic brown and black) are available, both with all-day longevity.

☺ **Intense i-Color Liquid Liner for Eyes** *($7.49)* has a brush and application that are nearly identical to Almay's Liquid Eyeliner above, except that each of the four shades are loaded with iridescence. The cool factor of this eyeliner is that the shades alter in changing light (for example, Raisin Quartz is a metallic purple but in certain light takes on a brownish cast). The negative is that this much shine so close to the lashes is distracting, and not flattering if wrinkles are noticeable. Still, teens and twenty-somethings will find this a fun departure, and it does last. ☺ **Eye Liner** *($6.39)* is a very good, automatic, retractable pencil with a smooth application that is only slightly prone to smudging. It won't outlast the gel-based eyeliners from Stila, Bobbi Brown, and Paula's Choice, but is a worthy contender if you prefer pencils. As claimed, this pencil is waterproof. In fact, it requires an oil- or silicone-based makeup remover to get it to come off completely.

☺ **Brow Defining Pencil** *($7.49)* is ultra-thin and does not require sharpening. It has a suitably dry texture that demands a soft touch while applying, but that's precisely what it takes to get the best results from this long-lasting brow enhancer. The three shades are terrific, including a great option for blonde (but not white-blonde) eyebrows.

😐 **Intense i-Color Liner** *($6.99)* is an automatic, retractable eye pencil with a stiff texture that makes smooth application difficult. The plus side is that once you apply it, it does indeed last, without smudging or smearing. Each shade is shiny, so this will make wrinkles on the eyelid or under-eye area look more noticeable (and I suspect enhancing those lines is not your intention).

😐 **Blendable Eye Pencil** *($7.49)* is a standard pencil with a creamy yet slightly stiff texture that is meant to be smudged (the opposite end of the pencil has a rubber-tip for smudging). If you're looking for long wear, this won't do, but does work to create dramatic, smoky eyes.

LIPSTICK, LIP GLOSS, AND LIPLINER: ✓😊 **Ideal Lipliner Pencil** *($7.49)* is an automatic, retractable Lipliner that includes a built-in sharpener. That's a nice touch (the sharpener is concealed in the base of the pencil component), but unless you like a fine, pointed tip you won't need to use it—that's the beauty of an automatic pencil! Although Almay created shades to coordinate with their lipsticks, the lipsticks are not recommended (though the Lipliner colors are great). By itself, this Lipliner has a smooth, easy-glide application that stays put and does a good job of preventing lipstick from feathering into lines around the mouth.

😊 **Truly Lasting Color** *($10.59)* is another contender in the category of paint-on, Lipfinity-like liquid lipsticks. This option has the same concept as its predecessors from Cover Girl and Max Factor, meaning that you apply it in a two-step process. The lip color goes on first. Allow it to dry for a minute or so, and then apply the glossy top coat for comfortable wear without disrupting the longevity of the color beneath. How does Almay's version measure up against those from Cover Girl, Max Factor, Lancome, and M.A.C., among others, in the contest to create the best long-wearing lipstick that really lasts? In most respects, Almay's option is at least comparable to its competitors. However, it doesn't improve on the wear time of Lipfinity or the smooth feel of M.A.C.'s Pro Longwear Lipcolor.

Almay's shade selection is a nice assortment of nudes and bright hues, all of which go on sheerer than you'd expect. Layering doesn't build color intensity—what you see from the first coat is pretty much what you'll get, and it's a softer look that lots of women prefer. Almay's glossy top coat is stickier than most, but for gloss lovers this feel probably won't be objectionable. Truly Lasting Color does not stay on for the 12 hours touted on the packaging, but, like others in this category, it lasts much longer than standard matte or cream lipsticks, although you will need to reapply the top coat regularly to maintain a creamy, lipstick-like feel.

😐 **Hydracolor Lipstick SPF 15** *($6)* claims to refresh lips with 100 times more water than regular lipsticks, yet that's easy for this water-based lipstick to do because most lipsticks do not contain any water! Water itself isn't enough to keep lips hydrated (it would just evaporate and leave lips feeling even drier), so it's a good thing Almay included emollients and moisturizing agents, too. Regrettably, the sunscreen does not include the UVA-protecting ingredients of titanium dioxide, zinc oxide, avobenzone, Tinosorb, or Mexoryl SX. That's disappointing, because Almay-owner Revlon's lipsticks with sunscreens get this critical part correct, and Almay has had lipsticks in the past that deliver sufficient UVA protection. Independent of the sunscreen, this lipstick feels water-light and, true to claim, refreshing upon application. The water content means this doesn't feel as creamy as standard lipsticks, so expect fairly frequent touch-ups to maintain a smooth, moist finish.

☹ **Ideal Lipcolor Lipstick SPF 17** *($7.49)* does not contain the UVA-protecting ingredients of titanium dioxide, zinc oxide, avobenzone, Tinosorb, or Mexoryl SX. That's shocking considering this essential element of sun protection is something Almay clearly knows about.

Making matters worse, the creamy formula contains peppermint oil, and for that reason is not recommended. ☹ **Ideal Lip Gloss** *($7.99)* has a smooth, non-sticky texture and high-shine finish, but the peppermint oil it contains will irritate and burn lips.

MASCARA: ✓☺ **One Coat Nourishing Mascara Triple Effect** *($7.99)* is marvelous. It has a dual-sided brush that maximizes length, curl, and thickness, although if you get too enthusiastic while applying, it can go on somewhat heavy and uneven. The brush side with the longer bristles quickly lengthens and separates lashes, while the opposite side has short, closely packed bristles to add thickness and drama. The formula keeps lashes soft and makes it easy to remove with a water-soluble cleanser, making this a top choice and one that rivals the best mascaras from L'Oreal. Of course, there is nothing in it that is nourishing for your lashes. ✓☺ **One Coat Nourishing Mascara Triple Effect Waterproof** *($7.99)* has the same dual-sided brush as the non-waterproof version above, but due to the formula changes necessary to create a waterproof mascara (which this is), the application is thinner. That means less drama, but otherwise there's no question that for a waterproof mascara, this maximizes lashes quickly and beautifully, and it wears without a hitch. ✓☺ **One Coat Nourishing Mascara Lengthening** *($5.99)* has a misleading name because not only does it take more than one coat to achieve results, but this superior mascara thickens as well as it lengthens! It applies cleanly, wears and removes well, and I for one am glad that, aside from the packaging graphics, Almay didn't choose to alter this long-standing great mascara.

☺ **One Coat Nourishing Mascara Thickening** *($5.99)* isn't as impressive as the One Coat Nourishing Mascara Lengthening above, but is still recommended. Again, the name is not accurate because this mascara lengthens better than it thickens. Slight clumping is apparent, but it brushes through easily, and this isn't a stubborn formula to remove. ☺ **One Coat Nourishing Mascara Thickening Waterproof** *($5.99)* applies beautifully and makes lashes noticeably longer and thicker, though I disagree with Almay's claim of "100% thicker lashes." Still, it wears well, is waterproof, and doesn't make lashes feel stiff or brittle. ☺ **Intense i-Color Lengthening Mascara** *($5.99)* builds OK length with minor clumps that can be combed through with successive coats. Thickness is minor, and in terms of overall performance this stops short of being genuinely impressive, but it's fine if you just want defined, longer lashes. By the way, this is not a gel-based formula as claimed. The main ingredients in this mascara are the same waxes and thickeners that show up in thousands of others.

✓☺ **Intense i-Color Mascara Volumizing Lash Color** *($7.49)* is an excellent mascara for length with appreciable thickness, but you can ignore the claims that the slight tint of each shade will somehow noticeably enhance your natural eye color. The aubergine tone of Raisin Quartz does little to make green eyes stand out, while Emerald Green will compete with, rather than enhance, green eyes. The Brown Topaz and Black Pearl shades are by far the winners. Best of all, this mascara goes on clump-free while offering long wear without flakes or smudges.

FACE AND BODY ILLUMINATING/SHIMMER PRODUCTS: ✓☺ **Face Brightener Sheer Shimmer SPF 15** *($12.49)* has a brilliant in-part titanium dioxide sunscreen, but, owing to the way in which shimmer products are generally used, this shouldn't serve as your only source of sun protection. Almay has created an amazingly silky, lightly moisturizing shimmer lotion that comes in three enticing sheer shades and leaves skin with a radiant glow. It's an ideal product to apply (sparingly) over a foundation with sunscreen—or save it for evening glamour when you want to make sure your skin has that lit-from-within quality. This product is definitely one of the more attractive ways to use shine to enhance your skin.

SPECIALTY PRODUCTS: ☹ **Bare-It All Legs** *($9.99)* sells itself (though not blatantly) as liquid hosiery in a can. This aerosol spray is designed to conceal minor skin flaws such as tiny veins. Essentially, it's a spray-on foundation that allows you enough time before drying to blend it thoroughly. After a couple of minutes it sets to a silky matte finish, although it's not transfer-resistant, as claimed. Fabric brushing against it will transfer the color and compromise wear, as will friction from skin (think of thighs brushing together as you walk), and it comes off on furniture. Lastly, the shades aren't all that convincing, at least not compared to the wealth of options you have when shopping for hosiery.

ALPHA HYDROX (SKIN CARE ONLY)

ALPHA HYDROX AT-A-GLANCE

Strengths: A good selection of well-priced, effective AHA products utilizing glycolic acid; also excels with skin-lightening and retinol products; a small but workable selection of cleansers; Alpha Hydrox is one of the only companies selling AHA products that is forthcoming about AHA percentage and pH level (both critical to ensuring you're getting an effective exfoliant).

Weaknesses: Problematic sunscreens and a couple of moisturizers with oxygenating ingredients; reliance on jar packaging for some products with antioxidants.

For more information about Alpha Hydrox, call (800) 552-5742 or visit www.alphahydrox.com or www.Beautypedia.com.

☺ **Facial Moisturizing Cleanser** *($6.99 for 5 ounces)* is a very good, water-soluble cleanser that is suitable for all skin types except very oily. It isn't much for moisturizing skin (and moisturizing in general is best left to leave-on products), but it won't make skin feel dry or tight either.

☺ **Foaming Face Wash** *($6.99 for 6 ounces)* is similar to but slightly more basic than the Facial Moisturizing Cleanser above. It is water-soluble with a slight foaming action. Expect this to do a sufficient job removing makeup and consider it recommended for all skin types except very oily. Foaming Face Wash is also fragrance-free.

☺ **Nourishing Cleanser** *($7.99 for 4.5 ounces)* contains a couple of vitamins and skin-conditioning agents that aren't all that helpful in a cleanser because they are rinsed from skin so quickly. This is otherwise a standard but good water-soluble cleanser suitable for all skin types except very oily. The tiny amount of corn and soybean oil should not pose a problem for those with blemish-prone skin.

☹ **Toner Astringent for Normal to Oily Skin** *($5.99 for 8 ounces)* lists alcohol as the second ingredient and that is followed by witch hazel and, shortly thereafter, menthol. This toner is not recommended (and, if you're curious, the pH is too high for the glycolic acid to function as an exfoliant).

☺ **AHA Souffle** *($15.99 for 1.6 ounces)* includes 12% glycolic acid formulated at a pH of 4, which makes this effective for exfoliation. The lightweight but substantial-feeling cream base is basic, but although a few antioxidants are included, the jar packaging will quickly render them ineffective. This is still an effective AHA option for normal to dry skin.

☺ **Enhanced Creme** *($10.89 for 2 ounces)* is nearly identical to the AHA Souffle above, minus the antioxidants (which is fine considering this product is also packaged in a jar) and with a slightly thinner texture. The other difference is the amount of glycolic acid, which is 10% in this product.

☺ **Enhanced Lotion** *($10.89 for 6 ounces)* remains the best AHA bargain Alpha Hydrox offers. The standard lotion formula contains 10% glycolic acid at a pH of 4, making it an effective option for exfoliating normal to dry skin. There isn't much else of note to discuss, but if you're looking for a good AHA product with a lotion texture, this is one to try.

☺ **Intensive AHA Revitalizing Peel** *($15.99 for 6 masks)* steeps a 14% solution of glycolic acid onto face-shaped cloth masks. The pH of 3.7 ensures exfoliation, but you're better off using a leave-on AHA product rather than something like this that has short-term contact with skin. Alpha Hydrox did add a few bells and whistles to this formula, and it's fine for occasional use—but for best results, use it in tandem with a leave-on AHA product.

☺ **Oil-Free Formula** *($10.89 for 1.7 ounces)* features 10% glycolic acid at a pH of 4 in a lightweight gel base that is indeed oil-free. This is an excellent option for those with oily to very oily skin seeking an AHA product. Keep in mind that if your oily skin is accompanied by blackheads and blemishes, BHA (salicylic acid) offers a greater benefit.

☹ **Moisturizing Daily Lotion SPF 15** *($9.29 for 4 ounces)* does not contain the UVA-protecting ingredients of titanium dioxide, zinc oxide, avobenzone, Tinosorb, or Mexoryl SX, and is not recommended.

😐 **Night Replenishing Crème for Normal to Dry Skin** *($9.29 for 2 ounces)* is a very basic, emollient, fragrance-free moisturizer for dry to very dry skin. Alpha Hydrox recommends this for use around the eyes, and it is suitable for that purpose.

☹ **Oxygenated Moisturizer** *($14.99 for 2 ounces)* claims to oxygenate skin while stimulating collagen production, but providing oxygen to intact, otherwise healthy skin is detrimental because it causes free-radical damage (Source: *Aging Cell*, June 2007, pages 361–370; *Journal of Pharmaceutical Sciences*, September 2007, pages 2181–2196; and *Human and Experimental Toxicology*, February 2002, pages 61–62). Alpha Hydrox used peroxidized corn oil in the form of TriOxygen-C, a patented ingredient that is also used in the Neoteric line for treating diabetic skin ulcers (Neoteric is the parent company of Alpha Hydrox). Although this ingredient's function is beneficial for supplying oxygen and promoting healing of ulcers, the physiological process that skin enacts to heal wounds is vastly different from treating wrinkles or supplying oxygen to non-wounded skin. Both repeated use of any peroxidized substance and delivering extra oxygen to skin are damaging (Sources: *Journal of Reconstructive Microsurgery*, May 2007, pages 225–230; *Plastic and Reconstructive Surgery*, May 2007, pages 1980–1981; and *Cell Tissue Bank*, 2000, volume 1, issue 4, pages 261–269).

☹ **Sheer Silk Moisturizer SPF 15** *($15.99 for 1 ounce)* contains an in-part zinc oxide sunscreen, which is excellent. However, the peroxidized corn oil is cause for concern because oxidizing an oil can lead to free-radical damage when applied over intact skin.

✓ ☺ **Retinol Night ResQ** *($14.99 for 1.05 ounces)* ranks as one of the top retinol products available in any price range. Alpha Hydrox uses packaging that keeps the retinol stable and they also included antioxidant vitamins E and C along with an anti-irritant. The fragrance-free base formula is quite thick and preferred for normal to very dry skin not prone to blemishes. Overall, well done!

✓ ☺ **Spot Light Targeted Skin Lightener** *($15 for 0.85 ounce)* is a well-formulated, skin-lightening product that combines 2% hydroquinone with 10% glycolic acid in a base with a pH of 3.3, all in packaging that will keep the hydroquinone stable. The lightweight lotion base is suitable for normal to slightly dry or dry skin, and the only thing missing is a selection of state-of-the-art skin-identical ingredients and more antioxidants (vitamin E is included). Still, this remains one of the better options for those who want to lighten sun- or hormone-induced brown skin discolorations, and the glycolic acid works in tandem with the hydroquinone to improve skin's appearance and texture.

☹ **Fade Cream** *($10.99 for 3.5 ounces)* lists 2% hydroquinone as the active ingredient for lightening sun- or hormone-induced pigment discolorations, but the jar packaging will quickly render it ineffective, making this a poor choice, especially compared to Alpha Hydrox's Spot Light Targeted Skin Lightener above.

AMATOKIN
(SEE BREMENN RESEARCH LABS)

AMERICAN BEAUTY

AMERICAN BEAUTY AT-A-GLANCE

Strengths: Many state-of-the-art moisturizers, though they're not without their issues; Lauder's formulary expertise in the moisturizer category at a lower price point than most other Lauder-owned lines; good foundations without sunscreen; good powders; excellent powder blush; several lip-enhancing options, including a remarkable long-wearing lip paint.

Weaknesses: Problematic toners, lackluster scrub, sunscreens whose UVA-protecting ingredients are present but at questionable amounts. No skin-lightening, AHA, BHA, or effective anti-acne products; jar packaging; foundations and lipsticks with sunscreen that lacks sufficient UVA protection; poor concealer.

For more information about American Beauty, call (866) 352-8337 or visit www.americanbeautycosmetics.com or www.Beautypedia.com. Note: American Beauty is sold exclusively at Kohl's deparment stores.

AMERICAN BEAUTY SKIN CARE

☺ **Luxurious Lather Creamy Cleanser** *($12.50 for 5 ounces)* is a very good, though very standard, water-soluble cleanser for normal to slightly dry or combination skin. The cleansing agents make it too drying for dry to very dry skin.

☹ **Fabulous Froth Gel Cleanser** *($12.50 for 5 ounces)* is a standard, detergent-based, water-soluble cleanser that would work for someone with normal to oily skin. The drawback is that it might be too drying for most skin types and the inclusion of irritant menthyl lactate makes it a tough sell.

😐 **Barefaced Beauty Makeup Remover for Eyes and Lips** *($12.50 for 4.2 ounces)* is a decent, silicone-based makeup remover, but the inclusion of rose extract (relatively high up on the ingredient list) in a product for use around the eyes is not a good idea, especially when there are other similar versions that are fragrance free.

😐 **Soft Glow Gentle Face Polisher** *($14 for 3.4 ounces)* is a mildly abrasive scrub that uses a mixture of clays to exfoliate the skin. It has a rather thick, pasty feel on the skin, and is a bit tricky to rinse, but for someone with normal to oily skin it's an interesting change from the typical scrubs you find at cosmetic counters.

☹ **Extra Clean Balancing Tonic** *($11 for 6.7 ounces)* is mostly water and rose extract, and—strangely enough—it also contains menthol, which is irritating for skin, and not balancing or cleansing in any way. How disappointing, because it does contain some good ingredients for skin, too.

☹ **Extra Clean Soothing Tonic** *($11 for 6.7 ounces)* has several skin-helpful ingredients and would have been a slam-dunk recommendation for a toner, but the menthol is irritating for skin, not soothing in the least.

😐 **Beauty Boost Overnight Radiance Cream** *($27 for 1.7 ounces)* is an emollient moisturizer with a silky texture and a nice blend of antioxidants, ingredients that mimic the structure of skin, and anti-irritants. What a shame the jar packaging renders this all for naught.

☺ **Moisture-Wise Continuous Hydrating Lotion** *($22.50 for 1.7 ounces)* is a very good, silky-smooth moisturizer for dry skin, with a smattering of ingredients that mimic the structure of skin, plus some anti-irritants and antioxidants. Someone with dry skin would not be disappointed by this product.

😐 **Moisture-Wise Continuous Hydrating Cream** *($22.50 for 1.7 ounces)* is similar to the Moisture-Wise Continuous Hydrating Lotion version above, but the jar package means that the longevity of the impressive ingredients will be too fleeting.

😐 **Moisture-Wise Continuous Hydrating Eye Cream** *($21.50 for 0.5 ounce)* is almost identical to the Moisture-Wise Continuous Hydrating Cream above save for a slightly less silky texture. Otherwise, the same basic comments apply.

☺ **Uplifting Firming Face Lotion SPF 15** *($25 for 1.7 ounces)*. With less than 1% titanium dioxide (you should expect at least 2% or greater when another active is listed, as is the case here), this is not the most uplifting lotion for sun protection, as that small amount limits its ability to defend your skin against the sun's UVA damage. Thankfully, the rest of the formulation is a standout, with an excellent variety of antioxidants, ingredients that mimic the structure of skin, and a cell-communicating ingredient. The firming claim is dubious, but for healthier skin, add this one to your list.

😐 **Uplifting Firming Face Cream SPF 15** *($25 for 1.7 ounces)* is similar to the Uplifting Firming Face Lotion SPF 15 reviewed above, but this cream version comes in a jar and the ingredients can't stand up to the kind of exposure to the air that type of packaging allows.

😐 **Uplifting Firming Eye Cream** *($22.50 for 0.5 ounce)* contains more rose extract than it does some of the more exciting ingredients that appear toward the end of the ingredient list. Still, it does have all the usual bells and whistles, even if (as with most eye creams) none of them are special for the eye area. In the final analysis, it's the jar packaging that reduces the rating, not the formulation.

😐 **Youth-Full Anti-Aging Face Cream SPF 15** *($25 for 1.7 ounces)* covers the UVA spectrum with avobenzone, which is a good start for any sunscreen regardless of the claim on the label. It also has an enviable blend of antioxidants, ingredients that mimic the structure of skin, and a cell-communicating ingredient. All in all, that could have added up to a great rating, but the jar packaging won't keep these ingredients stable. It works as a sunscreen, but everything else is more empty than full.

☺ **Youth-Full Anti-Aging Lotion SPF 15** *($25 for 1.7 ounces)*, unlike its cream counterpart above, comes in packaging that gives the state-of-the-art ingredients it contains (and there are a lot of them) a fighting chance to stick around and actually help your skin. A disappointment, but not a disaster, is the small amount (only 0.98%) of titanium dioxide present. This falls a little short in the UVA-protecting department, but not enough to reduce the rating.

☺ **$$$ All Is Forgiven Skin Repair Concentrate** *($35 for 1 ounce)* contains many of the beneficial antioxidants and skin-identical ingredients the Estee Lauder Companies (of which American Beauty is one) use in their lotion-style serums. The difference here is the lack of silicone and the prominent use of the fragrant American Beauty plant extract. It coincides with the name of this line, but has no benefit for skin. That fact keeps this product from earning a higher rating, but it's still a good option for normal to slightly dry skin. It does contain fragrance and the mica/titanium dioxide blend lends a glow to skin.

😐 **Spare Moment Purifying Mask** *($14 for 3.4 ounces)* is a standard clay mask with some good absorbing properties, at least for sebum (oil)—that is, it won't suck impurities of any kind out of the skin. It contains a small amount of antioxidants, which is helpful, but all in all this is a product that isn't worth a spare moment, given how precious time is.

☺ **Spare Moment Moisture Mask** *($14 for 3.4 ounces)* is a very good emollient mask that is similar in many regards to the moisturizers in this line, containing antioxidants, ingredients that mimic the structure of skin, and anti-irritants. In fact, using this as a moisturizer for dry to very dry skin would be more helpful than using it as a mask, because you rinse the mask off, while you'd leave the moisturizer on.

☹ **Glowing Radiance Self-Tanner for an All-Over Glow** *($16 for 5 ounces)* is a below-standard self-tanner that distinguishes itself in a negative way with the inclusion of irritating lavender oil (and it's not present in a meager amount, either).

AMERICAN BEAUTY MAKEUP

FOUNDATION: ☺ **Perfectly Even Natural Finish Foundation** *($16.50)* goes on evenly and the coverage is light to medium, so it does look fairly natural on the skin. The silicone-based formula, best for someone with normal to dry skin, does separate, so you must shake it before you apply it. Of the 14 shades, Medium/Warm and Medium/Cool can appear too peach, and Light/Cool can look too pink on the skin. ☺ **Super Plush Powder Foundation** *($16.50)* is a standard, talc-based pressed powder that deposits enough color to be considered a foundation. There are 14 decent shades (Light/Cool may be too pink for some skin tones) worth a test run, but be careful: powder foundation can make dry skin look drier, and can look too thick on oily skin. ☺ **Perfect Mineral Powder Makeup** *($25)* is American Beauty's most expensive foundation, and unless you're convinced that mineral makeup is the ultimate option, the cost isn't justified. The mica-based loose powder has no sunscreen, something inherent to many other mineral makeups. It has a silky, weightless texture and soft, dry matte finish that imparts a subtle sparkling shine to skin. Coverage is ligher than similar mineral makeups, but can be built to medium if needed. Among the six shades, be aware that Bronzer (a sheer tan color) is very shiny, while Medium is too orange to look convincing on anyone. The best shades are for those with fair to light skin.

☹ **Perfect Lighting Line Smoothing Foundation SPF 15** *($17.50)*. Regrettably, the SPF 15 part of this foundation lacks the UVA-protecting ingredients of titanium dioxide, zinc oxide, avobenzone, Tinosorb, or Mexoryl SX, and so this is not recommended, despite the noteworthy color selection and smooth, even application and finish.

CONCEALER: ☹ **Perfecting Concealer** *($11.50)* goes on too sticky, is difficult to blend or smooth out (so it looks uneven and obvious), and, finally, creases endlessly during the day. The only thing perfect about this concealer is the name.

POWDER: ☺ **$$$ Perfect Lighting Line Smoothing Pressed Powder** *($16)* is a traditional talc-based powder with an excellent silky-sheer application. Your lines won't disappear, but the six shades are great and definitely natural-looking when applied.

☺ **Perfectly Even Natural Finish Pressed Powder** *($15)* provides slightly more coverage than the Perfect Lighting pressed-powder version above, but other than that, these two powders have more in common than they do differences. Both are worthwhile choices, but this won't absorb oil any better than lots of other pressed powders. Only Deep can be too orange on skin; all the other colors are very good.

BLUSH: ✓ ☺ **Blush Perfect Cheek Color** *($15)* is a pretty darn near perfect powder blush. There are 22 attractive shades with a mix of matte and subtle shine versions. The application is sheer and even.

EYESHADOW: ☺ **Luxury for Lids Eyeshadow Duo** *($14.50)*. Duo eyeshadows usually pose a problem because you almost always end up using one faster than the other, or you use only one because you don't really like the color it's paired with. Luxury for Lids has that basic problem too, although some of the duos, particularly some of the attractive matte duos, do work nicely together. You will also be impressed with the smooth, even application. Still, if you have wrinkled eyelids watch out for some of the shiny shades; they will make your wrinkles more noticeable.

EYE AND BROW SHAPER: ☺ **Ultra-Easy Automatic Eyeliner** *($11)* lives up to its name. It comes in a twist-up container (no sharpening) and has a soft, smooth application. You get a choice of eight basic colors. For a basic eye pencil, this is very, very good.

MASCARA: ☺ **Double Lush Mascara Plus Primer** *($12.50)* is a two-sided mascara. One side is a white gel mascara meant to prime your lashes, and the other is regular mascara. With or without the two-step process you can get long, thick lashes with just a few strokes. My only concern is that the primer tends to make the lashes look spiky after you're done applying the "real" mascara. Without the primer, you just get long, thick lashes, with only a slight amount of clumping. You get long lashes either way, so I guess you can decide which look you like best.

😐 **Softly Shaping Mascara** *($11)* produces decent, attractive, long lashes, but you have to be patient while applying enough layers to get there. It can flake slightly during the day, but not enough to warrant a poor rating.

LIPSTICK, LIP GLOSS, AND LIPLINER: ✓ ☺ **$$$ Super Plush 10-Hour Lipcolor** *($16.50)* is American Beauty's version of Estee Lauder's Double Wear Stay-in-Place Lip Duo ($24.50) and M.A.C.'s Pro Longwear Lipcolour ($19.50). All of these include a lip color "paint" and glossy top coat packaged in a dual-sided slim component. You apply the lip color, allow one minute for it to dry, then apply the glossy top coat, which ensures comfortable wear. As with the Lauder and M.A.C. versions, the lip color applies smoothly (many of the shades go on opaque and most have some degree of shimmer) and feels drier as it sets. The silicone-based top coat adds a beautiful sheen without feeling slick, sticky, or greasy and the duo wears beautifully. Mine stayed on through coffee, lunch, and a late afternoon snack. As expected, the eventual color fading began at the inner portion of the lips and moved outward. The only drawback to American Beauty's option is that you may find yourself applying the top coat more often than others due to its thinner texture.

☺ **Luxury for Lips Moisture Rich Lipcolor** *($12.50)* is a fairly standard, extremely emollient lipstick with an impressive color selection. Just watch out: This is greasy enough to easily move into lines around the lips if you are prone to that. ☺ **Fabulous Feel Liquid Lipcolor**

($12.50) is a unique lip color that is neither lipstick, nor lip gloss, nor lip stain. It is a sweep of somewhat sheer color that is more matte than glossy, but it doesn't feel dry on the lips. I was impressed by the uniqueness of this product and suggest you give it a test run because it is not your run-of-the-mill lip product. There are 12 shades waiting for you to experiment with.

☺ **Pretty Glossy Luscious Lipshine** *($12.50)* is a basic, but good, lip gloss with nine attractive shades. ☺ **Ultra-Easy Automatic Lipliner** *($11)* is no easier than a bevy of standard, twist-up Lipliners, but this is still an excellent one to consider. There are eight beautiful, albeit tame, colors on display.

😐 **Enduring Beauty Longwear Lipcolor** *($12.50)* is about as long-lasting as an ice cube in hot water. This is merely an extremely emollient, standard lipstick that isn't much different from the Luxury for Lips reviewed above.

☹ **Perfectly Lush Moisturizing Lip Tint SPF 15** *($13.50)* doesn't contain the UVA-protecting ingredients of titanium dioxide, zinc oxide, avobenzone, Tinosorb, or Mexoryl SX, and is not recommended. That's a shame, because this is otherwise a soft-textured creamy lipstick that imparts sheer, non-greasy color. The formula is loaded with antioxidants too, but without sufficient UVA protection, this is not a lipstick to slick on in the sun.

FACE AND BODY ILLUMINATING/SHIMMER PRODUCTS: ☺ **Luminous Liquid All Over Face Glow** *($15)* is a sheer liquid that can be applied over or under foundation to add an extremely subtle glow to the skin. It comes in two shades, and can be a bit tricky to apply without disturbing your foundation, but with practice this can create a nice effect.

ARBONNE

ARBONNE AT-A-GLANCE

Strengths: Most of the NutriMinC RE[9] products have merit and contain an exciting blend of antioxidants and ingredients that mimic the structure and function of healthy skin; a small selection of basic but effective cleansers and masks; good powder, eyeshadow, and blush; brush and color sets are worth a look.

Weaknesses: Consistent and pervasive use of volatile fragrant oils that are irritating, allergenic, and/or photosensitizing for skin; no effective AHA or BHA products; no skin-lightening or effective anti-acne products; only one sun-care product that does not contain problematic ingredients; average foundations and eye pencils; bad concealer and mascara; this direct sales line perpetuates false information about several cosmetic ingredients; overzealous sales representatives; returning a product is not easy or convenient.

For more information about Arbonne International, call (800) 272-6663 or visit www.arbonne.com or www.Beautypedia.com.

ARBONNE SKIN CARE

ARBONNE CLEAR ADVANTAGE PRODUCTS

☹ **Clear Advantage Acne Wash** *($15.50 for 4 ounces)* uses salicylic acid as its active ingredient, but in a cleanser its benefit for blemish-prone skin is wasted. Even if the salicylic acid may have an impact on skin before rinsing, this water-soluble cleanser is not recommended due to the peppermint it contains.

☹ **Clear Advantage Refining Toner** *($15.50 for 4 ounces)* lists witch hazel as its second ingredient and that, coupled with the peppermint and other plant extracts known for their allergenic potential (dandelion, anyone?), makes this a clear problem, not an advantage, for all skin types.

☹ **Clear Advantage Acne Lotion** *($16.50 for 2 ounces)* proved frustrating because it came so close to being a slam-dunk option. This lightweight lotion contains 1% salicylic acid and has a pH low enough to allow it to work as an exfoliant. However, because Arbonne insists on portraying a natural image, several plant extracts were included, too. The problem? Most of them are either irritating or allergenic for skin (Source: www.naturaldatabase.com). What a shame! Some soothing plant extracts are included, too, but their benefit is canceled out by the problematic extracts.

ARBONNE INTELLIGENCE PRODUCTS

☹ **Intelligence Daily Cleanser** *($22.50 for 4.3 ounces)* doesn't even make it to average intelligence thanks to its inclusion of a grocery list of irritating plant extracts (including comfrey), along with menthol and volatile citrus oils. It may smell divine, but what's creating the aroma isn't doing your skin any favors.

☹ **Intelligence Daily Balancer** *($22.50 for 6 ounces)* contains enough comfrey to be problematic (this is a leave-on toner), and the inclusion of irritating citrus oils makes matters worse by compromising skin's barrier properties.

☹ **Intelligence Daily Eye Cream** *($28 for 0.52 ounce)* likely contains too small an amount of comfrey to make it a problem for routine application, but it also contains the preservative methylisothiazolinone, which is contraindicated for use in leave-on products due to its potential to cause allergic contact dermatitis (Source: *Contact Dermatitis*, June 2006, pages 322–324).

☹ **Intelligence Daily Moisturizing Cream, Day & Night** *($38.50 for 4.3 ounces)* contains the problematic preservative methylisothiazolinone as well as irritating citrus oils and cardamom oil. These inclusions are as intelligent as brushing your teeth with a cotton swab.

☹ **Intelligence Rejuvenating Cream** *($35 for 2.2 ounces)* would have been an excellent, ultra-emollient moisturizer for someone with dry to very dry skin if it did not contain irritating citrus oils along with clary and cardamom oils.

☹ **Intelligence Skin Conditioning Oil** *($18 for 1 ounce)* has several oils that are incredibly beneficial to severely dry skin and even includes a hefty amount of antioxidant green tea oil in stable packaging. It's unfortunate such goodness has to be marred by adding irritating rosemary and geranium oils.

☹ **Intelligence Exfoliating Masque with Thermal Fusion** *($32 for 4.6 ounces)* may very well get its thermal qualities from the irritation incited by the volatile citrus oils contained in this exfoliating clay mask. It also contains benzyl nicotinate, which is most often seen in lip-plumping products because it is a vasodilator (an ingredient that increases circulation to the area of skin it is applied to), which can cause capillaries to surge and potentially break within the skin.

☹ **Intelligence Personalizer** *($25 for 0.25 ounce)* rounds out the not-too-smart Intelligence line and ends up being the most inane product in the bunch. This is a shiny loose powder you're directed to dust on before applying moisturizer, in an effort to keep skin matte. Didn't anyone at Arbonne realize that applying almost any moisturizer after this powder will immediately negate its matte finish? Then there's the balm mint this product contains and the silly color-correcting claims that make no visible difference, all equaling a product that redefines the question "Why bother?"

ARBONNE NUTRIMINC RE^9 PRODUCTS

☺ **$$$ NutriMinC RE^9 REnewing Gelée Crème Hydrating Wash** *($35 for 3.15 ounces)* is a very good, water-soluble cleanser but one whose price should give you serious pause. Of course, the cost supposedly has to do with the bevy of antioxidants and other high-tech ingredients in this cleanser, but your money is better spent on leave-on products that contain these ingredients. The tiny amount of orange oil adds fragrance and may prove problematic for use around the eye area. Otherwise, this is best for those with large budgets and normal to slightly dry or slightly oily skin.

😐 **$$$ NutriMinC RE^9 REveal Facial Scrub** *($28 for 4 ounces)* is an OK but very overpriced topical scrub that uses walnut shell powder as the abrasive agent. Walnut shells are an option, but one that is not preferred to synthetic exfoliating beads because the shell pieces are uneven and may cause micro-tears in the skin. The oil in this scrub should offset this possibility, and also makes it preferred for those with normal to dry skin.

☹ **NutriMinC RE^9 REstoring Mist Balancing Toner** *($30 for 3.15 ounces)* lists witch hazel as its second ingredient and also contains a significant amount of comfrey extract, which is a problem in products meant to be left on skin.

☺ **$$$ NutriMinC RE^9 REactivating Facial Serum, Day & Night** *($40 for 1 ounce)* lists several fruit extracts in the hopes that you'll think they exfoliate skin, but they don't. Arbonne also included lactic acid at about 2%, an amount that's below ideal for exfoliation although the pH of this product is in the correct range. The tiny amount of salicylic acid has no exfoliating action on skin. Although not worthy as an exfoliant, this stably packaged serum is packed with helpful ingredients for skin, from antioxidants to nonirritating plant oils and (mostly) soothing plant extracts. Although the tiny amount of comfrey extract is not likely cause for concern, it keeps this product from earning a Paula's Pick rating. This product is best for normal to slightly dry or slightly oily skin.

☹ **NutriMinC RE^9 REality SPF 8 Day Creme** *($45 for 1.5 ounces)* costs way too much for a product that offers skin an inadequate SPF rating and lacks sufficient UVA-protecting ingredients. It also contains a high amount of comfrey extract, making it even more problematic. For details on why comfrey is a problem for skin, please refer to Chapter Seven, *Cosmetic Ingredient Dictionary*, at the end of this book.

😐 **$$$ NutriMinC RE^9 REcover Night Creme** *($72 for 1 ounce)* is a marvelously formulated moisturizer that is loaded with antioxidants and contains the cell-communicating ingredient lecithin as well as nonvolatile plant oils and emollients to make dry skin look and feel healthy. What a shame the potency of over a dozen ingredients in this product is hindered by the choice of jar packaging!

☹ **NutriMinC RE^9 REpair, Corrective Eye Creme** *($44 for 0.60 ounce)* lists comfrey extract (*Symphytum officinale*) as its second ingredient and contains significant amounts of other potentially problematic plant extracts, making it a non-contender. Please refer to Chapter Seven, *Cosmetic Ingredient Dictionary*, for more information on comfrey.

☺ **$$$ NutriMinC RE^9 REversing Gelee Transforming Lift** *($38 for 1.5 ounces)* is made to sound like a face-lift in a bottle, and claims to promote the production of collagen, elastin, and ground substance. The latter refers to the intercellular material in which the cells and fibers of connective tissue are embedded, and is part of the lowest layer of the dermis. This product isn't likely to make your skin's ground substance stronger, but it contains many beneficial ingredients that help restore a healthy barrier and allow skin to make collagen, something it does quite well on its own when not impeded by sun damage and topical irritants. This water-based, silicone-free serum is best for normal to oily skin. It does not rank a Paula's Pick due to the inclusion of a small amount of comfrey extract.

☺ **$$$ NutriMinC RE⁹ RElease Deep Pore Cleansing Masque** *($26 for 5 ounces)* is a standard clay mask that is overpriced for what you get, and the amount of comfrey extract is a cause for concern (though less so in a product such as this that would be used infrequently and only left on skin briefly). It's an OK option for normal to oily skin, but calling this "super-strength" is stretching things to the point of snapping.

ARBONNE SUN PRODUCTS

☹ **Damage Control Water Resistant SPF 30** *($28 for 6 ounces)* has the ability to protect skin from UVA and UVB rays while remaining water-resistant (though even water-resistant sunscreens require reapplying after swimming or perspiring). It's also loaded with a selection of skin-friendly ingredients, which is why it's so disheartening to find that this otherwise stellar sunscreen also includes so many irritating fragrant oils. In addition to their irritating properties, bergamot and lime oils can cause a phototoxic reaction (Source: www.naturaldatabase.com) and topical application of lavender oil causes skin cell death (Source: *Cell Proliferation*, June 2004, pages 221–229).

☹ **Glow With It After Sun Lotion** *($32 for 8 ounces)* contains several fragrant, volatile oils that are irritating to skin and problematic when applied to skin that may be exposed to sunlight. Whether pre- or after-sun, this product is not recommended.

☹ **Liquid Sunshine Tan Enhancer SPF 15** *($28 for 6.3 ounces)* features an in-part zinc oxide sunscreen but has troublesome claims (such as increasing the duration of your tan) while assaulting skin with irritants including bergamot, lime, lavender, cedarwood, and geranium oils.

☹ **Made In The Shade Self-Tanner SPF 15** *($28 for 6 ounces)* lacks sufficient UVA-protecting ingredients and contains a litany of irritating fragrant oils, none of which are helpful for skin. Countless self-tanners exist that turn skin brown without this risk of irritation.

☹ **Save Face & Body SPF 15** *($26 for 6 ounces)* wins points for its in-part avobenzone sunscreen, but then its score drops to zero due to the inclusion of the same volatile fragrant oils that all of the Arbonne sun products above include. Save your face and body by not purchasing this product!

☺ **Lip Saver SPF 30** *($8 for 0.17 ounce)* is the only product in Arbonne's sun line worth trying. This oil-based lip balm protects with an in-part avobenzone sunscreen and also contains two forms of antioxidant vitamin C. The amount of arnica extract is likely too low to be a concern for irritation, but it keeps this product from earning a Paula's Pick rating.

OTHER ARBONNE PRODUCTS

☺ **$$$ Cleansing Cream** *($16 for 2 ounces)* is a standard, cold cream–style cleanser that uses safflower oil to dissolve and help remove makeup. It's an option for dry to very dry skin but will require a washcloth for complete removal.

☺ **$$$ Cleansing Lotion** *($15 for 3.25 ounces)* is a thinner version of the Cleansing Cream above and the same review applies, except this is preferred for normal to dry skin. The tiny amount of witch hazel is not enough to cause irritation.

☺ **Wipe Out Eye Makeup Remover** *($19.50 for 3.7 ounces)* is a water- and glycerin-based eye-makeup remover whose cleansing agents are very mild. As such, this isn't effective for removing waterproof mascara or long-wearing eyeliner, but if that doesn't apply to you, using this is an option.

☹ **Facial Scrub** *($17.50 for 2 ounces)* stays true to Arbonne's natural theme by using less-than-ideal walnut shell powder and oat kernel meal as the exfoliating agents. However, staying natural also leads to the inclusion of peppermint oil, which makes this scrub too irritating for all skin types.

☹ **Freshener** *($19 for 8 ounces)* lists witch hazel as its second ingredient and that makes this anything but fresh; it also contains some plant extracts whose problems for skin outweigh their potential benefit.

☹ **Toner** *($19 for 8 ounces)* shares almost the same negative traits as the Freshener above, except this product adds peppermint to the list. It contains some soothing plant extracts, but the irritants that precede them win out.

😐 **Moisture Cream, Normal to Dry** *($19 for 2 ounces)* is a standard emollient moisturizer whose jar packaging will compromise the effectiveness of the antioxidants it contains. The plant extracts are mix of soothing (althea, licorice) and potentially irritating (dandelion, rosemary), and as such cancel each other out.

☹ **Moisture Cream, Normal to Oily** *($19 for 2 ounces)* contains enough comfrey extract to make it a problem for all skin types, and the peppermint oil causes irritation.

☹ **Night Cream, Normal to Dry** *($21.50 for 2 ounces)* is very similar to the Moisture Cream, Normal to Dry above except this version contains an appreciable amount of comfrey extract, making it too potentially problematic to consider.

☹ **Night Cream, Normal to Oily** *($21.50 for 2 ounces)* won't balance oils while simultaneously moisturizing skin, as claimed, but the amount of comfrey extract and the inclusion of peppermint oil are cause for concern and reasons enough to avoid this moisturizer.

😐 **$$$ PhytoProlief** *($30 for 2.5 ounces)* contains mostly water, plant oils, thickeners, glycerin, progesterone, anti-irritants, and a blend of helpful and potentially irritating plant extracts. Applying progesterone to the skin raises medical concerns and it should not be promoted under the guise of skin care from a sales team that has no medical expertise whatsoever. There is no way to know how much progesterone you are applying and whether or not it is even needed. Although this product has good moisturizing abilities, it deserves a neutral face rating because of the health concerns regarding the random topical application of hormones, and their effect on the body (Source: *Journal of Clinical Pharmacology*, June 2005, pages 614–619; and *Journal of Steroid Biochemistry and Molecular Biology*, April 2002, pages 449–455). However, to be fair, a small, controlled study showed topical application of progesterone increased skin firmness in peri- and postmenopausal women, although the amount used in that study is far above the small quantity Arbonne includes in its PhytoProlief (Source: *The British Journal of Dermatology*, September 2005, pages 626–634).

😐 **$$$ Prolief Natural Balancing Cream** *($30 for 2.5 ounces)* is similar to the Phyto Prolief moisturizer above and the same review applies.

☺ **$$$ Extra Strength Masque** *($17.50 for 4.5 ounces)* is a very standard clay mask that also contains corn-cob meal, which makes its texture somewhat rough and inelegant. It's an option for normal to oily skin, and the tiny amount of jojoba oil is not a cause for concern.

☺ **$$$ Mild Masque** *($17.50 for 4.5 ounces)* is nearly identical to the Extra Strength Masque above, minus the corn-cob meal and with apricot kernel oil instead of jojoba oil. Otherwise, the same review applies.

☹ **$$$ Thermal Fusion Enzyme Masque** *($20.50 for 3 ounces)* uses benzyl nicotinate to stimulate circulation and create a thermal (warming) effect. It doesn't really benefit skin but some may like the sensation. The papaya/papain enzyme in this mask is supposed to improve skin texture, clarity, and firmness. Enzymes are unstable exfoliants and no match for a well-formulated AHA or BHA product. Papain has limited research demonstrating its exfoliating prowess, but nothing to indicate it makes skin firmer or enhances clarity. It does, however, have research showing its worth for helping wounds (including burns) heal (Sources: *Journal of Wound Care*, November 2004, pages 424–426; *Journal of the International Society for Burn Injuries*, November 1999, pages 636–639). Wounds and burns are not related to wrinkles, so at best this mask may feel good and give skin a temporary rosy glow (something anyone dealing with rosacea should avoid entirely).

ARBONNE MAKEUP

FOUNDATION: ☹ **$$$ About Face Line Defiance Makeup SPF 8** *($26)* is an ultra-silky foundation that offers a natural matte finish and light to medium coverage. The in-part titanium dioxide–based sunscreen is present in too low an amount to provide adequate daytime protection, which is why it received a neutral face rating. However, if you're willing to pair this with a higher-number SPF product and have normal to slightly dry skin you should be pleased. Of the 15 shades, the following are too pink, peach, or rose for most skin tones: 3N, 4C, 5C, 6N, 10N, 11C, and 12C. ☹ **$$$ About Face Luminous Color Wand SPF 8** *($24)* also contains an in-part titanium dioxide–based sunscreen, but why Arbonne stopped at SPF 8 is a frustrating mystery, given that SPF 15 is the minimum for daytime protection according to countless medical and dermatologic organizations. This stick foundation has a smooth, creamy texture that blends wonderfully and provides sheer to light coverage and a natural satin finish that those with normal to dry skin will appreciate. The 15 shades showcase some great light and dark options, and are identical to the ones above, including the shades to avoid.

CONCEALER: ☹ **About Face Concealer** *($16)* replaces Arbonne's former concealers, both of which were incredibly poor options. Unfortunately, this version, housed in a bottle with a wand applicator, isn't much better. It provides excellent coverage and has a smooth texture, but because it never really sets you'll find creasing, fading, and slipping into lines under the eye to be constant problems. Two of the four shades (Fair and Dark) resemble real skin tones; Light and Medium are too peachy-pink, but not as dramatically so as Arbonne's previous concealers. The drawbacks are considerable enough to warrant an unhappy face rating.

POWDER: ☹ **$$$ About Face Translucent Finishing Powder** *($22)* is a soft, sheer, talc-based loose powder packaged in a tube with a powder brush on the end. Pressing a button on the opposite end shoots a small amount of powder onto the brush; a cap is also included to make this a practical on-the-go option. If only the two fairly peach shades were better, this would be easier to recommend. As is, this is one to test on your skin before buying.

☺ **$$$ About Face Translucent Loose Powder** *($24)* comes in a standard jar with a sifter and enclosed powder puff (though loose powder looks best when applied with a brush). The talc-free formula has a silky, light texture and slightly dry finish, suitable for normal to oily skin. The two shades available appear too pink and peach, but apply so sheer the color becomes inconsequential. ☺ **$$$ About Face Translucent Pressed Powder** *($18)* is talc-free and has a smooth, dry texture that makes it preferred for normal to oily skin. Among the four shades, Fair and Light are noticeably pink and peach. Medium and Dark are much more attractive colors, though Dark may turn slightly orange on someone with very oily skin.

BLUSH: ☺ **About Face Blushers** *($14 for pan; $3 for Custom Color Compact)* have an exquisite texture that applies evenly and imparts soft color that can be built up for more intensity. However, every shade is shiny and sparkling cheeks don't communicate sophisticated daytime makeup. For evening glamour, these are contenders, and there are some good choices for women of color.

EYESHADOW: ☺ **About Face Eye Shadows** *($12 per shade; $3 for Custom Color Compact)* have an enviable texture that is identical to the About Face Blushers above. These cling well, blend smoothly, and build color with ease. Again, the shine speaks louder than the wonderful texture, and most of these shades are shiny enough to emphasize wrinkles or crepey skin, making most of the shades best for younger eyes. The almost-matte options include Shy, Subtle, Suede, Diva, Reckless, Linen, and Sugar Beet.

EYE AND BROW SHAPER: 😐 **About Face Eye Pencil** *($12)* is a standard, but very good, pencil that glides on and tends not to smudge or smear. If only the colors weren't so iridescent or, in some cases, just plain tacky. On older skin the iridescence will only exaggerate an imperfect lash line, and the odd colors will serve to detract, rather than enhance. Eclipse, Urban, and Hepburn are the most workable shades. 😐 **About Face Brow Wax** *($18)* contains the same basic ingredients used to create a brow pencil, but this is a hard wax, poured into a compact. It's an OK option to fill in and define brows, but not nearly as efficient or elegant as the best brow pencils and powders because it tends to go on heavy and the finish isn't as long-lasting. The enclosed brush is uncomfortably stiff and scratchy, and best discarded in favor of a softer option. All three shades are good, including Auburn.

LIPSTICK, LIP GLOSS, AND LIPLINER: ☺ **About Face Lipstick** *($16.50)* features a gorgeous selection of shades (those who prefer a bevy of coral or peach-toned colors will be delighted), each with a creamy texture and slight glossy finish.

☺ **About Face Sheer Shine Duos** *($15)* is a dual-ended wand-type lip gloss that has a decent, minimally sticky feel and soft, sheer colors. There are less expensive, equally good lip glosses available, but at least with Arbonne's option you get two shades in one component.

😐 **About Face Lip Pencil** *($12)* is a standard pencil whose colors are decidedly vivid, but the texture is too creamy to prevent lipstick from feathering, and the bold colors tend to bleed.

MASCARA: ☹ **About Face Lash Duos** *($22)* is a dual-ended mascara that has Lash Colour Mascara on one end and Thick-It Lash Enhancer on the other. The mascara itself is unspectacular and makes lashes feel brittle, while the Enhancer is nothing more than a colorless lash primer that does make a difference, just not nearly enough to make this worth choosing over dozens of other less-expensive mascaras.

BRUSHES: ☺ **$$$ 10-Piece Precision Brush Set** *($35)* is a jaw-dropping value when you consider that most other lines charge two to three times more for similar makeup brush sets. The essential brushes that make up the bulk of this collection are all soft and well-shaped, though the Powder and Blush brushes could be a bit softer and more dense. The nonessential brushes serve as extras you likely will not use, but these can be removed so you can store preferred additional brushes in the attractive non-leather pouch.

SPECIALTY PRODUCTS: ☺ **$$$ About Face Colour Sets** *($116.50)* are preselected color kits that feature two eyeshadows, one blusher, and a lipstick, lip pencil, lip gloss, eye pencil, and mascara. If you're sold on Arbonne makeup, these kits may prove irresistible, and Arbonne now offers some improved color combinations, including Neutral Dramatic, Neutral Natural, and Cool Natural. If you're unsure of whether or not you'll use all (or even most) of the shades, you're better off buying individual colors.

☹ **Custom Colour Palette** *($18)* is a faux leather tri-fold makeup carrier that has room for every single Arbonne blush and eyeshadow. If the holders could be adapted to fit different sized colors from other lines, this would make sense. As is, you'd have to be completely devoted to Arbonne makeup to make this a useful purchase.

ARTISTRY BY AMWAY

ARTISTRY BY AMWAY AT-A-GLANCE

Strengths: One of the few cosmetics companies that offers complete ingredient lists on their Web site; features some excellent moisturizers, serums, and sunscreens; several foundations without sunscreen; good concealer, powder, lipstick, and eyeshadow options; excellent liquid eyeliner.

Weaknesses: Expensive for what you get (especially the Time Defiance products); lacks an effective disinfectant for blemishes; no viable skin-lightening options; some problematic toners and masks; foundations and lipstick with either low SPF ratings or a lack of sufficient UVA protection; OK makeup brushes; difficult online shopping platform.

For more information about Artistry, call (800) 253-6500 or visit www.artistry.com or www.Beautypedia.com.

ARTISTRY SKIN CARE

ARTISTRY TIME DEFIANCE PRODUCTS

Time Defiance is Artistry's premiere collection of skin-care products for those concerned with aging and wishing to forestall the trip to a cosmetic surgeon. Each product tempts you to defy age while bypassing medical procedures. Yet all of them use high-tech ingredients as mere window dressing—meaning not much of the good stuff is in here—while charging exorbitant prices. The company's Defense 4 blend of antioxidants claims to provide the "most complete defense against free radical damage," something I'd love to see proof of, because that would be no small miracle. We don't even know how much free-radical damage can be prevented, though it is accepted that topical application (and oral consumption) of antioxidants can mitigate its effects to some extent. Given that free-radical damage is pervasive and all around us, how can any product claim to be the solution for total protection unless you're in the dark without any light or oxygen... oops, wouldn't that mean you'd be dead? It cannot, so consider Artistry's boast a bogus one (though the products do contain an array of antioxidants, each barely present).

The Time Defiance products are approved by "nationally honored" dermatologist Dr. Indira Misra-Higgins, yet her statements about the line are not that the products are better than cosmetic corrective procedures but that they serve as an adjunct to them by keeping skin healthy, hydrated, and protected from environmental stressors, which is true of any well-formulated product, which Artistry does have. Despite Artistry's marketing spin (perhaps Dr. Higgins didn't see it), clearly she isn't encouraging any of her patients to forgo Botox or dermal fillers in favor of Artistry's solutions to aging skin. All told, the Time Defiance products end up being some of the weakest the company offers. Considering the steep prices, that's incredibly disappointing.

☺ **$$$ Time Defiance Cleansing Treatment** *($39 for 4.4 ounces)* is one of the most basic cleansers around, although it seems more impressive than it is because of the long list of fancy ingredients, all appearing in minuscule amounts after the fragrance and preservatives. For almost forty dollars, is it at all surprising that this cleanser claims to "defy age beyond procedures"? It absolutely cannot do that—all the state-of-the-art ingredients are going to be rinsed down the drain, and even sitting on your skin they can't stop aging. Still, this remains a good, water-soluble cleanser for normal to dry skin, if the price doesn't make your skin wrinkle!

😐 **$$$ Time Defiance Conditioning Toner** *($39 for 8.45 ounces)* is far from the ultimate anti-aging toner it claims to be. This consists primarily of water, slip agent, thickening gum, a couple of skin-identical ingredients, and preservative. The really interesting ingredients are present in amounts too small to impact skin; for the money they should be much more prominent.

😐 **$$$ Time Defiance Day Protect Creme SPF 15** *($74.20 for 1.76 ounces)* is outrageously priced for an in-part avobenzone sunscreen that doesn't offer skin much more than sun protection and moisture. As is the pattern for the Time Defiance products, the intriguing ingredients are present in minor amounts, so they're of little consequence to skin. Further, the jar packaging means the antioxidants will become ineffective shortly after the product is opened.

😐 **$$$ Time Defiance Day Protect Lotion SPF 15** *($74.20 for 1.7 ounces)* is the lotion version of the Time Defiance Day Protect Creme SPF 15 above, and other than having packaging that keeps the antioxidants stable (vitamin E is the only one present in a significant amount), the same comments apply.

✓ ☺ **$$$ Time Defiance Derma Erase** *($45.55 for 0.14 ounce)* is a water- and silicone-based serum that contains some excellent skin-identical ingredients, a cell-communicating ingredient, and a couple of good antioxidants, plus an anti-irritant. This product is Artistry's injection-free alternative to Botox treatments but the ingredient purporting to accomplish this (acetyl hexapeptide-3) isn't present in the amounts the company that offers this ingredient maintains is necessary for efficacy. Moreover, there is no substantiated proof this peptide has muscle-relaxing qualities, and not even Botox works like Botox when it's applied topically rather than injected. This is still a worthwhile, fragrance-free option for normal to slightly oily skin, but don't expect your expression lines to vanish.

☹ **Time Defiance Intensive Repair Serum** *($230.85 for 14-0.05 ounce vials)* does not even provide one ounce of product for its jaw-dropping price, and based on the mundane formula, expecting "revolutionary results" is assuredly going to leave you disappointed (and poorer). Each vial (you're directed to use one per evening for two weeks) contains mostly water, slip agents, thickener, and preservative. All of the state-of-the-art ingredients are present in amounts too small to matter, and for what Artistry is charging they should be front and center for maximum potency. This isn't intensive in the least, and is not recommended for reversing aging, though it could well reverse your bank account balance!

😐 **$$$ Time Defiance Night Recovery Creme** *($74.20 for 1.76 ounces)* consists primarily of water, glycerin, several thickeners, vitamin E, preservative, and fragrance. It is preposterously priced, and the jar packaging means the vitamin E will be ineffective shortly after the product is opened. Oodles of skin-friendly ingredients are present, but altogether they amount to no more than a dusting, and your skin deserves better than that.

😐 **$$$ Time Defiance Night Recovery Lotion** *($74.20 for 1.7 ounces)* rates as another unexciting formula whose look-younger-now claims are off the charts. It contains mostly water, thickener, film-forming agent, slip agent, vitamin E, and preservative. Although this is a well-packaged moisturizer for normal to slightly dry or slightly oily skin, it is vastly overpriced for what you get.

☹ **Time Defiance Vitamin C + Wild Yam Treatment** *($41.35 for the set)* claims to reduce the appearance of wrinkles by 58% with vitamin C "instead of a needle." You get a bottle of ascorbic acid fluid to mix with a water-based moisturizer that contains a considerable amount of wild yam extract. The wild yam doesn't have any antiwrinkle prowess on its own, and the form of vitamin C used (ascorbic acid) requires an acidic pH to be effective, but that's not the case here. Furthermore, the clear glass packaging renders the light-sensitive vitamin C ineffective (Sources: www.naturaldatabase.com; *International Journal of Pharmaceutics*, October 1999, pages 233–241).

Other Artistry Products

☹ **Clarifying Foaming Cleanser** *($18.30 for 4.4 ounces)* lists TEA-lauryl sulfate as its main detergent cleansing agent, which makes this cleanser too drying for all skin types.

☺ **$$$ Delicate Care Cleanser** *($18.30 for 4.3 ounces)* is a good, lotion-style cleanser for normal to dry skin. It contains neither detergent cleansing agents nor fragrance, and as such is suitable for sensitive, easily irritated skin.

☺ **$$$ Moisture Rich Vitalising Cleanser** *($18.30 for 4.4 ounces)* isn't as emollient as the Delicate Care Cleanser above, but its thinner texture and detergent-free formula is suitable for normal to slightly dry or slightly oily skin that is also sensitive. This cleanser does contain fragrance, and its oil content may be problematic for those with blemish-prone skin.

✓☺ **Eye & Lip Makeup Remover** *($13.95 for 4 ounces)* is an outstanding, sensibly priced water- and silicone-based makeup remover whose fragrance-free formula is laced with soothing agents. This is a well-formulated product that works beautifully.

☺ **$$$ Polishing Scrub** *($25.75 for 4.4 ounces)* is a cleanser/scrub hybrid product that uses polyethylene (plastic) as the abrasive agent. It is a good option for normal to slightly dry or slightly oily skin and it rinses well.

☹ **Clarifying Oil Control Toner** *($19.80 for 8.45 ounces)* lists alcohol as the second ingredient and that is followed by witch hazel, which only increases the alcohol content of this irritating toner.

😐 **$$$ Delicate Care Toner** *($19.80 for 8.45 ounces)* contains mostly water, slip agents, preservative, plant extracts, and water-binding agent. It is overpriced for what you get, and functions as a very basic toner for normal to dry skin.

☺ **$$$ Moisture Rich Refreshing Toner** *($19.80 for 8.45 ounces)* is a somewhat unique moisturizing toner that contains some very good skin-identical ingredients as well as a cell-communicating ingredient. The sugarcane, citrus, and sugar maple extracts do not function like AHAs and should not be considered as exfoliants.

☺ **$$$ Alpha Hydroxy Serum Plus** *($46.30 for 1 ounce)* ends up being an effective, though pricey, AHA product. With a sufficient amount of lactic acid and a pH of 3.6, this water-based serum will exfoliate skin and prompt a smoother texture. The only drawback is the inclusion of irritating guarana extract, though there are enough soothing agents in this product to cancel out the potential for irritation.

☺ **$$$ Clarifying Balancing Moisturizer SPF 15** *($28.65 for 2.6 ounces)* features an in-part zinc oxide sunscreen in a lightweight lotion base that contains some antioxidants and good skin-identical ingredients. Although not for oily or blemish-prone skin, this deserves consideration as a well-formulated daytime moisturizer for normal to slightly dry skin.

✓☺ **Delicate Care Calming Moisturizer** *($28.65 for 2.5 ounces)* is a bit short on antioxidants, but is otherwise an exceptional moisturizer for normal to dry skin. The fragrance-free formula contains an effective blend of emollients, skin-identical ingredients, cell-communicating ingredients, and antioxidants, all in stable packaging.

☺ **$$$ Extra Dry Hydration Oil** *($24.45 for 0.49 ounce)* ends up being an effective though costly way to supply dry to very dry skin with a blend of nonvolatile plant oils. Although this is an useful product, you could save money by applying plain safflower, olive, or evening primrose oil to dry areas (all of those oils are available in most health food stores).

✓☺ **Moisture Rich Protective Moisturizer SPF 15** *($28.65 for 2.5 ounces)* is a well-formulated, in-part avobenzone sunscreen in a moisturizing base suitable for normal to dry skin. Inside stable packaging are antioxidants, anti-irritants, and several ingredients that mimic the structure and function of healthy skin. Well done!

☺ **$$$ Replenishing Eye Creme** *($27 for 0.5 ounce)* does not contain ingredients that research has shown capable of reducing puffiness or dark circles, but if you can look beyond the claims this is a good moisturizer for slightly dry skin, just not around the eyes. The amount of bitter orange extract will likely prove too irritating for delicate eye-area skin.

✓☺ **$$$ Skin Refinishing Lotion** *($48.85 for 1 ounce)* contains mostly water, silicones, anti-irritant, thickener, several skin-identical ingredients, vitamin E, cell-communicating ingredients, antioxidants, slip agents, film-forming agents, preservatives, and fragrance. This serum-type moisturizer is an excellent (though costly) choice for normal to oily skin and is in packaging that keeps its light- and air-sensitive ingredients stable.

☹ **Blemish Control Acne Treatment Gel** *($13.80 for 0.5 ounce)* would have been a great option for a lightweight 1% BHA gel due to its pH of 3.5 and several soothing agents; however, the nonaqueous formula's alcohol base makes this too drying and irritating for all skin types.

😐 **$$$ Bright Idea Illuminating Essence** *($59.25 for 1 ounce)* claims to make skin 116% brighter in two weeks—which, depending on your skin's condition, may require others in your presence to wear protective glasses. All kidding aside, this is nothing more than a light-textured lotion that contains a tiny amount of *Uva ursi* leaf extract. Also known as bearberry, this ingredient has a tiny amount of research showing it can have skin-lightening properties (Source: *International Journal of Dermatology*, February 2003, pages 153–156). Bearberry extract's potential efficacy is derived from its active components of hydroquinone and arbutin (Sources: *Phytochemical Analysis*, September–October 2001, pages 336–339; and http://supplementwatch.com/suplib/supplement.asp?DocId=1306). However, if pigment discolorations are a concern, choosing a product with 1%–2% hydroquinone is a more reliable solution. For the money, there is no compelling reason to champion this product.

☹ **Moisture Intense Masque** *($20.65 for 3.6 ounces)* is a fairly emollient moisturizing mask but its soothing ability is compromised by the inclusion of menthol derivative menthyl lactate, making this too irritating for all skin types.

☹ **Pore Cleansing Masque** *($20.65 for 3.6 ounces)* is a substandard clay mask due to the menthyl PCA it contains. This derivative of menthol cools without the minty smell, but is still irritating to skin.

ARTISTRY MAKEUP

FOUNDATION: ☺ **$$$ Time Defiance Hydroplenish Foundation** *($22.45; $13.40 for refillable compact)* is similar to Vincent Longo's Water Canvas Creme-to-Powder Foundation ($52.50). This water-based compact makeup feels light and soothing, and provides sheer coverage that doesn't layer well. In other words, the initial coverage you see is pretty much what you'll get, so this isn't the best if you have flaws to soften or hide. If you don't need much coverage, have normal to oily skin, and desire a natural-looking matte finish, this is an excellent option. The 16 shades offer something for all skin tones, from fair to very dark, though some should be avoided: Shell Bisque is too pink and Fawn Beige is too peach for most medium skin tones. One last point: Artistry claims this is "the only foundation to stop aging where it starts." Don't believe it for a second. With no sunscreen included, it's ridiculous to make such a claim. Although this foundation contains several antioxidants, they are present in very tiny amounts, not to mention that their stability will be compromised every time this product is opened and exposed to air. ☺ **$$$ Absolute Oil Control Foundation SPF 15** *($27.35)* has a liquid texture and comes in packaging which, thankfully, allows for controlled dispensing. It blends on smoothly, providing medium coverage and a soft matte finish that those with normal to oily skin will appreciate. Someone with very oily skin will find this doesn't hold back shine in an "absolute" fashion, but it's a plus that the sunscreen is in-part zinc oxide. Among 16 shades, the colors to avoid because they are too peach, pink, or rose are True Beige, Shell Bisque, Fawn Beige, and Cappuccino. There are some excellent options for fair and dark skin alike. ☺ **$$$ Featherlight Maximum Foundation SPF 15** *($26.15; $13.80 for refillable compact)* is a powdery foundation that is inaccurately described as a cream-to-powder makeup. Yes, the powder feels creamy, but the formula lacks the ingredients necessary to create a true cream-to-powder texture. If you're thinking the "maximum" part of the name refers to this product's coverage, that's also false. This applies smoothly and offers light coverage with a satin matte, nonpowdery finish. Sufficient UVA protection is provided by an in-part zinc-oxide sunscreen, though this must be applied liberally to net the full SPF 15, which is why powders with sunscreen are best when matched with another product sporting sun protection. The range of 16 shades presents numerous very good options for fair to light skin. The darkest shades are decent, but some suffer from being too ash, including Fawn Beige. Bronzed Auburn and Deep Mahogany are good, but best applied with a brush because sponge application tends to make the color look a bit gray.

😐 **$$$ Self-Defining Sheer Foundation SPF 15** *($25.25)* loses points because it doesn't contain the UVA-protecting ingredients of titanium dioxide, zinc oxide, avobenzone, Tinosorb, or Mexoryl SX, so you can't rely it for sufficient sun protection. This slightly greasy liquid foundation goes on sheer and leaves a moist finish that ends up feeling lighter than anticipated. The 15 shades are mostly excellent, with the only missteps being Shell Bisque, Honey Creme, and Fawn Beige. It's a shame the sunscreen element is incomplete, because this foundation has a lot going for it. 😐 **$$$ Flawless Coverage Powder Foundation SPF 10** *($21.90; $13.90 for refillable compact)* is an amazingly silky, talc-based pressed-powder foundation with an in-part zinc-oxide sunscreen. It blends exceptionally well and provides sheer to light coverage with a soft matte (in feel) finish. Each shade features a subtle amount of shine, but definitely not enough to be distracting in daylight. Speaking of the shades, with one exception they are impeccable. Among 14 choices, only Flawless Cameo is a problem. Otherwise, this is a gorgeous range of neutrals with options for all skin tones from porcelain to ebony. Regarding the sunscreen, SPF 15 is preferred and the lower number is the sole reason why this foundation was not rated a Paula's Pick. However, it would work well over a moisturizer with sunscreen rated SPF 15 or higher.

CONCEALER: ☹ **$$$ Enhancing Concealer** *($16.45)* comes in a twist-up stick, and although its creamy texture makes application smooth, creasing is a problem because the creaminess stays that way. It's an OK option, but provides no more than medium coverage and doesn't last unless it is set with powder.

☺ **$$$ Ultimate Coverage Concealer** *($18.60)* has a liquid texture and provides much better coverage than the Enhancing Concealer above. It works well to camouflage blemishes and doesn't contain waxes or heavy thickeners that can prolong acne's stay. Three shades are available, but, with the exception of Light, they're a bit tricky to work with. Light-Medium is OK but may be too yellow for some skin tones, while Dark is only suitable for bronze to very dark skin. This concealer's strong matte finish makes it less desirable to use around the eyes if wrinkles are present, but it definitely has staying power and is worth considering if you have breakouts or very oily skin.

POWDER: The ☺ **$$$ Loose Powder** *($20.55)* is a standard, talc-based powder with three good color choices, though three is definitely a limited selection considering the number of foundation shades Artistry offers. It has a silky texture and satin-smooth finish appropriate for normal to dry skin. ☺ **$$$ Bronzing Powder** *($20.55)* is available in two realistic tan shades for light to medium skin, and its formula is identical to the Loose Powder above. It features a small amount of shine, not enough to make it a problem for daytime makeup—though in general, bronzing powder is best for casual and weekend use, rather than professional or office makeup.

BLUSH: The ☹ **$$$ Powder Blush** *($12.40 for blush pans; $13.80 for refillable compact)* colors have a reasonably smooth but drier than usual texture that manages to apply evenly, with each shade having a satin finish (courtesy of the shine each shade has). The ultra-shiny Innocence shade feels grainy due to the glittery particles it contains, and is not recommended. Price-wise, Artistry compares their blush to similar options from Estee Lauder, Lancome, and Bobbi Brown, yet there is no comparison: all three of the competing companies offer powder blushes that feel silkier and apply better than this.

EYESHADOW: Artistry's ☺ **$$$ Eye Colour** *($8.35 per pan)* comes in individual pans that are placed into a sold-separately **Four-Pan Compact** *($13.80)*. The compact can hold four eyeshadows, or you could arrange two eyeshadows with an Artistry Powder Blush. The eyeshadows have an ultra-smooth texture and silky application that blends and builds well. Every shade has some amount of shine, though there are some very good almost-matte options, including Chic, Veil, Wheat, Shell, and Misty. If you opt for the shades with noticeable shine, they do cling well so flaking shouldn't be an issue.

EYE AND BROW SHAPER: ✓ ☺ **$$$ Control Eyeliner** *($19.90)* is aptly named because this liquid liner's thin but short brush allows for precise control and makes it easier to draw a continuous line. The formula applies evenly, dries quickly, has incredible staying power, and yet it's easy to remove. You can find equally outstanding liquid liners for less money, but this still remains a prime choice from Artistry.

☺ **$$$ Eye Define** *($18.75)* is a very good automatic, retractable pencil that provides a smooth application with a soft, non-greasy finish. This tends to stay in place well but fades slightly before the day is done. Lunar is a navy blue shade that is dark enough to be a worthwhile alternative to classic black. ☺ **$$$ Brow Define** *($18.75)* has a dry, stiff texture but this allows for a softer application and the powdery finish really lasts. If you don't mind the dry application, this is recommended as a good, no-sharpening-needed retractable brow pencil. The opposite end of the pencil houses a dual-sided brow brush that does its job well.

😐 **$$$ Effortless Eye Pencil** *($18.60)* is a dual-sided, automatic, retractable pencil. One end is a very shiny cream eyeshadow; the other is a smooth eyeliner in standard colors. The cream eyeshadow portion stays creamy and is prone to creasing, but the pencil side is nice. This is an item that tends to come and go in the Artistry line, but the consultant I dealt with mentioned that this product is reintroduced with different color combinations as trends dictate.

LIPSTICK, LIP GLOSS, AND LIPLINER: ☺ **$$$ Matte Sheen Lip Colour** *($16)* is another in-and-out, trend-based lipstick, although it doesn't leave a sheen, and isn't matte in the least. It's a good, lightweight lipstick with a soft shimmer finish.

☺ **$$$ Effortless Lip Pencil** *($18.90)* features a creamy lipstick and coordinating, retractable Lipliner packaged in one automatic pencil unit. It's pricey for what you get, but does the job without anything spectacular to extol. ☺ **$$$ Mini Lip Rouge Set** *($19.45)* offers ten of the Perfect Moisture Lip Colours in one credit card–sized compact. You get a tiny amount of each shade, but for experimenting or travel this set is a handy option (note that you'll need a lip brush, too).

☺ **Perfect Moisture Lip Colour** *($14.55)*. These have a classic creamy texture (meaning not too dry, not too greasy) with a slight glossy finish. The color selection is decent, though nothing about this lipstick will promote younger-looking lips in one month, as claimed.

😐 **SoftSticks for Lips** *($13.60)* are just standard lip pencils with a creamy application and a good color selection, and they do require sharpening. 😐 **Jumbo Lip Pencil** *($14.10)* is a very soft lipstick in pencil form. It feels great and the opaque, versatile colors are sure to please, but it's too soft to use as Lipliner and you'll find these get used much faster than most lipsticks because of the constant sharpening and softness of the pencil. 😐 **Sheer Lip Colour SPF 15** *($14.55)* is a collection of standard, glossy finish lipsticks that feel great, but the SPF 15 doesn't include the UVA-protecting ingredients of titanium dioxide, zinc oxide, avobenzone, Tinosorb, or Mexoryl SX.

😐 **$$$ Glossy Lip Shine** *($19.45)* is an expensive gloss and the formula doesn't justify the cost. It is a standard tube-with-wand-applicator product that feels light and is non-sticky, but the shimmer each shade contains feels slightly grainy on lips. Revlon, Cover Girl, and Neutrogena make similar glosses without this side effect, and for half the price.

MASCARA: ☺ **$$$ Definitive Lash Mascara** *($18.75)* makes its mark as an all-around pleasing mascara. It produces length and thickness in equal measure, and the tiny brush allows you to easily reach every lash. It can go on a bit heavy, but combs out well so clumps aren't a problem.

😐 **$$$ Waterproof Mascara 200** *($16.30)* provides below-average length and minimal thickness but it wears well without flaking or smearing, is waterproof, and comes off with a water-soluble cleanser, all pluses. If you're looking for a minimalist effect yet need a waterproof formula, you may want to give this a try.

FACE AND BODY ILLUMINATING/SHIMMER PRODUCTS: ☺ **$$$ Light Reflective Lotion SPF 15** *($26.50)* is a lightweight moisturizer with tinted shimmer and an in-part zinc oxide sunscreen. The directions indicate to apply it liberally, as you would any sunscreen. However, the amount of shimmer is too intense for all-over application, with each ethereal color adding a strange hue to skin. It's a good option for spot highlighting or mixing with your foundation, but not for use as your sole sunscreen.

☹ **$$$ Shimmer Powder** *($26)* is pressed and comes in an attractive compact. The amount of shine is noticeable, and more sparkly than a soft glow. As with many shiny powders, this doesn't cling well to skin and tends to migrate.

BRUSHES: The ☹ **$$$ Artistry Brush Set** *($61.80)* includes six full-sized brushes that, for the money, aren't as exceptional as they should be. The Powder Brush is soft but should be fuller for easier application; the Blush Brush is too small to sweep blush over the cheek area, though it is dense. The Eyeshadow, Liner/Brow, and Lip Brush are fine but not nice enough to make splurging on this set a smart idea. The most intriguing part of this set is the brush case, because it includes a separate zippered pouch to store smaller makeup items as well as additional slots to hold other makeup brushes. The pouch isn't large enough to hold all your makeup essentials, but I can see its value for some women.

SPECIALTY PRODUCTS: The Artistry line offers several products to organize and conveniently transport your cosmetics. The items are priced from $35–$82, and are, for the most part, well made. If you're sold on Artistry makeup, consider the ☺ **$$$ Artistry Signature Organizer** *($58; $13.50 for replacement trays)*, a day planner–type book that has detachable pages to hold blushes, powders, and eyeshadows as well as a small, zippered bag to house loose items and a pouch for brushes. It's incredibly convenient and a portable way to have all your makeup with you. The ☺ **$$$ Artistry Cosmetics Case** *($82)* works well to store numerous cosmetics but you can find larger, more functional cases in this price range (and that would be of more interest to a professional makeup artist).

AUBREY ORGANICS

AUBREY ORGANICS AT-A-GLANCE

Strengths: None.

Weaknesses: Too numerous to list, but major issues include a lack of sunscreens without a problematic active ingredient; consistent use of ingredients proven to be irritating to skin while offering no substantiated benefit; a complete lack of products to address common skin-care concerns, from acne to pigmentation problems; the makeup is abysmal; the company's ingredient lists are mostly in violation of FDA guidelines, and they have been cited for these labeling errors.

For more information, call (800) 282-7394, or visit www.aubrey-organics.com or www.Beautypedia.com.

AUBREY ORGANICS DRY SKIN 1

☹ **Seaware with Rosa Mosqueta Facial Cleansing Cream, for Dry Skin** *($15.48 for 8 ounces)* lists the second ingredient as alcohol, and that can be drying and irritating for all skin types. The typical detergent-based cleanser in this product is standard in the industry, only here it has a less technical (and mislabeled) name, "coconut fatty acid." Coconut fatty acid goes by many less-friendly names, from tridecyl cocoate to cocamidopropylamine oxide, but if they were on the label, then it would start sounding like everyone else's products and it would be so much harder to convince people that you were all natural. This cleanser can be drying for most skin types.

☹ **Rosa Mosqueta & English Lavender Facial Toner, for Dry Skin** *($9.28 for 8 ounces)* lists alcohol as the second ingredient, followed by witch hazel. All the plants in the world can't change how irritating that is for skin. However, several of the plant extracts in this product are either skin irritants or have potential photosensitizing or toxic reactions on skin, including peppermint, coltsfoot, nettle leaf, St. John's wort, watercress, horsetail, arnica, and lemon.

☹ **Rosa Mosqueta Rose Hip Moisturizing Cream, for Dry Skin** *($16.28 for 4 ounces)* contains problematic plant extracts and an incomplete ingredient listing that doesn't follow FDA or CTFA regulations.

☹ **Jojoba Meal & Oatmeal with Rosa Mosqueta Mask & Scrub, for Dry Skin** *($8.98 for 4 ounces)* lists alcohol as its second ingredient and an unknown detergent cleansing agent as its first. This cleanser/scrub hybrid is too irritating for all skin types. If you want a natural scrub for dry skin, try mixing some cornmeal with a teaspoon or so of plain jojoba oil.

AUBREY ORGANICS COMBINATION DRY SKIN 2

☹ **Sea Buckthorn & Cucumber with Ester-C Facial Cleansing Cream, for Combination Dry Skin** *($12.98 for 8 ounces)* is similar to the Seaware with Rosa Mosqueta Facial Cleansing Cream, for Dry Skin, above, but with less alcohol. If you think that makes this a gentler cleansing option, think again: the geranium and lavender oils in this product are troublesome for skin and for use around the eyes.

☹ **Sea Buckthorn & Cucumber with Ester-C Facial Toner, for Combination Dry Skin** *($9.28 for 8 ounces)* lists alcohol and witch hazel as part of this toner's herbal base; and contains several other ingredients that, while natural, are also very irritating to skin.

☺ **Sea Buckthorn & Cucumber with Ester-C Moisturizing Cream, for Combination Dry Skin** *($16.28 for 4 ounces)* appears to be a good moisturizer for normal to dry skin, though the way Hampton lists some of the ingredients leaves you to wonder exactly what he's using. The good news is this product does not contain irritants. Instead, it uses beneficial, nonvolatile plant oils that have antioxidant activity, and plant extracts with proven soothing properties.

😐 **Sea Buckthorn & Cucumber with Ester-C Moisturizing Mask, for Combination Dry Skin** *($8.98 for 4 ounces)* works better as a topical scrub for normal to dry skin than a mask, and it contains some good anti-irritants, including chamomile oil. The questionable aspects include the mysterious "coconut fatty acid cream base" and the nut meals used as abrasive agents (these tend to be unevenly shaped particles that can be damaging to skin if used too aggressively).

AUBREY ORGANICS NORMAL SKIN 3

☹ **Green Tea & Ginkgo Facial Cleansing Lotion, for Normal Skin** *($15.48 for 8 ounces)* is almost identical to the Seaware with Rosa Mosqueta Facial Cleansing Cream, for Dry Skin, above, only this one is in lotion form. The same concerns apply.

☹ **Green Tea & Ginkgo Facial Toner, for Normal Skin** *($9.28 for 8 ounces)* follows the pattern set by all of the toners in this line: it's an alcohol and witch hazel base coupled with several irritating plant extracts. The anti-irritant plant extracts in this product don't have a flower's chance in a blizzard of helping skin.

☹ **Green Tea & Ginkgo Moisturizer SPF 15, for Normal Skin** *($16.28 for 4 ounces)* lists padimate-o (PABA) as its active ingredient, which is too irritating for skin and leaves it vulnerable to UVA damage. Several of the plant extracts are a problem, too, making this a sunscreen that won't keep normal skin in that state for long.

😐 **Green Tea & Green Clay Rejuvenating Mask, for Normal Skin** *($8.98 for 4 ounces)* is a standard clay mask that includes glycerin, plant extracts, and thickeners. It's an OK option for normal to slightly oily skin, but its oil content isn't encouraging for anyone battling blemishes.

AUBREY ORGANICS COMBINATION/OILY SKIN 4

☹ **Blue Green Algae with Grape Seed Extract Facial Cleansing Lotion, for Combination/Oily Skin** *($15.48 for 8 ounces)* has a cleansing base consisting of castile soap, and although this version uses olive oil instead of animal fat it can still be drying for skin. The lavender oil also contributes to making this cleanser problematic for any skin type.

☹ **Blue Green Algae with Grape Seed Extract Facial Toner, for Combination/Oily Skin** *($9.28 for 8 ounces)* lists alcohol and witch hazel as its main ingredients, making this not recommended for any skin type. This is as soothing for stressed skin as walking barefoot on a hot sidewalk.

☹ **Blue Green Algae with Grape Seed Extract Moisturizer SPF 15, for Combination/Oily Skin** *($16.28 for 4 ounces)* is nearly identical to the Green Tea & Ginkgo Moisturizer SPF 15, for Normal Skin, above and the same review applies.

☹ **Blue Green Algae with Grape Seed Extract Soothing Mask, for Combination/Oily Skin** *($8.98 for 4 ounces)* is similar to the Green Tea & Green Clay Rejuvenating Mask, for Normal Skin, above except this adds lavender oil, which makes it too irritating.

AUBREY ORGANICS OILY SKIN 5

☹ **Natural Herbal Facial Cleanser, for Oily Skin** *($12.98 for 8 ounces)* is painful to even write about! This very irritating cleanser exposes skin to soap, witch hazel, alcohol, eucalyptus, camphor, and menthol, among other problematic ingredients. Ouch!

☹ **Natural Herbal Facial Astringent, for Oily Skin** *($9.28 for 8 ounces)* is similar to all of the toners from Aubrey Organics, and harms skin more than it could possibly help. This is a classic example of why natural ingredients aren't inherently better for skin.

☹ **Natural Herbal Maintenance Oil Balancing Moisturizer, for Oily Skin** *($13.48 for 2 ounces)* cannot balance oil in the least but does subject skin to many irritating ingredients, including witch hazel, balsam oil, horsetail, balm mint, and coltsfoot, with the latter containing compounds that are carcinogenic (Source: *Toxicology and Industrial Health*, September 2006, pages 321–327).

☹ **Natural Herbal Seaclay with Goa Herb Oil Balancing Mask, for Oily Skin** *($8.98 for 4 ounces)* contains peppermint oil, which sabotages an otherwise effective but average clay mask. Goa herb oil (also known as ringworm oil) is very irritating to skin and mucous membranes, and is also easily absorbed, where it can cause systemic problems (Source: www.naturaldatabase.com).

AUBREY ORGANICS SENSITIVE SKIN 6

☹ **Vegecol Facial Cleansing Lotion, for Sensitive Skin** *($15.48 for 8 ounces)* contains several ingredients that are completely inappropriate for sensitive skin, or any skin type for that matter, including St. John's wort, coltsfoot, and lemon peel oil.

☹ **Vegecol with Aloe Alcohol-Free Facial Toner, for Sensitive Skin** *($9.28 for 8 ounces)* is preferred for sensitive skin compared to Aubrey Organics' other toners, but the witch hazel and lavender water still make it a poor choice for most skin types, particularly sensitive skin.

☹ **Vegecol with Aloe Moisturizing Cream, for Sensitive Skin** *($13.48 for 2 ounces)* contains several ingredients that are completely inappropriate for sensitive skin, or any skin type for that matter, including St. John's wort, coltsfoot, and lemon peel oil.

☹ **Vegecol with Aloe & Oatmeal Soothing Mask, for Sensitive Skin** *($8.98 for 4 ounces)* contains several ingredients that are completely inappropriate for sensitive skin, or any skin type for that matter, including alcohol, St. John's wort, coltsfoot, and lemon peel oil.

OTHER AUBREY ORGANICS PRODUCTS

☹ **Herbessence Makeup Remover** *($6.95 for 2 ounces)* is mostly nonvolatile plant and nut oils, but there's enough lavender oil in here to make it potentially problematic, especially if used to remove makeup around the eyes. Any of the non-volatile oils in this product will help break down makeup without risking irritation, so stick with that approach if you have dry skin and prefer an oil cleanser.

☹ **Sparkling Mineral Water Herbal Complexion Mist** *($7.48 for 4 ounces)* isn't akin to San Pellegrino in a bottle, though misting that on your face would be a far gentler option. This product is not recommended due to a list of irritants that includes balm mint, mistletoe, yarrow, and fragrant oak musk oil.

☹ **Collagen TCM Therapeutic Cream Moisturizer** *($13.48 for 2 ounces)* claims to deliver 100% pure, soluble collagen and elastin onto the skin, rather than *into* it. That's an accurate statement because the molecular structure of these ingredients is too small to penetrate into skin, so they do not act to replenish your skin's supply. It's interesting that a company that is so gung-ho to let its customers know it doesn't test on animals resorts to using animal-derived ingredients (at least they're being true to their natural roots). All told, the grain alcohol as the second ingredient and the lackluster formula make this a moisturizer to ignore.

☹ **Lumessence Rejuvenating Eye Creme with Liposomes** *($23.50 for 0.5 ounce)* contains many ingredients that are beneficial for dry skin, though few of them are listed correctly (there's no such ingredient as "humectant liposomes," though at least they indicate what the complex consists of). Unfortunately, lavender is present in an amount significant enough to make it a problem for skin.

☹ **Natural AHA Fruit Acids with Apricot Toning Moisturizer** *($19.95 for 4 ounces)* does not contain AHAs in any form but instead uses several plant extracts that are irritating for skin, including whole extracts of lavender, peppermint, and coltsfoot. Fragrant oils of jasmine and lavender only make matters worse.

😐 **Rosa Mosqueta Night Creme with Alpha Lipoic Acid** *($21.50 for 1 ounce)* contains a tiny amount of alpha lipoic acid (listed as such, though it should be listed as thioctic acid). But even if it was brimming with it, or other antioxidants, the translucent glass bottle won't hold them stable. This is a decent moisturizer for dry to very dry skin and, thankfully, lacks any of the problematic plant extracts found in most of Aubrey Organics' moisturizers. The amount of grain alcohol is too small to cause irritation.

☺ **Rosa Mosqueta Rose Hip Seed Oil** *($12.98 for 0.36 ounce)* contains nothing more than organic rose hip seed oil. It is a soothing, nonvolatile plant oil that is often touted for its vitamin C content. Although fresh rose hip seed oil is rich in this vitamin, most of this nutrient is destroyed during the drying and processing necessary to create products like this. Still, this product can be a good spot treatment for patches of very dry skin.

😐 **Sea Buckthorn with Ester-C Antioxidant Serum** *($15.98 for 0.36 ounce)*. Assuming that the ingredient list is somewhat accurate, this is mostly jojoba oil and some form of vitamin C. That can be helpful for dry skin. Sea buckthorn oil has antioxidant capability, but not in the type of packaging this product has.

☹ **Vegecell Nighttime Hydrator with Green Tea** *($18.75 for 1 ounce)* is similar to many of the products Aubrey sells, with no mention of skin type. The alcohol, lavender, peppermint, coltsfoot, nettle, sage, St. John's wort, watercress, lemon, ivy, sage, and lemon are all serious problems for skin.

😐 **White Camellia Oil** *($15.98 for 0.36 ounce)* contains exactly what the name indicates, and nothing more. Aubrey claims this is "a superb complexion oil" but that's either just his opinion or based on anecdotal evidence; there is no substantiated proof. Moreover, white camellia oil is primarily used for fragrance, not skin care, so this product is best dabbed on the wrist, if used at all.

AUBREY ORGANICS SUN PRODUCTS

☹ **After Sun Body & Face Maintenance Moisturizer** *($10.75 for 8 ounces)* contains too many problematic ingredients to make it worthwhile, whether skin is dealing with sun-induced dryness or not.

☺ **Pure Aloe Vera, Certified Organic** *($7.78 for 4 ounces)* consists of organic aloe vera and natural preservative. Aloe can be soothing to sun-exposed or reddened skin, but I disagree with the company's claim that it is the best ingredient for skin that has endured too much sun exposure. The company might disagree too if they sold a single effective sunscreen that didn't contain PABA.

☹ **Gone! Safe and Natural Outdoor Spray SPF 10** *($6.58 for 4 ounces)* uses only padimate-o (PABA) as its active ingredient, which leaves skin vulnerable to UVA damage, not to mention the substandard SPF rating. This actually qualifies as one of the most irritating skin-care products in this book due to the litany of irritants it contains, from eucalyptus oil and alcohol to menthol and lavender oil. The essential oils may naturally repel insects, but I'd save your skin by donning protective clothing instead.

☹ **Natural Sun SPF 8 Deep Tanning Sunscreen** *($7.25 for 4 ounces)* has an SPF rating that's too low, an active ingredient that is severely outdated and provides insufficient UVA protection, and still encourages users to get a deep tan. Talk about the fast track to wrinkles and, potentially, skin cancer!

☹ **Natural Sun SPF 12 Protective Tanning Butter** *($7.25 for 4 ounces)* does contain an in-part titanium dioxide sunscreen, but an SPF 15 is critical and basic to good skin care, and the padimate-o (PABA) can still be a problem for most skin types.

😐 **Natural Sun SPF 20 Tinted Sunscreen, for Face & Body** *($8.50 for 4 ounces)* is similar to but has a lighter texture than the Natural Sun SPF 12 Protective Tanning Butter above. Although the SPF rating is ideal, the inclusion of padimate-o still makes this not worth considering over the many effective sunscreens without it. Iron oxides give this lotion a sheer tint, but that's more to offset the whitening effect of the titanium dioxide than to add color to skin.

😐 **Natural Sun SPF 20 Unscented Sunscreen, for Face & Body** *($7.75 for 5 ounces)* is nearly identical to the Natural Sun SPF 20 Tinted Sunscreen, for Face & Body above, minus the iron oxides that give the previous sunscreen its "tint."

😐 **Natural Sun SPF 25 Green Tea Protective Sunscreen, Ideal for Children** *($8.50 for 4 ounces)* isn't ideal for children (or adults) because one of the active ingredients is padimate-o (PABA), though it is joined by titanium dioxide to provide broad-spectrum sun protection. This ends up being a decent, oil-rich sunscreen for dry to very dry skin. The jasmine oil is present in a tiny amount, but may still cause problems for those with sensitive skin (if the PABA doesn't stir things up first).

😐 **Natural Sun SPF 25 Sunscreen, Ideal for Active Lifestyles** *($8.50 for 4 ounces)* is a repackaged and renamed version of the Natural Sun SPF 25 Green Tea Protective Sunscreen, Ideal for Children, above and the same review applies.

☹ **Nature's Balance Unscented SPF 15 Hand & Body Lotion** *($12.95 for 8 ounces)* lacks the UVA-protecting ingredients of titanium dioxide, zinc oxide, avobenzone, Tinosorb, or Mexoryl SX, and is not recommended. Even with sufficient UVA protection, the St. John's wort oil in this product contains several components that are toxic when skin is exposed to sun (Sources: *Planta Medica*, February 2002, pages 171–173; *International Journal of Biochemistry and Cell Biology*, March 2002, pages 221–241).

☹ **Saving Face SPF 10 Sunscreen Protection Spray** *($8 for 4 ounces)* won't save your face from anything but will encourage wrinkles due to its lack of UVA-protecting ingredients and possibly a phototoxic reaction from the St. John's wort oil it contains.

☹ **Ultimate Moist Morning Meadow Hand & Body Lotion SPF 15** *($9.95 for 8 ounces)* conjures up images of a peaceful dawn when the grass is still wet with dew, but don't let that cloud your judgment of this sunscreen, whose problems are identical to the Saving Face SPF 10 Sunscreen Protection Spray above.

☹ **Amino Derm Gel Clear Skin Complex** *($7.95 for 2 ounces)* is said to help keep skin clear, but what's reliable about this product is how efficiently it causes irritation from the witch hazel, alcohol, and several problematic plant extracts.

☹ **Natural AHA Fruit Acids with Apricot Exfoliating Mask** *($19.95 for 4 ounces)* lists alcohol as the second ingredient and also contains lemon and jasmine oils to further complicate matters for your skin.

AUBREY ORGANICS MAKEUP

Perhaps the two best words to describe the small assortment of makeup from Aubrey Organics are "Don't bother"—but "What were they thinking?" is a close second. What you'll find here, available as single products or in preselected kits, is a selection of loose powders and sheer lip tints. The ☹ **Natural Translucent Base** *($18.65)* and ☹ **Silken Earth** *($6.05, or $19.38 for the kit)* powders are designed to be used as foundation, highlighter, contour, and blush, but the gritty texture of each and the incredibly dry finish make them all poor candidates—not to mention that each one contains cinnamon powder. That certainly is natural and may smell nice, but it's nevertheless problematic for skin.

☹ **Natural Lips** *($6.95, or $14.68 for the kit)* products are simply sheer lip tints that come packaged in glass jars. The colors are very soft and pretty, but they all contain enough peppermint oil to sound the irritation alarm for lips.

☹ **Natural Cosmetic Brush** *($3.95)* is inferior to almost any other powder brush you'll find for sale, and although it comes in two sizes (one for powder application and a smaller version for contouring), you're better off ignoring both. If you're intent on supporting a cosmetics company espousing natural ingredients, consider the vastly superior brushes from Aveda or The Body Shop.

AVAGE (SEE RETINOIDS)

AVEDA

AVEDA AT-A-GLANCE

Strengths: Effective use of beneficial plant oils and extracts in some products; one of the few lines that offers a lip balm and sheer lip tint whose sunscreen includes adequate UVA protection; superior tinted moisturizer with sunscreen; good concealer; terrific brushes and refillable compacts; Aveda takes its environmental commitments seriously.

Weaknesses: Several products contain irritating essential oils or fragrance components known to cause sun sensitivity or skin cell death; substandard cleansers and irritating toners; so-called treatment products that can irritate skin; foundations whose SPF rating falls below the minimum of 15; average to poor blush options; several lip color products contains irritating fragrant oils.

For more information about Aveda, call (866) 823-1425 or visit www.aveda.com or www.Beautypedia.com.

AVEDA ALL SENSITIVE PRODUCTS

☺ **All Sensitive Cleanser** *($18 for 5 ounces)* is a lotion-style cleanser that contains several plant extracts, including cardamom, which isn't the best for someone with sensitive skin. The good news is that Aveda has redone the plant aspect of this product, and most of them here now have soothing, anti-irritant properties. This does not contain detergent cleansing agents and you may need to use a washcloth for complete makeup removal. It's an option for normal to dry skin.

😐 **All Sensitive Toner** *($18 for 5 ounces)* contains too many fragrant plant extracts to make it appropriate for sensitive skin. Nonfragrant, anti-irritant plant extracts are included too, and this spray-on toner has some good skin-identical ingredients in it, too. Still, the fragrant plants and rose geranium oil make it an iffy proposition.

😐 **All Sensitive Moisturizer** *($32 for 5 ounces)* remains a bland, ordinary moisturizer that would be much better for sensitive skin without the fragrant plant extracts it contains. Cardamom and vetiver are problematic ingredients for someone dealing with skin sensitivity, and may cause sensitivity in otherwise normal skin. That makes this a tough recommendation though it's not a terrible product.

AVEDA BOTANICAL KINETICS PRODUCTS

😐 **$$$ Botanical Kinetics Purifying Creme Cleanser** *($17 for 5 ounces)* would be a much better lotion-style cleanser without the witch hazel extract, but the emollient ingredients keep it from being a significant problem for the normal to dry skin types this cleanser is best for.

☹ **Botanical Kinetics Purifying Gel Cleanser** *($17 for 5 ounces)* has a considerable amount of lavender and rosemary, two irritants that tarnish this otherwise standard and effective water-soluble cleanser. Several fragrant components (including eugenol and geraniol) are a problem when used around eyes or mucous membranes.

😐 **Botanical Kinetics Skin Firming/Toning Agent** *($17 for 5 ounces)* is a simple rose water toner with a couple of good skin-identical ingredients and a tiny amount of alcohol. It's more akin to misting skin with fragrance rather than with helpful ingredients.

☹ **Botanical Kinetics Toning Mist** *($17 for 5 ounces)* lists peppermint as the second ingredient and also contains witch hazel and alcohol, along with fragrant plant extracts with no established benefit for skin. This toner is not recommended.

☹ **Botanical Kinetics Exfoliant** *($17 for 5 ounces)* has a workable pH of 3, but the amount of salicylic acid it contains is too small for it to function as an exfoliant. This liquid contains several irritating plant extracts, including lavender, witch hazel, and balm mint.

☹ **Botanical Kinetics Hydrating Lotion** *($30 for 5 ounce)* is a basic moisturizer fraught with problematic ingredients, including significant amounts of lavender, rosemary, and comfrey, along with lesser amounts of fragrance components (such as eugenol) that are skin irritants. Eugenol is particularly egregious. It is a major component of clove oil, and research has shown the eugenol content of clove causes skin cell death, even when low concentrations of clove (0.33%) were applied to cultured skin cells (Source: *Cell Proliferation*, August 2006, pages 241–248).

AVEDA OUTER PEACE PRODUCTS

Aveda recommends that their clients with acne use all of the new Outer Peace products because—according to their research—the system resulted in a 92% success rate after just four weeks. The details of this study and how they came to their conclusion are not available and as such shouldn't be taken seriously. You have to ask yourself, Why is it that only the results are public information, but not the actual study itself? What's the big secret? It could be that one side of the face had nothing on it and the other had their products. Both would achieve some pretty good comparative results for Outer Peace, but it wouldn't answer the question of how the products compare to truly well-formulated blemish-fighting products.

For Aveda's system, rather than using a well-researched and proven antibacterial agent, such as benzoyl peroxide (Source: *Lancet*, December 2004, pages 2188–2195), the company chose to rely on plant extracts with an unproven history of anti-acne benefits. To their credit, most of the plant extracts included at least have soothing rather than irritating properties. Still, that doesn't help deal with the bacteria, the buildup of skin cells, and the excess oil production that are causing the problem in the first place.

☺ **$$$ Outer Peace Foaming Cleanser** *($24 for 4.2 ounces)* is a liquid-to-foam, water-soluble cleanser that contains gentle detergent cleansing agents along with several anti-irritant plant extracts. Salicylic acid is also present, but only a tiny amount, which is rinsed off before it has a chance to work. The amount of alcohol is insignificant, but the salicylic acid means this should not be used around the eyes. This cleanser contains tamanu seed oil, which is reputed to contain a fatty acid (calophyllic acid) said to have an antimicrobial action on skin. There is no substantiated information about tamanu oil's effect on acne, although there is some research showing it has wound-healing effects (Source: *International Journal of Cosmetic Science*, December 2002, pages 341–348), but fighting blemishes is completely different from healing wounds. All other claims about tamanu oil's benefit for skin are anecdotal, but its polyphenol content makes it a suitable antioxidant—just not in a cleanser where it is rinsed down the drain, along with the salicylic acid, before it has a chance to work.

☹ **Outer Peace Acne Relief Pads** *($30 for 50 pads)* contains 1.5% salicylic acid, but the pH of the base is too high for it to exfoliate skin. Also, the amount of alcohol in this solution is too irritating for all skin types, not to mention that the alcohol cancels out the anti-irritant effect of the much smaller amounts of plant extracts.

😐 **$$$ Outer Peace Acne Relief Lotion** *($38 for 1.7 ounces)* is a lightweight, matte-finish BHA lotion that contains 0.5% salicylic acid and has a pH of 3.9, meaning that exfoliation will occur, but not very much. With the 0.5% concentration, this product is only marginally effective. It would be better for blemish-prone skin if the salicylic acid were present in at least a 1% concentration, and for more stubborn acne 2% would be preferred. This also contains cornstarch (which contributes to this lotion's matte finish), but as a food-based ingredient, that isn't the best for dealing with the bacterium that triggers blemishes.

☹ **$$$ Outer Peace Acne Spot Relief** *($28 for 0.5 ounce)* ranks as an effective, but needlessly expensive, BHA lotion that comes with a frustrating balance of positives and negatives. It's great that the 2% salicylic acid is in a base with a pH of 3.7, which will allow exfoliation to occur. It's not so great that Aveda included alcohol and cornstarch, both of which can exacerbate problems for those battling acne. The amounts of the offending ingredients aren't large, but this product would have earned a Paula's Pick rating without them (even though I still have reservations about the price tag for the tiny amount of product provided).

☹ **$$$ Outer Peace Cooling Masque** *($35 for 4.2 ounces)* is a needlessly expensive clay mask, which doesn't contain anything that brings peace to acne-prone skin. Like all clay masks, this can absorb excess oil and leave skin feeling smooth and looking, at least for the short term, matte. There is more alcohol and preservative in this formula than potentially beneficial plants, and the fragrance is potentially irritating due to the volatile components it is composed of.

AVEDA TOURMALINE PRODUCTS

☺ **$$$ Tourmaline Charged Exfoliating Cleanser** *($28 for 5 ounces)* is a rich, foaming cleanser that uses jojoba beads to gently polish the skin as you wash. This cleanser contains a skin-friendly assortment of nonirritating plant and nut oils, making it a great choice for parched, flaky skin during the winter months. It does contain fragrance and fragrant components along with salicylic acid, but those ingredients would be more of a problem if this product was used around the eyes, and a scrub-type cleanser shouldn't be used in that area anyway. By the way, the antioxidants included are a nice touch, but are needless in a rinse-off product as they end up down the drain instead of being absorbed into your skin where they are needed.

✓☺ **$$$ Tourmaline Charged Eye Creme** *($30 for 0.5 ounce)* is a brilliantly formulated moisturizer for the eye area or any other place where skin is slightly dry. It contains mostly silicone, water, glycerin, thickeners, tourmaline, skin-identical ingredients, antioxidants, cell-communicating ingredient, slip agents, fragrance, and preservatives. Tourmaline is a crystalline mineral that Aveda maintains increases the energy (and, therefore, the potency) of the ingredients it is blended with. Although there is research proving tourmaline's worth for removing heavy-metal ions from water (Source: *Journal of Environmental Sciences*, 2006, pages 1221–1225), it has no established benefit for skin, so it's a good thing several other ingredients in this eye cream do!

☹ **$$$ Tourmaline Charged Hydrating Creme** *($32 for 1.7 ounces)* has a frustrating blend of beneficial and problematic ingredients, and the most helpful ingredients (the many antioxidants in this moisturizer) are hindered by jar packaging. This is an OK moisturizer for normal to dry skin, but the tiny amount of eugenol is potentially problematic. By the way, there's only a dusting of tourmaline in this product, though that's just fine since it has no effect on skin.

☺ **$$$ Tourmaline Charged Protecting Lotion SPF 15** *($38 for 2.5 ounces)* would rate a Paula's Pick if only the amount of titanium dioxide wasn't so low. As is, the amount (less than 1%), even coupled with octinoxate, is sketchy in terms of reliable UVA protection, especially if you don't apply this product liberally. That said, this moisturizing lotion has an excellent assortment of antioxidants, skin-identical ingredients, and cell-communicating ingredients. It is also free of problematic plant extracts and fragrance components.

☹ **Tourmaline Charged Radiance Fluid** *($37 for 1 ounce)* would have been a worthwhile serum-type moisturizer for all skin types were it not for the inclusion of alcohol (it's the second ingredient) and clary extract, along with a list of unnecessary irritants—oils of peppermint, lavender, geranium, marjoram, orange, and lemon peel. When you combine all of these it's quite an assault on the skin, and not what comes to mind when Aveda states that this product "energizes skin with new, visible life." This does contain tourmaline, which has no proven benefit for skin. If Aveda's statements that tourmaline increases the efficacy of the other ingredients combined with it were true, that would mean the many problematic ingredients in this product would be even more irritating.

✓☺ **$$$ Tourmaline Charged Radiance Masque** *($26 for 4.2 ounces)* is a very good moisturizing mask for normal to dry skin. It contains mostly water, glycerin, thickener, plant oil, emollients, slip agents, nonirritating plant extracts, tourmaline, lycopene (an antioxidant), more emollients, skin-identical ingredients, preservatives, and titanium dioxide (for opacity). Although this mask's claims of boosting skin's radiance due to the tourmaline it contains are unproven, it isn't a problem for skin. As with all moisturizing masks, the longer it is left on the skin the better your results will be, especially if your skin is dry.

OTHER AVEDA PRODUCTS

☺ **Pure Comfort Eye Makeup Remover** *($15 for 4.2 ounces)* is a water-based, gentle makeup remover that's essentially a modified version of a water-soluble cleanser. This isn't too effective for removing long-wearing makeup, but it's good news that all of the plant extracts used have soothing rather than irritating qualities.

☹ **Dual Nature Face Protection SPF 15** *($25 for 1.7 ounces)* combines titanium dioxide and zinc oxide for outstanding broad-spectrum sun protection in a lotion base that has a substantially matte finish, something normal to oily skin not prone to breakouts will appreciate. It's a shame that these positive traits are mixed with fragrant plant oils, including geranium, jasmine, and orange, all of which are potential irritants. In addition, orange oil is phototoxic, which means it can cause adverse reactions on skin that is exposed to sunlight (Source: www.naturaldatabase.com), although there is debate about how much orange oil is needed to cause such a reaction. Many aromatherapy Web sites recommend not using orange oil if skin will be exposed to sun, while others recommend using less than 1.4%, though I could not find research documenting why this specific amount or less is deemed acceptable, so I advise playing it safe and avoiding orange oil altogether.

😐 **$$$ Firming Fluid** *($32 for 1 ounce)* won't firm skin but instead functions as a lightweight, water-based moisturizer. It contains enough witch hazel to have constricting properties, but that ends up being irritating to skin when this fluid is applied regularly. The saving grace for this product would have been its antioxidant vitamins, but the translucent glass bottle won't keep them stable unless it is constantly kept away from light.

☹ **Brightening Essence** *($45 for 1 ounce)* contains nothing that can brighten (or lighten) skin discolorations, including "age and sun spots," as Aveda claims. This water-based formulation contains several potent skin irritants, including a hefty amount of alcohol and essential oils of grapefruit peel, lemon peel, rosemary, orange, and peppermint, and none have any ability to "brighten" skin. Some anti-irritants and antioxidants are included as well, but it's all for naught because they are paired with so many irritating ingredients. This is not the product to consider if you have any type of skin discoloration.

☹ **Brightening Moisture Treatment** *($40 for 2.5 ounces)* is the lotion version of the Brightening Essence above, and although this product omits the alcohol present in the Essence, it contains the same group of irritating essential oils. What a shame, because without the irritants this would have been a good anti-inflammatory moisturizer for normal to slightly dry skin. It cannot, however, work to diminish the appearance of sun-induced skin discolorations.

😐 **$$$ Night Nutrients** *($35 for 1 ounce)* has a sumptuous, silicone-enhanced texture and contains several plant oils that are terrific for dry skin, along with some antioxidants. The problem? Translucent glass packaging won't hold the vitamins (nutrients) stable for long. Additionally, the rosemary leaf oil is present in an amount that may cause irritation, further making this a tough sell.

😐 **$$$ Pure Vital Moisture Eye Cream** *($25 for 0.5 ounce)* doesn't hold a candle to the myriad eye creams other Lauder-owned lines offer, though many of those products (like this one) still suffer from reliance on jar packaging. This is an average moisturizer for the eye area or elsewhere, and it's unfortunate that the really intriguing ingredients show up too late in the game to be significant players.

☹ **Daily Light Guard SPF 15** *($16.50 for 5 ounces)* has an in-part titanium-dioxide sunscreen but its lavender content is cause for concern due to its reaction to sun, which makes this otherwise well-formulated sunscreen a problem for all skin types.

☺ **Sun Source** *($16.50 for 5 ounces)* contains dihydroxyacetone, the ingredient used in most self-tanners to turn skin brown. Although it would be easy to dismiss this self-tanner on its similarity to so many others, Aveda has concocted a thoughtful, irritant-free product that features an elegant moisturizing base that includes antioxidants (and in stable packaging, too). The tiny amount of balsam won't be a problem for skin and likely just contributes to this product's fragrance.

😐 **$$$ Balancing Infusion for Dry Skin** *($18 for 0.34 ounce)* is mostly meadowfoam seed oil and fragrance, along with tiny amounts of vitamins and other plant oils. The fragrance can be a problem for all skin types; you're better off moisturizing with plain olive or jojoba oil than this chancy product.

☹ **Balancing Infusion For Sensitive Skin** *($18 for 0.34 ounce)* contains some plant oils and extracts with established soothing properties, but fragrance is the second ingredient, and the fragrant components in this serum (including linolool and limonene) are an unnecessary pitfall for anyone with sensitive skin.

☹ **Balancing Infusion Salicylic Acid Acne Treatment** *($18 for 0.33 ounce)* is completely inappropriate for someone dealing with acne or blackheads, not only because the concentration of salicylic acid (0.5%) is too low, but also because of the plant oils this product contains. Jojoba, sunflower, and soybean oils are great for dry skin, but readily cause problems for someone with oily or blemish-prone skin. Last but not least, the fragrant plant extracts in this product (centered on rosemary) are potent irritants.

☺ **$$$ Deep Cleansing Herbal Clay Masque** *($19 for 4.4 ounces)* is as standard a clay mask as it gets. Although this masque has enough emollients to make it more "comfortable" than many other clay masks, the emollients are more suited to normal to dry skin than oily skin. Clay is not cleansing in the least, though it can absorb oil from skin.

☹ **Intensive Hydrating Masque** *($19 for 5 ounces)* brings the skin a mixed bag of helpful and potentially harmful ingredients and, despite the name, isn't all that hydrating (you won't think so if your skin is dry to very dry). The amount of lavender extract is likely too problematic to make this worthwhile for even occasional use, especially given the selection of moisturizing masks whose formulas best this one without troublesome ingredients.

☺ **Lip Saver SPF 15** *($8 for 0.15 ounce)* includes an in-part avobenzone sunscreen and is an outstanding emollient lip balm that's packaged ChapStick-style. The ratio of plant oil and jojoba esters to wax produces a softer-texture lip balm that leaves an attractive sheen on lips. The only drawback is the flavor, which is composed of cinnamon and clove. The amounts of these ingredients aren't enough to warrant avoiding the product, but it would have received a Paula's Pick rating without them. One more point: Aveda claims this is waterproof, but a more accurate term is "water-resistant." This balm will need to be reapplied after swimming or perspiring.

AVEDA MAKEUP

FOUNDATION: ✓☺ $$$ Inner Light Tinted Moisture SPF 15 *($25)* is an outstanding tinted moisturizer that uses titanium dioxide as its sole sunscreen active. It has a smooth, creamy texture that hydrates skin while leaving a satin finish, and is suitable for normal to dry skin, offering sheer coverage and a hint of color. Six shades are available and they are all excellent. Burl is an excellent shade for dark (but not very dark) skin, conveying deep color without turning ashy, while Aspen is a real find for someone with fair skin.

😐 **$$$ Inner Light Dual Foundation SPF 12** *($20.50)* is a pressed-powder foundation that contains a titanium dioxide–based sunscreen. Although SPF 15 would have been better—and would comply with the American Academy of Dermatology recommendations—this is still a consideration, as long as you understand that (as for any sunscreen product) it must be applied liberally to achieve the stated SPF. And since this is only SPF 12, to truly protect your skin you also need another sunscreen product, such as a moisturizer, to get sufficient protection. In contrast to its predecessor (Dual Base Minus Oil), this powder foundation is talc-free and instead contains mica, which creates a slightly drier texture and imparts noticeable shine, something that's not the best for a natural look in daylight. It maintains a smooth finish and is easy to blend, providing sheer to light coverage when used dry. Aveda claims it can be used wet, too, but as with most powder foundations, this method of application can promote streaks and look uneven. Nine mostly beautiful shades are offered, with options for light (but not very light) to dark skin tones. Ginger may turn peach on some medium-tan skin tones, but the rest of the colors are soft and neutral.

😐 **$$$ Inner Light Liquid Foundation SPF 12** *($20.50)* doesn't have a liquid texture, and in fact is so thick that it can be difficult to dispense from the bottle (if any foundation could benefit from a pump applicator, it's this one!). Out of the bottle, this does blend on smoothly and thins out before setting to a soft matte (in feel) finish. A slight amount of shine is apparent, but not enough to make this a problem for daytime wear. The all titanium dioxide sunscreen is great, though SPF 15 is preferred; the lower number keeps this foundation from earning a happy face rating. Twelve mostly exemplary shades are available, with some great neutrals for fair to light skin and non-ashy shades for African-American skin tones. The only shades to approach with caution are Sesame and Cinnamon, as both have a tendency to turn slightly peach. This foundation is best for normal to slightly oily skin.

CONCEALER: 😐 Inner Light Concealer *($15)* is a liquid concealer with an initially moist texture that quickly sets to a matte finish, so it must be blended quickly. But if you try to apply this in a sweep of color, it goes on somewhat choppy, providing spotty, rather than smooth, even coverage. It works far better if you apply it in dots over the areas where you need it, and then buff it out so you can get natural-looking coverage capable of concealing dark circles (without creasing) and minor redness. Among the six shades, only Bamboo is questionable because it has a slight orange cast. The others are winning neutrals, with Mahogany a standout for dark skin. Although this concealer has a matte finish, a slight amount of shine is evident. It's a minor issue, but one you should be aware of if you want to avoid shine.

POWDER: ☺ **$$$ Inner Light Pressed Powder** *($19)* is a talc-free pressed powder with a silky texture that feels creamier than most yet remains sheer on skin. Three very good shades are available; however, there are no options for dark skin tones. Keep in mind that because the minerals that comprise this powder have shine, their effect on skin is quite prominent—not really what you want if you're using powder to control or minimize shine.

😐 **$$$ Inner Light Loose Powder** *($19)* comes in only two shades, which is extremely limiting given Aveda's multicultural foundation and concealer colors. Compared to the top loose powders, this talc-free option, while decidedly light, is drier and has way too much shine to look convincing in daylight. It's an option for evening shimmer powder, but given the shine it imparts—just what someone with oily skin is trying to avoid—anyone considering this powder to keep oily areas in check won't be thrilled with the result.

BLUSH: 😐 **Petal Essence Cheek Color** *($14)* has a decently smooth texture but its application imparts almost as much shine as color, and tends to be somewhat uneven. The palette of mostly warm-toned (copper, peach) colors is limiting and, considering the price, this blush isn't in the same league as many others.

☹ **Petal Essence Cheek Tint** *($22)* is blush in stick form, and its stiff, waxy texture must be warmed on the skin prior to applying, which is inconvenient. The vivid yet sheer colors (all have shimmer) blend well and leave a moist finish appropriate for dry skin. The unhappy face rating is due to the inclusion of lavender oil, which is an irritant and a problem for the health of skin cells. ☹ **Uruku Cheek-Lip Creme** *($14)* presents an all-in-one option for quick lip and cheek color, but the creamy texture and slightly moist finish of this product mean it will fare best as a faint wash of color on the lips. Due to the inclusion of the irritants peppermint and cinnamon (along with fragrant components such as eugenol), this product is not recommended for cheeks or lips.

EYESHADOW: ☺ **Petal Essence Single Eye Color** *($11; various compacts sold separately)* retains its silky texture and smooth, flake-free application (quite a feat considering every shade has some amount of shine). The range of colors has been reduced, likely so Aveda can launch seasonal eyeshadow colors, but most of the mainstays are workable, depending on how much shine you want. Only Vinca is too purple to work for anything other than pulling focus from what eyeshadow is meant to enhance: the eyes.

😐 **Petal Essence Eye Color Duo** *($15)* shares the same texture and smooth, even application as the Petal Essence Single Eye Color above. Each Duo has some degree of shine, with most having an obvious shimmer. The main problem is that all but one pairing is either too blue, green, purple, or contrasting to consider, unless your intent with eyeshadow is to color (rather than shape and shade) the lid and underbrow area. Gobi Sand/Haze is the least shiny and most workable Duo. 😐 **$$$ Petal Essence Triple Accent** *($18)* is a dual-sided pencil meant for use on eyes, cheeks, and lips. One side is more pigmented and works for creamy cheek or lip color, while the opposite side works best as a shimmery highlighter. If you don't mind regular sharpening and like the shade pairings, this is an option, but not one that's easy to blend or long-lasting.

☹ **Uruku Eye Accent** *($14)* has a creamy, slick texture that glides over the eye area but doesn't set, so it remains movable and will definitely crease. There is no reason to put up with these drawbacks when companies such as Benefit and Revlon offer superior cream eyeshadows that have a powder finish to enhance wear. In case you're wondering, uruku is a natural reddish-orange pigment derived from the urukum palm tree, and although Aveda plays up its presence as a natural colorant in this product, other unnatural cosmetic pigments are used as well, such as manganese violet, which is derived from an inorganic source.

EYE AND BROW SHAPER: 😐 **Petal Essence Eye Definer** *($12)* is nothing special, just a nice selection of standard, needs-sharpening pencils with an appropriate dry finish that is minimally prone to smudging. Avoid Moss (green) and Indigo (blue). 😐 **Uruku Eye-Lip Color Liner** *($12)* is a standard pencil with three colors that work much better for lips than eyes. The uruku pigment lends an orange cast that just isn't that attractive for eye lining.

LIPSTICK, LIP GLOSS, AND LIPLINER: ✓☺ **Lip Tint SPF 15** *($11)*, in contrast to many of Aveda's lip products, is free of irritants and contains an in-part titanium dioxide sunscreen! The formula is wholly impressive, containing an excellent array of soothing, non-volatile plant oils, antioxidants, and ingredients that mimic the structure and function of healthy skin. Each sheer shade is wearable and contains a touch of shimmer for an attractive, slightly creamy finish.

😐 **Uruku Lip Pigment** *($14; $17 with refillable color case)* is a sheer and somewhat greasy lipstick that tends to drag over lips but does eventually settle into an agreeable creamy texture. The shades are subdued, each having a brownish undertone due to the natural pigmentation of uruku. 😐 **Lipliner** *($12)* is a standard, needs-sharpening pencil that is nicely creamy and available in mostly workable colors. Nice, but not extraordinary.

☹ **Lip Color Concentrate SPF 15** *($14; $17 with refillable color case)* wins major points for its titanium dioxide– and zinc oxide–based sunscreen and a creamy texture that feels comfortably smooth on the lips. The formula also happens to contain more antioxidants than I have ever seen in a lipstick, including cranberry and astaxanthin (a carotenoid pigment). So why the unhappy face rating? Aveda added peppermint oil to this product, and you'll feel the tingling from the moment you apply it. I wish that tingle were a positive sign, but alas, it isn't. All the antioxidants and the outstanding sunscreen (not to mention some beautiful colors) don't mean much if peppermint is there causing irritation. ☹ **Lip Color Sheer SPF 15** *($14; $17 with refillable color case)* is nearly identical to the Lip Color Concentrate above, except this is a collection of softer colors. The peppermint used for fragrance and flavor (you'll feel the minty tingle upon application) is what keeps this from earning a happy face rating.

☹ **Lip Glaze** *($15)* is a standard tube-type lip gloss with a moderately thick texture and a slightly sticky feel on the lips. Although the shades are gorgeous, this product contains peppermint and ginger oils, which combine to produce a warm, tingling sensation that you should read as a signal that your lips are being seriously irritated. There are so many other excellent choices for lip gloss that share the same positive traits as this one but don't assault your lips with irritants. ☹ **Lip Shine** *($13.50)* is a tube-type lip gloss with a light, slick texture. It leaves a smooth, glossy sheen and offers some great colors, but the inclusion of peppermint, anise, cinnamon, and basil oils add up to lip irritation, which dims this gloss's otherwise polished prospects. ☹ **Lip Replenishment** *($14)* is just a colorless lip balm in lipstick packaging. It feels very greasy and, although the emollients included will definitely make dry, chapped lips feel better, the peppermint tends to make chapped lips worse due to its irritating properties.

MASCARA: ☺ **Mascara Plus Rose** *($12)* produces copious length and decent thickness without clumping or smearing. It still goes on wetter than most mascaras, but if you're careful not to blink too much this is definitely worth considering as an all-purpose mascara.

😐 **Mosscara** *($14)* claims its conditioning formula is helped by the inclusion of Iceland moss, yet there is not enough moss in it to cover a twig, let alone condition lashes. This is an ordinary mascara formula that produces average length and minimal thickness, but it's hardly exciting or worth considering over the best Maybelline or L'Oreal mascaras.

✓ ☺ **BRUSHES:** Aveda has redone all of its brushes and each is now made with unbelievably soft and functional synthetic hair. Ever the environmentally conscious company, Aveda has provided brush handles that are composed of recycled wood and flax. I found the handles to be a bit awkward due to their squared edges, but that's a minor quibble for an overall superior brush collection. In the **Flax Sticks** collection *($11–$32.50)*, the best brushes include the **#5 Eye Smudger** *($13)*, **#6 Eye Contour Brush** *($17)*, **#8 Complexion Brush** *($20)* (which is best for eyeshadow application), and **#9 Blush Brush** *($28)*. The only misstep is the **#7 Brow and Lash Brush** *($16)*. This dual-sided brush features a brow shaper that is not firm enough for controlled color application, while the Lash Brush is too scratchy.

FACE AND BODY ILLUMINATING/SHIMMER PRODUCTS: ☺ **$$$ Petal Essence Face Accents** *($17)* combine three stripes of shimmer powder in one pressed-powder pan. The various color combinations are all workable whether applied separately or blended together, and each goes on sheer, imparting more shimmer than pigment. This product is remarkably similar to Bobbi Brown's Shimmer Brick Compact ($35), which is also a Lauder-owned company, but Brown's costs twice as much.

SPECIALTY PRODUCTS: ☺ **Eco-Brush Pouch** *($18)* is composed of 100% cotton and has space to hold every Aveda brush (or brushes from another company, depending on your preferences). It's functional but somewhat bulky once closed, which makes it less convenient for travel. However, it's fine for at-home brush storage. ☺ The **Eco Overnight Pack** *($23)* is a sensibly designed travel bag with space for skin care, makeup, and brushes. No bigger than most standard makeup bags, it allows you to pack the essentials and then some, and includes a detachable bag for smaller items. Well done!

☺ **Essentials Environmental Compact** *($18)* is a sleek metal compact that can hold two Aveda eyeshadows and one powder blush, or it can house a single pressed powder or powder foundation. The hinge element extends out a bit and can house an Aveda lipstick, making this a clever, portable way to carry your (Aveda) makeup.

☺ **$$$ Professional Environmental Compact** *($25)* is a large compact that can house up to 16 Aveda eyeshadows or numerous, other combinations of any Aveda makeup product sold in a pan. It's best for someone who uses several colors or who routinely alternates between various blush and eyeshadow combinations.

☺ **Total Face Environmental Compact** *($14)* is a happy medium between the smaller and larger Environmental Compacts above. This midsize option houses just the essentials: powder, blush, and eyeshadow. If you're sold on Aveda makeup and like the idea of customizing a palette, this is recommended.

AVEENO (SKIN CARE ONLY)

AVEENO AT-A-GLANCE

Strengths: Very good range of sunscreens that include avobenzone for UVA protection, and one outstanding sunscreen with retinol.

Weaknesses: Well-intentioned but ineffective anti-acne products; reliance on a single showcased ingredient (typically soy) that makes their anti-aging products less enticing than the competition; no products to address hyperpigmentation; and no toners.

For more information about Aveeno, call (866) 428-3366 or visit www.aveeno.com or www.Beautypedia.com. Aveeno is owned by Johnson & Johnson.

AVEENO CLEAR COMPLEXION PRODUCTS

😐 **Clear Complexion Cleansing Bar** *($3.39 for 3.5 ounces)* contains 1% BHA in a soap-free bar cleanser, but the pH is too high for the BHA to be effective as an exfoliant and it would be rinsed down the drain before it could have an effect on skin anyway. Bar cleansers can be drying, though this one is gentler than most; it could work for someone with normal to oily skin who doesn't have blemish-prone skin.

☹ **Clear Complexion Cream Cleanser** *($6.49 for 5 ounces)* is medicated with 2% salicylic acid, but it will be rinsed down the drain before it can penetrate pores and help with blemishes. There is a lot of fragrance in this cleanser, and it contains the irritating menthol derivative menthyl lactate, making it not recommended.

☹ **Clear Complexion Daily Cleansing Pads** *($6.99 for 28 pads)* contain a mere 0.5% salicylic acid (BHA), which isn't enough to combat blemishes or stubborn blackheads, plus the pH of the solution is too high for the BHA to exfoliate. These pads are best for cleansing oily to very oily skin because of their detergent cleansing agent, sodium C14-16 olefin sulfonate, which is more drying than most and generally should be avoided. Although it's present here with milder detergent cleansing agents, it is still too potentially drying for most skin types.

😐 **Clear Complexion Foaming Cleanser** *($6.99 for 6 ounces)* is a standard, detergent-based, water-soluble cleanser that contains 0.5% salicylic acid. Such a small amount of salicylic acid (BHA) is only somewhat effective against breakouts, though even if it could have an effect, it would be rinsed down the drain before it had a chance to do anything. This cleanser contains enough of the drying cleansing agent sodium C14-16 olefin sulfonate to make it a problem for almost all skin types. It also contains fragrance.

☹ **Clear Complexion Astringent** *($6.99 for 6.7 ounces)* lists sd-alcohol as the second ingredient, which makes this otherwise gentle toner an affront to anyone concerned with not irritating their skin. The 0.5% concentration of salicylic acid is too low to effectively exfoliate although the pH is in the correct range. Nothing about this toner will "help prevent breakouts," but it will likely make the redness and inflammation that accompanies them worse.

😐 **Clear Complexion Daily Moisturizer** *($13.99 for 4 ounces)* has enough enticing claims to fulfill the wish list of anyone suffering from bouts of dryness and breakouts. However, this 0.5% BHA lotion shortchanges blemish-prone skin with too little salicylic acid despite an effective pH of 3.7. That's discouraging, and things don't perk up since this is also an extremely ordinary lightweight moisturizer with nary an antioxidant or state-of-the-art water-binding agent to be found. This fragranced product won't do a thing to keep skin clear or help with blemishes you may already have.

☺ **Clear Complexion Correcting Treatment** *($13.99 for 1 ounce)* is a 1% salicylic acid (BHA) treatment, but it has a pH of 5, which means it is less effective than it could be for exfoliating skin or dislodging stubborn blackheads. Its only redeeming quality is the inclusion of retinol, backed up by opaque, airless packaging that will keep it stable. As a retinol product for normal to slightly oily or slightly dry skin, this is recommended.

AVEENO POSITIVELY AGELESS PRODUCTS

☺ **Positively Ageless Daily Exfoliating Cleanser** *($8.99 for 5 ounces)* is a standard, detergent-based cleanser that also contains polyethylene (plastic beads) for a topical scrub action. That's about all there is to this product, and it's an option for all but very dry skin—as long you don't expect to look ageless after using it.

☺ **Positively Ageless Daily Moisturizer SPF 30** *($19.99 for 2.5 ounces)* is a well-formulated daily moisturizer whose sunscreen features avobenzone. It is difficult to assess the relative quantities of the interesting ingredients in this sunscreen because Aveeno chose to list the inactive ingredients alphabetically. This is permitted by the FDA for over-the-counter drug products, but isn't as helpful for the consumer as listing ingredients in descending order would be. The mushroom extracts in this product won't take the years off, but, assuming they're present in sufficient quantities, they can have an anti-inflammatory effect.

😐 **Positively Ageless Eye Serum** *($17.99 for 0.5 ounce)* is a very basic, boring lightweight serum for slightly dry skin anywhere on the face. All of the intriguing ingredients add up to less than a dusting, making this pale in comparison to the superior serums from Olay and Aveeno's sister brand Neutrogena.

😐 **Positively Ageless Night Cream** *($19.99 for 1.7 ounces)* makes the tired claim of going beyond being "just" a moisturizer to visibly reduce the signs of aging. It's a basic but effective moisturizer suitable for normal to slightly dry skin, and Aveeno is banking on the mushroom extracts to produce ageless results. Both species used, reishi (*Ganoderma lucidum*) and *Lentinula edodes*, better known as shiitake, have research concerning their benefits when consumed as food, but there is no research showing them to be effective when used topically on skin (Source: *Natural Medicines Comprehensive Database*, www.naturaldatabase.com). Both mushrooms have antioxidant properties (Source: *Journal of Agricultural and Food Chemistry*, October 2002, pages 6072–6077), but that benefit will be short-lived because of this product's jar packaging.

😐 **Positively Ageless Rejuvenating Serum** *($19.99 for 1.7 ounces)* cannot self-adjust to an individual's skin and does not contain ingredients that stimulate exfoliation (Aveeno uses the term "cell renewal"). This is a water- and silicone-based serum that contains a tiny amount of water-binding agent and thickener along with mushroom extracts and the mold *Mucor miehei*. This mold is said to have enzymatic action that causes exfoliation, but there is absolutely no research to support the claim. At best, expect this serum to make skin feel silky and regain its softness. It isn't worth choosing over the similarly priced serums from Olay and Neutrogena, which both offer better formulations with bells and whistles that have an established track record as being good for skin.

AVEENO POSITIVELY RADIANT PRODUCTS

☺ **Positively Radiant Cleanser** *($6.99 for 6.7 ounces)* is a very good, water-soluble cleanser for all skin types except very dry. The soy sterol and soy protein look good on the label, and they do have water-binding properties, but their benefit is negligible in a product that is quickly rinsed from skin.

😐 **Positively Radiant Cleansing Bar** *($3.29 for 3.5 ounces)* is a soap-free bar cleanser that is an OK option for someone with normal to dry skin. It does contain fragrance.

😐 **Positively Radiant Daily Cleansing Pads** *($6.99 for 28 pads)* are a convenient way to cleanse skin gently. Aveeno boasts about the soy in these dual-textured pads, but there isn't enough of it to amount to a single bean. The water-based formula is composed of mild detergent cleansing agents. However, the cleansing agents' mildness means they won't do a thorough job of dissolving makeup and removing excess surface oil. Unlike several other cleansing cloths/wipes, this product does need to be rinsed. Left on the skin, it leaves a slightly sticky finish, and the strong fragrance from these pads isn't what you'd want to leave on your skin all day or night. The textured side of the pads allows for exfoliation during cleansing, and I am pleased to report this aspect of the pads is also gentle and fairly nonabrasive. These pads are best for someone with normal to dry skin who does not wear much makeup, or who is prepared to use these pads with a separate makeup remover.

☹ **Positively Radiant Anti-Wrinkle Cream** *($13.99 for 1.7 ounces)* is a product whose magazine ads proclaimed, "Wake up and see fewer wrinkles," a promise many consumers would love to come true. The reality is that this relatively standard moisturizer is only capable of (temporarily) reducing the appearance of wrinkles, and that's about all you can expect from any moisturizer making antiwrinkle claims. Aveeno is convinced that their "Soy Vitamin Complex" is chiefly responsible for this product's alleged age-diminishing ability. I keep searching for substantiated, independent research pertaining to soy (specifically, soybean seed extract) as an effective topical agent for warding off the signs of aging, but it still doesn't exist. What we do know is that soybean seed extract, which is prominent in this product, is a good antioxidant and anti-inflammatory agent for skin. That's positive, but it's also true of myriad ingredients in skin-care products, and in this one it just won't significantly get rid of wrinkles. This moisturizer would be a much better formulation had Aveeno not stuck with soy as the center-stage antioxidant, because the meager amount of vitamin E it also contains is not of any consequence for skin. Moreover, their choice of jar packaging renders both ineffective, making this a nearly do-nothing moisturizer not worth considering over many others.

😐 **Positively Radiant Daily Moisturizer** *($13.99 for 4 ounces)* carries the claim that it is clinically proven to even-out skin tone, though the results of this study aren't available and an even skin tone often comes down to subjective assessment, which isn't saying much. Besides, it would also be nice to know what this product was being compared to in the clinical test, and whether or not skin was irritated before the product was applied. Regardless of the relatively meaningless statement "clinically proven," this is another one-note moisturizer whose only noteworthy ingredient is soy extract. As mentioned, soy has antioxidant and anti-inflammatory benefits for skin, but it would be better if Aveeno's products included more than soy because it is not the be-all and end-all antioxidant. The mica and titanium dioxide add a soft shine to skin (for radiance) and this lotion is best for normal to slightly dry or slightly oily skin. This is only recommended for daytime use if your foundation contains UVA-protecting ingredients and is rated SPF 15 or greater.

😐 **Positively Radiant Daily Moisturizer SPF 15** *($14.99 for 4 ounces)* shares the same claims and general formulary traits as the Positively Radiant Daily Moisturizer above, except this one is preferred for daytime because of its in-part avobenzone sunscreen.

😐 **Positively Radiant Daily Moisturizer SPF 30** *($14.99 for 2.5 ounces)* has a lighter-weight, drier-finish formula than either of the Positively Radiant Daily Moisturizers above, as well as offering longer sun protection, still with an in-part avobenzone sunscreen. It's an OK option for normal to slightly oily skin, assuming you don't mind the soft shine it leaves on skin.

☺ **Positively Radiant Eye Brightening Cream** *($13.99 for 0.5 ounce)* is one of the best products Aveeno offers, though not because it reduces dark circles and puffiness around the eyes, as claimed. Praise is warranted because of its excellent combination of silicones, glycerin, emollients, soy-based antioxidants, vitamins, and skin-identical ingredients, all in packaging that keeps the vulnerable ingredients stable during use. The mineral pigments in this cream produce a slightly reflective (what Aveeno refers to as "brightening") effect on skin, which can cosmetically blur dark circles—but the effect is gone if you stop using the product. This works best when paired with a good concealer.

☺ **Positively Radiant Triple Boosting Serum** *($13.99 for 1.7 ounces)* has a texture that is more like a lotion than a serum, but the prominence of silicones lends it a silky-smooth finish. Aveeno claims that this product has their highest concentration of Total Soy Complex, listed as soybean seed extract. They maintain soy will even skin tone, diminish discolorations, and shield skin against further wrinkles. It would be great if soybean extract could accomplish all of that, but it isn't possible. The good news is that research has shown that soy and its components, when taken orally in supplement form (particularly the antioxidants genistein and other isoflavones), have protective properties, such as shielding skin from UV light–induced damage and reducing inflammation (Sources: *Carcinogenesis*, March 7, 2006; and *Archiv der Pharmazie*, December 2005, pages 598–601). In addition, limited in vitro and in vivo studies have shown that topically applied soybean seed extract increases collagen and hyaluronic acid synthesis in aging skin (Sources: *Photochemistry and Photobiology*, May–June 2005, pages 581–587; and *Journal of Cosmetic Science*, September–October 2004, pages 473–479), but that is true of lots of antioxidants, not just soy. Plus, none of that means soy will forestall wrinkles; you'll still need to wear an effective sunscreen every day and practice smart sun behavior, eat lots of antioxidants, and use skin-care products that are loaded with lots of antioxidants. This product would have been rated higher if Aveeno had included additional antioxidants and perhaps a cell-communicating ingredient or two. As is, it's an option if you're curious to see what soy does for your skin all on its own, but that makes it a one-note product. Ultimately your skin deserves and can reap greater benefit from a variety of beneficial substances. This product does contain fragrance.

☺ **Positively Radiant Lip Enhancer** *($6.99 for 0.12 ounce)* is accompanied by claims that make it sound like more than just a standard lip balm, but that's exactly what it is. Consisting of mostly castor oil, thickeners, and waxes, Positively Radiant Lip Enhancer contains nothing that can enhance the shape and contour of lips, nor can it restore plumpness. On the plus side it can be somewhat moisturizing, and it does not contain irritating ingredients such as menthol or peppermint as so many other lip balms do. It is also fragrance- and preservative-free.

AVEENO ULTRA-CALMING PRODUCTS

😐 **Ultra-Calming Foaming Cleanser** *($6.99 for 6 ounces)* uses feverfew extract, which Aveeno maintains will reduce facial redness and calm skin. However, according to published research, feverfew is a problem for skin because it causes contact dermatitis (Sources: www.naturaldatabase.com; *Medicinski Pregled*, January–February 2003, pages 43–49; and *Contact Dermatitis*, October 2001, pages 197–204). Feverfew is a plant producing pollen and also a must to avoid if you suffer from pollen-related allergies (Source: *Journal of the British Society for Allergy and Clinical Immunology*, January 1991, pages 55–62). This cleanser contains only a tiny amount of feverfew extract and so poses less of a problem, especially because it isn't left on the skin. With a gentle base and an array of skin-identical ingredients (though these are not particularly helpful for skin in a cleanser), this is a good option for normal to slightly dry skin. When complete makeup removal is an issue, a stronger cleanser would be needed. This cleanser is fragrance-free.

☹ **Ultra-Calming Moisturizing Cream** *($14.99 for 1.7 ounces)* contains a significant amount of feverfew extract, which is irritating, not calming, to skin. In addition, it is an exceedingly basic formula that lacks significant amounts of state-of-the-art ingredients.

😐 **Ultra-Calming Daily Moisturizer SPF 15** *($14.99 for 4 ounces)* is recommended for its in-part avobenzone sunscreen, though I wouldn't call that or the other active ingredients in this moisturizer "ultra-calming." Many people tolerate the sunscreen agents in this product well, but a product positioned as "calming" would be better with just titanium dioxide and/or zinc oxide for sun protection. These mineral sunscreens have almost zero risk of causing irritation, which is what someone dealing with facial redness or rosacea should be considering. Because this sunscreen's base formula is listed in alphabetical order (which is within FDA regulations because it is an over-the-counter drug, not a cosmetic), the relative amounts of the different ingredients are not as clear as when ingredients are listed in descending order. However, it does contain fragrance—another faux pas for an "ultra-calming" product—and lacks antioxidants. If calming isn't your expectation, this sunscreen is an option, just not an exciting one.

OTHER AVEENO PRODUCTS

😐 **Balancing Bar for Combination Skin** *($2.99 for 3.5 ounces)* is a non-soap, fragrance-free bar cleanser that is an OK option for combination skin, assuming blemishes and blackheads aren't a concern, because the ingredients that keep bar cleansers in their bar form can clog pores. The oat-flour base does convey a soothing benefit to skin.

😐 **Moisturizing Bar** *($3.39 for 3.5 ounces)* is a richer version of the Balancing Bar for Combination Skin, above, and although it is decent for normal to dry skin it is not preferred to a moisturizing, water-soluble cleanser.

☺ **Skin Brightening Daily Scrub** *($6.99 for 5 ounces)* doesn't entice with lots of needless frills. Instead, this standard, effective scrub goes about its business of allowing you to polish your skin while also providing a cleansing action. It is suitable for all skin types except very dry.

😐 **Positively Smooth Facial Moisturizer** *($13.99 for 4 ounces)* should, based on its claims, be renamed "Positively Does Everything Moisturizer"! Aveeno maintains that this positively standard facial moisturizer not only reduces the appearance of unwanted hair, but also improves skin tone, texture, and clarity, and visibly reduces fine lines. The ingredients these claims are hinged on are soybean seed extract and soy protein. Other than its antioxidant and anti-inflammatory properties, all other traits attributed to topical application of soy are questionable. There's nary a single published, substantiated study to support the notion that soy extract can minimize the appearance of unwanted hair—and it certainly does not have bleaching effects. Soy has volumes of published research on its effects when taken internally (or consumed in the diet), but reliable information to support soy's hair-minimizing properties is nonexistent. Beyond the soy, this is a mundane formulation that lacks other interesting antioxidants and skin-identical ingredients. It's basically water, thickeners, silicone, soy, glycerin, film-forming agents, and preservatives.

✓☺ **Skin Brightening Daily Treatment SPF 15** *($19 for 1 ounce)* remains a sleeper product from Aveeno, so don't overlook it because it's not part of one of their larger categories of products. This in-part avobenzone sunscreen comes in a lightweight moisturizing base that includes several antioxidants (more than any other Aveeno product), along with the cell-communicating ingredient retinol. It is an ideal sunscreen/daily moisturizer/treatment product for normal to slightly dry skin and the packaging will keep the light- and air-sensitive ingredients stable.

☹ **Intense Relief Medicated Therapy** *($3.49 for 0.15 ounce stick or 0.25 ounce pot)* comes in two formulas: The stick version uses 1% menthol as one of the active ingredients; the balm portion contains 1% camphor. Both serve their purpose as counter-irritants. What that means is the menthol and camphor in these products cause greater irritation on their own than the irritation or itching you may be feeling on your lips or skin. That's not healthy for skin, and this product is not recommended.

😐 **Continuous Radiance Moisturizing Lotion, for All Skin Tones** *($13.99 for 7.5 ounces)* is a moisturizer for body or face that contains the self-tanning ingredient dihydroxyacetone. The point of difference here is the dial-type dispensing system, which allows you to control how much self-tanning ingredient is dispensed into the lotion (half the product is self-tanner, the other half an ordinary lotion moisturizer). So you can control the amount of self-tanner that gets mixed into the lotion. It's a clever concept, but has its pros and cons. If you want a faster, darker tan, you would use this product up pretty quickly and be left with just the lotion portion, which has no special benefit. For subtle differences in lighter shades this is an option. The key point is that all self-tanners, regardless of how they are dispensed (lotion, gel, spray, mousse, and others) are more about application technique than anything else.

😐 **Continuous Radiance Moisturizing Lotion** *($8.69 for 8 ounces)* is nearly identical to the Continuous Radiance Moisturizing Lotion, for All Skin Tones, above, except without the separate dial-dispensing mechanism. Aveeno has an option for fair or medium skin tones, both with the same basic formula but with differing amounts of the self-tanning ingredient dihydroxyacetone. For facial use, this is best for normal to slightly dry skin.

AVEENO SUN PRODUCTS

☺ **Continuous Protection Sunblock Lotion SPF 30** *($9.99 for 4 ounces)* is an effective sunscreen. The standard base formula is suitable for normal to dry skin, and avobenzone is on hand to provide UVA protection. Just don't take the "continuous protection" part of the name seriously. Although an SPF 30 product provides longer protection than an SPF 15 product, you still need to reapply this after swimming, perspiring, or exercising if you want to maintain protection or plan for a full day out in the sun. Aveeno knows this or they wouldn't mention that this product maintains its SPF rating for only 40 minutes in water. After that you should reapply it rather than rely on the misleading name that implies longer protection than competing sunscreens rated at SPF 30.

☺ **Continuous Protection Sunblock Lotion SPF 30, for Face** *($9.99 for 3 ounces)* is similar to the Continuous Protection Sunblock Lotion SPF 30 above. Although it does have a few more bells and whistles than the "body" version, it doesn't contain any ingredients that make it better suited for use on the face. Many manufacturers of facial sunscreens today are responding to current research that indicates a complementary and positive effect when antioxidants are included in sunscreens. That includes Aveeno, because this product features vitamins A and E as well as soybean seed extract. As for the "continuous protection" claim in the name, the same comments above apply here, too.

☺ **Continuous Protection Sunblock Lotion SPF 45** *($9.99 for 4 ounces)* is nearly identical to the Continuous Protection Sunblock Lotion SPF 30 above, and the same review applies. The only difference of note is the slightly higher amount of active ingredients required to net an SPF 45 rating. If you're wearing this under the assumption that you'll get all-day protection, think again. For a full day in the sun, this will need to be reapplied regularly, especially after swimming or if you're perspiring.

☺ **Continuous Protection Sunblock Lotion SPF 55** *($9.99 for 3 ounces)* is similar to the Continuous Protection Sunblock Lotion SPF 30 above, except this product contains a higher amount of active ingredients necessary to achieve its SPF rating. An SPF 55 product won't be needed for most people because there simply aren't enough daylight hours to warrant it. Plus, the greater amount of active ingredients needed to reach such an SPF rating increases the chance of causing skin sensitivity and irritation. Still, this deserves credit for providing excellent broad-spectrum protection, and it includes antioxidants.

☺ **Continuous Protection Sunblock Lotion SPF 55, for Baby** *($9.99 for 4 ounces)* distinguishes itself from the Continuous Protection Sunblock Lotion SPF 55 above, in name and with the inclusion of anti-irritant oat flour. A sunscreen with this many active ingredients is ill-advised for babies, whose skin is not developed enough to tolerate them. Babies under six months of age should be shielded from sunlight rather than treated with sunscreens of any kind; beyond six months, the best sunscreen actives for a baby's skin are titanium dioxide and/or zinc oxide (Source: www.cancercare.ns.ca/media/documents/sunexposurebrochurefinal.pdf). This is worth considering by adults.

☹ **Continuous Protection Sunblock Spray SPF 30** *($9.99 for 4 ounces)* includes avobenzone for sufficient UVA protection as well as the antioxidant vitamin A and soy extract. Despite those positives, the alcohol content of this spray-on sunscreen, coupled with the high percentage of active ingredients, makes it too irritating for all skin types.

☹ **Continuous Protection Sunblock Spray SPF 45** *($9.99 for 5 ounces)* is nearly identical to the Continuous Protection Sunblock Spray SPF 30 above, save for the greater amount of active ingredient needed to achieve a higher SPF rating. Otherwise, the same review applies.

☹ **Essential Moisture Lip Conditioner SPF 15** *($3.39 for 0.15 ounce)* does not contain the UVA-protecting ingredients of titanium dioxide, zinc oxide, avobenzone, Tinosorb, or Mexoryl SX. Aveeno clearly recognizes the importance of UVA protection or they wouldn't be using avobenzone in their Continuous Protection sunscreens above.

AVITA (SEE RETINOIDS)

AVON

AVON AT-A-GLANCE

Strengths: Consistent UVA protection from almost all of the products with sunscreen; a few state-of-the-art moisturizers (some with sunscreen) at near-bargain prices; some good lip-protecting options; Avon Solutions cleansers; a couple of extraordinary foundations with sunscreen; a selection of formidable concealers, powders, blushes, and lipsticks; the company provides complete ingredient lists on its Web site and offers some of the most helpful Customer Service associates in the industry; deep discounts on makeup products are the rule rather than the exception.

Weaknesses: The Clearskin and True Pore-Fection products are mostly irritating and poor choices for anyone battling blemishes; the Anew Clinical lineup won't make you cancel that upcoming appointment for whatever cosmetic corrective procedure you've booked; an over-reliance on jar packaging diminishes the antioxidants found in many Avon moisturizers; the marriage of insect repellant with sunscreen is an imperfect union; endless, unnecessarily repetitive moisturizers with exaggerated, outlandish claims; several of the foundations look decidedly unnatural or have SPF ratings that are too low; average eyeshadows and pencils; mostly average to disappointing mascaras.

For more information about Avon, call (800) 500-AVON or visit www.avon.com or www.Beautypedia.com.

AVON SKIN CARE

AVON ANEW SKIN CARE

☺ **Anew Ultra Cream Cleanser** *($12 for 5.1 ounces)* is a good detergent cleansing agent– and soap-free, lotion-style cleanser for normal to dry skin. It contains mostly water, thickeners, emollients, skin-identical ingredients, film-forming agent, preservatives, and fragrance. It removes makeup but will leave a residue unless used with a washcloth.

😐 **Anew Clarifying Essence** *($12 for 5.1 ounces)* is a very basic toner consisting primarily of water, glycerin, and preservative. It's a functional option for normal skin, but countless toners deliver greater benefits than this limited formula.

😐 **Anew Advanced All-in-One Max SPF 15 Cream** *($16.50 for 1.7 ounces)* is an intriguing way to combine broad-spectrum sunscreen (including avobenzone for UVA protection) along with approximately 2% glycolic acid and the AHA ammonium glycolate. That amount is barely enough for sufficient exfoliation, though the product's pH is low enough for some to occur. The product is also loaded with antioxidants and contains retinol, but the jar packaging means they will be ineffective shortly after the product is opened. This is worth a look if you're curious to try a low-level AHA with sunscreen, and the formula is best for normal to slightly dry skin.

✓ ☺ **Anew Advanced All-in-One Max SPF 15 Lotion** *($16.50 for 1.7 ounces)* is similar to the Anew Advanced All-in-One Max SPF 15 Cream above, except for two important differences: packaging that keeps the retinol and antioxidants stable, and larger amounts of glycolic acid and ammonium glycolate. It is an excellent daytime moisturizer for normal to slightly oily skin. The inclusion of enzymes is interesting, but the exfoliation and smoothing benefits this product provides are from the AHAs; the enzymes are too unstable to function in that capacity.

😐 **$$$ Anew Alternative Intensive Age Treatment** *($32 for 1.7 ounces)* was heavily advertised in magazines and on television as a revolutionary new way to undo the signs of aging. Avon's use of words such as "herbaceutical" and phrases like "let the healing age begin" inspired much curiosity, but, as is often the case in the cosmetics industry, the ad slogans and hype don't equal fact. What Avon has produced is a good AHA product, using ammonium glycolate and glycolic acid (at a pH of 3.6) for exfoliation. The AHAs are in a decent moisturizing base of glycerin, thickeners, film-forming agent, and silicone. Plenty of antioxidants are included, but Avon's choice of a jar container means they'll be ineffective shortly after the product is opened.

One other ingredient of note in this product is 2-amino-4,5 dimethylthiazole HBR. In order to use this ingredient in their product, Avon signed a nonexclusive licensing agreement with Alteon, a biotech company. It is one of several ingredients Alteon has developed that they claim has an effect on advanced glycation end-products (AGEs). AGEs are abnormal, cross-linked, oxidized proteins that might play a role in the aging process.

Here's how AGE affects skin. Sugars, particularly in the form of glucose, are one of the primary ways the body gets its fuel for producing energy and get up and go. Yet glucose, through an enzymatic trigger, can also attach itself to proteins anywhere in the body and form "glycated" substances (advanced glycation end-products or AGEs) that damage tissue by making it stiff and inflexible. AGEs directly affect the surface layers of skin as well as structures beneath the surface such as collagen and elastin.

At this point, we don't know whether AGEs can be stopped, or even inhibited, and there is no published research pertaining to 2-amino-4,5-dimethylthiazole HBR (also known as alagebrium or ALT-711) and its effect on wrinkles or skin. The research that does exist, from Johns Hopkins University, involved 13 elderly men and women with systolic hypertension. The study participants took either daily doses of alagebrium for eight weeks or a placebo. The results showed an improvement in the stiffness of the arteries. At best, this was a small study, and whether that result relates to skin is an even bigger leap of faith. But it does at least show that Avon is making attempts to be more cutting-edge than many of its high-priced competitors.

The plant extracts in this product lend an intense fragrance that tends to linger on skin, so if you're considering purchasing this item, ask your Avon lady for a sample first! (Sources: *Journal of Investigative Dermatology*, December 2005; *Annals of the New York Academy of Science*, June 2006, pages 529–532; *Journal of Biological Chemistry*, April 2005, pages 12087–12095; and *Archives of Biochemistry and Biophysics*, November 2003, pages 89–96).

☺ **$$$ Anew Alternative Intensive Age Treatment SPF 25 Day** *($32 for 1.7 ounces)* makes much ado about the fusion of Eastern and Western technology to create a product that reactivates the skin's healing process, but the big—legitimate—news is that this is an exceptionally well-formulated daytime moisturizer with UVA protection (it contains avobenzone). Although somewhat thick, it has the feel of a lightweight lotion and a soft finish appropriate for someone with normal to slightly oily or slightly dry skin. Housed in stable packaging featuring an airless pump applicator, the formula is loaded with antioxidants, anti-irritants (including several forms of curcumin—an Avon specialty), and ingredients that mimic the structure of healthy skin. The only drawback is the pervasive fragrance. I generally don't comment on a skin-care product's specific scent (it would be best for skin if there weren't any fragrance), but this one is perfume-like to the max, and definitely something to take into consideration before you purchase this otherwise outstanding product.

☹ **Anew Alternative Intensive Eye Cream** *($25 for 0.5 ounce)* continues Avon's march into their created category of "herbaceutical" skin care. Claiming to "attack the major signs of dark circles," this won't work beyond making them look less apparent if eye-area skin is dry (something any moisturizer applied to this area will do). Although Avon included over a dozen state-of-the-art ingredients, most are rendered ineffective once this jar-packaged product is opened. Further, Avon's idea of herbaceuticals for this product included a host of irritating fragrant oils, including peppermint, geranium, frankincense, and West Indian sandalwood. Lastly, this contains a high amount of neem extract (listed as *Melia azadirachta* flower extract) from a plant whose profile is a mix of positive and negative effects, and it has no research showing it is a panacea for dark circles (Source: www.naturaldatabase.com).

😐 **Anew Force Extra Triple Lifting Day Cream SPF 15** *($22 for 1.7 ounces)* comes with claims that your face "will see a 60% improvement in fine lines and wrinkles in one week." If that happens in just a week, in two to three weeks you should be wrinkle-free, and that's not possible! Aside from the hype, this ends up being a decent moisturizer with a good SPF that includes avobenzone as one of the active ingredients. What makes this product unique, along with a few other Anew products, is Avon's trademark ingredient trioxaundecanedioic acid (also known as oxa acid). A patented ingredient, oxa acid is supposed to be effective as an exfoliant and to perform better than AHAs, without irritation. The only research supporting this notion is a very long, rambling patent held by Avon. What makes it confusing is that while one complaint about AHAs is that the low pH required to make them effective for skin can cause irritation, it seems that oxa acid, according to the patent, has the same problem: "in treating skin conditions [oxa acid] has been found to be affected by the pH of the composition… preferably in the pH range between 3.5 and 4.0." That's the same range that makes for effective use of AHAs. Nonetheless, if you wanted to give another exfoliant a try, this is one to consider, though the pH is definitely higher than the patent for this ingredient suggests. The lightweight lotion contains some good antioxidants, but the jar packaging is a problem.

😐 **Anew Force Extra Triple Lifting Night Cream** *($22 for 1.7 ounces)* won't lift anything and this isn't the best product in the Anew lineup, but it is a good basic moisturizer for normal to dry skin. It contains mostly water, silicone, thickeners, glycerin, Vaseline, more thickeners, Avon's patented oxa acid (see the preceding review for Anew Force Extra Triple Lifting Day Cream SPF 15 above), preservatives, skin-identical ingredients, antioxidant vitamins, and fragrance. The jar packaging won't help keep the antioxidants stable, so they cannot be relied on.

😐 **Anew Force Extra Eye Cream** *($16 for 0.5 ounce)* contains Avon's patented oxa acid (see the review for Anew Force Extra Triple Lifting Day Cream SPF 15 above). The pH of this product is above 4, which is borderline for accomplishing any exfoliation, based on their own research. There isn't much else of note in this product; the antioxidants would be beneficial if this product did not use jar packaging.

😐 **$$$ Anew Luminosity Ultra Advanced Skin Brightener SPF 15** *($22 for 1 ounce)* is an in-part avobenzone-based sunscreen in a decent moisturizing base that contains mostly water, thickeners, slip agent, water-resistant agent, a long list of plant extracts, antioxidants (unfortunately unstable due to the jar packaging), preservatives, and fragrance. This is a good option for someone with normal to slightly dry skin. Contrary to Avon's claims, Anew Luminosity does not contain any reliable amounts of ingredients known to inhibit melanin production or to lighten skin discolorations, other than the sunscreen itself. This does contain a tiny amount of uva-ursi leaf extract, although how much of this arbutin-containing plant is needed to produce satisfactory results, if any, is undetermined.

😐 **$$$ Anew Ultimate Day Transforming Lift Cream SPF 15** *($30 for 1.7 ounces)* includes an in-part avobenzone sunscreen and comes in a silky, moisturizing lotion base complete with some good skin-identical ingredients and a smattering of antioxidants. The antioxidants are rendered ineffective due to jar packaging, but this is still an OK daytime moisturizer for normal to slightly dry skin. As you may have guessed, its lifting ability is pure fantasy.

😐 **$$$ Anew Ultimate Transforming Lift Eye Cream** *($22 for 0.5 ounce)* is advertised as ultra-firming and "behaves like an invisible net that tightens, tones, and uplifts the look of skin." Yet if this is to be believed, then this same assertion would apply to just about every standard moisturizer on the market. There are some unique ingredients in this product (which I'll get to in a moment), but none of them are ultra-firming. Further, without sunscreen, any effect of an anti-aging ingredient would be defeated, sort of like Superman's response to kryptonite.

This product contains mostly water, glycerin, thickener, silicone, film-forming agent, emollients, several more thickeners, plant extracts, antioxidants, plant oils, preservatives, and mineral pigments (for shine). Among the unique ingredients are salmon egg extract (which has no special benefit for skin), xymenynic acid (a water-binding agent), *Punica granatum* extract (from pomegranate, a potent antioxidant, though Avon's choice of jar packaging quickly diminishes its potency once the product is opened), and zeolite (a mineral shown to have anti-cancer properties, but with no known research for topical application). This also contains a tiny amount of retinol, but with the translucent jar packaging, it won't remain stable. All told, this is a good moisturizer for normal to dry skin around the eyes or anywhere on the face, but it will not create lasting firmness, eliminate wrinkles, or reduce puffiness.

Avon Anew Clinical Products

This subcategory is Avon's self-proclaimed "innovative line of cosmetic, dermatological treatments that plump, resurface and firm skin with clinical precision." Reading the descriptions for these products, you wonder how any dermatologist offering cosmetic corrective procedures is staying in business. The reality is they are not only staying in business but they (and plastic surgeons) are thriving, because products such as these cannot replace what is possible with in-office treatments, be they Botox, lasers, or facial peels.

☹ **$$$ Anew Clinical Micro-Exfoliant** *($20 for 2.5 ounces)* is meant to take the place of in-office microdermabrasion treatments. Kits like this sprang onto the market between 2005 and 2006. They are marketed as being as effective as the microdermabrasion treatments performed at doctors' offices and by aestheticians. However published research has questioned the efficacy of microdermabrasion. A review of these treatments in the June 2006 issue of *Dermatological Surgery* (pages 809–814) stated that "Most of the literature based on subjective and patient-dependent assessment parameters [of microdermabrasion] points toward a marginal improvement in skin appearance following repeated procedures."

Another study, in *Dermatological Surgery*, March 2006, pages 376–379, showed that after three and four treatments "the ceramide level returned to baseline and then decreased." The researchers concluded that repeated treatments could have diminishing results. So it turns out that if the At-Home Kits really can work like professional microdermabrasion, it means they have problems that can be a problem for skin.

☹ **$$$ Anew Clinical Advanced Retexturizing Peel** *($25 for 30 pads)* used to be sold as a part of a two-step system involving glycolic acid-steeped disposable pads followed by neutralizing pads (formulated at a higher pH to stop the exfoliating action of the AHA). Clearly consumers didn't like the two steps or Avon wouldn't have changed it. Besides, the neutralizing step was a waste of time anyway, since just splashing skin with tap water will stop the acidic action of chemical exfoliants. These pads are supposed to be akin to a 35% AHA peel, but don't count on it. The water-based pads contain about 10% ammonium glycolate with glycolic acid, at a pH of 4, so exfoliation will occur. However, alcohol is the fourth ingredient listed, and that increases the potential for irritation. Although effective (just not to the extent of a physician-administered AHA peel), there are better, less-expensive AHA products available.

☹ **$$$ Anew Clinical Deep Crease Concentrate with Bo-Hylurox** *($32 for 1 ounce)* debuted with a name not only reminiscent of Botox, but also with claims that are intended to make you wonder why anyone would subject themselves to an injection when they can achieve the same (or at least similar) results with this water-based serum. Sold with the scare-tactic tag line "Look stunning, not stunned," Avon's alternative claims to "reduce the overall length, depth and number of deep expression lines around your eyes, mouth and forehead, the areas that are in motion whenever you show emotion." Well, when done correctly, Botox injections absolutely do not make a person look stunned—the list of Hollywood celebrities who have had them is what's really stunning, and they don't look "stunned"! In fact, unlike genuine Botox injections, this product absolutely cannot get rid of wrinkles, at least not better than any other well-formulated moisturizer.

The results from Botox are so impressive it's no wonder it has become the most commonly performed cosmetic procedure, and why so many cosmetics companies are launching "works like Botox" products. In 2005, more than 3.8 million Botox treatments were administered, making it the number-one nonsurgical cosmetic corrective procedure (Source: www.plasticsurgery.org). The statistics for Botox injections are increasing year-to-year, which has to make you wonder if any of the numerous creams claiming to mimic the effect of this procedure work at all. My answer is, basically they don't.

Anew Clinical Deep Crease Concentrate contains two showcased ingredients supposedly responsible for the crease-filling and wrinkle-smoothing claims. The first is *Portulaca oleracea*, a plant extract. Avon maintains it "helps you lose those hard-to-treat creases while keeping your facial expressions, naturally." However, there is no substantiated or published research showing *Portulaca oleracea* has that (or any) antiwrinkle effect. Research has shown that it may have anti-inflammatory or analgesic properties, and it is also believed to be effective topically for wound healing (Sources: *Journal of Ethnopharmacology*, October 2003, pages 131–136, and December 2000, pages 445–451). But none of that is related to treating expression lines in any way, shape, or form. Numbing muscles, which is how Botox works, doesn't prevent you from using them. One study did examine portulaca's effect on brain activity and resulting muscle relaxation, but the substance was used in a 10% concentration and injected into pigs' stomachs, quite a different thing from applying lesser amounts of this ingredient to skin (Source: *Journal of Ethnopharmacology*, July 2001, pages 171–176).

The second showcased ingredient is acetyl hexapeptide-3 (trade name: argireline), an ingredient I have discussed (and warned about) before. You may recall that Centerchem, the company that manufactures argireline, is the only source of information for this ingredient's effect on skin. That automatically means their antiwrinkle claims are suspect, but it also casts doubt on their statement that argireline works by moderating substances in your body that stimulate muscle movement. If that were true, it could lead to serious biological problems. In addition, the clinical studies for argireline revealed that this ingredient was (surprise!) not as effective as Botox (Source: www.cremedevie.com/clinical_details.htm). There are still too many unknowns about acetyl hexapeptide-3's effect on biological processes, not to mention the lack of research demonstrating it to be a worthy topical successor to Botox injections.

After all this, you may be wondering just what this product can do for your skin. Like any alcohol-free, serum-type moisturizer, it will provide light hydration and make skin appear temporarily smoother and feel a bit more firm. These effects are not permanent, nor do they have an impact on muscle movement; your expression lines will still be plainly visible regardless of how often you use Anew Clinical Deep Crease Concentrate. There are some soothing and skin-identical ingredients in this product, and so it's worth considering if you have normal to oily skin and need a lightweight moisturizer.

☺ **$$$ Anew Clinical Eye Lift** *($28 for 0.66 ounce)* is a two-part product packaged in one jar, and it's made out to be nothing short of an eye-area miracle (Avon sells lots and lots of miraculous products if you believe even a portion of their outlandish claims). If you need to give your eyes a lift or get rid of puffiness, dark circles, or a loss of firmness, Avon insists you should look no further than this product, and they have impressive-looking statistics to back their assertions. However, there are no details of how they came to their conclusions or how many women were involved in their tests. ("Dermatologist-supervised" may sound official, but that doesn't mean that even one iota of their claims is true—since without the study in hand the claims are all embellishment with no substance.) The product consists of an Upper Eye Gel and an Under Eye Cream. The Gel is supposedly responsible for the lifting and tightening actions, yet it doesn't contain ingredients that have that effect. Along with water, glycerin, and slip agents are numerous plant extracts (including several antioxidants, but the jar packaging will make these air-sensitive ingredients ineffective shortly after opening), skin-identical ingredients, film-forming agents, preservatives, and coloring agent. It's a good, lightweight moisturizer with a gel texture, but sagging or drooping skin won't do an about-face.

The Cream part is marketed as being able to "accelerate cellular metabolism" and alleviate under-eye darkness and puffiness. In contrast to the Gel, the Cream has a truly emollient texture with many beneficial ingredients for skin. None of them, however, will make dark circles or puffiness things of the past, and it's a shame that the many antioxidants are stalled by the product's jar packaging, though the Cream will unquestionably make dry skin around the eyes look and feel better. In addition, as with all well-formulated moisturizers, it will temporarily reduce the appearance of wrinkles. Cosmetically, the mica and titanium dioxide in the Under Eye Cream will help reflect light, diminishing the appearance of dark circles. Again, the effect is temporary and not as convincing as camouflaging dark circles with a good, neutral-toned concealer. The Cream does not list fragrance on the label, but it does contain fragrance components, so be careful about getting it too close to the lash line.

☹ **Anew Clinical Instant Face Lift** *($28 for 1 ounce)* lists alcohol as the third ingredient, which makes this too potentially irritating for all skin types. The lifting portion comes from the amount of PVP (a film-forming agent commonly used in hairstyling gels) in this water-based serum. When it sets on skin, you may notice a tightening effect, but no actual "lifting" is taking place. This contains tiny amounts of water-binding agents and antioxidants, but the alcohol's presence and the inclusion of menthol derivative menthoxypropanediol makes this a no-go.

☺ **$$$ Anew Clinical Line and Wrinkle Corrector** *($32 for 1.7 ounces)* is a product Avon positioned as "the painless, revolutionary new alternative to collagen injections." Anew Clinical Line and Wrinkle Corrector promises that it's a "painless way to inject youth" into the skin. Avon's Derma-3X technology supposedly rebuilds elastin, recreates collagen, and regenerates the skin's hydro-proteins. (Exactly what "hydro-proteins" are they don't explain, but all that term means is "water proteins," in essence an oxymoron.)

Avon states that their Derma-3X technology involves naturally derived ingredients, consisting primarily of coconut juice, hydrolyzed wheat protein, and extracts of carrot, apple root, fennel, alfalfa, and olive root. Can any of these ingredients (regardless of how they are blended or how many patents are pending) have even a mild effect on your skin's collagen and elastin? Beyond serving as skin-identical ingredients and antioxidants, there's not much more these natural ingredients can do, nor are they any more special than the other antioxidants and skin-identical ingredients found in many other Avon moisturizers or moisturizers from hundreds of other companies.

Anew Clinical Line and Wrinkle Corrector advertising makes it sound like the benefits you'd gain by using this product are preferred to what you'd get from collagen injections. Collagen injections work by filling in wrinkles. Although collagen injections typically last four to nine months before touch-ups are necessary, the results are far more dramatic and complete than any topical cream could possibly create, including this one. Avon's statement that "collagen injections do not build or promote collagen, elastin, and hydro-protein renewal. Derma-3X Technology™ found in Anew Clinical Line and Wrinkle Corrector does" is bizarre. And especially if you know that collagen injections do not stimulate collagen production (though other dermal fillers can—something Avon forgot to mention). Even if they could, that isn't the reason people get collagen injections. Millions of dermal injections are done each year because antiwrinkle creams can't come close to reproducing the kind of results obtainable from injections.

You may be wondering just what ingredient in Anew Clinical might let it even approach the results possible from collagen injections. For an allegedly advanced moisturizer making breakthrough claims, Avon's formulation is surprisingly similar to its other Anew products. It has a water and silicone base (so it feels very silky on the skin) and contains about 4% glycolic acid with ammonium glycolate, all at a pH of 3.5, so some exfoliation will occur. Interestingly, this also contains Avon's patented oxa acid, which they position as a "cutting-edge, next generation AHA." Yet Avon's own patent for this ingredient indicates that for it to be effective it requires the same pH as other AHAs (between 3 and 4). If Avon is counting on these acids to stimulate collagen production, then the same skin-plumping claims can be attributed to all the other Anew products that also contain these ingredients. Aside from the AHAs, there is nothing in this product that can create new collagen or elastin, any more than any other well-formulated moisturizer can. Anew Clinical does contain a smattering of antioxidants, but the amounts are negligible, and the jar packaging won't keep them stable once the product is opened.

☹ **$$$ Anew Clinical ThermaFirm Face Lifting Cream** *($32 for 1 ounce)*. Let's see, Avon has skin-care products in their Anew Clinical line that claim to work like Botox, mimic the effect of laser treatments, replace the need for collagen injections or liposuction, and on and on. Keeping up with this theme of you-don't-need-to-see-a-plastic-surgeon type of products is Anew Clinical ThermaFirm Face Lifting Cream. In case the name wasn't obvious enough, this product is designed as an alternative to Thermage treatments. Thermage uses radiofrequency energy to heat skin, causing a controlled, nonablative wound that stimulates new collagen production. It is a viable option for tightening skin and smoothing the appearance of wrinkles, and the results continue to improve as more is learned about how to perform the procedure to get the best results.

Does Avon's alternative even come close to mimicking the effect of Thermage? Not in the least. This is a surprisingly lackluster formula for a cream advertised as having "potent ingredients." It consists primarily of water, slip agents, triglyceride, several thickeners, shea butter, film-forming agent, preservatives, a menthol derivative, several plant extracts, minerals, and a tiny amount of vitamin E. Avon refers to this as their "most advanced and powerful facial lifting product ever." Well, it isn't, at least not from any published research, or any research Avon is willing to part with, and not in comparison to other products Avon sells. At best, this is a decent moisturizer for someone with normal to slightly dry skin, but the menthol derivative (used in a small amount to create the impression that the product is doing something) isn't the best for any skin type.

😐 **$$$ Anew Clinical Laser System** *($32 for the set—Anew Clinical Laser 0.5 ounce; Post-Laser Protector SPF 30 1.5 ounces)* continues Avon's trend of launching products claiming to forestall the need for (or work as well as) such effective cosmetic corrective procedures as Botox or collagen injections, or surgical procedures such as liposuction. The Anew Clinical Laser System purports to "correct and protect with all the precision of a professional laser." Anyone with even a passing understanding of how lasers work would realize Avon's claims are not just exaggerated, but border on ludicrous. There are at least 200 studies documenting the use of lasers for eliminating or reducing wrinkles and skin discolorations, but there's not even one for this product. The notion that a cosmetic can mimic what lasers do is sheer fantasy.

Two different products are included here, the first being the **Anew Clinical Laser**, an alcohol-based serum packaged in a ceramic vial with a metal roller-ball-tip applicator. That may well be enough to fool some women into thinking they are actually getting something akin to a laser treatment. The second product is a lightweight sunscreen with SPF 30 that provides UVA protection via avobenzone as one of the active ingredients. It has a silky finish and is suitable for most skin types. However, for the money, it lacks significant levels of antioxidants or intriguing skin-identical ingredients.

The attention-getting part of this set, however, the Clinical Laser, is a waste of your time and money, especially if you are hoping to get any laserlike skin improvements. The first five listed ingredients are utterly ordinary; the ones that follow (including vitamin C, several plant extracts, antioxidants, and skin-identical ingredients) have some benefit for skin, but nothing approaching what a laser does. And because this product is alcohol-based, it is inherently drying and irritating for skin, somewhat canceling out any potential benefit from the antioxidants and other skin-friendly ingredients. Not a single ingredient in either product has substantiated research proving it can "zap away" signs of aging, though it is well established that using an effective sunscreen daily can prevent further skin damage. The sunscreen portion of this set is recommended, while the serum is not. Therefore, the pairing earns a neutral face rating.

😐 **$$$ Anew Clinical Plump & Smooth Lip System** *($25 for 2 ounces)* mentions fuller lips in its description but really plays up the "youthful" results this two-step system provides. Housed in a dual-sided, pen-style component, both steps provide a silicone-enhanced texture coupled with lip-smoothing emollients and some good antioxidants plus retinol. The plumping action doesn't come from those ingredients. Rather, just like most lip plumpers, this version uses irritants (peppermint oil and menthoxypropanediol) to incite fullness and increase circulation to lips, resulting in a rosier color. It's a temporary effect, but too irritating for routine use, so consider this only for special occasions (or consider going with longer-lasting, less irritating lip injections such as collagen).

AVON ANEW RETROACTIVE+ PRODUCTS

☹ **Anew Retroactive+ 2-in-1 Cleanser** *($12 for 4.2 ounces)* has merit as a water-soluble cleanser and it contains several interesting ingredients (including a cell-communicating ingredient), but their contact with skin is too brief to exert a benefit. This would be still be recommended if it did not contain the irritant menthyl lactate. Although its contact with skin is brief, it is problematic when used around the eyes—and why choose a cleanser with an irritant when there are so many good ones without that problem?

✓ ☺ **Anew Retroactive+ Day Defense SPF 15** *($25 for 1.7 ounces)* includes avobenzone for UVA protection and features an elegant, lightweight lotion texture loaded with skin-identical ingredients. The formula also includes a great selection of antioxidants, anti-irritants, and a cell-communicating ingredient. It is an excellent daytime moisturizer option for normal to slightly oily skin, and is unlikely to pose a problem for those prone to blemishes.

☹ **Anew Retroactive+ Youth Extending Cream SPF 25, Day** *($27 for 1.7 ounces)* gets a lower rating because jar packaging is this brilliant formula's undoing. It won't keep the retinol and many antioxidants stable during use, and that won't extend anyone's youth. The sunscreen element includes avobenzone, and the base formula is suitable for normal to slightly oily skin. Avon, rethink your packaging for an otherwise state-of-the-art product!

☺ **Anew Retroactive+ Repair Eye Serum** *($18 for 0.4 ounce)* contains mostly water, film-forming agent, slip agents, antioxidants, skin-identical ingredients, anti-irritant, a cell-communicating ingredient, plant oil, more film-forming agents, and preservative. It's a good lightweight serum for slightly dry skin, but the claims about what its cell-communicating ingredient is capable of go beyond what this class of ingredients is known to do for skin.

☺ **Anew Retroactive+ Skin Optimizer** *($22 for 1 ounce)* may pique interest as an alternative to AHAs, but the papaya enzymes are notoriously unstable and not preferred to the even results possible from a well-formulated AHA or BHA product. This is still worth considering as an ultra-light moisturizer for those with normal to oily skin. It contains some very good antioxidants, skin-identical ingredients, and a cell-communicating ingredient. The titanium dioxide and mica add a subtle radiant glow to skin.

☹ **Anew Retroactive+ Youth Extending Cream, Night** *($27 for 1.7 ounces)* is a very elegant formula whose silky, slightly creamy texture is tailored to those with normal to mildly dry skin. It's a shame jar packaging was chosen; it won't keep the hefty amount of retinol stable nor keep the many antioxidants in this moisturizer potent during use. That means any youth-extending benefit is incidental, though this will make dry areas look and feel better.

AVON BASICS PRODUCTS

☹ **Rich Moisture Face Cream** *($4.99 for 3.4 ounces)* is hardly rich, not with alcohol as its third ingredient. This is a very dated, very basic moisturizer that is barely passable for normal skin.

☹ **Vita Moist Face Cream** *($4.99 for 3.4 ounces)* is a bit more interesting than the Rich Moisture Face Cream above, and is better suited to dry skin. However, it's still a boring formula whose vitamins are compromised by jar packaging.

☺ **Care Deeply with Aloe Lip Balm** *($0.99 for 0.15 ounce)* is a standard, effective petrolatum-based lip balm that does its job of making dry, chapped lips feel better. For under one dollar, that's not such a bad deal!

AVON SOLUTIONS PRODUCTS

☺ **Clean Cloths Facial Cleansers** *($7.50 for 25 cloths)* are gentle, basic cleansing cloths that can be used by all skin types for on-the-go face-freshening or makeup removal. While not an ideal substitute for a water-soluble cleanser, they are a convenient secondary option for occasional use.

☺ **Clean Cream Cold Cream Cleanser** *($8 for 5 ounces)* is accurately named, because this is similar to, but with a thinner texture than, a standard cold cream. This will work as well as any to dissolve makeup, but it does not rinse well without the aid of a washcloth. It is best for someone with dry to very dry skin. Avon included an array of antioxidants, and in a cleanser that is not water-soluble, that's not a bad idea, since some amount of the antioxidants will indeed stay on the skin.

☺ **Keep It Clean Vitamin Charged Cleanser** *($6 for 6.7 ounces)* is an excellent, gentle, water-soluble cleanser for all skin types. It lathers slightly (though the lather itself isn't what does the cleansing) and rinses clean, leaving skin smooth and soft.

☺ **Keep It Quick 3-in-1 Cleanser, Toner, Moisturizer** *($6 for 6.7 ounces)* is a lightweight lotion cleanser similar to Cetaphil Gentle Skin Cleanser. It contains a tiny amount of detergent cleansing agent, and, unlike Cetaphil, is fragranced. It's still a good option for normal to slightly dry skin, as long as you aren't using it to remove much makeup. And unless you have normal skin with very basic needs, you'll still at least want to consider a separate moisturizer and, of course, sunscreen.

☹ **Keep It Fresh Vitamin Charged Toner** *($6 for 6.7 ounces)* won't keep skin fresh but its alcohol content will keep it irritated. It contains some AHAs and is formulated at the right pH to allow exfoliation, but the amount of alcohol is too problematic to make this toner worth considering.

☹ **Advanced Eye Perfector with Peptides** *($9.50 for 0.5 ounce)* is a minimally moisturizing serum that contains enough witch hazel to be irritating for all skin types. Avon included a significant amount of a peptide, but its beneficial properties are compromised by the witch hazel.

😐 **Ageless Results Overnight Renewing Cream** *($14.50 for 1.7 ounces)* contains mostly water, glycerin, silicone, thickeners, film-forming agent, absorbent, skin-identical ingredients, vitamins, ingredients that mimic the structure and function of healthy skin, more silicone, fragrance, and preservatives. The jar packaging hinders the stability of the vitamins (antioxidants) but this is still a good moisturizer for normal to dry skin.

✓☺ **Ageless Results Renewing Day Cream SPF 15** *($14.50 for 1.7 ounces)* is an outstanding daytime moisturizer for normal to slightly oily skin. It contains an in-part avobenzone sunscreen and covers every base in terms of what skin needs to look and feel healthy, all in stable, hygienic packaging. Well done, and this is noticeably less expensive than some of Avon's pricier but less impressive moisturizers.

😐 **Ageless Results Renewing Eye Cream** *($12.50 for 0.5 ounce)* suffers from jar packaging, which is a shame because it contains several antioxidants. It is otherwise an emollient moisturizer for dry skin anywhere on the face. The mineral pigments titanium dioxide and mica are what's making the eye area appear "brighter."

☺ **Ageless Results Intensive Line Filler SPF 15** *($12.50 for 0.06 ounce)* includes titanium dioxide and zinc oxide for sun protection, and these mineral ingredients plus mica are what help "blur the look of fine lines." Avon claims this product reduces the look of deep wrinkles in two weeks, but that isn't possible. The base of this product is mostly heavy-duty thickeners and waxes. An intriguing ingredient in this product is retinoxytrimethylsilane. Also known by its trade name of SilCare 1M75, it's an Avon-patented blend of retinol, silicone, and soybean oil that is supposed to be as effective as "straight" retinol without the potential for irritation (Source: www.freepatentsonline.com/7074420.html). There is no published research substantiating the claims for this ingredient, so you're left to take Avon's word for it. However, in theory it should work similarly to retinol, though neither ingredient is capable of making deep, etched lines look significantly better. Avon wisely uses packaging that keeps this retinol derivative stable. This is worth trying for its value as a sunscreen and temporary line-filling effect—but don't expect results that turn back the clock to your pre-wrinkle days.

☺ **Beautifully Protected Daily UV Moisturizer SPF 30** *($12 for 1.7 ounces)* is recommended as a good sunscreen for normal to oily skin. UVA protection is achieved via avobenzone, and the only sore point for this product is the inclusion of a few fragrant plant extracts that have no established benefit for skin. It is not as impressive as the Ageless Results Renewing Day Cream SPF 15 above, but if you need a higher SPF rating it is worth considering.

☹ **Dramatic Firming Cream for Face and Throat** *($8.50 for 1.7 ounces)* is an emollient moisturizer that isn't firming in the least and is not recommended because of the amount of arnica it contains. Arnica is associated with a high incidence of skin sensitization (Source: *American Journal of Contact Dermatitis*, June 1996, pages 94–99).

😐 **Healthy Boost Skintrition Moisture Lotion** *($12.50 for 4 ounces)* contains enough vitamins and minerals to rival any multivitamin! What a shame they are present in such tiny amounts, leaving this to be an ordinary, lightweight lotion for normal to slightly oily skin.

✓ ☺ **Hydra-Radiance Moisturizing Day Lotion SPF 15** *($12 for 4 ounces)* may have gotten your attention because it claims that it "Moisturizes better than the #1 department store moisturizer—how brilliant!" However, Avon doesn't tell us which department-store moisturizer they are comparing this one with, so it's essentially an empty claim because the comparison could have been with a really bad product. For example, Clinique's Dramatically Different Moisturizing Lotion (a dated, unacceptable formula if there ever was one—it was even ordinary when it was first launched) is the likely candidate for that sales position, and comparing this state-of-the-art product with Clinique's option is like comparing a boom box to an iPod.

Avon has crafted a daytime moisturizer with an in-part avobenzone sunscreen and lotion base suitable for normal to slightly dry or slightly oily skin. The formula contains a balanced array of antioxidants and cell-communicating ingredients along with ingredients that mimic the structure and function of healthy skin, all in opaque packaging to keep the light- and air-sensitive ingredients stable. This would be even better without the fragrance, but all in all it's one of the best moisturizers with sunscreen from Avon in years.

😐 **Hydra-Radiance Moisturizing Night Cream** *($12 for 1.7 ounces)* meets the needs of those with normal to dry skin with its mix of glycerin, shea butter, silicone, plant oil, and petrolatum. It's a shame that the jar packaging will undermine the effectiveness of the many antioxidants in this product. Opaque, airless packaging would have made this a slam-dunk recommendation.

☹ **Hydrofirming Bio6 Eye Cream** *($10.50 for 0.5 ounce)* contains several antioxidants, but the jar packaging won't keep them stable. An even bigger offense is the inclusion of eucalyptus extract, present in an amount greater than all of the antioxidants in this poorly executed eye cream.

☹ **Hydrofirming Bio6 Night Cream** *($12.50 for 1.7 ounces)* is similar to but more emollient than the Hydrofirming Bio6 Eye Cream above, yet the same review applies because of jar packaging and a lot of eucalyptus.

☹ **Hydrofirming-Lift Day Cream SPF 15** *($12.50 for 1.7 ounces)* lacks the UVA-protecting ingredients of titanium dioxide, zinc oxide, avobenzone, Tinosorb, or Mexoryl SX, and is not recommended. This is one of Avon's only sunscreen missteps; the amount of eucalyptus is also a cause for concern.

😐 **Moisture 24** *($10 for 1.7 ounces)* is a simple but effective formula whose gel-cream texture is ideal for normal to dry skin. What a shame the many antioxidants in this product won't remain stable due to the poor decision of jar packaging.

😐 **Nurtura Replenishing Cream** *($8 for 1.7 ounces)* contains mostly water, thickener, antioxidant plant oils, sunscreen agent, glycerin, more thickeners, preservatives, fragrance, and coloring agents. The jar packaging will keep the plant oils from exerting an antioxidant benefit, but this still addresses the basic needs of dry skin.

😐 **Banishing Cream Skin Discoloration Improver** *($8.50 for 2.5 ounces)* used to contain hydroquinone as its active ingredient, but Avon opted to remove this controversial, yet effective skin-lightening agent. Unfortunately, they did not replace the hydroquinone with anything that can produce the same results, so any lightening effect from this product is purely coincidental! Without the hydroquinone, this is a ho-hum moisturizer whose tiny amount of antioxidants is rendered insignificant thanks to jar packaging.

☺ **Banishing Cream Skin Tone Perfector SPF 15** *($8.50 for 2.5 ounces)* is the sunscreen version of the Banishing Cream Skin Discoloration Improver above. It contains avobenzone for UVA protection, but is otherwise lacking ingredients with significant research proving their skin-lightening potential. At least this version stands on its own as a good daytime moisturizer with sunscreen with packaging that keeps its antioxidants stable.

☺ **Lighten Up Plus Undereye Treatment** *($15 for 0.5 ounce)* won't lighten under-eye circles, but is a well-formulated lightweight moisturizer for slightly dry skin. Its silicone content promises a silky finish (great for prepping the eye area for concealer) and it contains vitamin-based antioxidants and some good skin-identical ingredients.

AVON CLEARSKIN PRODUCTS

☹ **Clearskin Cleansing Pads for Normal to Oily Skin** *($4.29 for 42 pads)* lists alcohol as the second ingredient, followed by witch hazel and, further down, menthol. Ouch!

☹ **Clearskin Deep Cleansing Cloths** *($5.29 for 20 cloths)* are deeply irritating due to their alcohol and witch hazel content. These cleansing cloths are not recommended.

☹ **Clearskin Purifying Gel Cleanser for Normal to Oily Skin** *($4.29 for 5.1 ounces)* ends up being too drying for all skin types because the main detergent cleansing agent is sodium C14-16 olefin sulfonate. The 2% salicylic acid in this cleanser won't work on blackheads because it is quickly rinsed from the skin and the pH is too high for exfoliation to occur.

☹ **Clearskin Blackhead Clearing Cleanser** *($4.99 for 5 ounces)* is similar to the Clearskin Purifying Gel Cleanser for Normal to Oily Skin above, and the same review applies.

☹ **Clearskin Invigoration Cleansing Scrub** *($4.29 for 2.5 ounces)* contains menthol and eucalyptus; these may feel invigorating but are primarily irritating and have nothing to do with creating clearer skin.

☹ **Clearskin Purifying Astringent Blackhead Clearing Formula** *($4.29 for 8 ounces)* lists alcohol as the main ingredient, which makes this astringent too irritating for all skin types. The 2% salicylic acid is coupled with a pH above 4, so exfoliation will not occur.

😐 **Clearskin Balanced Cycle Cleanser/Mask** *($5.29 for 5 ounces)* is a standard clay mask with a detergent cleansing agent. It contains a tiny amount of salicylic acid at a pH that is incorrect for exfoliation to occur. The amount of alcohol in this mask is potentially problematic, but this is an OK option for oily to very oily skin that needs an absorbent cleanser.

☹ **Clearskin Immediate Response Spot Treatment** *($5.29 for 0.5 ounce)* has 2% salicylic acid and is formulated at an effective pH of 3.8. What a shame the base for this spot treatment contains enough alcohol to make it an irritating prospect for all skin types.

☹ **Clearskin Correct & Fade Peel** *($5.29 for 30 pads)* lists alcohol as the second ingredient, which makes this 1% salicylic acid product too irritating and drying for all skin types. The amount of AHAs is less than 2%, though the pH of these pads is too high to permit either the AHAs or the BHA to exfoliate, much less, in Avon's verbiage, "peel" skin.

AVON TRUE PORE-FECTION PRODUCTS

☹ **True Pore-Fection Skin Clearing Gel Cleanser** *($7.50 for 6.7 ounces)* has more bells and whistles than the Clearskin Purifying Gel Cleanser for Normal to Oily Skin above, but shares the same problem of using a drying detergent cleansing agent. It is not recommended for any skin type.

☹ **True Pore-Fection Skin Refining Cleanser** *($7.50 for 6.7 ounces)* is a fairly drying lotion-style foaming cleanser that contains menthol, which makes it a problem for all skin types.

☹ **True Pore-Fection Skin Refining Toner** *($6.50 for 6.7 ounces)* lists alcohol as the second ingredient, which makes this toner too irritating for all skin types. The combination of glycolic and salicylic acids amounts to around 2%, but the pH of 4.1 keeps them from being effective as exfoliants.

☺ **True Pore-Fection Oil-Free Skin-Clearing Lotion** *($9.50 for 2 ounces)* contains 0.5% salicylic acid and has a pH of 3.9, which makes this a viable, if not too effective, option for blemished skin. Why Avon kept the irritants out of this product but loaded irritants into all their other products in this group is a mystery, but it's also something they should have done for all of their anti-acne products.

☹ **True Pore-Fection Skin Refining Mask** *($8.50 for 3.4 ounces)* lists alcohol as the second ingredient and also contains pumice, making this mask more abrasive and irritating then refining.

OTHER AVON PRODUCTS

☺ **Moisture Effective Eye Makeup Remover Lotion** *($4 for 2 ounces)* is a very basic, but effective, water- and oil-based makeup remover. It is fragrance-free and gentle enough to use around the eyes, though it is best used prior to washing with your regular cleanser.

😐 **Moisture Therapy Intensive Extra Strength Cream** *($5.99 for 5.3 ounces)* is a very basic and rather boring moisturizer for dry skin that contains mostly water, mineral oil, Vaseline, thickeners, plant oils, silicone, preservatives, and fragrance.

☹ **Moisture Therapy Intensive Moisturizing Lip Treatment SPF 15** *($1.49 for 0.15 ounce)* lacks sufficient UVA protection, so it is not a good choice for daytime wear if your goal is sun protection for the lips. This is otherwise a fairly standard, emollient lip balm that also contains some good antioxidants and emollient oils, which makes the lack of UVA protection that much more disappointing.

AVON SUN PRODUCTS

☺ **Avon Sun Kids Disappearing Color Sunscreen Lotion SPF 40** *($9.99 for 6.7 ounces)* doesn't have any extras going for it, though its blue tint slowly disappears on skin as you apply it, which does make it more kid-friendly and parent-reassuring. Avobenzone is included for UVA protection and the formula is water-resistant (though keep in mind it still needs to be reapplied after your child swims, towels off, or perspires heavily).

☺ **Avon Sun General Protection Sunscreen Lotion SPF 40** *($9.99 for 6.7 ounces)* is nearly identical to the Avon Sun Kids Disappearing Color Sunscreen Lotion SPF 40 above, minus the blue coloring agent. Otherwise, the same review applies.

☺ **Avon Sun Self-Tanning Spray** *($9.99 for 6.7 ounces)* is a very good self-tanning spray that, while not absorbing as quickly as claimed, still feels light and supplies skin with helpful ingredients like lecithin and cholesterol. It uses the same ingredient (dihydroxyacetone) most self-tanners have, and does contain fragrance.

☹ **Avon Sun Sport Sunscreen Spray SPF 30** *($9.99 for 6.7 ounces)* contains avobenzone for UVA protection, but there's nothing sporty about the amount of alcohol in the base formula, and it winds up being too irritating for all skin types.

☹ **Skin So Soft Bug Guard Plus IR3535 Expedition Gentle Breeze SPF 15 Pump Spray** *($12 for 4 ounces)* is a combination insect repellant and sunscreen, but it is not recommended due to the absence of UVA-protecting ingredients and the presence of a high amount of alcohol (which doesn't create "skin so soft").

☹ **Skin So Soft Bug Guard Plus IR3535 Insect Repellent Unscented SPF 15 Sunscreen Spray** *($10 for 4 ounces)* may work to keep mosquitoes and flies away, but fails to provide sufficient UVA protection, while the amount of alcohol is irritating to skin, especially when paired with the chemical insect repellant.

☹ **Skin So Soft Bug Guard Plus IR3535 SPF 15 Sunscreen Cooling Gel** *($12 for 4 ounces)* is similar to the Skin So Soft Bug Guard products above, only in gel form. The same concerns about the lack of UVA-protecting ingredients and high amount of alcohol apply here, too.

☹ **Skin So Soft Bug Guard Plus IR3535 SPF 15 Sunscreen Spray** *($10 for 4 ounces)* contains a different blend of active ingredient to repel insects, but its sunscreen actives and the presence of alcohol match those of the Skin So Soft Bug Guard products above, and it is not recommended.

AVON MAKEUP

FOUNDATION: ✓ ☺ **Visual Perfection Tint Releasing Moisturizer SPF 20 UVA/UVB** *($12.50)* comes in one shade and features an in-part avobenzone sunscreen for sufficient UVA protection. The product dispenses looking grayish-white, but morphs into a sheer, flesh tone as soon as you begin blending. The color is so soft and translucent it will work for a variety of skin tones, though very dark skin may find it slightly ash. It has a smooth, moist finish that's not at all heavy, though formula-wise this is best for normal to slightly dry skin. A nice surprise is the inclusion of several antioxidants, and the product is packaged to keep these light- and air-sensitive ingredient stable. If only Avon's other foundations provided higher SPF numbers, they would be categorically recommended without reservation. ✓ ☺ **Beyond Color Line Softening Mousse Foundation** *($12)* makes a big deal about the vitamins it contains, but they're barely present in this silicone-based foundation—plus the jar packaging won't keep them potent once the product is opened. Despite that bit of bad news, this foundation has an amazing, almost otherworldly texture that, true to claim, is "light as air" and blends flawlessly. It provides sheer to medium coverage with a silky-soft matte finish, which makes this appropriate for normal to very oily skin. Someone with any degree of dry skin won't appreciate this foundation's finish, though it is far from being a flat, dulling matte. The nonaqueous formula is long-lasting and will require more than a standard water-soluble cleanser for complete removal. Among the 12 mostly beautiful shades, only Warmest Beige suffers from being too peach. The remaining shades include excellent options for fair to dark (but not very dark) skin.

☹ **Personal Match Natural Liquid Foundation SPF 10** *($10)* has an amazingly smooth texture, a near-flawless application that blends impeccably, and a gorgeous soft matte finish. It provides light to medium coverage, and the sunscreen is pure titanium dioxide. How frustrating that it did not rate SPF 15 or higher, because that is so essential the lower number alone keeps this from earning a better rating. The claims for this foundation are far-fetched (you can't absorb oil and provide moisture with one formula). In fact, the amount of absorbent ingredients (including dry-finish silicones, talc, and kaolin) is much greater than the lightweight moisturizing agents included. That makes this foundation ideal for normal to very oily skin. Twelve shades are available, with options for fair to dark skin. The shades to avoid due to being slightly to strongly peach are Porcelain, Buff, Warmest Beige, and Honey. Chestnut is also problematic due to its reddish cast, though it may work for certain ethnic skin tones.

☹ **Personal Match Matte Liquid Foundation SPF 10** *($10)* has a pure titanium dioxide sunscreen, though Avon would have been wise to offer SPF 15 instead of 10. Compared to Personal Match Natural Liquid Foundation SPF 10 above, this version is less silky and, despite the name, offers a weaker matte finish—it actually leaves behind a slightly moist feel, although it does look smooth and natural on skin, providing light to medium coverage. Among the 12 shades are great options for fair to dark skin, but avoid Porcelain, Buff, Warmest Beige, and Beautiful Bronze due to their pink and peach tones.

☺ **Beyond Color Radiant Lifting Foundation SPF 12** *($12)* purports to make skin "look lifted and radiant instantly," but that statement is only partially true. This foundation's fluid, silky texture blends smoothly, provides medium coverage, and sets to a soft satin-matte finish that does indeed look radiant. It's the lifting claim that's empty. Nothing in this product will lift skin in the slightest, though the pure titanium dioxide sunscreen provides broad-spectrum sun protection (SPF 15 is the minimum daily protection to strive for). Fourteen shades are offered, with options for very light to dark skin tones. Almost all of them are beautiful, but be careful with the slightly pink Porcelain, and avoid Chestnut due to its copper overtone, Beige because of its rosy color, and Beautiful Bronze, which is slightly peach. This foundation is best for normal to slightly dry or slightly oily skin. Cocoa and Mahogany are excellent shades for women of color. Two final comments: This foundation has a strong fragrance, and the state-of-the-art ingredients Avon touts are listed long after the preservatives and fragrance.

☹ **Personal Match Dewy Souffle Foundation SPF 10** *($10)* includes an in-part titanium dioxide sunscreen but shortchanges your skin by not providing the recommended SPF 15 protection. This has a moist, somewhat thick texture that has lots of movement on skin, so it takes longer than usual to blend. It maintains its creamy feel and offers a dewy finish capable of medium coverage, and is an option for dry to very dry skin willing to pair it with an effective sunscreen rated SPF 15 or higher. Twelve shades are available, with many good options. Avoid Honey, Buff, Warmest Beige, and Porcelain—all are strongly peach and don't resemble real skin tones in the least.

☹ **Personal Match Cream-to-Powder Foundation SPF 10** *($10)* has, like all of the other Personal Match foundations above, a sunscreen rating that's too low for daytime protection (though it does include titanium dioxide for UVA protection). It has a somewhat greasy yet lightweight application that sets to a satin finish capable of sheer to light coverage. It's not the most elegant cream-to-powder foundation around, and as such not really worth seeking out since better versions are readily available at drug and department stores. The collection of 12 shades leans a bit toward peaches and pinks, but there are some suitably neutral shades for fair to light skin. These shades are too peach to consider: Porcelain, Buff, Warmest Beige, Honey, and Toffee.

☹ **Perfect Wear Foundation SPF 10** *($10)* has a pure titanium dioxide sunscreen but the amount used (2.5%) here is not enough to achieve the minimum recommended SPF of 15. That's a shame, because this is otherwise a great liquid foundation for those with normal to oily skin. It has a smooth, even application that provides medium coverage and a natural matte finish. Avon claims it lasts for 12 hours; many other foundations say the same thing (and this definitely won't maintain its matte finish over oily areas for that long). The 12 shades are mostly quite good, except for the usual peach-tinged suspects: Porcelain, Honey, Warmest Beige, and Buff. The darkest shades are a bit coppery and have limited use for African-American skin tones. However, they may work for some Indian or Polynesian skin tones.

☹ **Personal Match Smooth Mineral Powder Makeup** *($10)* is Avon's contribution to the mineral makeup craze. Unlike most loose mineral powders, this one lists kaolin (clay) as the main ingredient. Because it has a clay base, this powder provides an extremely matte finish without a hint of shine (except for the Warmth and Mineral Veil shades). It applies smoothly, feels surprisingly silky, and offers medium to almost full coverage that can look more apparent than you might like yet doesn't feel heavy. The downside is that most of the nine shades don't resemble real skin tones. Warmest Beige, Warmth, Buff, Almond, and Mineral Veil all have issues associated with being too peach, red, or ash. Bisque, Ivory, Toffee, and Beautiful Bronze are options, but that shuts out anyone with a medium skin tone. I wouldn't choose this over mineral powders from Laura Mercier or L'Oreal, but it's worth a look if you have oily to very oily skin and can find a shade that matches.

☹ **Anew Beauty Age-Transforming Foundation SPF 15** *($16)* is a beauty first! This silky liquid foundation not only provides an in-part titanium dioxide sunscreen, but contains approximately 3% glycolic acid at a pH of 3.4, which permits exfoliation. It blends smoothly and offers light to medium coverage with a satin finish that feels moist. So why didn't this innovative foundation receive a Paula's Pick rating? Because, for all its positive traits, it looks very much like a layer of makeup sitting on top of your skin. The formula settles easily into lines, large pores, and facial crevices, and trying to soften this effect noticeably diminishes the coverage it provides. If you decide the benefit of sun protection and AHA exfoliation is worth the tradeoff, there are some suitably neutral colors among the 14 shades. The following shades are best avoided due to peachy overtones: Porcelain, Natural, Warmest Beige, and Toffee.

CONCEALER: ☺ **Beyond Color Radiant Lifting Concealer** *($7)* makes lifting claims similar to the Beyond Color Radiant Lifting Foundation above, but this one also cannot lift skin anywhere, anymore than any cosmetic can. This liquid concealer is outfitted with a precision brush applicator to facilitate application. It does indeed make application convenient, but this product provides such sheer coverage it doesn't do a respectable cover-up job on even minor flaws. If your camouflaging needs include dark circles, broken capillaries, or blemishes, this won't make you happy. For those with near-perfect skin and barely noticeable imperfections that need only minor coverage, this product is worth checking out. It takes longer than usual to set, but once it does the satin-matte finish lasts well. Five mostly excellent shades are available—watch out for the too-peach Medium, and use caution with Deep, which women of color may find too dark for most African-American skin tones (though it's a great, non-ashy shade).

☺ **Anew Beauty Age-Transforming Concealer SPF 15** *($10)* provides the benefits of an illuminating concealer, an in-part titanium dioxide sunscreen, and glycolic acid in one concealer. The pH of 3.6 allows the glycolic acid (present at about 3%) to exfoliate, but such exfoliation isn't needed for the under-eye area, which is precisely where this concealer is likely to be applied. The click-pen applicator dispenses the product onto a brush, and although initially too slippery, it sets quickly to a matte (in feel) finish that has a soft shimmer. Coverage is moderate; this hides minor redness and dark circles, but requires layering for more pronounced flaws. Six shades are available: Natural Golden is slightly peach but may work for some medium skin tones; Natural Deep turns slightly ash due to the amount of titanium dioxide it contains; Natural Medium is too pinky-peach and best avoided. Based on the formula, this will make skin smoother and protect it from sun damage—just be cautious about using it too close to the eye due to the acidic pH.

😐 **Clearly Flawless Treatment and Concealer** *($10)* is a dual-sided automatic, retractable pencil that includes a clear treatment stick on one end and a creamy concealer on the other. The treatment stick includes 2% salicylic acid, but the pH is too high for it to function as an exfoliant. Another drawback is that it leaves an odd white cast on skin. The concealer portion fares better, but the oils and thickeners it contains are inappropriate for use over blemishes. It provides decent coverage, but you must set it with powder to avoid slippage and creasing. All four shades are good, yet to reiterate, this is not for use over blemishes.

☹ **Personal Match Natural Concealer Stick** *($6)* does have a natural finish on skin, but in this case it doesn't translate to significant coverage, and the highly fragranced formula tends to slip and slide throughout the day, eventually fading and leaving your imperfections exposed. Five reasonably good shades are available, but I don't recommend putting up with this concealer's inadequacies even if you have little to hide.

POWDER: ✓ ☺ **Personal Match Pressed Powder** *($9)* has an enviably silky texture that applies smoothly and makes skin look perfectly polished. The talc-based formula comes in six neutral shades, all excellent and including options for fair to dark (but not very dark) skin. Ignore Avon's claim that this powder adds moisture while it absorbs excess oil "where needed." Such disparate ingredients don't mesh well in one product.

☺ **Personal Match Loose Powder** *($9)* won't perfectly match 98% of skin tones, as Avon claims, because most of the six shades have a subtle peach cast, which doesn't represent the majority of skin tones. But this talc-based loose powder does have a wonderfully silky texture and natural finish. The silica and calcium silicate in this product make it best for normal to very oily skin, and there are some worthwhile shades for fair and dark skin.

☺ **Personal Match Matte Pressed Powder** *($9)* is talc-based with a smooth texture and dry finish suitable for oily to very oily skin. It keeps skin matte without looking thick or caked, and comes in six superb shades for fair to dark skin. Avon really does well with their powder shades—too bad this doesn't translate to all of their foundation colors!

BLUSH: ✓ ☺ **Split Second Blush Stick** *($8)* promises "just-flushed perfection" and delivers! This is one of the smoothest cream-to-powder blushes around, and it blends impeccably. Note that blending is required because it sets quickly. It works best if you dab on the color in dots and then blend with a sponge or clean fingers. The color selection is slightly marred by one too many iridescent shades, but there are enough great colors so that it's worth a test run if you prefer this type of blush.

✓ ☺ **Beyond Color Mousse Blush** *($9)* is described as "silky, light, and blendable" and that sums it up! Housed in a glass jar, this is an intriguing, well-executed way to use blush. The shades are beautiful and apply sheer, so there's no chance of overdoing it on the first try. Even better, the formula lasts—though if your cheek area is very oily, you'll do better with powder blushes.

☺ **True Color Blush** *($8)* has a smooth, dry texture and soft, non-powdery application. The palette offers enough enticing options to make this a worthwhile option, but bear in mind that every shade has at least a slight shine. Rose Lustre and Golden Glow Light/Medium have the most shine, though the latter is an acceptable shimmer powder for evening. Earthen Rose is a great tan color for contouring.

EYESHADOW: ☺ **Heavenly Soft Eyeshadow Trio** *($7)*. This has a silky softness that's almost creamy and an application that's smooth, even, and nearly flake-free. The question of whether to purchase this comes down to sheerness: every trio deposits minimal color that is too soft for a classic eye design. That is, none of the colors are dark enough for use as liner and the potential crease colors need lots of layering to show up. You'll get sparkling shine that's not too distracting, but that's the most impact these shadows make. If you desire very sheer color for eye makeup, the best sets to consider are Brown Trio, Nude Trio, and Plum Trio.

😐 **True Color Eyeshadow Duo** *($5)* has a smooth texture but the finish on skin isn't as nice as many others, with the colors tending to apply unevenly and lose intensity as the day goes by. Additionally, most of the duos are too blue, purple, or green to recommend, and all have shine. If you're intent on trying this, the best duos are Rich Mauve, Bronze, Steel Grey, Classic Neutral Light, and Classic Neutral Medium.

😐 **True Color Eyeshadow Quad** *($6.50)* has the same smooth texture and wear issues as the True Color Eyeshadow Duo above. Every shade in these quads is shiny (and the shine tends to flake), making for an overall eye design that's shine overload, not to mention that most of the color combinations are unworkable or predominantly blue, green, or purple.

😐 **Loose Powder Eyeshadow Pot** *($7)* must be an attempt by Avon to put a new spin on pressed-powder eyeshadow, but it holds no advantage over that format besides cute packaging. This is housed in an inkwell-type bottle, and you use the sponge-tip wand applicator to sweep loose color onto the eye area. Yes, it's messy—but the colors do apply smoother than expected, and each is sheer. More gimmicky than practical, this isn't an essential addition, nor does it replace standard powder eyeshadows, Avon's included.

😐 **Shimmer Shadow & Liner Duo** *($9)* offers a liquid-to-powder eyeshadow on one end and a coordinating shade of liquid eyeliner on the other. Both products are shiny, and the eyeshadow portion blends on sheer, leaving mostly sparkles behind. It's an intriguing concept, but handling this amount of shine demands a smooth, firm eye area.

😐 **Pure Shimmer All Over Color Stick** *($5)* is a twist-up stick that is meant for eyes, cheeks, and lips with most of the colors being best for the latter two. The creamy but lightweight texture is prone to creasing when worn as eyeshadow or liner, yet that's how Avon has been advertising this product in its catalogs.

😐 **Eyeshadow Trio** *($6)* has a cream-to-powder application, and each of the three shades is very shiny. In fact, using this is more about adding lots of glistening shine rather than color. Avon instructs you to use the lightest shade to highlight, the medium shade to contour, and the darkest for shading. That makes sense, but doesn't work with this product because the colors are so sheer you can't create any depth or shadow—all you're left with is lots of shine. These do stay in place and pose minimal risk of creasing, but please consider this type of look for evening only, and definitely not if you have wrinkles around the eye.

😐 **Shadowstix Eyeshadow Stick** *($8)* has a talc- and pumice(!)-based formula that applies smooth but dry and can be difficult to blend. This is best for adding a hint of color or shading to a small area, and what little blending can be done must be done immediately. All of the shades have some degree of shine, and most are so pale or pastel they're best reserved for highlighting the brow bone. The shine is slightly prone to flaking.

☹ **Beyond Color Radiant Lifting Eyeshadow** *($7)* doesn't just add color to eyes, it also claims to reduce lines, wrinkles, and crepey skin while providing a "lifted appearance." Should you cancel your cosmetic surgery appointment? No way! The anti-aging ingredients include a selection of B-vitamin polypeptides along with antioxidant vitamins A, C, and E—all listed after the preservative, meaning their presence is insignificant. As an eyeshadow, this product has a thick texture that applies unevenly; it tends to get chunky and then thinner as it is blended. The mostly pastel and pale neutral colors have shimmer, and enough of it to make less-than-smooth eyelids look wrinkled, plus the formula creases slightly. None of this is great news, and makes this difficult to recommend.

EYE AND BROW SHAPER: 😐 **Ultra Luxury Eye Liner** *($5)* has an attractive price for a standard pencil that applies easily and offers a smooth, dry finish. This is still prone to mild smearing as the day wears on. 😐 **Big Color Eye Pencil** *($6)* is a standard chunky pencil with a smooth, silicone-enhanced application and a soft, slightly creamy finish. Every color is quite shiny and most are pastel, but if that's your thing these do hold up reasonably well. 😐 **Ultra Luxury Brow Liner** *($5)* is an ordinary brow pencil that has a typical dry texture, but it is easier to apply than most. The price is right, and this is one to consider if you prefer brow pencil to powder and don't mind routine sharpening.

☺ **Glimmersticks Brow Definer** *($6)* has been improved and now this automatic, retractable brow pencil is a strong contender for enhancing brows. Its four colors (including a good option for blonde brows) go on smoothly and evenly, each with a soft powder finish that lasts.

☺ **Glimmersticks Waterproof Eye Liner** *($6)* applies easily and the retractable pencil doesn't require sharpening, which is always a plus. These glide so well you'll need to be extra careful to not over-apply, and each slightly to moderately shiny shade sets to a fairly immovable finish. True to the name, this is a waterproof formula, though it does come off with a water-soluble cleanser.

☺ **Glimmersticks Waterproof Brow Definer** *($6)* is a great automatic, retractable brow pencil that comes in four very good colors (no options for redheads). Application is smooth and the waterproof finish is long-lasting. The drawback is the slightly tacky, waxy finish that doesn't dissipate. That's not a deal-breaker, but this trait keeps it from earning a higher rating.

☺ **Color Glide Liquid Eye Liner** *($7)* applies smoothly without skipping or sheering out, though its longer brush demands precise control (it's tricky to draw a thin line). Still, this is a much better liquid liner than it once was due to its quick drying time and enhanced wear. ☺ **Feeling Fine Ultra Thin Liner** *($6)* is an ultra-thin, automatic, nonretractable eye pencil that applies effortlessly and sets to a long-wearing finish. It's easy to create a thin or thick line with this pencil, but note that every shade is shiny, and will leave either a shimmer or metallic finish. That won't make a less-than-taut or wrinkled eyelid look any better, but if that doesn't apply to you, this remains a terrific pencil to consider.

☹ **Glimmersticks Eye Liner** *($6)* is an automatic, retractable pencil with a texture that's too creamy to last for long, particularly as eyeliner. If you prefer pencils, there are better ones available in this price range from Revlon, L'Oreal, and others. ☹ **Perfect Wear Liquid Eyeliner Pen** *($7)* has a short, stubby brush that doesn't make application easier, though the formula dries quickly. The problem is that the colors tend to fade, and it's also difficult to build much intensity. Almay's liquid eyeliners have a similar price point and near-flawless performance.

LIPSTICK, LIP GLOSS, AND LIPLINER: ✓☺ **My Lip Miracle Lipcolor** *($8)* promises up to eight hours of wear without fading, plus lots of moisture and shine. What this silicone-based lipstick has is definitely different from traditional lipsticks, though it's hardly a miracle. Rather, it glides on smoothly and sets to a semi-matte finish, which manages to feel creamy enough that you won't be reaching for your lip balm or gloss shortly after application. Each shade goes on opaque, and the palette of saturated colors is beautiful. This lipstick does have longevity, but won't last eight hours without needing a touchup, especially if you eat or drink anything. However, it is a very good option for semi-matte lipstick and worthy of a Paula's Pick rating. ✓☺ **Glazewear Liquid Lip Color** *($6)* is a very good, medium-coverage lip gloss that has a slick application and a non-sticky, glossy finish. The color range is extensive and gorgeous, owing to this product's deserved popularity. ✓☺ **Glazewear Metallics Lip Gloss** *($6)* differs little from Glazewear save for its metallic finish. ✓☺ **Glazewear Lipstick** *($8)* is positioned as a high-performance gloss and luxury lip color in one, and it is. Essentially it's a lip gloss in lipstick form; what sets it apart (aside from some riveting sheer colors) is its smooth, moisturizing yet non-slippery texture and a glossy finish that's free of stickiness. Another plus: These last longer than a standard lip gloss, so frequent touch-ups aren't necessary. This isn't a foolproof product for anyone prone to lip color bleeding into lines around the mouth, but it is a must-try if you love the high shine many lip glosses provide but dislike their brevity.

☺ **Beyond Color Quick Pen Plumping Lip Gloss** *($7)* is a glossy, non-sticky liquid lip color housed in a click-pen component with an angled, sponge-tip applicator. The sheer colors are easy to use (Dolled Up is practically colorless) and many have an enticing shimmer, which creates the illusion of fuller lips (the retinol in this product does not plump lips at all). ☺ **Beyond Color Plumping Lipliner with Retinol** *($7)* is a standard, automatic lip pencil that goes on smoothly and does a reasonably good job in keeping creamy lipsticks from feathering into lines around the mouth. The shade selection is modest but good, especially if you're looking for more neutral, versatile colors. As for the retinol, it is present (listed as retinoxytrimethylsilane), but in such a minuscule amount it is just wasted in this product, and the packaging isn't the best for keeping it stable anyway. ☺ **Ultra Color Rich Lipstick** *($6.50)* is a traditional creamy lipstick with a large selection of full-coverage colors, most with a satin finish. The ☹ **Sheer SPF 15** colors are not recommended due to their lack of sufficient UVA protection. ☺ **Kissable Lip Frost** *($6)* comes in a tin and is basically an emollient lip balm with a hint of color. Each shade has a shimmer finish, and nicely protects lips from getting chapped, and everyone knows chapped lips are no fun to kiss!

☺ **Fruity Juice Lip Gloss** *($6)* comes in a squeeze tube and is a fairly thick, sticky but shiny lip gloss. The shades are so sheer it doesn't matter which one you choose, and each has sparkles. ☺ **Topcoat Lip Gloss** *($6)* is a tube lip gloss with your choice of a glitter or pearly shimmer finish. Both shades go on clear, leaving their respective sparkles to steal the spotlight. The glitter version feels grainy as it wears off, but the shimmer version is good.

☺ **Perfect Wear Ever Glaze Lip Ink & Gloss Duo** *($10)* is Avon's contribution to the lip paint and top-coat system originally launched by Procter & Gamble via Max Factor Lipfinity and Cover Girl Outlast. Just as with all the other two-step, all-day lip colors, you apply a base color, allow it to dry, then top with a gloss so the color below feels smooth and comfortable. Avon's base color, referred to as **Lip Ink**, applies well but takes longer than usual to dry, and as it does your lips feel parched. That's remedied by applying the **Lip Gloss** (top coat), which has an extremely shiny finish and feels slightly sticky. Unlike competing products, the Lip Gloss intensifies the base color, making it much brighter (not to mention looking nothing like the base color you see in the container). The good news is this product does have excellent staying power, even when used with other lipsticks and glosses. See if you like the effect the gloss has on the color, and if not, you can customize it with other lipsticks or glosses of you own.

☺ **Glimmersticks Lipliner** *($6).* If it weren't for this automatic, retractable lip-liner's somewhat tacky finish, it would be among the best for smooth application and ability to keep lipstick from feathering into lines around the mouth. As is, it's recommended for those willing to tolerate the finish, though that becomes less of an issue when paired with a lipstick.

😐 **Beyond Color Plumping Lipcolor SPF 15** *($8)* lacks the UVA-protecting ingredients of titanium dioxide, zinc oxide, avobenzone, Tinosorb, or Mexoryl SX, but its opacity does provide some element of sun protection. This creamy, full-coverage lipstick feels moist but not too slick, and comes in a color range with something to please everyone. As for the lip-plumping claim, don't count on it—there is nothing in the formula that has this effect.

😐 **Shine Supreme Lip Color** *($8)* is a lipstick/lip gloss hybrid that provides near-opaque coverage and a glossy finish. Although workable, it doesn't apply as evenly as it should, tending to deposit more color, then less, then more. I thought it was a fluke, but color after color exhibited this frustrating application. The shade range is attractive, though the formula is slick enough to creep into any lines around the mouth. 😐 **Perfect Wear All-Day Comfort Lipstick SPF 12** *($8)* comes so close to an SPF 15 rating it's disheartening to rate this with a neutral face. However, there is no question that SPF 15 is the minimum standard for sun protection, and anything that falls short of that isn't a smart choice for daytime wear. What's ironic is that Avon's other lipstick, Ultra Moisture Rich Lipstick SPF 15 (rated below), has no UVA-protecting ingredients, yet this one includes an in-part titanium dioxide sunscreen! This opaque, silicone-based lipstick goes on quite slick and initially feels greasy. However, it sets to a soft matte finish that feels light and wears better than a standard creamy or glossy lipstick. The shade range is stunning, and, as I mentioned earlier, it's a shame to rate this below a Paula's Pick because of the too-low SPF number.

😐 **Ultra Moisture Rich Lipstick SPF 15** *($6.50)* lacks the UVA-protecting ingredients of titanium dioxide, zinc oxide, avobenzone, Tinosorb, or Mexoryl SX, so forget about it for sufficient sun protection. As a lipstick, it feels light yet creamy without being too slippery, and the colors are indeed rich (each has a good stain). Contrary to claim, this lipstick doesn't contain special ingredients that seek out dry patches of lips and go to work softening them. Rather, applying this or any other creamy lipstick will make dry lips look and feel better all over. Just keep in mind that if chapping or flaking is apparent, the time to eliminate it is before applying lipstick.

😐 **Ultra Luxury Lipliner** *($5)* has a great price for a standard pencil that isn't too dry or too creamy for precise application. The fact that it needs sharpening prevents it from earning a happy face rating.

☹ **Beyond Color Lip Recovery Cream SPF 15** *($8)* contains a small (very, very small) amount of retinyl palmitate, a combination of palmitic acid with retinol that's not considered the most effective form of vitamin A. But in any form, retinol won't plump lips, nor will anything else in this product. What's operating here to make lips appear fuller is a combination of light-reflecting shimmering pigments made long-lasting with film-forming agents, and several emollient oils, including jojoba. The effect is subtle, but there is no question lips look fuller with shimmery, glossy lip products than without, although that effect isn't unique to this product.

Otherwise, this liquid lipstick housed in a click-pen-with-brush applicator is good, but nothing special. Disappointingly, the sunscreen does not provide sufficient UVA protection and the colors are sheer enough to not provide much protection on their own.

MASCARA: ☺ **Superfull Mascara** *($8.50)* joins the group of mascaras (such as those from Cover Girl and Chanel) that exchange standard nylon bristles for spiky, variegated rubber bristles. Although this style of brush takes some getting used to (take it from someone who has tested thousands of mascaras), with practice you can get really impressive results. Avon's contribution is aptly named; it takes some time to build, but with effort lashes end up full, thick, and appreciably long. Clumping is minimal, and the only issue involves the manner in which the rubber bristles deposit mascara—they tend to leave the tips of your lashes with little balls of mascara. These require a lash comb to eliminate, and doing so is a must or you run the risk of flaking during wear. Aside from that caveat, this mascara is enthusiastically recommended.

☺ **Extreme Volume Mascara** *($6.50)* acquits itself nicely as an all-purpose lengthening and thickening mascara. It doesn't do either dramatically, but is a good option for enhancing lashes without producing anything too over-the-top. The name isn't accurate, because nothing about this mascara is extreme, but it is a commendable option nonetheless.

☺ **Defining Curves Waterproof Mascara** *($7.50)* allows you to quickly create long, curvaceous lashes that are defined and separated and that just keep getting longer the more you apply, all without clumping. Thickness is minor, even with successive coats, but the formula is waterproof and recommended if you prefer a lengthening mascara and don't need much volume. This requires an oil- or silicone-based makeup remover.

😐 **Daring Definition Mousse Mascara** *($7.50)* does have a lightweight, mousse-like texture, but that doesn't make for a better mascara. If anything, the texture of this mascara makes it more prone to clumping during application. It produces impressive length quickly, but loses points for making lashes feel dry and flaking throughout the day.

😐 **Daring Curves Mascara** *($7.50)* does create softly curled lashes that last all day, but its lengthening prowess is moderate and thickness is scant. It's a good choice if you don't need much lash enhancement beyond a bit of length and curl, but is otherwise unremarkable.

😐 **Wash-Off Waterproof Mascara** *($6.50)* is oddly named, because you don't expect a mascara to wash off, right? This one does, though as with most waterproof mascaras, you'll need more than a water-soluble cleanser to remove it completely. The real question is why anyone would bother with this lackluster mascara. It provides some length without clumps or smears, but no thickness. That's not terrible, but far better waterproof mascaras are available for the same amount of money from L'Oreal, Rimmel, and Maybelline New York.

😐 **Astonishing Lengths Waterproof Mascara** *($7.50)* is about as astonishing as seeing someone wear red, white, and blue on the Fourth of July. This utterly boring mascara goes on thin, minimally emphasizing lashes but eventually making them noticeably longer. It's waterproof, but so are many other mascaras superior to this one.

😐 **Lash Designer Mascara** *($7.50)* warns you to "stand back: you'll have lashes that go from 'where?' to lush, luxurious lengths"—but they must be joking. This lackluster mascara builds minimal length and absolutely no thickness, all while taking its time to produce such modest results.

☹ **Beyond Color Lash Fortifying Mascara** *($7.50)* is not worth considering, even if you're shopping for a middle-of-the-road mascara for modest length and thickness. That's because this uninspired product tends to flake, depositing mascara flecks on the upper and lower lash-lines throughout the day, no matter how careful you are during application. With the wealth of truly awesome mascaras available, there is no reason to consider this poor contender.

☹ **Astonishing Lengths Mascara** *($7.50)* produces copious length and does so quickly! What's not so astonishing about this mascara is its tendency to flake and not make it through the day without some smearing.

☹ **Perfect Wear Long Lasting Mascara** *($7.50)* is anything but perfect, which makes the name embarrassing. While it builds decent length and minimal thickness, you'll notice that lashes feel slightly tacky and tend to stick together. Neither trait is attractive, so even though this mascara does wear well, keep in mind many others can leave lashes soft and separated.

BABOR (SKIN CARE ONLY)

BABOR AT-A-GLANCE

Strengths: A handful of well-formulated, stably packaged, antioxidant-rich products; good to above average moisturizing masks for dry to very dry skin; and self-tanners that have nice textures and are not exorbitantly priced.

Weaknesses: Overreliance on jar packaging and redundant moisturizer formulas; many products (even those with few ingredients) containing more than eight preservatives, which increases the potential for irritation; no sunscreens recommended as part of a daily routine; no products to treat blemishes; and, as usual for the cosmetics industry, pricey products that don't have research to support their claims or make them worth the investment; "spa-quality" is a bogus claim because there are no established standards for this market.

For more information about Babor, call (888) 222-6791 or visit www.babor.com or www.Beautypedia.com. Note: All Babor products contain fragrance unless otherwise noted.

BABOR ADVANCED BIOGEN LINE

☹ **Advanced Biogen Concentrate** *($52 for 1 ounce)* lists isopropyl alcohol as the fourth ingredient, and what precedes it is nothing more than water, castor oil, and a slip agent. How is this supposed to energize skin and boost its regenerative process? If anything, that much alcohol will irritate and hurt skin. This serum is a pricey waste of time and not good for your skin.

😐 **$$$ Advanced Biogen Day Cream** *($53 for 1.7 ounces)* is an emollient moisturizer for dry to very dry skin that contains some outstanding antioxidants and cell-communicating ingredients, but they're undermined by the jar packaging, which makes this less impressive.

😐 **$$$ Advanced Biogen Decollete Cream** *($50 for 1.7 ounces)* is similar to, but slightly less emollient than, the Advanced Biogen Day Cream above. Nothing in this product is specific to the neck and décolleté; skin is skin and it deserves the same beneficial ingredients wherever it is on your body.

😐 **$$$ Advanced Biogen Intensive Repair** *($68 for 1.7 ounces)* is primarily water, plant oils, thickener, alcohol, and Vaseline. The oils and Vaseline are intensely moisturizing, but you don't need to spend even a fraction of Babor's price to gain their benefit. The company maintains that this rich moisturizer is "ideal for problem skin once blemishes have subsided," but if you're blemish-prone, this formula may well encourage blemishes to return or at the very least feel greasy on your skin.

😐 **$$$ Advanced Biogen Night Cream** *($68 for 1.7 ounces)* will work wonders to make dry to very dry skin feel smooth and comfortable, but the ingredients responsible for this are commonplace, consisting of plant oils, thickeners, shea butter, and beeswax. Small amounts of several antioxidants could have added up to a nice boost for skin, if it were not for the jar packaging.

☺ **$$$ Advanced Biogen Mask** *($32 for 1.7 ounces)* is so similar to all of the Advanced Biogen moisturizers above that there's no need to consider adding it. However, if you're curious to try Babor and have dry skin, this mask can certainly be used as a leave-on moisturizer—and the opaque tube packaging works much better than a jar to keep the antioxidants stable.

BABOR B. YOUNG LINE

😐 **$$$ B. Young Balance Cream** *($32 for 1.7 ounces)* is a lightweight yet creamy moisturizer for normal to dry skin. It contains several antioxidants, but they lose their potency shortly after this jar-packaged product is opened.

😐 **$$$ B. Young Combination Cream** *($32 for 1.7 ounces)* contains some emollients and nut oil that should not be used by anyone with oily skin, as this product recommends. However, the rice starch provides a temporary mattifying effect. What's most disappointing is the copious amount of antioxidants, which will be rendered unstable once this jar-packaged product is opened.

☺ **$$$ B. Young Moisture Gel** *($25 for 1.7 ounces)* has potential as a good but basic ultralight moisturizer for those with normal to oily or blemish-prone skin. It contains some very good water-binding agents, with lesser amounts of antioxidants, and the cell-communicating ingredient lecithin.

😐 **$$$ B. Young Sensitive Cream** *($32 for 1.7 ounces)* is nearly identical to the B. Young Balance Cream above, except this version is fragrance-free. Otherwise, the same review applies.

☺ **$$$ B. Young Tinted Day Cream 01** *($23 for 1.7 ounces)* and **B. Young Tinted Day Cream 02** *($23 for 1.7 ounces)* have the same formula. Both are sheer, tinted moisturizers whose oil-heavy formula is best for dry to very dry skin. Of course, without sunscreen, these are not for daytime wear unless you're willing to layer with a product that offers reliable sun protection (and that would prove too much for most skin types, except those with very dry skin).

✓☺ **B. Young Lip Balm** *($11 for 0.5 ounce)* can be a good alternative to traditional Vaseline- or oil-based lip balms. This lotion-textured lip moisturizer contains some lightweight hydrating agents along with more substantial emollients. It also has a high concentration of vitamin E and features other antioxidants, all in stable packaging.

BABOR CALMING SENSITIVE LINE

😐 **$$$ Calming Sensitive Bi-Phase Moisturizer** *($48 for 1 ounce)* contains some intriguing ingredients for sensitive skin, including sea buckthorn oil. However, the preservative-free formula may spell trouble because several ingredients in this water-based lotion won't last long without a stable preservative system, and I'd be concerned about bacterial contamination (although the pump-bottle packaging helps minimize exposure). Despite some commendable ingredients, the inclusion of orange flower oil makes it not suitable for sensitive skin, and it may cause photosensitivity in fair-skinned persons (Source: *The Medical Journal of Australia*, April 2003, pages 411–412).

☺ **$$$ Calming Sensitive Concentrate** *($40 for 0.8 ounce)* is a standard moisturizing gel that contains the soothing agents calendula and allantoin. It is fragrance-free and an option for normal to oily skin that is sensitive or reddened. Note: If you have ragweed (or similar plant) allergies, topical application of calendula is not recommended because of the risk of an eczematous allergic reaction (Source: www.naturaldatabase.com).

☺ **$$$ Calming Sensitive Couperose Serum** *($44 for 1 ounce)* is described as being a product that can camouflage varicose veins, but it isn't capable of providing this benefit. (*Couperose* is a French term often used to describe rosacea.) This water-based serum provides no coverage (it isn't makeup, and it takes a heavy-duty foundation to hide varicose veins). It contains horse chestnut and escin, a component of the horse chestnut plant. Although both of these ingredients have research about their benefit for varicose veins (especially when consumed orally), the research does not study the effects of the small amounts contained in cosmetic products like this (Sources: *Pharmacological Research*, September 2001, pages 183–193; *Phytotherapy Research*, March 2002, number S1, pages 1–5; and *Archives of Dermatology*, 1998, volume 134, pages 1356–1360). Although this product has no discernible effect on veins, it is a lightweight, water-based serum that can be helpful for normal to oily or blemish-prone skin.

😐 **$$$ Calming Sensitive Day Cream** *($53 for 1.7 ounces)* claims to offset the effects of light- (sun) induced aging, but this isn't something to slather on before heading outdoors because it does not contain active sunscreen ingredients. It's a standard emollient moisturizer for normal to dry skin whose antioxidants are compromised by the jar packaging. It is fragrance- and colorant-free.

😐 **$$$ Calming Sensitive Night Cream** *($65 for 1.7 ounces)* includes some beneficial soothing agents and antioxidants, but they are rendered unstable once this jar-packaged moisturizer is opened. Even if this were in airtight packaging, this mundane formula is overpriced for what you get.

☺ **$$$ Calming Sensitive Mask** *($32 for 1.7 ounces)* doesn't contain copious amounts of calming ingredients, but it's still a well-formulated moisturizing mask for normal to dry skin that is not prone to blemishes. The fragrance-free, well-packaged product contains mostly water, plant oil, thickener, slip agents, nut oil, glycerin, plant-based fatty acids, antioxidants, plant extracts, emulsifiers, and preservatives.

BABOR HIGH SKIN REFINER (HSR) LINE

😐 **$$$ HSR Lifting Cream** *($94 for 1.7 ounces)* differs little from the emollient moisturizers Babor offers in their Advanced Biogen line, but it costs considerably more. I take particular issue with their claim that this product helps delay light-induced aging. Without sunscreen, that claim is completely bogus and potentially harmful to skin if you mistakenly use this alone to protect your skin during the day. It looks impressive that this moisturizer for dry to very dry skin contains many antioxidants, but it's all for naught thanks to the jar packaging.

😐 **$$$ HSR Lifting Cream Rich** *($105 for 1.7 ounces)* is a thicker but not necessarily richer version of the HSR Lifting Cream above, and this formula contains fewer antioxidants (and also uses jar packaging). Otherwise, the same basic comments apply.

😐 **$$$ HSR Lifting Eye Cream** *($68 for 1 ounce)* is remarkably similar to the HSR Lifting Cream above, and the same review applies, with one notable change: this product is fragrance-free.

✓☺ **$$$ HSR Lifting Decollete Cream** *($84 for 1 ounce)* is overpriced, but there's no denying it is a beautifully formulated moisturizer for dry to very dry skin. It contains non-volatile plant oils, lots of antioxidants (and in airtight packaging to keep them stable), elegant water-binding agents, and a tiny amount of film-forming agent. Although this is described for application to your chest, it can be used anywhere on your face (except around the eyes because of the fragrance).

☺ **$$$ HSR Lifting Gel** *($84 for 1 ounce)* won't lift skin, but will make it softer and smoother while also supplying well-known, effective water-binding agents. This product lacks significant amounts of antioxidants, which is why it didn't receive a higher rating. The mica and iron oxides add a sheer, shimmering tint to skin, but that isn't about skin care, just about glitter.

☺ **$$$ HSR Lifting Serum** *($126 for 1 ounce)* is a water-based serum that contains some good water-binding agents and a couple of antioxidants, including potent tannic acid. This won't lift skin, but it can be a lightweight moisturizer for oily skin, although some may not appreciate its slightly tacky finish.

☹ **HSR Lifting Foam Mask** *($50 for 2.5 ounces)* doesn't need to foam (foam has no effect on performance, it just creates an airy texture and reduces the efficacy of any antioxidants that may or not be present), and it contains too much alcohol to make it worth recommending.

☺ **$$$ HSR 28 Perfect Effect** *($157 for 28 0.02-ounce ampoules; total of 0.56 ounce)* is all about promoting and safeguarding skin's elasticity. There are some good antioxidants in these ampoules, but nothing worth the expense or special dose packaging. Further, although antioxidants can help repair skin to some extent, applying them topically won't result in renewed elasticity or a noticeable shoring-up of what age and sun damage have destroyed.

BABOR PERFECT COMBINATION LINE

😐 **$$$ Perfect Combination Day Cream** *($53 for 1.7 ounces)* is an OK emollient moisturizer for normal to dry skin. It doesn't feature a "perfect combination" of ingredients, however, and the effectiveness of the antioxidants is limited by the jar packaging.

😐 **$$$ Perfect Combination Concentrate** *($52 for 1 ounce)* contains mostly water, castor oil, slip agents, water-binding agent, witch hazel, soothing agents, thickener, fragrance, alcohol, and preservatives. It's hardly perfect, and the witch hazel prevents it from being too calming, but it's an OK option for normal to slightly dry skin.

😐 **$$$ Perfect Combination Night Cream** *($65 for 1.7 ounces)* continues Babor's pattern of spinning off the same basic emollient moisturizer formula within its subcategories. The plant and nut oils may vary, but the benefit remains about the same and the recommendation restricts its use to those with dry to very dry skin, but that's assuming you don't mind that the antioxidant's potency will be diminished as soon as the product is opened.

☹ **Perfect Combination T-Zone Control** *($48 for 1 ounce)* lists alcohol as the second ingredient and is too drying and irritating for all skin types.

😐 **$$$ Perfect Combination Mask** *($32 for 1.7 ounces)* redefines boring thanks to its dull (if somewhat confusing) blend of water, slip agent, castor oil, rice starch, plant extracts, fragrance, and preservatives. I don't know who this mask is supposed to be for: it's too rich for oily or blemish-prone skin and it's too absorbent for dry skin.

☹ **Perfect Combination Purifier Gel** *($28 for 0.5 ounce)* contains a lot of alcohol along with the allergenic plant extract *Plantago lanceolata leaf* (buckhorn plantain). It is not recommended for any skin type.

BABOR PHYTOACTIVE PRODUCTS

☹ **Phytoactive Base** *($25 for 3.4 ounces)* is designed for dry skin, but it irritates all skin due to its alcohol content and other problematic ingredients such as peppermint and rosemary.

☹ **Phytoactive Combination** *($25 for 3.4 ounces)* is similar to the Phytoactive Base above, but with a longer ingredient list and a different set of irritating plant extracts. It also contains a very good soothing agent, but any positive effect is canceled out by the effect of the irritating ingredients.

☹ **Phytoactive Reactivating** *($25 for 3.4 ounces)* lists alcohol as the second ingredient, and Babor recommends using it after their oily Hy-Oil cleanser. The alcohol will help remove the oil residue, but why bother with either product when a water-soluble cleanser works so much better without confusing the skin by first greasing it up and then drying it up?

☹ **Phytoactive Sensitive** *($25 for 3.4 ounces)* is similar to the Phytoactive Reactivating above, but adds oil and problematic melissa leaf extract to the list.

BABOR PURE LINE

☹ **Pure Day Cream** *($32 for 1.7 ounces)* is an average moisturizer that won't endear itself to your skin because it contains irritating horsetail, witch hazel, and volatile fragrance components.

☹ **Pure Night Cream** *($37 for 1.7 ounces)* is pure potential irritation due to the irritating horsetail extract and bevy of volatile fragrance components, including problematic eugenol.

☹ **Pure Fluid** *($37 for 7 0.07-ounce ampoules)* is purely irritating due to its alcohol content along with the potentially drying preservative sodium shale oil sulfonate.

☹ **Pure Mask** *($26 for 1.7 ounces)* is mostly water, clay, and alcohol. The absorbent and drying qualities of this mask are countered somewhat by the oils and waxes. It is neither clarifying nor calming, and contains many volatile fragrance components that can irritate skin.

☹ **Pure Clear & Cover Stick** *($17)* is an oil-, triglyceride-, and wax-based concealing pencil for blemishes that is little more than an eyeliner or lipliner with a clever name. The ingredients are a problem for breakouts, and the teeny amount of salicylic acid included won't exfoliate skin. Plus, the sheer peach tint does a poor job of camouflaging blemishes.

BABOR SELECTION PRODUCTS

😐 **$$$ Selection Ultimate Care Cream** *($84 for 1.7 ounces)* barely differentiates itself from most of Babor's other moisturizers for dry to very dry skin, unless you believe that champagne yeast is an epidermal sealer (it isn't, but the corn oil is). Once again, some very good antioxidants will become ineffective once this jar-packaged product is opened.

☹ **Selection Ultimate Concentrate** *($105 for 1 ounce)* contains a yeast extract from wine, but there is no proof anywhere that this ingredient is active or that it promotes skin's natural defenses. Even if it could, the prevalence of volatile fragrance components in this product, including linalool and eugenol, present a problem for skin.

😐 **$$$ Selection Ultimate Gel Spray** *($84 for 1 ounce)* is a spray-on moisturizer that doesn't contain anything unique or interesting for skin. The mineral pigments add a soft glow, but this cosmetic effect can be achieved with other products and without this expense.

😐 **$$$ Selection Ultimate Foam Mask** *($44 for 5 ounces)* uses propellants to produce a foaming texture, but it's hardly "ultimate" for skin, or even necessary for that matter. The non-propellant ingredients in this mask are standard emollients and moisturizing agents suitable for normal to dry skin; the champagne yeast has questionable benefit for skin, but may function as a water-binding agent.

BABOR SENSATIONAL EYES PRODUCTS

☹ **$$$ Sensational Eyes Cream** *($42 for 0.5 ounce)* features some great emollients to make dry skin around the eyes look and feel better. What a shame the antioxidants won't last long once this jar-packaged product is opened. This moisturizer is fragrance-free.

☺ **$$$ Sensational Eyes Fluid** *($32 for 0.14 ounce)* is a good, lightweight moisturizing fluid for slightly dry skin anywhere on the face. It contains a couple of antioxidants and some efficient water-binding agents, but it is not, as claimed, "masterful at eliminating lines and wrinkles."

☹ **$$$ Sensational Eyes Gel** *($42 for 0.7 ounce)* is a very basic gel moisturizer that provides a slight soothing benefit and is an OK option for smoothing barely dry skin.

☹ **Sensational Eyes Hydro Pads** *($15 for 5 sets of 2)* contains too much polyvinyl alcohol (a plastic-like alcohol usually seen in peel-off facial masks) to recommend its use around the eyes, and the witch hazel doesn't make this problematic product any better.

BABOR VITA BALANCE LINE

☹ **$$$ Vita Balance Day Cream** *($53 for 1.7 ounces)* would be a much better choice for normal to slightly dry skin if it contained a sunscreen for daytime protection and had packaging that kept the many antioxidants protected from light and air exposure. As is, this is a lot of money for what amounts to another basic emollient moisturizer.

☹ **$$$ Vita Balance Concentrate** *($52 for 1 ounce)* is a lightweight hydrating serum that infuses skin with a few standard water-binding agents, but that's about it.

☺ **$$$ Vita Balance Lipid Plus** *($68 for 48 capsules)* is an oil-based moisturizer for dry to very dry skin that contains antioxidants, and the capsule packaging will keep them stable per single use.

☹ **$$$ Vita Balance Night Cream** *($68 for 1.7 ounces)* is another emollient, jar-packaged moisturizer from Babor. The antioxidants won't have a lasting impact, but the nonvolatile plant oils, glycerin, and wax-based thickeners are good for dry to very dry skin.

☺ **$$$ Vita Balance Mask** *($32 for 1.7 ounces)* is very similar to the Advanced Biogen Mask above, and the exact same comments apply.

BABOR WHITE EFFECT LINE

☹ **$$$ White Effect Enzyme Cleanser** *($38 for 3.4 ounces)* is a talc-based cleanser that turns into a creamy foam when mixed with water. The enzymes it contains are notoriously unstable (not to mention that they will just be rinsed down the drain before they have any effect). Those features mean that this product cannot match the polishing that your skin can get with a standard topical scrub or gentle washcloth—or better yet, a well-formulated AHA or BHA product left on the skin.

☹ **$$$ White Effect 24h Lotion Combination SPF 8** *($40 for 3.4 ounces)* does not list active ingredients and thus should not be relied on for daytime sun protection; plus the SPF 8 is woefully below the SPF 15 or greater that is recommended by the American Academy of Dermatology and the Skin Cancer Foundation. This is a very boring moisturizer that doesn't contain a single ingredient capable of whitening skin, and the couple of antioxidants it does contain are listed well after the fragrance.

☹ **$$$ White Effect 24h Lotion Sensitive** *($40 for 3.4 ounces)* is similar to the White Effect 24h Lotion Combination SPF 8 above, minus the SPF rating. Otherwise, the same review applies. The only white effect this product offers is the wool it pulls over your eyes trying to convince you that it can do what it really can't do.

☺ **$$$ White Effect Cream Mask** *($37 for 1.7 ounces)* is a very good moisturizing mask for dry to very dry skin, but it has no whitening ability. Three forms of vitamin C are present, but not in high enough concentrations to inhibit melanin production (although each has antioxidant ability). The lactic and glycolic acids function as water-binding agents because the pH is above 4, which limits their effectiveness as exfoliants.

☺ **$$$ White Effect Intensive Concentrate** *($47 for 1.7 ounces)* does not contain any ingredients that can inhibit "the renewed formation of melanin." It's just a basic, water-based serum with some plant extracts that have no research establishing their benefit for skin.

OTHER BABOR PRODUCTS

☹ **Cleansing Gel** *($26 for 6.7 ounces)* contains irritating peppermint oil, so there is no reason to consider this overpriced option over countless other water-soluble cleansers.

😐 **$$$ Cleansing Gel & Tonic 2 in 1** *($32 for 6.7 ounces)* is a water-soluble cleanser that contains way too much alcohol to make it beneficial for skin, and it should definitely be kept away from the eyes.

😐 **$$$ Hy-Oil** *($29 for 6.7 ounces)* is an oil-based liquid cleanser that does a good job dissolving makeup, but you will still need to use a washcloth for complete removal. Why spend this much money for oil when soybean oil (the main ingredient) from the grocery store would do the same thing?

😐 **$$$ Mild Cleanser** *($26 for 6.7 ounces)* is a less oily version of the Hy-Oil above. This water- and corn oil–based liquid is an OK option for normal to dry skin not prone to blemishes; it will take off makeup, but you will need to use a washcloth for complete removal.

☺ **$$$ Mild Cleanser Foam** *($26 for 6.7 ounces)* is a standard water-soluble cleanser for normal to oily skin. It foams prodigiously, but the foam isn't what's cleansing your skin.

😐 **$$$ Hy-Pads Eye Make Up Remover** *($17 for 100 pieces)* are cotton pads presoaked with a blend of oils, emollients, alcohol, fragrance, vitamin C, and water. They remove eye makeup, but not without leaving a greasy film that must be rinsed or wiped away. This type of makeup remover is not preferred to water-soluble options or to those without fragrance and alcohol.

😐 **$$$ Mild Peeling** *($21 for 1.7 ounces)* is a creamy scrub that contains peach seed powder as the abrasive agent. It's a novel approach and a decent option for normal to dry skin not prone to blemishes—but it's overpriced.

☹ **Cleansing Tonic** *($26 for 6.7 ounces)* irritates skin with alcohol, horsetail, and peppermint oil. How this concoction is supposed to clarify the complexion is anyone's guess, but it's a problematic formula and should not be used.

☹ **$$$ Rose Toning Lotion** *($26 for 6.7 ounces)* is basically a classic rose-water toner that is little more than eau de cologne, and that is not good skin care in any way, shape, or form.

😐 **$$$ Algae Active** *($38 for 7 0.07-ounce ampoules; total of 0.49 ounce)* attempts to seduce you with the algae-and-thermal-plankton-from-the-deep-sea-are-essential hype, but they're none of that. Algae have water-binding and anti-inflammatory benefits for skin, but there are no species of algae in this "intensive" product, only plankton (which has no established benefit for skin). This gimmicky product isn't bad for skin; it's just not worthy of your time or money.

☺ **$$$ Cell Energy Fluid** *($38 for 7 0.07-ounce ampoules; total of 0.49 ounce)* provides a teeny amount of product in each ampoule; the fluid contains a blend of water, slip agents, a cell-communicating ingredient, antioxidant caffeine, soothing agent, thickening gum, plant oil, stabilizers, fragrance, and lots of preservatives. This can be a helpful hydrating serum for all skin types except sensitive, but the packaging makes it look more impressive than it is.

☹ **$$$ Complex C Cream** *($58 for 1.7 ounces)* contains vitamin C along with several other vitamins and various antioxidants, which makes it a shame that jar packaging was chosen. It has potential for normal to dry skin, but, for the money, the packaging disappoints.

☺ **$$$ Complex C Lotion** *($47 for 1 ounce)* is a lighter-weight, lotion version of the Complex C Cream above, but the translucent glass bottle won't keep the vitamin C or other antioxidants stable unless it is consistently kept away from sources of light. The overall formula is best for normal to slightly dry skin not prone to blemishes.

☹ **$$$ Express Relief Fluid** *($38 for 7 0.07-ounce ampoules; total of 0.49 ounce)* is mostly water, almond oil, thickeners, glycerin, panthenol, and plant extracts with no established benefit for skin. Labeling this as first aid for extremely stressed skin is sort of like considering a Twinkie and a Diet Coke a balanced nutritional meal. At best this will moisturize dry skin and keep it protected from further dryness—something any basic moisturizer can do.

☹ **$$$ Face Contour Fluid** *($38 for 7 0.07-ounce ampoules; total of 0.49 ounce)* is said to contain ingredients that flush out waste material from skin tissue, which is absurd. Skin cannot be flushed of wastes from the outside; while the process of sweating helps to do this, most other waste products are filtered by the liver and kidneys. And how anything in this lightweight serum is supposed to contour the face isn't explained—I guess once the wastes are flushed you'll stop looking so puffy? It isn't possible, at least not with this product. These ampoules contain some helpful ingredients for all skin types, but nothing that cannot be found elsewhere at a lower price and without the false claims.

☺ **$$$ HydraPlus Active Fluid** *($50 for 14 0.07-ounce ampoules; total of 0.98 ounce)* brings us more special ampoules, this time filled with a lotion that contains some great ingredients to help skin look and feel better. Although the ampoules are well sealed, the clear glass packaging will render the antioxidants ineffective if they are exposed to natural light for any length of time.

☹ **$$$ Mimical Control Cream + Q10** *($75 for 1.7 ounces)* is similar to almost every other Babor moisturizer. It's a good emollient option for someone with dry to very dry skin, but any potential benefit from the many antioxidants is stopped short by the jar packaging. This option contains peptides, which have water-binding and, theoretically, cell-communicating ability.

☹ **$$$ Moist & Vitality Fluid** *($38 for 7 0.07-ounce ampoules; total of 0.49 ounce)* is an OK, lightweight moisturizer for normal to slightly oily skin not prone to blemishes. The ampoule packaging is unnecessary, but if you want to keep the single antioxidant, in this case pomegranate extract, stable they should be kept away from natural light.

☹ **$$$ Moist Intense Cream** *($37 for 1.7 ounces)* is a good moisturizer for normal to slightly dry skin, but again the jar packaging poses a problem for the antioxidants.

☹ **$$$ Multi Active Vitamin Fluid** *($50 for 14 0.07-ounce ampoules; total of 0.98 ounce)* contains a few antioxidant vitamins in a water-based fluid whose ampoule packaging is unnecessary, although it may make you think you're getting something extraordinary. This can be helpful for normal to slightly dry skin, but is easily replaced by serums that come in larger containers, and that are much more economical.

☹ **$$$ Re-Beauty Fluid** *($25 for 7 0.07-ounce ampoules; total of 0.49 ounce)* continues Babor's endless, exceptionally gimmicky offerings of lightweight moisturizing serums packaged in ampoules. This version is nearly useless because most of the plant extracts have no established benefit for skin. You're left to take Babor's word for it that what's inside these ampoules is a "unique dermal rejuvenator." And I ask you, what are all the other endless Babor products for if this is the one that can rejuvenate skin?

☺ **$$$ Re-Generation Fluid** *($38 for 7 0.07-ounce ampoules; total of 0.49 ounce)* easily replaces the Re-Beauty Fluid above because it contains better ingredients, whose antioxidant activity or other helpful abilities for skin have been proven. If you like the ampoule setup, this is recommended for all skin types.

☺ **$$$ Re-Solution Fluid** *($25 for 7 0.07-ounce ampoules; total of 0.49 ounce)* won't regulate the skin's natural bacterial flora as claimed, but it will moisturize and soothe thanks to the well-selected ingredients.

😐 **$$$ Sea Creation Concentrate** *($250 for 1 ounce)* is sold as Babor's "smart cream" because it defends against free radicals at the cellular level. Never mind that even the top layer of dead skin can be considered the "cellular level" (after all, it is composed of cells). If this moisturizer is so smart, you may wonder why Babor sells dozens of other moisturizers. Do all those others lack intelligence?

The company claims that "*Thermus thermophilus* ferment" is the anti-aging miracle worker in this product. (But if it's such a miracle why isn't it included in other Babor products?) Supposedly, the ferment is harvested at 7,500 feet below sea level (because, of course, nothing that exciting for skin ever washes up on the shore), but *Thermus thermophilus* is merely a gram-negative strain of bacteria found both in shallow and deep water, and at varying temperatures. There is no research anywhere (aside from "statistics" from Babor, which are just wordplay) demonstrating that this bacteria has any benefit for skin, but I suppose it could function as a water-binding agent. It is known to be a stable source of enzymes and as such may also function as a topical exfoliant, but that's assuming that the active enzymes survive the manufacturing process of creating this product. It's a leap of faith to assume they do, however, and it will cost you a lot to find out. I recommend sticking with an antioxidant-rich serum paired with a well-formulated AHA or BHA product (and daily application of sunscreen rated SPF 15 or greater) as a far more sensible, proven anti-aging plan, rather than what this questionable, overpriced product offers.

😐 **$$$ Sea Creation Cream** *($400 for 1.7 ounces)* has claims that go even further than those of the Sea Creation Concentrate above. Supposedly, this product can reverse the aging process—but how far back do you want to go? 25 years? 4 decades, a week or two? And it's all due to the blending of the *Thermus thermophilus* discussed above with silk proteins. This is yet another emollient moisturizer from Babor that is incapable of reversing anything, except the look and feel of dry, flaky skin. The jar packaging won't keep the antioxidants and other air-sensitive ingredients stable and the volatile fragrance components may be a source of irritation. For $400, you should expect and receive legitimate proof that this really works as claimed. As is, you're left to believe that Babor's deep-sea exploration has unearthed the fountain of youth, though even the statistics they use to tout this aren't that impressive.

😐 **$$$ Sea Creation Eye Cream** *($175 for 0.5 ounce)* is very similar to the considerably less expensive (but still overpriced) HSR Lifting Eye Cream above and the same basic comments apply. The only reason to consider this one would be if you happened to believe that combining *Thermus thermophilus*, protein from mollusks, and algae extract can create a stress-activated eye cream capable of not only lifting eye-area skin but also regenerating its deepest layers. That's a drug-like claim, but not to worry—this cream won't penetrate past the superficial surface layers of skin.

☹ **$$$ Skin Guard Fluid** *($38 for 7 0.07-ounce ampoules; total of 0.49 ounce)* doesn't deserve consideration unless you like the idea of getting a standard moisturizing lotion formula out of scientific-looking ampoules. The plant extracts included have soothing benefits, but that alone doesn't make this worth the splurge.

☺ **$$$ Skin Revival Fluid** *($47 for 7 0.07-ounce ampoules; total of 0.49 ounce)* is a water- and oil-based moisturizing fluid that contains the cell-communicating ingredient lecithin along with ceramides and other ingredients that work to restore a healthy barrier function.

☹ **$$$ Wrinkle Filler** *($60 for 1 ounce)* is Babor's alternative to medical dermal filling injections. They claim that their microspheres of hyaluronic acid infuse into skin to plump up wrinkles. The problem is that instead of hyaluronic acid they've substituted the ingredient's salt form, sodium hyaluronate, which is not the same thing. Hyaluronic acid does have a plumping effect when applied topically because it can bind to many times its weight in water. However, the topical effect is minuscule and even when present it amounts to nothing more than moisturizing when compared to what injecting the pure substance can do, making Babor's claim more comical than factual. It's odd that Babor chose packaging for this moisturizer that will keep antioxidants stable, because there aren't many of them in here to preserve.

☺ **$$$ Express Protect Mask** *($21 for 1.7 ounces)* is lightweight but also a richer-than-you-might-think cream-gel mask for normal to dry skin. It contains some good water-binding agents as well as antioxidants, though these work best when left on skin rather than rinsed off. But there's no reason you can't leave this mask on as a moisturizer.

✓☺ **Fruitaction Mask** *($21 for 1.7 ounces)* isn't suitable for all skin types due to its oil content, but it is a fantastic moisturizing mask for anyone with dry to very dry skin not prone to blemishes. It contains antioxidant-rich fruit and plant oils, emollients, and some vitamin-based antioxidants. The price is reasonable and Babor keeps the claims realistic, making for an all-around treat because this product delivers exactly what it claims it does.

☹ **$$$ Intelli-Zyme** *($46 for 3.5 ounces)* is a very confused product, especially if you believe all the claims. This nonaqueous product has a powder texture (talc is one of the main ingredients) and its detergent is activated when you mix it with water, as you're directed to do. The product foams a bit and has a mild abrasive action on skin, but less so than a standard topical scrub. Babor maintains that the enzymes in this product are "intelligent" because they target only dead skin cells. (Interestingly, that's the case with all other exfoliants as well, because none of them reach below the top layer of skin, and the cells in the top layer are all dead; living cells exist only far below the skin's surface, so the claim is nonsense.) Further, enzymes are notoriously unstable ingredients, so how does Babor expect them to remain active when they've been mixed with a detergent whose action involves the breakdown of substances, including enzymes? Moreover, when this powder is mixed with water, the pH goes above 6, far beyond the range where chemical exfoliation can occur. Another claim Babor makes is that exfoliating with this product won't cause "upper layer thinning." However, if that were true, then the product wouldn't be an exfoliant; any mechanical scrub (even just a plain washcloth on skin) causes upper layer thinning because it removes superficial layers of dead skin cells—exactly what you want an exfoliant to do. This product isn't intelligent in the least, but it's still an option if you need a mild mechanical scrub that also has some cleansing ability, though a washcloth and gentle cleanser will do the exact same thing for far less money.

BABOR SUN PRODUCTS

😐 **$$$ After Sun Care Shimmer Gel** *($21 for 6.7 ounces)* adds a soft shimmer to skin, but in terms of providing what skin needs after sun exposure this formula falls short. It contains mostly water, aloe, slip agent, castor oil, and fragrance, which adds up to boring but okay for skin. Pure aloe from the health food store would be a far better option.

☺ **$$$ After Sun Care Soothing Balm** *($21 for 6.7 ounces)* is a slightly emollient body lotion that contains some good ingredients to restore a smooth, soft feel to dry skin. However, this doesn't beat the less-expensive body lotions available at the drugstore from Neutrogena, Olay, or Dove. Most of the really intriguing ingredients are listed after the alcohol, so they don't amount to much (the small amount of alcohol is unlikely to be irritating).

😐 **$$$ After Sun Care Soothing Mask** *($17 for 1.7 ounces)* is similar to, but less impressive than, the Fruitaction Mask above. The Fruitaction Mask would be a much better choice for soothing weatherbeaten skin, especially if dryness is a concern.

☺ **$$$ Medium Protection Sun Spray SPF 15** *($21 for 6.7 ounces)* contains avobenzone for UVA protection in a lightweight, water-resistant, spray-on formula. Babor recommends this for sensitive skin, but the synthetic active ingredients and the fragrance don't jibe with that directive. This is best for normal to oily skin.

☺ **$$$ Maximum Protection Sun Lotion SPF 30** *($29 for 6.7 ounces)* provides UVA protection from titanium dioxide and avobenzone (these actives are permitted for use in sunscreens manufactured outside the United States, and Babor products are made in Germany). This water-resistant moisturizing sunscreen is best for normal to dry skin not prone to breakouts. The amount of alcohol is unlikely to be problematic for skin.

☺ **$$$ Moderate Protection Sensitive Sun Cream SPF 20** *($27 for 1.7 ounces)* is nearly identical to the Maximum Protection Sun Lotion SPF 30 above, except this contains a smaller amount of active ingredients. Otherwise, the same review applies. This product is listed on Babor's Web site as High Protection Sensitive Sun Cream SPF 20.

☺ **$$$ Self-Tanning Cream** *($19 for 1.7 ounces)* is a good self-tanner for normal to dry skin not prone to breakouts. It contains the same self-tanning agent (dihydroxyacetone) present in most self-tanners, along with erythrulose, which builds a sunless tan over a longer period of time.

☺ **$$$ Self-Tanning Fluid** *($21 for 7 0.07-ounce ampoules; total of 0.49 ounce)* is a liquid self-tanner that contains dihydroxyacetone and erythrulose to turn skin brown. It's suitable for all skin types except those prone to blemishes, but the amount you get is ridiculously small. In addition, the ampoule packaging is just gimmicky, making it not only very difficult to apply evenly, but also very expensive to get an all-over self-tan.

☺ **$$$ Self-Tanning Lotion** *($32 for 6.7 ounces)* does not contain sunscreen so it will not protect against premature, light-induced aging as claimed. It's a standard, lightweight self-tanning lotion that contains dihydroxyacetone and erythrulose to turn skin brown. The antioxidants this contains are barely there compared with the amount of fragrance, so they're not an added benefit.

☺ **$$$ Self-Tanning Summer Effect** *($26 for 5 ounces)* provides instant sheer bronze color via cosmetic pigments and your "tan" develops over a couple of hours as the dihydroxyacetone goes to work. This formula is best for normal to oily skin.

BANANA BOAT (SUN CARE ONLY)

BANANA BOAT AT-A-GLANCE

Strengths: Inexpensive and widely distributed; various textures to please a wide variety of skin types and preferences; great selection of self-tanning products; some good sunscreen options with avobenzone or titanium dioxide (check labels carefully).

Weaknesses: Several sunscreens lack sufficient UVA-protecting ingredients; several sunscreens carry SPF ratings that are miserably low; a selection of products that promote tanning; no sunscreens for sensitive skin; problematic sunscreens for kids and babies.

For more information about Banana Boat, call (800) 723-3786 or visit www.bananaboat.com or www.Beautypedia.com. Note: All Banana Boat products contain fragrance unless listed otherwise.

BANANA BOAT KIDS AND BABIES PRODUCTS

☹ **Baby Tear-Free Sunblock Spray Lotion SPF 50** *($10.89 for 8 ounces)* makes much ado about being the first no-more-tears sunscreen spray for babies. This is a point that I, along with any cosmetics chemist familiar with sunscreen formulations, will beg to differ with. The active ingredient list is based around synthetic sunscreen agents (including avobenzone for UVA protection) that will indeed sting and cause tearing if this mist gets into the eyes. Further, this contains the preservatives methylisothiazolinone and methylchloroisothiazolinone (Kathon CG), which are contraindicated for use in leave-on products because they are strong skin sensitizers (Sources: *Contact Dermatitis*, November 2001, pages 257–264; and *European Journal of Dermatology*, March 1999, pages 144–160). This is absolutely not a safe product to use on babies.

☺ **Baby Tear-Free Sunblock Lotion SPF 50** *($8.99 for 8 ounces)* makes the same no-stinging, no-tearing claim as the Baby Tear-Free Sunblock Spray Lotion SPF 50 above, but at least this omits the problematic preservatives. The almost 30% active ingredients necessary to create the high SPF rating are not "as mild as water," though they're certainly effective at protecting skin from sun damage. Titanium dioxide is on hand for sufficient UVA protection and the silicone and wax-based, fragrance-free formula applies smoothly—but this is not a great option for use on babies.

☺ **Kids Dri-Blok Sunblock SPF 30** *($5.99 for 6 ounces)* is a lightweight, dry-finish lotion with nearly 3% avobenzone for UVA protection. The powdery finish is said to keep sand from sticking to skin and for the most part that's true (sand sticks much more readily to a moist finish, which this sunscreen lacks). This is a good sunscreen option for kids (or adults) who find most high-SPF products feel too thick or goopy on skin.

☺ **Kids Quik Blok Sunblock Spray Lotion SPF 35** *($9.99 for 8 ounces)* is a thin lotion in spray-on form that includes avobenzone for UVA protection. The amount of film-forming agents supports the waterproof claim, but "water-resistant" is the more accurate term. This will need to be reapplied after periods of swimming or toweling off. The tiny amount of aloe is of no consequence for skin.

☹ **Kids Sunscreen Stick SPF 30** *($5.89 for 0.55 ounce)* does not contain the UVA-protecting ingredients of titanium dioxide, zinc oxide, avobenzone, Tinosorb, or Mexoryl SX, and is not recommended.

☺ **Kids Tear-Free Sunblock Lotion SPF 30** *($8.49 for 8 ounces)* is absolutely not "as mild as water" (that's like saying soda pop is as good for you as a glass of milk), but this in-part titanium dioxide lotion has a silky texture and smooth finish that is water-resistant. The tiny amount of antioxidants included here is better than nothing, but they likely convey minimal benefit to skin.

☹ **Kids Tear-Free Sunblock Lotion SPF 50** *($9.49 for 8 ounces)* does not contain the UVA-protecting ingredients of titanium dioxide, zinc oxide, avobenzone, Tinosorb, or Mexoryl SX. This product is not recommended.

☹ **Ultra Mist Kids Tear-Free Sunblock SPF 50 Continuous Lotion Spray** *($9.99 for 6 ounces)* is, save for the name change, identical to the Baby Tear-Free Sunblock Spray Lotion SPF 50 above. As such, the same review applies.

BANANA BOAT SPORT PRODUCTS

☹ **Quick Dry Sport Sunblock SPF 30 Spray** *($8.59 for 6 ounces)* dries quickly because of the amount of alcohol it contains, yet that—coupled with the active sunscreen ingredients that include avobenzone—can prove too irritating for all skin types.

☺ **Sport Dri-Blok Sunblock SPF 30 Lotion** *($8.99 for 6 ounces)* is identical to the Kids Dri-Blok Sunblock SPF 30 above, and the same review applies.

☺ **Sport Quik Blok Sunblock Spray Lotion SPF 35** *($8.49 for 8 ounces)* is identical to the Kids Quik Blok Sunblock Spray Lotion SPF 35 above, and the same review applies.

☹ **Sport Sunblock Lotion SPF 15** *($8.99 for 8 ounces)* does not contain sufficient UVA protection and is not recommended for any amount of sun exposure.

😐 **Sport Sunblock Lotion SPF 30** *($8.99 for 8 ounces)* is a very basic, in-part titanium dioxide sunscreen in a creamy, moisturizing base suitable for normal to dry skin. The product needs to be reapplied, as all sunscreens do, while you are engaging in sporting activities outdoors.

☹ **Sport Sunblock Lotion SPF 50** *($8.99 for 8 ounces)* does not contain the UVA-protecting ingredients of avobenzone, titanium dioxide, zinc oxide, Tinosorb, or Mexoryl SX, and is not recommended.

☹ **Sport Sunscreen Stick SPF 30 ($5.79 for 0.55 ounce)** does not contain the UVA-protecting ingredients of avobenzone, titanium dioxide, zinc oxide, Tinosorb, or Mexoryl SX, and is not recommended.

☹ **Ultra Mist Sport Sunblock SPF 15 Continuous Clear Spray** *($9.99 for 6 ounces)* deserves credit for its broad-spectrum blend of sunscreen actives that includes avobenzone, but the amount of alcohol it contains will prove too irritating and drying to skin.

☹ **Ultra Mist Sport Sunblock SPF 30 Continuous Clear Spray** *($9.99 for 6 ounces)* is similar to the Ultra Mist Sport Sunblock SPF 15 Continuous Clear Spray above, and the same review applies.

☹ **Ultra Mist Sport Sunblock SPF 50 Continuous Clear Spray** *($9.99 for 6 ounces)* is, save for a higher percentage of active ingredient, similar to the Ultra Mist Sport Sunblock SPF 15 Continuous Clear Spray above, and the same review applies.

BANANA BOAT SUNLESS TANNING PRODUCTS

☺ **EveryDay Glow Daily Moisturizer** *($5.79 for 7.5 ounces)* is a standard self-tanning lotion that uses a lower amount of dihydroxyacetone than most, so color takes longer to develop and isn't too dark. Erythrulose is also included to develop subtle color after several days. Versions are available for fair or medium skin tones.

☺ **EveryDay Glow Face Daily Moisturizing Lotion SPF 20, For All Skin Tones** *($4.97 for 3 ounces)* is similar to the EveryDay Glow Daily Moisturizer above, except for the addition of sunscreen that includes avobenzone for UVA protection. Otherwise, the same review applies, and this is the one to choose if you're going to apply this minimal-color self-tanning lotion in the morning.

☺ **EveryDay Glow SunDial Face Self-Tanning Moisturizer, For All Skin Tones** *($9.57 for 3.4 ounces)* is a dual-chambered product that allows you to control how much self-tanner and moisturizer it dispenses per use. If you want a darker tan, dispense more of the water- and glycerin-based self-tanner. Less color? Dispense more of the emollient lotion to mix with the self-tanner. It takes experimentation to see how the ratios work for you, and dialing the component so it dispenses just self-tanner will leave you with more lotion which you may not need (and adding it may cause the self-tanner portion to streak). Still, this is a clever way to try self-tanning, and both formulas are suitable for normal to dry skin.

☺ **EveryDay Glow SunDial Self-Tanning Moisturizer, For Darker Skin Tones** *($9.57 for 6.7 ounces)* has the same packaging and application methods (and caveats) as the EveryDay Glow SunDial Face Self-Tanning Moisturizer, For All Skin Tones above, but the self-tanner portion contains a greater amount of dihydroxyacetone for darker color. Otherwise, the same comments apply.

☺ **EveryDay Glow SunDial Self-Tanning Moisturizer, For Lighter Skin Tones** *($9.57 for 6.7 ounces)* is identical to the EveryDay Glow SunDial Face Self-Tanning Moisturizer, For All Skin Tones above, and the same review applies. Lighter skin tones should notice the same self-tan results with either product.

☺ **Summer Color Self-Tanning Mist, For All Skin Tones** *($6.77 for 5 ounces)* is an alcohol-free, fine-mist self-tanning spray. It uses dihydroxyacetone (DHA), the same ingredient found in most self-tanners to turn skin dark. This option is well-suited for those with oily or breakout-prone skin.

☺ **Summer Color Sunless Tinted Lotion, Deep Dark** *($7.69 for 6 ounces)* is a very standard self-tanner that uses dihydroxyacetone to turn skin color darker. It's the second ingredient in this product, and as such is capable of producing a darker tan that's best for medium to dark skin tones.

☺ **Summer Color Sunless Tinted Lotion, Light/Medium** *($7.69 for 6 ounces)* is similar to the Summer Color Sunless Tinted Lotion, Deep Dark above, except this lotion has slightly less dihydroxyacetone for a less intense tan.

BANANA BOAT TANNING PRODUCTS

☹ **Dark Tanning Lotion SPF 4** *($9.69 for 8 ounces)* not only encourages tanning, which is unethical, but contains only a single sunscreen ingredient, one that is primarily capable of protecting skin only from UVB radiation. Using this is the fast track to wrinkles and future skin discolorations.

☹ **Dark Tanning Oil, Contains No Sunscreen** *($7.69 for 8 ounces)* has a name that says it all. This mineral oil–based product smells like a day at the beach, but the deleterious effects of the sun on unprotected skin are no picnic.

☹ **Dark Tanning Oil SPF 4** *($7.69 for 8 ounces)* is infused with all kinds of food ingredients and smells divine, but it encourages tanning, lacks UVA protection, and is an all-around disingenuous product.

☹ **Indoor Tanning Lotion** *($9.39 for 8 ounces)* is recommended for those who prefer to use tanning beds or booths, and is a very basic lotion that's wholly incapable of protecting skin from the up-close, concentrated doses of UVA radiation used in tanning parlors. Using this would be like smoking while receiving radiation treatments for lung cancer.

☹ **Protective Tanning Oil SPF 8** *($7.79 for 8 ounces)* lacks sufficient UVA-protecting ingredients, has a poor SPF rating, and promises a "deliciously dark" tan, and so paves the way for the damaged skin that those who tan will seek help for later in life from cosmetic corrective procedures.

☹ **Protective Tanning Oil SPF 15** *($7.79 for 8 ounces)* lacks the UVA-protecting ingredients of titanium dioxide, zinc oxide, avobenzone, Tinosorb, or Mexoryl SX, plus it encourages tanning. This mineral oil–based product is not recommended.

☹ **Sunscreen Lotion SPF 8** *($7.99 for 8 ounces)* has a too-low SPF rating and uses active sunscreen ingredients that leave skin vulnerable to UVA damage, making it one to leave on the shelf.

☹ **Ultra Mist Dark Tanning Lotion SPF 4 Continuous Lotion Spray** *($9.99 for 6 ounces)* and **Ultra Mist Tanning Dry Oil SPF 8 Continuous Clear Spray** *($9.99 for 6 ounces)* both sport SPF ratings that are too low and leave skin vulnerable to UVA damage while irritating it with alcohol. Avoid this at all costs!

BANANA BOAT GENERAL PROTECTION PRODUCTS

☹ **Maximum Sunblock Lotion SPF 50** *($10.39 for 8 ounces)* and **Sunblock Lotion SPF 15** *($9.04 for 8 ounces)* both invite you to celebrate the sun, but the merriment comes without sufficient UVA protection, making these two sunscreens not recommended.

☹ **Sun Wear Daily Sunblock Lotion SPF 50** *($6.77 for 6 ounces)* is a good, in-part avobenzone sunscreen in a silky, matte-finish base that contains some very good antioxidants and skin-identical ingredients. What a shame the Kathon CG preservative system makes an otherwise fine sunscreen ill-advised due to its potential for causing a sensitized reaction.

☹ **Sun Wear Faces Daily Sunblock Lotion SPF 30, Oil-Free** *($8.99 for 3 ounces)* contains the preservatives methylisothiazolinone and methylchlorothiazolinone (Kathon CG), which are contraindicated for use in leave-on products.

☹ **Ultra Mist Ultra Sunblock SPF 30 Continuous Clear Spray** *($9.99 for 6 ounces)* includes avobenzone for UVA protection but irritates skin with its strong alcohol base, making it a poor choice for all skin types.

😐 **Ultra Sunblock Lotion SPF 30** *($7.99 for 8 ounces)* is identical to the Sport Sunblock Lotion SPF 30 above, and the same review applies.

BANANA BOAT AFTER SUN PRODUCTS

☹ **Aloe After Sun Gel** *($5.89 for 8 ounces)* lists alcohol as the second ingredient and contains a mere token amount of aloe, making this a bad choice for after sun or any other time.

😐 **Aloe After Sun Lotion** *($5.99 for 16 ounces)* contains a hint of aloe and is primarily a standard, creamy lotion composed of water, thickener, mineral oil, coconut oil, slip agents, lanolin, and preservatives. It does contain fragrance and coloring agents. Skin deserves more after sun exposure than this average product.

☹ **Sooth-A-Caine Aloe Vera Spray Gel with Lidocaine** *($5.99 for 8 ounces)* contains the topical anesthetic lidocaine as the active ingredient, which is helpful. What's not helpful is the amount of alcohol in this product and the inclusion of irritating menthol.

☹ **Ultra Mist Aloe After Sun Continuous Spray Gel** *($6.99 for 8 ounces)* cools skin with a fine mist of alcohol, but the overall effect is more irritating than soothing, and truly beneficial ingredients are a foreign concept for this poorly formulated product.

OTHER BANANA BOAT PRODUCTS

☹ **Aloe Vera with Vitamin E Sunscreen Lip Balm SPF 30** *($1.99 for 0.15 ounce)* lacks the UVA-protecting ingredients of titanium dioxide, zinc oxide, avobenzone, Tinosorb, or Mexoryl SX, and is not recommended.

☹ **Faces Plus Sunscreen Stick SPF 30** *($5.49 for 0.55 ounce)* leaves skin vulnerable to UVA damage because it lacks titanium dioxide, zinc oxide, avobenzone, Tinosorb, or Mexoryl SX. The heavy wax base is not "ideal under makeup" as claimed.

BARE ESCENTUALS

BARE ESCENTUALS AT-A-GLANCE

Strengths: A well-formulated BHA product; good makeup removers (unless you wear waterproof formulas); a good loose powder and some impressive mascaras; several elegant brush options; not too expensive.

Weaknesses: One problematic BHA product; self-tanner with unidentified essential oils; the mineral makeup has its share of pros and cons and isn't for everyone; several of the loose powder products with shine have a grainy feel and cling poorly; greasy lipstick; farfetched claim that theirs is the healthiest, purest makeup in the world.

For more information about bare escentuals, call (800) 227-3990 or visit www.bareescentuals.com or www.Beautypedia.com.

BARE ESCENTUALS SKIN CARE

BARE ESCENTUALS BAREVITAMINS PRODUCTS

✓☺ **bareVitamins Skin Rev-er Upper** *($21 for 2.3 ounces)* rates as a very good 1% BHA (salicylic acid) product and its pH of 3.5 ensures exfoliation will occur. The lightweight lotion formula contains an effective blend of anti-irritants and antioxidants, while being fragrance-free. This is highly recommended for normal to oily skin battling blemishes or blackheads.

☺ **$$$ bareVitamins Eye Rev-er Upper** *($21 for 0.45 ounce)* claims to make you look like you got 12 hours of sleep, but this rather basic moisturizer doesn't adequately substitute for a good night's rest, or for a better formulated product. It contains mostly water, slip agent, occlusive agent, emollient, thickeners, silicone, antioxidant vitamins, plant extracts, skin-identical ingredients, preservatives, and mineral pigments (that's what creates the cosmetic brightening effect). This is a decent choice for those with normal to slightly dry skin.

☺ **bareVitamins Prime Time** *($21 for 1 ounce)* is a standard, silicone-based, waterless primer. Like others cut from the same cloth, it makes skin feel very silky and can improve foundation application. However, many lightweight moisturizers do this too, and supply skin with more of what it needs to look and feel its best. This product contains vitamin-based antioxidants in stable packaging, and that makes it a step above some other primers, though it's not a must-have if you're already using a silicone-enhanced moisturizer pre-makeup.

☺ **$$$ bareVitamins Lip Rev-er Upper** *($16 for 0.06 ounce)* is a stick lip balm based on macadamia nut oil. It applies smoothly and the amount of film-forming agent (it's the second ingredient) has some ability to keep lipstick in place, though it's not foolproof. This isn't the best for very dry or chapped lips, but is worth testing if you want something lighter to wear under lipstick.

OTHER BARE ESCENTUALS PRODUCTS

☺ **i.d. bareEyes Eye Makeup Remover** *($14 for 4 ounces)* is a standard, fragrance-free, detergent-based eye-makeup remover that does the job, but is best used prior to cleansing the face since the ingredients are best rinsed from the skin.

☺ **i.d. On The Spot Eye Makeup Remover** *($5 for 24 swabs)* provide a very gentle eye-makeup remover inside the hollow center of a cotton swab. Snapping the swab at the indicated point feeds the fluid onto the cotton tip, making for quick, convenient application. This isn't the most economical way to remove makeup, and the formula is too mild for stubborn or waterproof makeup, but it's an option.

😐 **Faux Tan** *($22 for 4.5 ounces)* contains dihydroxyacetone, the same ingredient found in most self-tanning products. This works as well as any, but gets a cautious recommendation because of the fragrance in its blend of essential oils. Without knowing which oils comprise this fragrance, you could be applying irritants to skin whose only benefit is smelling pleasant.

☹ **i.d. Blemish Repair** *($24 for 2.5 ounces)* has 1% salicylic acid at a pH that permits exfoliation, but it also contains alcohol, which makes this otherwise well-formulated BHA product too irritating for all skin types.

😐 **$$$ RareMinerals Skin Revival Treatment** *($60)* is reviewed below in the "Foundation" section for bare escentuals makeup because, despite the claims, this is not skin care, it is merely a powder foundation.

☺ **Buzz Latte Lip Balm** *($8 for 0.25 ounce)* is a good emollient lip balm in stick form. It contains helpful emollients and waxes along with token amounts of antioxidants.

☹ **Soy Mocha Lip Balm SPF 15** *($8 for 0.15 ounce)* does not contain the UVA-protecting ingredients of titanium dioxide, zinc oxide, avobenzone, Tinosorb, or Mexoryl SX, and is not recommended. The peptide in this lip balm won't help lips reach their "fullest pout potential."

BARE ESCENTUALS MAKEUP

FOUNDATION: 😐 **$$$ RareMinerals Skin Revival Treatment** *($60)*. The list of claims for this product make it sound like Nirvana for the skin. For all intents and purposes the showcased ingredient in this product is, well, dirt. (Dirt is my term, bare escentuals uses the term "Jurassic, virgin soil," but by any name, soil is just another term for dirt, although I have to agree soil does sounds less, well, dirty). I have to admit that seeing dirt advertised as skin care is a first!

RareMinerals Skin Revival Treatment is supposed to contain 72 organic "macro" and "micro" minerals. However, you won't find 72 minerals listed on the ingredient label, just Organic Soil Mineral Concentrate—so you have to take their word that these 72 minerals are present in the "virgin" dirt. According to the company, this mixture, along with the other ingredients, will produce firmer, smoother, and brighter skin while at the same time prompting exfoliation and reducing pore size. Essentially, this is being sold as a one-size fits all "skin-care" product "feeding" skin with everything it needs to look its best and function optimally. That part is definitely a stretch because, first and foremost, this powder-based product isn't moisturizing in the least (minerals aren't moisturizing, if anything they absorb oil), nor does it provide sun protection. Its mica base is there for the shine, and while other absorbent minerals are included they also prevent the skin-identical ingredients in the product from having much, if any, benefit for skin. Actually, the formula isn't too far removed from the original bareMinerals Foundation SPF 15. Both are loose powders that go on smoothly and impart a radiant glow to skin, the latter the result of those shiny particles of mica.

RareMinerals Skin Revival Treatment comes in four shades, including a Clear option that still imparts some color, and most of them provide enough coverage to camouflage minor flaws and redness, so you will perceive that your skin looks better. The recommendation to wear this at night is just shocking to me. Be forewarned that sleeping with this product on your face will result in makeup stains on your pillowcase, and that leaving this stuff on overnight would most likely be drying and irritating. Minerals on the skin, even plain talc or chalk or soil of any kind, aren't soothing in the least, and need to be washed off, not worn to bed, and this product is no exception.

Getting back to the mineral claims—is there anything to them? Does this "pure mineral concentrate" hold the secret to revitalized, youthful skin? Regardless of the purity of the soil, minerals cannot be absorbed by skin (their molecules are just too big), so any effect would be entirely superficial. Moreover, while there hasn't been much research on topical application of minerals, we do know that whether they are applied topically or ingested, minerals depend on other factors (most notably coenzymes) to work, and even when that happens the benefits aren't all that exciting (Sources: Cosmeceuticals, Elsner & Maiback, 2000, pages 29–30; and *International Journal of Cosmetic Science*, 1997, page 105). There is no substantiated research proving that minerals, whether concentrated or not, exfoliate skin or have any effect on pore size. Any perceived reduction in pore size from using this product is solely from its reflective quality and natural opacity, the same as any other powder foundation. It can work to temporarily fill in large pores, but when it's washed off any potential benefit is washed away at the same time.

You may be wondering about the vitamin C (ascorbic acid) in this product. According to the chemists I spoke with, ascorbic acid tends to remain stable in an anhydrous (waterless) product, which this powder certainly qualifies as. How much of the vitamin C reaches the skin is a question, however, along with whether RareMinerals uses an effective amount.

The bottom line is that although RareMinerals may be unique in terms of its extraction process and its use of virgin soil, those elements won't translate into skin care. It's just another form of powder, and a rather expensive one at that.

☹ **$$$ bareMinerals Foundation SPF 15** *($25)* is the loose-powder foundation that put bare escentuals on the map and it is the backbone of this makeup line. This talc-free, mica-based powder has a soft, almost creamy texture and an undeniably shiny finish (not a good look for someone with oily skin). The titanium dioxide and bismuth oxychloride lend this powder its opacity, medium to full coverage, and slightly thick finish. In addition, with 25% titanium dioxide listed as an active ingredient, broad-spectrum sun protection is assured. This foundation can be tricky to blend, and is best applied with a powder brush. Twelve 12 shades are available, with the best options being for fair to light skin. There are plenty of shades for women of color, but the high amount of titanium dioxide causes them to look or turn ashy on darker skin. The Tan shade is an excellent choice for loose bronzing powder.

☺ **$$$ Multi-Tasking Minerals** *($18)* are sold as colors to use as an eyeshadow base or as a concealer to be used with the bareMinerals Foundation SPF 15 above. These loose powders have less shine than the foundation, but are far from matte. A small but good selection of neutral shades (best for fair to light skin) is available. The Summer Bisque and Honey Bisque shades have 20% zinc oxide as an active ingredient, rating an SPF 20.

POWDER: ☺ **$$$ Mineral Veil** *($19)* is a talc-free loose powder with a softer and much lighter consistency than the bareMinerals Foundation SPF 15 above, and it applies matte. The two sheer colors have a dry finish that's best for someone with normal to oily skin. This is cornstarch-based, so avoid it if you're prone to or are battling blemishes.

BLUSH: 😐 **$$$ bareMinerals Blush** *($18)* has the same basic texture as the loose foundation, and the comments about its being messy and hard to control apply here, too. There are some matte shades of this product, and the application is soft and relatively even once you've mastered how much loose color to pick up on your brush for best results. Although it's hard for me to encourage this option, I'm sure some women will love it. 😐 **$$$ All Over Face Color** *($20)* is in this category because most of the shades are suitable as blush, not colors you'd want to dust all over the face. This is another loose powder with a shiny finish comparable to the bareMinerals Foundation SPF 15 above. Even the least shiny shade, Soft Focus True, has enough shine to make someone with oily skin nervous. 😐 **$$$ bareMinerals Blush Compatibles** *($22)* provides two loose powder blushes in one jar, with the colors separated by a divider. The sifter twists so you can more easily control how much powder is dispensed, but this still remains a messy way to apply blush. One shade is almost matte while the other is sparkling, and both have a dry texture that can go on somewhat thick but will blend better than you'd expect. Among the duos, use caution with the odd pairing of Pink Ice and Ginger Spice.

EYESHADOW: 😐 **bareMinerals Glimpse** *($13)* is a small collection of loose-powder eyeshadows with more emphasis on sparkling shine than pigment. They're for "whisper soft" eye effects, but the amount of shine these leave isn't more than a whisper amount, and it doesn't stay in place. 😐 **bareMinerals Eye Shadow** *($13)* has a much silkier, lighter texture than the bareMinerals Foundation SPF 15 above. They apply and blend well, with most of the shades going on softer than they look. Some of the shades appear matte in the container, but their noticeable shine is revealed on application. Speaking of shine, it runs the gamut here, from a "you're glowing" to a "you're blinding me" finish. This is still a messy way to apply eyeshadow, and the shiniest shades don't cling as well as they should.

☹ **bareMinerals Glimmer** *($13)* is an ultra-shiny loose shimmer powder with a grainier texture than the other bareMinerals powders due to the high amount of mica. Any flaking (and this powder does flake) will be extremely obvious. With almost 30 shades, this is clearly a star attraction of the line, but there are less messy, longer-lasting ways to add intense shine to your routine. ☹ **Foiling Glimmers** *($46)* offer four bareMinerals Glimmer shades in one kit and include a wet/dry eyeshadow brush. This is a lot of money for a lot of flaky shine, but it is eye-catching, and the teens I observed in the bare escentuals store were all abuzz over this kit.

EYE AND BROW SHAPER: 😐 **bareMinerals Brow Powder** *($11)* is loose powder for the brows that comes in six suitable colors, though this is an incredibly untidy way to shape and define your brows. Why anyone would choose this over a pressed matte brow powder (or eyeshadow) or even a good, standard brow pencil is a mystery. In addition, all of the colors have a subtle shine.

😐 **bareMinerals Liner Shadow** *($13)* would indeed work as eyeliner, and these intensely pigmented loose powders function wet or dry. They're not as grainy as they used to be, though every shade is imbued with shine, some featuring a metallic or glittery finish (and yes, the glitter flakes). Just as with the Brow Powder, this is a messy way to line your eyes, but if you're willing to tolerate that and have a smooth, wrinkle-free eyelid and lower lash line, go for it—with one caveat: avoid the obvious blue and green shades, which have nothing to do with shaping and defining the eye.

LIPSTICK, LIP GLOSS, AND LIPLINER: ☹ **Lip gloss** *($14)* is a standard non-sticky wand lip gloss with some attractive sheer colors. The same type of gloss can be found for less, and the minty fragrance this has makes me nervous. It's convenient that the ☹ **Lipliner** *($11)* does not need sharpening and is retractable, but the texture is too creamy to draw a defined line, not to mention the short wear time. ☹ **Quick Stick** *($14)* is an automatic, retractable lipstick/lip pencil combination. Almost as greasy as the Lipstick above, this isn't for anyone prone to lip color bleeding into lines around the mouth. It's an OK option if this type of product appeals to you.

☹ **Buxom Lips** *($18)* pledges to naturally create the look of fuller lips, something most lip glosses with light-reflecting shimmer can do. These sheer, sparkling glosses contain menthone glycerin acetal, which can be irritating, but the amount used doesn't even cause a tingling sensation, which means it's not doing much. That's not such a bad thing; as is this is an OK lip gloss whose stickiness doesn't make it preferred to many others, and the plumping effect just doesn't happen.

The ☹ **Lipstick** *($15)* offerings have some nice colors, but the formula is very greasy and won't last long, not to mention it will quickly migrate into lines around the mouth. How disappointing!

MASCARA: ☺ **Magic Wand Brushless Mascara** *($15)* doesn't have a brush, so the name is accurate. Instead, you get a stick with grooves that grab and coat the lashes, providing dramatic length in the process. It can go on heavy and wetter than usual, which sticks lashes together rather than creating a separated, fringed look. Still, the results are impressive if you're looking for a lengthening mascara. ☺ **Weather Everything Waterproof Mascara** *($15)* stays on no matter how wet lashes get, and manages to make lashes look decently longer with a soft fullness and clean separation. Unlike several waterproof formulas, this one doesn't make lashes feel dry or brittle, though it takes some effort to remove completely.

☹ **Big Tease Mascara** *($15)* really is a tease because this is not a mascara that will "get even the most timid lashes noticed." After considerable effort, this builds merely average length and minimal thickness. The dual-sided brush appears useful, but neither the long, thin bristles nor short, thick bristles produce anything resembling big, flirtatious lashes. ☹ **Mascara** *($15)* produces respectable length and some thickness, but not enough to distinguish itself from many less expensive mascaras at the drugstore. It's an OK mascara, but for the money, OK isn't enough.

☹ **$$$ Double-Ended Mascara & Lash Builder** *($26)* is a dual-sided mascara that includes a colorless lash primer and the same (original) bare escentuals Mascara reviewed above. As usual, the Lash Builder (primer) does little to impress. Actually, two coats of the mascara alone produced longer-looking lashes. If you're curious to try this type of product, L'Oreal and Maybelline New York have much better, less expensive options.

BRUSHES: The **Brushes** *($10–$28)* in this line are impressive, with almost as many options as makeup artist-driven lines such as M.A.C. Unfortunately, many of them use hair that isn't as soft as it could be, or they aren't shaped as well as others. Among the best options are the ☺ **Precision Liner Brush** *($12)*; the retractable, synthetic hair ☺ **Soft Focus Face** *($30)*, ☺ **Soft Focus Liner**, and ☺ **Soft Focus Eyeshadow** *($22)*; and the ☺ **Covered Lip Brush** *($14)*, ☺ **Double Ended Precision Brush** *($28)*, ☺ **Blending Brush**

($16), ☺ **Flawless Application Face Brush** *($22)*, ☺ **Eye Defining Brush** *($16)*, ☺ **Tapered Shadow Brush** *($14)*, ☺ **Wet/Dry Shadow Brush** *($18)*, ☺ **Eyeliner Brush** *($12)*, **Heavenly Eyeshadow Buffing Brush** *($16)*, and ☺ **Crease Defining Brush** *($18)*.

😐 **Maximum Coverage Concealer Brush** *($20)* is synthetic and works well to apply liquid products, but is too large for applying concealer to small areas, such as the inner corner of the eye. 😐 **Flathead Shadow Brush** *($15)* is cut straight across, which doesn't really have an advantage other than for applying a thick line of powder eyeshadow, a feat other, more versatile brushes can accomplish. 😐 **Angled Shadow Brush** *($12)* is too small for all but the tiniest amount of shading, but other brushes allow you to get the same effect while having other advantages.

The 😐 **Heavenly Eyeliner Blending Brush** *($14)* has enough firmness for eyeliner application, but tends to only draw a thick line and plenty of other tools can be used to soften or smudge eyeliner if smoky eyes are the goal.

Avoid the ☹ **Lash Comb** *($10)*, which features metal teeth that can be severely damaging if you inadvertently scratch your eye. If you prefer using a lash comb, stick with the safer versions that have plastic teeth. I'd also advise against the ☹ **Full Coverage Kabuki Brush** *($28)*, which is hard to hold and, for the manner in which it is used, not soft enough, and the too-stiff, scratchy ☹ **Brow Brush** *($12)*.

SPECIALTY PRODUCTS: ☺ **$$$ Quick Change** *($18 for 3.7 ounces)* has its place as a spray-on brush cleanser, especially if you're using the same brushes on multiple people or using one brush to apply very different colors. Those scenarios don't apply to most women, but the fact remains that this product works, albeit the dry time is a bit slow due to the glycerin it contains. For cleaning and sanitizing makeup brushes quickly and easily, I prefer Brush Off ($13.50 for 4 ounces), available from www.brushoff.com. Keep in mind that such products are alcohol-based, and consistent use can make natural brush hairs feel dry and brittle, and so are best for occasional use.

☹ **Weather Everything Liner Sealer** *($18)* is a tiny bottle of a liquid solution meant to make any bareMinerals powder last through all manner of wet weather or swimming. The formula contains mostly water, alcohol, and film-forming agent (the same type used in hairsprays). It smells medicinal, feels sticky, and although it does work to keep the powder colors in place when wet, the textural (and irritation) tradeoffs aren't worth it.

BECCA (MAKEUP ONLY)

BECCA AT-A-GLANCE

Strengths: The foundation and concealer shade range is spectacular; excellent eyeshadows; good lip gloss; several outstanding brushes; the bronzing gel and one of the shimmer powders are exemplary.

Weaknesses: Foundations with sunscreen that do not list active ingredients; the loose shimmer powders; poor cream eyeshadows; average mascaras.

For more information about Becca, call 415-553-8972 or visit www.beccacosmetics.com or www.Beautypedia.com.

FOUNDATION: ☺ **$$$ Stick Foundation SPF 30+** *($39)* is a traditional, creamy stick foundation with decent slip that can drag slightly due to the product's high wax content. Once warmed to skin temperature it blends quite well, and sets to a satin cream finish suitable for normal to dry skin. Coverage is in the medium range but it can be sheered out or made more opaque if needed. This foundation's sunscreen is one of the few with a higher SPF that contains avobenzone. Perhaps most impressive is the range of 27 shades, most of which are beautifully neutral. Whether your skin is very fair, very dark, or somewhere in between, chances are one of these colors will work for you. The only shades to consider carefully are the slightly peach Mallow and Pecan.

The Reviews B

☹ **$$$ Luminous Skin Color SPF 20+** *($40)* would have rated a happy face if the active ingredients were listed (a requirement of the Therapeutic Goods Association, Australia's version of the FDA here in the U.S.). Because they're not, this foundation shouldn't be relied on for sun protection, even though it does contain sunscreen ingredients, including avobenzone. The semi-fluid texture has almost too much slip, which makes blending take longer than it should. However, the reward is a sheer, natural finish that feels slightly moist and is best for normal to slightly dry skin. This is a great example of how natural a foundation can look while still blurring minor imperfections. Among the 14 mostly terrific shades, the only colors to avoid are Nut and Sepia, both of which are strongly peach and tricky to soften. The remaining shades present great options for fair to dark skin tones. Note that, as this book goes to press, some shades are labeled as SPF 20 while others list SPF 25. However, in the absence of designated active ingredients, such distinctions don't matter.

CONCEALER: ✓☺ **$$$ Compact Concealer** *($35)* contains two concealers in one compact. Both formulas are mineral oil–based and have smooth, thick textures that must be warmed (with fingers) prior to application. The Medium Cover version has a slightly softer consistency and provides nearly opaque coverage on its own. If you need still more camouflage, you can dab on the Extra Cover formula, which does provide a bit more coverage. In spite of the oil-based formula, both concealers set to a soft matte finish that is minimally prone to creasing. Unlike many other concealers that provide this level of coverage, Becca's version works without looking thick or obvious on skin (of course, blending is key, too). The range of 34 (yes, 34) shades is nothing short of remarkable because almost all of them are outstanding and present options for the fairest to the darkest skin tones. The ones to avoid due to peach, orange, or copper overtones are Brulee, Mallow, Toffee, Pecan, and Fudge. The Butterscotch shade is slightly peach but may work for some medium skin tones. If you're curious, Compact Concealer is much easier to work with than Laura Mercier's Secret Camouflage ($28).

POWDER: ☺ **$$$ Fine Pressed Powder** *($38)* has a beautifully smooth texture and natural, seamless finish. The talc- and rice starch–based formula is best for normal to oily skin, and applies evenly. Twelve shades are available, including several choices for very fair to light skin. The Carob and Cocoa shades have a slight tendency to turn ash on darker skin, so consider those carefully. ☺ **$$$ Pressed Bronzing Powder** *($34)*. With shade names such as Flamenco and Calypso, this bronzing powder is all about feeling energized, and it delivers a soft tan glow that makes you look as if you've been dancing the day away outdoors. The slightly grainy texture manages to apply evenly and sheer, and it's easy to build more intensity if needed. This is one of the better bronzing powders with shine because the result is glow rather than glitter.

☹ **$$$ Fine Loose Finishing Powder** *($35)* is talc-based and feels silky, yet its dry finish looks too powdery and, dare I say, too matte. Perhaps the flat finish is why sparkles were added to this powder, but even so there are more natural-looking powders in this price range, and below it, too. The only reason to consider this is the range of shades for very fair skin (Eggshell,

Bisque, Sesame, and Ginger are so close in color as to be indistinguishable on skin). The Carob and Cocoa shades are too ash for dark skin tones.

BLUSH: ☺ **$$$ Beach Tint** *($22)* appears at first glance to be a liquid-to-powder blush in a tube, but instead this has a lotion-like texture that's easy to blend, imparting translucent color and a slightly moist finish. Only one shade is available (best for medium skin tones) but this may be worth a try if you're looking for an alternative to powder blush. ☺ **$$$ Creme Blush** *($27)* is a modern interpretation of traditional cream blush. The smooth, slightly slick and creamy texture applies evenly though blending must be methodical due to the amount of slip (which can push product where you don't want it). The sheer to light-intensity colors are attractive, and each leaves a creamy finish suitable for normal to dry skin. Byzantine and Frangipani have noticeable shimmer and are best used for evening glamour.

😐 **$$$ Soft Touch Blush** *($29)* is a dry-textured yet soft pressed powder blush that comes in just two sheer colors and leaves its mark more with sparkling shine than pigment. The shine doesn't cling as well as it should, and overall this isn't a great powder blush.

EYESHADOW: ✓☺ **$$$ Eye Color Powder** *($20)* ranks as a standout product from Becca. This powder eyeshadow has an awesome silky texture and supremely smooth application that is highly blendable. Every shade has shine (including those labeled Demi-Matte) but it doesn't flake and the pigmentation in most of the shades allows for its use by many of skin tones. Although Chintz and Chiffon are both too green to use alone, they work mixed with other shades, particularly the many brown-toned options here.

☺ **$$$ Eye Tint** *($29)* is a liquidy eyeshadow packaged in a tube. Application is surprisingly good; it isn't as slippery as many others, but still demands careful blending. The formula sets to a slightly moist satin finish, and is waterproof as claimed. In fact, this is difficult to remove without an oil- or silicone-based cleanser. There is only one shade available, but at least the soft brown hue has broad appeal (except for darker skin tones).

☹ **Creme Eye Colour** *($25)* proves Becca's developers may have run out of creative steam after producing such stellar powder eyeshadows. These traditional cream shadows have enough slip to blend nicely, but they stay creamy and as such quickly crease and the intensity fades throughout the day. All of the colors are shiny, so keep that in mind if you decide to pursue this. Yet why anyone would opt for these over Becca's Eye Color Powder is beyond me.

EYE AND BROW SHAPER: ☺ **$$$ Brow Gel** *($16)* is a very basic, but good, clear brow gel that maintains a slightly sticky finish courtesy of the film-forming agent it contains. It has a bit more hold than most brow gels, making it worth considering if the kindest word used to describe your brows is "unruly." ☺ **$$$ Eye Liner & Water Proof Sealer Set** *($27)* is a powder eyeliner that is meant to be applied wet, and it works brilliantly in that regard, imparting rich, even color that lasts. Both shades (black and light brown) are matte. For enhanced longevity and waterproofing, Becca includes a tiny bottle of Waterproof Sealer. This alcohol-free fluid is basically water with several film-forming agents, and it works as stated to keep the powder eyeliner waterproof, as well as making it smear-proof. Although pricey, this is a well-done duo.

😐 **$$$ Brow Powder** *($20)* has a sheer application with a drier texture that's mildly prone to flaking during application. The formula would be better if the talc preceded the clay (kaolin), because that's primarily what contributes to the flaking. Still, applied sparingly, each of the five very good colors softly fills in the brow with natural-looking results. A tiny amount of shine is noticeable in the compact but doesn't really register on skin (or brow hairs). 😐 **$$$ Line and Illuminate Pencil** *($22)* is a dual-sided pencil with half being a standard, creamy black eyeliner and half being a soft-textured, thicker bronze color infused with chunks of glitter. The eyeliner portion applies well and is relatively smudge-proof, but the glitter on the other side of the pencil separates from the bronze color and flakes. Both sides need sharpening, but only half of this pencil is recommended, which makes it a tough sell.

LIPSTICK, LIP GLOSS, AND LIPLINER: As this book goes to press, Becca does not sell regular lipsticks. Instead, shoppers may wish to consider her ☺ **$$$ Glossy Lip Tint** *($22)*. This wand-applicator lip gloss has an emollient feel that's neither too thick nor sticky. You'll find most of the shades have a glossy finish with shimmer, and that the intensity varies from sheer to light. Although it would be easy to dismiss this as another lip gloss, what really sets it apart are the many attractive yet unusual shades.

☺ **$$$ Lip & Cheek Creme** *($27)* looks terrible on the lips because the formula tends to just sit on them and get cakey. However, it's fine as a pigmented cream blush with a finish that's almost powdery. A little goes a long way and it doesn't have too much movement, so blend swiftly.

MASCARA: 😐 **$$$ Water Resistant Mascara** *($19)* is, for the money, pretty darn boring. Lash emphasis never ratchets past midlevel on the wow-factor dial, and there are plenty of similar, average mascaras at the drugstore (you'll also find some truly extraordinary mascaras there). 😐 **$$$ Water Proof Mascara** *($19)* shares the same basic comments as the Water Resistant Mascara above, except that this formula is waterproof and takes more effort to remove (as most waterproof formulas do). It's OK if you aren't expecting much other than a mascara that stays on through tears or whatever tearjerker is being broadcast on *Lifetime*.

FACE AND BODY ILLUMINATING/SHIMMER PRODUCTS: ✓☺ **$$$ Pressed Shimmer Powder** *($34)*. These feel lusciously smooth and have a beautifully even application. The level of shine is moderate to high depending on the shade you choose (all of the shades are gorgeous and versatile), and it not only meshes well with skin but also doesn't flake. This is highly recommended for evening makeup or to highlight specific features.

☺ **$$$ Brazilian Bronzing Sheen** *($26)* comes in a compact and casts a sultry, sheer bronze sheen on skin. The slick formula demands controlled blending, and it sets to a dewy finish best for normal to dry skin. This won't last all day, but is good for casual, outdoorsy makeup. ☺ **$$$ Bird of Paradise Gloss** *($26)* is best described as a face gloss with subtle iridescence. A semi-solid delivered in a compact, it applies well and has a soft, creamy finish that does make skin look glossy. This isn't for anyone with oily areas, but is suitable for dry skin. ☺ **$$$ Jewel Dust** *($22)* are pots of highly pigmented, shiny loose powders. The colors are striking and allow for a variety of dramatic looks, though you have to want a theatrical flair to your makeup or be in full-on diva mode. Although the shine flakes a bit, the pigment stays and that's what provides most of the impact anyway.

😐 **$$$ Shimmering Skin Perfector SPF 20+** *($38)* does not list any active ingredients and as such should not be relied on for any amount of sun protection. This has a lotion-like texture with lots of slip, and provides a slightly moist, glowing finish that would be appropriate for normal to dry skin looking for a radiance boost. The shades are attractive and may be used alone or with a foundation, and each imparts very sheer color and a soft shimmer.

☹ **Loose Shimmer Powder** *($20)* comes in a tiny jar with a built-in sifter, and although that helps keep this weightless, shiny powder from being too messy, it clings poorly and leaves sparkles everywhere. I would have been less critical of this if the Pressed Shimmer Powder above wasn't so much better in every respect.

☹ **Fiesta Bronzing Dust** *($34)* is a very sheer loose bronzing powder with lots of gold shine. The color is beautiful but the shine clings poorly, and that makes application and wear too messy.

BRUSHES: The ✓☺ **$$$ Brushes** *($19–$64)* are another standout in this line. Almost all of them work expertly for their intended purpose, are well-shaped, full, and soft enough to warrant the splurge. The brushes are composed of natural or synthetic hair, with the synthetic-hair options being preferred for use with moist products. Particularly great are the ✓☺ **$$$ Powder/Blush 15 Brush** *($54)*, ✓☺ **$$$ Eye Colour Wash 36 Brush** *($37)*, ✓☺ **$$$ Brow/Liner Brush 09** *($25)*, ✓☺ **$$$ Eye Colour Blender Brush 35** *($30)*, and the versatile ✓☺ **$$$ Medium Tapered Brush 10** *($32)*. The only superfluous brush is the 😐 **$$$ Bronzer/Shimmer Fan Brush 39** *($35)*, and some may find the 😐 **$$$ Creme Blush/Bronzer Brush 34** *($37)* too firm for a smooth application.

SPECIALTY PRODUCTS: ✓☺ **$$$ Translucent Bronzing Gel** *($34)* has a cream-gel texture that blends easily and provides a truly translucent bronze color that's appropriate for light to medium skin tones. It isn't the least bit orange nor is it shiny, making it a prime pack if you're a fan of this type of product.

☺ **$$$ Line and Pore Corrector** *($30)* is similar in formula to most foundation primers, but Becca went the extra mile by including a few antioxidants (and in packaging to keep them stable, too). This sheer, flesh-toned product leaves a silky matte finish on the skin. That doesn't correct pores in the least but it feels soothing and soft.

😐 **$$$ Silky Hydrating Primer** *($35)* has a lightweight, thin lotion texture and is a very basic formula that contains a bit of silicone for a smooth finish. Unlike many foundation primers that are nonaqueous and silicone-based, this product is essentially a fluid moisturizer that isn't necessary pre-foundation if you're already using a similar product (with or without sunscreen).

😐 **$$$ Mattifying Primer** *($35)* doesn't contain significant levels of the type of ingredients that keep skin matte. It feels and performs very similarly to the Silky Hydrating Primer above, though it does set to a soft matte finish. Overall this isn't any different from prepping skin with a lightweight moisturizer, and there are plenty of those with formulas that are more state-of-the-art than this one.

BENEFIT

BENEFIT AT-A-GLANCE

Strengths: One of the few cosmetic lines that tries to bring fun back to skin-care, but succeeds more with their makeup; a good BHA product; Lipscription deserves an audition if you're prone to chapped lips; all of the foundations are good; two of the concealers are exceptional; well-deserved reputation for liquid blush and bronzer; Dallas, Hoola, Dandelion, and Georgia are all impressive; good brow-enhancing options; several good lip glosses; excellent shimmer products; enthusiastic sales staff that encourages customers to play with the products, all of which are accessible.

Weaknesses: No sunscreens in the skin-care lineup; mostly irritating anti-acne products; clever names and product descriptions are much more interesting than product contents; mostly unimpressive eyeshadows; the chunky pencils; lip-plumping products disappoint; mostly average mascaras.

For more information about Benefit, call (800) 781-2336 or visit www.Benefitcosmetics.com or www.Beautypedia.com.

Benefit Skin Care

☺ **$$$ Wooosh** *($22 for 5 ounces)* is a liquid-to-foam, fragrance-free cleanser that contains 2% salicylic acid (BHA) to "battle that one roaming boo boo," but it is rinsed off before it can be of benefit for skin. Still, if you avoid using this product around the eyes, its base is gentle and it rinses clean. The happy face rating pertains to this cleanser's base formula, not to its blemish-busting prowess.

☺ **You Clean Up Nice Face Wash** *($23 for 8 ounces)* is a fairly standard water soluble cleanser for normal to oily skin, but would be better without the peppermint extract. Still, there is very little of it in here and it's not likely to be a problem because this is a product that's rinsed from skin (and the peppermint is the extract rather than more potent oil form).

☺ **Gee...That Was Quick! Oil-Free Makeup Remover for Eyes & Face** *($19 for 8 ounces)* is a basic, gentle, fragrance-free makeup remover that makes quick work of most types of makeup. It's not the best for waterproof or long-wearing formulas, but is otherwise great to use before cleansing.

☺ **$$$ Honey... Snap Out of It Scrub** *($26 for 5 ounces)* is marketed as a dual-purpose scrub and mask, but is really just a thick-textured scrub that uses polyethylene (plastic beads) as the main abrasive agent. The plant oil and thickeners make this preferred for normal to dry skin, and the tiny amount of honey won't make skin snap to attention.

😐 **$$$ Dear John** *($30 for 2 ounces)* Dear Benefit: While I think many of your skin-care products have imaginative names and cute stories, I wish your formulas were just as beguiling and enticing. In most cases, they're not, and Dear John is no exception. This facial cream is described as having "brains and beauty," but in truth this product doesn't have an intelligent formulation. An impressive moisturizer would include recognized, state-of-the-art skin-care ingredients and technology. Instead, this is a paltry mix of water, castor oil, thickeners, a tiny amount of vitamin E, and preservative. Everything else is present in amounts too small to matter, so you have to ask: How beneficial is that? Not in the least. This moisturizer isn't terrible, just really disappointing. It would be OK for normal to dry skin, but it isn't anything I would encourage you to consider over countless other more elegant formulations.

😐 **$$$ Dr. Feelgood** *($27 for 0.85 ounce)* is supposed to be worn either alone or over makeup to smooth skin and fill in fine lines and noticeable pores. I guess you could also call this product spackle, because that is exactly how it works. The waxlike formula melts over the skin and then fills in the flaws (at least somewhat). You won't notice much difference in wrinkles or pore size, but long-term use may lead to clogged pores because of the waxlike thickening agents in this product. The first ingredient is cornstarch, and while this offers a dry finish, it isn't optimum for use over blemish-prone skin because food-based ingredients can feed the bacteria that promote acne. By the way, the tiny amounts of vitamins A, C, and E won't nourish skin and the packaging chosen for this product won't keep them stable.

😐 **$$$ Eyecon** *($28 for 0.5 ounce)* promises to fade dark circles—a phrase that is a surefire clue that you're reading a science fiction story designed to make you fall for the hope that dark circles can actually be alleviated. However, before you pull out your credit card, you should know that there is nothing in this basic, ordinary moisturizer that can fade dark circles—or even be any real benefit for skin. The hyped ingredients in this product—sweet almond and apple fruit extract—are barely present, but even if they were there in greater amounts, they come up short in comparison to countless other skin-care ingredients. So what you're left with is a moisturizer whose high concentration of film-forming agents may make eye-area skin look smoother and perhaps feel a bit firmer. But the effect is merely temporary, and it should be noted that at these levels the acrylate-based film-forming agents may pose a risk of irritation (Source: *International Journal of Toxicology*, November 15, 2002, Supplement 3, pages 1–50).

😐 **$$$ Firmology** *($30 for 1.7 ounces)* is sold as being "so sexy you'll be tempted to call it 'complexion lingerie,' " but it's all talk. This is a standard, water- and silicone-based serum that contains light-reflecting pigments for a nice glow. The silicone makes skin feel silky, but you can find it in lots of other products—including many body lotions at the drugstore—so there's no reason to consider this sounds-exciting-but-is-really-underwhelming product. By the way, the fragrance components in this product may cause a skin reaction if you're not using it with an effective sunscreen.

☺ **$$$ Sisters Ford Depuffing Action Eye Gel** *($26 for 0.5 ounce)* attempts to send under-eye bags packing, and is accompanied by a very cute description that makes it seem like a cure-all for puffy eyes. Not to burst anyone's bubble, but your puffiness won't recede one bit with this simple formulation that contains nothing unique or special. Given that the primary sources of puffiness and bags around the eye have to do with fat pads, muscles, and edema (swelling), there just isn't a cosmetic that can affect those biological causes. This lightweight, water- and silicone-based gel feels soothing and contains good antioxidants and anti-irritants, and it comes in opaque tube packaging that will keep them stable during use. The hydrolyzed soy flour, which Benefit claims will firm and lift skin, is chiefly used as a thickening agent, and won't lift skin anywhere. But if you think soy is the answer, Aveeno includes a better form of it in their products. As a lightweight gel moisturizer for around the eyes (it can be used on the rest of the face, too), this is an option. It does contain fragrance.

☹ **Boo-Boo Zap** *($20 for 0.20 ounce)* contains an unknown amount of salicylic acid and has a pH of 2. The pH encourages exfoliation, but coupling the salicylic acid with the alcohol and camphor in this product makes this exceedingly irritating to skin. Benefit's directive to apply this "several times a day" is akin to repeated slaps in the face.

😐 **$$$ Ka-Pow** *($20 for 0.08 ounce)* is sold as a before-bed treatment product to banish blemishes while you sleep. It contains 2% salicylic acid formulated in a surprisingly nonirritating base, but it includes plant oils, which don't belong in an anti-acne product. It would be great if dabbing this solution on blemishes was all it took to eliminate them, but that's not the case. Specifically, this product's pH of 4 is borderline for the salicylic acid to have value as an exfoliant, though it's not a throwaway product.

✓☺ **$$$ Lipscription** *($32 for two-piece set)* features a tube of **Buffing Lip Beads** that are a gentle, effective way to remove dry, flaky skin from lips. The plant oils provide some moisture, but the **Silky Lip Balm** is the real savior for dry lips. This Vaseline-based balm contains a film-forming agent to help it stay around longer, and enough silicones to warrant the silky portion of the name. Although pricey, this duo will keep your lips smooth, soft, and flake-free.

☺ **$$$ Smoooch** *($20 for 0.25 ounce)* makes mention that the vitamin E in this water-based lip balm will "cure, comfort and heal your lips while you sleep." Vitamin E alone isn't a star ingredient for lips—and pure vitamin E can be sensitizing for them—but more to the point, the amount of it in this product is next to nothing. The emollients, mineral oil, and waxes are what's working to keep lips smooth and soft, though this is a very expensive way to supply lips with those commonplace ingredients.

☹ **$$$ Jiffy Tan** *($24 for 6.7 ounces)* is a good alternative to traditional self-tanners for those who want an instant tan with no commitment. This tinted bronzing lotion does not contain dihydroxyacetone, the standard ingredient used in almost every self-tanning product on the market. Instead, it provides a tan tint to skin that you can remove with a cleanser, though it tends to stain skin and you must use a washcloth to remove it completely. More akin to body makeup, the flattering color looks convincing on light to medium skin tones. It would be better if the second ingredient weren't alcohol, but that is what gives it its quick dry-down. Still, this is an OK option for occasional use; just note that it does leave skin with a sheer layer of sparkles.

☹ **Jiggle Gel** *($26 for 6.7 ounces)* should be renamed "Irritation Gel" because that's about all this alcohol- and menthol-based product will do to your skin, jiggly or not. Not a single ingredient in this product will help reduce sagging or flabby areas of skin, regardless of how often it is applied, and it can cause significant irritation.

BENEFIT MAKEUP

FOUNDATION: ☺ **$$$ PlaySticks** *($32)* is one of the few foundation sticks left and it remains a very good choice. It must be blended quickly because it dries to a powder finish almost immediately, and the finish does have longevity. Coverage can go from light to medium and the drier finish makes this suitable for normal to slightly oily skin only; it won't hold up as the day goes by for those with very oily skin. Each of the ten colors is soft and neutral, and options for fair and dark skin are included.

☺ **$$$ Nonfiction** *($30)* has a beautiful, smooth texture that glides over skin and feels lighter than you'd expect given the product's slightly moist finish. It provides light to medium coverage and is suitable for normal to dry skin. The ten shades aren't as impressive when compared to the PlaySticks foundation above, but enough of them are good to make this worth considering. Avoid Volumes 3, 5, and 10 due to overtones of pink, peach, and copper.

☺ **$$$ You Rebel SPF 15** *($28)* is Benefit's only foundation-with-sunscreen option and although the sunscreen is in-part avobenzone, only one sheer shade is available. This qualifies more as tinted moisturizer than foundation, and its creamy texture leaves a slightly moist sheen, making it suitable for normal to dry skin.

☺ **$$$ Some Kind-A-Gorgeous** *($26)* is meant to be one-shade-fits-all sheer foundation that "evens skin tone without the look or feel of makeup." Although this is indeed lightweight thanks to its silicone-enhanced cream-to-powder texture, it isn't translucent enough to work on any skin tone. Some Kind-A-Gorgeous is best for fair to almost medium skin tones, and provides minimal coverage with a satin matte finish.

CONCEALER: ✓☺ **$$$ Lyin' Eyes** *($18)* is the clever name for this click-pen concealer that you apply with a built-in synthetic brush. Each of the three skinlike shades applies with ease and provides medium coverage while setting to a smooth matte finish. It does a great job of convincingly concealing minor flaws without looking like you're hiding something—and that's the truth! ✓☺ **$$$ Galactic Shield!** *($20)* is a pencil-style concealer in a twist-up container (no sharpening needed), and includes 2% salicylic acid (BHA) for blemish-fighting. The pH is not low enough to allow the BHA to function as an exfoliant. Still, while it isn't the best for battling blemishes, it does provide outstanding coverage of blemishes and red spots. Also, the pencil format allows pinpoint application, and it blends well without having too much slip. The three neutral shades provide a smooth matte finish and make this a great option for normal to oily skin.

☹ **$$$ Boi-ing** *($18)* is billed as "the world's best concealer," which makes me wonder why Benefit sells several other (better) concealers. If this is the best, then wouldn't everything else pale in comparison? Regardless, this cream-to-powder concealer (which leans toward being creamier) provides almost complete coverage and blends easily. It layers well if you need to camouflage very dark circles, but won't last through the day unless it's set with powder, which can make the under-eye area look dry and cakey. Among the three shades, only Medium is too peach to strongly consider.

☹ **You're Bluffing** *($22)* is a twist-up cream concealer meant to camouflage redness, but its single yellow shade would add a strange, obvious hue to most skin tones unless it is blended on very sheerly. Of course, doing so means that blotchy or ruddy spots would receive minimal coverage, so the result is almost no effect at all. You're Bluffing is too slick and creamy to use over blemishes. ☹ **It-Stick** *($18; $4 for sharpener)* is a thick pencil concealer intended to "cease the crease" and fade expression lines. There is only one color, a fleshy peach, which won't work on most skin tones, and the creamy texture dries to an unflattering finish that looks heavy and tends to crease in your creases. ☹ **Eye Bright** *($18; $4 for sharpener)* is a pale pink, slightly greasy pencil meant to be used on the dark inner corners of the eyes. It is completely unnecessary because any neutral-shade concealer can do the same without the unflattering pink tint.

POWDER: ☺ **$$$ Get Even** *($28)* has gotten better. This talc-based pressed powder used to tint skin with its yellow to cantaloupe-orange shades, but now the three colors are toned down and go on sheer. That means less coverage, but the payoff is smooth skin that looks polished, not powdered. The shade range still isn't that neutral, but these apply so softly, it's hardly an issue. ☺ **$$$ Hoola** *($28)* is a pricey, but excellent, bronzing powder. If you don't mind parting with this much moola, you'll find that Hoola has a smooth texture, minimally shiny finish, and a believable tan color that is very flattering on fair to medium skin.

☹ **Bluff Dust** *($22)* just doesn't look convincing on skin, no matter how sheerly you apply it (or how good your bluffing skills are). This is yet another yellow-toned product meant to conceal redness, but it is so intense that skin ends up looking more yellow. None of this is attractive, and you will find that a natural-looking, skin-tone foundation does a much better job of evening out your own skin tone.

BLUSH: ✓☺ **$$$ BeneTint** *($28)* has become a beauty classic, though it's not for everyone. This simple, rose-tinted, liquid cheek color only looks good on flawless, smooth skin. It can be used as a lip stain, and is relatively long-lasting in that capacity. If you prefer liquid blush, this is deservedly one of the best. ✓☺ **$$$ Glamazon** *($26)* is virtually identical to the BeneTint, but this is a sheer, believable bronze tint. If your skin is perfectly smooth and even, it will work well. Note: this product and BeneTint dry quickly, so blending must be fast and precise.

☺ **$$$ Dandelion** *($28)* is positioned as a highlighting powder but works best as a pale pink blush. It has a very soft gold undertone and a sheer amount of shine. This has a nice, smooth texture and the pressed powder is finely milled, so application is even, if a bit sheer. Color-wise, Dandelion is best for those with fair to light skin tones who want a touch of shine. Although it's pricey, the good news is that the shine is muted enough to not be distracting when worn for daytime makeup. ☺ **$$$ Dallas** *($28)* promises an "outdoor glow for the indoor gal" and it delivers this via shine that leaves skin with a healthy glow. The nude pink shade has a soft tan undertone and is bound to become a Benefit favorite because this color is foolproof for many skin tones.

☺ **$$$ Georgia** *($28)* is a lovely pressed powder blush that comes in one shade, a soft, pink-peach. It goes on smoothly and offers more shine than Dallas or Dandelion, making it trickier (but still an option) for daytime wear.

☹ **Powder Blush** *($22)* is pricier than ever but doesn't have an outstanding formula to support it. This is a disappointing blush due to its dry texture and uneven, spotty application. Almost all department store lines (and many at the drugstore) have powder blushes whose texture and application best this product.

EYESHADOW: ☺ **Powder Eyeshadow** *($14)* sports an enviably silky texture that glides onto skin and blends easily. All of the shades go on sheer and have at least a slight amount of shine, with the almost-matte options being Pass the Potatoes and Don't Rock the Boat. Those names are a kick, and by far the most entertaining aspect of this product. By the way, Benefit describes their eyeshadow palette as "trendy neutrals," but there are far too many green and blue hues to qualify the collection as neutral!

😐 **Creme Eyeshadow** *($14)* has a creamy, slick feel and a minimal powder finish. The formula now creases, which explains why Benefit dropped an earlier portion of the name. Only six shades remain, all very shiny, and since most are pastel to soft colors these are best for highlighting the brow bone, assuming yours is smooth and firm.

😐 **$$$ F.Y...eye!** *($22)* is an overpriced, peach-toned eyeshadow base that adds a subtle, strange tone to the eye area. This stays slick on the skin but has a powdery finish. Your foundation or matte-finish concealer will work better. 😐 **$$$ Lemon-Aid** *($18)* is an unnecessary pale yellow eyeshadow base that has a thick, creamy texture; it does not work as well as a neutral foundation for minimizing discoloration. 😐 **$$$ High Brow** *($20; $5 for sharpener)* is a creamy, chunky pencil whose pastel pink color is designed to highlight and *visually* "lift" the underbrow area. It can do that, assuming you apply it sparingly and blend well. This pencil's texture makes it relatively easy to apply and soften, but it stays slightly moist and so is prone to smearing and fading. The highlighting concept this pencil espouses is an important part of a classic eye makeup design, but the effect is as achievable—and longer-lasting—when created with a light-toned traditional powder eyeshadow. Not only is this pencil unessential, it also requires sharpening.

EYE AND BROW SHAPER: ☺ **$$$ Speed Brow** *($16)* works well as a sheer brow tint while helping to groom and keep stray hairs in place. A Clear Speed Brow option is available, as are shades for dark blonde to light brown and medium to dark brows. Speed Brow dries quickly and the brush is small enough to allow for precision grooming of thin or sparse brows. If you're considering the Clear version, keep in mind that a container of Maybelline New York's Great Lash Clear Mascara costs one-third the price and has four times as much product. ☺ **$$$ Brow Zings** *($30)* have been improved and are now more thoughtfully assembled. Included in one compact are two coordinated brow colors (in a creamy wax and powder cake) along with two tiny but functional brushes and a mini pair of tweezers. The non-greasy, wax-based color is good for tinting and grooming unruly brows, while the powder is for softer accenting or less dramatic shading. It's true that brushes this size are no match for those of standard length, but for travel or purse, what's included here is workable and not scratchy or flimsy.

😐 **$$$ Sketching Pencils Eyes** *($16)* are standard pencils that have a soft, creamy, ready-to-smudge texture. Application is easy, but you might as well use the included smudger before the pencil does so on its own. 😐 **$$$ Babe Cakes** *($22)* is a standard cake eyeliner that is applied wet and then dries to a liquid liner–like finish, though not as intense. One pairing of brown and deep black is available, and is an OK option if you prefer this method for eyelining. ☹ **$$$ She-Laq** *($28)* is meant as a sealant for lipstick, eyeliner, or brow color. It's a thick, alcohol-based liquid with hairspray ingredients that should not go anywhere near the eye, as the irritation potential is just too high. Otherwise, it's just an expensive variation on brow gel, and the supplied applicators and tools are inferior to professional brushes.

☹ **Bad Gal, Gilded, and Mr. Frosty** *($18; $5 for sharpener)* are standard chunky pencils that are all creamy enough to consistently smear and fade. It may seem impressive that all of these pencils are heralded by major fashion magazines, but remember, such publications applaud many products that are mediocre to poor, or just plain irritating.

LIPSTICK, LIP GLOSS, AND LIPLINER: ☺ **$$$ BeneTint Lip Balm** *($20)* is a standard, but good, castor oil–based lip gloss with a texture that is not too sticky and a sheer, cherry-red color that would work well on a variety of skin tones.

☺ **$$$ BeneTint Pocket Pal** *($20)* is a dual-sided wand that features a vial of BeneTint liquid on one end and a clear lip gloss on the other. You brush the BeneTint on lips, allow it to dry, and then top it with the lip gloss (which is necessary because BeneTint on its own does not moisturize lips). If you like the way BeneTint colors your lips and want a glossy finish, this is recommended!

☺ **$$$ Her Glossiness V.I.P. Lip Gloss** *($16)* is a standard lip gloss with a thick texture, slightly sticky finish, and selection of sheer colors with classic Benefit names such as "Life on the A-List." It is inaccurately described as "impossibly shiny," but I can think of several glosses that offer a shinier finish than this, so although there is nothing wrong with this gloss the expense is considerable compared to what's available at the drugstore.

☺ **The Gloss** *($14)* isn't different from most other glosses, at least those that have a smooth application and relatively non-sticky texture, which is good. The translucent (and extensive) selection of colors features mostly safe options—meaning nothing too bright, bold, or garish. A colorless option is available, too.

☹ **$$$ Color Plump Plumping Lip Color** *($22; $4 for special sharpener)* is the return of the chubby lip pencil, a trend I thought had finally and thankfully gone the way of other extinct and out-of-date makeup dinosaurs. Why Benefit brought it back is a good question, because the constant sharpening these pencils require is a pain. Gripes aside, the product does have a smooth, easy-to-apply texture that feels creamy without being slippery. As for Benefit's claim that their tripeptide complex enhances lip volume, don't bet on it. The amount of peptides in this pencil is minimal (it's the very last ingredient listed) and there is no substantiated proof that peptides in minor amounts, or for that matter even in large amounts, prompt fuller lips—and they are in no way comparable to the results you get from collagen injections. What's making lips look fuller is the soft, reflective shimmer each light-coverage shade has, and that's a benefit you can get from many lipsticks. Benefit's ☹ **$$$ Lipstick** *($16)*, much like their eyeshadows, is all about the playful to humorous shade names. Favorites (for names) include "But Officer," "One Hit Wonder," and "Luck Be a Lady." The lipstick itself is rather ordinary, with a texture that's more waxy than creamy and that supplies medium coverage. Despite the fun names, these feel old-fashioned compared to the ultra-smooth, often lightweight lipsticks from lines such as Estee Lauder and Lancome.

☹ **$$$ California Kissin'** *($16)* is a sheer, blue-tinted lip gloss that's also mint-flavored and said to brighten your smile. The blue tint is soft enough to not interfere with whatever lipstick it is paired with, but that also means it won't make teeth look any whiter. It is otherwise a standard emollient lip gloss that's pricey for what you get.

☹ **$$$ Sketching Pencils Lips** *($16)* has a less creamy texture than most standard lip pencils and glides on easily without smearing. If only it didn't need sharpening—a part of the picture that keeps it from earning a happy face rating. ☹ **$$$ D'finer D'liner Clear Lipliner** *($18)* beckons you to "conquer the feather factor," meaning that this needs-sharpening pencil, meant to be applied on the border of your lips, will keep lipstick locked in place for hours. It works marginally well, but the oil-based formula doesn't hold up as long as similar products whose base is made up of stay-put silicones. Although described as clear, this product has a faint pink color and leaves a subtle shimmer finish, so it sort of looks like you missed your lips a bit. Those with a consistent problem of lipstick feathering into lines around the mouth will likely be disappointed by this product's brief staying time.

MASCARA: ☺ **$$$ Get Bent Wonder Lifting Mascara** *($19)* does have a bent brush, and if you like the concept, you can manipulate any mascara brush head in this manner. This "whole new angle" on mascara is more gimmicky than anything else, but that's forgivable because this quickly produces long, lifted, beautifully separated lashes without clumps or smearing. The mascara formula keeps lashes softer than most, and allows you to apply multiple coats without incident—though this does eventually reach the point of diminishing returns.

☹ **$$$ Plush Mascara** *($18)* takes a long time to build what amounts to minimal length and no thickness. It doesn't clump during application or flake during wear, but if you're looking for a product that delivers on its promise of sexy lashes, this one will leave you disappointed. ☹ **$$$ Bad Gal Lash Mascara** *($19)* is not, in the words of Benefit, "like wearing a set of false eyelashes without the glue." From the box to the oversized brush, everything about this mascara is big except the results. It does apply cleanly and evenly, with no clumps in sight, but after much effort for moderate length and minimal thickness, I wasn't ready to put on a black leather jacket and ride off into the night on the back of a motorcycle. I was ready for a nap!

FACE AND BODY ILLUMINATING/SHIMMER PRODUCTS: ✓☺ **$$$ 10** *($28)* tempts you to "be a perfect 10," and although it takes more than this cosmetic to go from bland to glam, without question you'll be pleased with the wonderfully silky texture and smooth application. This pressed shimmer powder is housed in a large cardboard box and includes a pale pink and sheer bronze shade with no divider in between. The concept is to bronze and highlight but this is best for highlighting by adding soft touches of shine because the bronze shade is so sheer. The shine clings well and is glow-y without being too show-y, making for an attractive, though pricey, evening look.

☺ **$$$ High Beam** *($24)* comes in a nailpolish bottle and is applied to the face with a brush (or you can use a sponge or your fingers). It is a silvery-pink shimmer lotion that dries to a matte finish, leaving the shine behind. ☺ **$$$ Moon Beam** *($24)* is identical to High Beam except for its golden pink color. Both products tend to stay put and are much easier to control than shimmer powders with their minimal ability to cling. ☺ **$$$ Flamingo Fancy** *($24)* is a shimmering body lotion whose shine is an attractive mix of peach, pink, gold, and bronze. This is too fragranced for use on the face, especially the eye area. However, from the neck down and for special occasions, it's a fun option.

☹ **$$$ Hollywood Glo** *($24)* is another bottle of liquid shimmer lotion with a pale golden pink shimmer. Compared to High Beam and Moon Beam above, the shine is subtle and works under or over foundation or moisturizer to highlight skin, but only if your nose can tolerate the potent rosy fragrance of this product (it's strong enough to clash with your regular perfume). ☹ **$$$ Hollywood Glo Body Lustre** *($26)* is a shimmer-infused body balm that leaves skin shiny but is also over-scented. It's a decent option, but make sure you like the fragrance, because it really lingers.

☹ **Show Offs** *($16)* are small jars of iridescent loose powder that are pretty to look at but messy to apply. The shine from most of the shades is intense and sparkling, but this flakes off easily so don't count on its lasting or staying in place.

BRUSHES: As this book goes to press Benefit had discontinued all their brushes. They are expected to be relaunched late 2007.

☺ **Bluff Puff** *($20)* is a powder brush with a stubby handle that fits easily into the palm of your hand for dusting the face with powder. The brush head is firm but soft, and the densely packed bristles hold powder well and distribute it evenly. I wouldn't use this with Benefit's too-yellow Bluff Dust above, but it is a suitable alternative to traditional brushes for applying loose or pressed powders that come in true skin-tone shades.

SPECIALTY PRODUCTS: ☺ **$$$ Rush Hour** *($20)* is sold as an instant makeover for lips and cheeks, promising to refresh your look in ten seconds or less. Packaged like a standard slim lipstick, this has a creamy but light texture that's closer to a lipstick than a cream-to-powder blush. The single shade was designed to be so versatile that anyone can use it, and for the most part that's true. It's a medium rosy pink with a hint of mauve that complements many skin tones—just don't expect it to show up well on very dark skin. Rush Hour is comfortable to wear on lips and has a nearly opaque, creamy finish. On cheeks, the shade definitely works for blush and can be sheered out to create a soft flush of color.

😐 **$$$ Ooo La Lift** *($20)* feels like an "instant eye lift!"—or so Benefit would like you to believe. This is just a pale pink liquid highlighter with a smooth texture and a slight shine. There is absolutely nothing in it to support the "depuffing and firming" claims, though using this under the eyes to banish dark areas will make puffiness less apparent.

☹ **Lip Plump** *($20)* has been around for too long when you consider its lackluster performance, inconvenient application, and price. It supposedly smooths and builds the contour of the lips, but is really just a lightweight, flesh-toned concealer that minimally fills in lip lines and takes too long to set. Even the Benefit counter personnel agreed this is a product that is difficult to work with, messy to apply, and, perhaps most importantly, doesn't really work. It's not that often I get such candid comments from a line's representatives, but I think they sum up this product exactly!

☹ **De-groovie** *($28)* is supposed to prevent lipstick from feathering and to some extent this thick, wax-based product works. However, the formula contains lavender oil, which poses problems for lips and skin.

BIORE (SKIN CARE ONLY)

BIORE AT-A-GLANCE

Strengths: Provides complete ingredient lists for every product on the company Web site; improved cleansers.

Weaknesses: Known for their pore strips, which aren't as helpful as they seem; lots of products that contain alcohol and/or menthol, neither of which improve the look or function of pores; the sole sunscreen option lacks the proper UVA-protecting ingredients.

For more information about Biore, call (888) BIORE-11 or visit www.biore.com or www.Beautypedia.com.

Biore Shine Control Products

☺ **Shine Control Cream Cleanser** *($5.99 for 6.25 ounces)* doesn't contain advanced oil absorbers as claimed but acquits itself nicely as a water-soluble foaming cleanser for normal to slightly dry or slightly oily skin. It does contain fragrance.

☺ **Shine Control Foaming Cleanser** *($5.99 for 6.7 ounces)* is a standard, gel-based, water-soluble cleanser that foams, but without the cushiony lather produced by the Shine Control Cream Cleanser above. The amount of alcohol is too small to matter, making this a good option for normal to oily skin.

☹ **Shine Control Moisturizer** *($5.99 for 1.7 ounces)* lists alcohol as the third ingredient. That, coupled with no other genuinely redeeming qualities, make this a moisturizer (and I use that term loosely) to ignore.

☹ **Shine Control Clay Mask** *($5.99 for 4 ounces)* doesn't deserve consideration because it is a below-standard clay mask due to several irritating plant extracts and menthol. Lots of clay masks omit these offending ingredients, so there's no need to try this one.

😐 **Shine Control Oil Blotting Sheets** *($5.99 for 65 sheets)* are just thin pieces of paper impregnated with talc. They reduce shine by absorbing excess oil, but leave a powdery film that may interfere with your existing makeup. Blotting papers without powder are preferred, but those who don't wear makeup may appreciate Biore's version.

Other Biore Products

☹ **Blemish Fighting Cleansing Cloths** *($5.99 for 30 cloths)* have a barely interesting formula featuring 0.5% salicylic acid, an amount that is really too low to have a significant effect on blemishes. Moreover, the cloths are soaked in alcohol, which is far too irritating for the skin. And Biore recommends using these cleansing cloths to remove waterproof mascara. Ouch!

☹ **Blemish Fighting Ice Cleanser** *($5.99 for 6.7 ounces)* gets its icy feeling from menthol, the sole ingredient that sabotages this otherwise very good, water-soluble cleanser. The 2% salicylic acid is useless against blemishes in this product, not only because of a too-high pH but also because of its brief contact with skin.

☹ **Daily Deep Pore Cleansing Cloths** *($5.99 for 30 cloths)* lists alcohol as the second ingredient and is not preferred to almost every other cleansing cloth being sold at the drugstore (Pond's, Olay, and Dove have much better options).

☺ **Pore Minimizing Foaming Face Wash** *($6.99 for 4 ounces)* is a non-minty cleanser from Biore, making this truly a surprise from a line that has a preponderance of irritating skin-care ingredients in so many of their products. Aside from a couple of potentially problematic plant extracts (though the amounts are negligible), this is a very good, water-soluble cleanser for normal to oily or combination skin. It removes makeup well and contains fragrance. Don't count on any discernible minimizing of pores. This product is no more capable of that than any other water-soluble cleanser.

😐 **Warming Anti-Blackhead Cream Cleanser** *($5.99 for 6.25 ounces)* contains the mineral zeolite, which causes an exothermic (heat-generating) reaction when mixed with water. That may feel interesting but it has no benefit for the skin, so this ends up being more gimmicky than anything else and isn't preferred to other cleansers in the Biore line. The 2% salicylic acid is rinsed down the drain before it can impact skin, and the lack of cleansing agents makes this a poor choice to remove makeup. It's a mediocre cleanser for normal to dry skin.

☹ **Pore Unclogging Scrub** *($5.99 for 5 ounces)* is a cleanser, not a scrub, and its wax content impedes rinsing. More of an issue than the name and wax is the menthol, which makes this product too irritating for all skin types.

☺ **Pore Minimizing Refining Exfoliator** *($12.49 for 3 ounces)* is a creamy, somewhat abrasive scrub that contains alumina particles for exfoliation. This is not a "professional grade" product and won't replace the results from an in-office microdermabrasion treatment, but if used gently it is a good option for a topical scrub for all but very oily skin types. As far as scrubs go, keep in mind that no scrub will work much better than a clean washcloth used with a good cleanser.

☹ **Triple Action Astringent** *($6.09 for 8.5 ounces)* contains two types of drying alcohols along with witch hazel and menthol, making this a problem product for all skin types.

☹ **Pore Minimizing Lightweight Moisturizer SPF 15** *($12.49 for 1.7 ounces)* does not contain the UVA-protecting ingredients of titanium dioxide, zinc oxide, avobenzone, Tinosorb, or Mexoryl SX, and is absolutely not recommended. That's unfortunate, because the lightweight, matte-finish base formula would have been ideal for oily skin.

☺ **Self Heating Mask** *($5.99 for 2.08 ounces)* claims to open pores and provide "an intensive deep clean," but this relatively standard clay mask does no such thing. Pores cannot be opened (and if they closed we would lose the ability to sweat, which would cause us to overheat), and a mask like this cannot go deeper than the superficial surface layer of skin. This is a good option for oily skin, and the heating effect is primarily a tactile sensation, not a unique benefit. Heat is a problem for blemished or inflamed skin too, so avoid this mask if that describes your skin's condition.

☹ **Deep Cleansing Pore Strips** *($8.99 for 7 nose & 7 face strips)* is the gimmicky product that put Biore on the map several years ago. Now available in a single package that includes removable strips for the nose and face, the concept remains the same: you place a piece of cloth with an incredibly sticky substance on it over your nose or elsewhere on the face, as you might do with a Band-Aid, wait 15 minutes for it to dry, and then rip it off. Along with some amount of skin, blackheads are supposed to stick to it and come right out of the skin. The main ingredient on the strips is polyquaternium-37, a film-forming, hairspray type ingredient—so it's basically a piece of gauze with a form of hairspray on it. You may at first be impressed with what comes off your nose. (Well, there is no question: you will be impressed.) Most people do have some oil sitting at the top of their oil glands, and most of the face's oil glands are located on the nose. So whether you use these strips or a piece of tape, black dots and some skin will be removed. Is that helpful? Only momentarily, although if you use the Biore product, the plastic-forming agent can get into the pores and possibly cause breakouts and irritation. The way these strips adhere, they can absolutely injure or tear skin and cause spider veins to surface. They are especially unsafe if you've been having facial peels; using Retin-A, Renova, AHAs, or BHA; or are taking Accutane; or if you have naturally thin skin or any skin disorder such as rosacea, psoriasis, or seborrhea.

Biore claims this product can pull an entire blackhead plug out of the skin. It can't. If you could grab a blackhead out of the skin, your skin would be left with an empty hole (and there is nothing in this product that will close it up), but that's not what happens. Instead, just the top layer of the blackhead is removed, and then the blackhead returns because the source of the problem was never corrected. Nothing was done to reduce irritation, exfoliate skin cells, help keep oil flow normal, or close the pore. Without question, this product is not preferred to a well-formulated BHA product, which, in most cases, effectively dissolves and controls blackheads (in addition to its other positive traits).

☹ **Ultra Deep Cleansing Pore Strips** *($5.99 for 6 nose strips)* are nearly identical to the Deep Cleansing Pore Strips above, but here tea tree oil and irritating menthol have been added, too. These are designed for the nose only, and the act of tearing off the strip is irritating enough without adding troublesome ingredients to the mix.

BLISSLABS

BLISSLABS AT-A-GLANCE

Strengths: Good selection of cleansers; a lip balm with sunscreen featuring zinc oxide; fantastic gel blush.

Weaknesses: A preponderance of products whose claims raise hopes but that don't work even remotely as described; several sunscreens without sufficient UVA protection; no effective anti-blemish or skin-lightening products; Eyeshadow Fastener is a bust.

For more information about Blisslabs, call (888) 243-8825 or visit www.blissworld.com or www.Beautypedia.com. Note: Blisslabs is owned by Starwood Hotels and Resorts, and their products are included in virtually all of this company's guest rooms.

BLISSLABS SKIN CARE

BLISSLABS SLEEPING PEEL PRODUCTS

☺ **$$$ Sleeping Peel Cleansing Cream** *($32 for 5 ounces)* isn't a true cream cleanser, but is instead more like a water-soluble cleanser with a slightly creamy texture, making it suitable for normal to dry skin not prone to breakouts. The appreciable amount of wax in this cleanser makes it somewhat difficult to rinse, but also offers a cushion to protect drier skin during use. The many amino acids in this cleanser may look nice on the label, but they are rinsed down the drain before they can exert any action on skin—and they do not help boost the absorption of other Sleeping Peel products.

😐 **$$$ Sleeping Peel Resurfacing Gel** *($30 for 4.2 ounces)* just isn't a very exciting formula. It's a water-based gel that contains a good amount of sodium hyaluronate (a beneficial water-binding agent and skin-identical ingredient), but additional state-of-the-art ingredients are either in short supply or are listed after the alcohol and fragrance. Clinique's Advanced Stop Signs Visible Anti-Aging Serum bests this product, as do Olay's Regenerist and Total Effects Serum or Neutrogena's Visibly Firm Serum. Nothing in this Blisslabs product is capable of relaxing facial muscles, a claim that shows up frequently in the cosmetics industry despite any proof of efficacy. 😐 **$$$ Sleeping Peel Age-Minimizing Eye Gel** *($52 for 0.5 ounce)* has no peeling effect on the skin, nor is it essential to use it before you sleep, so the name is a bit odd. What this water- and silicone-based serum does is make skin feel silky smooth and lightly moisturized. It is fragrance-free and contains antioxidants, but the jar packaging will undermine their effectiveness once the product is opened. A less expensive, generously sized product with a better formulation is Clinique's Advanced Stop Signs Visible Anti-Aging Serum ($38.50 for 1.7 ounces).

😐 **$$$ Sleeping Peel Serum** *($60 for 1 ounce)* bills itself as an amino acid antioxidant and the ingredient statement does list alpha amino acid, which supposedly can exfoliate the skin without causing irritation. However, Blisslabs seems to be the only one proclaiming the benefit of alpha amino acid, because there doesn't seem to be a single published study to support their claims that this product "levels fine lines in less than a week." A cosmetics chemist I interviewed was familiar with the ingredient, but wouldn't consider using it as an AHA or BHA alternative because the research to support the claim is nonexistent. Further, he mentioned that any chemical exfoliant, regardless of its gentle attributes or natural-sounding name, would need to be present in a low pH base in order for exfoliation to occur. Of course, that would negate the element of gentleness, because a pH of 3 to 4 (considered the effective range for AHAs, BHA, and PHA) can be a problem for some skin types.

Of greater concern is the ingredient statement, which does not appear to be complete or in compliance with FDA regulations. "Alpha amino acid" is not listed in the latest edition of the *International Cosmetic Ingredient Dictionary and Handbook*, and this formula does not list any stabilizing ingredients (including preservatives). Yet it does contain alcohol, which may cause just the irritation this product is supposedly meant to avoid.

☹ **Sleeping Peel Mask** *($52 for 1 ounce)* is recommended for use once per week, as a five- to ten-minute treatment to combat large pores, fine lines, and a dull skin tone. Sounds impressive, as if this were a quick fix for skin flaws, but the formula is likely to keep your skin awake at night from irritation. This product contains mostly innocuous ingredients, yet the inclusion of aluminum chlorohydrate (yes, the same ingredient used in antiperspirants) can cause irritation, especially over abraded skin—and that includes skin that has been subjected to chemical peels or microdermabrasion treatments. This mask dries very quickly, and can feel constricting on the skin, which is not a good sign; nor something necessary in order to achieve a more even skin tone. Nothing in this product can help eliminate blackheads, though the clay can absorb some of the oil that can make them look darker and more pronounced. Finally, there is no substantiated evidence that alpha amino acid can exfoliate the skin. Until there is, I wouldn't choose this product over a well-formulated AHA or BHA product, or even a mechanical scrub.

☹ **Sleeping Peel Liver Spot Lifter** *($52 for 0.5 ounce)*, supposedly developed by an "overachieving dermatologist," uses a proprietary amino acid antioxidant along with asafoetida extract to lighten pigment discolorations. First, whoever this "overachieving dermatologist" is, he or she must have underachieved in the class on skin physiology 101 because the liver has nothing to do with brown skin discolorations. These discolorations (technically referred to as solar lentigo, melasma, and cholasma) are caused by sun damage or hormone-related changes, not the liver (Sources: *Clinical & Experimental Dermatology*, October 2001, page 583; and *Medline Plus*, National Institutes of Health, www.nlm.nih.gov/medlineplus/ency/article/001141.htm). In fact, the primary way to combat and potentially eliminate these brown pigment changes is with an effective, well-formulated sunscreen.

Aside from that bit of ineptitude, asafoetida, also known as *Ferula foetida*, has no research proving it has skin-lightening properties. According to www.naturaldatabase.com, this plant is used topically to treat corns and calluses. (It is also used as a seasoning in Indian cuisine, but clearly that doesn't impact skin color.) Otherwise, there's insufficient information to support its topical effectiveness for other conditions. As for the amino acid antioxidant, it is simply a water-binding agent that can't affect skin discolorations. The only ingredient in this water-based serum that has skin-lightening potential is ascorbic acid, but the amount present is too low for it to exert an effect, and the type of packaging won't keep it stable, making this product a waste of time and money.

BLISSLABS STEEP CLEAN PRODUCTS

☹ **Steep Clean Professional-Strength Facial Mask, for All Skin Types** *($54 for 3.4 ounces)* is supposed to be the next best thing to having a facial, and claims to "transform even a permanently-clogged T-zone into a scene of extreme clean," all while exfoliating and lightening dark spots. It's all false because there is nothing in this product that will positively impact blackheads nor fade discolorations. It is mostly glycerin, water, cleansing agent, film-forming agent, and thickener, along with shea butter and castor oil (emollient ingredients that should be kept away from blemish-prone areas). The only miracle about this mask is that anyone would benefit from it as described, or spend their money on such a waste-of-time product. If I were seeing an aesthetician who used this product as a means of combating blackheads and discolorations, I'd cancel my next appointment.

☺ **$$$ Steep Clean Cleansing Milk** *($30 for 8.28 ounces)* has lots of bells and whistles coupled with claims of banishing acne and reducing the inflammation it causes. However, this is just a mild (almost too mild) water-soluble cleanser that's best for normal to slightly oily skin. The tiny amounts of salicylic acid, fruit extracts, and alpha arbutin won't clear a single blemish or even minimize it. Anti-acne ingredients are best used in leave-on products, but that doesn't make this a poor cleanser—just a misguided, overpriced one.

☹ **Steep Clean Toner Pads** *($35 for 50 pads)* lists alcohol as the second ingredient, which makes these pads too irritating for all skin types. Salicylic acid is on hand at about 1% concentration with an effective pH of 3.8. However, the alcohol content is too high to overlook.

☹ **Steep Clean Moisture Lotion** *($48 for 1.7 ounces)* has some intriguing ingredients and includes a silky silicone base suitable for normal to oily skin. However, it's not worth considering because it contains menthol and the menthol derivative menthyl lactate, both in higher concentrations than most of the antioxidants in this moisturizer.

OTHER BLISSLABS PRODUCTS

☹ **Clog Dissolving Cleansing Milk** *($28 for 8.28 ounces)* cannot dissolve clogs of any kind. Does Blisslabs really believe that this concoction of thickeners, plant oils, film-forming agents, and emollients (all rather pore-clogging on their own) can reach into pores and break up the dead skin cells, bacteria, and sebum hiding inside? If anything, this cleanser can easily make matters worse. This product does have merit as a cleansing lotion for dry skin, but absolutely not for those prone to breakouts. The marketing and claims are completely inaccurate and misdirected and, therefore, I'm giving it a very unhappy face rating.

☺ **Fabulous Foaming Face Wash** *($18 for 8.28 ounces)* is a standard, water-soluble cleanser that is a good option for all skin types. Supposedly, this product can also exfoliate skin, but it doesn't contain any ingredients that can accomplish that. It does contain acetyl hexapeptide-3, an ingredient included in several products from an array of cosmetics companies all making claims that it can work like Botox, but this ingredient doesn't work that way in the least (even Botox doesn't work like Botox when rubbed on the surface of skin). Even if acetyl hexapeptide-3 could work like Botox, it's in a cleanser, so it would just be rinsed down the drain before it could have an effect.

☺ **Lid + Lash Wash** *($22 for 8.5 ounces)* is a very standard makeup remover that contains mostly water, slip agents, cleansing agent, film-forming agent, more cleansing agents, preservatives, and fragrance.

☺ **$$$ Pore Perfecting Facial Polish** *($28 for 4.2 ounces)* is a pricey but good topical scrub that uses calcium carbonate (chalk) as the abrasive agent. It is best for normal to dry skin; the thickeners and wax aren't ideal over blemish-prone skin.

😐 **$$$ Daily Detoxifying Facial Toner** *($26 for 6.7 ounces)* claims it is amped up with antioxidants, but instead uses fragrant and irritating *Rosa centifolia* flower extract and plantain extract, which can be anti-inflammatory but also allergenic (Source: www.naturaldatabase.com). This is otherwise a very standard toner that is not "one giant leap for your skin" as described.

☹ **All Around Eye Cream** *($26 for 0.5 ounce)* is short on antioxidants and long on standard thickening agents that, while helpful, don't replace the need for more state-of-the-art ingredients. The plant oils and antioxidants in this moisturizer are eclipsed by the high amount of orange oil, which can be irritating when used around the eyes. This is absolutely not "the most eye cream bang for your buck."

☹ **An Ounce of Prevention AM** *($48 for 1 ounce)* would have been a much better moisturizer (far-flung claims notwithstanding) if the amount of *Iris florentina* root extract (also known as orris root) was not present. This plant extract is used primarily as a fragrance ingredient and has no benefit for skin. It can, however, cause allergic or sensitizing reactions (Source: *Botanical Dermatology Database*, http://bodd.cf.ac.uk/BotDermFolder/BotDermI/IRID.html). There are many moisturizers available that supply skin with much more than this product provides, without fragrant irritants. Besides, without sunscreen, this isn't any savvy skin-care consumer's idea of an ounce of prevention!

😐 **$$$ An Ounce of Prevention PM** *($48 for 1 ounce)* contains tiny amounts of several antioxidants, but they're compromised by this product's jar packaging. This is otherwise a standard moisturizer for normal to slightly dry skin that includes acetyl hexapeptide-3, the "works like Botox" peptide that has no research substantiating its antiwrinkle claims (never mind the fact that not even Botox works like Botox when applied topically rather than injected).

☺ **$$$ Baggage Handler** *($26 for 1 ounce)* deserves an accolade for its eminently clever name, but it's clear more thought went into what to call the product than what to put in it. In short, Baggage Handler cannot keep under-eye bags (or dark circles or puffiness) in check. This fragrance-free, water-based gel contains a slip agent, several skin-identical ingredients, soothing plant extracts, film-forming agents, thickener, and preservatives. It's not a bad combination, at least if your only goal is to lightly moisturize the under-eye area without causing irritation. However, that's not how this product is sold, and if you were banking on the claims about reducing the appearance of drooping or baggy areas around the eyes, this won't impress, and your money would be better spent elsewhere. Therefore, the smiling face rating pertains to this gel's ability to hydrate and soften normal to slightly dry skin, not for performing as claimed.

😐 **$$$ Crease Police** *($52 for 1 ounce)* is a roll-on product that is supposed to renovate wrinkles. It doesn't contain anything capable of turning back the clock on aging skin. Beyond water, the main ingredient is something called polyamino sugar condensate. There is no information on this ingredient other than a description of it as a skin-conditioning agent, and absolutely no research to support even a shred of its antiwrinkle claims. At best, it is a water-binding agent. The other ingredients of note in this product are the moisturizing agent urea and the antioxidant vitamin C. Although worthwhile, neither can do much when it comes to vanquishing wrinkles, though each has beneficial properties for skin.

☺ **$$$ Instant Mattification** *($35 for 0.5 ounce)* consists of a blend of silicones and silicone polymers with salicylic acid, fragrant plants, and zinc oxide (used as an absorbent ingredient, not a sunscreen). It leaves skin feeling silky and to some extent will absorb excess oil. Because a pH cannot be established in a nonaqueous product, the salicylic acid is useless as an exfoliant. Consider this a good makeup primer if you have oily skin, but that's about it.

☹ **No-Motion Lotion** *($35 for 1 ounce)* is another "works-like-Botox" product, and, like its pals, is completely ineffective at preventing muscle contractions to "relax facial tension ... and prevent future wrinkling." What a joke! This lotion contains sodium polystyrene sulfonate, a resin-based film-forming agent that is considered a skin irritant (Source: *Handbook of Cosmetic and Personal Care Additives*, Second Edition, volume 2, 2002, page 1513). Peppermint oil and menthol are included so you'll think this do-nothing product is doing something. This is a poorly formulated product and it's not even worth going through the motions of ordering it.

😐 **$$$ The Youth As We Know It** *($79 for 1.7 ounces)* is "Formulated with the ten most effective anti-aging ingredients we've found over ten years of giving 'great face', The Youth As We Know It is a one-stop shop for wrinkle renovation, exfoliation, oxygenation, binding hydration, surface line relaxation, cellular respiration, and collagen and elastin regeneration." Wow! If any of this were true, you'd have to wonder why Blisslabs is still selling its numerous other antiwrinkle products. This water- and silicone-based moisturizer contains more antioxidants than any other Blisslabs moisturizer, but the choice of jar packaging won't keep them stable once the product is opened. That leaves you with an OK moisturizer for normal to dry skin and the unfortunate fact that many of the beneficial substances not affected by light and air exposure are barely present. Lastly, I don't know where Blisslabs got their ten most effective anti-aging ingredients because no research has established any such directive, but I can think of dozens and dozens they did not include.

😐 **$$$ Thinny Thin Chin** *($48 for 1.7 ounces)* is sold as being the most exciting thing to happen to your neck since your first hickey (if you consider a bruised red spot on your neck exciting) because of its alleged effect on jowls and loose skin on the chest. This is nothing more than a standard emollient moisturizer for dry skin; it has no special benefit whatsoever for sagging skin, nor is it a "liquid bra for your V-zone." More ridiculous claims from Blisslabs wrapped up in a very ordinary product. Great name, though.

☹ **Wrinkle Twinkle** *($42 for 0.5 ounce)* is a product whose description basically amounts to "apply, and POOF! your wrinkles are gone." But that's not all! After two months this also makes short work of bothersome dark circles while continuing to relax wrinkles formed by facial expressions. In fact, this product is basically a water- and silicone-based serum whose antiwrinkle, line-smoothing ingredient is aminobutyric acid. Please refer to Chapter Seven, *Cosmetic Ingredient Dictionary*, at the end of this book for a definition of this ingredient, which does not work as claimed here. A major problem this product has that won't put a twinkle in anyone's eye is the inclusion of lavender oil, which has been shown to cause skin cell death when applied topically (Source: *Cell Proliferation*, June 2004, pages 221–229).

☹ **Ray of Hope SPF 20** *($36 for 8.5 ounces)* gets its sun-protection credibility from its effective blend of active ingredients, which include avobenzone for UVA protection. Beyond that, however, this product enters fantasyland when it claims that slathering it on allows you to "fight fat while lying on the beach!" (With this claim, Bliss has won a spot in my how-low-can-you-go-to-market-a-product award!)

Ray of Hope supposedly contains spheres of cellulite-busting ingredients that burst open upon exposure to sunlight, going to work to minimize dimpled skin. It contains caffeine and esculin, two ingredients that show up in many anti-cellulite products, but neither has substantiated research proving such an effect for this condition. Further, esculin is considered toxic and is not recommended for topical application by some experts (Source: *Ellenhorn's Medical Toxicology: Diagnoses and Treatment of Human Poisoning*, 2nd Edition, Baltimore, MD: Williams & Wilkins, 1997). That alone makes this sun-worthy but cellulite-bogus product not worth considering.

☹ **Sunban Lotion for the Body SPF 20, Oil-Free** *($32 for 6 ounces)* does not contain the UVA-protecting ingredients of titanium dioxide, or zinc oxide, avobenzone, Tinosorb, or Mexoryl SX, and is not recommended. Even if it did contain them, for this amount of money, this is a truly basic, no-frills sunscreen.

☺ **$$$ Sunban Lotion for the Face SPF 30, Oil-Free** *($32 for 1.7 ounces)* lists titanium dioxide as its only active ingredient and it is formulated in a silky lotion base that sets to a nearly imperceptible matte finish. Antioxidants are in very short supply, which is a shame given the cost of this product, but this one aces it for nonirritating sun protection if you have normal to oily skin. This sunscreen does contain fragrance.

☹ **The Big Screen SPF 30** *($25 for 8.5 ounces)* is more like the big letdown, since it does not include the UVA-protecting ingredients of titanium dioxide, zinc oxide, avobenzone, Tinosorb, or Mexoryl SX. That's unfortunate, because the base formula contains appreciable levels of antioxidants.

😐 **$$$ A Tan For All Seasons** *($36 for 4.4 ounces)* is a very basic self-tanning mist that uses dihydroxyacetone to bronze skin and contains coloring agents for an immediate sheer bronze glow. The amount of alcohol and fragrance in this mist makes it a risk for sensitive skin, but it is an OK option for oily to very oily, breakout-prone skin.

☹ **Change Your Spots** *($30 for 0.5 ounce)* was originally known as See Spots Run, and the formula basics remain the same. This is essentially an expensive version of many of the anti-acne gels sold at the drugstore. It contains 2% salicylic acid, and although its pH is low enough to allow exfoliation, the alcohol and several plant irritants prevent this product from being a slam-dunk solution for blemished skin because it can cause dryness and irritation. Salicylic acid (BHA) definitely plays a role in helping post-inflammatory hyperpigmentation fade, but irritation can counteract that benefit.

☹ **Instant Mattification 10-Minute Deep Cleaning Treatment** *($36 for 1 ounce)* debuted as a product that took Blisslabs over two years and 57 fine-tunings before they had what they believe is the best oil controlling, pore-tightening mask possible. I couldn't disagree more, but doubt that going back to the drawing board one more time would have produced anything that was a logical improvement. It contains mostly water, glycerin, thickener, clay, titanium dioxide, plant extracts (none of which have research proving they adeptly control oil or tighten pores), and preservative. The tiny amount of salicylic acid is too low to matter, since the pH of the product is above 4. This product is not only ineffective for its intended purpose but also contains rosemary and mint oils that will irritate skin. This is not recommended for any skin type.

☹ **Triple Oxygen Instant Energizing Mask** *($52 for 3.4 ounces)* brings us a "complexion brightening" formula that claims to use "every technology in the book to work to furnish you with a fresher, younger-looking face"—but that doesn't explain why the backbone of this formulation is closer to a cleanser than any age-erasing treatment product. The second ingredient is methyl perfluorobutyl ether, a mild solvent used most often for industrial, not cosmetic, purposes, and it can release oxygen in the presence of water. But the issue this fails to address is that supplying oxygen to otherwise healthy skin isn't beneficial—after all, oxygen is a prime source of free-radical damage. Further, if Bliss is pro-oxygen, why did they include antioxidants in this product that would in effect block the oxygen from having any impact? This product is a waste of time and a bigger waste of money at the ludicrous price of $52.

😐 **Breath Freshening Lip Balm: Mint** *($14 for 0.45 ounce)* is a standard Vaseline- and wax-based lip balm that works to keep chapping and dryness at bay. It contains a tiny amount of menthyl PCA, a menthol derivative that can be irritating, though considering the amount this product includes it's not likely to be an issue.

☹ **Poutrageous Lip Plumper** *($20 for 0.15 ounce)* is a lip gloss-type product that contains retinol, which is good. What is definitely irritating (and causes lips to appear temporarily plump) is the menthol this balm contains, and with repeated use that can add up to chapped lips.

😐 **$$$ Spiff Upper Lip** *($48 for 0.5 ounce)*. Sigh. Here is yet another Blisslabs product claiming to target an age-apparent area with a multi-pronged approach designed to address every perceivable concern. This time it's for the lips, and this product is supposed to tackle vertical lines, unwanted hair growth, darkness, and the loss of collagen that "leaves your previously pouty lips limping along." By now it won't surprise you when I report there is nothing in this water-, thickener- and silicone-based lip product that can accomplish even a fraction of the claims that accompany it. The plant oils provide moisture and an antioxidant benefit, but the aminobutyric acid isn't effective against lip lines, and there isn't enough alpha-arbutin in this product to lighten a dark upper lip (assuming it's dark from pigment, not hair growth). As for dealing with "man-worthy moustache hair," well, there's nothing in the formula that can eliminate that concern either. The amounts of peptide and retinol are too low to register a benefit, and at most this product will temporarily fill in lines around the mouth and keep that area soft and smooth. This is not recommended over Estee Lauder's Perfectionist Correcting Concentrate for Lip Lines ($35 for 0.08 ounce). That won't take the place of lip injections or smoothing treatments performed by a dermatologist, but it's a better formulation than what Blisslabs offers.

✓☺ **Super Balm Lip Conditioner with SPF 15** *($10 for 0.5 ounce)* has an in-part zinc oxide sunscreen and an emollient, slightly slick base formula packed with ingredients capable of keeping dry lips soft and smooth. The antioxidants are a thoughtful touch (though most are included in meager amounts) and the salicylic acid does not have an exfoliating effect, but everything else about this lip balm really is super!

BLISSLABS MAKEUP

✓☺ **$$$ Ink Pink Blushing Balm** *($22)* is quite a find for those who prefer gel blush. This sheer, long-lasting formula is easier to spread and apply than liquid versions such as Benefit's famed BeneTint ($28). The name is a bit misleading, because the translucent wash of color is more red than pink, but it nicely approximates a flushed appearance, especially for light skin tones. Applying a tiny dab produces very sheer "I just returned from a brief walk" blush effect, and it can be layered (without streaking) for more color. This type of blush is best for those with smooth, even skin.

☹ **Eyeshadow Fastener** *($22)* purports to enhance eyeshadow application and wearability, but this is just an overpriced, substandard concealer. It has a slightly matte finish that feels a bit tacky, but it blends well, if too sheer for eyelid coverage. A bigger problem is the high amount of synthetic sunscreen ingredient (no SPF number is on the label) and fragrance. Neither ingredient is recommended for use on eyelids, yet that is precisely where you're supposed to apply this misguided product. For less money, less potential irritation, and better results, consider one of the matte finish concealers from Revlon, L'Oreal, or Maybelline New York.

☺ **Fabulips** *($9)* is a smooth, slightly creamy lipstick that comes in a small assortment of nude colors. It's a good option for a subdued lipstick that feels comfortable and doesn't easily migrate into lines around the mouth.

☺ **$$$ Blisslash** *($16)* goes on heavy and clumps slightly, but with patience (and a lash comb) you can build incredibly long, reasonably thick lashes with a soft curl. The formula wears well and removes easily—just be careful not to overdo it while applying!

BLISTEX (LIP CARE ONLY)

BLISTEX AT-A-GLANCE

Strengths: Includes complete ingredients for all of its products on the company Web site; a couple of lip balms with excellent UVA protection and above-average formulas.

Weaknesses: The majority of lip balms with sunscreen lack sufficient UVA-protecting ingredients, leaving lips vulnerable to sun damage; many contain irritants such as menthol, phenol, or camphor.

For more information about Blistex, call (888) 784-2472 or visit www.blistex.com or www.Beautypedia.com.

✓☺ **Clear Advance SPF 30** *($1.89 for 0.15 ounce)* includes avobenzone for sufficient UVA protection in an emollient Vaseline base that's ideal for dry lips. This twist-up stick lip balm is marketed to men but is ideal under lipstick (or alone) for women too, and it contains some good antioxidants.

✓☺ **Pro Care SPF 30** *($2.49 for 0.16 ounce)* gets the UVA protection right by including 3% avobenzone. This smooth-textured stick lip balm contains standard waxes along with beneficial ingredients such as borage seed oil, cholesterol, ceramide, lecithin, and glycolipids. It's an excellent formula and one Blistex should have modeled most of their other lip balms on.

☹ **Complete Moisture SPF 15** *($1.89 for 0.15 ounce)* is a standard lip balm that pales in comparison to the Clear Advance SPF 30 above because it lacks the UVA-protecting ingredients of titanium dioxide, zinc oxide, avobenzone, Tinosorb, or Mexoryl SX. Complete moisture is nice, but a lip balm sporting an SPF rating should offer complete UVA protection as well.

☹ **Daily Conditioning Treatment SPF 20** *($1.89 for 0.25 ounce)* lacks the UVA-protecting ingredients listed for the Complete Moisture SPF 15 above, and is not recommended. This also contains camphor and menthol, which only serve to irritate chapped lips.

☹ **Fruit Smoothies SPF 15** *($2.99 for 3 pack of 0.10-ounce sticks)* may taste like various fruits, but flavored lip balms encourage lip-licking, which removes the product and leaves lips vulnerable to further chapping. Even without the flavors, this lip balm lacks sufficient UVA protection and is not recommended.

☺ **Gentle Sense** *($2.19 for 0.15 ounce)* is a very basic, but very good, lip balm containing mostly petrolatum (Vaseline) along with cocoa and shea butters. It is fragrance-free and less greasy than using plain Vaseline, not to mention being in portable stick form.

☹ **Herbal Answer Stick SPF 15** *($1.89 for 0.15 ounce)* lacks sufficient UVA-protecting ingredients, so this isn't the answer for daytime sun protection. It is otherwise a standard ChapStick-style lip balm that contains a smattering of natural (not herbal) ingredients.

☹ **Herbal Answer Tube SPF 15** *($2.19 for 0.35 ounce)* is a less waxy version of the Herbal Answer Stick SPF 15 above, but also lacks the right UVA-protecting ingredients to protect lips from sun damage.

☹ **Lip Balm SPF 15** *($1.09 for 0.15 ounce)* lacks sufficient UVA-protecting ingredients and irritates lips with camphor and menthol, regardless of whether you choose the Regular, Berry, or Mint varieties. Padimate O, one of the sunscreen actives, is one of the more irritating, infrequently used sunscreens.

☹ **Lip Infusion Sheer Liquid Balm SPF 15 Moisture Splash** *($3.19 for 0.14 ounce)* has a roller-ball applicator for its liquid formula, and although it feels less thick and waxy on lips than many lip balms in stick form, the lack of sufficient UVA-protecting ingredients makes it a poor choice for daytime use.

☹ **Lip Infusion Sheer Liquid Balm SPF 15, Cherry Splash** *($3.19 for 0.14 ounce)* is nearly identical to the Lip Infusion Sheer Liquid Balm SPF 15 Moisture Splash above, except for its cherry flavor. Otherwise, the same comments apply.

☹ **Lip Medex** *($1.59 for 0.38 ounce)* can only possibly relieve sore lips by virtue of being so irritating, you'll forget whatever was irritating your lips before applying this product! Camphor and menthol are the active ingredients, and the potent menthol derivative menthoxypropanediol is also included just in case lips weren't pushed past the brink of irritation.

☹ **Lip Ointment** *($1.89 for 0.21 ounce)* contains camphor, menthol, and phenol, which means that the tiny amount of soothing allantoin will be powerless to keep lips from becoming very irritated. There are far more effective treatments for cold sores than the active ingredients in this product.

☹ **Lip Revitalizer** *($1.89 for 0.25 ounce)* contains carvone, an essential oil used as a flavoring agent that can be a significant skin sensitizer and allergen (Source: *Planta Medica*, August 2001, pages 564–566; and *Contact Dermatitis*, June 2001, pages 347–356).

☹ **Lip Tone SPF 15** *($1.89 for 0.15 ounce)* is a sheer, tinted lip balm whose sunscreen lacks sufficient UVA-protecting ingredients; it is not recommended.

☺ **Pro Relief** *($2.49 for 0.16 ounce)* lists the topical anesthetic pramoxine hydrochloride. This can provide temporarily relief to painful lip conditions such as cold sores, but is most often used to quell itchy areas such as can occur with psoriasis. It's only an option if lips are in need of treatment for cracked, dry skin that has led to itching, and use should be discontinued if lips show further signs of irritation.

☹ **Silk & Shine SPF 15** *($2.49 for 0.13 ounce)* contains hydrolyzed silk and ingredients that make lips feel silky, but it's a poor choice for daytime protection because it lacks the UVA-protecting ingredients of titanium dioxide, zinc oxide, avobenzone, Tinosorb, or Mexoryl SX, and is not recommended.

☹ **Spa Effects SPF 15** *($3.49 for 3 pack of 0.10 ounce sticks)* has some intriguing ingredients, including some vitamin-based antioxidants, but it's all for naught since this is yet another flavored Blistex lip balm that lacks sufficient UVA-protecting ingredients.

☹ **Ultra Protection SPF 30** *($1.89 for 0.15 ounce)* lacks the UVA-protecting ingredients listed in the review of Silk & Shine SPF 15 above, and is not recommended.

BOBBI BROWN

BOBBI BROWN AT-A-GLANCE

Strengths: Some good cleansers; a few stably packaged products loaded with advanced ingredients to keep skin in top shape; an easy-to-use, lightweight self-tanner; one of the best neutral shade ranges for foundation; foundation options for all skin types and preferences; very good blush and eyeshadows (powder and cream), including several matte shades; the Gel Eyeliner, Shimmer Brick and Matte Lip Stain; mostly excellent brushes; several refillable compact options and other useful accessories; counter personnel are typically well-trained as makeup artists.

Weaknesses: As with most Lauder-owned companies, the well-formulated moisturizers are hindered by jar packaging, which compromises the effectiveness of light- and air-sensitive ingredients; several otherwise effective products marred by irritating fragrant oils or fragrance components; some of the foundations without sunscreen lack sufficient UVA-protecting ingredients; concealers are a mixed bag; mostly unappealing lip glosses, and none of those with sunscreen provide sufficient UVA protection.

For more information about Bobbi Brown, owned by Estee Lauder, call (877) 310-9222 or visit www.bobbibrowncosmetics.com or www.Beautypedia.com.

BOBBI BROWN SKIN CARE

BOBBI BROWN EXTRA PRODUCTS

☹ **Extra Balm Rinse** *($20 for 1.7 ounces)* is a very rich, luxurious cleansing balm for dry to very dry skin, but the olive oil prevents it from rinsing well without the aid of a washcloth. That's not a big deal, but the amount of the fragrant component limonene in this product is. Limonene is a volatile compound found in most citrus fruits, and its topical application causes contact dermatitis (Source: www.naturaldatabase.com).

☹ **Extra Eye Balm** *($55 for 0.45 ounce)* is an extremely emollient, rich moisturizer that would have been a slam-dunk for those with dry skin (and an imposing skin-care budget) if it did not include appreciable levels of potent irritants like mint oil, orange oil, and galbanum oil, among others. None of these ingredients should go anywhere near the eye. What a shame, because aside from those irritants this is an exceptionally well-formulated product.

☹ **Extra Face Oil** *($55 for 1 ounce)* contains some highly effective oils for dry to very dry skin, including olive, sesame, and jojoba. Not willing to leave well enough alone, this product also contains the irritants neroli, patchouli, lavender, and sandalwood, along with problematic fragrance components such as geraniol and linalool. Using plain olive oil would be preferred to this well-intentioned but faulty product.

☹ **Extra Moisturizing Balm** *($80 for 1.7 ounces)* ends up being a very expensive way to supply skin with Vaseline and silicone, the main ingredients (next to water) in this rich balm. The antioxidant plant oils are rendered ineffective by this product's jar packaging, and the geranium oil, while smelling nice, can cause skin irritation (Sources: *Contact Dermatitis*, June 2001, pages 344–346; and *Journal of Applied Microbiology*, February 2000, pages 308–316). Choosing plain Vaseline not only costs considerably less but spares your skin an irritant response.

☹ **Extra Moisturizing Balm SPF 25** *($80 for 1.7 ounces)* has avobenzone for UVA protection, but contains irritating bitter orange oil and angelica oil, which is photosensitizing (Source: www.naturaldatabase.com). What's that type of ingredient doing in a product whose intention is to protect skin while outdoors? And even if it didn't include these problem ingredients, how liberally are you going to apply a sunscreen with a price like this?

☹ **Extra Soothing Balm** *($55 for 0.5 ounce)* contains triglycerides, waxes, emollients, and plant oils that can protect and restore dry skin to a healthier-looking and smoother-feeling state. What's not the least bit soothing is the inclusion of ginger root and bitter orange oils. Both can be irritating to skin and they keep this product from being a worthwhile purchase (Source: www.naturaldatabase.com).

Other Bobbi Brown Products

☺ **$$$ Lathering Tube Soap** *($22 for 4.2 ounces)* isn't a true soap, but the name is apropos for the apothecary-style packaging chosen for this product. This is a standard foaming cleanser that uses the soap derivative potassium myristate as the main cleansing agent, one that can be drying and sensitizing for some skin types. However, this cleanser also contains a battery of nonirritating plant oils for extra cushioning while cleansing. There are minute amounts of lavender, jasmine, and grapefruit for fragrance, but likely not enough to be problematic. Though pricey, this is still a decent cleansing option for normal to slightly dry skin.

☺ **$$$ Rich Cream Cleanser** *($22 for 4.2 ounces)* is an emollient cleansing cream for dry to very dry skin. It doesn't rinse well without the aid of a washcloth, and would be better without the fragrant additives, but it's still an option if you want to splurge on a cleanser.

☺ **$$$ Eye Makeup Remover** *($20 for 3.4 ounces)* is a very standard, detergent-based eye-makeup remover that contains fragrant rose water and soothing cornflower extract. It works well, but so do many similar removers that cost much less than this one and skip the fragrance.

☺ **$$$ Buffing Grains for Face** *($40 for 0.99 ounce)* are made to sound special because you can add these loose grains to any cleanser to create a custom scrub. The novelty may be fun, but this concoction is simply polyethylene beads (plastic beads) with adzuki bean powder and tiny amounts of plant oils, plus a detergent cleansing agent that is activated by water. Polyethylene is used in most topical scrub products; you don't need to spend this much money for its benefit. Still, for the money-is-no-object among us, this is a viable option. Still, for many reasons, a soft washcloth works just as well if not better than a scrub.

☹ **Exfoliating Cream Wash** *($22 for 4.2 ounces)* is minimally exfoliating but does provide a potent dose of irritation with each use from a who's who of offenders, including menthol, arnica, peppermint oil, eucalyptus oil, and camphor.

😐 **$$$ Brightening Facial Water** *($28 for 6.7 ounces)* has a huge ingredient list for a toner and, as expected, it's not all good news for your skin. Several fragrant ingredients are included among some impressive antioxidants and skin-identical ingredients. The licorice extract is said to help even skin tone, but there is limited research showing it can deliver on that promise (Source: *Planta Medica*, August 2005, pages 785–787). Moreover, the amount of it in this toner is likely insignificant for skin-lightening. This ends up being an OK toner for normal to dry skin.

😐 **$$$ Soothing Face Tonic** *($22 for 6.7 ounces)* is a very good toner for all skin types, though its clear glass packaging hinders the effectiveness of the antioxidants present. Still, this supplies skin with some excellent water-binding and soothing agents, and the tiny amount of lavender is unlikely to be a problem.

😐 **$$$ Brightening Essence** *($60 for 1 ounce)* doesn't contain any ingredients with substantial research proving their effectiveness for lightening skin discolorations. However, Brown's product is about brightening, a cosmetic effect that should not be (but often is) confused with lightening products that work to inhibit melanin production. This well-formulated water- and silicone-based moisturizer has some intriguing ingredients, including some potent antioxidants, but they're less effective than they could be because of this product's clear glass packaging. It's a decent moisturizing lotion for normal to slightly dry skin.

😐 **$$$ Brightening Moisturizer SPF 25** *($45 for 1.7 ounces)* contains titanium dioxide, but the amount is less than 1%, which may leave skin vulnerable to UVA damage. This is otherwise a well-formulated moisturizer that contains most of the skin-beneficial ingredients that are a hallmark of Lauder-owned companies. The problem in this case is that the translucent glass packaging won't keep the antioxidants stable unless the product is stored away from natural light. If you're willing to store this properly, it is recommended for normal to dry skin, but there are better sunscreens available from Estee Lauder and Clinique. By the way, Bobbi Brown claims the bamboo extract technology in this product provides antioxidant benefits, but there is no research substantiating this claim.

😐 **$$$ Hydrating Eye Cream** *($35 for 0.5 ounce)* definitely contains ingredients that can hydrate skin around the eyes or elsewhere on the face, but it's an overall lackluster formula whose antioxidant vitamins are compromised by jar packaging. This eye cream is fragrance-free.

😐 **$$$ Hydrating Face Cream** *($40 for 1.7 ounces)* contains mostly water, silicone, slip agent, thickeners, plant oil, algae, vitamins, fragrant plant extracts, film-forming agent, a cell-communicating ingredient, and preservatives. It's a good option for normal to dry skin but would be much better in packaging that keeps the antioxidant vitamins stable once it's opened.

✓ ☺ **$$$ Intensive Skin Supplement** *($55 for 1 ounce)* has some impressive ingredients and a lightweight, water-based serum texture built around slip agents and silicones. The amounts of vitamin C and mulberry root extract are probably not enough to have an effect on melanin production, but between them, the other antioxidants, and a cell-communicating ingredient, this is a well-formulated product that can be used by all skin types. For less money, an equal product to consider, also from a Lauder-owned company, is Clinique's Advanced Stop Signs ($38.50 for 1.7 ounces).

😐 **$$$ Overnight Cream** *($55 for 1.7 ounces)* is sold as a "technologically advanced repair product for nighttime use," and although it does use ingredients that can repair skin's barrier and improve its appearance, the choice of jar packaging renders the many antioxidants in this product unstable shortly after you open it. This still has merit for dry to very dry skin; it does contain fragrant plant extracts.

☹ **Protective Face Lotion SPF 15** *($40 for 1.7 ounces)* wins points for its in-part titanium dioxide sunscreen and a silky lotion base laced with soothing chamomile, several antioxidants, and cell-communicating ingredients. The problem is the inclusion of fragrance components of linalool, limonene, and cinnamyl alcohol, the latter of which is a known skin sensitizer and inappropriate for use in a product meant to protect skin from sun damage (Source: *Chemical Research in Toxicology*, March 2004, pages 301–310). It's interesting that cinammyl alcohol and its aldehyde form are part of a standard fragrance mix used by dermatologists to determine whether a patient is suffering allergic contact dermatitis from fragrance (Source: www.dermatologytimes.com/dermatologytimes/article/articleDetail.jsp?id=396332).

😐 **$$$ Vitamin Enriched Face Base** *($45 for 1.7 ounces)* lists many antioxidant vitamins but what's not explained is the choice of jar packaging, which won't hold them stable once this moisturizer is opened. It contains some good anti-irritants, but these are countered by fragrant geranium oil and lesser amounts of potentially sensitizing fragrance components, further making this product a tough sell, especially given its price.

☺ **$$$ Sunless Tanning Gel for Face and Body** *($30 for 4.2 ounces)* is a water- and silicone-based self-tanner that uses the same ingredient (dihydroxyacetone) found in almost all self-tanning products. Brown offers two versions, based on whether you have a light to medium or medium to dark skin tone. This does contain volatile fragrance components, and is best used in the evening and rinsed in the morning to avoid the potential for irritation when skin is exposed to sunlight.

☹ **Beach Sunscreen Body Spray SPF 15** *($25 for 6.7 ounces)* may smell like Brown's popular Beach fragrance, but the formula lacks the UVA-protecting ingredients of titanium dioxide, zinc oxide, avobenzone, Tinosorb, or Mexoryl SX, and is not recommended. This also contains several fragrant components that aren't the best to put on skin before a day at the beach.

☹ **Beach Sunscreen for Face SPF 25** *($25 for 1.7 ounces)* holds much promise as an in-part avobenzone sunscreen with a great lightweight but creamy texture. However, it contains several problematic fragrant essential oils, including limonene, a strong skin irritant and sensitizer. This product also contains geraniol, a volatile component of many essential oils that can cause allergic reactions. Given the active nature of sunscreen ingredients and the increased odds that synthetic sunscreen agents can cause a sensitizing reaction (especially as the SPF number rises), adding other sensitizing ingredients to a formulation like this is a genuine disservice to consumers trying to protect their skin. Without these unnecessary additives, this sunscreen would have received a much better rating.

☹ **Beach Sunscreen Gel for Body SPF 30** *($25 for 3.7 ounces)* contains the same problematic essential oils present in the Beach Sunscreen for Face SPF 25 above, and that's just too much potential for irritation from a product meant to protect skin.

☹ **Overnight Blemish Paste** *($15 for 0.59 ounce)* contains less than 1% salicylic acid, which isn't much, but even so the pH of this product is too high for it to be effective as an exfoliant. The main ingredient in this Paste is calcium carbonate (chalk or limestone), which has a rather high pH of over 9 in its pure form. While it does have absorbing properties, the negative effect of a high pH on the skin is of concern, especially for breakouts.

☺ **$$$ Blotting Papers** *($20 for 100 sheets)* are powder-free, tissue paper–style blotting papers that work well to absorb excess oil before you touch up with powder. The only issue is cost; you definitely don't have to spend this much to get an identical product.

☹ **Lip Balm SPF 15** *($15 for 0.5 ounce)* lacks the UVA-protecting ingredients of titanium dioxide, zinc oxide, avobenzone, Tinosorb, or Mexoryl SX, and is not recommended.

BOBBI BROWN MAKEUP

FOUNDATION: ✓☺ $$$ Oil-Free Even Finish Compact Foundation *($40)* is a silicone-based creamy compact makeup that applies and blends beautifully. In fact, along with Prescriptives' Liquid Touch Compact Makeup ($37) and Clarins Soft Touch Rich Compact Foundation ($36), it raises the bar for next-generation cream-to-powder makeups. Brown's version has a natural, slightly moist finish that isn't really powdery—it actually leaves skin with a soft glow that only those with oily skin will want to avoid. It provides light to medium coverage but if you layer it you can net nearly full coverage, a feature that also makes it an option for use as concealer. Fifteen shades are available, and the only ones to consider carefully are Golden, Chestnut, and Honey. Brown's lightest shade (Alabaster) is not offered in this foundation, which leaves those with very fair skin at a bit of a loss, but Porcelain may work for some.

✓☺ $$$ SPF 15 Tinted Moisturizer *($40)* has an in-part titanium dioxide–based sunscreen, and the silicone-based formula has a light but noticeably moist feel on the skin. The eight colors are exceptional, making this an outstanding tinted moisturizer for normal to dry skin. As expected, coverage is sheer and even.

☺ **$$$ Smooth Skin Foundation** *($40)* has a creamy-smooth, slightly thick texture with a nice amount of slip, so application is easy, though this takes longer to set than similar foundations. It leaves skin with a dewy finish and provides medium coverage. A major selling point of this foundation is that it can supposedly control oily areas while moisturizing dry areas. As I have written several times in the past, it is not possible for the same ingredient to keep oil at bay in one place while intuitively sensing where skin is dry and releasing moisturizing agents only over those areas. Moisturizing and oil-absorbing ingredients can (and often do) coexist in the same product, but once everything is uniformly mixed together, the moisturizing agents and oil-absorbers cancel each other out, since neither is able to exert its full benefit on skin. Don't believe the disparate claim, but do consider this foundation if you have normal to dry skin. The 16 shades are mostly gorgeous, but they're not all aces. Avoid Golden (too yellow) and Almond (slightly red; Warm Almond is much better). Walnut is slightly red, but may be an option for some darker skin tones.

☺ **$$$ Luminous Moisturizing Foundation** *($45)* has an elegant, fluid texture with just enough slip to make blending over normal to dry skin a pleasure. This does indeed have a luminous, satin-like finish, casting a healthy glow (rather than obvious shine) on skin. Coverage goes from light to medium and, as usual, almost all of the ten shades are flawlessly neutral. There are several good options for fair to light skin, but the palette doesn't extend toward deeper skin tones as it does for Brown's other foundations (I was told she may launch darker shades in the future). I wouldn't label this foundation "super-moisturizing" as the company does, but it will hydrate. Just don't expect it to firm or lift the skin as the showcase ingredient with that alleged benefit (acetyl hexapeptide-3) is barely present and doesn't work in that manner anyway. The only thing keeping this from earning a Paula's Pick rating is the inclusion of lavender extract, which lends a noticeable lavender fragrance to this otherwise top-notch foundation.

☺ **$$$ Foundation Stick** *($38)* was the debut foundation from Bobbi Brown, and it's interesting (and worthwhile) to note that the shade range has improved considerably over the years. Initially, the small lineup was very yellow, though it was clear Brown was heading in the right direction—there wasn't a pink or rose-toned shade to be found. Today's assembly of 17 mostly neutral shades runs the gamut from fair to very dark, with just a few missteps along the way. Warm Natural and Honey are slightly peach, but may work for some skin tones, while Chestnut has enough red so it may be problematic for some dark skin tones. Golden is still too yellow, and not recommended. Espresso is a brilliant shade for very dark African-American skin tones, while Alabaster should please those who feel no foundation is light enough for their skin. Texture-wise, this remains creamy, is surprisingly easy to blend, and provides medium coverage that can be sheered if desired. I disagree with the company's "for all skin types except very oily" claim, because this is not the type of foundation someone with blemishes should use, nor does it have a matte quality to please someone with an oily T-zone. It is best for normal to dry skin.

😐 **$$$ Oil-Free Even Finish Foundation SPF 15** *($40)* does not contain the UVA-protecting ingredients of titanium dioxide, zinc oxide, avobenzone, Tinosorb, or Mexoryl SX. That's a shame (and a near-insult at this price level) because this liquid foundation has a smooth, fluid texture that blends beautifully and sets to a soft, natural matte finish. Coverage runs from light to medium, and the formula is best for those with normal to slightly oily skin. Sixteen shades are available, including options for darker skin tones, and almost all of them are praiseworthy. The only ones to consider avoiding are Golden (the lone shade that suffers from being too yellow), and the slightly peach but still passable Almond.

😐 **$$$ Moisture Rich Foundation SPF 15** *($40)* has a wonderfully soft, fluid-but-creamy texture that blends beautifully and dries to a natural, soft glow finish. Coverage is in the light to medium range and the 17 shades are almost impeccable—the only ones to watch out for are Golden, which is quite yellow, and Walnut and Almond, both being slightly red. Warm Natural is borderline peach and has a brightness to it that's not exactly skin-true, but it may work for some Asian skin tones. African-American skin tones are well-served here, as are those with skin in the very fair range. Lamentably, the sunscreen is without sufficient UVA-protecting ingredients, which means this must be paired with another product that provides that critical protection. How shortsighted—because this is otherwise a formidable foundation for someone with normal to dry skin.

☹ **Extra SPF 25 Tinted Moisturizing Balm** *($48)* includes an in-part avobenzone sunscreen. But for this greasy tinted moisturizer, that benefit is negated by the many fragrant oils, all of which are irritating to skin and that counteract the anti-irritants present in the formula. Without them, this would have been a good option for those with very dry skin, and all seven shades are impeccably neutral.

CONCEALER: ☺ **$$$ Eye Brightener** *($32)* is a slightly fluid, jar-packaged concealer hybrid designed less for coverage and more for highlighting and brightening shadowed areas. The texture has just the right amount of slip if you blend delicately, and it sets to a satin matte finish with a slight hint of shine. When this is layered you can achieve medium coverage, but, as described, this product is not intended to conceal dark circles. Each of the four shades has a pink to peach cast, though the only one that doesn't resemble real skin tones is the Medium to Dark option. Eye Brightener may be used with or without an additional concealer and it can also serve as a late-day touch-up instead of adding more of your regular concealer (which, depending on the formula, may result in a heavy or caked look). A similar version of this product that is easier to work with because it includes a built-in brush is Estee Lauder Ideal Light Brush-On Illuminator ($24.50).

😐 **$$$ Blemish Cover Stick** *($20)* has a creamy, slightly greasy texture that is not what I would recommend using over a blemish. This stick concealer contains too many ingredients that can be problematic for use on breakout-prone skin, though it is oil-free. However, its natural finish and good coverage make it a winner for use on dark circles or other discolorations. The six shades nicely represent light to dark skin tones, and all of them are worth considering if you prefer this type of concealer.

😐 **$$$ Creamy Concealer Kit** *($32)* is a two-part product, with a creamy, thick, crease-prone concealer nestled on top of a small jar of loose powder. I suppose this will seem handy for some, but it adds little to the appeal of this product. The pros for the concealer are excellent coverage, reasonably smooth application, and reliable colors—only Beige and Almond are too pink and peach to pass muster. The lightest shade, Porcelain, is a great color for very fair skin, but it is coupled with a Pure White powder that can look ghostly. The rest of the ten shades come paired with Brown's Pale Yellow powder, which isn't as yellow as it used to be, but it's not a one-shade-fits-all deal either. The **Creamy Concealer** *($22)* is also available alone, though it offers one less shade than the Creamy Concealer Kit above. Powder is absolutely needed with this concealer; without it, expect to see creasing into lines and fading by the end of the day.

☹ **Corrector** *($22)* has the same texture, application, and level of coverage as the Creamy Concealer above, but this version is meant for those with very dark circles. The six shades are almost all strongly peach or pink, but the logic from Brown is that such hues cancel the purple tinge dark circles have. They do cancel it, but the effect is not nearly as flattering or neutral as it is from a neutral- to yellow-toned concealer. If anything, using a noticeably pink or peach-toned concealer over purple skin discolorations just replaces one discoloration with another. Regardless of what you need to conceal, no one's skin is this pink or peach. If you're intent on trying this product, the least problematic shades are Deep Bisque and Very Deep Bisque.

POWDER: ✓☺ **$$$ Sheer Finish Loose Powder** *($32)* is a talc-based powder that has a light, silky texture and smooth, slightly dry finish thanks to the cornstarch it contains. It feels weightless and looks very natural, yet makes skin look polished. Among the seven shades, avoid White (which really is pure white), and Golden Orange. Sunny Beige is slightly peach, but may work for some medium skin tones. ✓☺ **$$$ Sheer Finish Pressed Powder** *($30)* is also talc-based and shares the silky, lightweight texture and beautiful finish of the Sheer Finish Loose Powder above. The same shade cautions apply, here, too, but there are good choices for fair to dark skin.

Bobbi Brown's loose ☺ **$$$ Face Powder** *($32)* is a standard, talc-based powder that has an airy, silky texture and a dry finish. It's not quite as silky as the Sheer Finish Loose Powder above, but you get more product for your money (1 ounce vs. 0.25 ounce). The colors have been improved, and are not as yellow and orange as they once were, though Golden Orange is still one to check in natural light and carefully consider to make sure it doesn't look too bright. The ☺ **$$$ Pressed Powder** *($30)* is virtually identical to the loose powder, with the same colors and same caution about the Golden Orange shade, and, in this case, avoid Sunny Beige, which is too orange. ☺ **$$$ Bronzing Powder** *($32)* shows Brown knows what she's doing when it comes to creating believable tan shades for fair to medium skin tones. All of the shades are attractive and convincing, each possessing a smooth application and soft finish with a tiny amount of visible shine. Those with fair skin should apply this sparingly and build as needed—a little goes a long way.

BLUSH: ✓☺ **$$$ Pot Rouge for Lips and Cheeks** *($22)* is an above-average sheer cream blush for dry to very dry skin. Pot Rouge looks greasier than it is. You may be surprised how easily it applies because there's no heavy feel and it's free of excess slip. Its semi-moist finish makes it great for dry skin, but not the best for solo use on the lips or if you have an uneven skin texture or breakouts. If you opt to use this as timesaving lip-and-cheek makeup, you may want to follow up with a lip gloss, particularly if your lips are routinely dry or chapped. This is recommended over Stila's similar, but slightly too greasy, Convertible Color ($20).

The pressed powder ☺ **$$$ Blush** *($20)* features gorgeous colors that apply and blend evenly with a smooth matte finish (a few shades have a negligible amount of shine). This blush has a good color payoff on the skin, so if you want a sheer look, apply sparingly. ☺ **$$$ Cream Blush Stick** *($25)* is a sheer, slightly greasy cream blush that remains creamy on the skin. Blending takes some time, and this is really best for flawless normal to dry skin, as it is too creamy for oily skin types. The shade selection is a nice mix of understated brown-based colors and pastel brights.

EYESHADOW: ✓☺ **$$$ Long-Wear Cream Shadow** *($22)* takes a cue from Brown's successful Long Wear Gel Eyeliner and merges that technology into a silky, cream-to-powder eyeshadow collection. Application is surprisingly easy, but you better be fast because the formula sets quickly. It also doesn't have as much initial movement as powder eyeshadows, which can make blending difficult to nearly impossible. In terms of long wear, this passes with flying colors and absolutely refuses to crease—though you may notice slight fading at the end of the day. All but two of the shades have shimmer, but the shine level is mostly subtle to moderate. Bone and Suede are completely matte, with the former being a great all-over shade and the latter good for softly defining the crease. All told, this is a very good option if you're looking for a departure from powder eyeshadows, or something novel to use with a powder eyeshadow. And because the two formulas go together easily, you can apply powder eyeshadow over or under Long-Wear Cream Shadow, if you are careful not to rub too hard.

Bobbi Brown's ☺ **$$$ Eye Shadows** *($19)* have a silky, smooth-blending texture and most of the colors are beautifully matte (those that aren't true matte have a very soft, nonintrusive shine). There are some great choices for darker skin tones, and many of these shades would work well for lining the eyes or defining the eyebrows. The lighter shades apply sheerer than the medium to deep shades, which isn't necessarily advantageous but can make blending colors a bit easier. ☺ **$$$ Shimmer Wash Eye Shadow** *($19)* is how Brown chose to separate her matte Eye Shadows from the obviously shiny powder ones. These have the same smooth texture and even application, except every shade has a non-flaky shimmer finish. There are shine-enhancing options for all skin tones.

☹ **Cream Shadow Stick** *($20)* is a creamy eyeshadow in a roll-up stick form. There is only one color left (Vanilla, a soft nude) but it goes on choppy and can be difficult to blend out evenly. Plus, the texture of this starts smooth yet remains sticky once it has set! I'm a bit surprised this hasn't improved.

EYE AND BROW SHAPER: ✓☺ **$$$ Long Wear Gel Eyeliner** *($19)* is a cream-gel eyeliner that is applied with a brush. It goes on like a liquid liner, and quickly sets to a long-wearing, budge-proof finish. It's truly an extraordinary product for lining the eyes, especially for anyone who finds powders or pencils fade or smear by the end of the day (or sooner). Brown's selection of shades often sees high-shine options rotated in seasonally, but the core assortment of blacks, charcoal brown, and steely grays are perfect.

✓☺ **$$$ Natural Brow Shaper** *($17)* is essentially a lightweight mascara for brows. You can groom and shade your eyebrows with natural-looking color and a soft, natural-looking finish. This is truly best for the brows only; it applies well and dries quickly, yet the bristles on the brush aren't long enough to reach down to the roots of any gray hair you may wish to conceal. The colors aren't the best for very dark brown or black hair, but there is a nice range for lighter hair shades, while the Auburn shade is a neutral tan best for someone with light brown or dark blonde brows. A Clear version is also available. One caution: Overapplying this can cause flaking, so use it sparingly until you adjust to how much is needed to achieve the desired effect.

☹ **Creamy Eye Pencil** *($20)* is a standard, needs-sharpening pencil that definitely has a creamy texture. It tends to have a sticky finish, and smudges easily. Check out Brown's excellent matte eyeshadows for lining instead.

LIPSTICK, LIP GLOSS, AND LIPLINER: This is where Bobbi Brown began in 1991, and although the color palette is exceptional the formulas are standard and not as differentiated as those from other Lauder-owned lines such as Clinique and Prescriptives.

✓☺ **$$$ Matte Stain for Lips** *($20)* doesn't meet the true definition of matte, but its creaminess and lightweight feel on lips will doubtless win more customers than many other matte lipsticks with a drier texture. Packaged in a compact and designed to be applied with a lip brush, each shade is pigment-rich, creating a stain that lasts once the initial creaminess wears off. It applies smoothly and, as usual, Brown's palette of shades is beautiful, with options from nude pink to opulent reds. Think of this product as a modern matte with a velvety finish, and if the price doesn't deter you, check this out the next time you're at the Bobbi Brown counter.

The ☺ **$$$ Lip Color** *($21)* is a traditional cream lipstick with nice opaque coverage and great colors, including less conventional but still attractive options. Regardless of depth, the shades have minimal stain, so don't expect long wear. ☺ **$$$ Lip Shimmer** *($21)* has the same texture and application as the Lip Color above, only with a shimmer finish, slightly less pigment, and a comparatively small selection of shades. ☺ **$$$ Lip Sheer** *($21)* has a smooth, creamy feel that isn't as greasy as many other sheer lipsticks. It's actually not that sheer either, though its definitely softer than the Lip Color and Lip Shimmer above. The Brown makeup artist was raving about how these go on slick, then transform to a matte finish, which they absolutely do not. They remain glossy, which I pointed out to her, but she nevertheless insisted the matte finish was coming. It never did. ☺ **$$$ Tinted Lip Balm** *($17)* comes in a glossy black ChapStick-style component and imparts translucent, moisturizing color to lips. This petrolatum-based balm doesn't feel overly thick or greasy and leaves a soft sheen. Although pricey, the colors are versatile and wear is comfortable. You may find this is worth the splurge, although it works best worn alone rather than applied over lipstick.

The 😐 **$$$ Lip Gloss** and 😐 **$$$ Shimmer Lip Gloss** *(both $19)* are extremely overpriced, standard, thick, sticky glosses with a poor brush that tends to splay after a few uses; the Shimmer version just adds sparkle. 😐 **$$$ Crystal Lip Gloss** *($16)* is a very thick, sticky and syrupy gloss that comes in a squeeze tube. This will provide a high shine to the lips, but the thick feel is less than pleasant. 😐 **$$$ Brightening Lip Gloss** *($19)* has a thick, syrupy texture that ends up being quite sticky, and also tenacious. The brightening part comes from the noticeable shimmer in each shade of this sheer gloss. The brush applicator is a nice touch, but with repeated use it can splay (when is Brown going to change this inelegant feature?), which makes for a messy application if you're not careful.

😐 **$$$ Shimmer Lip Tint SPF 15** *($17)* does not contain the UVA-protecting ingredients of titanium dioxide, zinc oxide, avobenzone, Tinosorb, or Mexoryl SX, and is not recommended for sun protection. It acquits itself nicely as a standard tube lip gloss, and has a smoother, less sticky texture than Brown's regular Lip Gloss 😐 **$$$ Lip Tint SPF 15** *($17)* has the same texture and sheer, glossy finish as the Shimmer Lip Tint SPF 15 above, but also lacks sufficient UVA-protecting ingredients. It remains an OK, needlessly overpriced gloss option. 😐 **$$$ SPF 15 Lip Shine** *($19)* is a lightweight but too-slick sheer lipstick that is overpriced for what you get, and the sunscreen offers incomplete UVA protection, leaving lips vulnerable to sun damage.

😐 **$$$ Lipliner** *($20)* is a standard creamy lip pencil that features a smooth application and beautiful shade range, but the pencil has limited longevity compared to many others, including those that need sharpening, as this does.

MASCARA: ✓ ☺ $$$ No Smudge Mascara *($20)* really doesn't smudge but its performance goes beyond that. You'll enjoy how quickly this mascara lengthens lashes without clumping, and it provides more thickness than most waterproof mascaras. It stays on all day whether you're swimming or getting caught in the rain, and doesn't make lashes feel dry or brittle. Removing it requires more than a water-soluble cleanser, but that's par for the course. This is one to try if you prefer shopping for mascara at the department store.

☺ **$$$ Everything Mascara** *($20)* is a great all-purpose mascara, but it doesn't excel in any particular area. Moderate length and thickness are both present in equal proportion, so if you're looking to build amazingly long or dramatically thick lashes, this mascara won't bring you "everything." However, it does nicely separate lashes, doesn't clump or smear, and leaves lashes feeling soft rather than stiff or brittle.

😐 **$$$ Lash Glamour Lengthening Mascara** *($20)* is only glamorous if your definition of the word as it pertains to mascara is "minimal length and no thickness after much effort." This mascara is best for a natural look, and it applies cleanly without flaking.

FACE AND BODY ILLUMINATING/SHIMMER PRODUCTS: ☺ **$$$ Shimmer Brick Compact** *($38)* could almost be considered a value-priced item, even though the price tag for what amounts to pressed shimmer powder may raise some eyebrows. The value comes from the fact that you get five individual shades of powder (which resemble stacked bricks, hence the name), and all of them are viable options for adding a soft shine to the skin. The powder applies well, despite the fact that it feels drier than most, but the shine tends to migrate and dissipate after a few hours of wear. If the colors appeal to you, go for it—just don't expect the shimmer effect to go the distance. Interestingly, this product was originally intended to be a limited edition holiday item in 2002. Because of its popularity, it was permanently added to the line and continues to be a favorite.

BRUSHES: Brown's **Brushes** *($20–$55 for single brushes; $85–$225 for brush sets)* are quite nice, with well-tapered edges and dense bristles, though the prices are on the high side. Many of the brushes are available in either a travel (4-inch) or professional (6-inch) length. There are some to carefully consider, and some to ignore altogether. One to ignore is the ☹ **Powder Brush** *($55)*; for this amount of money it should be perfect, but it's too floppy and soft to apply powder well. The 😐 **$$$ Blush Brush** *($45)* is also somewhat difficult to control due to its softness. The ☹ **Brow Brush** *($20)* is very stiff and scratchy, and the ☹ **Bronzer Brush** *($35)* is also scratchy. The ☹ **Eye Shader Brush** *($25)* is too big for most women's eye area, again making control and placement of color an issue. The rest of the collection is worth considering, with the best, most useful brushes being the ☺ **$$$ Ultra Fine Eyeliner Brush** *($20)*, ☺ **$$$ Eye Shadow Brush** *($25)*, ☺ **$$$ Eye Contour Brush** *($25)*, the fabulous ✓☺ **$$$ Eye Smudge Brush** *($25)*, the ☺ **$$$ Foundation Brush** *($30)*, ✓☺ **$$$ Concealer Brush** *($20)*, ☺ **$$$ Touch Up Brush** *($25)*, and ☺ **$$$ Retractable Lip Brush** *($20)*.

SPECIALTY PRODUCTS: ✓☺ **$$$ All Over Bronzing Gel SPF 15** *($25)* is a brilliant, easy-to-blend option for bronzing skin, and contains an in-part avobenzone sunscreen for additional sun protection wherever it is applied. More a lotion than a gel, this single shade is a gorgeous sheer golden tan color without overtones of copper, orange, or peach. The shade works best on fair to medium skin tones, and offers a soft, moist finish without any shine (an all-too-common trait of bronzing products). If you're looking for this type of product, All Over Bronzing Gel SPF 15 should be on your short list of contenders.

😐 **$$$ Conditioning Brush Cleanser** *($16.50 for 3.4 ounces)* is nothing more than standard shampoo that will nicely clean your brushes, but it can easily be replaced with much less-expensive options from L'Oreal, Johnson & Johnson, or Neutrogena. The formula contains peppermint, which is a strange addition, and not an ingredient you'd want to remain on your brushes, especially those used near the eyes. The 😐 **$$$ Brush Case** *($35)* is available in sizes to fit Brown's short or professional-length brushes, but the cases themselves aren't anything special, especially for the money. The 😐 **$$$ Face Palette** *($15)* has six compartments in a portable compact. It comes empty, and you fill it with chunks of cream-based products, such as lipsticks or Brown's Foundation Stick (a spatula is included to smush things down). This isn't the best way to travel with makeup, but if you're up for slicing and dicing your full-size cosmetics for on-the-go use, check this out.

The ☺ **$$$ 3-Pan Palette** *($15)* and ☺ **$$$ 6-Pan Palette** *($25)* don't involve slicing pieces of your makeup up for travel. Instead, these clever, well-designed palettes hold either three or six powder-based products in their original containers. It's quick and easy to slip products in and out, and both versions are worth considering if you use several shades of Bobbi Brown eye shadow or powder blush. The palettes include a built-in mirror but do not have extra room to stow brushes. ☺ **Blotting Papers** *($20 for 100 sheets; $5 for refill packs of 100 sheets)* are standard blotting papers, the kind that do not deposit extra powder on skin but do mop up excess oil and perspiration. The price seems unreasonable, but the extra initial investment gets you a chic faux leather case to conceal and carry the papers. The refill pack comes in a soft cardboard container, so go for that if you don't want the special case.

THE BODY SHOP

THE BODY SHOP AT-A-GLANCE

Strengths: One of the few cosmetic companies that lists complete product ingredients on its Web site; affordable; the Aloe Products for Sensitive Skin are appropriate for that skin condition; good selection of eye makeup removers; one of the best pressed-powder foundations around; great pressed powder; liquid eyeliner; lip gloss; nice selection of affordable makeup brushes and specialty products; the entire makeup collection is laid out well, with testers, mirrors, and tissues readily available, plus a low key sales staff.

Weaknesses: The Tea Tree Oil and Kinetin collections; subcategories that focus on one beneficial ingredient (grape seed, vitamin C, etc.) to the exclusion of others, making for several collections of one-note products; no effective routine to address blemishes; poor skin-lightening products; surprisingly lackluster to poor foundations and concealers; poor long-wearing lip product.

For more information about The Body Shop, owned by L'Oreal, call (800) 263-9746 or visit www.thebodyshop.com or www.Beautypedia.com.

Postscript: The Body Shop's founder, Anita Roddick, passed away in September 2007 at the age of 64. Although through the years I have had my issues with several of her company's products, it must be said that her business acumen and worldwide humanitarian efforts deserve accolades. She was a unique, passionate businesswoman and I have no doubt her input will be sorely missed.

THE BODY SHOP SKIN CARE

THE BODY SHOP ALOE PRODUCTS FOR SENSITIVE SKIN

☺ **Aloe Calming Facial Cleanser, for Sensitive Skin** *($12 for 6.75 ounces)* is a good, gentle cleansing lotion for normal to dry or sensitive skin. It is fragrance-free and does not contain detergent cleansing agents. The oil content may require the use of a washcloth for complete removal.

✓☺ **Aloe Gentle Facial Wash, for Sensitive Skin** *($14 for 4.2 ounces)* is a very good, fragrance-free, gentle water-soluble cleanser for its intended skin type. In fact, this is great for all but very oily skin and rinses cleanly while removing makeup easily.

☺ **Aloe Gentle Exfoliator, for Sensitive Skin** *($12 for 2.5 ounces)* exfoliates skin with a small amount of mildly abrasive diatomaceous earth derived from tiny sea creatures. This ingredient is cushioned in a slightly creamy base of water, aloe, slip agents, and thickeners. It is a workable option for dry skin and is fragrance-free.

☹ **Aloe Calming Toner, for Sensitive Skin** *($10 for 6.75 ounces)* doesn't contain any skin irritants, including fragrance, but it's also a really boring concoction of just water, aloe, slip agents, and glycerin. It doesn't provide much benefit to skin other than slight moisture and helping to remove last traces of makeup.

☹ **Aloe Soothing Day Cream, for Sensitive Skin** *($12 for 1.7 ounces)* isn't the most soothing moisturizer around, and the tiny amount of oat flour in this fragrance-free moisturizer will barely register on skin. It's just a basic moisturizer for normal to slightly dry skin.

☺ **Aloe Soothing Moisture Lotion SPF 15, for Sensitive Skin** *($16 for 1.7 ounces)* is worth considering as a fragrance-free daytime moisturizer for normal to slightly dry skin. It includes an in-part avobenzone sunscreen and lightweight moisturizing ingredients plus a tiny amount of anti-irritants.

☹ **Aloe Soothing Night Cream, for Sensitive Skin** *($14 for 1.7 ounces)* is a more emollient version of the Aloe Soothing Day Cream, for Sensitive Skin, above, and contains an additional soothing agent, though not in an amount great enough for irritated skin to notice.

THE BODY SHOP GRAPESEED PRODUCTS FOR NORMAL/DRY SKIN

☺ **Grapeseed Facial Wash, for Normal/Dry Skin** *($10 for 3.4 ounces)* is a slightly water-soluble cleanser due to its plant oil content. Although this is a fine option for normal to dry skin not prone to blemishes, you will need to use a washcloth for complete removal.

☹ **Grapeseed Hydrating Toner, for Normal/Dry Skin** *($10 for 6.75 ounces)* contains more alcohol and fragrance than its namesake grape seed oil and extract, but there's not enough alcohol to make this toner an irritating experience for skin. It's a standard formula that provides an extra cleansing step and softening benefit, but that's about it.

☹ **Grapeseed Daily Hydrating Moisture Cream, for Normal/Dry Skin** *($12 for 1.7 ounces)* contains appreciable amounts of antioxidant grape seed and sesame seed oils, but the jar packaging hinders their effectiveness. This is otherwise a standard moisturizer whose few other bells and whistles are present in token amounts.

☹ **Grapeseed Extra Rich Night Cream, for Normal/Dry Skin** *($14 for 1.7 ounces)* is a more emollient version of the Grapeseed Daily Hydrating Moisture Cream, for Normal/Dry Skin, above, and although it's preferred for dry skin, the same basic comments apply.

☺ **Grapeseed Hydrating Moisturizer SPF 15, for Normal to Dry Skin** *($12 for 1.7 ounces)* is a very good in-part titanium dioxide sunscreen that contains antioxidant grape seed oil as its main antioxidant. There's not much else to extol about this product, but it's an affordable daytime moisturizer with sunscreen for its intended skin type.

THE BODY SHOP KINETIN PRODUCTS

All of The Body Shop's kinetin products contain varying amounts of kinetin, which is the trade name for N6-furfuryladenine. This is a plant hormone responsible for cell division. As a "natural" skin-care ingredient it is primarily being promoted as having been clinically proven to reduce the signs of aging, improve sun damage, reduce surfaced capillaries, and offer many other skin benefits of particular interest to aging baby boomers. There is a good deal of research on kinetin when it comes to plants or in test tubes (in vitro), with cells, or even with flies, but there is no published research on kinetin's topical effect on either animal or human skin (Source: *Dermatologic Clinics*, October 2000, pages 609–615).

Recent studies indicate that kinetin can help increase cell differentiation (turnover rate) and that it works best in the presence of calcium as an inducing agent, but that combination isn't what's being used in skin-care products that contain kinetin (Source: *Annals of the New York Academy of Sciences*, May 2006, pages 332–336). Kinetin may have benefit as a cell-communicating ingredient, but this has only been demonstrated in vitro (Source: *Proteonomics*, February 2006, pages 1351–1361). Please refer to the "Cosmetic Ingredient Dictionary" at the end of this book for more information about this ingredient.

☹ **24 Hour Treatment Lotion with Kinetin** *($26 for 1 ounce)* contains kinetin and the antioxidant vitamin E, but also has a lot of spearmint and orange oils, both of which are irritating to skin and would offset any potential benefit from kinetin.

☹ **Daily Eye Treatment with Kinetin** *($20 for 0.4 ounce)* isn't that much of a treatment. It's a relatively standard moisturizer that contains a significant amount of *Paullinia cupana* extract. Also known as guarana, this ingredient's caffeine content has constricting effects on skin and can be an irritant. If you were hoping to get your money's worth from the kinetin in this product, you're out of luck because it is barely present.

☹ **Facial Day Treatment SPF 15 with Kinetin** *($24 for 2 ounces)* covers the UVA spectrum with its in-part titanium dioxide sunscreen and contains a lot of kinetin (though exactly how much is needed in topical products has not been established), but it irritates skin with an appreciable concentration of spearmint and orange oils.

☹ **Illuminating Eye Treatment with Kinetin** *($16 for 0.25 ounce)* contains *Paullinia cupana* (guarana) extract, which has no effect on dark circles, though its constricting effect is irritating to skin. The illuminating effect this gel-textured product provides is from mineral pigments, not a dramatic change in skin as a result of kinetin.

☹ **Illuminating Face Treatment with Kinetin** *($26 for 1.4 ounces)* is a boring, jar-packaged moisturizer that spells trouble for skin in the form of irritating spearmint and orange oils.

THE BODY SHOP MOISTURE WHITE PRODUCTS

😐 **$$$ Moisture White Cleansing Powder** *($22 for 1.67 ounces)* is a nonaqueous, talc-based foaming cleanser that has no whitening effect on skin whatsoever. It's basically a novel way to cleanse skin, and talc has a very mild exfoliating effect. For the money, this doesn't compare favorably to most water-soluble cleansers.

☹ **Moisture White Toning Essence** *($22 for 5 ounces)* lists alcohol as the second ingredient, making this toner too drying and irritating for all skin types.

☹ **Moisture White Moisture Cream Plus** *($28 for 1.3 ounces)* is a below-standard moisturizer that contains irritating clove leaf oil and is not recommended. The tiny amounts of vitamin C and licorice extract have no ability to lighten skin.

☹ **Moisture White Night Treatment Cream** *($36 for 1.3 ounces)*. The form of vitamin C in this product is magnesium ascorbyl phosphate, which research has shown to be an effective skin-lightening agent in concentrations of 3% and above (Source: *Skin Research and Technology*, May 2002, pages 73–77). Although this product appears to meet that percentage, the jar packaging won't keep the vitamin C stable once it's exposed to air and light. It contains the fragrant components of linalool, geraniol, limonene, and eugenol, all of which are problematic for skin.

☺ **Moisture White Brightening Serum** *($36 for 1.5 ounces)* contains mostly water, glycerin, emollients, silicone, slip agents, vitamin C, plant oils, thickeners, preservatives, and fragrance. It's a good lightweight moisturizer for normal to slightly dry skin types curious to try a vitamin C product.

THE BODY SHOP SEAWEED PRODUCTS FOR COMBINATION/OILY SKIN

☹ **Seaweed Deep Cleansing Facial Wash, for Combination/Oily Skin** *($10 for 3.3 ounces)* has merit as a water-soluble cleanser for its intended skin type but doesn't make it across the finish line because it contains irritating menthol.

☺ **Seaweed Purifying Facial Cleanser, for Combination/Oily Skin** *($12 for 6.76 ounces)* is a good cleansing lotion that omits detergent cleansing agents in favor of silicone and emollients. It is best for normal to slightly dry skin and rinses surprisingly well without the aid of a washcloth. This cleanser isn't more purifying than any other, so ignore that claim.

☺ **Seaweed Pore-Cleansing Facial Exfoliator, for Combination/Oily Skin** *($12 for 2.5 ounces)* is a cleanser and topical scrub in one that uses olive seed powder as the abrasive agent. The jojoba oil is inappropriate for oily areas, but this is an acceptable scrub for normal to slightly dry skin.

☹ **Seaweed Clarifying Toner, for Combination/Oily Skin** *($10 for 6.76 ounces)* contains menthol and that additive is made more irritating by the presence of fragrant components such as linalool and citronellol.

☹ **Seaweed Clarifying Night Treatment, for Combination/Oily Skin** *($16 for 1 ounce)* is one of the most boring moisturizers in this entire book. Despite enticing claims, this product is primarily water, thickener, and preservative. Lots of ingredients follow these basics, but none of them are intriguing for skin and leave it shortchanged yet highly fragranced.

😐 **Seaweed Mattifying Day Cream, for Combination/Oily Skin** *($14 for 1.7 ounces)* offers skin slightly more than the Seaweed Clarifying Night Treatment for Combination/Oily Skin, above, but that's not saying much. This is an average water- and silicone-based moisturizer for its intended skin type.

😐 **Seaweed Mattifying Moisture Lotion SPF 15, for Combination/Oily Skin** *($16 for 1.69 ounces)* provides an in-part avobenzone sunscreen in a lightweight lotion base suitable for its intended skin type. What's missing are several essential elements necessary to create a great moisturizer, making this an effective, though average, sunscreen.

THE BODY SHOP TEA TREE OIL PRODUCTS

Tea tree oil, also known as melaleuca, has disinfecting properties that have been shown to be helpful for breakouts. According to *Healthnotes Review of Complementary and Integrative Medicine* (www.healthwell.com/healthnotes/Herb/Tea_Tree.cfm) and the *Medical Journal of Australia*, October 1990, pages 455–458, 5% tea tree oil and 2.5% benzoyl peroxide are both effective in reducing the number of blemishes, though the benzoyl peroxide showed significantly better results than the tea tree oil. Skin oiliness was lessened significantly in the benzoyl peroxide group versus the tea tree oil group. However, the tea tree oil had somewhat less irritating side effects. Regrettably, while tea tree oil is an option for treating blemishes, all of The Body Shop's products have less than a 1% concentration, which means they are unlikely to have an effect on breakouts.

☹ **Tea Tree Oil Daily Cleansing Wipes, for Normal, Oily or Blemished Skin** *($12 for 25 wipes)* initially have a lot going for them in terms of being a good option for normal to oily and/or blemish-prone skin, but the presence of peppermint oil makes these wipes too irritating for all skin types. In addition, the fragrant compounds limonene (found in citrus peels) and linalool (from lavender) magnify the irritation factor and are not ingredients you'd want to use to remove makeup around the eyes.

☹ **Tea Tree Oil Daily Foaming Facial Wash, for Normal, Oily or Blemished Skin** *($11.50 for 5 ounces)* is a liquid-to-foam cleanser that contains a hefty amount of tea tree oil but also includes peppermint oil, making it too irritating for any skin type.

☺ **Tea Tree Oil Facial Wash, for Normal, Oily or Blemished Skin** *($10 for 8.4 ounces)* is a very good water-soluble cleanser whose tiny amount of denatured alcohol is unlikely to be a problem for skin. The amount of tea tree oil is minor, though this ingredient isn't of much benefit in a cleanser because it is rinsed from skin before it can exert an antibacterial effect. Still, this is appropriate for its intended skin type.

☹ **Tea Tree Oil Soap, for Normal, Oily or Blemished Skin** *($6 for 3.5 ounces)* is standard-issue bar soap, and although it contains tea tree oil, the ingredients that keep this in bar form can clog pores because they do not rinse well from skin.

😐 **Tea Tree Oil Facial Scrub, for Normal, Oily or Blemished Skin** *($10.50 for 3.7 ounces)* has minimal scrub abilities and is more of a cleanser than anything else. Its wax content can impede rinsing, and it's not ideal for use on blemished skin. However, this is an OK cleanser/scrub option for normal to dry skin not prone to blemishes.

😐 **Tea Tree Oil Freshener, for Normal, Oily or Blemished Skin** *($10 for 8.4 ounces)* offers minimal benefit for skin beyond an extra cleansing step, and contains just a trace of tea tree oil. It is primarily water, surfactant, and preservative.

😐 **Tea Tree Oil Mattifying Moisture Gel, for Normal, Oily or Blemished Skin** *($11.50 for 1.7 ounces)* temporarily mattifies skin due to its dry-finish silicone base, but unless you're excited about tea tree oil (and there's less than 1% of it in this product), there are more intriguing mattifying products to consider from Smashbox or Clinique.

☹ **Tea Tree Oil, for Normal, Oily or Blemished Skin** *($7.50 for 0.33 ounce)* lists alcohol as the second ingredient and, despite the name, doesn't appear to contain the requisite amount of tea tree oil to have an anti-blemish effect.

😐 **Tea Tree Oil Blemish Fade Night Lotion, for Oily/Blemished Skin** *($18 for 1 ounce)* contains barely any tea tree oil, instead relying on laurelwood oil (listed as *Calophyllum inophyllum* and also known as tamanu oil) for its alleged anti-blemish properties. I wrote "alleged" because there is insufficient evidence available to gauge the effectiveness of this oil for blemishes (Source: www.naturaldatabase.com). It might work to some extent against blemishes, but wouldn't you rather spend your money experimenting with proven anti-acne ingredients?

😐 **Tea Tree Oil Blemish Stick, for Normal, Oily or Blemished Skin** *($7 for 0.08 ounce)* contains more alcohol than tea tree oil, though neither is present in amounts large enough to impact skin for better or worse. That makes this merely a water- and glycerin-based solution that provides minimal hydration and won't help heal blemishes (though it won't make them worse either).

☺ **Tea Tree Oil Face Mask, for Normal, Oily or Blemished Skin** *($14 for 4.8 ounces)* has a tiny bit of tea tree oil, so the name isn't nonsense, but is otherwise a standard clay mask that's a good option for normal to oily skin. Some of the thickening agents in this mask may be problematic for use on blemished skin.

☹ **Tea Tree Oil Nose Pore Mask, for Normal, Oily or Blemished Skin** *($8 for 1 ounce)* is a standard, alcohol-based, peel-off mask, the same kind that has been around for years. You're supposed to believe that once this solution of alcohol, silica, and glycerin has dried, the peeling process can pull surface impurities from pores. But if your intent is to improve the lining of the pore, you need something (such as salicylic acid) that goes deeper than this superficial mask. The alcohol makes this mask too irritating to use regularly.

☺ **Tea Tree Oil Facial Blotting Tissues, for Normal, Oily or Blemished Skin** *($10 for 65 sheets)* are standard oil-blotting papers that omit the powder in favor of tea tree oil and fragrant limonene. They're a good option, but the tiny amount of tea tree oil doesn't offer a special benefit for blemished skin.

THE BODY SHOP VITAMIN C PRODUCTS

☹ **Vitamin C Hydrating Facial Cleanser** *($14 for 8 ounces)* would have been a great cleansing lotion for normal to dry skin, but it contains grapefruit oil, which is irritating to skin and eyes, and this isn't made better by the orange oil that's also present (Source: www.naturaldatabase.com).

☹ **Vitamin C Cleansing Face Polish** *($14 for 3.38 ounces)* contains grapefruit and orange oils, making this substandard scrub too irritating for all skin types.

☹ **Vitamin C Micro Refiner** *($21 for 2.5 ounces)* contains grapefruit and orange oils, making this substandard scrub too irritating for all skin types.

😐 **Vitamin C Energising Face Spritz** *($14 for 3.3 ounces)* omits the grapefruit oil but leaves the fragrant orange oil, and its vitamin C content is paltry. This average toner is more akin to spraying perfume on the face than anything really helpful.

😐 **Vitamin C Eye Reviver** *($18 for 0.5 ounce)* isn't much for vitamin C but is still a decent water- and silicone-based moisturizer for slightly dry skin anywhere on the face. The orange flower water just provides fragrance and can be a problem for use around the eyes, though there's only a tiny amount present.

😐 **Vitamin C Intensive Night Treatment** *($22 for 1 ounce)* contains a significant amount of vitamin C (ascorbic acid) in a nonaqueous base with a silky finish. Vitamin E is on hand as well, and the only detriment is the inclusion of orange oil. A more robust ingredient listing would have made the name "intensive" really mean something.

☹ **Vitamin C Moisturizer SPF 15** *($16 for 1.7 ounces)* has the right stuff when it comes to broad-spectrum sun protection, but also contains grapefruit oil. The chemical constituents of grapefruit oil are known to cause contact dermatitis and phototoxic reactions when skin is exposed to sun. Although this product provides sun protection, why risk a reaction when so many effective sunscreens are available without problematic extras?

😐 **Vitamin C Plus Time Release Capsules** *($25 for 28 capsules)* isn't pure vitamin C as claimed because there are several ingredients in these silicone-filled capsules, including fragrant orange oil and fragrance components, that aren't the best for skin. This is an intriguing way to supply skin with stable doses of vitamin C (ascorbic acid) but overall it's not as elegant as Elizabeth Arden's Ceramide Time Complex Capsules ($45 for 30 capsules), which, while without vitamin C, supply skin with a greater array of beneficial ingredients than this product, and without adding potential irritants.

☹ **Vitamin C Re-Texturizing Peel** *($20 for 1.7 ounces)* lists alcohol and polyvinyl alcohol as main ingredients, making this peel-off peel too drying and irritating for all skin types. This also contains several citrus oils that only add to the irritation from the alcohol.

☹ **Vitamin C Skin Boost** *($22 for 1 ounce)* contains grapefruit and orange oils, neither of which provides a positive boost for skin. This serum is not recommended.

☹ **Vitamin C Lip Care SPF 15** *($5 for 0.15 ounce)* lacks the UVA-protecting ingredients of titanium dioxide, zinc oxide, avobenzone, Tinosorb, or Mexoryl SX, and is not recommended.

THE BODY SHOP VITAMIN E PRODUCTS

☺ **Vitamin E Cream Cleanser** *($11 for 6.75 ounces)* is a very standard, cold cream–style cleanser that can work well for someone with normal to dry skin. It does contain fragrance and fragrance components that are potentially irritating, though less so in a rinse-off product like this. The amount of vitamin E is insignificant.

☹ **Vitamin E Gentle Cleansing Wipers** *($12 for 25 wipes)* are water- and castor oil–based cleansing wipes that, while effective for removing makeup, contain fragrant irritants of linalool, eugenol, and limonene, among others. With the abundance of cleansing wipes available, most for less money, there is no reason to use these and subject skin to irritation.

☹ **Vitamin E Soap** *($6 for a 4.5-ounce bar)* is standard bar soap, and no amount of vitamin E will make it less drying for any skin type.

😐 **Vitamin E Cream Exfoliator** *($12.50 for 2.5 ounces)* contains some problematic fragrant components (eugenol among them) that downgrade an otherwise excellent topical scrub for dry to very dry skin. This is still worth considering since it is rinsed from skin so quickly.

😐 **Vitamin E Face Mist** *($12 for 3.2 ounces)* is a very basic toner with a minor amount of vitamin E, almost to the point of making the name embarrassing. It's an OK option for normal to dry skin, and contains fragrance in the form of rose water.

😐 **Vitamin E Eye Cream** *($14 for 0.5 ounce)* is a basic but decent moisturizer for slightly dry skin around the eyes or elsewhere on the face. Vitamin E makes more than a cameo appearance in this product, and in this amount is much more likely to be effective as an antioxidant. This eye cream is fragrance-free.

😐 **Vitamin E Facial Day Lotion SPF 15** *($14.50 for 2.5 ounces)* has an in-part titanium dioxide sunscreen in a rather boring base formula that's mostly aloe and thickeners. The vitamin E content is minuscule and no other antioxidants are included.

😐 **Vitamin E Illuminating Moisture Cream** *($15 for 1.7 ounces)* is an average moisturizer for normal to dry skin that's mostly water, thickener, water-binding agent, shea butter, pH adjuster, and wax. The jar packaging won't help keep the meager amount of vitamin E stable.

😐 **Vitamin E Moisture Cream** *($12.50 for 1.8 ounces)* is nearly identical to the Vitamin E Illuminating Moisture Cream above, and the same review applies. The fact that this product is a Body Shop best-seller means a lot of people aren't giving their skin everything it needs to look and feel its healthy best.

😐 **Vitamin E Nourishing Night Cream** *($14.50 for 1.7 ounces)* covers some of the basics in terms of what makes a great moisturizer, but some isn't enough, and the jar packaging won't keep the tiny amount of vitamin E in here stable once the product is opened.

😐 **Vitamin E Moisture Mask** *($15.50 for 3.38 ounces)* is worth considering by those with dry to very dry skin due to its effective blend of glycerin, silicone, plant oils, and skin-identical ingredients. It's a shame the jar packaging doesn't help keep the vitamin E stable, but without question this will make dry skin look and feel better, and it does not need to be rinsed from skin.

☹ **Vitamin E Lip Care Stick SPF 15** *($5 for 0.15 ounce)* does not contain the UVA-protecting ingredients of titanium dioxide, zinc oxide, avobenzone, Tinosorb, or Mexoryl SX, and is not recommended.

THE BODY SHOP WISE WOMAN PRODUCTS

☺ **Wise Woman Luxury Cleanser** *($15.50 for 6.75 ounces)* is primarily a blend of water with several nonvolatile plant oils. The detergent cleansing agents are present in minor amounts, though the oils certainly work to remove makeup. This is a good option for dry to very dry skin not prone to blemishes; you may need a washcloth for complete removal.

☹ **Wise Woman Softening Toner** *($15.50 for 5.4 ounces)* has some fancy-sounding ingredients and some of them are beneficial for dry skin, but not in the tiny amounts used in this overall boring toner. It contains mostly water, slip agents, witch hazel, castor oil, and preservative.

😐 **$$$ Wise Woman Eye Cream** *($22 for 0.5 ounce)* is an aloe-based moisturizer that contains more witch hazel than beneficial ingredients, though not enough to be irritating. This is an OK, slightly emollient formula whose most intriguing ingredients are listed after the preservative, so they don't count for much.

😐 **$$$ Wise Woman Regenerating Day Cream** *($30 for 1.7 ounces)* isn't suitable for daytime because it does not carry an SPF rating (though sunscreen agents are the second- and fifth-listed ingredients). Why The Body Shop included broad-spectrum protection without going through the testing necessary to establish an SPF rating is a mystery, and leaves this as an unwise choice for any woman. Moisturizer-wise, it doesn't break any new ground and is best suited for normal to dry skin. The antioxidants are sullied by jar packaging.

☹ **Wise Woman Regenerating Night Cream** *($34 for 1.7 ounces)* would have been a slam-dunk for dry to very dry skin were it not for jar packaging that hinders the effectiveness of the antioxidant-rich plant oils and the inclusion of irritating lavender oil.

😐 **$$$ Wise Woman Vitality Serum** *($34 for 1.7 ounces)* is built around the ingredient lactobacillus clover flower extract. Lactobacillus is a type of aerobic bacteria that produces large amounts of lactic acid as it ferments with carbohydrate sources. There is some research indicating that taking supplements of lactobacillus (it is also considered a probiotic) may help reduce skin allergies and forms of dermatitis. However, substantiated research on topical application of lactobacillus is nonexistent, though it likely functions as a water-binding agent. Clover flower has no research proving its mettle for aging skin, though it may be sensitizing. There is little reason to consider this serum compared to superior options from Olay, Neutrogena, Clinique, and Paula's Choice.

☺ **Wise Woman Intensive Firming Mask** *($18.50 for 3.4 ounces)* is a very good moisturizing mask for normal to dry skin. It is not ultra-creamy or lush, so it will leave those with very dry skin wanting more. The film-forming agent in this mask can make skin look firmer temporarily, but this is a minor cosmetic improvement; no one will think you've had anything lifted. Still, in terms of moisturizing ability and some elegant ingredients, this is worth considering.

OTHER BODY SHOP PRODUCTS

☺ **Camomile Gentle Eye Make-Up Remover** *($12.50 for 8.4 ounces)* combines silicone with standard gentle detergent cleansing agents, and works well to remove makeup, including waterproof formulas. The amount of chamomile is likely too small to have a soothing effect, but it's a plus that this makeup remover is fragrance-free.

☺ **Camomile Gentle Eye Make-Up Remover Gel** *($10.50 for 3.4 ounces)* is similar to the Camomile Gentle Eye Makeup Remover above, only in gel rather than liquid form. Otherwise, the same review applies.

✓☺ **Camomile Waterproof Eye Make-Up Remover** *($12.50 for 3.3 ounces)* doesn't contain much chamomile, but is in fact an excellent lotion-type eye-makeup remover. It works swiftly to remove even stubborn waterproof mascara, and is fragrance-free. This is best applied before washing with a water-soluble cleanser.

☹ **Skin Focus Re-Texturizing Peel** *($20 for 1.67 ounces)* has a low enough pH to allow the salicylic acid to exfoliate (peel) skin, but the amount in this product is 0.5% or less, meaning the results are limited. More of an issue is that alcohol is the second ingredient—and there's enough bergamot oil on hand to cause irritation without any benefit for skin.

☹ **Blue Corn 3 in 1 Deep Cleansing Scrub Mask, for Normal/Oily Skin** *($14 for 4.2 ounces)* has been around for years and, although it has some positives (the convenience of an absorbent mask that has a slightly abrasive quality so you can exfoliate as you rinse), it's more harmful than helpful for skin because of the volatile fragrant oils it contains.

☺ **Natural Oceanic Clay Ionic Mask** *($18 for 4.2 ounces)* is about as basic as a clay mask can get, containing mostly clay, water, preservative, and fragrance. Whether clay comes from the ocean or land isn't important; all clay has absorbent qualities that can be helpful for controlling oily skin (albeit temporarily).

☹ **Warming Mineral Face Mask** *($14 for 5.1 ounces)* contains a mineral that warms when it is mixed with water, but that has no special benefit for skin beyond feeling pleasant. That's fine, but what's not is the inclusion of irritating ginger oil and cinnamon bark oils, joined by several fragrance components, including problematic eugenol.

☹ **Lavender Camomile Facial Blotting Tissues** *($10 for 65 Sheets)* are blotting tissues steeped in plant oils, which is odd because who needs oil on oil blotting papers? Odd becomes irksome when you see that one of the oils is lavender, and that's a problem for skin.

☺ **Natural Powder Facial Blotting Tissues** *($10 for 65 sheets)* work to mattify skin by depositing a sheer layer of talc, clay, and absorbent minerals each time you blot. The finish may need some slight blending to avoid a too-powdered look, but these certainly work to tame shine.

☺ **Powder-Free Facial Blotting Tissues** *($10 for 65 sheets)* are standard, powder-free blotting papers that are a quick, convenient way to absorb excess oil before touching up your makeup.

😐 **Rose Powder Facial Blotting Tissues** *($10 for 65 sheets)* are not preferred to the blotting papers above because these use wood pulp rather than refined tissue paper and aren't as absorbent.

☹/☺ **Born Lippy Balms** *($5 for 0.3 ounce)* are standard castor oil– and lanolin-based lip balms that are available in a variety of fruit flavors. Rather than dwell on the fact that fruit-flavored balms encourage lip-licking and create the need to reapply the product frequently, not all of the flavors are recommended. The ones to avoid due to irritating fragrance components are Mango Peach and Strawberry. Exotic Passionfruit, Raspberry, and Watermelon do not contain these problematic ingredients and are recommended.

✓☺ **Cocoa Butter Lip Care Stick** *($5 for 0.15 ounce)* is an excellent lip balm that contains a thoughtful blend of nut oils, wax, olive oil, and, as the name states, cocoa butter. An added bonus is several anti-irritants, which makes this lip balm a step above most others.

✓☺ **Hemp Lip Care Stick** *($5 for 0.15 ounce)* has a different assortment of beneficial ingredients for dry lips than the Cocoa Butter Lip Care Stick above, but is just as effective and equally recommended.

☹ **Hemp Lip Protector Tin** *($6.50 for 0.3 ounce)* contains clary oil, which is irritating to skin and likely even more so to lips. It is not worth considering over either of the lip balms above.

☹/☺ **Lip Butter** *($6 for 0.3 ounce)* has a buttery-smooth texture and can ably take care of dry, chapped lips. However, it is available in several flavors and all but one of them contain irritating fragrance components. The flavor to consider is Coconut. None of the others are recommended, which explains the split-face rating.

☹ **Stop Violence in the Home Lip Care Stick** *($5 for 0.15 ounce)* should be renamed "Stop the Irritation," because that's what your lips are subjected to once this peppermint oil–infused stick balm is applied. The proceeds from this product support a good cause, but there are ways to be charitable without irritating your lips.

☺ **Fake It! Self-Tan Lotion for Body, Light Medium Shade** *($16.50 for 6.75 ounces)* turns skin tan thanks to dihydroxyacetone, the same ingredient used in most self-tanning products. This option has a silky-smooth lotion texture and the only reason to not consider it over countless others is the addition of fragrance components, including limonene and linalool.

☺ **Fake It! Self-Tan Lotion for Body, Medium Dark Shade** *($16.50 for 6.75 ounces)* is nearly identical to the Fake It! Self-Tan Lotion for Body, Light Medium Shade above, except this version has a greater concentration of dihydroxyacetone. Otherwise, the same review applies.

☺ **Fake It! Self-Tan Lotion for Face** *($16.50 for 1.69 ounces)* has a silkier texture and a soft matte finish compared to the Fake It! self-tanners above, but also shares the same concern about fragrance components, including linolool and limonene. It works as well as any self-tanner, but isn't preferred to those that omit the fragrant irritants.

☺ **Fake It! Self-Tan Mousse for Body** *($16.50 for 4.2 ounces)* has the lightest texture of all the Fake It! self-tanners, but shares the same concern over fragrance components.

THE BODY SHOP MAKEUP

FOUNDATION: ✓☺ **All in One Face Base** *($16.50)* has been reformulated and is better than ever! This talc-based, pressed-powder foundation has an amazingly silky application that provides a natural matte finish and light coverage. Few powders look this natural on skin, and it does a great job of minimizing pores and controlling excess oil. The one caution is that the third ingredient is cornstarch, which can contribute to breakouts by "feeding" the bacteria that trigger them. However, your skin may not react in that manner, so don't let that stop you from trying this. The six shades are best for fair to medium skin tones and all of them are soft and neutral. All in One Face Base is best for normal to slightly dry or slightly oily skin.

☺ **Ultra Smooth Foundation** *($18.50)* is aptly named because this is indeed one smooth foundation! The initially thick texture blends well, leaving a powdery matte finish. Unfortunately, the finish, while feeling matte, remains slick on the skin. That means someone with oily skin or oily areas will find this foundation easily slips, fades, and may make large pores more apparent. What a shame, because the shade selection has some very good choices for those with fair and dark skin. This is a potential option for someone with normal to dry skin, but those skin types may not like the matte feel.

☺ **Oil-Free Foundation SPF 15** *($20)* gets its sunscreen partly from titanium dioxide. Although that's great news for this matte finish foundation, the high amount (and likely the grade) of titanium dioxide used lends a slightly chalky finish that is difficult to soften. If you want an oil-free, medium to full coverage foundation and are amenable to this one's finish (the chalkiness is coupled with a soft shimmer) it may be worth a look. The predominantly yellow-based shades are quite good and include options for fair to dark skin tones. Shades 05 and 06 may be too gold for medium skin tones but are still worth testing.

CONCEALER: ☺ **Ultra Smooth Liquid Concealer** *($12)* has an accurate name because this silicone-enhanced liquid concealer dispensed from a tube is very smooth. Its ultra-light texture blends to a silky finish that, unfortunately, never sets completely. That leads to slippage into lines under the eyes and less than ideal coverage that fades before it should. It comes in three excellent neutral shades, but this is only one to consider if you need minor coverage and are willing to tolerate some creasing. ☹ **Tea Tree Oil Cover Stick** *($8)* has an emollient texture that is a problem for use over blemishes. The ingredients that keep this concealer in stick form can easily clog pores, while the amount of tea tree oil is too low to function as a disinfectant. The two shades are workable, but this has limited appeal.

☹ **Concealer Pencil** *($10)* is a thick, creamy concealer packaged as a thick pencil that needs regular sharpening. This covers well and blends better than expected, but the greasepaint-like texture creases easily and the shades aren't anything to get excited about. Considering the number of amazing concealers available in all price ranges, this isn't worth an audition.

POWDER: ✓☺ **Pressed Face Powder** *($14)* has an admirably silky, talc-based texture that is minimally dry. In fact, the oils in this pressed powder and the smooth, non-powdery finish it provides make it a good choice for those with normal to dry skin. The four shades are remarkably neutral and meant for light to medium skin tones only.

☺ **Loose Face Powder** *($12.50)* has a silky, airy, talc-based texture and a drier-than-usual finish that is ideal for normal to very oily skin. Shades 01, 02, and 03 are neutral flesh tones perfect for fair to medium skin, while shade 05 is a sheer bronze color with gold shimmer, which tends to flake. Apparently The Body Shop hasn't had a loose powder for years, and customer demand made them reconsider—and what they produced is well worth an audition! ☺ **Bronzing Powder** *($14)* possesses a wonderfully smooth texture that applies evenly—a critical point for bronzing powder. Even better, both of the shades allow you to create a convincing tan effect. The 01 shade is matte and best for fair to light skin, while shade 02 is for light to medium skin and has a subtle amount of shine.

☹ **$$$ Brush-On Beads** *($17.50)* has been part of The Body Shop makeup line for years, but I don't understand why these shiny powder beads have maintained such an indispensable status in this line. In any event, this is still the same as it ever was, and it works well for a sparkling peachy brown effect, or use Brush-on Buff as a soft highlighting powder. The beads allow for very sheer color application, but if they break you're left with an uneven application with chunks of powder.

☹ **$$$ Brilliance Powder** *($18.50)* comes in a self-contained component that houses a loose powder in a tube, which is attached to a built-in brush. Pushing a button at the base shoots powder onto the brush, ready for application to skin. Regrettably, that's the most exciting aspect of this barely there powder. Application is extremely sheer, and two of the three shades impart noticeable shine that doesn't stay put. A matte bronzing powder is also available, but you have to brush on a lot to get even a hint of color, making this a costly investment.

BLUSH: ☺ **Cheek Blush** *($12.50)* is an odd product. It begins slick and so is tricky to blend, and then stays that way, so it always has some movement. Here's the odd part: The sheer, shimmer-laced colors have a stain effect on skin, so the color itself stays where you blend it. This product is best for normal to dry skin types that don't mind shimmering cheeks.

☹ **Cheek Color** *($12.50)* is a large-size traditional powder blush, reminiscent of the size and packaging of M.A.C.'s powder blushes. This has a soft texture and a dry but smooth application that imparts very sheer, see-through color. All of the shades shine, but Golden Pink and Hazelnut are ultra-shiny and are not recommended for daytime. The shine among the remaining understated shades is, well, understated!

EYESHADOW: ☺ **Cream Eye Color** *($10)* is a find if you want a sheer, shimmer-infused eyeshadow that has a soft, lightweight, cream-to-powder texture and a silky, creaseless finish that stays put (so does the shine). The shade selection favors warm nudes and steely silver-to-blue cool tones, but if you find an appealing hue and want to experiment beyond powder eyeshadows, why not?

The collection of over 20 ☺ **Eye Colors** *($9.50)* feels silky and blends beautifully, but here's the frustration: All of the shades, even the dark ones, go on extremely sheer. Talk about subtle color! And these do not build that well, so you're pretty much stuck with no intensity and a light wash of color that stands a good chance of fading even before you leave your house. If you're looking for very soft color, these are worth a peek, but watch out for the glittery shades because they do not apply as smoothly and the glitter tends to flake. The non-glittery but still shiny shades don't have this trait. If you're shopping for matte options, you'll need to look elsewhere. ☺ **Eye Shimmer** *($9.50)* doesn't apply as smoothly as the Eye Colors above, but it's not worth downgrading to an unhappy face rating. The small selection of shades is all about shine, and they serve their purpose with minimal flaking despite slightly uneven application.

EYE AND BROW SHAPER: ✓☺ **Liquid Eyeliner** *($11.50)* has an excellent soft, but firm, brush that is adept at drawing a thin, continuous line and a fast-drying formula that minimizes the risk of smearing, plus its wearability has improved since it was last reviewed, making it deserving of a Paula's Pick rating.

☺ **$$$ Brow & Liner Kit** *($16)* combines a brow powder and powder eyeshadow to use as liner in one petite compact. The circular component houses a cleverly designed dual-sided brush, but regrettably the brow brush is too stiff (and deposits too much product if your brows are thin) and the eyeliner brush is too floppy for precise control. Still, both powders go on smoothly and are pigment-rich. Each also has a touch of shine, but it's barely noticeable on skin. The three duos include options for all brow colors except shades of red or auburn.

☺ **Eye Definer** *($8.50)* is a routine pencil in terms of the inevitable sharpening, but it does glide on and is minimally creamy, which means there's a low risk of smudging or fading. Avoid shade 07, which is blue. ☺ **Brow & Lash Gel** *($12)* is a standard clear gel that works to groom brows and barely enhance lashes. It will feel sticky unless applied lightly, but it doesn't take much to achieve a groomed look.

☹ **Brow Definer** *($8.50)* has a smooth, not-too-stiff texture but applies unevenly, depositing even color followed by dots and specks of color, plus the tip breaks off quickly. Under the assumption that I was experimenting with old testers, I used this pencil at other Body Shop stores, all with the same result. That's reason enough to avoid it.

LIPSTICK, LIP GLOSS, AND LIPLINER: ☺ **Lip Color** *($12)* feels smooth, goes on light, and is truly a very nice opaque, mildly creamy lipstick. There are some striking nude and attractive bright colors available, although the overall shade selection isn't huge. ☺ **Sheer Lip Shine** *($12.50)* is moderately sheer, imparting less color than traditional lipstick but more than many lip glosses (and similarly-textured sheer lipsticks). It offers an emollient feel and glossy finish without excess slickness, and the shades are mostly inviting. ☺ **Hi-Shine Lip Treatment** *($11.50)* is billed as a treatment because it contains marula oil, but this plant oil isn't a special or essential ingredient for lip care, it's just another emollient plant oil. This is otherwise a standard viscous gloss and offers a wet-looking, high-shine finish with a slightly sticky feel. All of the colors are very sheer. The ☺ **Shimmer Hi-Shine Lip Treatment** *($11.50)* is identical in every respect to the original version above, except that a couple of shades have a shimmer finish that may be more to your liking. ☺ **Liquid Lip Color** *($13)* feels smooth yet slippery and offers a glossy, minimally sticky finish. The shades go on softly but build well if more intensity is desired; think of it as a lip gloss with a bit more pigment than the norm.

😐 **Lip Gloss Dots** *($8.50)* has a strange name for what amounts to a standard, thick lip gloss packaged in a pot. The color intensity is deceptively sheer, even for the deepest shades, and it is sticky enough to be bothersome (assuming sticky lip gloss bothers you). 😐 **Lip Care** *($12)* is a very ordinary, but nevertheless emollient, lipstick-type lip balm that has a particularly glossy finish. It will soothe dry skin quite nicely. 😐 **Lipliner** *($9)* is a standard, but quite workable, lip pencil that features some versatile colors. If this did not need to be sharpened it would earn my Paula's Pick rating for its texture and application, but convenience is important too when it comes to makeup application.

☹ **Stay On Lip Color** *($14.50)* doesn't measure up to the estimable Max Factor Lipfinity or M.A.C.'s Pro Longwear Lipcolour. The dual-sided packaging includes a lip color applied with the wand applicator and a clear gloss at the other end to add shine (and comfort). The shades have been whittled down to two, and each goes on opaque and takes too long to dry. Once the lip color has set, you will immediately feel your lips become dry and tight, which is where the clear top coat comes in. It provides the requisite glossy finish, but it can't overcome the dry, slightly grainy feel of the lip color underneath. After a short time (less than an hour in my case, but your experience may vary) the glossy effect and the smooth feel were gone, and the lip color began to flake and peel off—and I hadn't even tried to eat with this on yet! I rarely refer to a makeup product as "abysmal," but the word is applicable here. ☹ **Lip & Cheek Stain** *($12)* is an exceptionally sheer, gel-based stain that comes in one pink-berry color. This stays sticky on the skin, and is not preferred to similar versions from Origins or Benefit.

MASCARA: ☺ **Super Volume Mascara** *($12)* is a reworking of The Body Shop's former Volumizing Mascara, and although it is a distinct improvement this mascara's performance doesn't fall into the "super" category. It builds average length and thickness in equal measures, and has a slightly uneven application that requires a bit more patience—but the results may be worth it if you want a reliable mascara that doesn't take lashes too far. The ☺ **Waterproof Mascara** *($12)* was redone as well, and it lengthens lashes and provides a hint of thickness without clumps, leaving lashes with a soft curl. It is waterproof.

😐 **Define and Lengthen Mascara** *($12)* is the same as it was when I last reviewed it: a boring mascara that builds minimal length and definition even after considerable effort. It's OK for a natural look, but that's about it.

BRUSHES: The Body Shop's ☺ **Brushes** *($8.50–$24.50)* are each composed of synthetic hair and most of them are supremely soft and beautifully shaped. The best of the bunch (notable for their ability to hold and accurately deposit color) include: **Eyeliner Brush** *($10.50)*, **Face & Body Brush** *($24.50)*, **Foundation Brush** *($22.50)*, **Slanted Brush** *($16.50)*, **Retractable Blusher Brush** *($18.50)*, and **Blusher Brush** *($22.50)*. The less appealing or unnecessary brushes include the rubber-tipped **Line Softener** *($8.50)*, **Brow & Lash Comb** *($8.50)*, **Lipstick/Concealer Brush** *($12.50)*, and **Eyeshadow Blender Brush** *($16.50)*, which is nicely shaped but doesn't have enough give to apply color evenly. The **Mini Brush Kit** *($14.50)* is a small, portable brush set that includes a built-in mirror and a brush to apply powder, blush, eyeshadow, and lipstick. It's not the best to tote for applying a full makeup, but is ideal to keep in your purse or office for quick touch-ups.

FACE AND BODY ILLUMINATING/SHIMMER PRODUCTS: ☺ **Glow Enhancer** *($12.50)* is a liquid shimmer that casts an ethereal pink glow that is apparent but still understated. It is easy to apply and control, and dries to a matte (in feel) finish. ☺ **Tinted Glow Enhancer** *($12.50)* has the same basic characteristics as the Glow Enhancer above, but comes in four sheer, flesh-toned tints. Each imparts a very soft glow to skin that would actually be acceptable even in daylight. However, this works best applied over or mixed with a foundation to delicately highlight skin. ☺ **Shimmer Waves** *($17.50)* presents "waves" of shiny pressed powder colors in one compact. Although the powder has a dry, grainy feel, it goes on smoothly and clings better than expected. The finish is best described as moderate shimmer, and is an option for evening glamour. ☺ **Shimmer Sun Gel** *($12.50)* has a different formula than the Sheer Sun Gel reviewed under Specialty products below. It has more slip so blending doesn't have to be as quick, and instead of getting a bronze color you get a sheer medium gold that leaves a very shiny finish. The best news is the shine lasts, though it can rub off a bit on clothing.

😐 **Lightening Touch** *($12)* has been around for years and is available in two sheer shades. It's an OK highlighting option with a soft shimmer finish, but doesn't illuminate the skin in the same beguiling way as superior options from Revlon Skinlights, Giorgio Armani, and Lorac.

😐 **$$$ Brilliance Powder** *($18.50)* packages loose shimmer powder in a cylindrical component with an attached brush. A push button shoots powder onto the brush, ready for application. Although the powder adds lots of shine to skin and clings well, the brush is somewhat stiff and uncomfortable to use.

☹ **Shimmer Cubes** *($17.50)* are described as "four cute blocks of earthy, shimmery color" but end up being anything but cute. The blocks are not fastened to the main component, which is a poor choice given how easily these could break if dropped. In addition, each shade is grainy and the shine tends to flake. ☹ **Shimmer Cubes Sparkle** *($17.50)* is nearly identical to the Shimmer Cubes except the shine comes from multicolored, prismatic pigment. Otherwise, the same negatives apply.

SPECIALTY PRODUCTS: ✓☺ **Lip Line Fixer** *($9)* marks the return of a former Body Shop favorite, though the name has been changed. Lip Line Fixer was No Wander in its first incarnation, and this remains a very good automatic, retractable lip pencil whose colorless formula puts an invisible border around the mouth that stops lipstick from feathering into lines. It worked brilliantly as No Wander, and works just as well today. Keep in mind that as effective as this pencil is, it won't completely stop greasy, overly slick lipsticks or lip glosses from traveling into lines around the mouth.

✓☺ **Lipscuff** *($10)* has been reformulated and no longer abrades lips with walnut shells and irritates them with mint. Instead, the emollient lipstick formula is blended with smooth polyethylene (ground-up plastic) beads, and works well to remove dry, flaky skin from chapped lips. It can still feel a bit abrasive unless used gently, so please heed that advice if you decide to try this.

☺ **Sheer Sun Gel** *($12.50)* is a very standard but good bronzing gel that feels light and dries fast, so blending must be quick. The translucent color is convincing and relatively long-lasting. It is best for medium skin tones looking for a touch of sun without the damage actual tanning causes.

😐 **Matte It Face & Lips** *($12.50)* is a basic silicone serum that contains a tiny amount of aloe and chamomile to reinforce The Body Shop's natural persona. This has a silky finish and will allow for smooth application of foundation, but the type of silicone used is too slick to provide significant shine control.

BOOTS

BOOTS AT-A-GLANCE

Strengths: Inexpensive; some great cleansers, including a few without fragrance; all sunscreens provide sufficient UVA protection; a couple of good scrubs; well-formulated self-tanning lotions; a smoothing, soothing lip balm; the only mass-market makeup line with testers for almost every product; great return policy on makeup at Target, if you save your receipt; mostly impressive foundation shades; very good powders; powder blush; great sheer lipstick; the Botanics Gloss; a handful of good mascaras.

Weaknesses: Abundance of ordinary formulas; Botanics line products contain few botanical ingredients; Time Dimensions line lacks sunscreen and provides more shine than proven anti-aging formulas for skin; repetitive formulas and a penchant for including the good stuff in amounts too small to be all that helpful; majority of products are surprisingly average; no AHA or BHA products; no products to help battle blemishes or lighten skin discolorations; jar packaging; foundations are more expensive than the competition, but do not best them; No7 and Botanics makeup products have several similarities, except the Botanics include plant extracts that have no impact on performance; mostly disappointing eyeshadows; average to poor eye, brow, and lip pencils; inferior makeup brushes; superfluous or just plain unattractive specialty products.

For more information about Boots, call (866) 752-6687 or visit www.boots.com or www.Beautypedia.com.

Note: Boots No7 and Botanics brands (only) are sold in Canada at Shoppers Drug Mart stores.

BOOTS SKIN CARE

BOOTS BOTANICS

☺ **Botanics Complexion Refining Deep Clean Mousse** *($8.99 for 5 ounces)* is a basic but good water-soluble cleanser for all skin types except very oily. The liquid-to-foam action may be your preference, but it has no advantage over nonfoaming cleansers.

☺ **Botanics Moisturising Deep Clean Foam** *($6.99 for 5 ounces)* is similar to the Botanics Complexion Refining Deep Clean Mousse above, but the higher concentration of glycerin makes it more moisturizing and best for normal to dry skin. The tiny amount of sodium lauryl sulfate in both of these cleansers is not cause for concern.

😐 **Botanics Quick Fix Cleansing Wipes** *($6.99 for 30 wipes)* work very well to remove makeup and leave skin refreshed, but they're not the best for on-the-go cleansing without water because one of the preservatives can be irritating if left on skin. The same goes for the fragrance components linalool and benzyl salicylate. These are recommended only if you rinse your skin after using them.

😐 **Botanics Skin Brightening Cleanser** *($6.99 for 8.4 ounces)* won't brighten skin, but it can be a good cleansing lotion for normal to very dry skin. The mineral oil doesn't rinse easily without the aid of a washcloth.

☺ **Botanics Skin Brightening Deep Clean Gel** *($6.99 for 5 ounces)* is a very good water-soluble cleanser for normal to oily skin. It removes makeup and won't leave skin feeling stripped.

☺ **Botanics Soothing Eye Make-Up Remover** *($5.99 for 5 ounces)* is a silicone-in-water dual-phase makeup remover that works well to take off all types of makeup. This is labeled as suitable for even the most sensitive skin, but the preservative 2-bromo-2-nitropropane-1,3-diol can be problematic (Source: *Handbook of Cosmetic and Personal Care Additives*, 2nd Edition, volume 1, *Synapse Information Resources*, 2002). Almay and Neutrogena sell the same type of makeup remover with more gentle preservatives.

☺ **Botanics in Shower Facial Polish** *($7.99 for 3.3 ounces)* is an OK scrub with cleansing ability for normal to oily skin. It loses points for the amount of ginger root it contains, along with several potentially irritating fragrance components.

☺ **Botanics Purifying Face Scrub** *($7.99 for 2.5 ounces)* is a greasy scrub that contains apricot seeds and walnut shells as the abrasive agent. These are not preferred to polyethylene beads, but the mineral oil helps protect skin from their rough edges.

☺ **Botanics Complexion Refining Toner** *($7.99 for 5 ounces)* is a water-based toner that contains two kinds of clay, which allows it to have a matte finish. Including castor oil is inappropriate, but the amount is small, making this an OK option for normal to oily skin.

☹ **Botanics Skin Brightening Toner** *($6.99 for 8.4 ounces)* contains enough alcohol to be irritating, and the sole plant extract, horsetail, has constricting properties that are not helpful for skin. The amount of AHAs is too low for exfoliation to occur.

☺ **Botanics Complexion Refining Day Moisturising Lotion SPF 12** *($12.99 for 2.5 ounces)* has merit due to its in-part avobenzone sunscreen, but the SPF rating is below the benchmark set by most major medical organizations, and the base formula for normal to dry skin is, well, really basic. This does contain potentially irritating fragrance components.

☺ **Botanics Complexion Refining Light Night Cream** *($13.99 for 1.69 ounces)* is an unremarkable lightweight moisturizer for normal to dry skin. The jar packaging won't keep the two antioxidants in it stable during use.

☺ **Botanics Day Moisture Cream SPF 12** *($8.99 for 1.69 ounces)* improves slightly on the Botanics Complexion Refining Day Moisturising Lotion SPF 12 above, but the similarities still keep it from earning a happy face rating.

☺ **Botanics Day Moisture Lotion** *($8.99 for 2.5 ounces)* is similar to the Botanics Complexion Refining Light Night Cream above, but this version comes in better packaging. That's a plus, but still doesn't elevate this above average status.

☺ **Botanics Eye and Lip Correction Serum** *($14.99 for 0.5 ounce)* claims to make dark circles and puffiness around the eyes "a thing of the past in just 4 weeks," but you're in for a disappointing experience if you believe it. This is a simple blend of mostly water, glycerin, mineral oil, slip agent, emollient, silicones, film-forming agent, and preservative. These ingredients cannot fade dark circles or reduce puffiness any more than an accountant can perform laser eye surgery.

☺ **Botanics Face Defence Moisture Cream SPF 15** *($12.99 for 1.69 ounces)* is worth considering if you have normal to slightly dry skin and are OK with a basic daytime moisturizer that includes avobenzone for UVA protection. Jar packaging won't keep the lone antioxidant in this moisturizer stable during use.

☺ **Botanics Face Lift Firming Cream SPF 10** *($13.99 for 1.69 ounces)* has a better base formula than any of the Boots Botanics sunscreens above; what a shame the SPF 10 with avobenzone is too low for daytime use. This is an option if you have normal to dry skin and are willing to pair this with a foundation rated SPF 15 or greater.

☺ **Botanics Face Renewal Cream SPF 15** *($13.99 for 1.69 ounces)* is nearly identical to the Botanics Face Lift Firming Cream SPF 10 above, except that this one has a better SPF rating and a change in antioxidants. Unfortunately, jar packaging won't keep them stable during use, though this is an option for normal to dry skin.

☺ **Botanics Hydrating Serum Capsules** *($9.99 for 30 capsules)* are filled with a blend of silicones, thickener, antioxidant plant oils, and potentially irritating plant extracts, including narcissus and horsetail. This is an option for normal to dry skin, and it leaves a silky finish, but the mixed bag of good and problematic plant extracts is disappointing.

☺ **Botanics Moisturising Eye Cream** *($13.99 for 0.84 ounce)* is a very basic moisturizer for normal to dry skin anywhere on the face. The amount of mica leaves a noticeable shine on skin. Grape seed oil is a great antioxidant, but the jar packaging won't let it maintain its potency during use.

☹ **Botanics Night Facial Treatment Oil** *($11.99 for 1 ounce)* contains far too many irritating fragrance components to make it a treatment for anyone's skin. You'd be better off massaging plain olive, grape, or soy oils on dry skin.

☺ **Botanics Night Moisture Cream** *($13.99 for 1.69 ounces)* is an OK lightweight moisturizer for normal to slightly dry skin. The amount of grape seed oil is impressive, but the jar packaging won't keep its antioxidant elements stable during use.

☺ **Botanics Radiance Beauty Balm** *($11.99 for 1.3 ounces)* provides a visual pick-me-up because the mica leaves a shiny finish. That can help make dull, dry skin look livelier, but the main ingredients in this balm are standard, and what's lacking makes this nothing more than an average option.

☺ **Botanics Radiance Renewal Night Serum** *($15.99 for 1 ounce)* is a very good, ultra-light moisturizer for normal to oily skin. It contains bilberry extract as the main antioxidant, and it does have anti-inflammatory benefits. The citrus extracts and sugarcane do not function as AHAs, but do contribute to this serum's water-binding properties. However, the citrus is potentially irritating, and that keeps this serum from earning a Paula's Pick rating.

☺ **Botanics Responsive Moisture Lotion** *($9.99 for 2.5 ounces)* claims to be responsive in the sense that it moisturizes where needed, but also helps minimize excess oil to keep skin shine-free. Don't bet on it; moisturizing and absorbent ingredients don't separate on skin, each going to where they're needed most (how would they know where to go?). The amount of zinc oxide this contains does lend a soft matte finish, but that also keeps the emollients from being as moisturizing as they could be. One of the antioxidants has a positive effect on skin while the other has a negative effect (not every plant with antioxidant ability is great for skin), so they cancel each other out. That leaves you with an unimpressive moisturizer for normal to slightly dry or slightly oily skin not prone to blemishes.

☺ **Botanics Smoothing Facial Serum** *($14.99 for 1 ounce)* contains one "botanic," which in this case is a tiny amount of horse chestnut extract. I can think of several other botanical ingredients that would have made this silicone-based serum for all skin types more intriguing, but it does contain a dusting of antioxidant vitamins. Nothing in this serum can purify skin or make it feel clearer. Skin can look clearer, but how can it feel clearer?

☺ **Botanics Soothing & Calming Eye Base** *($8.99 for 0.27 ounce)* contains a tiny amount of soothing licorice extract, but is otherwise a bland blend of thickeners, mineral oil, aluminum starch, and several waxes. The iron oxide pigments provide a bit of sheer color and coverage, but I wouldn't choose this over a great liquid or cream concealer.

☺ **Botanics Ultimate Lift Eye Gel** *($13.99 for 0.5 ounce)* is so basic and boring that the name is embarrassing. This won't lift skin in the least; it's just water, slip agents, plant extract, film-forming agent, and preservatives. It's not even exciting that this is one of the only Boots products that is fragrance-free.

☹ **Botanics Complexion Refining Clay Mask** *($8.99 for 1.69 ounces)* is a below-standard clay mask due to the amount of irritating isopropyl alcohol. It cannot draw out "even the most deep-rooted impurities"—you won't see a marvelously clear complexion after use, and your skin may feel uncomfortably dry.

☺ **Botanics Conditioning Clay Mask** *($8.99 for 4.2 ounces)* is a very standard but good clay mask that is an option for oily to very oily skin. It is fragrance-free and the sole plant extract, burdock root, has soothing properties.

☺ **Botanics Quenching Face Mask** *($8.99 for 2.5 ounces)* is an average mask with slight moisturizing qualities for normal to dry skin. A blend of interesting water-binding agents and some antioxidant plant oils would have made this a much better contender.

☺ **Botanics Refining Sauna Mask** *($8.99 for 5 0.27-ounce masks)* is a gel-textured mask that contains a zeolite mineral. Upon mixing with water, the zeolite causes a warming sensation (Boots describes it as "self-heating"), while the clay helps absorb surface oil. It ends up being pricey for what you get, but is an option for normal to oily skin (and the warming sensation is just that, a sensation).

☺ **Botanics Vitamin Recovery Mask** *($7.99 for 1.69 ounces)* contains an inconsequential amount of vitamin E, and lacks significant amounts of ingredients that allow dry skin to recover (that is, restore a healthy barrier function so skin can repair itself). This is barely passable as a decent mask for normal to slightly dry skin.

BOOTS NO7

☺ **No7 Quick Thinking 4 in 1 Wipes** *($6.99 for 30 wipes)* are nearly identical to the Boots Botanics Quick Fix Cleansing Wipes above, and the same review applies. The tiny amount of witch hazel included is not cause for concern.

✓☺ **No7 Beautifully Balanced Purifying Cleanser, for Oily/Combination Skin** *($7.99 for 6.6 ounces)* is a slightly fluid, fragrance-free, water-soluble cleanser that is suitable for its intended skin type. The smaller amount of detergent cleansing agent doesn't allow for complete removal of makeup, but this is an option as a morning cleanser or for those who wear minimal makeup.

☺ **No7 Gentle Foaming Facial Wash, for All Skin Types** *($8.99 for 5 ounces)* is similar to the Boots Botanics Moisturising Deep Clean Foam above, but with fewer bells and whistles (which just end up being rinsed down the drain anyway). Otherwise, the same review applies.

✓☺ **No7 Soft & Soothed Gentle Cleanser, for Normal/Dry Skin** *($7.99 for 6.6 ounces)* is a good detergent-free cleansing lotion for its intended skin types. The fragrance-free formula is very gentle, yet removes makeup easily (though you may need a washcloth to avoid leaving a residue of mineral oil).

☺ **No7 Cleanse & Care Eye Make-Up Remover** *($7.99 for 3.3 ounces)* is nearly identical to the Boots Botanics Soothing Eye Make-Up Remover above, save for a smaller size and the addition of some plant extracts, none of which help remove makeup. Otherwise, the same review (and concern) applies.

☺ **No7 Radiance Revealed Exfoliator, for All Skin Types** *($10.99 for 2.5 ounces)* is a good fragrance-free scrub for dry to very dry skin. The water- and mineral oil–based formula contains a small amount of polyethylene beads for a gentle polishing, but this doesn't rinse as well as water-soluble scrubs.

☺ **No7 Total Renewal Micro-Dermabrasion Exfoliator** *($14.99 for 2.5 ounces)* has a similar base and is recommended for the same skin types as the No7 Radiance Revealed Exfoliator, for All Skin Types above. However, the abrasive agent is alumina, and as such this scrub can be grittier and potentially too abrasive unless used with great care. This does rinse better than the aforementioned scrub above.

☹ **No7 Beautifully Balanced Purifying Toner, for Oily/Combination Skin** *($7.99 for 6.6 ounces)* lists alcohol as the second ingredient, which makes this toner too drying and irritating for all skin types; plus alcohol can cause free-radical damage.

😐 **No7 Soft & Soothed Gentle Toner, for Normal/Dry Skin** *($7.99 for 6.6 ounces)* provides skin with a tiny amount of soothing agents, but is otherwise a lackluster fragrance-free formula that merely helps remove the last traces of makeup and leaves normal to dry skin soft.

😐 **No7 Advanced Hydration Day Cream SPF 12** *($14.99 for 1.69 ounces)* provides sufficient UVA protection via its in-part avobenzone sunscreen, but the SPF rating is disappointing because you cannot use this as your only source of daily sun protection. Another letdown is that this day cream for normal to dry skin contains just a dusting of several state-of-the-art ingredients, including ceramides and phytosphingosine.

😐 **No7 Advanced Hydration Day Fluid** *($14.99 for 1 ounce)* is an OK moisturizing lotion for normal to slightly dry or slightly oily skin. It lacks antioxidants, and the amounts of skin-identical ingredients found in healthy skin are in very short supply.

😐 **No7 Advanced Hydration Night Cream** *($15.99 for 1.69 ounces)* is a standard lightweight moisturizer for normal to slightly dry skin. Jar packaging is irrelevant because this does not contain any air- or light-sensitive ingredients. The truly elegant ingredients round out the ingredient list, but that's not where you want to see them, especially in a moisturizer labeled "advanced."

😐 **No7 Lifting & Firming Day Cream SPF 8** *($19.99 for 1.69 ounces)* tries to seem more state-of-the-art than it is, but doesn't get off to a grand start because of its low SPF rating (though avobenzone is included for UVA protection). Boots claims this will firm skin in just two weeks, but this product doesn't contain ingredients that will restore youth, and the low amount of peptides and antioxidants is a letdown, as is the choice of jar packaging. And this is supposed to be their most advanced formula?!

😐 **No7 Lifting & Firming Eye Cream** *($19.99 for 0.5 ounce)* provides moisture to slightly dry skin and has a silky texture, but that's the extent of this jar-packaged eye cream's abilities. Once again, the amount of intriguing ingredients is depressingly small.

😐 **No7 Lifting & Firming Night Cream** *($19.99 for 1.69 ounce)* is nearly identical to the No7 Lifting & Firming Eye Cream above, except this is more emollient for dry skin. Otherwise, the same review applies.

😐 **No7 Moisture Quench Day Cream, for Normal/Dry Skin** *($12.99 for 1.69 ounces)* fails to impress because the majority of its formula is ho-hum, and the good stuff that shows up at the end of the ingredient list is too little, too late. Consider this a decent choice for dry skin, but realize that there are several superior formulas available elsewhere.

😐 **No7 Moisture Quench Day Fluid, for Normal/Dry Skin** *($12.99 for 3.3 ounces)* is the lotion version of the No7 Moisture Quench Day Cream for Normal/Dry Skin, above, and other than being better suited for normal to dry skin and not using jar packaging, the same review applies.

☺ **No7 Moisture Quench Night Cream, for Normal/Dry Skin** *($12.99 for 1.69 ounces)* is a standard emollient moisturizer for dry to very dry skin. Someone with normal skin will likely find this too rich. And someone shopping for a brilliantly formulated moisturizer not packaged in a jar will be disappointed.

☺ **No7 Radiant Glow Beauty Lotion** *($15.99 for 1 ounce)* is a respectable lightweight moisturizer with shine for normal to slightly dry skin. It is fragrance-free and works well under makeup, but comparably speaking, doesn't best several moisturizers from Olay or Dove.

😐 **No7 Rebalancing Day Gel, for Oily/Combination Skin** *($12.99 for 1.69 ounces)* will not revitalize skin with green tea and seaweed because those ingredients are barely present. This is merely a boring gel moisturizer that's suitable for its intended skin types. It's nice that fragrance was omitted, but why aren't more beneficial ingredients added?

😐 **No7 Rebalancing Night Fluid, for Oily/Combination Skin** *($12.99 for 3.3 ounces)* is a skin-confusing mix of slip agent, silicone, zinc oxide, emollients, clay, talc, and wax. It's too light and absorbent for dry skin, yet too potentially troublesome for oily skin or oily areas. I suppose it's OK for normal skin, but overall it's an unimpressive formula.

😐 **No7 Refine & Rewind Intense Perfecting Serum** *($19.99 for 1 ounce)* is said to work little miracles on your skin day by day, but the only miracle is how amazingly silky the silicones in here can make your skin feel. Silicones are hardly unique to this serum, and while it should be loaded with antioxidants, skin-identical substances, and cell-communicating ingredients, it either comes up short or contains such a tiny amount that your skin (and wrinkles) won't notice. The form of vitamin C is sodium ascorbyl phosphate. Although it has antioxidant ability like other forms of vitamin C, research has shown that it is not as effective as ascorbic acid (pure vitamin C) despite being more stable (Sources: *Skin Pharmacology and Physiology*, July-August 2004, pages 200–206; and *International Journal of Pharmaceutics*, April 2003, pages 65–73). That's not to say it does not have benefit for skin; it most certainly does. It's just that this doesn't appear to be the ideal form of vitamin C to include in a serum with claims like those Boots is making. By the way, the pro-retinol referred to is not retinol, but rather retinyl palmitate, which is not the same thing.

😐 **No7 Restore & Renew Beauty Serum** *($19.99 for 1 ounce)* reigns above every other Boots product in terms of reader curiosity. It seems there is intense interest in whether or not the claims made for this product and the media attention paid to it are true. Why the hullabaloo? A television documentary that aired in the United Kingdom in March 2007 featured the results of a blind test that compared the efficacy of this serum to tretinoin, the active ingredient in Retin-A and Renova. The research was carried out by scientists at the University of Manchester, with the conclusion that this Boots serum was just as effective at stimulating collagen production as tretinoin, yet costs considerably less. That sounds great until you learn that Boots paid for the research, which means they had a vested interest in making sure the study made their product look great. Also, because the study was done blind instead of double-blind, the researchers knew who was getting which treatment. This type of study isn't as reliable as double-blind studies because, especially when money is at stake, there is a natural bias toward making sure the product in question comes out in the best possible light. That fact was lost on consumers in England, however, who lined up at Boots stores for hours when word hit that the product was back on shelves (after selling out country-wide) again. Apparently, Boots had waiting lists that stretched into the triple digits and their production team worked around the clock to ensure that adequate supplies of the serum were available. This is a great example of how media hype can generate tremendous interest in (and resulting sales of) a product. It reminds me of the frenzy after ads for StriVectin-SD appeared in *Parade* magazine, with the tag line "Better than Botox!" Beauty chat rooms were quick to crown this serum as an anti-aging powerhouse, simply on the basis of media attention alone. It's not that this serum isn't worth purchasing, but I wouldn't recommend anyone consider it over tretinoin or several other serums whose formulas outpace this one.

Restore & Renew Beauty Serum is silicone-based and contains a small amount of vitamin C as sodium ascorbyl phosphate (which research has shown is not as effective as ascorbic acid, though it is more stable). A nearly insignificant amount of vitamin A (as retinyl palmitate, not retinol as claimed) and other antioxidants hardly makes this an anti-aging product worth any amount of frenzy. Its vitamin C content and other attributes are not even worth mild enthusiasm when you consider that several companies offer serums that are infinitely more state-of-the-art. Examples include serums from Estee Lauder Perfectionist, Clinique Repairwear, Olay Regenerist, MD Skincare by Dr. Dennis Gross, Dr. Denese's Hydroshield products, and various options from Skinceuticals. And if you're looking for peptides (or hope that the ones used in this Boots serum will spell certain doom for your wrinkles), this isn't the product that will flood your skin with them. In fact, there are more preservatives than peptides in this fragrance-free serum. Despite my dispelling the hype this product generated (and remember, it all began with funding from Boots, and no one else has reproduced the results from their "study"), it can be a good serum-type moisturizer for all skin types, and the silicones make skin feel wonderfully silky. This product is sold in England under the name No7 Protect and Perfect Beauty Serum, and except for the name change is identical to the version sold in the United States and Canada. Both feature translucent glass packaging that will compromise the stability of the vitamin C and vitamin A unless this is constantly kept away from light. One more thing: There is plenty of substantiated, published research indicating that topically applied vitamin C can stimulate collagen production, as can tretinoin (Sources: *Journal of Cosmetic Dermatology*, June 2006, pages 150–156; *Pharmaceutical Development and Technology*, November 2006, pages 255–261; *Dermatologic Surgery*, July 2005, pages 814–817; and *Experimental Dermatology*, June 2003, pages 237–244). Tretinoin is more potent, but instead of choosing one over the other, why not treat aging skin to both, along with an array of antioxidants and cell-communicating ingredients?

😐 **No7 Reviving Eye Gel** *($11.99 for 0.5 ounce)* is nearly identical to the Boots Botanics Ultimate Lift Eye Gel above, except this version adds a couple of silicones for a silky texture. It remains an unexciting product that is minimally helpful for slightly dry skin. The amount of witch hazel and horse chestnut are too small for skin to notice, for better or worse.

No7 Time Resisting Day & Night Eye Care *($19.99 for 0.66 ounce)* offers two products for the eye area. 😐 **Night Eye Cream** promises youthful beauty but can only minimize dryness with its standard blend of glycerin and emollients. The amount of bells and whistles is so small as to be inconsequential for skin. The ☹ **Day Eye Gel** is a lightweight formula with a silky texture and tiny amount of water-binding agent. The cooling sensation comes from the menthol derivative menthyl PCA, and it makes this not recommended because of its potential to cause irritation.

😐 **No7 Time Resisting Day Cream SPF 12** *($19.99 for 1.69 ounces)* deserves credit for its in-part avobenzone sunscreen, but the base formula for normal to slightly dry skin offers little of substance for skin. The mica provides a soft shine finish and while Boots talks up this sunscreen's antioxidant complex, the amount of antioxidants is likely too small for skin to gain any benefit.

😐 **No7 Time Resisting Night Cream** *($19.99 for 1.69 ounces)* does not contain retinol as claimed (retinyl palmitate is not the same thing), and ends up being another plain emollient moisturizer for normal to dry skin. It is far less elegant than the moisturizer options from many other drugstore lines, including Olay, Dove, Pond's, and Neutrogena.

☺ **No7 Sunless Tanning Quick Dry Tinted Lotion, for Face and Body** *($14.99 for 6.6 ounces)* is available in two formulas. The Light/Medium version is a water-based lotion with a tiny amount of emollients, while the Medium/Dark formula is silicone-based and omits the emollient. The latter is best for normal to oily skin, while the former is preferred for normal to dry skin. Both self-tanners turn skin color via dihydroxyacetone and the slower-acting erythrulose, and are tinted so you can see where they've been applied. Each also contains soothing chamomile oil, though in an amount that's likely too small to have much, if any, effect on skin. Still, these are good, inexpensive self-tanning lotions.

😐 **No7 Deep Cleansing Purifying Mask, for All Skin Types** *($11.99 for 4 0.33-ounce masks)* is similar to the Boots Botanics Refining Sauna Mask above, except this version contains a much smaller amount of non-volatile plant oil, which helps it make good on the claim of leaving skin shine-free. Otherwise, the same review applies.

😐 **No7 Intensive Line Filler** *($17.99 for 0.67 ounce)* is very similar to the No7 Refine & Rewind Intense Perfecting Serum above, except here you get less product and it is packaged in a tube instead of a bottle with built-in pump applicator. This formula differs because it has a slightly thicker texture and it includes mineral pigments (what the company refers to as "light-diffusing particles"), but otherwise the same comments apply. I can think of many other products whose state-of-the-art formulas are a better way to treat aging skin.

😐 **No7 Intensive Moisture Face Mask** *($19.99 for 3.3 ounces)* is an exceptionally standard moisturizing mask for dry to very dry skin. What you get for your money isn't worth the cost, but this will cover the basics in terms of making dry skin feel smoother and comfortable.

☹ **No7 Pamper & Peel Radiance Mask** *($19.99 for 1.69 ounces)* is a traditional peel-off mask that contains polyvinyl alcohol, which means it is too irritating for all skin types.

☺ **No7 Deeply Moisturising Lipcare** *($6.99 for 0.33 ounce)* is a somewhat sticky but emollient lip balm that is an option if you need such a product and prefer a glossy finish. Including several ceramides was a good idea, but the amounts in this product—well, they don't amount to much.

TIME DIMENSIONS

✓☺ **Time Dimensions Conditioning Cleansing Cream** *($8.99 for 6.7 ounces)* is nearly identical to the No7 Soft & Soothed Gentle Cleanser, for Normal/Dry Skin above, and the same review applies.

☺ **Time Dimensions Deep Cleansing Wipes** *($6.99 for 30 wipes)* work well to cleanse normal to very dry skin, and are fairly adept at removing makeup (waterproof formulas will withstand these wipes). The amount of plant extracts is very small, and they won't reduce the visible signs of aging any more than a steady diet of cheesecake will encourage weight loss.

☺ **Time Dimensions Clarifying Facial Exfoliator** *($9.99 for 5 ounces)* is very similar to the No7 Radiance Revealed Exfoliator for All Skin Types, above, except this version has greater cleansing ability because it contains sodium laureth sulfate. Otherwise, the same review applies. This version ends up being a better value than the No7 scrub.

☹ **Time Dimensions Refining Toning Water** *($8.99 for 6.7 ounces)* offers too few beneficial ingredients for skin and the amount of alcohol is likely to cause irritation. The amount of AHA is too low and the pH too high for exfoliation to occur.

☹ **Time Dimensions Brightening Facial Balm** *($16.99 for 1 ounce)* is a fluid moisturizer whose silicone content will make all skin types feel silky while the mica imparts a noticeable shine. The amount of antioxidants and peptides is disappointing, and certainly doesn't make this a top choice for improving skin of any age.

☹ **Time Dimensions Instant Eye Reviver** *($14.99 for 0.33 ounce)* is similar to but with more ingredients than the Boots Botanics Moisturising Eye Cream above, and the same basic comments apply. The addition of petrolatum makes this product more moisturizing than the Botanics version, but the amounts of the extra ingredients are mere dustings, so cannot be counted on for a healthy skin boost.

☹ **Time Dimensions Intensive Restoring Treatment** *($18.99 for 1 ounce)* is neither intensive nor restorative. This is a simple, light-textured lotion with a lot of mica for a shiny finish. Vitamin A and peptides are supposed to be major players here, but their presence amounts to a non-speaking, walk-on part in a movie, not the "top billing" your skin needs to look and feel its best.

☹ **Time Dimensions Nourishing Eye Cream** *($18.99 for 0.5 ounce)* is a below-standard lightweight moisturizer for slightly dry skin anywhere on the face. The mica leaves a soft shine finish, but this has nothing to do with boosting collagen or elastin, or reducing fine lines or puffiness in the eye area.

☹ **Time Dimensions Rejuvenating Day Moisturiser** *($16.99 for 1.69 ounces)* is a thicker version of the Time Dimensions Nourishing Eye Cream above, except this version doesn't contain mica. Otherwise, the same basic comments apply.

☹ **Time Dimensions Restoring Night Moisturiser** *($17.99 for 1.69 ounces)* contains a teeny-tiny amount of antioxidants and peptides, features jar packaging, and is otherwise very similar to the Time Dimensions Rejuvenating Day Moisturiser above.

☹ **Time Dimensions Softening Line Smoother** *($15.99 for 0.5 ounce)* is merely a blend of silicones and slip agents whose texture is meant to serve as a sort of spackle for superficial lines and wrinkles. It works marginally well, but how long the effect lasts depends on how much you move your face. At least this is an option for those who want to try such a product but don't want a shiny or sparkling finish.

☹ **Time Dimensions Instant Lip Plumper** *($9.99 for 0.27 ounce)* is perhaps the most irritating lip plumper being sold today. Most such products contain one or two irritants that cause lips to swell slightly by virtue of irritation. Boots uses menthol (a lot of it), spearmint oil, eugenol, clove oil, pepper extract, methyl eugenol, and cinnamon. All I can say, besides "Buyer beware," is "Ouch!" And Boots calls this product a "special treat"!?

OTHER BOOTS PRODUCTS

☹ **Feel the Difference Detox Face Mask** *($7.99 for 1.69 ounces)* is a substandard clay mask for oily skin. It is more drying than most others because of the amount of isopropyl alcohol—but that's not a difference your skin really wants to feel.

☹ **Mediterranean Olive, Almond & Sage Wonderbalm** *($8.99 for 0.84 ounce)* is a petrolatum (Vaseline)-based balm that contains some very helpful non-volatile plant oils as well as emollient cocoa butter. Sage oil makes this an imperfect choice, but the amount is small enough so it's not a concern for irritation (the product doesn't even have a hint of sage aroma). Still, this would've received a happy face rating without it.

BOOTS MAKEUP

FOUNDATION: ✓☺ No7 Soft & Sheer Tinted Moisturiser SPF 15 *($11.99)* is a great find for those with normal to dry skin! Titanium dioxide is partially responsible for UVA protection, while the creamy-smooth texture applies and blends beautifully, providing sheer coverage and a fresh, moist finish. All three shades are recommended.

✓☺ No7 Stay Perfect Foundation SPF 15 *($15.99)* makes reference to the skin-strengthening ceramides it contains, but the amount of them in this silky liquid foundation is barely a dusting. Although this isn't skin care disguised as makeup, it contains an in-part titanium dioxide sunscreen, feels nearly weightless, and sets to a smooth matte finish. Sheer to light coverage is obtainable and the overall formula is best for normal to very oily skin. Among the eight mostly great, neutral shades, the only one to avoid (due to its orange tone) is Truffle.

☺ No7 Lifting and Firming Foundation SPF 15 *($15.99)* gets its sun protection partly from titanium dioxide, though it would be better if a higher percentage were included (1.6% is low). This is otherwise a very silky liquid foundation for those with normal to oily skin seeking medium coverage and a non-powdery matte finish. Seven of the eight shades are recommended; Truffle is too peach for its intended range of skin tones. Do I need to state that this won't lift or firm skin in the least? **☺ No7 True Identity Foundation** *($15.99)* is a foundation no superhero should be without, lest their true identity be revealed! OK, not really, but the attempt at humor was a lead-in to what is an amazing foundation—if you need barely any coverage. The silicone- and talc-based formula feels silky, provides a real-skin finish, and has a hint of color. It is best for normal to oily skin, and all four shades are great (but again, this is not one to pick if you need coverage beyond what strategically placed concealer provides). **☺ No7 Radiant Glow Foundation SPF 15** *($13.99)* is remarkably similar to the No7 Lifting and Firming Foundation SPF 15 above, right down to the number of shades and advice to avoid Truffle. This version doesn't contain as much mica, which is strange because that pigment provides a "glow," but the Lifting and Firming Foundation isn't shiny.

☺ No7 Intelligent Balance Foundation SPF 12 *($13.99)* contains octinoxate and titanium dioxide for broad-spectrum sun protection, and is one of those foundations that claims to know where skin is oily and where it is dry, releasing the appropriate moisturizing or absorbent ingredients where needed most. The claim is bogus, but the fluid texture has a smoothness that makes blending a pleasure, though you don't have much time before this sets to a true matte finish. Best for normal to oily skin, this provides light to medium coverage without looking artificial, and among the six shades, only Walnut is suspect for being slightly peach (but it's still worth a try). This would be rated a Paula's Pick if the SPF rating were 15 or greater.

☺ Botanics Fresh Face Tinted Moisturiser *($8.99)* is a fragrant tinted moisturizer whose omission of sunscreen is odd, given that its competitors typically include this for the 3-in-1 benefit many women love. Still, it has a great lightweight but creamy texture, very sheer coverage, and a natural finish from either of its two shades.

☺ No7 Stay Perfect Foundation Compact SPF 15 *($15.99)* is a traditional cream-to-powder makeup with an in-part titanium dioxide sunscreen. The creamy texture sets quickly to a powder finish, owing to the fact that aluminum starch is the second ingredient. This is best for normal to slightly oily skin not prone to blemishes, and provides light to medium coverage.

Each of the six shades is soft and neutral, though options for fair and dark skin tones are lacking. The crescent-shaped sponge accompanying this foundation is almost useless; a full-size circular sponge works much better.

☹ **Botanics Complexion Refining Foundation** *($12.99)* begins slightly creamy, but sets to a nearly weightless matte finish suitable for normal to oily skin. Coverage goes from sheer to light, and each of the eight shades is a winner (there are options for someone with fair skin, too). The only drawback is the inclusion of volatile fragrance components, which can cause irritation.

☹ **Botanics Quench Your Face Foundation SPF 12** *($11.99)* provides an in-part avobenzone sunscreen, though its SPF rating should be higher for sufficient daytime protection. Further downgrading this creamy liquid foundation is its heavy appearance on skin. This is one of those foundations that tends to settle into every pore and line, which isn't flattering. What a shame, because all six shades are worthwhile.

CONCEALER: ☺ **Botanics Totally Concealed** *($7.99)* is a good liquid concealer available in three workable shades. It has enough slip for targeted blending, and sets to a matte finish that remains slightly tacky and only minimally creases into lines. This does not provide total coverage as the name implies, but offers enough camouflage for minor imperfections. ☺ **Botanics Complexion Refining Concealer Stick** *($9.99)* is a find for those who prefer lipstick-style concealers and are not using them to cover blemishes (because the ingredients that keep this in lipstick form can contribute to clogged pores). It blends very well, leaves a satin-smooth finish, and poses just a slight risk of creasing into lines around the eye. Only two shades are available, one of which (Sweet Ginger) will be too peach for some, so this is recommended only if you have light skin.

☹ **No7 Radiant Glow Concealer** *($12.99)* functions best as a highlighter because it brightens shadowed areas, but provides minimal coverage. The finish feels matte but has a slight shine to it, which works to a subtle extent to reflect light away from dark areas. You push a button at the bottom of the pen-style component, and the product is fed onto a built-in synthetic brush. There are better versions of this product from Estee Lauder (Ideal Light) and Yves St. Laurent (Touche Eclat Radiant Touch), but both cost twice as much.

☹ **No7 Quick Cover Blemish Stick** *($9.99)* lists its first ingredient as chalk and, as expected, looks chalky on skin. This lipstick-style concealer contains wax-like ingredients that are not recommended for use on blemishes, though it does provide sufficient coverage. Still, each of the four shades tends toward pink and peach tones, and overall this has more strikes than positives.

POWDER: ✓☺ **No7 Perfect Light Loose Powder** *($12.99)* has a feather-light texture and seamless, dry finish. The aluminum starch– and talc-based formula is excellent for normal to oily skin because it absorbs well without looking chalky or thick. Although Boots advertises four shades on their Web site, the Target stores I visited consistently sold only two, both of which are sheer and recommended. Bonus points are deserved because the packaging for this loose powder works great to minimize mess.

✓☺ **No7 Perfect Light Portable Loose Powder** *($12.99)* has the same formula and review as the No7 Perfect Light Loose Powder above, except this comes in a portable container that includes a built-in brush. Powder is dispensed onto the brush for quick touch-ups on-the-go, and the brush itself is quite nice; not incredibly dense, but soft and shaped well for its intended purpose.

☺ **No7 Sun Kissed Bronze Shimmer Powder Compact** *($11.99)* is a dual-sided powder bronzer that features a light and medium color, both with a soft shine. This has a good, smooth texture but works best as blush because neither shade has enough depth to register as a bronze-y color on skin.

😐 **Botanics Complexion Refining Pressed Powder** *($11.99)* has a silky, almost creamy-feeling texture and natural matte finish that would be suitable for normal to slightly dry or slightly oily skin. This would've earned a happy face rating if each of the three shades did not go on slightly peach.

☹ **No7 Perfect Light Pressed Powder** *($11.99)* has a texture that feels waxy and dry at the same time. That not only makes application with a brush difficult (the powder doesn't pick up easily) but also creates a heavy appearance on skin. The finish is made even more obvious because each of the shades has a slight pink or peach tone. ☹ **Botanics Lighter Than Air Loose Powder** *($12.99)* has an accurate name, but although the feel is weightless, the finish is unnaturally dry and lends a flat, overly powdered appearance to skin, even when applied sheer. Moreover, this powder has a strong scent and contains volatile fragrance components. Why consider this when there are so many great powders without this one's drawbacks?

BLUSH: ☺ **No7 Blush Tint Cream Blush** *($9.99)* presents cream blush in stick form, and you get a surprisingly small amount of product. Still, this goes on easily, blends well, and provides a sheer wash of translucent color with a slightly moist finish. It is best for normal to dry skin not prone to blemishes.

☺ **No7 Natural Blush Cheek Colour** *($9.99)* isn't the silkiest powder blush around, but is a definite option for those who prefer soft colors that apply sheer, build well (if more color is desired), and come in a selection of very good matte shades.

☺ **Botanics Cheek Colour** *($8.99)* is very similar to the No7 Natural Blush Cheek Colour above, except each shade has a soft shine and the formula includes walnut shell powder and apple extract. Neither additive makes a big difference in performance, so the same review applies.

EYESHADOW: 😐 **No7 Stay Perfect Eyeshadow Single** *($5.99)* has a smooth but dry texture that applies better than expected but can be tricky to blend with other colors (it doesn't have much movement after the initial application). The range of colors allows for some good pairings, but every one has strong shine, so these aren't for women with wrinkles or a sagging eye area.

☹ **No7 Stay Perfect Eye Shadow Palette** *($7.99)* products have a different formula that's inferior to that of the No7 Stay Perfect Eyeshadow Single above. It is unusually dry, flakes all over the place, and tends to sit on top of skin rather than mesh with it (owing to its lack of smoothness). Further, most of the color combinations either lack depth, are too pastel, or are contrasting.

😐 **No7 Stay Perfect Eye Mousse** *($7.99)* has a light-as-mousse texture but so much slip that controlled blending becomes an issue. Once set, these tend to last with minimal creasing, though because the shine is intense they're not for the wrinkled set. Only a tiny dab is needed, and again, blending must be done carefully or this will slide all over the eye area.

☺ **Botanics Eye Colour** *($4.49 each; $4.99 for refillable compact)* has a much smoother, silkier texture and application than either of the No7 eyeshadow products above. The shade selection includes some almost matte nude and brown tones alongside shiny blues and greens that are best left alone. The Botanics Personal Eyes Magnetic Compact is sold separately and can house three eyeshadows. Colors can be rotated as needed because they are held in place by a magnet.

EYE AND BROW SHAPER: ☺ **No7 Amazing Eyes Pencil** *($6.99)* needs sharpening but other than that this is quite good, and preferred to the Botanics Eye Definer below. It glides on swiftly, deposits strong color (which is what you want for eye lining) that can be softened with the built-in sponge tip, and stays in place. The only issue is minor fading, which will be a deal-breaker only for those with oily eyelids.

😐 **No7 Liquid Eye Liner** *($9.99)* comes in inkwell packaging and features a thin, flexible brush that works well; if only the color deposit weren't so sheer. That means successive layers are needed to build color, which increases the chance of smearing. This dries quickly, but will fade before long, so overall it doesn't compare favorably with liquid liners from L'Oreal and Almay, to name just two.

😐 **Botanics Eye Definer** *($6.99)* is a very standard eye pencil that needs routine sharpening and is available in classic colors. This applies easily and feels almost powdery but is still slightly prone to smudging.

☹ **No7 Beautiful Brows Pencil** *($6.99)* won't create beautiful brows unless your definition of that includes flaking color and matted brow hairs from this substandard pencil's waxy texture and finish. This is one of the worst brow pencils I've ever come across. Great colors, though.

LIPSTICK, LIP GLOSS, AND LIPLINER: ✓☺ **No7 Sheer Temptation Lipstick** *($9.99)* feels rich and emollient, and while the colors look quite bold in the tube, each goes on sheer, as the name states. This has a glossy finish yet isn't too slippery, and the colors are great. If you want sheer lip color, what more could you ask for?

✓☺ **Botanics Lip Gloss** *($8.99)* earns its rating because it has a superior smooth texture, moisturizes lips without feeling goopy, isn't sticky, and provides a beautiful selection of sheer to moderate colors, each with a sexy gloss finish and subtle shimmer.

☺ **No7 Stay Perfect Lip Lacquer** *($9.99)* is Boots' version of the long-wearing lip paint first made famous by Max Factor. Just like that company's Lipfinity, this two-part product includes a lip paint and a clear top coat to ensure a glossy finish and comfortable wear (the lip paint used by itself makes lips feel dry). Although this version doesn't have the same impressive longevity as Max Factor's (or Cover Girl's, or those from Estee Lauder and M.A.C.), I was pleasantly surprised that not once in several hours of wear did I feel compelled to apply more top coat. Perhaps I should have, as this might have "protected" the color from fading so much; but at least when that occurred it did so evenly rather than peeling or flaking off. All in all, this is worth a look despite the fact that it does not keep color looking perfect for eight hours, as claimed. ☺ **No7 Moisture Drench Lipstick** *($9.99)* is a standard, but good, cream lipstick. Each of the attractive colors provides moderate coverage and a soft, moisturizing finish. Several shades provide a dimensional shimmer, which can create the illusion of fuller lips.

☹ **Botanics Lipstick** *($8.99)* has an unappealingly thick, waxy texture that's a far cry from the elegantly smooth creaminess of countless other lipsticks. This isn't much for color either, requiring several coats to register beyond sheer, but that only makes this lipstick feel worse.

☺ **No7 Stay Perfect Lipstick** *($9.99)* feels much better and more modern than the Botanics Lipstick above. It has a lightweight texture and smooth, creamy finish that remains a bit slick, so this will migrate into lines around the mouth. If that is not a concern, this is definitely worth auditioning.

☺ **No7 Lip Glace** *($9.99)* comes in a tube and is a standard, thick lip gloss with a slightly sticky finish and wet, glossy shine. Some of the colors go on sheer, while others go on more intense and imbue lips with sparkles. That's why it's good that the Boots display includes testers.

☺ **No7 High Shine Lip Gloss** *($7.99)* is a traditional sheer lip gloss applied with a sponge tip attached to a wand. It feels smooth and is non-sticky and has a less extreme gloss finish than the No7 Lip Glace.

😐 **Botanics Lipliner** *($6.99)* applies easily but has an emollience that makes it prone to smearing and traveling into lines around the mouth. This needs-sharpening pencil works best when applied all over lips and blended with a gloss for a soft, stained effect.

☹ **No7 Line & Define Lip Pencil** *($6.99)* is a decent automatic, retractable lip pencil available in a small assortment of mostly versatile shades. Although this applies easily, the finish feels (and stays) tacky, and the colors, while initially rich, fade too quickly.

MASCARA: ☺ **Botanics Volumising Mascara** *($7.99)* ranks as the best non-waterproof mascara from Boots. You'll enjoy equal parts length and thickness without clumps or smearing, resulting in moderately dramatic, beautifully separated lashes.

☺ **No7 Natural Definition Mascara** *($9.99)* was the first Boots mascara I tried, and although it didn't knock my socks off, I liked it well enough to hope it was a harbinger of things to come. As it turns out, this is one of only a few good mascaras from Boots. It doesn't thicken, but it does make lashes noticeably longer and defines each lash without a clump.

☺ **No7 Maximum Volume Waterproof Mascara** *($9.99)* is much better than its non-waterproof partner below, but its one drawback is that it is minimally waterproof (your eyes getting misty won't cause this to budge, but don't go into the pool with the expectation this will stay put). It is otherwise a very good lengthening and thickening mascara that builds well without getting too dramatic, and it doesn't clump. Removing this takes just a water-soluble cleanser.

☺ **No7 Super Sensitive Mascara** *($9.99)* has fewer ingredients than most mascaras, although that's not a guarantee that someone with sensitive eyes won't have a problem (and the bulk of this formula consists of ingredients found in most mascaras). Still, this has a very clean application that lets you build impressive length and some thickness with zero clumps. As a bonus, it leaves lashes very soft and doesn't flake.

☺ **No7 Lash & Brow Perfector** *($8.99)* is a clear mascara that works best as a lightweight brow gel. Although application is wetter than most, this does not feel sticky or stiff once it dries, yet it holds brows neatly in place. Used as mascara, you'll get a smidgen of emphasis, but that's it.

😐 **No7 Ultimate Curl Mascara** *($9.99)* has a great name but the performance of this boring mascara is far from "ultimate." You'll get negligible length, no thickness whatsoever, and minimal curl.

😐 **Botanics Lash Defining Mascara** *($7.99)* winds up being merely average and is an option only if you want to barely enhance your lashes because you're already satisfied with they way they look minus mascara. 😐 **No7 Longer Lashes Mascara** *($9.99)* is a decent lengthening mascara that doesn't do a thing to build even a hint of thickness. It wears well and removes easily, but this is an option only if slightly longer lashes are your sole requirement.

😐 **No7 Longer Lashes Waterproof Mascara** *($9.99)* has an overly wet application, which causes some smearing during application. Several coats produce nicely elongated lashes without thickness, and this is tenaciously waterproof.

😐 **No7 Maximum Volume Mascara** *($9.99)* is below average if you were banking on the name translating into copiously thick lashes. This does little to enhance lashes in any respect, but is OK if you want a minimalist look.

☹ **Botanics Waterproof Mascara** *($11.99)* is Boots' most expensive mascara, but is not recommended at any price unless you want minimal length, sparse definition, and no thickness regardless of how many coats you apply. It is waterproof and comes off with a water-soluble cleanser, but so what?

FACE AND BODY ILLUMINATING/SHIMMER PRODUCTS: ☺ **No7 Sun Kissed Bronze Shimmer Pearls** *($11.99)* are multicolored powder beads packaged in a jar. You swirl a brush over the beads and apply a sheer layer of powder, which creates a peachy tan color and provides a radiant finish. Although gimmicky, this is a good way to perk up a sallow complexion and add a soft, non-sparkling shine.

☺ **Botanics Shimmer Pearls** *($12.99)* are identical to the No7 Sun Kissed Bronze Shimmer Pearls above, except there are more pink and peach beads, so the result is a soft blush color that applies sheer and leaves a subtle shine.

☺ **No7 High Lights Illuminating Lotion** *($12.99)* is a standard lightweight shimmer lotion that applies easily and sets to a matte (in feel) finish that stays put. The shine is moderate and not sparkling or glittery, making it a good choice for evening makeup. The pale, opalescent pink color works best on fair to light skin tones.

BRUSHES: 😐 **No7 Powder Brush** *($8.99)* is an OK powder brush that isn't as soft as most others, but isn't terrible either. Its floppiness doesn't make for controlled application, but it works in a pinch. 😐 **No7 Blusher Brush** *($7.99)* should be softer, but it is the appropriate shape and, for the money, works well. Spending a bit more for Sonia Kashuk's brushes (also sold at Target) will get you better performance and higher quality. The 😐 **No7 Eye Brush** *($5.99)* is also inferior to those from Kashuk's line, but is still functional and preferred to the sponge-tip applicators that accompany most powder eyeshadows.

The ☹ **No 7 Retractable Lip Brush** *($6.99)* has the retractable benefit, but so do many other lip brushes whose brush heads aren't so ridiculously small. It would take way too long for someone to apply lip color with this, even if they have thin lips.

SPECIALTY PRODUCTS: ☺ **No7 Mattifying Makeup Base** *($9.99)* creates a solid, long-lasting matte finish with silicones, clay, and a tiny amount of alcohol (likely too low to cause irritation). This is a very good (colorless) option to use prior to foundation if you have oily to very oily skin. It is not rated a Paula's Pick because other companies (including mine) sell better versions of this product; better because they mattify skin and control excess shine while supplying oily skin with beneficial ingredients it needs.

☹ **No7 Stay Perfect Smoothing & Brightening Eye Base** *($6.99)* is a pink-tinted cream meant to function as an anchor so eyeshadow lasts longer. The thick, creamy formula does just the opposite—your eyeshadows won't make it to lunch without fading, creasing, or smearing, and the pink color is obvious enough to interfere with any eyeshadow color used over it. Stay away from this product if you want your eye makeup to stay perfect!

☹ **No7 Colour Calming Makeup Base** *($9.99)* has a strong green tint that doesn't correct a reddened complexion; it just substitutes one problem for another, and the light lotion texture, while easy to apply, doesn't do a thing to make the green color less apparent.

BOTOX COSMETIC

BOTOX COSMETIC AT-A-GLANCE

Strengths: An injection procedure that genuinely works to eliminate expression lines and minor wrinkles due to the effect it has on muscles that control facial movement; far superior to any topical product claming to work like Botox.

Weaknesses: Cost; the procedure needs to be repeated every 3-6 months to maintain results; some people have a fear of the needle; Botox parties, where women gather to drink alcohol and get injections of Botox, are never a good idea.

For more information about Botox, call Allergan at (800) 433-8871 or visit www.botox-cosmetic.com or, for my extensive report, www.Beautypedia.com.

Note: Further pros and cons of Botox injections (and there are far more pros) should be discussed at length with the physician who will perform the procedure.

BREMENN RESEARCH LABS
ALSO DOING BUSINESS AS:
BASIC RESEARCH, LLC; VOSS LABORATORIES; AND KLEIN-BECKER

BREMENN RESEARCH LABS AT-A-GLANCE

Strengths: Some state-of-the-art ingredients wrapped up in fantastic claims that are too good to be true.

Weaknesses: Because of Basic Research's sketchy history and ongoing government and legal issues, I don't recommend any of their products, even if they are well formulated (the face ratings below indicate which of their products fall into that category) because too many regulatory and ethical issues remain unresolved.For more information about Bremenn Research Labs, call (800) 621-9553 or visit www.bremennlabs.com or www.Beautypedia.com.

AMATOKIN

unrated **Amatokin** *($173 for 1 ounce)* is marketed by Voss Laboratories, another umbrella company that is headed by Klein-Becker, which markets StriVectin-SD, Hylexin, and Idebenol, all products that use questionable marketing tactics to make their formulas sound like miracles (the FDA has been trying with little success to curtail their advertising). The only miracle about these products is the number of women who buy into the hype, a response that only encourages other companies to continue their own misleading advertising campaigns. After all, if StriVectin-SD is the antiwrinkle breakthrough of the decade that is supposed to replace Botox (that's how Klein-Becker advertises their product), how do they explain away the claim that Amatokin is "the most profound advancement in the skin-care sciences in more than three decades"? Clearly they hope you won't notice that these two companies are distorting the same information in several different products.

The attention-getting concept with this product is the use of stem cells. Amatokin is supposed to enhance the expression of stem cells in the skin, which the company claims will reduce deep and superficial wrinkles and discolorations from sun damage. The problem is that there is no published, independent research to prove that claim.

Here's how Amatokin explains their formula: "Skin is the largest reservoir of stem cells in the human body. Amatokin is the first and only topical compound shown to highlight the expression of stem cell markers in skin.... Amatokin's functional isolates have been clinically shown to dramatically reduce the appearance of both deep and superficial wrinkles, as well as skin coloration associated with photo-aging." Give me a break!

The ingredient list is incredibly ordinary. The name Amatokin is the trade name for the polpypeptide 153 ingredient in this product, and the company claims it is THE ingredient that makes Amatokin special. Yet since Amatokin is almost entirely wax and water, and isn't even as nicely formulated as StriVectin is, the ad copy is really smoke and mirrors. The phrase "highlights expression of stem cell markers in skin" has no meaning. What does highlighting mean anyway? The ad copy is so vague that it nicely gets around any risk of FDA attention because there is no medical or structural change in the body termed "highlighting." "Functional isolates" also has no meaning. What isolates are they referring to? Isolates can refer to any number of substances—they're not a specific group of ingredients. So the claim just alludes to the product's effects on stem cells without actually saying that it does or contains anything that can affect them.

What is even more absurd about this claim is that stem cell research is in its infancy, and in terms of wrinkles and skin care for humans it is nonexistent (Klein-Becker itself doesn't have even one published study). This is a classic example of how a cosmetics company can take serious science and manipulate it to sell products. Scientific literature is clear that stem cells are indeed the basis for every organ, tissue, and cell produced in the human body, and it is possible that stem cells **may be able to repair or replace damaged tissue,** thereby reversing diseases and injuries such as cancer, diabetes, cardiovascular disease, and blood diseases, to name a few. But notice the wording, *may be*. We just don't know, and neither does Amatokin.

Research on adult stem cells, as well as on embryonic stem cells (though the latter is far more controversial), holds great potential. In fact, adult blood-forming stem cells from bone marrow have been used in bone marrow transplants for over 30 years. Certain kinds of adult stem cells seem to have the ability to differentiate into a number of different cell types, given the right conditions. If this differentiation of adult stem cells can be controlled in the laboratory, these cells may become the basis for therapies for many serious common diseases, and they could solve the important problem of immune rejection. Scientists are experimenting with different research strategies to generate tissues that will not be rejected.

Many complicated questions remain to be answered about stem cells. The following are a few I learned from www.wikipedia.com, the National Institutes of Health (www.nih.gov), and other Web sites on stem cell research: How many kinds of adult stem cells exist, and in which tissues do they exist? What are the sources of adult stem cells in the body? Are they "leftover" embryonic stem cells, or do they arise in some other way? Why do they remain in an undifferentiated state when all the cells around them have differentiated? Do adult stem cells normally exhibit plasticity, or do they only transdifferentiate when scientists manipulate them experimentally? What are the signals that regulate the proliferation and differentiation of stem cells that demonstrate plasticity? Is it possible to manipulate adult stem cells to enhance their proliferation so that sufficient tissue for transplants can be produced? Does a single type of stem cell exist—possibly in the bone marrow or circulating in the blood—that can generate the cells of any organ or tissue? What are the factors that stimulate stem cells to relocate to sites of injury or damage? As you can see, there are far more questions than answers, and the answers certainly aren't found in this $173 cosmetic product sold by a company known for its deceptive advertising.

HYLEXIN

☺ **$$$ Hylexin** *($95 for 0.78 ounce)* was a heavily advertised product that quickly became one of the products my readers most urgently requested me to review. I initially held on to my belief that my readers would dismiss the ads and claims as too good to be true. OK, I was wrong. You may have noticed that the full-page magazine ads for Hylexin are similar in design and content to those for Klein-Becker's StriVectin-SD. Hylexin is from Bremenn Research Labs, but the customer-service contact number that appears on Hylexin and StriVectin-SD is identical. Calls to this number revealed that Hylexin and StriVectin are manufactured by different companies, but both are distributed by Customer Service Distribution in Salt Lake City, Utah. Both products also seem to have the same marketing team behind them, and the ad for Hylexin does make for entertaining reading. That's because its tone is conversational, and it reads as if it were written by an enthusiastic, but uninformed, college student, with statements such as "Science is soooo cool!" and "See you at the Hylexin counter!" All I can say is that, based on the volume of questions I have received, the ads are working.

So is there anything to Hylexin? Although it contains some state-of-the-art ingredients that make it worthwhile as a lightweight moisturizer, none of them can affect the oxidation of hemoglobin in capillaries lying beneath the surface of the skin in the eye area (or anywhere else), nor do they have an impact on the enzyme activity that supposedly controls this function, as claimed. The ingredient associated with this potential effect is the citrus bioflavonoid called hesperidin methyl chalcone. There is research supporting its internal use as an aid to venous (vein) problems. One study documented that it lowers the filtration rate of capillaries; less blood flowing though capillaries close to the surface of skin potentially means less hemoglobin would oxygenate to cause a dark bluish discoloration under the eyes. However, there is no substantiated research proving that hesperidin methyl chalcone will have this effect when applied topically.

Another study detailed this ingredient's use when combined with the root of the *Ruscus aculeatus* plant and vitamin C, but again it was about oral consumption for alleviating symptoms of varicose veins and helping prevent them from becoming a chronic disease (Source: *International Angiology*, September 2003, pages 250–262). It is clear from published research that hesperidin methyl chalcone does have various benefits for the body, but diminishing severe dark circles via topical application is not one of them (Source www.pdrhealth.com/drug_info/nmdrugprofiles/nutsupdrugs/hes_0295.shtml).

The "scientific" study mentioned in the ads for Hylexin is not published, so consumers are left to take the company's word for it (and it's anyone's guess how reliable and "scientific" their study is). Because Hylexin is a cosmetic, not a drug, it does not have to prove its claims, although Bremenn Research Labs comes very close to making Hylexin sound like it has druglike benefits, especially with their statements about strengthening the capillary matrix to prevent leakage of oxidized hemoglobin into the under-eye area. There is absolutely zero proof that hesperidin methyl chalcone can affect blood vessels when applied topically (Source: www.naturaldatabase.com). However, as a bioflavonoid, it has antioxidant and anti-inflammatory properties, so it is still a potentially good ingredient for skin, provided you aren't hoping for a dark circle–eliminating miracle. Hylexin is fragrance-free.

LUMEDIA PRODUCTS

☹ **Lumedia Facial Brightener** *($90 for 3 ounces)* claims to be a hydroquinone-free way to reduce hyperpigmentation and restore a healthy, pink glow to skin. Its "active" ingredient is listed as Lumenase-3HF Concentrate. However, designating an ingredient as an "active" ingredient is something controlled by the FDA for over-the-counter drugs, and Lumedia is absolutely not in that category. I'm curious as to how Bremenn slipped this bogus "active" ingredient past the FDA. Or perhaps the FDA hasn't gotten to it yet. It took three years for the FDA to get StriVectin-SD to change their grossly deceptive advertising practices (Source: www.fda.gov).

So what is Lumenase? I have no idea, nor does anyone else, except maybe Bremenn, and as you can well imagine they didn't want to talk to me. There is not a shred of information about this "active" ingredient, which the company claims is actually a "proprietary blend composed of many ingredients." As far as cosmetic ingredient lists go, the FDA requires all ingredients, proprietary or otherwise, to be listed on the packaging, so the lack of that is just one more example of how unethical this company is. There are many reasons not to buy this product, but at the top of the list are lack of efficacy, unknown ingredients, absurd pricing, and over-the-top claims. In case you're curious, the base formula lists a drying, alcohol-based film-forming agent as its second ingredient, and one of the preservatives (methylisothiazolinone) is not meant for use in leave-on products due to its irritating properties (Source: *Archives of Dermatological Research*, February 2007, pages 427–437).

☹ **Lumedia, for Hyperpigmented Age Spots** *($90 for 1 ounce)* at least has the courtesy to use hydroquinone, a tried-and-true active ingredient that offers real hope and help for those dealing with pigmentation issues. However, the price is out of line for what you get and there is enough alcohol to make this irritating and drying for skin, whether used as a spot treatment (as recommended) or all over the face. For the money, Alpha Hydrox Spot Light Targeted Skin Lightener ($15 for 0.85 ounce) runs circles around this overhyped product.

STRIVECTIN PRODUCTS

☹ **StriVectin-SD** *($135 for 6 ounces)*. Quite a few of you have written (and continue to write) asking about the rather prominent newspaper and magazine ads for this product. With a headline that reads "Better than Botox?" along with the increasing number of topical products hitting the market claiming they can mimic the effects of Botox without "painful injections," I certainly understand the curiosity.

I had previously written about StriVectin-SD, when a reader asked about its ability to repair stretch marks. That was StriVectin's original marketing claim to fame, though the fame was all self-promoted, as there is not a single independent, peer-reviewed study to prove that StriVectin is an effective option for repairing stretch marks. The studies that do exist about StriVectin's benefits for stretch marks were paid for by Klein-Becker, the company that distributes StriVectin (and is associated with Bremenn Research Labs).

According to the company's ads, they were surprised to find that not only was StriVectin-SD getting rid of women's stretch marks, but also that somehow their facial wrinkles were going away, too. For that reason, we now have the astounding "antiwrinkle breakthrough of the decade." Regrettably, no supportive research needs to be available to sell this kind of hyperbole. All it takes is to promise women that a product will get rid of their wrinkles and they will buy it in droves, no matter how many other product lines, infomercials, advertisements, or cosmetics salespeople pledge the exact same thing. According to results from the marketing firm NPD Group, StriVectin-SD has been the top-selling product in department stores since November 2003 (Source: *The Rose Sheet*, June 7, 2004, page 3).

StriVectin's ad continues, "The active formula in StriVectin-SD has recently been shown in clinical trials to significantly reduce that category of fine lines and facial wrinkles that can add 10–15 years to your appearance … and even reduce the dark circles under your eyes ... without irritation, painful injections, or surgery." One more flourish is the statement that "in fact, [StriVectin-SD] is the only topical formulation clinically proven to effectively confront every aspect of wrinkle reduction." It is easy to debunk all of this overblown nonsense by pointing out the product's lack of sunscreen. Perhaps StriVectin overlooked the research about sun exposure's deleterious, wrinkling, and discoloring effects on skin.

Klein-Becker has parlayed these claims into what appears to be nothing less than an effort to spin off the popularity of Botox to its own benefit. StriVectin-SD is supposedly preferred because of its alleged long-term results, versus the short-term results (and repeated treatments) of Botox. A Dr. Nathalie Chevreau is quoted in the ad, saying "The cumulative effects of using a product like StriVectin become more noticeable every day, and ultimately last longer than Botox." Chevreau is hardly an impartial source, as she works for Klein-Becker. Further, Dr. Chevreau is licensed as a dietician in Utah, a fact that is conveniently left out of StriVectin's ad because it would conflict with her credibility as a medical doctor speaking about the legitimate benefits of an antiwrinkle cream.

The final Botox comparison comes from the ad's statement that StriVectin not only addresses the expression lines Botox treats, but also the lines Botox doesn't affect. However, the only lines Botox wouldn't affect are the ones not injected.

So is StriVectin better than Botox? The short answer is no—and that means no way, and no how. It isn't even better than the daily use of an effective sunscreen! StriVectin is merely a moisturizer with some good emollients and antioxidants, though the addition of peppermint oil is extremely suspect—the tingle is probably meant to lead women to believe that the product is doing something to their skin. It is doing something: causing irritation without a benefit. Botox prevents the use of facial muscles, and that instantaneously smooths out the skin. StriVectin-SD won't alter the wrinkling on any part of your face, not in the long term, and not in the short term. A recent study supports this conclusion. Researchers recruited 77 women who were divided into five groups. One group received Botox injections, one used a placebo product, and the other groups applied either StriVectin-SD, Hydroderm, or DDF Wrinkle Relax. Only the group that received Botox injections reported satisfaction with the results; wrinkle depth measurement parameters established for this study proved Botox produced the best results. And StriVectin-SD? It was deemed NOT better than Botox. Actually, three test subjects using StriVectin-SD had to drop out due to "adverse reactions," likely from the peppermint oil in the product (Source: *Dermatologic Surgery*, February 2006, pages 184–197).

Incidentally, the two studies quoted in StriVectin's ads for "Better than Botox" were supposedly from information presented at the 20th World Congress of Dermatology, held in July 2002. These examined the effects of palmitoyl pentapeptide-3 (trade name: Matrixyl, but also known as Pal-KTTKS, which is the term used in StriVectin's ads) and compared it to vitamin C and retinol. However, there is no published research substantiating the results, and StriVectin declined (and continues to decline) to send us any documentation. The FDA issued a warning letter to Basic Research, LLC, the umbrella company of Klein-Becker, challenging the validity of and druglike claims made for several products, including StriVectin-SD and the Eye Cream below (Sources: www.casewatch.org/fdawarning/prod/2005/basicresearch.shtml; and www.cfsan.fda.gov/~dms/cos-skin.html). The final word on the matter is that StriVectin-SD has a great story, but this time the fairy tale doesn't come true. Your wrinkles have a much better chance of living happily ever after with Botox than any of its imitators.

☹ **StriVectin-SD Physicians' Formula SPF 15** *($63 for 2 ounces)* makes a medical association via its name, but this in-part zinc oxide sunscreen is not what the doctor ordered. Not only is it unnecessarily pricey, but—just like the original StriVectin-SD formula above—it contains peppermint oil. Further, there is no substantiated research proving that the company's

Striadril compound (consisting of glycerin, butylene glycol, peptides, plant extracts, and some good skin-identical ingredients) is the preferred anti-aging blend because of its superior stability, tolerability, and effectiveness. The peptides in this complex are beneficial for skin, but whether or not they exert a noticeable effect on wrinkles is undetermined.

☺ **$$$ StriVectin-SD Eye Cream** *($59 for 1.3 ounces)* is a surprisingly good moisturizer for dry skin around the eyes, and the price is better than the original StriVectin-SD. It contains olive-based emollients, nonvolatile plant oils, skin-identical ingredients, and, further down on the list, some very good anti-irritants and antioxidants. Because this is for use around the eyes, manufacturer Klein-Becker wisely omitted the peppermint oil found in the original StriVectin-SD product. Interestingly, the company mentions this on their Web site, stating that "since the original StriVectin-SD formula was designed as a stretch-mark reducer, it contains aromatic agents (such as peppermint) which cause some users' eyes to water when applied to the delicate skin in the orbital eye area…." How thoughtful of them to let us know, though they left out the part about the irritation it can cause skin, and never mind the fact that peppermint oil and other "aromatic compounds" have absolutely no effect on stretch marks!

The real question is whether this Eye Cream is the antiaging breakthrough it's made out to be. But it's no surprise the answer is "No!"—though as mentioned above, it is a good moisturizer. Klein-Becker claims the patented pentapeptides in this product are the wrinkle-reducing, dark circle–diminishing wonders, but independent research does not correlate with this claim because there are no independent, peer-reviewed studies analyzing the effects of palmitoyl pentapeptide-3 on wrinkles. The studies that do exist were paid for by Sederma (now owned by Croda), the ingredient's manufacturer and distributor. Such company-sponsored studies are not a reliable source of information because the company has a vested interest in making sure that whatever tests they conduct show their ingredient performs as intended. Lastly, Sederma's own research mentions that in order to gain maximum benefit from palmitoyl pentapeptide-3, it must be used at a 3% to 5% concentration, yet the amount in StriVectin-SD Eye Cream is unknown, and a look at the ingredient list indicates that it's far less than 3% (Klein-Becker would not reveal the exact percentage when we called). If you still want to know if this ingredient is the miracle the ads claim, Olay Regenerist serums and moisturizers contain the exact same thing, and more of it, for a fraction of this price.

☹ **StriVectin-HS Hydro-Thermal Deep Wrinkle Serum** *($153 for 0.9 ounce)* is a cosmetics rip-off that is a must to avoid. That's not only because it doesn't work as claimed, but because it includes an inaccurate ingredient statement (there's no such ingredient as "Tripeptide"; it should be followed by a number). For over $150, you're getting a water-based serum that temporarily tightens skin because of the amount of sodium polystyrene sulfonate (a film former) and egg white (albumen) it contains. It cannot penetrate to the dermal/epidermal junction and plump deep wrinkles from the bottom up. Wasting money on a few bottles of this would only match the cost for a series of facial peels or Intense Pulsed Light (IPL) treatments, options proven to make a positive difference in skin. (Though even so, neither of these treatments will significantly improve the appearance of deep wrinkles—for that, more invasive procedures are needed.)

SOVAGE DERMATOLOGIC LABORATORIES PRODUCTS

☹ **Idebenol** *($109 for 3.4 ounces)* was launched (via double-page ads in leading fashion magazines and newspaper ads) to capitalize on the success of Allergan's Prevage product, which contains the synthetic antioxidant idebenone. Sovage's name for this product is nearly identical to idebenone, but here's the kicker: This moisturizer does not contain any idebenone (after all, idebenol isn't idebenone)! Ads for this product state as much, but in very small print outside the main text. The formula contains mostly water, silicone, film-forming agent, slip agents, barley extract, thickeners, plant oil, fragrant plant extracts, ingredients that mimic the structure and function of healthy skin, antioxidants, fragrance, and preservatives. The irony here is that the claims for this product go above and beyond the already too-good-to-be-true (and unproven) claims being made for Prevage MD as well as the version of Prevage being sold by Elizabeth Arden, which do contain idebenone.

Sovage claims their antioxidant miracle worker can "reverse the hands of time," making the skin-renewal rate of a sixty-something woman revert to that of a woman in her late 20s. I'd love to see the studies that support this claim, but they are unpublished and the company would not furnish them. Needless to say, the age-reversing claims are pure fantasy. If they were true, hundreds of well-formulated moisturizers (that's essentially all idebenol is) would have the same effect, and we'd all enjoy wrinkle-free faces that would never require cosmetic surgery or Botox treatments.

The ad text for Idebenol had the same tone as ads for Klein-Becker's StriVectin-SD and Bremenn Research Lab's Hylexin. I have suspected for some time that all three companies were under the same umbrella because their ad copy, packaging, and even their Web sites and product packaging graphics are remarkably similar. As it turns out, my suspicion was correct: All three of these companies are part of Basic Research, LLC, a Provo, Utah–based company which, at least according to Web sites devoted to legal issues and rip-off alerts, is as duplicitous and unethical as a company can be. Its CEO, Dennis Gay, has received warning letters from the FDA for many unscrupulous products as well as for the ads that promote them (Source: www.fda.gov/foi/warning_letters/g5195d.htm). The name of Klein-Becker's Director of Scientific Affairs, Dr. Daniel Mowrey, is all over the literature for idebenol, but he is not a medical doctor. According to the company, he has his Ph.D. in psychology (Source: www.businessweek.com/bwdaily/ dnflash/nov2004/nf20041130_2214_db042.htm). All of this makes for fascinating reading, and offers a lesson in how quickly a company can seize consumers' dollars with outlandish, unsubstantiated promises (StriVectin's sales topped $30 million in five months!).

☹ **Instant Lip Plumper** *($39 for 0.22 ounce)* contains menthol, which plumps lips by virtue of its irritating properties. The strong film-former base of this product promises to keep the menthol around longer than it would be in an ordinary emollient base, and in case that isn't long enough, camphor is also included to add to the irritation.

BURT'S BEES

BURT'S BEES AT-A-GLANCE

Strengths: One good, nonirritating lip balm; budget-priced (it's always a letdown when you pay too much for lackluster to ineffective products); good lip gloss; the oil-blotting papers; complete ingredient lists for every product are available on the company's Web site; honest about claims of being all-natural, though that's not without its drawbacks.

Weaknesses: Pervasive use of irritating ingredients, all of which have documentation proving their problematic nature for skin (and lips); only one sunscreen and it has fragrant oils that can cause a phototoxic reaction; no effective anti-blemish products; poor selection of cleansers; antioxidants sullied by reliance on jar packaging; most of the makeup has either unappealing textures or is loaded with irritating fragrant oils.For more information about Burt's Bees, call (866) 422-8787 or visit www.burtsbees.com or www.Beautypedia.com.

BURT'S BEES SKIN CARE

☹ **All-In-One Wash** *($5 for 4 ounces)* is sold as a gentle formula suitable for cleansing face, hair, and body—yet this is as gentle for skin as exfoliating with sandpaper thanks to the inclusion of irritating fragrant oils including lime, peppermint, and spearmint.

☹ **Baby Bee Buttermilk Soap** *($5 for a 3.5-ounce bar)* has some gentle ingredients, including oatmeal flour, but this is still standard-issue bar soap and is not recommended over cleansing baby's skin with a water-soluble, fragrance-free body wash.

☹ **Garden Carrot Complexion Soap** *($8 for a 4 ounce bar)* is standard-issue bar soap that also contains irritating cinnamon powder, and is not recommended for any skin type.

☹ **Garden Tomato Complexion Soap** *($8 for a 4 ounce bar)* has tomato powder but that's of little consequence in a drying bar soap, and lycopene (the red pigment in tomatoes) has no ability to balance skin's pH as claimed.

☹ **Orange Essence Facial Cleanser** *($8 for 4.34 ounces)* has more than orange essence; it irritates skin with orange and rosemary oils and is not recommended. It isn't even a very good cleanser, making it a waste of time and money.

☹ **Soap Bark & Chamomile Deep Cleansing Cream** *($8 for 6 ounces)* contains several problematic ingredients for skin, especially for use around the eyes, and is not recommended.

☹ **Poison Ivy Soap** *($6 for a 2-ounce bar)* is standard, drying bar soap that adds irritation to its drying base thanks to pine tar and balsam leaf. Both will lessen the itch of poison ivy, but they do so as counter-irritants (meaning their stimulus is more irritating than the poison ivy itself).

☹ **Wild Lettuce Complexion Soap** *($8 for a 4-ounce bar)* is standard bar soap and not recommended, either for that or for the irritating comfrey extract it contains.

☹ **Citrus Facial Scrub** *($7.50 for 2 ounces)* is an inelegant scrub whose abrasive agents are composed of nutshells whose uneven shape can cause tiny tears in the skin during use (in contrast, perfectly rounded polyethylene beads polish skin without this effect). Although the nutshells aren't the best, they don't make this product a poor contender. What does are the nutmeg and clove powders, which only serve to provide fragrance and irritate skin.

☹ **Citrus Spice Exfoliating Shower Soap** *($5 for a 4-ounce bar)* contains a bevy of irritating volatile oils, including bay, fir needle, clove, and sage. This is akin to paying money to hurt your skin and then having nothing positive to show for it.

☹ **Lemon Poppy Seed Facial Cleanser** *($8 for 4 ounces)*. Lemons and poppy seeds make for good muffins, but adding lemon oil to a cleanser is only asking for trouble, and there's a significant amount of it in here, too.

☹ **Peach & Willowbark Deep Pore Scrub** *($8 for 4 ounces)* contains an appreciable amount of sodium borate. Also known as borax, this ingredient has a drying effect on skin due to its alkaline pH. It is fine in small amounts, but that's not the case here, making this a scrub to avoid.

☹ **Carrot Seed Oil Complexion Mist** *($10 for 4 ounces)* contains several fragrant oils that are irritating to skin, including rose, sandalwood, and patchouli.

😐 **Cucumber Chamomile Complexion Mist** *($10 for 4 ounces)* is a simple spray-on toner that contains merely water, cucumber and chamomile extracts, and fragrance. It's an OK option for normal to dry skin.

☹ **Garden Tomato Toner** *($12 for 8 ounces)* lists alcohol as the second ingredient, which makes this toner too drying and irritating for all skin types.

☹ **Grapefruit Complexion Mist** *($10 for 4 ounces)* contains lime, lemon, and grapefruit oils, making this a mist that's more suited to flavoring citrus-based cocktails than smart skin care.

☹ **Lavender Complexion Mist** *($10 for 4 ounces)* contains lavender, bergamot, and cedar oils, all of which are irritating, not nourishing, to skin.

☹ **Rosewater & Glycerin Toner** *($12 for 8 ounces)* lists alcohol as the second ingredient, which makes this toner too drying and irritating for all skin types.

😐 **Baby Bee Skin Creme** *($11 for 2 ounces)* is a basic, oil-based moisturizer for dry skin of any age, though its jar packaging compromises the stability of the antioxidant vitamin E.

😐 **Beeswax & Royal Jelly Eye Creme** *($12 for 0.25 ounce)* contains a tiny amount of royal bee jelly (in powder form), but this ingredient, despite tempting folklore, has no established benefit for skin. It can cause contact dermatitis, though the amount of it in this product likely negates that possibility (Source: www.naturaldatabase.com). This is otherwise a boring moisturizer consisting mostly of plant oil, glycerin, and beeswax. It's an OK option for dry skin anywhere on the face.

😐 **Beeswax Moisturizing Creme** *($12 for 2 ounces)* is described as a lightweight formula but it contains too much oil to make that claim a reality. This is a good, basic moisturizer for dry skin but definitely lacks state-of-the-art ingredients.

😐 **Beeswax Moisturizing Night Creme** *($12 for 1 ounce)* is primarily plant oil, water, wax, and aloe. It serves its purpose for dry skin, but also leaves skin wanting more.

☹ **Carrot Nutritive Day Creme** *($12 for 2 ounces)* doesn't make sense for daytime because it lacks sun protection; it also contains enough balsam peru to cause irritation and has the potential to cause a phototoxic reaction due to its volatile components (Source" www.naturaldatabase.com).

😐 **Carrot Nutritive Night Creme** *($12 for 1 ounce)* contains a much smaller amount of balsam than the Carrot Nutritive Day Creme above, but its jar packaging compromises the effectiveness of the antioxidant plant oils that compose the bulk of this moisturizer.

☹ **Evening Primrose Overnight Creme** *($15 for 1 ounce)* has more problematic than beneficial oils for skin, including lavender, rose, and ylang ylang. Otherwise it differs little from the Carrot Nutritive Night Creme above.

☹ **Marshmallow Vanishing Creme** *($15 for 1.5 ounces)* contains too many emollients to vanish immediately into skin as claimed. Although this has ingredients that are great for very dry skin, the rosemary oil makes it too irritating to consider over better formulations.

☹ **Radiance Day Creme** *($15 for 2 ounces)* contains several irritating or problematic ingredients, including comfrey, spearmint, and lemon oil. It is not recommended.

☹ **Radiance Eye Creme** *($15 for 0.5 ounce)* contains the same offending ingredients as the Radiance Day Creme above and is also not recommended. Using lemon oil around the eyes is never a good idea.

☹ **Radiance Night Creme** *($15 for 2 ounces)* contains the same offending ingredients as the Radiance Day Creme above and is also not recommended.

☹ **Repair Serum** *($15 for 1 ounce)* won't repair skin but will damage skin cells due to its high content of lavender oil. Components in lavender oil have been shown to cause skin-cell death when applied topically (Source: *Cell Proliferation*, June 2004, pages 221–229).

😐 **Royal Jelly Eye Creme** *($15 for 0.5 ounce)* shares the same basic formula as most of the Burt's Bees moisturizers above that combine a nonvolatile plant oil with glycerin and beeswax to benefit dry skin. The amount of royal jelly is minuscule, but that's fine because it isn't a must-have ingredient for skin.

☹ **Aloe & Linden Flower After Sun Soother** *($10 for 6 ounces)* has more irritating than soothing properties for skin thanks to the comfrey extract and citrus oils it contains. Pure aloe vera gel would be a much better option.

☹ **Chemical-Free Sunscreen SPF 15** *($15 for 3.46 ounces)* leaves out synthetic sunscreen actives (though there's nothing wrong with those ingredients) and relies on titanium dioxide for sun protection. That's great, but the many fragrant volatile oils in this product are a considerable problem. Of particular concern is the balsam oil, which can cause a phototoxic reaction (Source: *The British Journal of Dermatology*, September 2002, pages 493–497).

☹ **Dr. Burt's Herbal Blemish Stick** *($8.50 for 0.3 ounce)* proves without a doubt that Burt should stick to beekeeping instead of doctoring. With alcohol as the main ingredient and irritating fragrant oils of juniper, lemon, and eucalyptus, this only serves to make blemished skin look worse and to impede skin's healing process.

☹ **Parsley Blemish Stick** *($8 for 0.26 ounce)* is nearly identical to the Dr. Burt's Herbal Blemish Stick above, and the same review applies (though at least the doctor reference was dropped here).

☹ **Pore-Refining Mask** *($8 for 1 ounce)* is just clay with fragrance and fragrant plant extracts, including peppermint. It has absorbent properties, but is too potentially irritating to make it worth considering over numerous other clay masks.

😐 **Dr. Burt's Herbal Defense Ointment** *($8 for 3.2 ounces)* contains some fragrant oils and plant extracts that can be irritating to skin, but is primarily zinc oxide, almond oil, and beeswax. As such, it has a thick, protective texture even though it's not cosmetically elegant. It isn't something you'd want to use routinely, and for those occasions when a protective ointment is needed, plain Desitin is preferred to this product.

😐 **Dr. Burt's Res-Q Ointment** *($5 for 0.6 ounce)* is a rich, oil-based balm that contains some restorative ingredients for dry to very dry skin. The tiny amounts of fragrant plant extracts don't add to the benefit, but they're on target with the natural image this company espouses. The jar packaging hinders the antioxidant properties of the olive oil and vitamin E.

☹ **Beeswax Lip Balm Tin** *($3 for 0.3 ounce)* is the company's most popular product, but it isn't one I'd recommend because it contains irritating peppermint oil.

☹ **Beeswax Lip Balm Tube** *($3 for 0.15 ounce)* is a waxy version of the Beeswax Lip Balm Tin above, and also contains peppermint oil.

☺ **Honey Lip Balm** *($3 for 0.15 ounce)* is a shea butter–based lip balm that contains a nice array of ingredients to make dry, chapped lips look and feel better. The comfrey root is of minor cause for concern, so this is overall a very good lip moisturizer.

☹ **Lifeguard's Choice Weatherproofing Lip Balm** *($3 for 0.15 ounce)* contains peppermint oil, and the lifeguard who chooses this is in for lip irritation along with sun damage since this balm lacks active ingredients (the titanium dioxide is not listed as such).

☹ **Replenishing Lip Balm With Pomegranate Oil** *($3 for 0.15 ounce)* has pomegranate oil, which is great, but it's downhill from there because this also contains irritating cinnamon, sage, mandarin, anise, and cassia oils.

BURT'S BEES MAKEUP

FOUNDATION: ☺ **Tinted Facial Moisturizer** *($11)* is contradictory, because it's for someone who "doesn't want to load up their face with heavy foundation." Yet this tinted moisturizer has a thick, creamy texture that definitely makes its presence known. It is indeed sheer, but it blends unevenly and keeps skin feeling moist, almost greasy. Four shades are available, and all except Light (which is ghostly white) are acceptable. This product doesn't contain any irritants, but is only appropriate for those with dry skin (and those with a willingness to tolerate this product's shortcomings).

POWDER: ☹ **Vanishing Facial Powder** *($16)* is a talc-free loose powder available in only one color, which goes on chalky-looking due to the high amount of calcium carbonate. This powder has an ultra-dry texture and its finish doesn't look attractive on skin, even when applied sheer.

BLUSH: ☹ **Blushing Creme** *($9)* is definitely creamy for dry to very dry skin. The translucent colors would have been a good sheer cream blush option for dry skin, but the rosemary oil in this product makes it too irritating to consider.

EYESHADOW: ☹ **Eye Shadow** *($9)* is only available in an oil-based, creamy formula that is tricky to apply, difficult to blend with other colors, and creases (though not as quickly as you might think). The final straw is that the pastel-metallic colors end up looking more ghastly than pretty.

EYE AND BROW SHAPER: ☺ **Eyeliner and Eyebrow Pencil** *($9)* needs sharpening (and a sharpener is included), but otherwise this is a perfectly good eyeliner whose smooth, easy-glide texture and light application make it suitable as a brow pencil too. It is available in three authentic colors, though not for light blonde or auburn/red brows.

LIPSTICK, LIP GLOSS, AND LIPLINER: ☺ **Lip Gloss** *($3.50)*. The grape seed oil–based formula moisturizes while feeling light and leaving a minimal gloss finish. Each gloss contains natural fruit flavors, and none of them contain irritants.

☹ **Lip Shimmers** *($4)* are sheer, glossy lipsticks that apply well but irritate lips with a potent mix of peppermint and rosemary oils.

SPECIALTY PRODUCTS: ☺ **Vanishing Facial Powder Tissues** *($3 for 65 sheets)* work well to absorb excess shine prior to touching up with powder. These thin rice-paper sheets deposit a bit of absorbent cornstarch and zinc oxide on skin, which is fine if you are not absorbing oil over blemished skin. As a food ingredient, cornstarch can feed the bacteria that contribute to blemishes, and zinc oxide, though a skin protectant, isn't the best ingredient to press over blemished areas.

CELLEX-C (SKIN CARE ONLY)

CELLEX-C AT-A-GLANCE

Strengths: A worthwhile line to consider if you want to zero in on topical vitamin C; some effective AHA products that feature a blend of acids within the correct pH range.

Weaknesses: Irritating anti-acne products; lackluster sunscreens; expensive; pervasive use of jar packaging, which completely ignores the stability issues critical to the efficacy of vitamin C; mostly boring moisturizers that, for the money, should be brimming with state-of-the-art ingredients; Cellex-C is still mostly a one-trick pony compared to competing lines that offer more to skin than just vitamin C.

For more information about Cellex-C, call (800) 235-5392 or visit www.cellex-c.com or www.Beautypedia.com.

CELLEX-C BETAPLEX PRODUCTS

☺ **$$$ Betaplex Gentle Cleansing Milk** *($29 for 6 ounces)* is a standard, plant oil–based cleanser that also includes a small amount of detergent cleansing agent. It is an option for someone with normal to dry skin. It contains lactic acid as the third ingredient, but the pH of the product isn't low enough for it to have exfoliating properties.

✓☺ **$$$ Betaplex Gentle Foaming Cleanser** *($29 for 6 ounces)* is a very good, water-soluble gel cleanser with mild foaming properties. Suitable for all skin types, it contains some good soothing agents (remember, though—it's a cleanser, so the soothing agents will be there only briefly, and so can't provide much of a benefit) and is fragrance-free.

☹ **Betaplex Facial Firming Water** *($29 for 6 ounces)* lists alcohol and witch hazel as its second and third ingredients, making this toner too drying and irritating for all skin types. The amount of glycolic acid is less than what's considered best for exfoliation, although the pH is within the correct range.

☹ **Betaplex Fresh Complexion Mist** *($29 for 6 ounces)* is designed to "gently stimulate" your skin, but there's nothing gentle about the irritation caused by the witch hazel and alcohol, especially when they're coupled with oils of lavender, peppermint, and thyme. The amount of lactic acid is too low for significant exfoliation, although the pH is in the correct range.

☺ **$$$ Betaplex Line Smoother** *($59 for 1 ounce)* is a basic, though very effective AHA serum that contains a blend of glycolic, lactic, and malic acids at a pH of 3.1. The willow bark extract is meant to be a natural alternative to BHA (salicylic acid), but its active constituents cannot be converted to salicylic acid when used topically. It does, however, have anti-inflammatory properties.

☺ **$$$ Betaplex New Complexion Cream** *($59 for 2 ounces)* contains a blend of glycolic, lactic, and malic acids at about a 5% concentration in a pH of 2.9. That makes this a good AHA cream for normal to dry skin, but the jar packaging won't keep the antioxidants stable. Still, it deserves a happy face rating for its exfoliating ability, which is the main reason to consider it.

☺ **$$$ Betaplex Smooth Skin Complex** *($59 for 2 ounces)* is nearly identical to the Betaplex New Complexion Cream above, except this version is more emollient due to the amount of mineral oil it contains and a slightly higher pH (but it's still effective). Otherwise, the same review applies.

☹ **Betaplex Clear Complexion Mask** *($40 for 2 ounces)* contains several thickening agents that won't promote clear skin, and the pH above 4 means the glycolic acid won't exfoliate skin as effectively as it would if the pH were lower. Although the thickening agents are reason enough to skip this mask, the clincher is the peppermint oil it contains.

CELLEX-C CORE FORMULATIONS

😐 **$$$ Eye Contour Cream Plus** *($70 for 1 ounce)* is an emollient moisturizer whose jar packaging will quickly compromise the effectiveness of the vitamin C. What a shame, because there are some very good ingredients in here for dry skin anywhere on the face.

😐 **$$$ Eye Contour Gel** *($51 for 0.5 ounce)* is a basic but effective vitamin C gel that contains a couple of skin-identical ingredients. However, there's enough astringent zinc sulfate in here to cause irritation around the eyes, especially given the acidic nature of this product.

☹ **High-Potency Serum** *($90 for 1 ounce)* lists zinc sulfate as the first ingredient, which makes this serum highly irritating to skin. Topical application of zinc sulfate has not been shown to promote skin healing, and it is of very little benefit to skin (Source: *Acta Dermato-Venereologica*, supplemental, 1990, pages 1–36).

☺ **$$$ Serum for Sensitive Skin** *($90 for 1 ounce)* contains much less zinc sulfate than the High-Potency Serum above, and is a good way to supply skin with stabilized vitamin C. There isn't much else of note to report, other than that this product is fragrance-free.

😐 **$$$ Skin Firming Cream Plus** *($114 for 2 ounces)* is nearly identical to the Eye Contour Cream Plus above, and the same review applies.

☹ **Sun Rescue Gel** *($55 for 3 ounces)* has a lot of vitamin C, but there are no established guidelines to show what amount is needed to reduce wrinkles—plus, higher percentages can be irritating in an acidic base like this. Although the vitamin C content is considerable, the amount of peppermint oil makes this incapable of rescuing skin or treating it to anything other than irritation.

😐 **$$$ Fade Away Gel for Sun & Age Spots** *($38 for 0.85 ounce)* contains ascorbic acid (vitamin C) to lighten skin discolorations. There is some convincing research proving this ingredient has skin-lightening benefits, but it still isn't as effective as hydroquinone, and the ascorbic acid has difficulty penetrating the skin sufficiently to impact the cause of the discoloration (Sources: *International Journal of Dermatology*, August 2004, pages 604–607; and *Dermatologic Surgery*, July 2005, pages 814–817). The amount of zinc sulfate has the potential for causing irritation, and the inclusion of thyme extract (which the company accurately describes as a "powerful antiseptic") isn't going to lessen that potential any. That leaves you with a potentially effective skin-lightening product that may cause undue irritation, though this may be worth trying if your skin has not responded favorably to products with hydroquinone.

CELLEX-C CORRECTIVES PRODUCTS

☹ **Fresh Complexion Foaming Gel** *($38 for 6 ounces)* contains several irritating plant extracts including peppermint, thyme, eucalyptus, and cajeput (a form of melaleuca). It is not preferred to the Betaplex Gentle Foaming Cleanser above, and its price is ridiculous for what you get.

☹ **Clear Complexion Complex** *($38 for 6 ounces)* is claimed to be of significant benefit to oily or teenaged skin prone to occasional breakouts, but all you can count on from this faulty toner is irritation. Peppermint, thyme, lavender, and witch hazel won't help breakouts any more than topping a piece of pie with whipped cream will reduce the number of calories.

☹ **Speed Peel Facial Gel** *($33 for 3 ounces)* is a moisturizing scrub product whose abrasive agent is the ground-up peel of bitter oranges. It does a poor job of exfoliating and is difficult to rinse from the skin because of the high amount of plant oil. Yet what is most problematic about this scrub is the needless inclusion of irritating peppermint oil. I suppose that with a substandard topical exfoliant like this, Cellex-C needed to add something so a consumer would think the product is "working." By the way, the company claims that the jojoba oil helps unclog pores, a notion that is completely false (like thinking gasoline will extinguish a fire). Jojoba oil is excellent for dry skin, but its molecular makeup is similar to our own oil (sebum), and that oil, while helpful for dry skin, is a causative, not combative, factor where blemishes are concerned.

☹ **Clear Complexion Seboregulator** *($55 for 3.3 ounces)* is supposed to inhibit the inflammatory process that leads to acne while controlling "the synthesis of comedoes-inducing skin lipids." What that means is that this product claims to interfere with the process that causes acne. This process, briefly, involves acne-causing bacteria that feed on the oil in the pore and then release free fatty acids that elicit an inflammatory response by the skin, leading to an acne eruption and reddened skin. This product is supposed to interrupt that process, but this unbalanced concoction of water, jojoba esters (a fatty acid chemically similar to our own oil), witch hazel, and castor oil–based thickener does no such thing. It's actually a problem product for acne-prone skin and contains some potentially irritating plant extracts that won't help control bacteria or do anything to change the way oil is broken down in the pore lining.

☹ **Skin Perfecting Pen** *($24 for 0.34 ounce)* contains herbal ingredients chosen for their healing properties, but there is no research demonstrating that peppermint, lavender, rosemary, and thyme heal acne lesions. All of these ingredients can cause irritation that can make acne look worse, although the tingling sensation from this product may convince you it's "working."

☹ **Under-Eye Toning Gel** *($35 for 0.34 ounce)* has some very good, plant-based soothing agents as well as skin-identical ingredients, but the inclusion of irritating zinc sulfate and lavender oil is a mistake, not to mention the lesser amounts of peppermint, thyme, and eucalyptus. And we're supposed to apply this around the eye? Yikes!

CELLEX-C ENHANCERS

😐 **$$$ G.L.A.** *($58 for 2 ounces)*. The "G.L.A." in the name stands for gamma linolenic acid, a fatty acid used in cosmetics as an emollient and considered to promote healthy skin growth, which is great and similar to what many effective antioxidants do. However, there is no research showing G.L.A. to be effective in the treatment of wrinkles (Sources: *British Journal of Dermatology*, April 1999, pages 685–688; and *Dermatology*, 2000, volume 201, number 3, pages 191–195). G.L.A. has been shown to have some anticancer properties when taken orally, but there is no research showing that effect translates to products applied to the skin. Even if the research were there to support the antiwrinkle ability of G.L.A., the choice of jar packaging will render it and the other antioxidants in this product unstable shortly after the product is opened.

😐 **$$$ G.L.A. Extra Moist** *($58 for 2 ounces)* is nearly identical to the G.L.A. product above and the same comments apply. Both of these moisturizers are helpful for normal to dry skin, but would be more so with better packaging.

😐 **$$$ G.L.A. Eye Balm** *($54 for 1 ounce)* is similar to the G.L.A. moisturizers above, save for a couple of thickeners, which create a different texture. Once again, the jar packaging hinders the effectiveness of the antioxidants.

😐 **$$$ Hydra 5 B-Complex** *($66 for 1 ounce)* does not contain hyaluronic acid, which would help justify this product's price if it were present. Instead, Cellex-C uses the less expensive, but still beneficial, salt form of hyaluronic acid. Although this gel-like serum has merit for slightly dry to slightly oily skin, it's basically a one-note product, and your skin deserves more.

☺ **Sea Silk Oil-Free Moisturizer** *($49 for 2 ounces)* contains plankton, algae, and other sea extracts, but these don't have any special benefit for skin beyond being good skin-identical ingredients. That's what this jar-packaged, antioxidant-free moisturizer is all about, and it's a very good option for normal to slightly oily skin not prone to blemishes. The jojoba esters can be problematic for blemish-prone skin.

😐 **$$$ Seline-E** *($58 for 2 ounces)* contains a good mix of antioxidants in a rather ordinary moisturizing base that would be OK for someone with normal to dry skin, though the jar packaging won't keep the antioxidants stable.

CELLEX-C PROFESSIONAL FORMULATIONS

☹ **$$$ Advanced-C Eye Firming Cream** *($90 for 1 ounce)* contains mostly water, vitamin C, emollient, thickeners, wax, silicone, zinc sulfate, plant oil, and antioxidants. The vitamin C and other antioxidants will lose potency because of the jar packaging, making this a subpar and yet very expensive moisturizer for normal to dry skin.

☹ **$$$ Advanced-C Eye Toning Gel** *($70 for 0.5 ounce)* is nearly identical to the Eye Contour Gel above, except this pricier version contains additional antioxidants. That makes it a better product, but the amount of irritating zinc sulfate is still cause for concern for use around the eyes.

☹ **$$$ Advanced-C Neck Firming Cream** *($115 for 2 ounces)* loses points for jar packaging that will quickly degrade the effectiveness of the vitamin C and other antioxidants in this product. This is otherwise an ordinary moisturizer that's mostly thickeners and wax. It has no unique benefit for skin on the neck, and it won't reduce sagging or minimize the appearance of neck cords.

☺ **$$$ Advanced-C Serum** *($115 for 1 ounce)* is similar to the Serum for Sensitive Skin above except this version contains more antioxidants. The amount of zinc sulfate is potentially irritating and keeps this serum from earning a Paula's Pick rating.

☹ **$$$ Advanced-C Skin Tightening Cream** *($135 for 2 ounces)* is so similar to most of the Cellex-C moisturizers above that all of those must be able to tighten skin too. Vitamin C (which this product has in spades) can stimulate collagen production, resulting in "tighter" (I think a better word is "firmer") skin, but not when jar packaging is used, as it is here.

☹ **$$$ Advanced-C Skin Toning Mask** *($55 for 8 ounces)* is mostly cornstarch and egg white along with vitamin C and some soothing agents. It's an OK option for normal to slightly dry skin, but it's hardly essential and not worth its price. The only things advanced about this product are the exaggerated marketing claims.

☹ **$$$ Skin Hydration Complex** *($79 for 1 ounce)* is a modified version of the Hydra 5 B-Complex above because it contains antioxidants. What a shame the clear glass bottle packaging won't protect them from light degradation. That disappointment doesn't make swallowing the cost of this water-based serum any easier.

CELLEX-C SUN-CARE PRODUCTS

☺ **$$$ Bio Tan** *($110 for 8 ounces)* tries to make itself seem like a revolutionary advance in self-tanners, but it contains the same ingredient (dihydroxyacetone) found in most self-tanning products. The only part that is revolutionary is the absurd cost for such a standard product. This does contain erythrulose, an ingredient chemically similar to dihydroxyacetone, and because erythrulose takes longer to develop, that can make it easier to fine-tune the amount of color you get. Still, that doesn't justify the price, and you don't have to spend this much to see if a self-tanner with erythrulose is for you; Jergens Natural Glow Daily Moisturizer ($6.99 for 7.5 ounces) or Hawaiian Tropic Island Glow Moisturizer Medium Skin Tones ($8.99 for 8 ounces) also contain it and are recommended.

☹ **$$$ Sun Care SPF 15** *($36.30 for 5 ounces)* contains an in-part titanium dioxide and zinc oxide sunscreen, but how odd that Cellex-C left vitamin C out of this sunscreen. Plenty of research has demonstrated vitamin C's protective ability when skin is exposed to sunlight. Maybe the thinking was you'd be using all of their other products with vitamin C, so why add it to the sunscreen too? Although this is effective when outdoors and is best for dry skin, it ends up being an expensive sunscreen considering what was left out.

😐 **$$$ Sun Care SPF 30** *($38.50 for 5 ounces)* gets its UVA protection from titanium dioxide and zinc oxide, but is otherwise a lackluster formula for normal to dry skin.

😐 **$$$ Sun Care SPF 30+** *($30.80 for 3.4 ounces)* is nearly identical to the Sun Care SPF 15 above save for higher percentages of some of the active ingredients (necessary to achieve a greater SPF rating). Otherwise, the same comments apply.

✓😊 **$$$ Sunshade SPF 30+** *($45 for 2 ounces)* is a very good sunscreen for normal to very dry skin not prone to blemishes. It features an in-part zinc oxide sunscreen in an emollient base that contains a nice selection of skin-identical ingredients and a few antioxidants. Cellex-C claims this was formulated specifically for acne-prone skin, but the jojoba ester base and the other thickening agents are nearly guaranteed to make acne worse.

CERAVE

CERAVE AT-A-GLANCE

Strengths: Affordable, gentle, and fragrance-free; an impressive delivery system for skin-identical substances.

Weaknesses: Cleanser does not remove makeup well on its own; formulas are effective but don't go the extra mile to supply dry skin with a wider complement of beneficial ingredients.

For more information about CeraVe, call Coria Laboratories at (866) 819-9007 or visit www.cerave.com or www.Beautypedia.com.

😊 **Hydrating Cleanser** *($11.99 for 12 ounces)* deserves serious consideration by anyone with normal to dry skin that's also sensitive, including those dealing with rosacea. It is an exceptionally gentle, soothing cleanser that contains several ingredients that mimic the structure and function of healthy skin. These are a good, but not essential, addition to a cleanser (ideally, they are ingredients that should be left on your skin). But when you're dealing with an impaired barrier, which is a hallmark of consistent dryness, every little beneficial extra helps. This cleanser is fragrance-free; its only drawback is its limited ability to remove makeup unless used with a washcloth.

😊 **Moisturizing Cream** *($14.99 for 16 ounces)* is a basic but thoughtfully formulated fragrance-free body moisturizer that contains several helpful ingredients for restoring and maintaining skin's barrier function, including glycerin, ceramides, and cholesterol. This product's jar packaging isn't such a bad thing this time given that it contains no antioxidants, a fact that keeps this from being downgraded to a neutral face rating. This will work quite well if you have normal to dry or sensitive skin.

😊 **Moisturizing Lotion** *($12.99 for 12 ounces)* is the lotion version of the Moisturizing Cream above, and other than having a lighter texture and smoother dry-down, the same formulary comments apply. The blend of glycerin, ceramides, cholesterol, and hyaluronic acid will help normal to dry skin look and feel very good. However, even better performance would be possible if CeraVe had added antioxidants. Other than that, every other aspect should make your skin very happy.

CETAPHIL (SKIN CARE ONLY)

CETAPHIL AT-A-GLANCE

Strengths: Inexpensive; their original, often-recommended Gentle Skin Cleanser; mostly fragrance-free products; affordable and widely available; offers complete ingredient lists on its Web site.

Weaknesses: Only one sunscreen; no anti-acne products; no state-of-the-art moisturizers.

For more information about Cetaphil, call (817) 961-5000 or visit www.cetaphil.com or www.Beautypedia.com.

☺ **Gentle Skin Cleanser** *($6.99 for 8 ounces)* has remained the same for years, and that's a good thing! This fragrance-free, ultra-gentle cleanser is very good for normal to dry skin that is sensitive or prone to skin conditions such as eczema or psoriasis. The non-lathering, lotion formula rinses well without the aid of a washcloth, and the tiny amount (less than 1%) of sodium lauryl sulfate does not cause dryness or irritation (a question I'm often asked). The only significant drawback of this cleanser is it does not remove makeup very well. However, it has its place as a morning cleanser or for those who use minimal makeup.

☺ **Daily Facial Cleanser for Normal to Oily Skin** *($6.99 for 8 ounces)* is a standard, detergent-based cleanser that can work for most skin types except for dry to very dry skin. It removes makeup nicely, far better than the original Cetaphil Gentle Skin Cleanser, and doesn't irritate the eyes or dry out the skin. It does contain fragrance, which seems a misguided idea for this company.

☹ **Antibacterial Gentle Cleansing Bar** *($3.89 for 4.5 ounces)* is a standard bar cleanser with the antibacterial active ingredient triclosan. Please refer to Chapter Seven, *Cosmetic Ingredient Dictionary*, for details on this ingredient. The limited research on triclosan as a topical disinfectant for acne is dated and wasn't all that impressive; plus, even those scarce studies looked at the effectiveness of triclosan in leave-on products, not in a rinse-off product like this one (Sources: *European Journal of Pharmaceutics and Biopharmaceutics*, November 2003, pages 407–412; and *The British Journal of Clinical Practice*, March 1976, pages 37–39). This bar cleanser contains ingredients that impede rinsing and that won't make breakouts any better. It is not preferred to Cetaphil's water-soluble cleansers.

😐 **Gentle Cleansing Bar** *($3.89 for 4.5 ounces)* is similar to Dove's original Beauty Bar and is a soap-free bar cleanser. It's an OK option for use from the neck down, but the sodium tallowate and sodium palm kernelate may clog pores and exacerbate breakouts.

☺ **Daily Facial Moisturizer SPF 15 with Parsol 1789** *($10.64 for 4 ounces)* is a good, avobenzone-based sunscreen in a standard moisturizing base that is OK for someone with normal to dry skin. The product is fragrance-free; adding antioxidants and a broader array of ingredients that mimic the structure and function of healthy skin would make this good daytime moisturizer superior.

😐 **Moisturizing Lotion** *($5.99 for 8 ounces)* claims to be fragrance-free but it contains farnesol, an ingredient whose chief function is adding fragrance to a product (Source: *International Cosmetic Ingredient Dictionary and Handbook*, 11th edition, 2006, page 864). This is a good, basic moisturizer for normal to dry skin anywhere on the body. It contains mostly water, glycerin, thickeners, nut oil, silicone, vitamin E, preservatives, fragrance, and film-forming agent.

😐 **Moisturizing Cream** *($11.99 for 16 ounces; also available in a 3-ounce tube)* is a thicker version of the Moisturizing Lotion above, although this product really is fragrance-free; it's an excellent choice for dry to very dry skin that is sensitive. The tiny amount of vitamin E is likely inconsequential for skin, and this moisturizer would be rated higher if it contained more antioxidants and a cell-communicating ingredient such as lecithin.

CHANEL

CHANEL AT-A-GLANCE

Strengths: Hmmmm... sleek and occasionally elegant packaging; almost all of the sunscreens contain avobenzone for UVA protection; one very good Age Delay serum; a handful of good cleansers and topical scrubs; two fantastic foundations with sunscreen; some very good concealers; pressed powder with sunscreen; several good mascaras; a sheer lipstick with sunscreen that includes avobenzone; all of the powder eyeshadows have superb textures; some elegant shimmer liquids.

Weaknesses: Expensive, with an emphasis on style over substance; overpriced; overreliance on jar packaging; antioxidants in most products amount to a mere dusting; terrible anti-acne and oily skin products; almost all of the Micro-Solutions products are hardly what the doctor ordered, yet priced to be in line with professionally administered cosmetic corrective treatments; no products to address sun- or hormone-induced skin discolorations; mediocre to poor eye pencils and brow-enhancing options; extremely limited options for eyeshadows if you want a matte finish.

For more information about Chanel, call (800) 550-0005 or visit www.chanel.com or www.Beautypedia.com.

CHANEL Nº 1 SKINCARE PRODUCTS

😐 **$$$ Concentre Nº 1, Skin Recovery Concentrate** *($275 for 14 0.06-ounce vials)* is supposed to increase skin's oxygen consumption as a way to improve the appearance of wrinkles and create a vibrant, healthy look. Did everyone in Chanel's lab overlook the fact that oxygen is a key, if not the main, source of free-radical damage we encounter each day? What about the Oxygen Paradox, which states that oxygen is dangerous to the very life forms for which it has become an essential component of energy production (including human beings)?

The first defense against oxygen toxicity is the sharp reduction in the amount of oxygen present in cells, from the level present in air of 20% to a tissue concentration of only 3% to 4% oxygen. These relatively low oxygen levels in tissue prevent most oxidative damage from ever occurring. Cells, tissues, organs, and organisms have multiple layers of antioxidant defenses, plus damage-replacement and repair systems to cope with the stress and damage that oxygen engenders (Source: *Journal of the International Union of Biochemistry and Molecular Biology*, October–November 2000, pages 279–289). Using a product that adds to the body's oxidative stress load won't do a thing to create younger-looking skin.

However, the good news is that there is nothing in this outrageously expensive product that can increase skin's oxygen consumption. It's a terribly boring concoction of water, glycerin, almond protein, plasticizer, skin-identical ingredients, silicone, plant oil, film-forming agent, and fragrance. The price and the precisely measured vials go a long way toward convincing consumers this is a specialized scientific treatment for aging skin, but the reality is this product, while an OK moisturizer for slightly dry skin, is not worth even a fraction of its price.

☹ **$$$ Creme N° 1, Skin Recovery Cream** *($200 for 1.7 ounces)*. If this is "the world's most luxurious treatment," as claimed, then by comparison a room at Motel 6 should be just as well-appointed as a suite at the Waldorf-Astoria! That's not the case in either situation, and this is merely a standard moisturizer for normal to slightly dry skin, and its meager antioxidant content is diminished by jar packaging. The name is misleading, because in terms of what it takes to create a state-of-the-art moisturizer, this formula wouldn't even crack the top 50.

☹ **$$$ Emulsion N° 1, Skin Recovery Emulsion** *($160 for 1.7* ounces*)* costs a lot of money for what amounts to mostly water, thickeners, glycerin, almond extract, slip agents, more thickeners, anti-irritant, and film-forming agent. The effectiveness of the tiny amount of antioxidants is compromised by this product's translucent glass packaging. Although not worth the price, it's a suitable formula for normal to dry skin.

☹ **$$$ Eye Cream N° 1, Skin Recovery Eye Cream** *($110 for 0.5 ounce)* contains such ordinary ingredients that it's almost shocking that other eye creams don't lay claim to Chanel's assertion that this product creates dramatically younger-looking skin. At best, this slightly emollient eye cream will make dry skin anywhere on the face look and feel better than it would if you used nothing. Lots of products can do this, and Chanel's jar packaging leaves the antioxidants in their formula vulnerable to degradation.

CHANEL PRECISION AGE DELAY PRODUCTS

☺ **$$$ Age Delay Eye, Rejuvenation Eye Gel** *($58.50 for 0.5 ounce)* comes with all sorts of beguiling claims that it can correct, prevent, and rejuvenate eye-area problems such as dark circles, puffiness, and fine lines. According to Chanel, the end result should be a wide-awake, luminous look. According to the ingredient list, this is a good, gel-based moisturizer that contains a sufficient amount of silicone to make the skin feel silky-smooth and also some interesting skin-identical ingredients, but it lacks any significant antioxidants. It will address normal to slightly dry skin, but nothing in this product is capable of lightening dark circles or reducing puffiness. It does showcase tamarind seed polysaccharide as one of its main ingredients. Tamarind doesn't perform well as an antioxidant (Source: *Phytotherapy Research*, March 1999, pages 128–132), but it does work well for wound healing and may be a useful addition to sunscreen because it seems to protect the skin's immune system from sun damage (Sources: *European Journal of Ophthalmology*, January–March 2000, pages 71–76; and *Cutis*, November 2004, pages 24–28). That can be helpful for skin, but no more so than many other ingredients, from vitamin E to copper, and none of that has anything to do with puffy eyes or dark circles.

☹ **$$$ Age Delay Nuit, Time-Fighting Rejuvenation Night Cream** *($65 for 1.7 ounces)* has a silky-smooth texture thanks to silicone, and also includes some good emollients for normal to dry skin. But the price is out of line for what you get, and all told this product is not preferred to any of the better-packaged moisturizers from Olay's Regenerist or Definity lines.

✓☺ **$$$ Age Delay Rejuvenation Serum** *($68.50 for 1 ounce)* promises to help skin achieve its youngest look possible, but how young are we talking? A week? A year? I suspect the consumer gets to decide because the claim is so vague, but it can lead to some intriguing, albeit incorrect, suppositions. This ends up being one of the better formulations from Chanel. The water-, glycerin-, and silicone-based serum contains some good skin-identical ingredients and several antioxidants in stable packaging. The mica and titanium dioxide lend a soft glow finish that those with oily skin may not like. It is otherwise recommended as an excellent serum-type moisturizer, but it will not cause your wrinkles to retreat; what's needed to truly delay the signs of aging is an effective sunscreen.

😐 **$$$ Age Delay Time-Fighting Rejuvenation Lotion SPF 15** *($55 for 1.7 ounces)* contains a tiny amount of apple fruit extract, a cell-communicating ingredient. The manner in which cell-communicating (also known as cell-signaling) ingredients like this work is still theoretical, but in this case the effect is likely improbable since such a tiny amount of the extract is present. Although this has worth as an in-part avobenzone sunscreen for normal to dry skin, it's pricey for what you get and the price may discourage liberal application, a critical element of getting the most benefit from your sunscreen.

CHANEL PRECISION MICRO SOLUTIONS PRODUCTS

😊 **$$$ Micro Solutions Refining Peel Program** *($250 for 0.63 ounce)* is shocking, and not in a good way—at least not if you're at all concerned about spending way more than you need to for an effective skin-care product. In what essentially amounts to a hamburger with Kobe beef pricing, Chanel has produced an 8% glycolic acid serum, packaged in three stacked plastic trays, each containing seven single-use mini-tubes of product. The product's pH of 3.8 does ensure exfoliation, and the water and silicone base feels exceptionally light and silky, but the price is outrageous!

Chanel positions this system as equivalent to a professional AHA peel, "without the drawbacks," but the amount of glycolic acid doesn't even come close to what is used in a professional setting, where AHA concentrations range from 20% to 40% and up. For what Chanel is charging, you could get a professional AHA peel and purchase one of the effective 8% AHA products from Alpha Hydrox, Neutrogena, or Paula's Choice, and end up with better results. Precision Micro Solutions Refining Peel Program deserves a happy face rating because it is an effective exfoliant, but it is absolutely not worth even a fraction of its price. In fact, it's almost insulting that Chanel didn't include other state-of-the-art ingredients in this formula, especially anti-irritants. By the way, Chanel's labeling of this product as "ultra-gentle" isn't accurate for many reasons, primarily due to the effective AHA component, which can be irritating for lots of women, and also because of the unnecessary amount of fragrance.

😊 **$$$ Micro Solutions Refining Peel Program Advanced** *($275 for 0.63 ounce)* is nearly identical to the Micro Solutions Refining Peel Program above, except this slightly more expensive version contains 10% glycolic acid. That will theoretically produce better results, but the tradeoff is increased risk of irritation. This kit will not approximate the results obtainable from a series of doctor-performed AHA peels, but it is a good, albeit exceedingly pricey, AHA product.

☹ **Micro Solutions Wrinkle Filler Program** *($250 for the set)* is made out to be the over-the-counter equivalent of injectable dermal fillers, but winds up (no surprise here!) paling in comparison, and the price is ridiculously inflated. Step 1 of this program involves an "in-depth wrinkle filler" that is supposed to offer "deep down wrinkle filling." Reviewing the formula, I can state with confidence that there is no way the water, thickeners, and talc (the third ingredient) that make up the bulk of this product can have any effect on filling in wrinkles, either in-depth or superficially. This cream does leave a smooth, dry finish on skin, but that won't come close to the results obtained from a collagen or hyaluronic acid injection, or even a better-formulated moisturizer from any number of companies.

Step 2 brings us the "wrinkle-filling treatment," which is to be applied after the cream in Step 1. This product's formula is composed primarily of different forms of silicone. It has the texture of soft spackle, and comes in single-dose packaging (providing three weeks' worth of usage). This is a waste of time and money. Whether applied over Step 1 or not, this silicone cream makes skin temporarily look smoother, and that includes softening the appearance of lines. How long the effect lasts depends on the depth of your lines and on how often you move your face. It's no more an alternative to injectable fillers or Botox treatments than looking at pictures of Hawaii compares to being there. As with all of the Chanel Micro Solutions products, this is labeled as a "dermatologist-based procedure," which is pure fiction; I have no idea what dermatologist would endorse this—and if yours does, it's time to seek a second opinion!

☹ **Micro Solutions Wrinkle Neutralizing Treatment** *($185 for 0.05 ounce)* is a kit that comes with a wrinkle massaging tool and a gel-texture serum that's applied afterward, left on overnight, and rinsed in the morning. I don't quite know how to describe the absurdity of this "treatment," but I'll do my best. Chanel's "tool" (a plastic device with a rubber massaging piece that resembles an inverted "C" similar to Chanel's logo) is supposed to relax expression lines and lift wrinkles before you apply the gel. The kit comes with instructions on how to carefully massage your wrinkles, depending on whether or not they are vertical or horizontal lines, or crow's feet around the eyes. These instructions are meaningless, because nothing about this tool (or massaging wrinkles in any possible way) will relax or change expression lines or prep wrinkles for treatment with the gel. If anything, manipulating or pulling the skin too much will eventually lead to sagging, and that certainly won't make a wrinkle less apparent!

You may be wondering, forgetting the inane massage tool for a moment, if there is something special about this gel. There isn't. It's a water- and alcohol-based liquid that also includes film-forming agents (like those found in hairstyling products), meager amounts of plant extracts, and a tiny amount of two forms of vitamin C. There is enough alcohol that it has a constricting effect on skin, not to mention its irritation potential. This and the tightening effect of the film-forming agents may make wrinkles look less obvious, but the effect is at best fleeting and in the long run problematic to the health of your skin. Like the Micro Solutions Wrinkle Filler Program above, Chanel labels this kit a "dermatologist-based procedure," but no self-respecting dermatologist would offer patients such a baseless, useless treatment under the guise of reducing the appearance of wrinkles.

CHANEL PRECISION PURETE IDEALE PRODUCTS

☹ **Purete Ideale Serum, Intense Refining Skin Complex** *($67.50 for 1 ounce)* gets its matte finish from silicone and alcohol, but the amount of alcohol here, along with witch hazel, makes this water-based serum too drying and irritating for all skin types. Alcohol won't balance oil production because oil production is controlled by hormones, and topically applied products like these have no effect on what's happening hormonally.

☹ **Purete Ideale T-Mat Shine Control** *($35 for 1 ounce)* lists alcohol as the second ingredient, followed by witch hazel. It is too drying and irritating for all skin types and not recommended over superior products such as Clinique Pore Minimizer Instant Perfector ($16.50 for 0.5 ounce).

☹ **Purete Ideale Blemish Control** *($35 for 0.5 ounce)* has enough beeswax and other thickeners to make blemishes worse; the salicylic acid is not present in an amount that's effective, and even if it were the pH of this lotion puts it out of its efficacious range.

CHANEL PRECISION RECTIFIANCE INTENSE PRODUCTS

☹ **Rectifiance Intense Retexturizing Line Correcting Fluid SPF 15** *($72 for 1.7 ounces)* is supposed to contain "a micro-protein complex [that] slows down the deterioration of the Extra-Cellular Matrix, the supporting cushion essential for skin firmness and elasticity." That's a fancy, scientific-sounding way to say that this product prevents the breakdown of collagen and other elements of skin's support structure, such as elastin and fibronectin; however, the minuscule amounts of amino acids, plant extracts, and protein in this fluid aren't up to that task. What is suspect about this product is the third ingredient, alcohol, which is problematic because it can break down skin, not reinforce it.

Chanel should have bragged that it is the in-part avobenzone sunscreen in this product that can benefit the underlying portion of your skin by preventing it from assault by ultraviolet rays from the sun—but it is the rare cosmetic company that brags about their sunscreens. An effective sunscreen with UVA-protecting ingredients can prevent the breakdown of collagen and other elements present in the extracellular matrix. The base formula is primarily water, silicones, and alcohol. All of the intriguing, state-of-the-art ingredients are listed after the preservative, so they are a mere dusting, which won't do your skin much good. Considering the formulary issues and the price, there's no logical reason to select this sunscreen over dozens of better-formulated, less expensive alternatives.

😐 **$$$ Rectifiance Intense Eye, Retexturizing Line Correcting Eye Cream** *($67 for 0.5 ounce)* has a secret: a unique microprotein complex designed to target three types of wrinkles, making telltale signs of aging "a thing of the past." Too bad this secret isn't one worth repeating! This ordinary, silicone-enhanced moisturizer is not capable of taking care of eye-area woes. The really interesting ingredients (including those that serve as a protein source for skin) are listed well after the preservatives, meaning they're barely present. All in all, this is just another average option for normal to dry skin for an above- average amount of money.

☺ **$$$ Rectifiance Intense Nuit, Retexturizing Line Correcting Night Cream** *($82 for 1.7 ounces)* works beautifully to keep dry to very dry skin moisturized and smooth. The jar packaging is inconsequential given the paltry amount of antioxidants in this product, but its blend of silicone, thickeners, nut oil, and proven emollients makes it worth considering if your budget allows (though to be clear, better moisturizers are available that cost much less). This does contain fragrance.

😐 **$$$ Rectifiance Intense Retexturizing Line Correcting Cream SPF 15** *($72 for 1.7 ounces)* makes claims identical to those of the Rectifiance Intense Retexturizing Line Correcting Fluid SPF 15 above, and contains the same in-part avobenzone sunscreen. It comes in a standard, but effective, moisturizing base suitable for normal to dry skin, but if you were hoping your $72 would buy you an appreciable amount of state-of-the-art ingredients, you would be mistaken. A relatively small number of antioxidants and skin-identical ingredients are here, but in amounts too tiny to matter for skin.

😐 **$$$ Rectifiance Intense Serum, Retexturizing Line Corrector** *($90 for 1 ounce)* contains Chanel's typical token amount of intriguing ingredients, and basically relies on fanciful claims to convince women they can "outsmart time" with this silicone-laden serum. Water and several forms of silicone comprise the bulk of the formula, followed by some slip agent and preservative. Silicone isn't a bad ingredient for skin, but it's not an anti-aging miracle and there is no reason to spend this much for it when Olay, Neutrogena, Clinique, Estee Lauder, and Aveeno offer similar but better serums for much less money.

CHANEL PRECISION ULTRA CORRECTION PRODUCTS

☹ **$$$ Ultra Correction Creme, Restructuring Anti-Wrinkle Firming Cream SPF 10** *($85 for 1.7 ounces)* has an SPF rating that falls short of the minimum recommended by the National Cancer Institute and the American Academy of Dermatology, although it does include an in-part avobenzone sunscreen. The base formula falls short, too, offering skin little more than a bland mixture of water, glycerin, plant extract, slip agents, canola oil, and silicone. It is an OK option for normal to slightly dry skin if you're willing to pair it with another sunscreen or foundation with sunscreen rated SPF 15 or greater.

☹ **$$$ Ultra Correction Eye, Restructuring Anti-Wrinkle Firming Eye Cream** *($75 for 0.5 ounce)* is just an emollient, creamy moisturizer that can moisturize dry skin anywhere on the face. An ingredient referred to as Adhesioderm (I am not making this up) is the alleged wrinkle reducer, but it's not listed as one of the ingredients, and there is no other information beyond what Chanel wants you to believe about it. I won't even get into the second part of this product, referred to as the Life Cycle Regenerator! Anyone who knows how to interpret an ingredient list would likely find these "pay no attention to the man behind the curtain" claims far-fetched, but there is no question that consumers are taken in by this, as are Chanel salespeople, who speak of this product so highly you would swear it was a packaged fountain of youth (Ponce de Leon should be pulling up to a counter any minute). This is not a bad product, and it will soften, smooth, and hydrate the skin. But anything beyond that is not within the realm of possibility, despite claims to the contrary. Chanel left the fragrance out of this product, but did add mica, which will add a subtle shimmer to the skin.

☹ **$$$ Ultra Correction Lip, Restructuring Anti-Wrinkle Lip Contour** *($50 for 0.5 ounce)* is said to contain, like the Firming Eye Cream above, the Adhesioderm complex, but Chanel doesn't explain what it is or what it does. Perhaps a surgical-sounding name is necessary when your anti-aging product contains nothing of significance to restore firmness or rejuvenate the lips. This is merely water, plasticizing thickener, talc, wax, silicone, and several thickeners, along with a tiny amount of vitamin E and lesser amounts of soothing plant extracts and antioxidants. At best, this is an overpriced lip balm, but the talc keeps it from being all that moisturizing.

☹ **$$$ Ultra Correction Nuit, Restructuring Anti-Wrinkle Firming Night Cream** *($95 for 1.7 ounces)* encourages you to be firm, look young, and, while you're at it, go ahead and use this product to "correct every sign of age." You're to believe this standard emollient moisturizer has the ability to resculpt and firm skin as you sleep while Chanel's exclusive "Life Cycle Regenerator" attacks wrinkles and restores "the look of youth." It's all fiction (someone on Chanel's marketing team must be a great storyteller), because all this product will do is restore a soft, smooth feel and appearance on normal to dry skin. The amount of vitamin E is next to nothing, so the jar packaging, which is attractive, doesn't really make a difference in this case (form over function is rarely a good idea, especially in skin care).

☹ **$$$ Ultra Correction Restructuring Anti-Wrinkle Firming Lotion SPF 10** *($85 for 1.7 ounces)* does contain an in-part avobenzone sunscreen, but providing the optimum SPF is as crucial for the skin as the UVA-protecting active ingredient, and SPF 10 just doesn't cut it. Apart from the low SPF, this product claims to have ingredients that firm and resculpt the skin "as if surface skin is bonded to its support system." Here's a news flash: Surface skin already is bonded to its support system—the dermis and subcutaneous layer of fat. It is the lower layers of skin (including facial ligaments, muscles, bone, fat, and collagen) that deteriorate with age and years of unprotected sun exposure, and none of those can be affected in any way by this product.

Along with the enticing claims comes Chanel's "unique resculpting massage," which supposedly relaxes facial muscles "contracted by aging." Yet facial muscles do not contract with age, they simply diminish in mass and lose their tension. It is this process, coupled with the fact that the skin continues to grow as the muscles and bone break down and the fat pads break through the lax muscles, that eventually leads to sagging. That can be corrected with plastic surgery, but not by massage of any kind. (If massage could build muscles then bodybuilders could forgo lifting all those heavy weights and just get massages all day long.) The aluminum starch in this product will leave a slight matte finish, and makes this best for normal to slightly dry skin.

☹ **Ultra Correction Serum, Restructuring Lift Complex** *($110 for 1 ounce)* lists alcohol as the second ingredient. That's not only irritating to skin, but, given the price of this product, insulting to consumers. It does not contain a single ingredient capable of firming skin—and definitely not in the paltry amounts Chanel used (as usual, there's more fragrance than anything genuinely intriguing).

😐 **$$$ Ultra Correction Total Eye Revitalizer** *($110 for the set)* comprises a roll-on serum and an eye patch, both designed to lift and firm eye-area skin. The serum is mostly water, glycerin, film-forming agents, and starch; the patches are basically a lightweight, water-based solution with ultra-small amounts of truly state-of-the-art ingredients. Used alone or as a pair, this gimmicky duo won't lift or firm in the least, though the amount of film-forming agent can have a temporary tightening effect. It's up to you to decide if that's worth more than $100, but don't say I didn't warn you.

OTHER CHANEL PRECISION PRODUCTS

😐 **$$$ Systeme Eclat La Mousse, Radiance Cleansing Foam, Rinse Off** *($36 for 5 ounces)* is a cream-textured foaming cleanser whose potassium content makes it a highly alkaline product (akin to standard bar cleansers) that can be too drying for most skin types. Chanel claims this rather standard cleanser can eliminate the effects of indoor and outdoor pollution, but unless they are referring to dirt or the daily accumulation of dead skin cells as the "pollutants," the claim is not justified. And how do you wash off carbon monoxide or smog when they don't stick to the skin? The answer is, you can't. Furthermore, the plant ingredient that can supposedly rid skin of pollutants (*Moringa pterygosperma* seed extract) is present in such a tiny amount (listed after the fragrance and preservatives) that its effect, if any, on the skin would barely register.

😐 **$$$ Systeme Hydration La Creme, Nourishing Cleansing Gel-Cream Rinse Off** *($36 for 5 ounces)* is a water- and silicone-based cleansing liquid that contains enough alcohol to make it problematic for use around the eyes. This product does not contain a cleansing agent. Instead it relies on silicones and plant oils to dissolve makeup, which does work—but why subject your skin to the alcohol and the intense fragrance of this product when Neutrogena, Almay, and my line, Paula's Choice, all make excellent, inexpensive, silicone-based makeup removers that work so much better?

☺ **$$$ Systeme Hydration Le Lait, Nourishing Cleansing Milk Face and Eyes** *($36 for 5 ounces)* is such a standard oil-in-water cleanser that the price is truly embarrassing. Although this is a good option for dry to very dry skin and removes makeup proficiently, I'd select any of the cleansing lotions from Pond's or Neutrogena before this one.

😐 **$$$ Systeme Purete La Mousse, Purifying Deep-Cleansing Foam, Rinse Off** *($36 for 5 ounces)* is a standard foaming cleanser that contains alkaline potassium stearate and potassium laurate as the main detergent cleansing agents, and they can be fairly drying, even for someone with oily skin. The deep-cleansing benefit refers to the polyethylene beads (plastic beads), which are a standard ingredient of many scrub products. All in all, this is a commonplace scrub with cleansing agents that may prove harsh for some skin types. Watch out for the potent fragrance.

☺ **$$$ Systeme Purete Le Gel, Purifying Cleansing Gel, Rinse Off** *($36 for 5 ounces)* is a very good, though very overpriced, water-soluble cleanser for all but very dry skin. The mushroom extract may seem exotic, but it's a superfluous ingredient in a cleanser because it is rinsed from skin before it can have any benefit, and its benefit is overhyped anyway, so either way it is extraneous and not worth its showcase position.

☺ **$$$ Demaquillant Yeux Intense, Gentle Biphase Eye Makeup Remover** *($28.50 for 3.4 ounces)* is a standard, but good, water- and silicone-based makeup remover. It makes short work of long-wearing makeup, including waterproof mascara, but so do similar removers from Neutrogena, Almay, Maybelline New York, and my line, Paula's Choice.

☺ **$$$ Gommage Microperle Eclat, Extra Radiance Exfoliating Gel** *($40 for 2.5 ounces)* is a minimally abrasive, fairly gentle topical scrub whose oil content makes it preferred for dry to very dry skin. The exfoliating agent is pearl powder, but that in and of itself has no special benefit for skin compared with other scrub ingredients. What a shame to grind up pearls for this effect when a washcloth would have the same benefit.

☺ **$$$ Gommage Microperle Hydration, Gentle Polishing Gel** *($40 for 2.5 ounces)* is similar to the Gommage Microperle Eclat, Extra Radiance Exfoliating Gel above, minus the prevalence of oil and some thickeners. It is preferred for normal to oily skin but still contains enough plant oil to be potentially problematic for blemish-prone skin.

☺ **$$$ Gommage Microperle Purete, Deep Purifying Exfoliating Mousse** *($40 for 2.5 ounces)* contains polyethylene beads as the abrasive agent, making it a more traditional exfoliating gel than those above. The oil content makes this best for normal to dry skin, and helps keep the witch hazel from causing irritation.

☹ **Activateur Eclat, Energizing Radiance Lotion** *($36 for 6.8 ounces)* lists alcohol as the second ingredient, and is otherwise a very boring, exceedingly overpriced toner that isn't worth consideration.

☹ **Activateur Hydration, Gentle Hydrating Lotion** *($36 for 6.8 ounces)* doesn't treat skin gently due to its alcohol content; without that, this would have been an interesting toner for normal to dry skin.

☹ **Activateur Purete, Oil-Controlling Purifying Lotion** *($36 for 6.8 ounces)* lists alcohol as the second ingredient, which makes this too drying and irritating for all skin types. What a shame, because there are some very good skin-identical ingredients and a cell-communicating ingredient in this toner.

☺ **$$$ Lotion Tendre, Soothing Toner** *($36 for 6.8 ounces)* is far and away Chanel's best toner. It contains a dry skin–friendly mix of water, aloe, water-binding and soothing agents, plant oil, and slip agents. Being Chanel, this also contains an extreme amount of fragrance and coloring agents. Because a brightly colored product is so important for good skin care?—NOT!

☹ **Eclat Originel, Maximum Radiance Cream** *($55 for 1.7 ounces)* lists alcohol as the second ingredient, and at that level it is one of the last things you want to apply to skin if your goal is to boost radiance. Looking past the water-and-alcohol base reveals a lightweight moisturizer that contains several worthy ingredients for skin, including silicones, shea butter, glycerin, and good skin-identical ingredients. However, they won't be as effective in a product that lists alcohol before them, and as such this moisturizer is not recommended. A superior, less-expensive option is Clinique's Advanced Stop Signs ($38.50 for 1.7 ounces).

☹ **$$$ Eclat Originel, Radiance Revealing Serum** *($67.50 for 1 ounce)* shortchanges skin of antioxidants and ends up being a basic, water-based serum with a gel-like texture and silicones for a silky finish. It contains a tiny amount of vitamin E and negligible amounts of other intriguing ingredients, making it a so-so option for normal to slightly oily skin.

☹ **$$$ Hydramax+, Moisture Boost Cream** *($55 for 1.7 ounces)* continues Chanel's tradition of offering beautifully packaged moisturizers that are long on claims that the formulas cannot live up to. This is a decent moisturizer for normal to dry skin, but vitamin E is the only significant antioxidant and elegant skin-identical ingredients are absent, so you're not getting your money's worth. The few intriguing ingredients are listed well after the preservatives and fragrance, making them inconsequential.

☹ **$$$ Hydramax+, Serum Intense Moisture Boost** *($68.50 for 1 ounce)*, according to Chanel, features a "powerful formula" that "performs at the source of dehydration," but somehow the ad copy didn't mention that this product contains a high amount of alcohol (it's the third ingredient). When alcohol is listed before such skin-identical ingredients as glycerin and sodium PCA, it means your dry skin won't get the moisture boost it deserves. Also, as with the Hydramax+, Moisture Boost Cream above, the unique, potentially beneficial ingredients are barely present, making this an expensive investment that guarantees relatively meager returns for skin. This product does contain a strong, lingering fragrance.

☹ **$$$ Lift Serum Extreme, Anti-Wrinkle Firming Complex** *($120 for 1.7 ounces)* is a cornerstone product of Chanel skin care and is recommended for use with almost all of their other serums and moisturizers. If the collagen and elastin in this product were so great for preventing wrinkles, why aren't they present in any of Chanel's other products? Collagen and elastin are basically just good water-binding agents when applied topically; they don't add in any way to the collagen and elastin in your skin. The amount of antioxidants is about the same as in most Chanel products, which is to say not much. Fragrance is more prominent than soothing and other beneficial ingredients, and that's not exactly money well spent.

☹ **$$$ Sublimage Essential Regenerating Cream** *($350 for 1.7 ounces)* is one of those products that causes me to throw up my hands and say "I give up!" We are asked to believe that the vanilla plant in Madagascar (where most of the world's vanilla comes from), coupled with Chanel's exclusive "polyfractioning" technique (polyfractioning isn't a word found in any dictionary—rather it is a term coined by Chanel), is the key to restoring firm, radiant, youthful skin. According to Chanel, polyfractioning is a new process that isolates the active ingredients from a plant, paring down millions of molecules to just a handful. Even if that were true, the concept of obtaining the active component from a plant is hardly new, and it's definitely not unique to Chanel.

Considering its price, this product contains a minuscule amount of vanilla oil (there's more fragrance and preservative in it than there is of the supposedly wrinkle-fighting ingredient). All in all, this ends up being just a very emollient moisturizer for dry to very dry skin. It contains several ingredients that make dry skin feel smoother and softer, but so do hundreds of other moisturizers that wouldn't dare charge this much. The air-sensitive ingredients in this product (antioxidants and the vanilla) will become almost instantly useless once you open it, thanks to the unwise choice of jar packaging. Putting your faith and dollars in this product won't bring you any closer to a wrinkle-free face—and personally I'd rather devote these funds to new shoes or a night at the theater or an investment toward my face-lift.

😐 **$$$ Sublimage Eye, Essential Regenerating Eye Cream** *($160 for 0.5 ounce)* doesn't carry the same sticker shock as the Sublimage Essential Regenerating Cream above, but is still outrageously priced for what amounts to a standard emollient moisturizer for dry skin anywhere on the face. It contains mostly water, glycerin, emollient thickening agents, canola oil, film-forming agent, wax, more film-forming agent, a cell-communicating ingredient, silicone, preservatives, and a tiny amount of vanilla oil and antioxidants (which are rendered ineffective due to jar packaging). You don't have to spend even one-third this much to get a good moisturizer, and in this case, unless you believe the claims, why would you?

☹ **Soleil Identite, Perfect Colour Face Self-Tanner SPF 8** *($38.50 for 1.7 ounces)* not only has a woefully low SPF rating, but also lacks the UVA-protecting ingredients of titanium dioxide, zinc oxide, avobenzone, Tinosorb, or Mexoryl SX, and is not recommended. Yes, this is a self-tanner, but the sunscreen means you're meant to apply it before venturing outdoors. Using this as your sole source of sun protection puts skin at risk for UVA damage and all that comes with it.

☺ **$$$ Soleil Identite, Perfect Colour Body Self-Tanner** *($45 for 5 ounces)* contains the same ingredient (dihydroxyacetone) found in most self-tanners. This has a lightweight lotion texture and tiny amounts of lily extract, which has no established benefit for skin but does add fragrance. Two shades are available: Bronze is darker and contains more dihydroxyacetone; Golden has less and is preferred for fair to light skin. Either shade may be applied to the face, too.

😐 **$$$ Eye Patch Total** *($67.50 for 1 set)* is a set of adhesive patches cut to fit the contours of the eye area. The formula is mostly water, glycerin, and several acrylate-based film-forming agents, which, in this amount, can have a temporary tightening effect on skin but also may prove irritating.

😐 **$$$ Eye Tonic Dark Circle Corrector** *($50 for 0.33 ounce)* cannot remedy dark circles, despite its name and price. This is nothing more than a moisturizer, and not a very impressive one at that. The presence of silicone and several film-forming agents can help make the eye area appear smoother, but not a single ingredient in this product can lighten dark circles, and the many antioxidants are present in such tiny amounts they're inconsequential. Chanel claims that "the intensity of dark circles is optically minimized by light-reflecting pigments." This product does contain mica (for shine) and titanium dioxide (for its highlighting effect), but that is the definition of a concealer, not a skin-care product. Using a slightly creamy concealer (some of the best are from M.A.C., Revlon, and Prescriptives) will lighten the under-eye area while leaving a natural finish, and all at a significant savings when compared to this ill-conceived product.

☹ **Masque Destressant Eclat, Anti-Fatigue Gel Mask** *($45 for 1.7 ounces)* lists alcohol as the second ingredient, which isn't exactly a "luxurious time-out for tired, lackluster skin." If anything, this gel mask will cause dryness and irritation while providing minimal benefit.

😐 **$$$ Masque Destressant Hydratation, Nourishing Cream-Gel Mask** *($45 for 1.7 ounces)* is said to imbue skin with a sense of serenity, but serenity is a state of mind, not something skin can experience, so the claim is silly. There are some great-for-dry-skin ingredients in this mask, but many of them are listed after the alcohol (and at least the amount of alcohol is not cause for concern). It's an OK mask but vastly overpriced for what you get.

☺ **$$$ Masque Destressant Purete, Purifying Cream Mask** *($45 for 2.5 ounces)* uses all manner of beguiling adjectives to make it sound like more than it is, which is a basic clay mask for normal to oily skin (those with very oily skin would want something more absorbent). The thickening agents (including beeswax) may be problematic for blemish-prone skin, but this does the job in terms of absorbing surface oils without overdrying the skin.

CHANEL MAKEUP

FOUNDATION: ✓☺ $$$ Double Perfection Fluide Matte Reflecting Makeup SPF 15 *($42.50)* has an amazing silky, light texture that blends incredibly well over the skin, but it dries quickly to a solid matte finish that will enhance any dry, flaky skin you already have, so it must be applied over smooth skin. The silicone-in-water emulsion and the in-part titanium dioxide–based sunscreen make this excellent for those with normal to oily skin who should ideally use as few products on the face as possible. Coverage is light to medium, and despite the foundation's matte finish it does not look or feel thick or heavy on the skin, and it has good staying power. There are nine mostly gorgeous shades, with nary an overtone of peach, pink, rose, or ash, although Natural Beige falls short due to its ashy pink tone. The colors offer options for light to dark (but not very dark) skin.

✓☺ $$$ Vitalumiere Satin Smoothing Creme Compact SPF 15 *($55)* is sold as being "exceptionally creamy," and that's an accurate description for this rich, compact-type foundation. Complete with a titanium dioxide sunscreen, this is an excellent foundation for dry to very dry skin that needs only sheer to light coverage. It moisturizes without feeling thick or greasy and leaves skin with a radiant finish that, if you truly have dry skin, needn't be set with powder. All but two of the nine shades are attractive options for fair to medium skin tones. Avoid Cool Beige (slightly peach) and Natural Beige (slightly pink) unless you will be applying this so minimally that an off shade is irrelevant. Just keep in mind that sheer application of a sunscreen means you will not be getting a reliable amount of sun protection. One last point: Contrary to claim, and as worthy as this foundation is, don't expect it to erase the look of wrinkles. Its non-powdery finish won't magnify them, but the most you can expect is a slightly softened appearance.

㊀ $$$ Pro Lumiere Professional Finish Makeup SPF 15 *($50)* has a strange name because nothing about this foundation makes it more "professional" than the others in Chanel's collection. If anything, this falls short due to its lack of sufficient UVA protection. It does have a smooth, fluid texture that applies creamy and sets to a soft satin finish providing medium to full coverage. Blending isn't difficult but, because this foundation doesn't set that quickly, it is more time-consuming than some others. Best for normal to dry skin, Pro Lumiere Professional Finish Makeup SPF 15 comes in 11 shades, with no options for dark skin tones. Most of the shades are quite good, but avoid Cool Beige and Natural Beige (both are too pink) and be wary of Caramel, which has a tendency to turn peach.

㊀ $$$ Teint Innocence Naturally Luminous Foundation SPF 12 *($42.50)* has an SPF rating that's below the benchmark for daytime protection, and lacks the UVA-protecting ingredients of titanium dioxide, zinc oxide, avobenzone, Tinosorb, or Mexoryl SX. That's a letdown, because this foundation has a beautiful silky texture that blends flawlessly to a soft matte finish suitable for normal to oily skin. It provides light to almost medium coverage, and layering doesn't net significantly more camouflage. The 13 shades present better options for fair to light skin tones than for dark skin tones, though the darkest shades are recommended. The following shades are slightly pink or peach and should be considered carefully: Naturel 4.5, Soft Bisque 2.5, and Soft Honey 7.0. Avoid Natural Beige 3.5; it is noticeably pink.

㊀ $$$ Teint Naturel Liquid Makeup SPF 8 *($57.50)* is now Chanel's oldest foundation, and I understand why it's still around: it has a beautifully smooth, creamy texture that blends exceptionally well and leaves a satin finish that gives a natural (meaning not sparkly) glow to skin. Capable of light to medium coverage and best for normal to dry skin, it is available in eight shades, of which two (Warm Beige and Natural Beige) are noticeably rose-toned. The bad news is that the woefully low SPF 8 lacks UVA protection and, if this is worn alone, will leave skin vulnerable to sun damage.

😐 **$$$ Double Perfection Compact Matte Reflecting Powder Makeup SPF 10** *($48.50)* has merit as a silky-feeling, easy-to-blend, talc-based pressed-powder foundation. Its sunscreen is pure titanium dioxide, but why Chanel stopped at SPF 10 is a frustrating mystery. The ultralight, non-powdery finish puts skin in its most polished light, but be aware that any dry spots will be magnified with this type of makeup. Ideal for normal to very oily skin, it comes in 12 superb shades for fair to dark (but not very dark) skin. If you opt to use this product as an adjunct to a foundation with sunscreen or regular sunscreen rated SPF 15 or higher, it earns a happy face rating.

😐 **$$$ Vitalumiere Satin Smoothing Fluid Makeup SPF 15** *($52)* had almost everything going for it, but Chanel inexplicably didn't include UVA-protecting ingredients. The liquid texture is irresistibly smooth, and blends with ease to a light to medium coverage satin finish. But using words like "vibrant" and "young" to describe this is disingenuous considering the incomplete sunscreen (and Chanel knows better because many of their sunscreens do include UVA-protecting ingredients). Still, for those with normal to dry skin willing to pair this with a good sunscreen, the 11 colors present some impressive options. The only shades to avoid due to rose or peach tones are Soft Bisque, Cool Bisque, Natural Beige, and Tawny Beige.

CONCEALER: ✓😊 $$$ Quick Cover *($35)* has a surprisingly light, silky texture and offers even, medium coverage with a smooth matte finish. It achieves an ideal balance, providing necessary camouflage without calling attention to what you're trying to hide. All three shades are workable, including Roselight, which does not go on as pink as it looks. One caution: This concealer's finish is not attractive over dry, flaky areas, so be sure to remedy that before application.

😊 **$$$ Pro Lumiere Correcteur** *($38)* has a texture that Chanel refers to as "velvety-smooth," and that's correct. This liquid concealer is housed in a pen-style container with a built-in synthetic brush applicator. It blends very well, with just enough slip, and sets to a satin matte finish that provides moderate but natural-looking coverage. The finish presents a small risk of creasing into lines around the eyes, but this is much less apparent if you set it with a loose or pressed powder. All five shades are recommended, and best for fair to tan skin tones. Overall, this is a good compromise if you think true matte-finish concealers are too dry and creamy concealers are too emollient.

😊 **$$$ Vitalumiere Satin Smoothing Creme Concealer** *($40)* has a lush, creamy texture and is presented in packaging that looks elegant on your vanity. A true cream concealer, it has sufficient slip and is easy to blend, while also providing substantial coverage that builds well without caking. The moist finish lends itself to creasing unless blended very well and set with powder, which is this concealer's only drawback (well, that and the steep price). All three shades are beautiful, though they only cover fair to barely medium skin tones.

☹ **Estompe de Chanel Corrective Concealer** *($30)* is a creamy, lipstick-style concealer with light coverage and poor colors that can easily crease into lines around the eye. Trying to achieve additional coverage creates a heavy, caked appearance and you have to wonder, after all these years, who is still buying such an inferior concealer?

POWDER: ✓😊 $$$ Natural Finish Loose Powder *($47.50)* has an extremely fine, sifted texture and a soft matte finish that looks beautiful on skin. It is talc-based and comes in three very good, sheer colors. Do you need to spend this much money for a superior loose powder? No, but if you're swayed by Chanel, this won't disappoint.

✓☺ **$$$ Purete Mat Shine Control Powder SPF 15** *($42.50)* is a smooth-as-silk pressed powder that helps absorb excess oil, doesn't look cakey or thick on skin, and includes an in-part titanium dioxide sunscreen for enhanced sun protection. Chanel has crafted a wonderfully light-textured, talc-based pressed powder with broad-spectrum sunscreen, and three of the four available shades are outstanding. The darkest shade, Warm Rose, is OK, but may be too peach for some medium skin tones. Each shade has a very slight shine that does not detract from this powder's best qualities. This is highly recommended for normal to oily skin, but only if your budget allows for such a splurge.

☺ **$$$ Natural Finish Pressed Powder** *($42.50)* has a finely milled texture and a sheer, dry finish. This talc-based powder comes in only two shades, suitable for fair to light skin, but they're both good.

☺ **$$$ Silky Bronzing Powder** *($46)* is pressed to appear quilted in its oversized compact, and comes complete with a decent brush to sweep this sparkle-laced bronzer over cheeks. The smooth texture allows for even application, and the two shades are believable, assuming your skin naturally sparkles as it tans!

😐 **$$$ Poudre Douce Soft Pressed Powder** *($50)* is a silky, slightly dry-textured, talc-based powder that imparts sheer color and a soft shine finish. Only two shades are available, but the color deposit is so minimal that it makes them versatile for fair to medium skin tones, assuming you don't mind the shiny finish. The included compact-sized brush is better than most, but that doesn't completely justify the price of this powder.

BLUSH: ☺ **$$$ Powder Blush** *($39.50)* goes on very smoothly without being dusty or flyaway, and has a dry finish. The selection of shades favors shine, with the sole almost-matte option being Cedar Rose. The rest of the surprisingly understated palette (brown-based shades outnumber the pastels and brights) would look better without the shiny finish, but if that's your preference these pigmented shades build well and really last.

😐 **$$$ Silky Cheek Color** *($40)* costs a bit more than Chanel's Powder Blush, and it isn't nearly as nice. The sheer, shine-infused colors are pretty but are pressed so tightly it is difficult to pick up much product on your blush brush. That means application is incredibly sheer and it takes a lot of effort to build visible color. For the money, there are dozens of sheer powder blushes whose application is quick and seamless by comparison.

EYESHADOW: ☺ **$$$ Ombre Essentielle Soft Touch Eyeshadow** *($26.50)* consists of single eyeshadows packaged lavishly in the typical Chanel style, complete with their logo embossed on the powder shadow. The formula is accurately described as a creamy-feeling powder, and it applies beautifully—though this is best applied in sheer layers to avoid flaking. You'll find these are pigment-rich, blend smoothly, and their intensity lasts through the day. The matte shades are few and far between (with Beige being the closest to true matte), but if shiny eyeshadows are what you want and the price doesn't faze you, this is highly recommended based on its application and longevity. Avoid the green-tinged Bambou, and Amethyst (which is too purple) unless you're wearing eyeshadow for shock value. ☺ **$$$ Quadra Eyeshadow** *($55)* has been the backbone of Chanel's eyeshadow collection for years, and they have maintained its enviably silky, utterly blendable texture and wonderfully even application. It is a pleasure to work with these shadows, but working with the colors is another story! In most of these quads, three of the four shades are intensely shiny. Either that, or the selected shades are too contrasting to create an attractive, enhancing eye design. The best neutral quad is Les Divines Matte (which isn't matte, but nearly so). The Fascination, Spices, Influences, and Dreams quads have stronger but workable colors. Without such intense shine, these would easily merit a Paula's Pick rating. For an equally impressive texture and application with less obvious shine, consider Dior's 5-Colour Eyeshadow ($49.50). ☺ **$$$ Silky Eyeshadow Duo** *($38.50)* has a beautifully smooth application with slightly softer colors than what you'll find in Chanel's quad and single eyeshadows. Shine is a fact of life with Chanel shadows, but at least they paired some good colors, including Matte-Velvet, Brun-Express, and Desert Rose.

😐 **$$$ Fluid Iridescent Eyeshadow** *($30)* really is a fluid eyeshadow that comes in a small glass bottle. The bi-phase formula must be shaken before use (the pigments settle to the bottom of the bottle), but it applies surprisingly easily and evenly. You have only a few seconds to blend this shadow correctly because the formula dries fast and, once dry, stays put—no smudging, flaking, or smearing. It really is an innovative formula and a fun new way to experiment with eyeshadow, but the colors! Only Sand and Source resemble shades that you could use to shape and shadow the eye. The other colors are so bright or pastel they would look out of place as part of a sophisticated eye design. Every shade is intensely shiny, so use these sparingly for evening makeup and avoid them altogether if you have any amount of wrinkling or crepey skin in the eye area.

😐 **$$$ Professional Eye Shadow Base** *($30)* is essentially a cream-to-powder concealer for the eyelids, sold with the claim that it prolongs eyeshadow wear while also brightening eyes. Eye Shadow Base is packaged in a click pen with a brush applicator, and comes in two shades, a fleshy peach tone and the shiny Lumiere Bright. This product does blend well and sets to a matte (in feel) finish, but so do many other concealers, most of which cost less than this.

EYE AND BROW SHAPER: ☺ **$$$ Long-Lasting Eyeliner Waterproof** *($26.50)* is indeed waterproof. In fact, this automatic, retractable pencil puts on eyeliner that is nearly budge-proof; it takes considerable effort to remove. However, it applies easily and it lasts, its creamy texture and finish belie its longevity, and it is best for creating a moderately thick rather than thin line. Avoid the various green, blue, and purple shades unless you're going for shock value.

😐 **$$$ Precision Eye Definer** *($27.50)* is a very expensive, utterly standard pencil that has a soft texture, a slightly dry finish, and an angled sponge tip for blending. Nothing is extraordinary here except the price, and it isn't justified by the performance.

😐 **$$$ Intense Eye Pencil** *($26)* is a standard pencil that's about as intense as reading the funny pages on Sunday morning. The pencil's creamy texture has a soft powder finish and the colors are quite soft, meaning you need several applications before you get what most consider an intense line. 😐 **$$$ Automatic Liquid Eyeliner** *($30)* is packaged in a click-pen applicator and has a decent, flexible brush. Problems arise when too much liquid liner is dispensed (which happens fairly often), so you wind up wasting a lot of product. It applies a bit too wet, so don't blink or it will smear, though dry time remains fast. Once set, this wears well but you have to be OK with the fact that each shade has a shiny finish. Given the price and the difficult-to-avoid dispensing of excess product, this is one to consider with caution. 😐 **$$$ Precision Brow Definer** *($27.50)* is a needs-sharpening pencil that has a texture and application that's a step above most brow pencils, and it includes a brush to comb through brows. This goes on softly, has a dry, smooth finish, and would have been rated a Paula's Pick if sharpening weren't required. If you decide to try this, the Taupe shade is great for blondes (but not platinum or very light blonde brows), while Auburn is suitable for redheads.

😐 **$$$ Professional Brow Duo** *($35)* comes in a compact and features complementary shades of a brow wax and brow powder. Also included are a mini angled brow brush and a mini toothbrush-style brush. It's a thoughtful set, but the wax tends to feel thick and slightly sticky and the pressed powder is a bit too sheer, but still workable. Inexplicably, the brow powder has shine. This set is an improvement over Chanel's previous all-in-one brow sets, but still doesn't compare to filling in brows with a full-size brush and soft matte powder eyeshadow or a tinted brow gel.

☹ **Aqua Crayon Eye Colour Stick** *($23.50)* is Chanel's only automatic eye pencil, but since it isn't retractable, winding up more than you need becomes an issue. The tip remains dull and rounded, making it impossible to draw a thin line. Yet it's the creamy, fleeting texture that is the main reason to skip this pencil altogether. ☹ **Brow Shaper** *($30)* is a brow gel with a very small color selection: Taupe and Clear. There are no shades for brunettes, light blondes, or redheads, and even though it does keep brows in place, it also tends to glob onto the hairs and flake once it's dried. Origins' Just Browsing *($12)* is a far superior option.

LIPSTICK, LIP GLOSS, AND LIPLINER: ✓☺ $$$ Aqualumiere Sheer Colour Lipshine SPF 15 *($24.50)* is one of a handful of lipsticks whose sunscreen offers adequate UVA protection. This features an in-part avobenzone sunscreen in a silky, weightless, but still creamy-feeling lipstick. All of the colors are gorgeous, though none are all that sheer. For a medium-coverage lipstick with an effective sunscreen, this wins high marks. If only the price weren't so "Chanel." Watch out for the shades with large glitter particles, as these tend to feel grainy as the lipstick wears off. However, to maintain sun protection, you should be reapplying it often anyway, especially if you are spending more than a couple of hours outdoors.

☺ **$$$ Rouge Allure Luminous Satin Lip Color** *($30)* promises alluring color and sensational comfort, and it does deliver—but so do many other creamy lipsticks that cost much less than this one. The semi-opaque, shimmer-infused shades slip over lips and feel comfortably light, but the slight amount of stain doesn't promote longevity, so frequent touch-ups are necessary. As usual, Chanel's shade range is an enticing blend of traditional and fashion-forward hues, so you won't be disappointed there. However, I'd think twice about spending this much on lipstick. Chanel made a considerable price leap here for no reason other than status.

☺ **$$$ Rouge Hydrabase Creme Lipstick** *($24.50)* has an excellent creamy, slightly greasy texture and a splendid variety of opaque colors. This traditional cream lipstick is not worth the price when compared with less-expensive options. But do women buy Chanel for performance or for the image it evokes?

☺ **$$$ Rouge Double Intensite Ultra Wear Lip Colour** *($30)* is poised as Chanel's answer to the question some women must be asking: "Max Factor's Lipfinity and Cover Girl's Outlast work really well, but isn't there a similar product that costs a lot more?" Mirroring the same concept introduced by the aforementioned products (i.e., a lip color that dries to a matte, unmovable finish, accompanied by a clear gloss that doesn't disturb the color to create a comfortable finish), Rouge Double Intensite Ultra Wear Lip Colour is a formidable option for those looking for long-wearing lip color. The shade selection is smaller than those of competing brands, but each shade is quite attractive, with colors that are complimentary to light and dark skin tones (the dark shades are very dark, so test them before purchasing). It does wear well throughout the day (and night), but as with similar products, it requires regular reapplication of the glossy top coat to keep lips from feeling dry and chapped.

☺ **$$$ Aqua Crayon Lip Colour Stick** *($23.50)* is an automatic, nonretractable lip pencil that applies well and has good pigmentation to ensure long wear. It's not as creamy as it used to be, and so is a better (though needlessly pricey) option than it once was.

☹ **$$$ Precision Lip Definer** *($27.50)* needs sharpening, and despite some versatile colors that are sure to please this doesn't distinguish itself from many other pencils that cost less. The built-in brush is a nice touch, but not enough to justify the expense.

☹ **$$$ Glossimer** *($25)* has a sumptuous name and a bevy of sparkling colors, but that does little to make this very standard, thick, and sticky gloss a top contender. Glossimer just isn't as nice as many newer glosses in all price ranges.

MASCARA: ✓☺ $$$ Inimitable Waterproof Mascara *($27)* impresses in every respect, which it should at this price! The rubber-bristled, spiky-looking brush quickly thickens and lengthens lashes for outstanding definition without clumps. It wears without flaking or smearing, and is very waterproof (you will need an oil- or silicone-based remover when it's time to take this off). **✓☺ $$$ Sculpte Cils Sculpting Mascara Extreme Length Fine Lashes** *($25)* has a thin brush with short, dense bristles. It's brilliant at making lashes extra long without a clump in sight, and the brush allows you to easily reach every lash for even application. This isn't much for thickness, but makes no such claims. Meanwhile, Chanel's "longest possible lashes" claim turns out to be true, at least to the lengthening limits of mascara!

☺ **$$$ Cils `A Cils Lash Building Mascara** *($25)* doesn't quite make it to Paula's Pick status, but it is still a very good lengthening and thickening mascara. It offers a clean, defining application, but it takes some effort to really show what it can do.

☺ **$$$ Inimitable Mascara Multi-Dimensionnel** *($26.50)* is the mascara that Jennifer Aniston allegedly loved so much that she had a case flown in from Paris before the official U.S. launch. Perhaps Aniston hasn't experimented with some of the superior mascaras at the drugstore, because although this is an impressive product its pre-release hype was a bit overblown. You'll achieve length and thickness in nearly equal measures, but neither is extraordinary and there are some clumps along the way (which can be brushed through without incident). This wears all day without a flake or smear, and keeps lashes remarkably soft and with a slight curl. Note: Based on the brush style and rubber bristles, you should know that similar results are obtainable from Cover Girl's Lash Exact Mascara ($6.99). ☺ **$$$ Mascara Base Beaute Lash Enhancing Base** *($24)* is one of the few pre-mascara lash primers that makes a noticeable difference. The formula differs from most mascaras, and it applies smoothly without making lashes look too coated. Applying mascara afterward allows for slightly enhanced definition and more length. I'd argue that you can get even better results by using a superior mascara, but for those who like the idea of primers, this is a good one to consider.

☹ **$$$ Cils Magiques Instant Lash Mascara** *($25)* doesn't provide instant lashes—it takes considerable effort to build moderate length and uneven thickness, plus the formula tends to clump along the way. For the money, most of Lancome's mascaras (and those from less-expensive Maybelline New York and L'Oreal) work better. ☹ **$$$ Extracils Super Curl Lengthening Mascara** *($25)*. They have to be joking with the "super" part of the name, but it isn't too funny considering the price of this below-average mascara. You will achieve some length and lashes will be cleanly separated, but curl is practically nonexistent, as is thickness. Chanel (and many other lines) have done better with their other mascaras.

FACE AND BODY ILLUMINATING/SHIMMER PRODUCTS: ✓☺ $$$ Sheer Brilliance *($42)* is a generous (for Chanel) sized bottle of liquid shimmer that can be used anywhere, though it's recommended for the face, with or without foundation. It imparts a subtle shine that makes skin look luminous rather than laced with sparkles, and remains one of the top liquid shimmer products around. **✓☺ $$$ Bronze Universel de Chanel Sun Illuminator** *($42.50)* is a gorgeous cream-to-powder bronzer housed in a large glass jar. It comes in one color—medium golden tan—and it meshes well with the skin, leaving a sheer, semi-matte finish and a healthy glow.

☺ **$$$ Blanc Universel de Chanel Sheer Illuminator** *($42.50)* is a thick, silicone-based primer meant to smooth skin texture and (minimally) fill in large pores. It does not leave a white cast on skin but does leave a very soft shimmer. Its matte (in feel) finish can, to some extent, help control excess oil. It will make your foundation go on smoother, but so will many lightweight, silicone-based moisturizers or serums, which makes this product an option, but not an essential.

BRUSHES: Chanel does its namesake proud with an attractive, satiny, and competitively priced collection of brushes *($25–$48.50)*. Many of them are very useful, with excellent shapes and sizes. The ☺ **$$$ #6 Powder Brush** *($48.50)* is the most expensive and is quite nice, but it could benefit from a more tapered head. ☺ **$$$ #8 Touch-Up Brush** *($32)* is wonderfully soft and dense, but without a handle (you hold onto a short, stubby base) it can be awkward to use, so try this at the counter if you're curious. Those fond of applying foundation with a brush should check out the excellent ✓☺ **$$$ #16 Foundation Brush** *($38)* because it is well-shaped and not as thick as many others, making it a little easier to get into tiny spaces. The synthetic ✓☺ **$$$ #11 Quick Shadow Brush** *($28)* is also commendable. 😐 **$$$ #10 Contour Face Brush** *($40)* applies a wider swatch of color than is needed for contouring, which sort of defeats the purpose of that step. 😐 **$$$ #12 Contour Shadow Brush** *($26)* is too floppy for more than a very soft wash of color, which won't do much to shape or shade the eye's contour.

Avoid the ☹ **#4 Shadow/Liner Brush** *($26)*, which is not only overpriced, but also poorly shaped for its intended purposes. I'd also avoid the ☹ **#9 Eyelash/Brow Definer Brush** *($25)* due to its metal lash comb and stiff, scratchy brow brush.

SPECIALTY PRODUCTS: ☺ **$$$ Base Lumiere Illuminating Makeup Base** *($38.50)* works to promote smooth skin and leaves a silky feel that isn't the least bit heavy. Sold as a foundation primer, it does facilitate application of makeup, but so do many other lightweight, silicone-based gels and serums. So, while the effect is nice, you don't necessarily need another step in your routine to achieve results. ☺ **$$$ Tinted Bronzing Gel** *($40)* turns out not to have the texture of a gel. Rather, it's an opaque lotion that feels very light and imparts sheer, peachy bronze color with a soft shimmer finish. The formula blends very well and leaves a bit of a glow that's perfectly suitable for daytime. The sole shade is best for fair to almost medium skin tones.

CLARINS

CLARINS AT-A-GLANCE

Strengths: Broad selection of effective, broad-spectrum sunscreens; excellent range of self-tanning products; some good cleansers and gentle topical scrubs; The makeup has improved considerably; superb foundations and powders; very good powder blush; an ideal brow pencil; wonderfully creamy lipsticks; great lipliner and mascaras.

Weaknesses: Overpriced; pervasive reliance on jar packaging; most products have more fragrance than beneficial plant extracts; poor toners; an overabundance of average moisturizers; no effective products for lightening discolorations or treating acne; no AHA or BHA products; the Anti-Pollution complex cannot protect skin as claimed; disappointing eye pencils; average eyeshadows and makeup brushes.

For more information about Clarins, call (866) 252-7467 or visit www.clarins.com or visit www.Beautypedia.com. Note: All Clarins products contain fragrance.

CLARINS SKIN CARE

CLARINS ADVANCED EXTRA-FIRMING & EXTRA-FIRMING PRODUCTS

☹ **$$$ Advanced Extra-Firming Eye Contour Cream** *($54 for 0.7 ounce)* is an extension of Clarins' previously released "extra firming" products, but this version is an "advanced" formula accompanied by a higher price tag, most likely due to the claim that it is specially designed for the eye area. If this is Clarins' idea of an advanced formula, then I assume their chemists are still using textbooks dating back at least a decade or two. Far from being a "revolutionary night-time treatment," this water-based moisturizer has a temporary tightening effect on skin, thanks to the amount of absorbent rice starch it contains and a significant amount of film-forming agent. (Neither of these ingredients is beneficial or helpful for dry skin.) The truly beneficial ingredients are few and far between, including tiny amounts of the plant extracts Clarins always boasts about, but that isn't unique to this product. For an absurd amount of money, you're getting mostly water, thickener, glycerin, rice starch, slip agent, film-forming agent, preservatives, and vitamin E. Not very exciting, and in no way should this be considered a state-of-the-art anti-aging moisturizer for the eyes or elsewhere.

☹ **$$$ Advanced Extra-Firming Eye Contour Serum** *($54 for 0.7 ounce)* makes the same claims and has the same non-advanced formulary issues as the Advanced Extra-Firming Eye Contour Cream reviewed above, except this has a serum texture and omits the rice starch. It still has enough film-forming agent to produce a temporary tightening effect on skin, and the silica lends a drier finish, but this type of effect can eventually make the eye area look dry and more wrinkled. This product does not contain anything that can lift or regenerate skin.

☺ **$$$ Advanced Extra-Firming Neck Cream** *($75 for 1.7 ounces)* claims to be the ultimate firming neck treatment, but that's about as true as saying Ivory soap is the ultimate cleanser. This product contains mostly water, silicone, thickeners, slip agent, preservative, and fragrance. None of it is firming, but it will make dry skin look and feel smoother. That's probably not what you were expecting for $75, but it's the truth.

☹ **$$$ Advanced Extra-Firming Day Lotion SPF 15, for All Skin Types** *($75 for 1.7 ounces)* doesn't disappoint with its in-part avobenzone sunscreen and silky, lightweight lotion base. However, for the money, this supplies skin with almost no extras beyond basic sun protection, and any firming benefit would have to be accidental, because none of the ingredients in this daytime moisturizer have that effect. It is best for normal to slightly oily or slightly dry skin.

☺ **$$$ Extra-Firming Concentrate** *($60 for 1 ounce)* is a water- and aloe-based serum that contains some interesting antioxidants, but none of them will promote extra-firm skin. Some of the plant extracts have astringent properties on skin, which can cause irritation with consistent use; others look exotic on the label, but their effectiveness is rooted in anecdotal rather than scientific evidence. I wouldn't call this "high performance age control," but it's an OK lightweight moisturizer for normal to slightly dry skin.

☺ **$$$ Extra-Firming Day Cream, for All Skin Types** *($70 for 1.7 ounces)* is a very boring, exceedingly overpriced concoction of water, emollients, glycerin, slip agents, aluminum starch, preservative, and fragrance. The amount of plant extracts (none of which have a firming effect) and peptide is so small as to be nearly inconsequential for skin. This is too emollient for all skin types; it is best for normal to dry skin not prone to breakouts.

😐 **$$$ Extra-Firming Day Cream, for Dry Skin** *($70 for 1.7 ounces)* is a more emollient version of the Extra-Firming Day Cream, for All Skin Types above, and as such is preferred for dry to very dry skin. That preference doesn't change the fact that this is an overall mundane formula with an undeserved price.

☺ **$$$ Extra-Firming Day Lotion SPF 15** *($72 for 1.7 ounces)* ends up being one of the better daytime moisturizers from Clarins thanks to its in-part titanium dioxide sunscreen and more interesting mix of lightweight emollients, silicones, and soothing plant extracts. This won't firm skin in any noticeable way, but is a good option for those with normal to slightly oily skin.

☺ **$$$ Extra-Firming Eye Contour Cream** *($52.50 for 0.7 ounce)* has more of a lotion than cream texture, but it contains some intriguing skin-identical ingredients, antioxidant soy, and emollient peanut oil. Antioxidants are present but in very limited supply, making this a not-quite state-of-the-art option for slightly dry skin anywhere on the face. The product contains fragrance in the form of orange fruit extract.

😐 **$$$ Extra-Firming Eye Contour Serum** *($52.50 for 0.7 ounce)* is a lighter, serum version of the Extra-Firming Eye Contour Cream above, but the amount of fragrant *Rosa gallica* flower extract and pineapple can be a problem for use around the eyes.

😐 **$$$ Extra-Firming Night Cream, for All Skin Types** *($80 for 1.7 ounces)* is the help Clarins maintains skin over age 40 needs (if you're 38 or 39 you'll have to stay away), and purports to lift, firm, and tighten skin each night. The formula is similar to, but more boring than, that of the Extra-Firming Day Cream, for All Skin Types above, and absolutely not worth the price. Any facial moisturizer from Nivea is better than this, and Nivea isn't all that great! This product is heavily fragranced.

😐 **$$$ Extra-Firming Night Cream, for Dry Skin** *($80 for 1.7 ounces)* contains a smattering of plants, but is primarily a water- and mineral oil–based moisturizer joined by several thickeners, glycerin, shea butter, and peanut oil. It will take good care of dry to very dry skin, but it won't make it firmer. It's interesting that although some Clarins products contain mineral oil, I have dealt with several salespeople from this line who love to speak of the alleged evils of this ingredient, ignoring (or oblivious to) the fact that Clarins uses it. Just to be clear, mineral oil is not harmful or suffocating to skin in the least and it doesn't deserve its reputation as a problematic ingredient.

😐 **$$$ Extra-Firming Facial Mask** *($44 for 2.7 ounces)* is sold to reinforce the benefits of the other Extra-Firming products, but is similar enough that using it will only do what the others products accomplish, which is the basic task of making skin softer and smoother. This is an OK mask for dry to very dry skin not prone to breakouts; it would be rated higher if it contained less fragrance and added some soothing ingredients.

😐 **$$$ Extra-Firming Age Control Lip & Contour Care** *($33 for 0.7 ounce)* is a lightweight lotion that contains mostly water, film-forming agent, silicone, glycerin, emollient, and more silicones. The peptide and plant extracts are barely present, and although this can provide moisture and a temporary smooth appearance to lips and the surrounding area, it won't firm them.

CLARINS BRIGHT PLUS CARE PRODUCTS

☺ **$$$ Bright Plus Brightening Cleansing Mousse** *($26 for 5.1 ounces)* cannot reduce the appearance of darks spots any more than drinking coffee will make teeth whiter. This is an overpriced but effective water-soluble cleanser that contains mostly water, several detergent cleansing agents, and lather agent. It is best for normal to oily skin.

☺ **$$$ Bright Plus Gentle Brightening Exfoliator** *($30 for 1.7 ounces)* has the properties of a cleanser, topical scrub, and clay mask all in one product, with the clay and its absorbency being the dominant quality. This is an interesting option for someone with normal to oily skin, but is best used in the morning because this much clay isn't going to help remove makeup. Nothing in this product will reduce the appearance or occurrence of dark spots.

☹ **Bright Plus HP Protective Brightening Day Lotion SPF 20** *($55 for 1.7 ounces)* promises radiant, matte skin all day long, but the amount of alcohol in this daytime moisturizer with an in-part avobenzone sunscreen is irritating. Further, the amount of soothing plant extracts is minimal while fragrance wafts, and none of this is helpful for skin or worth the expense.

😐 **$$$ Bright Plus HP Repairing Brightening Night Cream** *($58 for 1.7 ounces)* is a good moisturizer for normal to dry skin but does not contain a single ingredient that will work to fade sun-induced skin discolorations. It contains mostly water, emollient, glycerin, silicone, thickeners, antioxidant (vitamin C), slip agent, several more thickeners, preservatives, fragrance, film-forming agent, and plant extracts (none of which have any skin-lightening or brightening ability). This mundane, pricey formulation is a dim light for day or night, though the vitamin C will be preserved thanks to airless jar packaging.

😐 **$$$ Bright Plus HP Firming Brightening Serum** *($62 for 1.06 ounce)* is a lighter, less emollient version of the Bright Plus HP Repairing Brightening Night Cream above, and although it cannot fade a freckle or reduce the appearance of discolorations, it is an OK, ordinary moisturizer for normal to slightly dry or slightly oily skin.

☹ **Bright Plus HP On-The-Spot Brightening Corrector** *($31 for 0.34 ounce)* lists alcohol as the second ingredient, and that makes this product too irritating and drying for all skin types. In addition, none of the ingredients can fade sun or age spots, and the pH of the product is too high for the tiny amount of salicylic acid it contains to function as an exfoliant.

😐 **$$$ Bright Plus Intensive Age Control Brightening Program** *($145 for the 6 bottle kit)* is billed as an intensive, two-step system to use whenever your skin needs a boost because it appears dull. Step 1 is the **Brightening Concentrate** *(3 0.2-ounce bottles)*, whose formula isn't too far removed from the Bright Plus HP Repairing Brightening Night Cream above. It's a blend of water, emollient, silicone, glycerin, thickeners, vitamin C, slip agents, more thickeners, and preservative, along with token amounts of plant extracts, none of which are capable of lifting, firming, or brightening skin. Step 2 is the **Age-Control Concentrate** *(3 0.2-ounce bottles)*, but the only control this has over skin is the ability to make it feel temporarily tighter because of the amount of film-forming agent and the starch it contains. It's otherwise nothing special, and the forms of vitamin C present don't have research to support their alleged ability to lighten discolorations. This pricey program is essentially a moisturizer coupled with a serum-textured product, and together they exert minimal effects on skin beyond a slightly smoother appearance and temporary tight feel.

CLARINS LINE PREVENTION MULTI-ACTIVE PRODUCTS

😐 **$$$ Line Prevention Multi-Active Day Cream, for All Skin Types** *($63 for 1.7 ounces)* is supposed to "regulate daily stresses responsible for premature aging," but without sunscreen, that claim is as reliable as a snowstorm in Miami! This is yet another mundane moisturizer from Clarins whose formula follows their pattern of standard thickeners and emollients followed by fragrance and tiny amounts of several plant extracts (some beneficial, some problematic, and some with unknown or unproven properties). The helpful plant ingredients (antioxidants) are compromised by jar packaging, making this a lesser consideration and assuredly not one to choose if your concern is forestalling wrinkles.

☺ **$$$ Line Prevention Multi-Active Day Cream, for Dry Skin** *($63 for 1.7 ounces)* is an inappropriate choice for daytime unless you're willing to pair this standard moisturizer with an effective sunscreen. Calling this daytime product "Line Prevention" and not including a sunscreen is sort of like calling chocolate cake a diet food. This is a moisturizer you can easily pass up in favor of products with better formulations, though it has some benefit for normal to dry skin.

☺ **$$$ Line Prevention Multi-Active Day Cream-Gel, for All Skin Types** *($63 for 1.7 ounces)* is also an inappropriate option for daytime use unless you pair it with an effective sunscreen. This is a light-textured moisturizer that is an OK option for normal to slightly dry skin. Most of the plant extracts that Clarins plays up are listed after the preservatives, so they don't count for much. One of the main plant extracts (*Pinus lambertiana*) may have skin-sensitizing properties (Source: *Botanical Dermatology Database*, http://bodd.cf.ac.uk/index.html).

☺ **$$$ Line Prevention Multi-Active Day Lotion SPF 15** *($63 for 1.7 ounces)* has a price that is insulting when you consider that the only significant thing this moisturizer has going for it is an in-part avobenzone sunscreen. If no one else was using this UVA sunscreen in their products, Clarins would have a unique product on their hands—but that's not the case. If anything, Line Prevention Multi-Active Day Lotion SPF 15 is mundane and ordinary. And because this is Clarins, there are lots of plant extracts thrown in for show that are not very effective for skin care. What seems to be a priority is the fragrance. Aside from that, there are plenty of sunscreens available at the drugstore with far more in the way of state-of-the-art ingredients, and that cost much less, too.

☺ **$$$ Line Prevention Multi-Active Night Lotion** *($70 for 1.7 ounces)*. Clarins claims that using this will help avoid the appearance of first lines, but without a sunscreen that's a dubious claim. This lackluster formula consists primarily of water, film-forming agent, silicones, and fragrance. This has considerably more fragrance than most of the other ingredients, but no effective skin-identical ingredients or antioxidants. There is no reason to consider this moisturizer over the far more elegant options available from Estee Lauder, Clinique, or Chanel, to name just a few.

☺ **$$$ Line Prevention Multi-Active Night Cream** *($70 for 1.7 ounces)* is a better formulation than the Line Prevention Multi-Active Night Lotion above, and the fragrance is less prominent on the ingredient list. This is an OK moisturizer for normal to dry skin, but lacks any state-of-the-art ingredients that would help justify the price. It almost goes without saying that this product is not able to forestall the appearance of first lines, nor can it offer protection against free-radical damage, since it lacks significant antioxidants.

☹ **Line Prevention Multi-Active Serum** *($68 for 1 ounce)* lists drying, irritating alcohol as the second ingredient, while claiming to keep skin looking younger longer. How insulting, and to top that off there isn't a significant amount of a single interesting ingredient in this serum. Any of the serum options from Olay, Neutrogena, or Aveeno beat this one hands down.

CLARINS SUPER RESTORATIVE PRODUCTS

☺ **$$$ Super Restorative Day Cream** *($92 for 1.7 ounces)* is another fairly standard moisturizer from Clarins with the usual assortment of wow-factor claims, including smoothing wrinkles, helping skin feel "lifted," and restoring a youthful appearance. If you have dry, dehydrated skin, any moisturizer can make skin look younger and feel smoother, so where are the state-of-the-art ingredients to justify the hefty expense? There are barely enough to mention. To make matters worse, Super Restorative Day Cream isn't the best choice for daytime because it lacks a sunscreen, and there is no recommendation on the label to make sure you use sunscreen in addition to this product. It contains mostly water, emollient, glycerin, thickeners, silicone, slip agent, plant oil, fragrance, pH adjuster, plant extracts, film-forming agent, mica (for shine), several more plant extracts, vitamins, and preservatives. Given such a rather ordinary emollient moisturizer, your money is best saved for some other splurge.

☹ **$$$ Super Restorative Day Cream SPF 20** *($92 for 1.7 ounces)* has an in-part titanium dioxide sunscreen, but that's the only positive element of this vastly overpriced, overhyped moisturizer. Nothing about it is a restorative treatment for aging skin, and some of the fragrance components can be a problem on skin that's exposed to sunlight.

☹ **$$$ Super Restorative Night Wear** *($102 for 1.7 ounces)* is nearly identical in emollient feel and performance to the Super Restorative Day Cream above, and the same basic comments apply. There is no logical reason to charge $10 more for this product than for the Day Cream, but this would still be illogically priced even if it cost only $20. The various types (and tiny amounts) of algae it contains cannot promote a brighter, more even-toned complexion. Actually, all of the played-up plant extracts—and a few antioxidants too—are listed after the fragrance, so they don't add up to much of anything, and the jar packaging will reduce what little potency may be present.

☹ **$$$ Super Restorative Serum** *($118 for 1 ounce)* is one of Clarins' most expensive skin-care products, but this is also a classic case of a product's name, price, and marketing agenda not adding up to what's inside the bottle, which, for all intents and purposes, is just another moisturizer. The Clarins sales staff would no doubt blanch at that statement, as most of the counter personnel I spoke to treated this product as if it were the fountain of youth, yet they clearly must be entranced by their company's assertions, because nothing in this product can firm, lift, restore, or tone the skin. This product contains mostly water, slip agents, thickeners, emollient, silicone, film-forming agent, water-binding agent, fragrance (lots of fragrance), several plant extracts (all present in minute amounts), caffeine, preservatives, and coloring agents. Clarins tends to favor exotic-sounding plants over state-of-the-art skin-care ingredients such as antioxidants or anti-irritants. Obviously, although that is undeniably enticing to some consumers, it doesn't help skin and it often causes undue irritation. There is no reason to consider this product an anti-aging treatment option. If you're shopping for moisturizers at the department store and want a selection of modern, elegant formulas, your skin and pocketbook would be better off exploring the options from Estee Lauder, Chanel, or Clinique before just about anything Clarins offers.

☹ **$$$ Super Restorative Total Eye Concentrate** *($68 for 0.53 ounce)* promises to banish all manner of under-eye skin complaints, from puffiness to crow's feet. Yet all it can do is moisturize the skin, and at most temporarily reduce the appearance of wrinkles. Although this isn't what I would consider a cutting-edge formula, it will make skin look smoother and feel softer. It contains mostly water, silicone, glycerin, thickeners, emollient, preservative, plant extracts, and the tiniest amount of peptides you're likely to find in a skin-care product. Nothing in this eye cream will protect skin from pollution, a claim Clarins is fond of making for many of their moisturizers and specialty items.

OTHER CLARINS PRODUCTS

☹ **Cleansing Milk with Alpine Herbs, for Dry or Normal Skin** *($26 for 7 ounces)* is a basic cleansing lotion that rinses decently but contains some problematic plant extracts, including arnica, St. John's wort, and Melissa (balm mint), along with fragrance components that are irritating for skin, including eugenol and linalool. This is not recommended for any skin type.

☹ **Cleansing Milk with Gentian, for Combination/Oily Skin** *($26 for 7 ounces)* contains a lot of sage extract, way too much fragrance, and lesser but still potentially problematic amounts of fragrance components, including eugenol. This is not recommended because even without the irritants it is way too emollient for its intended skin type.

😐 **$$$ Extra-Comfort Cleansing Cream, for Dry or Sensitized Skin** *($39 for 7 ounces)* is a rich, cold cream–style cleanser for dry to very dry skin. It is not recommended for sensitized skin due to its fragrance and the presence of fragrance components. This requires use of a washcloth for complete removal.

☺ **$$$ Gentle Foaming Cleanser, for All Skin Types** *($25.50 for 4.4 ounces)* is one of Clarins' most popular products and remains a good, foaming, water-soluble cleanser for all but very dry skin. The amount of plant oils may be a problem for blemish-prone skin, but overall this is well-formulated and doesn't contain irritating fragrance components.

☺ **$$$ Gentle Foaming Cleanser, for Dry or Sensitive Skin** *($25.50 for 4.4 ounces)* has more detergent cleansing agents than the original Gentle Foaming Cleanser for All Skin Types, above, and its overall formula, while not bad, is not the best for its intended skin types. It is best for normal to oily skin not prone to blemishes.

☹ **One-Step Facial Cleanser** *($30 for 6.8 ounces)* lacks cleansing agents and is sort of a modified silicone-based makeup remover. The amount of orange-fruit water makes this ill-advised for use around the eyes, and several of the fragrance components will prove irritating because this product is not intended to be rinsed from skin.

☹ **Purifying Cleansing Gel** *($25.50 for 4.4 ounces)* lists witch hazel as its second ingredient, which makes this water-soluble cleanser too irritating for all skin types. The wintergreen extract doesn't help, either.

☺ **$$$ Water Comfort One-Step Cleanser, for Normal to Dry Skin** *($26 for 6.8 ounces)* is a water- and solvent-based cleanser that contains gentle cleansing agents and, aside from fragrance, no problematic ingredients. That's a positive step since this product is meant to be a convenient cleanser that does not require rinsing. It is an option for normal to slightly dry skin, but is not adept at removing long-wearing or waterproof makeup.

☹ **Water Purify One-Step Cleanser, for Combination or Oily Skin** *($26 for 6.8 ounces)* is a cleanser that doesn't require rinsing, but contains peppermint extract, which may feel refreshing but winds up irritating skin unless you rinse thoroughly, which isn't the point of this otherwise gentle cleanser.

😐 **$$$ Gentle Eye Make-Up Remover Lotion** *($23.50 for 4.2 ounces)* is an exceptionally standard water-based makeup remover that contains a lot of fragrant rose water along with soothing cornflower water. The rose water isn't the best for use around the eyes, making this not preferred to less costly options that omit fragrant additives.

☺ **$$$ Instant Eye Make-Up Remover** *($23.50 for 4.2 ounces)* is a standard, silicone-in-water, dual-phase fluid that works very well to remove stubborn makeup and waterproof mascara. The rose flower water is primarily fragrance, and doesn't make this preferred to less-expensive silicone-based removers from Almay or Neutrogena, among others.

☺ **$$$ Gentle Exfoliating Refiner** *($27 for 1.7 ounces)* is a good, basic creamy scrub that contains cellulose as the abrasive agent. That is indeed gentle and makes this a good, though pricey, scrub for normal to dry skin.

☺ **$$$ One-Step Gentle Exfoliating Cleanser** *($31 for 4.4 ounces)* is a standard, but good, water-soluble cleanser that contains gentle detergent cleansing agents. Plant cellulose provides a mild exfoliating effect, and is fine for occasional use by all skin types—just use caution and avoid massaging this over blemishes. Clarins claims this cleanser purifies and smooths the skin with natural botanicals, but their presence is sparse and mainly provides an orange-tinged fragrance. Actually, the ratio of synthetic to natural ingredients in this product is 5:1, which pretty much nullifies any credibility for the botanical claim.

😐 **$$$ Extra-Comfort Toning Lotion, for Very Dry or Sensitized Skin** *($26 for 6.8 ounces)* is a fairly basic toner but it does contain some decent ingredients for dry skin. The problem is that the really beneficial ingredients are listed after the preservative and the fragrant ingredients, so there's little chance this will be what sensitized skin needs.

☹ **Purifying Toning Lotion** *($23 for 6.8 ounces)* lists witch hazel as the second ingredient and also contains plenty of iris root (orris) extract, which can cause severe irritation on contact with skin.

☹ **Toning Lotion, for Combination or Oily Skin** *($23 for 6.8 ounces)* lists witch hazel as the second ingredient and contains a lesser but still worrisome amount of iris root extract.

😐 **$$$ Toning Lotion, for Dry or Normal Skin** *($23 for 6.8 ounces)* is an OK toner for normal to dry skin, but does not distinguish itself from several less-expensive options. It contains some good skin-identical ingredients, but leaving the fragrance components on the skin after daily use isn't the best idea.

😐 **$$$ Aromatic Plant Day Cream** *($42.50 for 1.7 ounces)* has aromatic qualities, as do most Clarins products, but that doesn't translate into superior skin care. This emollient, oil-rich moisturizer would be better for dry to very dry skin without the inclusion of potentially problematic plants, but the amounts used are unlikely to be an issue. Still, it's sad to see them take precedence over the antioxidants in this stably packaged moisturizer.

😐 **$$$ Beauty Flash Balm** *($40 for 1.7 ounces)* is an extremely average moisturizer that contains absorbent rice starch, which can be problematic for dry skin.

☹ **Contouring Facial Lift** *($62 for 1.7 ounces)* lists alcohol as the second ingredient, and that makes this serum too irritating for all skin types. Nothing in this product will minimize signs of slackened skin.

😐 **$$$ Double Serum Generation 6** *($90 for 0.5 ounce of each product)* is a dual-phase product that Clarins sells as "the complete answer to age-control." It certainly isn't complete—what about sunscreen, something that's key to anti-aging and not present in this serum? And what about the dozens of other products Clarins sells, all claming a subtle variation on that theme? Reading the ingredient list for both the **Hydro Serum** and **Lipo Serum**, neither one has any wow-factor ingredients. In fact, both contain mostly common ingredients that show up in hundreds of other moisturizers (and some serums), including other options from Clarins.

The Hydro (referring to water) serum is mostly water, glycerin, starch, slip agents, preservative, and film-forming agent. Plant extracts and a peptide are barely present, certainly not in an amount your skin will derive great benefit from.

The Lipo (lipid, as in fat) portion adds dry-finish solvents, oils, vitamin-based antioxidants, and emollients to the mix, along with a lot of fragrance, making it the more interesting of the two, but still not enough to warrant the investment. Of course, they're dispensed as one and applied to skin, so you're getting a mix of beneficial, questionable, and very fragrant ingredients. How this is the answer to age control is anyone's guess, but it's an OK moisturizing serum for dry skin—just keep it away from the eye area due to the potent fragrance.

⊜ **$$$ Energizing Morning Cream** *($56 for 1.7 ounces)* has a very long ingredient list, parts of which read like a trip through your grocer's produce department. Tiny amounts of pineapple, kiwi, and orange won't energize skin, and this remains another ho-hum, jar-packaged moisturizer that's a poor choice for daytime unless you're willing to pair it with a sunscreen or a foundation with sunscreen. The formula is suitable for normal to dry skin.

⊜ **$$$ Eye Contour Balm, for All Skin Types** *($45 for 0.7 ounce)* is an exceedingly ordinary moisturizer that would be OK for dry skin. However, it lacks any state-of-the-art ingredients for skin, and a couple of the fragrance components can be irritating for use around the eyes.

⊜ **$$$ Eye Contour Balm, Special for Dry Skin** *($45 for 0.7 ounce)* contains mostly water, mineral oil, thickeners, water-binding agent, silicone, plant oils, antioxidants, mica (adds shine), and preservatives. This is a good moisturizer for dry skin but it isn't special, although it is preferred to the All Skin Types version above.

⊜ **$$$ Eye Contour Gel** *($45 for 0.7 ounce)* is primarily water, slip agent, and the pH-adjusting and emulsifying ingredient triethanolamine. It is fragrance-free, but other than feeling refreshing due to its gel texture it has minimal benefit for skin around the eyes.

⊜ **$$$ Eye Re Vive Beauty Flash** *($43 for 0.7 ounce)* is supposed to be an emergency treatment to relieve dark circles, puffiness, and fine lines around the eyes. It's a basic moisturizer with a standard combination of mostly water, thickener, slip agents, glycerin, antioxidant olive leaf, emollient, film-forming agent, and preservative. It will take care of dry skin around the eyes, but calling this a "one-of-a-kind treatment" is akin to thinking tap water is a rare beverage.

☹ **Face Treatment Oil, Blue Orchid, for Dehydrated Skin** *($44 for 1.4 ounces)* contains a lot of irritating patchouli oil as well as irritating rosewood oil and several volatile fragrance components, making this about as good for dehydrated skin as massaging it with sandpaper!

☹ **Face Treatment Oil, Lotus, for Combination Skin** *($44 for 1.4 ounces)* contains rosemary, geranium, and clary oils, all of which are irritating to skin and do not provide a soothing or rebalancing benefit for combination skin. This oil-based product cannot tighten pores; if anything, this much oil can lead to clogged pores, which will enlarge their appearance.

☹ **Face Treatment Oil, Santal, for Dry or Extra Dry Skin** *($44 for 1.4 ounces)* contains a lot of sandalwood and lavender oils, along with more fragrance and problematic fragrance components. This is akin to applying perfume to your face and is not recommended.

☺ **$$$ Gentle Day Cream, for Sensitive Skin** *($55 for 1.7 ounces)* isn't more gentle than most Clarins moisturizers and the fact that it contains fragrance shows they're not taking the needs of truly sensitive skin seriously. Still, this can be a good moisturizer for normal to dry skin not prone to blemishes, and most of the plant extracts are soothing and anti-inflammatory, which is a nice change of pace.

⊜ **$$$ Gentle Day Lotion, for Sensitive Skin** *($55 for 1.7 ounces)* is similar to the Gentle Day Cream, for Sensitive Skin above, but less emollient. Fragrance components such as linalool, geraniol, and hexyl cinnamal are a potential problem for all skin types, and worth avoiding entirely if your skin is sensitive.

☺ **$$$ Gentle Night Cream, for Sensitive Skin** *($65 for 1.7 ounces)* is nearly identical to the Gentle Day Cream, for Sensitive Skin above, and its higher price isn't justified. Either option is best for normal to dry skin not prone to blemishes.

☹ **$$$ Hydra-Matte Lotion, for Combination Skin** *($38 for 1.7 ounces) is* a replacement for Clarins' former Hydra-Matte Day Lotion, and although it's not a really impressive moisturizer it's an improvement over its predecessor. This glycerin-enriched fluid does not contain skin-repairing ingredients, at least not any that can't be found in hundreds of other moisturizers. Fragrance and preservatives are listed before all of the plant extracts (some of which are soothing) and antioxidants, so the latter don't count for much.

☺ **$$$ Hydration-Plus Moisture Lotion** *($42.50 for 1.7 ounces)* is a well-formulated moisturizer for normal to slightly oily skin. It contains some good soothing ingredients and several skin-identical ingredients, although most of the antioxidants are listed after the fragrance. The mica and titanium dioxide add a radiant finish to skin.

☹ **$$$ Hydration-Plus Moisture Lotion SPF 15** *($42.50 for 1.7 ounces)* has an in-part titanium dioxide sunscreen, but is otherwise a much less interesting version of the Hydration-Plus Moisture Lotion above. There's more mica, preservative, and fragrance than beneficial substances for skin, and that doesn't justify the price.

☺ **$$$ Instant Shine Control Gel** *($22.50 for 0.7 ounce)* is a blend of silicones along with a silicone polymer and absorbent silica, plus fragrance. It creates a silky-smooth matte finish but isn't as absorbent as the mattifying products from Clinique's less expensive Pore Minimizer collection.

☹ **Moisture Quenching Hydra-Care Cream** *($55 for 1.7 ounces)* contains a significant amount of *Pinus lambertiana* wood extract, a pine extract that can have skin-sensitizing properties (Source: *Botanical Dermatology Database*, http://bodd.cf.ac.uk/index.html). It also contains the irritating fragrance component eugenol.

☹ **Moisture Quenching Hydra-Care Lotion** *($55 for 1.7 ounces)* has the same drawbacks as the Moisture Quenching Hydra-Care Cream above, and the same review applies.

☹ **$$$ Moisture Quenching Hydra-Care Lotion SPF 15** *($55 for 1.7 ounces)* contains much less of the offending pine extract noted in the two Moisture Quenching products above and has an in-part avobenzone sunscreen. However, the base formula is very ordinary for the money, and all of the unique beneficial ingredients are present at amounts too small for skin to notice.

☹ **Normalizing Night Gel, for Oily or Combination Skin** *($35 for 1.06 ounces)* is supposed to purify oily skin overnight, but instead contains several ingredients that cause irritation, while the truly helpful ingredients are barely present.

☹ **Pore Minimizing Serum** *($45 for 1 ounce)* leaves skin with a soft matte finish, but the amount of alcohol here means this isn't the best for any skin type. None of the plant extracts in this serum have any effect on pores. Even if they did, the amount of each is minuscule when compared with the amount of fragrance. Clinique's Pore Minimizer products are much better than this.

☺ **$$$ Renew-Plus Night Lotion** *($60 for 1.7 ounces)* is said to contain a retinol precursor activated by plant extracts, but retinyl palmitate is not the precursor to retinol, nor can it be activated by plants to become retinol; even if it could, they'd be moving in the wrong direction, since retinol and retinyl palmitate require special enzymes in skin to convert them to all trans retinoic acid. Even if this was a slam-dunk process, there's barely any vitamin A in this moisturizer. It is a decent formulation for normal to dry skin and contains some helpful plant oils and a couple of good antioxidants.

☹ **Skin Beauty Repair Concentrate for Sensitive Skin** *($57 for 0.5 ounce)* is an emollient fluid that contains irritating lavender and marjoram oils. Talk about adding fuel to the fire! Topically applied lavender oil can cause skin cell death (Source: *Cell Proliferation,* June 2004, pages 221–229).

☺ **$$$ Thirst Quenching Hydra-Care Serum** *($55 for 1 ounce)* is a lightweight serum with slight hydrating ability for normal to slightly dry skin. It contains more fragrance than intriguing ingredients, and the many fragrance components listed toward the end of the ingredient list may prove sensitizing for some. This is not the ideal drink for thirsty skin.

☹ **Ultra-Matte Day Concentrate** *($35 for 1.06 ounces)* contains significant amounts of irritating ingredients, including witch hazel, iris, and wintergreen. The silica helps to keep skin matte, but that ingredient is present in other (less expensive) products that don't irritate skin while absorbing excess oil.

☹ **Ultra-Matte Rebalancing Lotion, for Oily Skin** *($38 for 1.7 ounces)* lists alcohol as the second ingredient, which means this won't rebalance anything. This "lotion" also contains a significant amount of fragrance; the most helpful ingredient, green tea, is listed last.

☺ **$$$ UV Plus Protective Day Screen SPF 40** *($37 for 1 ounce)* contains titanium dioxide as its sole active ingredient and it's blended in a silky silicone base with absorbent ingredients that make it suitable for oily skin. The vitamin E and green tea are barely present (and incapable of blocking pollution as claimed), which is disappointing, but this is an option if you want a matte-finish daytime moisturizer that provides minimal hydration.

☹ **Aromatic Plant Purifying Mask** *($29.50 for 1.7 ounces)* has been around for years and remains an odd mix of water, talc, mineral oil, thickeners, and clay. The absorbency of the clay and talc are hindered by the oil, making this a mask that's too rich for normal to oily skin yet too absorbent for dry skin. There is far more fragrance in this mask than plant extracts, and none of those are a purifying experience for skin.

☹ **Blemish Control** *($19 for 0.5 ounce)* lists alcohol as the second ingredient, followed by irritating witch hazel and lesser amounts of problematic plant extracts. The salicylic acid is an afterthought, and the pH of this product prevents it from working as an exfoliant.

☹ **Expertise 3P** *($40 for 3.5 ounces)* contains mostly water, rosemary water, slip agent, salt, water-binding agent from bacteria, detergent cleansing agent, plant extracts, gum-based thickener, pH-adjusting agent, preservative, and more slip agents. Can any of these ingredients protect skin from the "accelerated aging effects of all indoor and outdoor pollution," especially electromagnetic waves? Not in the least. Such logic is on par with thinking that a steady diet of cheese pizza will fulfill all of your nutritional needs. Clarins is heralding this product as a worldwide first, and it is—though that doesn't mean it's an innovative, must-have product whose time has come. Rather, it just has an eccentric, something-else-to-be-afraid-of marketing angle.

Electromagnetic radiation (low- or high-frequency electrical currents, also called electromagnetic fields [EMF]) has been around since the birth of the universe; light is its most familiar form. Electromagnetic radiation includes radiation from magnets, the sun, cell phones, X-rays, radios, televisions, heat lamps, and on and on. Tiny electrical currents are even present in the human body due to the chemical reactions that occur as part of normal bodily functions, even in the absence of external electric fields. For example, nerves relay signals by transmitting electrical impulses. Most biochemical reactions, from digestion to brain activity, are associated with the rearrangement of charged (electric) particles. Even the heart is electrically active—an activity a doctor can trace with the help of an electrocardiogram. You have to wonder what would happen if Expertise 3P could protect us from all that!

There is concern about EMFs, though it's not so much from computer monitors, which are truly a minor source. However, the World Health Organization, after reviewing more than 25,000 research papers on the topic, concluded that there is no negative biological consequence associated with low-level electrical currents. Therefore, there is no need to "protect" skin with a "snake-oil" product like this one. The unhappy face rating has little to do with the product's formula, which ends up being that of a very ordinary toner. Rather, it pertains to the false claims that may stir a sense of unease in women who sit down in front of their computers every day.

😐 **$$$ Gentle Facial Peeling** *($29.50 for 1.4 ounces)* uses paraffin (a wax) to gently exfoliate skin. You apply this cream-textured product to skin, and as you massage it in the paraffin balls up, taking dead skin cells with it for a smooth result. Clarins maintains that regular use of this product helps skin "breathe better," but the wax can leave a film that clogs pores, so that claim is nonsense. A product like this is best for exfoliating dry trouble spots such as elbows, knees, and heels. A water-soluble topical scrub is better for the face.

😐 **$$$ Normalizing Facial Mask** *($25 for 1.7 ounces)* is a basic clay mask with enough witch hazel to make it potentially irritating, but it is an OK option for oily skin. This mask holds no advantage over any clay mask sold at the drugstore.

😐 **$$$ Pure and Radiant Mask** *($26 for 1.7 ounces)* contains more moisturizing ingredients than absorbents, which may leave combination to oily skin confused rather than purified. This mask is best for normal to slightly dry skin, but for the money it's a rather superfluous product. Contrary to claim, the thickening agents this mask contains can clog pores.

😐 **$$$ Skin-Smoothing Eye Mask** *($44 for 1.05 ounces)* does not contain ingredients unique to the eye area, and the amount of rice starch may prove too drying. Nothing in this product will minimize dark circles or puffiness either. This has moisturizing qualities, but is not preferred to Clarins Eye Contour Balm Special for Dry Skin above.

😐 **$$$ Thirst Quenching Hydra-Care Mask** *($32.50 for 1.7 ounces)* contains some good skin-identical ingredients and will feel soothing, but it also contains pine extract and fragrance components that can cause irritation. For the money, better moisturizing masks are available from other department-store lines.

😊 **$$$ Moisture Replenishing Lip Balm** *($23 for 0.7 ounce)* is a mineral oil–based lip balm that contains an effective blend of emollient thickeners and helpful plant extracts. It's a pricey way to care for dry, chapped lips, but will do the job if you decide to splurge. The amount of peptide is so small as to be inconsequential.

☹ **Total Body Lift** *($58 for 6.9 ounces)*. Every couple of years, Clarins revamps and relaunches its anti-cellulite product. Former versions have included Body Lift Advanced Cellulite Control and "Cellulite" Control Gel (quotation marks are from Clarins)—you sort of wonder, if those previous incarnations worked, why did they need to reformulate? Regardless of the name, every version of this product has made the same promise to quickly reduce cellulite and firm the skin. The selling point with Total Body Lift is right there in the product name: it claims to provide a "lifting action" for skin "for a firmer, more streamlined silhouette." Because this product absolutely cannot eliminate cellulite, Clarins skillfully uses the phrase "reduces the appearance of cellulite" in the ad copy. What they don't mention is that this product has a high amount of alcohol—it's the second listed ingredient—which is not helpful for skin. Rounding out the list of "actives" are caffeine (found in many anti-cellulite products, despite the lack of substantiated proof that it works) and menthol (to create a tingling reaction so you perceive the product is doing something). A half-dozen exotic plant extracts are also present, but in amounts so small that your thighs, dimpled or not, won't notice. If you refuse to believe that anti-cellulite products don't work (though if they did, who would have cellulite?), skip this product and seek out some of the similar options from Neutrogena or L'Oreal. Those don't work either, but at least they're less of a financial burn!

☹ **Stretch Mark Control** *($46 for 6.7 ounces)* purports to prevent stretch marks from forming and to reduce the appearance of stretch marks that are less than two years old. How it goes about doing this isn't explained, and rightly so, because it isn't possible. Stretch marks are broken elastin fibers in the subcutaneous (lower) layers of skin, coupled with collagen bundles trying to correct the damage. The problem happens because not all of the pieces of the "building materials" are there, resulting in the familiar white lines that, in most people, are slightly raised, though they may also be indented. Aside from topical application of prescription tretinoin, no other topical product is backed by any evidence it can prevent stretch marks or measurably reduce their appearance. And even tretinoin's results aren't that impressive, unless you consider a 20% length reduction wow-inducing (Source: *Advances in Therapy*, July/August 2001, pages 81–86). This product is principally body lotion with a selection of plant extracts, none of which have a shred of research proving their mettle against stretch marks. Clarins' use of *Empetrum nigrum* fruit juice is actually a problem for skin. This plant, also known as crowberry or pokeweed, has components (especially the root) that are toxic to skin cells. In fact, ingesting only ten crowberries can be fatal to an otherwise healthy adult (Source: www.naturaldatabase.com). This product will have zero effect on stretch marks, but may cause skin problems.

CLARINS SELF-TANNING TREATMENTS FOR FACE AND BODY

☺ **After Sun Moisturizer with Self Tanning Action** *($26.50 for 5.3 ounces)* is sold to prolong and enrich a natural tan, a choice that is infuriating from a company with so many products that claim to forestall aging and wrinkles, because getting a tan from the sun is what causes the wrinkles in the first place. (Well, perhaps that's job security for Clarins?) Despite the lack of ethics involved in encouraging tanning, this is a good self-tanning lotion that contains dihydroxyacetone (DHA) and a small amount of erythrulose, an ingredient similar to DHA that develops color at a slower rate.

☺ **Intense Bronze Self Tanning Tint, for Face and Decollete** *($28.50 for 4.2 ounces)* is a tinted self-tanner so you'll get instant sheer bronze color and a longer-lasting "tan" once the dihydroxyacetone has time to work its magic on skin. Alcohol is the third ingredient listed, but it's unlikely to cause irritation because of the small amount. This product's cotton-pad applicator is a nifty inclusion, but for best results you'll still want to blend it into your skin with your fingers.

✓☺ **Liquid Bronze Self Tanning, for Face and Decollete** *($28 for 4.2 ounces)* is a very silky self-tanning lotion that can be used anywhere on the body. It turns skin tan with dihydroxyacetone and a lesser amount of the self-tanning ingredient erythrulose.

☺ **$$$ Radiance-Plus Self Tanning Cream-Gel** *($50 for 1.7 ounces)* is a lightweight, silicone-enhanced moisturizer with a lesser amount of the self-tanning ingredient DHA. That means less color, so this can be a good option for fair skin tones or times when you want a hint of sunless tan rather than that "day at the beach" look.

☺ **Radiance-Plus Self Tanning Body Lotion** *($39 for 5.3 ounces)* has a color result similar to that of the Radiance-Plus Self Tanning Cream-Gel above, but in a more emollient lotion base. This version may be used on the face if desired, and is best for normal to dry skin.

✓ ☺ **Self Tanning Instant Gel** *($29.50 for 4.4 ounces)* contains dihydroxyacetone to turn skin tan, along with a tiny amount of erythrulose, all in a silky lotion base that doesn't feel thick or greasy. Clarins states there's no need to wait before dressing once this is applied, but I'd play it safe and wait at least 30 minutes to avoid streaks and stained clothing.

☺ **Self Tanning Milk SPF 6** *($29.50 for 4.4 ounces)* has an in-part avobenzone sunscreen, but the SPF rating makes it too low for daytime protection. Given that most people don't apply self-tanner daily, formulating one with a sunscreen is an odd choice. This product is recommended as a standard, creamy self-tanner, though its active ingredient, dihydroxyacetone, is found in many self-tanning products that cost less than this.

😐 **Sheer Bronze Self Tanning Hydrating Gel, for Face** *($28 for 1.7 ounces)* has a silky gel texture, but is otherwise an ordinary self-tanner that contains DHA, the same ingredient found in most self-tanners. This version is suitable for normal to oily skin, but is not preferred to the Clarins self-tanning products above because of its potentially irritating fragrance components.

☺ **Sheer Bronze Tinted Self Tanning, for Legs** *($29.50 for 4.4 ounces)* contains pigments to turn skin a sheer golden bronze color (with shimmer) instantly, while the self-tanning ingredient DHA develops a "tan" over a couple of hours. Although this is a good option from the neck down, it's basically a superfluous addition to the Clarins self-tanning lineup.

☹ **Tinted Self Tanning Face Cream Very High Protection SPF 15** *($28 for 1.7 ounces)* lacks the UVA-protecting ingredients of titanium dioxide, zinc oxide, avobenzone, Tinosorb, or Mexoryl SX, and is not recommended. It works as a self-tanner, but if it's going to encourage you to expose your skin to sunlight (which it should, because it has an SPF rating) it falls short.

CLARINS SUN PROTECTION TREATMENTS FOR THE FACE

☺ **$$$ Sun Control Stick Ultra Protection SPF 30, for Sun-Sensitive Areas** *($24.50 for 0.17 ounce)* is an emollient, oil-based sunscreen stick that includes titanium dioxide for UVA protection. It's a good choice for use over dry to very dry areas of skin, or areas such as the scalp or top of the ears, assuming you feel the need to overspend on sun protection.

☺ **$$$ Sun Wrinkle Control Cream Very High Protection SPF 15, for Face** *($27.50 for 2.7 ounces)* has a misleading name because no one familiar with sunscreen chemistry would consider SPF 15 to be "very high protection." This in-part titanium dioxide sunscreen has a smooth lotion base that lacks any bells or whistles (the antioxidants are window dressing only), but it is suitable for normal to dry skin.

☺ **$$$ Sun Wrinkle Control Cream Ultra Protection SPF 30, for Sun-Sensitive Skin** *($27.50 for 2.7 ounces)* is a good, though ordinary, in-part titanium dioxide sunscreen in a moisturizing cream base suitable for dry to very dry skin. It is oil-free as claimed, but the thickening agents are a poor fit for oily or blemish-prone skin. And by the way, all skin types and all skin colors are sun-sensitive!

☺ **$$$ Sun Wrinkle Control Eye Contour Care Ultra Protection SPF 30** *($24.50 for 0.7 ounce)* contains only titanium dioxide as the active ingredient, making this a gentle, non-stinging option to use around the eyes. The base formula isn't exciting, but it is fragrance-free—a rarity for Clarins!

CLARINS SUN PROTECTION TREATMENTS FOR THE BODY

☹ **Sun Care Cream-Gel Advanced Tanning SPF 6, for Tanned Skin** *($27 for 4.4 ounces)* lacks the UVA-protecting ingredients of titanium dioxide, zinc oxide, avobenzone, Tinosorb, or Mexoryl SX, and is not recommended.

☹ **Sun Care Cream Very High Protection SPF 15, for Outdoor Sports** *($27 for 4.4 ounces)* lacks the UVA-protecting ingredients of titanium dioxide, zinc oxide, avobenzone, Tinosorb, or Mexoryl SX, and is not recommended.

☺ **$$$ Sun Care Cream Very High Protection SPF 20, for Fair Skin** *($33.50 for 7 ounces)* has plenty of titanium dioxide (with other sunscreen actives) to keep any kind of skin protected from the sun, fair or not. The slightly creamy lotion base lacks beneficial amounts of antioxidants, and several of the fragrance components can cause sensitivity, but the small amount is unlikely to be a problem for most skin types.

☺ **$$$ Sun Care Cream Ultra Protection SPF 30, for Children and Sun Sensitive Skin** *($27 for 4.4 ounces)* is a good, in-part titanium dioxide sunscreen for normal to slightly dry skin. The synthetic actives are not the best for children (titanium dioxide and zinc oxide are preferred), but this is fine for adults with normal to dry skin looking for a water-resistant sunscreen. It also includes some good antioxidants.

☹ **Sun Care Oil Intensive Tanning Spray SPF 4** *($27.50 for 5.3 ounces)* contains avobenzone, but this product's SPF rating is embarrassingly low and it encourages users to get a deep tan, which is akin to an oncologist sending a patient off with a carton of cigarettes.

☹ **Sun Care Spray High Protection SPF 15, Oil-Free** *($27.50 for 5.3 ounces)* includes avobenzone for sufficient UVA protection, but the formula is alcohol-based and contains lots of fragrance, a combination that's just too troublesome for skin.

☹ **Sunscreen Cooling Gel Rapid Tanning SPF 8** *($34 for 6.8 ounces)* achieves sufficient UVA protection from its in-part avobenzone sunscreen, but the SPF rating, according to the American Academy of Dermatology and the Skin Cancer Foundation, is too low for daytime protection, and the base formula is primarily alcohol, which makes this drying and irritating.

☺ **$$$ Sunscreen Cream High Protection SPF 30, 100% Mineral Filters, for Children** *($28 for 4.8 ounces)* is indeed a good option for kids because it provides gentle, broad-spectrum protection with titanium dioxide and zinc oxide. The creamy lotion formula is fine for adults too, particularly those with normal to dry skin. This would be a slam-dunk for sensitive skin if it did not contain fragrance, and would be even better for all skin types if it contained some established antioxidants. However, it is still worth considering.

☺ **$$$ Sunscreen Cream High Protection SPF 30, for Sun-Sensitive Skin** *($28 for 4.4 ounces)* has too many synthetic active ingredients and too much fragrance to make it a safe bet for sensitive skin, but it does include titanium dioxide for sufficient UVA protection. This water-resistant sunscreen has a silky-smooth finish that doesn't feel too thick, and is best for normal to slightly dry or slightly oily skin.

☹ **Sunscreen Smoothing Cream-Gel Rapid Tanning SPF 10** *($34 for 7 ounces)* has a name that should not be taken seriously, because the sunscreen agents in this product, which include avobenzone, are not designed to allow skin to tan rapidly, nor do you want your skin to tan. Regardless of the ethical issue of a company selling dozens of antiwrinkle products alongside items like this that encourage tanning, the amount of alcohol in this sunscreen makes it a poor choice for skin of any color.

☺ **Sunscreen Soothing Cream Progressive Tanning SPF 20** *($34 for 7 ounces)* is said to ensure an even, long-lasting tan, which is an unethical claim for any cosmetics company to make, especially one with as many anti-aging products as Clarins. Still, this in-part titanium dioxide sunscreen is a great option for normal to slightly dry or slightly oily skin. It is very similar to the Sunscreen Cream High Protection SPF 30, for Sun-Sensitive Skin above.

☺ **Sunscreen Spray Gentle Milk-Lotion Progressive Tanning SPF 20** *($28 for 5.3 ounces)* leaves skin wanting more in terms of antioxidants (fragrance got higher priority in this sunscreen), but it's an easy-to-apply, alcohol-free sunscreen spray that includes 3% avobenzone for UVA protection. The water-resistant formula is best for oily to very oily or breakout-prone skin. It may be applied to face or body (but don't spray it directly on your face).

☹ **Sunscreen Spray Oil-Free Lotion Progressive Tanning SPF 15, for Outdoor Sports** *($28 for 5.1 ounces)*. Clarins should be ashamed of selling so many products that encourage tanning from the sun. Ignoring this issue (which I can't; I just want to scream!), this in-part avobenzone sunscreen suffers from an alcohol base that makes it too drying and irritating for all skin types.

😐 **$$$ Sunscreen Spray Radiant Oil Intensive Tanning SPF 4, for Body and Hair** *($28 for 5.1 ounces)* includes avobenzone for UVA protection, but SPF 4 is a pathetic rating unless your time outdoors is very brief. Ignoring the "intensive tanning" part of this product's name, it's a nonaqueous, triglyceride- and silicone-based spray that can make hair look greasy, and it's not recommended for skin unless you're willing to pair it with a sunscreen that meets trustworthy dermatology guidelines for daytime protection.

☹ **After Sun Gel Ultra Soothing** *($26.50 for 5.3 ounces)* lists alcohol as the second ingredient, which isn't the least bit soothing.

😐 **After Sun Moisturizer Ultra Hydrating** *($28.50 for 7 ounces)* doesn't improve Clarins' track record of producing average moisturizers. This is an OK option for dry skin, sun-exposed or not, but doesn't best what's available at the drugstore from Curel, Olay, or even Lubriderm.

😐 **$$$ After Sun Replenishing Moisture Care for Face** *($34.50 for 1.7 ounces)* should be loaded with antioxidants and ingredients that mimic the structure and function of healthy skin—but it's not, which makes this a poor choice for after-sun care. This is a lot of money, too, for what amounts to water, thickeners, silicone, and talc.

☺ **$$$ After Sun Shimmer Oil** *($26.50 for 5.3 ounces)* is a spray-on emollient moisturizer with oil-like ingredients. It adds a sheer, shimmering bronze finish to skin and can beautifully enhance the results of a self-tanner while at the same time smoothing and softening skin.

CLARINS MAKEUP

FOUNDATION: ✓☺ $$$ Express Compact Foundation Wet/Dry *($36)* replaces the Clarins Hydrating Powder Foundation, and improves on its predecessor in every respect. It has a supremely silky, talc-based texture that blends seamlessly to a natural matte finish that makes skin look dimensional, not dry and powdery. The eight outstanding shades provide sheer to light coverage, but there are no options for dark skin tones. It can be used wet for more coverage, but apply it carefully or you'll risk streaking.

✓☺ **$$$ Soft Touch Rich Compact Foundation** *($36)* can only be described as a next-generation cream-to-powder makeup. This amazingly silky, silicone-based foundation has one of the smoothst textures around, and blends impeccably to a soft powder finish that has just a touch of dewiness—so this is not the best choice for those with oily skin or oily areas. Those with normal to slightly dry skin who prefer this type of makeup should give this an audition. It provides medium to full coverage and comes in six excellent neutral shades, though options for darker skin tones are limited. Clarins claims this "sweeps on like a second skin," and for the most part they're absolutely correct.

✓☺ **$$$ Extra Firming Foundation** *($37.50)* doesn't contain a single ingredient capable of firming skin, extra or otherwise (tiny amounts of mushroom and algae extracts do not firm skin). That doesn't stop this foundation from being a top choice for someone with normal to dry skin. Its texture and application are creamy smooth, setting to a soft matte finish that remains slightly moist to the touch, which provides a healthy glow. You can attain medium to full coverage, but it looks best when blended on lightly (over a sunscreen if you're using it during daylight hours). The range of 11 shades has some impressively neutral options for fair to medium skin, as well as Clarins' only selection of truly dark foundation shades (Mahogany, Camel, and Chestnut).

✓☺ **$$$ Truly Matte Foundation SPF 15** *($34)* has an utterly accurate name! This fluid is a beautiful, silky liquid foundation that provides sun protection solely from titanium dioxide, which helps contribute to its powdery, long-wearing matte finish. Even better, this provides light to medium coverage while looking surprisingly skinlike. Someone with very oily skin will be pleased with the application and finish, not to mention the sun protection, because that means you wouldn't have to layer products. Drawbacks include a strong scent and the fact that the darkest shades tend to look a bit dull due to the amount of titanium dioxide and the dry finish of the silicones. Among the 15 shades (Clarins' largest selection) are options for fair to dark (but not very dark) skin tones. Most of the shades are very good; the ones to avoid are the slightly peach Ginger, Real Honey, and Hazelnut, the slightly pink Sunlit Beige, and the orange-tinged Nutmeg.

✓☺ **$$$ Colour Tint** *($34)* is more of a foundation than a tint because this provides light coverage that has enough opacity to improve the appearance of an uneven, reddened skin tone. The lotion-like texture and light matte finish make this ideal for normal to slightly dry or slightly oily skin, but it does have a subtle sparkle that is apparent in daylight. Clarins offers five shades, and although Warm Beige and Golden Beige initially appear too pink and peach, they both become more flattering as they're blended, and they are good options for medium skin tones. This foundation looks beautifully natural on the skin, and as long as you pair it with an effective sunscreen for daytime wear, it is highly recommended.

☺ **$$$ True Radiance Foundation** *($36)* supposedly distinguishes itself from other foundations with its gold pigments, which Clarins describes as "enhancing luminosity while maximizing the power of surrounding light." The only luminosity you will see is from the glittery gold particles in the foundation. You have to look closely to see them, but catch your skin in the right light, and there they are. That doesn't make this modestly creamy foundation a poor choice, but you should know you're getting shine, not maximizing the power of light.

Beginning moist and blending impeccably, this sets to a satin matte finish and provides light to medium coverage. It does an excellent job of enhancing skin tone rather than concealing it. Because of this feature, you shouldn't use True Radiance Foundation if you have many flaws to hide. But those with minor flaws (including redness) who also have normal to slightly dry or slightly oily skin should take a closer look. Ten shades are available for light to dark (but not very dark) skin, with only a few to avoid. Praline 06 and Tender Gold 10 are slightly peach, so consider them carefully. Sunlit Beige 08 can turn pink, but is still an option for light skin tones, while Tender Ivory 07 and Soft Ivory 03 are wonderful neutral shades. Clarins typically has take-home samples of this foundation, which gives you an excellent opportunity to audition it all day and in natural (not department-store) lighting.

☹ **$$$ True Comfort Foundation SPF 15** *($36)* would have been a great foundation in almost every respect except for sun protection—an omission that prevents it from earning a better rating. Without titanium dioxide, zinc oxide, avobenzone, Tinosorb, or Mexoryl SX listed as an active ingredient, you need to pair this makeup with another sunscreen that contains UVA-protecting ingredients. If you have normal to dry skin and don't mind the aforementioned pairing, you will be pleased with this foundation's lightweight yet creamy texture, its superb blendability, and its satin finish, which lends a radiant glow to skin. Coverage goes from light to medium and nine of the ten shades are remarkably neutral, although there are no options for darker skin. Only Tender Gold and Chestnut stand out as being a bit too peach, though they may be options for medium and tan skin tones.

☹ **$$$ Hydra-Balance Tinted Moisturizer SPF 6** *($38.50)* has an embarrassingly low SPF 6. This is a sheer, silicone-based moisturizer that would be fine for normal to dry skin. Of the four shades, the best are Bisque and Gold. Amber is too peach and Copper is too orange, but they may work for darker skin tones. This is absolutely not recommended as your sole source of daytime sun protection.

CONCEALER: ☺ **$$$ Instant Light Perfecting Touch Concealer** *($27)* is an agreeably smooth concealer that nicely diffuses dark circles and minor flaws. It is easy to blend, doesn't have too much slip, and sets to a soft matte finish (with sparkles) that poses only a minimal risk of creasing into lines around the eye. There are three shades (best for fair to light-medium skin), and although each starts out a bit pink they soften once the product dries. Use caution with the click-pen and brush applicator, because it is easy to dial up more concealer than you need, and there's no way to put it back.

POWDER: ✓☺ **$$$ Loose Powder** *($34)* comes in a generous container and has a silky, feather-light texture and a sheer, dry application that looks beautiful and feels weightless on the skin. The two sheer shades are good, each with a satin finish—meaning this is best for those with normal to dry skin who want to avoid a true matte finish. ☺ **$$$ Compact Powder** *($33; $21 for powder refills)* has a very silky, ultra-fine texture and a dry, nonpowdery finish. The talc-based formula comes in three sheer shades appropriate for fair to light skin. ☺ **$$$ Shine Stopper Powder Compact** *($29)* comes in only one shade, but this talc-based pressed powder applies nearly translucently, so it can work for a range of skin tones. It is adept at tempering shine without looking thick or powdery, and offers a sheer, dry finish. The only caution is the amount of rice starch it includes. Although not irritating, this food-based ingredient can feed the bacteria that cause blemishes. The salicylic acid in this powder cannot exfoliate skin (even if it could, the amount Clarins includes is nearly insignificant).

☺ **$$$ Bronzing Duo** *($34)* is a pressed-power bronzer that provides two shades in one compact. Without a divider, you need to be careful if you opt to use the lighter or darker shade alone. Both shades go on sheer and look more peachy gold than tan, and a soft shine is present. This isn't the best for creating a bronzed look, but works well as a warm-toned blush.

BLUSH: ✓☺ **$$$ Compact Powder Blush** *($26)* impresses with its finely milled silky texture and smooth application. The selection of sheer, warm-toned shades are quite flattering and matte, but it struck me as odd that some classic pink and rose colors are absent. ✓☺ **$$$ Multi Blush** *($26)* is an excellent option for cream-to-powder blush. The formula is very easy to blend, and all but one of the colors are beautiful, with Tender Chestnut being a great bronze tone. Avoid Tender Raspberry because it's intensely fuchsia and not easy to soften to a more flattering tone.

EYESHADOW: ☺ **$$$ Soft Shimmer Eye Colour** *($20)* has a soft texture and very smooth application that imparts more shimmer than color. This is a pricey but good eyeshadow for young women with unwrinkled eyes or for older women to use as a browbone highlighter, but please think twice before using the Forest or Cool Blue shades.

☺ **$$$ Deep Shimmer Intense Eye Colour** *($20)* is only "deep" because the colors have more pigment than the nearly identical Soft Shimmer Eye Colour above. Although more intense, the shades still apply sheer, so it will take effort if you want effective shading. Avoid Groovy Green (which is anything but groovy) and the aptly named Vibrant Violet—unless you want your eyeshadow color to be more noticeable than you, though of course that's always an option.

😐 **$$$ Colour Quartet for Eyes** *($38)* have an almost creamy powder texture but don't apply as smoothly as they feel, tending to look spotty and flake slightly due to the high amount of shine. In addition, all but one of the quads feature color combinations that are either too contrasting or too pale to create a complete eye design.

😐 **$$$ Soft Cream Eye Colour** *($17.50)* comes in aluminum tubes, each containing a concentrated amount of very shiny cream-to-powder eyeshadow. A little of this product goes a long way, and each shade blends out sheer, leaving a hint of color (and lots of shine) behind. Because this product remains somewhat slick, applying it evenly takes practice, and it does have a tendency to settle into creases. If this concept appeals to you, consider M.A.C.'s Paints ($16) first—you'll get a broader selection of shades and budge-proof, crease-resistant wear.

EYE AND BROW SHAPER: ✓☺ **$$$ Retractable Brow Definer** *($22.50; $10 for pencil refills)* isn't inexpensive, but for the money you get a very good, automatic, retractable brow pencil that applies smoothly and has a dry, powderlike finish that lasts. Three natural-looking shades are available (those with black brows are out of luck this time), and considering that refills are available for less than half the cost of the pencil itself, this ends up being a wise investment for anyone who prefers brow pencil to powder.

☺ **$$$ Liquid Eye Liner** *($22)* has a long, thin brush. That makes it harder to control, but once you get the hang of it the formula lays down color well (if a bit wet), and it dries quickly. Wear-time is more than respectable, but the more-trouble-than-it-needs-to-be brush keeps this from earning a Paula's Pick rating.

😐 **$$$ Waterproof Eyeliner Pencil** *($21.50)* has a tenacity that can survive swimming and tears, so it is waterproof—but you have to tolerate sharpening it, and a finish that remains tacky to the touch. It's an OK occasional-use option, but there are smoother, silicone-based eye pencils that are also waterproof, even though they may not advertise that fact.

😐 **$$$ Eyeliner Pencil with Sharpener** *($21.50)* is a black, standard, slightly creamy eye pencil that comes with its own sharpener. It's functional and has only a slight tendency to smear, but the price is prohibitive considering the equally good eye pencils available at the drugstore.

☹ **Eye Liner Pencil** *($21.50)* is a standard pencil with substandard attributes. This soft-textured pencil glides on but is too creamy for it not to smudge and smear, though the built-in sponge-tip applicator facilitates smudging and smearing if you use it. ☹ **Eye Shimmer Pencil** *($21)* is nearly identical to the Eye Liner Pencil above, except that the few available shades have a strong shimmer finish that detracts from rather than enhances the eyes.

LIPSTICK, LIP GLOSS, AND LIPLINER: ✓☺ **$$$ Le Rouge Lipstick** *($21.50)* has a sumptuous creamy texture, rich, opaque colors, and a satin-smooth finish. There are over 30 colors, numbered from the 200s to the 600s. The color intensity increases as the numbers go up, making it easy to zero in on the light, medium, and deep shades. Quite simply, this is one of the better cream lipsticks available at any price.

✓☺ **$$$ Colour Quench Lip Balm** *($19)* shows Clarins has its act together for lip gloss, too. This tube-packaged gloss feels wonderfully emollient and keeps lips smooth while leaving a non-sticky, wet-look finish. The juicy colors offer varying degrees of intensity, so those looking for sheer and more intense shades are well served. If you're going to splurge on lip gloss, this option is money well spent! ✓☺ **$$$ Retractable Lip Definer** *($22)* will make those prone to lipstick feathering into lines around the mouth happy because this automatic, retractable lipliner applies smoothly without smearing, setting up a solid boundary to keep traveling lipstick from crossing the border. As a bonus, it is minimally prone to fading. The only disappointment here is the small selection of shades, of which three are dark brown tones that won't work with softer lipstick colors.

☺ **$$$ Le Rouge Sheer Lipstick** *($21.50)* doesn't impress as much as the Le Rouge Lipstick above, but it is a pleasant enough sheer, glossy lipstick with a good selection of glitter-infused shades. ☺ **$$$ Le Rouge Pearl Shimmer Lipstick** *($21.50)* has a texture that's in-between the Le Rouge and Le Rouge Sheer lipsticks, and it feels nicely creamy and light. Each shade has a pearlized shimmer that's more becoming than the glitter finish of the Le Rouge Sheer Lipstick.

☺ **$$$ Lip Colour Tint** *($19)* works beautifully to impart soft color to lips along with a smooth texture that's creamy without being overly slick. The shade range is enticing, and many of them have a flattering soft shimmer finish to highlight lips. This is worth a look if you prefer shopping for lipsticks at the department store! ☺ **$$$ Colour Gloss** *($19)* is applied with a wand applicator and goes on thick but not sticky. Lips are left shimmering and definitely glossy, but overall this doesn't have the same sexy feel and finish of the superior Colour Quench Lip Balm above.

😐 **$$$ Lipliner Pencil** *($20)* is a standard pencil that has an easy-to-apply texture, but it needs sharpening and doesn't hold a candle to many other automatic lip pencils.

MASCARA: ✓☺ **$$$ Pure Volume Mascara** *($22)* is a formidable, Lancome-rivaling mascara that enables you to lengthen, thicken, and lightly curl lashes with minimal effort. A minor drawback is that this can clump a bit on the ends of lashes, but that can be remedied by lightly wiping down the brush before application or using a lash comb afterwards. ✓☺ **$$$ Pure Curl Mascara** *($22)* is a superior lengthening mascara, but no more so than any other good mascara (and there are many in this book and on www.Beautypedia.com for half the price). Where this mascara sets itself apart is in how well it lifts and curls lashes. You'll get even better results using it with an eyelash curler (though that's only needed if your lashes grow straight or slant down), but even on its own you will be impressed. ✓☺ **$$$ Wonder Volume Mascara** *($22)* provides substantial lash enhancement without being too dramatic, and the formula wears well without making lashes feel brittle. It is similar to Clarins Pure Volume Mascara, except it doesn't have the same curling effect and it goes on a bit heavier (but without clumps or smearing).

😐 **$$$ Fix Mascara Waterproofing Seal** *($18)* is sold as a waterproofing top coat for use with non-waterproof mascaras. It works, but applying this over mascara isn't always flattering because—depending on which mascara you're wearing—it either clumps lashes together, makes them look spiky, or creates a wet look that may not be to your liking. Why bother with this (and the extra expense) when there are dozens of excellent waterproof mascaras available?

BRUSHES: The majority of Clarins 😐 **$$$ Brushes** *($18.50–$28)* are decent, but they pale in comparison to what most makeup artistry lines sell for the same amount of money. The hair quality isn't up to par, nor are the brush shapes as elegantly functional as they could be, all of which makes this small brush collection one to consider carefully, if at all. The **Eye Definer Brush** *($24)* is good, but its shape and density make it ideally suited for applying brow powder. **The Brush** *($18.50)* is meant as a take-along powder applicator, but since it isn't retractable you're looking at a messy makeup bag or purse after a few uses.

SPECIALTY PRODUCTS: ☺ **$$$ Instant Smooth Perfecting Touch** *($26)* calls itself "the modern, magic makeup base" and has "innovative line-filling technology" that claims to do all sorts of astounding things for skin. Reading the description, you might be curious how you ever got away with wearing makeup before this jar of wonder arrived. As it turns out, this is nothing more than a multiple silicone primer whose spackle-like texture and silky finish does work (temporarily) to fill in superficial wrinkles and large pores. How long the effect lasts depends on your skin type and, in the case of wrinkles, in how expressive you are. The pale pink color adds a subtle luminous quality to skin, but that's camouflaged if you follow it with foundation. It's an option for a silky-feeling pre-makeup moisturizer, but not as impressive as silicone-based serums loaded with antioxidants and other skin-beneficial ingredients (and Clarins did not include any).

CLE DE PEAU BEAUTE

CLE DE PEAU BEAUTE AT-A-GLANCE

Strengths: None of note among skin-care items; even the best products are not worth the money when compared with superior versions from other lines that cost slightly to considerably less; foundations that provide excellent coverage without looking heavy; a magnificent concealer; good highlighting powder and eyeshadows; one good mascara.

Weaknesses: Too many to list, but major ones include: average to ineffective moisturizer and serum formulas; no sunscreens; no products to address acne; several products sold as nourishing or anti-aging that douse skin with alcohol or other irritants; makeup products rated as average that are definitely not worth the investment, particularly the lipsticks; no foundations that provide sunscreen (it's not essential for them to do that, but it's nice to have the option).

For more information about Shiseido-owned Cle de Peau, call (212) 751-6665 or visit www.cledepeaubeaute.com or www.Beautypedia.com. Note: Many of Cle de Peau's formulations are variations on what Shiseido itself offers for much less money. Shiseido doesn't necessarily have better formulas (although their sun-care line is formidable and worth a look), but they offer proportionately more products I feel comfortable recommending.

CLE DE PEAU BEAUTE SKIN CARE

☺ **$$$ Cleansing Cream (Creme Demaquillante)** *($62 for 4.2 ounces)* has a lot going for it in terms of being a cushiony-rich cleansing cream for dry to very dry skin. It removes makeup easily and rinses decently (a washcloth is needed for complete removal), but then look at the price! There's no reason to spend this much money on such a small amount of cleanser, but if you do this shouldn't disappoint.

☹ **Cleansing Lotion (Lotion Demaquillante)** *($62 for 6.7 ounces)* lists alcohol as the second ingredient, and that makes this shockingly basic cleanser a no-go for all skin types.

☺ **$$$ Deep Cleansing Oil (Huile Demaquillante)** *($60 for 1.3 ounces)* is a mineral oil–based cleanser that also contains silicones and a tiny amount of alcohol and vitamin E. I am almost speechless that a company is charging $60 for just over 1 ounce of mineral oil. This will remove makeup quickly, but regardless of your budget, so will plain Johnson's Baby Oil ($4.99 for 20 ounces). One more thing: Cle de Peau's claim that this oil diminishes the appearance of coarse or darkened pores is a falsehood.

☺ **$$$ Gentle Cleansing Foam (Mousse Nettoyante Tendre)** *($50 for 3.3 ounces)* is a basic foaming cleanser that is water-soluble and an option for normal to oily skin. Its name would make more sense without the fragrance.

☺ **$$$ Refreshing Cleansing Foam (Mousse Nettoyante Fraiche)** *($50 for 3.3 ounces)* is nearly identical to the Gentle Cleansing Foam above, and the same review applies. The fragrance might seem refreshing, but it won't do your skin any favors.

☺ **$$$ Absolute Eye Makeup Remover (Demaquillant Pour Les Yeux Absol)** *($39 for 2.5 ounces)* is a silicone-in-water makeup remover that is very similar to considerably less expensive options from Almay, Neutrogena, and Clinique. It works quickly and efficiently, but so do the others.

☹ **Micro-Refining Treatment (Soin Micro-Lissant)** *($195 for the kit)* begins the first of many examples of Cle de Peau's ludicrous pricing of mediocre to downright poor formulations. This two-step system includes **Exfoliator** and **Mask**. The Exfoliator uses silica beads and cellulose to function as a topical scrub, and contains enough alcohol to be problematic. The Mask (the kit includes six two-piece masks) is mostly water, glycerin, thickener, and alcohol. The tiny amount of plant extracts and silk powder have no research proving their benefit for skin, and that's the least you should expect at this price.

😐 **$$$ Gentle Balancing Lotion (Lotion Tendre)** *($85 for 5 ounces)* contains enough alcohol to be potentially irritating, and makes the price insulting. The sugar-based skin-identical ingredients are a nice addition, but the plant-based antioxidants are scant when they should be front and center.

☹ **Refreshing Balancing Lotion (Lotion Fraiche)** *($85 for 5 ounces)* lists alcohol as the second ingredient and otherwise takes a "too little" approach to adding truly beneficial ingredients for skin.

😐 **$$$ Clarifying Emulsion (Emulsion Eclat)** *($100 for 1.7 ounces)* is supposed to be an exfoliating moisturizer but does not contain ingredients that are capable of removing or dissolving dead skin cells. It barely passes as a moisturizer due to its lackluster formula, which is primarily water, slip agent, silicone, thickener, alcohol, and the water-binding agent xylitol. Antioxidants are present, but not in an amount your skin will notice.

☹ **Clarifying Serum (Serum Eclat)** *($100 for 2.5 ounces)* could not be a more mundane serum, which makes the price outrageous. It contains mostly water, glycerin, alcohol, slip agents, and preservative, and is not recommended unless you enjoy wasting money.

😐 **$$$ Energizing Cream (Creme Energisante)** *($148 for 3.3 ounces)* is an OK moisturizer for normal to dry skin, but the energizing element will only occur if you happen to get hyped from spending this amount of money on a single skin-care item (and an unexciting one at that).

😐 **$$$ Energizing Essence (Essence Energisante)** *($155 for 2.5 ounces)* is a water- and silicone-based serum whose truly interesting ingredients are barely present, so they don't count for much. Any serum from Olay, Clinique, Neutrogena, or Estee Lauder easily bests this formula.

😐 **$$$ Enriched Nourishing Cream (Creme Soyeuse)** *($120 for 1 ounce)* claims to improve the appearance of lines overnight, but does that no better than any other ordinary moisturizer, because that is what this product is—an extremely ordinary, standard moisturizer.

The ingredients responsible for the "enriched" name are present in such tiny amounts that your skin has every right to feel shortchanged, and what little potency they had will quickly deteriorate in the jar packaging.

😐 **$$$ Enriched Protective Cream (Creme Protectrice Soyeuse)** *($100 for 1 ounce)* contains appreciable amounts of sunscreen ingredients, but does not sport an SPF rating. You'd think Cle de Peau could bankroll the required SPF testing given what a skin-care routine from them costs the consumer, but that's not the case. This is otherwise another ho-hum, severely overpriced moisturizer that's an OK option for normal to slightly oily skin.

😐 **$$$ Enriched Protective Emulsion (Emulsion Protectrice Soyeuse)** *($120 for 1.7 ounces)* is similar to the Enriched Protective Cream above, but with a thicker texture better suited for normal to slightly dry skin. Otherwise the same comments apply.

☺ **$$$ Eye Contour Balm Anti-Wrinkle (Baume Contour Des Yeux Anti-Rides)** *($130 for 0.5 ounces)* is a very good emollient moisturizer that's suited for dry skin around the eyes or elsewhere. It contains more antioxidants, the cell-communicating ingredient retinol, and skin-identical ingredients than the products above, although the price is absurd given that better formulations are available from other companies for a lot less.

😐 **$$$ Eye Contour Essence Anti-Dark Circles (Essence Contour Des Yeux Anti-Cernes)** *($115 for 0.5 ounces)* does not contain any ingredients that improve the appearance of dark circles unless they are accompanied by dry skin. In that case, they'll look better—because the same benefit can be had by applying any emollient ingredient to dry skin around the eyes. It's a decent moisturizer for slightly dry skin, but once again the really intriguing ingredients are in very short supply.

😐 **$$$ Gentle Nourishing Emulsion (Emulsion Tendre)** *($120 for 2.5 ounces)* has a price that should reward the consumer with a moisturizer that goes above and beyond state-of-the-art, but ends up barely meeting minimum requirements. This isn't a problematic moisturizer, just unbelievably boring for the money. It's an OK option for normal to dry skin, but nothing I'd encourage you to choose over countless other options.

😐 **$$$ Gentle Protective Emulsion (Emulsion Protectrice Tendre)** *($96 for 1.7 ounces)* contains mostly water, slip agent, sunscreen, glycerin, skin-identical ingredients, avobenzone, and Vaseline. This lightweight lotion is not SPF-rated and so it cannot be relied on for daily sun protection. It is another lackluster moisturizer for normal to slightly oily skin (though the sunscreen agents don't coincide with the "gentle" portion of the name).

☹ **Intensive Wrinkle Correcting Cream (Creme Intensive Correctrice Rides)** *($160 for 1 ounce)* contains an insignificant amount of retinol, although the packaging will keep it stable. Even so, the alcohol and peppermint content of this no-action product are cause for concern. Oddly, a few of the plant extracts in this moisturizer are used medicinally to treat urinary tract infections and female reproductive organ anomalies. What that has to do with wrinkles is anyone's guess!

😐 **$$$ Massage Cream (Creme de Massage)** *($113 for 3.4 ounces)* promises a delightful sensation and magnificent result, both adjectives that don't accurately describe this substandard yet very emollient moisturizer for dry to very dry skin. The chief ingredients (squalane, water, and Vaseline) are found in dozens of moisturizers costing significantly less than this product.

☹ **Oil Balancing Essence (Essence Equilibrante)** *($52 for 2.5 ounces)* contains too much alcohol to balance oil, but it will help degrease oily skin (at the expense of causing irritation with no lasting benefit). The amount of astringent zinc phenosulfate is also cause for concern, as is the presence of sage oil.

☹ **Oil Balancing Gel (Gel Equilibrant)** *($52 for 1 ounce)* lists alcohol as the second ingredient, along with menthol and camphor. Oddly enough, this product does contain the anti-irritant dipotassium glycyrrhizate (from licorice), but that doesn't have a chance against the potent skin sensitizers included in this formulation.

☹ **Refreshing Nourishing Emulsion (Emulsion Fraiche)** *($120 for 2.5 ounces)* contains enough alcohol to be anything but nourishing for skin (when was the last time someone called a martini nourishment?). This is a poorly formulated moisturizer that provides minimal benefit at an insulting price.

☹ **Refreshing Protective Emulsion (Emulsion Protectrice Fraiche)** *($96 for 1.7 ounces)* is similar to the Refreshing Nourishing Emulsion above, except this adds some sunscreen ingredients to the mix, although it carries no SPF rating. Otherwise, the same review applies.

😐 **$$$ Revitalizing Emulsion (Emulsion Revivifiante)** *($136 for 1.3 ounces)* claims to protect the skin from signs of sagging, but it cannot do that. This water- and silicone-based moisturizer will feel silky and leave a lightweight smooth finish, but when it comes to beneficial skin-care ingredients, it didn't just miss the boat—it missed the dock, too.

☹ **Soothing Essence (Essence Apaisante)** *($86 for 5 ounces)* lists alcohol as the second ingredient and also contains menthol and its derivative menthyl lactate. And this is supposed to be soothing?!

☹ **The Cream (La Creme)** *($500 for 1 ounce)* is one of the growing number of prestige moisturizers with stratospheric prices. Before I get into the details of this product, suffice it to say that this product is poorly formulated and absolutely not worth even a fraction of the price. The former version of this product contained the skin-lightening agent arbutin, making it effective for those seeking an ultra-pricey product to handle discolorations. This version is arbutin-free and, considering the cost, free of anything else that justifies the price. The bulk of the formula is water, glycerin, slip agent, Vaseline, emollient thickeners, and jojoba oil. Does any of that sound like it can deliver "unparalleled age-defying benefits" to your skin? Hardly, and this is a poor choice for daytime because it doesn't provide sun protection. Further, the choice of jar packaging means the antioxidants (including a decent amount of vitamin C) will become ineffective shortly after the product is opened. This cream has an elegant texture, but its sensation on skin doesn't translate into a sensational formula that's worth parting with hundreds of dollars.

☹ **Anti-Age Spot Serum (Serum Anti-Taches Brunes)** *($140 for 1.3 ounces)* lists alcohol as the second ingredient, which is a real burn for skin and the pocketbook. All of the exotic-sounding plant extracts and the form of vitamin C included don't have an established track record of lightening skin discolorations. Cle de Peau wants you to think their cellular ion channel technology can inhibit the formation of melanin (skin pigment), but there is no research showing that to be the case.

😐 **$$$ Facial Contour Treatment (Traitement Visage Remodelant)** *($130 for the kit)* is a two-step kit designed to treat puffiness by "encouraging the skin's healthy fluid exchange balance," which in turn will make skin more resistant to becoming puffy. The **Anti-Puffiness Massage Gel** contains a blend of water, emollient squalane, slip agents, thickeners, and vitamin E, along with meager amounts of plant extracts, none capable of reducing puffy skin. The second portion is the **Cooling Mask**, which doesn't cool skin with menthol but does contain alcohol and a hairspray-like film-forming agent that can temporarily smooth skin and make it feel tighter. None of the ingredients in either product can control skin's fluid balance, although the alcohol in the Cooling Mask may cause some superficial dehydration. Although this duo won't work as claimed, I suppose it can be a somewhat soothing experience for those with money to burn.

☹/😐 **$$$ Intensive Treatment (Soin Intensif)** *($130 for the kit)* is sold as a weekly treatment to exfoliate and nourish skin instead of just using your usual nighttime skin-care lineup. The **Lotion Intensive** *(6 0.1-ounce bottles)* is an alcohol-laden toner with barely a dusting of intriguing ingredients for skin; the **Essence Intensive** *(6 0.1-ounce bottles)* is a slightly creamy moisturizer similar to most of those in the Cle de Peau line. It contains some antioxidants and cell-communicating ingredients, but not in amounts that are likely to benefit skin, making them relatively useless. Last is the **Intensive Mask**, which is mostly slip agent and film-forming agents with a small amount of absorbents and alcohol. Nothing in these products exfoliates skin, nor are any of them "intensive." It's just another gimmicky, superfluous kit that is dressed up as a specialized solution for aging skin.

☹ **Translucency Mask (Masque Transparence)** *($115 for 3.4 ounces)* is a standard, peel-off facial mask that lists polyvinyl alcohol (a hairspray fixative) as the second ingredient, followed by utterly ordinary ingredients that don't come close to offering anything to rationalize the product's price. This is an unsatisfactory choice for any skin type.

☹ **Lip Treatment (Soin Levres)** *($60 for 0.14 ounce)* reigns as one of the most expensive lip balms in existence. Although this emollient stick will moisturize and help keep dry, chapped lips protected, it will not prevent and correct signs of aging because it contains no sunscreen. Further, the orange and peppermint oils promote irritation, which promotes chapped lips, making this an expensive mistake.

CLE DE PEAU BEAUTE MAKEUP

FOUNDATION: Although several formulas are available, none of the Cle de Peau foundations are appropriate for dry to very dry skin unless it is sufficiently prepped with an emollient sunscreen or you happen to prefer a matte finish.

☺ **$$$ Teint Naturel Cream Foundation** *($110)* has its strong points but there is no doubt the price is out of line, and nothing in this foundation makes it exceptional or even remotely worth the money. (You'd think that for over $100 they would have included a sunscreen or some state-of-the-art ingredients.) It is just a very good silicone- and talc-based makeup that goes on very smoothly and dries to a silky matte finish.

What is unique about the formulation is that it's densely pigmented. That can be good in the sense that a little goes a long way, but it can also be problematic if you want sheer or light coverage. This can be mixed with a moisturizer to thin out the coverage if desired, and that may be a good idea, since using it at full strength results in such intense camouflage it isn't what anyone would call "natural." The formula is best for normal to oily skin, and comes in ten shades, of which the following are slightly pink or peach, but not worth dismissing altogether: B10, B20, and B30. In addition to the shades mentioned above, there are also two shades of ☺ **$$$ Color Control Foundation** *($90)*. This foundation includes white and bronze shades that Cle de Peau recommends using to deepen or lighten any of the foundation colors, or for contouring and highlighting the face. These two extras are an option (and much better than standard color correctors), but before you drop almost $200 for two bottles of foundation, please remember that the existing foundation colors should work just fine on their own and that any special shading or highlighting can be achieved with considerably less-expensive products. This formula is good for normal to oily skin. Using it over dry skin can be tricky because it tends to accentuate the dryness; however, an emollient sunscreen underneath can help it go on more easily.

☺ **$$$ Silky Cream Foundation** *($110)* was launched as a lighter alternative to the Teint Naturel Cream Foundation above. It has a similar consistency and comes in the same type of jar packaging, but provides less intense coverage for a more natural finish. "Natural" is a relative term here, because although this foundation feels exceptionally light and silky on skin, it still has enough pigment and opacity to provide medium coverage, and its somewhat powdery finish isn't the best if you have any dry areas—though its mica content does provide a soft glow. The water- and silicone-based formula contains enough absorbents (including talc) to keep oily areas matte for longer than usual. Eight shades are offered, with no options for tan to dark skin. The only colors to skip are P10, which is too pink, and the too-peach B10.

☺ **$$$ Liquid Foundation** *($110)* is Cle de Peau's lightest foundation in terms of its finish and level of coverage, which is sheer to light. Its smooth texture feels nearly weightless and it sets to a soft, slightly dry matte finish suitable for normal to oily skin. Among the five shades, only B10 is off due to its peachy tone. The rest are recommended for fair to medium skin, provided your cosmetics budget knows no limits.

☺ **$$$ Creamy Powder Foundation** *($75 for powder cake; $25 for compact; $10 for sponge)* is an incredibly standard but undeniably smooth, talc-based powder foundation. It applies easily and quite sheer, with a satin finish. The ten shades are very good, but B10, B20, B30, and B40 can turn peach if used on oily skin. For the money, this is not as impressive as the powder foundation options from Lancome, L'Oreal, Chanel, Estee Lauder, Clinique, and Laura Mercier.

CONCEALER: Cle de Peau's ✓ ☺ **$$$ Concealer** *($68)* is exceptional. This twist-up stick concealer has a light, smooth texture that glides over the skin and offers substantial but (almost) imperceptible coverage in three excellent shades, best for fair to light skin. The soft matte finish poses little risk of creasing, and the only thing that's disconcerting about this is the prohibitive price. As a suggestion, Maybelline's Instant Age Rewind Double Face Perfector works brilliantly for a fraction of the cost.

POWDER: ✓ ☺ **$$$ Luminizing Relief Powder** *($45 for powder cake; $30 for refillable case with brush)* is meant to "create great sculptural effects," but that's just a fancy way of saying these pressed powders can be used for contouring (shade 32) or highlighting (shade 31). Both have shine but also an enviably silky texture, and they apply flawlessly, with minimal flaking (of the shine, not the color itself—that goes on evenly). Although pricey, both shades work well for their intended purpose if you have fair to medium skin. The included brush is compact, but the hair is sable, so it's not your standard throwaway applicator.

Both the ☹ **$$$ Translucent Loose Powder** *($100; $70 for refill)* and ☹ **$$$ Translucent Pressed Powder** *($80; $20 for refillable compact; $70 for powder refill)* are talc-based, have superfine textures, and come in a single shade that is supposedly translucent but can look pink on light skin and ashen on dark skin. Both powders have a refined finish, although the Loose version is slightly shiny while the Pressed version has a noticeably drier feel. For a comparable texture and more than one shade, consider the powders from Sonia Kashuk, L'Oreal, or Laura Mercier.

☹ **$$$ Perfect Enhancing Powder** *($55)* is a product that has some versatility, but it shouldn't be used as an all-over finishing powder because the four colors aren't true skin tones. The pale pink and pale yellow pressed powders are workable for highlighting or using as eyeshadow base, while the pale gold and bronze tones can work as a blush combination or for eyeshadows. All have a silky texture, but aren't as smooth as the Luminizing Relief Powder above, and are not worth the money unless you can honestly see yourself using one of the shades over a standard blush or eyeshadow.

BLUSH: ☹ **$$$ Cheek Color** *($40 for powder cake; $30 for compact)* has a great silky feel and even application, but for the money, it is too sheer. For $70, you want a blush that will last and last, and this doesn't, though it will leave your cheeks with a soft sparkly finish.

EYESHADOW: ☺ **$$$** Each **Eye Shadow** *($17 per shade; $20 for duo case; $40 for palette to hold 9 eyeshadows; $10 for sponge-tip and/or brush tip applicators)* has a suede-smooth texture that applies well and doesn't flake. However, each of the 30+ shades has a decent amount of shine (either soft pearl or glaring metallic), and that can magnify any eye-area flaws, including the ones Cle de Peau's skin-care products claim to alleviate but cannot. If you choose to indulge, at least avoid the following shades, all of which are too blue, green, or purple to look sophisticated: 18, 19, 20, 55, 56, 57, 65, 68, and 70. ☺ **$$$ Creme Eye Shadow** *($45 for eyeshadow; $20 for regular compact; $40 for palette)* has the strangest texture! It feels almost gelatinous, but applies slightly creamy and sets to a sheer powder (in feel) finish. Each of the six shades is shiny, imparting more sparkles than pigment to the eye area. That's fine if you're young and wrinkle-free, but I don't think that describes the typical Cle de Peau customer. For a cream eyeshadow, these pose minimal risk of creasing. Avoid the Green and Violet shades.

EYE AND BROW SHAPER: ☺ **$$$ Eyebrow Liner** *($25 for cartridge; $30 for pencil case)* is a very good, automatic brow pencil that has the standard hard texture but goes on well without being greasy or looking thick. This has a powder finish and comes in three workable colors, but none for blondes or redheads. ☺ **$$$ Eyebrow Shadow** *($16 per shade; $33 for compact)* is much easier to use and its intensity is much easier to control. Each of the four excellent shades applies smoothly, and all are suitably named for their intended brow color.

☹ **$$$ Eyebrow Cake Liner** *($16 for color; $33 for compact)* is a brow wax that can be paired with the Eyebrow Shadow above or another Eyebrow Cake Liner for a customized brow compact. It applies well for a wax, and doesn't leave brow hairs sticky or matted. The automatic, retractable ☹ **Eyeliner** *($25 for cartridge; $30 for pencil case)* has a soft, cream-wax texture that is eminently easy to work with, but it applies color too softly and tends to smudge and fade before too long, so it ends up being a costly disappointment. ☹ **Liquid Eyeliner** *($40)* has a brush that applies color in a thick line, and since the formula can apply a bit chunky, you'll need another brush to get smooth results. Couple this with a drying time that will test your patience, plus uneven wear, and it quickly becomes one to avoid.

LIPSTICK, LIP GLOSS, AND LIPLINER: ☺ **$$$ Lip Gloss** *($45)* doesn't have any issues other than its price, which becomes ridiculous when you consider the number of equally good non-sticky glosses that impart sheer color without feeling thick. This lip gloss includes a brush applicator. ☺ **$$$ Lipliner** *($25 for cartridge; $30 for pencil case)* is an automatic, retractable lip pencil that has a creamy, just-right texture, although precise application is hindered by the wider-than-usual pencil tip. The pencil case includes a very good lip brush; the only oddity is the small selection of shades, most of which don't easily complement Cle de Peau's lipsticks.

Cle de Peau's ☹ **$$$ Lipstick** *($55)* is available in Cream or Sheer formulas, and in the previous edition of this book I recommended them. This time, they're different. I'm not certain if the formula changed (the counter personnel I asked were too new to know) or if the last few years have brought enough improved lipsticks on the market so that these slick, greasy-feeling lipsticks are less than desirable by comparison. Either formula, but especially the glossy Sheer, will make a beeline into lines around the mouth. A review of the ingredients shows that your money isn't buying anything not found in hundreds of other lipsticks.

MASCARA: The regular ☹ **$$$ Mascara** *($40)* beautifully lengthens lashes without a trace of clumping, no matter how many coats you apply. But therein lies this mascara's weakness: The formula dries so fast that subsequent coats tend to drag through lashes, diminishing the positive results.

In contrast, the ☺ **$$$ Volume Mascara** *($40)* has a bit more gusto and ably builds noticeable length and some thickness without clumping or smearing. You absolutely do not have to spend this much money for a good mascara, but if you're set on Cle de Peau, this is the one to purchase. One last point: With either mascara, avoid the blue and violet shades, which are none too subtle.

SPECIALTY PRODUCTS: ☹ **$$$ Refreshing Smoothing Pre-Makeup Emulsion SPF 22** *($70)* and ☹ **$$$ Gentle Smoothing Pre-Makeup Emulsion SPF 20** *($70)* have nearly identical formulas, with each boasting a titanium dioxide sunscreen that leaves a soft, nearly translucent white cast on skin. The lightweight lotion texture leaves a silky finish that does indeed prep skin for foundation, but so do many other moisturizers, sunscreens, and serums that cost significantly less. If you're banking on the higher cost netting you a state-of-the-art formula chock full of antioxidants, this won't come through for you.

☹ **$$$ Refining Corrector for Lines** *($50)* is sold as "a translucent, hydrating concealer," which is sort of like wearing sunglasses that are minimally tinted. In other words, what's the point? This isn't a concealer at all; it's an eye cream that has an emollient feel and noticeably dewy finish. Applying makeup over this can cause it to slip into wrinkles around the eye, not to mention shorten its wear time. If you're looking for an eye cream, consider the non-jar-packaged options from Estee Lauder before this moisturizing but lackluster formula. ☹ **$$$ Translucent Corrector for Pores** *($50)* is said to provide a flawless, smooth skin tone that "envelops rough or enlarged pores." Before you reach for your credit card, you should know this silicone-based twist-up stick won't make pores less visible, at least not any more than a matte-finish foundation or concealer. It is very silky and easy to apply, but the "fill-in" effect it has on pores is fleeting, primarily due to the wax and jojoba esters in this product (which, ironically, can clog pores). These ingredients help keep the stick texture in solid form, but aren't too far removed from the sebum your skin produces. If you have oily skin and large pores, you don't want to apply anything with ingredients that make matters worse. This corrector is a superfluous option for smoothing skin, but doesn't really correct anything.

CLEAN & CLEAR (SKIN CARE ONLY)

CLEAN & CLEAR AT-A-GLANCE

Strengths: Inexpensive; an excellent 10% benzoyl peroxide product; some very good cleansers.

Weaknesses: The majority of products contain irritating fragrant extracts, alcohol, menthol, menthyl lactate, or other problematic ingredients; no broad-spectrum sunscreens; below-average moisturizers; not at all a one-stop shopping experience for someone battling blemishes.

For more information about Clean & Clear, owned by Johnson & Johnson, call (877) 754-6411 or visit www.cleanandclear.com or www.Beautypedia.com.

CLEAN & CLEAR ADVANTAGE PRODUCTS

☹ **Advantage Acne Cleanser** *($6.49 for 5 ounces)* contains 2% salicylic acid in a base with a pH of 4, but because this cleanser is quickly rinsed away, the BHA will have little to no impact on the skin. In addition, this cleanser contains sodium C14-16 olefin sulfonate as its main cleansing agent, which makes it too drying for all skin types, plus the cinnamon and cedar extracts are irritating. For an "advanced formula," this is quite a letdown.

☹ **Advantage Daily Cleansing Pads** *($6.29 for 70 pads)* are below-standard, alcohol-based pads whose 2% salicylic acid won't be effective because the pH is to high; even so, your skin ends up irritated from the menthol derivative menthyl lactate.

☹ **Advantage Acne Clearing Astringent** *($4.49 for 8 ounces)* lists alcohol as the main ingredient, and also contains irritating cinnamon and cedar bark extracts. None of this is helpful for acne-prone skin, or for any skin for that matter.

😐 **Advantage Oil-Free Acne Moisturizer** *($6.99 for 4 ounces)* is an OK lightweight moisturizer for normal to oily skin. The 0.5% concentration of salicylic acid isn't that helpful for blemishes, and it's not effective in this product given that its pH is above 4. The cinnamon and cedar bark extracts pose a risk of irritation.

☹ **Advantage Acne Spot Treatment** *($6.49 for 0.75 ounce)* is a 2% salicylic acid gel with a pH of 3.2, so it can exfoliate the skin's surface and inside the pore lining. That's great, but the alcohol base is problematic, especially when combined with the cinnamon and cedar bark extracts here. You would fare better with Neutrogena's BHA products.

☹ **Advantage Daily Acne Clearing Lotion** *($6.49 for 1 ounce)* contains 1% salicylic acid, but a pH of 4.9 greatly reduces the likelihood of exfoliation. It contains cinnamon and cedar bark extracts, which do nothing but irritate already inflamed, reddened blemishes.

☹ **Advantage Invisible Acne Patch** *($9.99 for 0.07 ounce)* seems a convenient way to zero in on blemishes and zap them overnight with 2% salicylic acid. However, the BHA is suspended in a solution of alcohol along with irritating cedar and cinnamon bark extracts, making it a problem product for all skin types.

😐 **Advantage Concealing Treatment Stick** *($5.99 for 0.07 ounce)* contains 1% salicylic acid and has a pH of 3.8, but it can be irritating to skin because of the amount of cedar and cinnamon bark extracts it contains. The single shade is good for light skin tones and provides moderate coverage with a matte finish.

☹ **Advantage Acne Control Kit** *($19.99 for the kit)* is supposed to make fighting acne as easy as 1-2-3, but each of the products in this misguided kit has its share of problems. The **Advantage Acne Control Cleanser** contains 10% benzoyl peroxide, a concentration that can be quite drying, although it won't have time to work because it is rinsed quickly from your skin. A larger problem is the drying detergent cleansing agent sodium C14-16 olefin sulfonate along with menthol, neither of which helps combat blemishes, and which just add irritation and inflammation to skin. Step 2 is the **Advantage Acne Control Moisturizer**, which is nearly identical to the Advantage Oil-Free Acne Moisturizer reviewed above. Last is the **Advantage Fast Clearing Spot Treatment**, which contains 2% salicylic acid, but also enough alcohol to cause irritation, and that problem is not reduced by the inclusion of cinnamon and cedar bark extracts. In short, there is little reason to expect relief from acne with this kit, and every reason to expect irritated, reddened skin.

CLEAN & CLEAR BLACKHEAD CLEARING PRODUCTS

☹ **Blackhead Clearing Daily Cleansing Pads** *($4.99 for 70 pads)* contain almost 40% alcohol along with menthol derivative menthyl lactate, making these pads too irritating for all skin types.

😐 **Blackhead Clearing Facial Cleansing Bar** *($2.99 for a 3.5-ounce bar)* is a soap-free bar cleanser with 0.5% salicylic acid and a pH above 4 that permits it to work as an exfoliant. This is an OK option for those who prefer bar cleansers, but the ingredients that keep this in bar form won't clear blackheads and may make them worse.

☹ **Blackhead Clearing Scrub** *($4.99 for 5 ounces)* is a standard scrub that contains polyethylene (ground-up plastic) as the abrasive agent. This also contains 2% salicylic acid, which can help eliminate blackheads, but not when used in a scrub that is rinsed off the skin after only a moment or two. Even if this brief exposure to salicylic acid were beneficial, the pH of this product is too high for effective exfoliation. This product contains menthyl lactate, which is irritating and offers no benefit to skin.

☹ **Blackhead Clearing Astringent** *($4.99 for 8 ounces)* contains too much alcohol and menthyl lactate (a form of menthol) to be anything but irritating to the skin. The 1% salicylic acid is formulated at an effective, though considerably irritating, pH of 2.5.

CLEAN & CLEAR DAILY PORE PRODUCTS

☺ **Daily Pore Cleanser, Oil-Free** *($4.99 for 5.5 ounces)* is a very good, water-soluble cleanser/scrub hybrid for oily to very oily skin. The tiny amount of witch hazel is unlikely to cause irritation. This does contain fragrance.

☺ **Daily Pore Cleansing Cloths** *($5.99 for 25 wipes)* won't clean pores better than other water-soluble cleansers, but if you prefer cloths for their convenience, these are recommended for their gentle yet effective water-soluble formula. They remove most makeup, but you'll need a separate remover or washcloth for long-wearing or waterproof formulas.

☹ **Daily Pore Cleansing Pads** *($7.59 for 24 pads)* are similar to the Daily Pore Cleansing Cloths above, except that these pads are textured instead. The inclusion of irritating menthyl lactate means that these are not recommended.

CLEAN & CLEAR DEEP ACTION & DEEP CLEANING PRODUCTS

☹ **Deep Action Cleansing Wipes, Oil-Free** *($4.99 for 25 wipes)* list alcohol as the second ingredient, and also contain menthol; these wipes are an irritation waiting to happen.

☹ **Deep Action Cream Cleanser, Oil-Free** *($4.99 for 6.5 ounces)* contains menthol and is not recommended for any skin type.

☹ **Deep Action Cream Cleanser, Sensitive Skin** *($4.69 for 6.5 ounces)* contains menthol and is not recommended for any skin type. Without it, this would be an appropriate cleanser for sensitive skin.

☹ **Deep Cleaning Astringent** *($4.49 for 8 ounces)* makes me hurt just to write about it because this toner's blend of 42% alcohol, eucalyptus, peppermint, and clove oils—plus camphor—is, quite simply, an assault on skin. Avoid this product at all costs!

☹ **Deep Cleaning Astringent, Sensitive Skin** *($4.49 for 8 ounces)* contains a significant amount of alcohol, plus eucalyptus, peppermint, and clove oils at a pH of 2.7. "Ouch!" is an understatement!

CLEAN & CLEAR MORNING BURST PRODUCTS

☹ **Morning Burst Cleansing Bar** *($2.99 for a 3.5-ounce bar)* is a standard bar soap that contains a lot of fragrance. It is too drying for all skin types.

☹ **Morning Burst Facial Cleanser** *($5.99 for 8 ounces)* is a below-standard, water-soluble cleanser that "wakes you up" with an irritating dose of menthol, which leaves your face tingling after rinsing.

☹ **Morning Burst Shine Control Facial Cleanser** *($5.99 for 8 ounces)* wants you to wake up radiant, but after washing with this problematic cleanser you'll only be waking up irritated. It contains menthol and menthyl lactate along with irritating citrus extracts, and is not recommended.

☹ **Morning Burst Energizing Astringent** *($3.99 for 8 ounces)* lists alcohol as the second ingredient, followed closely by fragrance and a form of menthol. Once again, a Clean & Clear toner strikes out.

☹ **Morning Burst Facial Scrub** *($5.99 for 5 ounces)* is a standard scrub that contains polyethylene (plastic) beads as the scrubbing agent. It also contains methyl lactate, a form of menthol that instantly makes this scrub too irritating for all skin types.

☹ **Morning Burst Shine Control Facial Scrub** *($6.99 for 5 ounces)* has the same problem as the Morning Burst Facial Scrub above, and the same review applies. Johnson & Johnson–owned Neutrogena makes better scrubs than this (although some of J&J's also contain menthol derivatives).

😐 **Morning Glow Eye Brightening Cream** *($5.99 for 0.5 ounce)* creates a glow thanks to the mineral pigments it contains. This is a relatively standard moisturizer that lacks significant amounts of helpful ingredients for skin, but it's an OK option for slightly dry skin anywhere on the face.

☹ **Morning Glow Moisturizer SPF 15, Oil-Free** *($5.99 for 4 ounces)* contains a form of menthol that can cause skin to tingle (not glow) with irritation, and that is unquestionably a problem. Without it, this in-part avobenzone sunscreen would have been highly recommended as a basic, lightweight, affordable sunscreen for normal to slightly oily skin.

😐 **Morning Burst Oil-Absorbing Sheets** *($5.19 for 50 sheets)* are thin plastic polypropylene sheets. They work decently to absorb excess oil and perspiration, but the mineral-oil additive won't keep skin as shine-free as other options. These are fragranced, too.

CLEAN & CLEAR OXYGENATING PRODUCTS

☺ **Oxygenating Fizzing Cleanser** *($6.79 for 5 ounces)* is a fairly standard liquid-to-foam cleanser that is a good option for all but very dry skin. It rinses cleanly and removes all but the most stubborn makeup (such as waterproof mascara or long-wearing foundation). It contains fragrance.

All of the Clean & Clear Oxygenating products contain *Corallina officinalis* extract from a form of red algae that is a source of bromoperoxidase, an enzyme that catalyzes the oxidation of a substance by releasing peroxide. Peroxide is a potent source of free-radical damage (Sources: *Endocrine*, February 2006, pages 27–32; and *Biotechnology and Bioengineering*, September 2001, pages 389–395). For many reasons, getting oxygen into the skin is an ill-conceived concept, mainly because it can cause free-radical damage. Thankfully, the likelihood that these products will ever get a bit of oxygen into the skin is practically nil. Overall, the enzyme's capability to provide oxygen or peroxide is doubtful, and that's a good thing.

☹ **Oxygenating Facial Scrub** *($6.79 for 5 ounces)* doesn't do anything to "oxygenate" the skin. It does, however, contain a derivative of menthol that makes this otherwise standard scrub too irritating for all skin types. In addition, the wax content makes this difficult to rinse completely, and a scrub is not something you want lingering on your skin all day.

☹ **Oxygenating Ultra-Light Moisturizer SPF 15, Oil-Free** *($6.99 for 4 ounces)* does not contain the UVA-protecting ingredients of titanium dioxide, zinc oxide, avobenzone, Tinosorb, or Mexoryl SX, and is absolutely not recommended. Even if UVA-protecting ingredients had been included, the menthol and menthol derivative in this product make it needlessly irritating.

OTHER CLEAN & CLEAR PRODUCTS

☹ **Continuous Control Acne Cleanser** *($4.99 for 5 ounces)* contains 10% benzoyl peroxide, but this topical disinfectant is of little use to skin because it is quickly rinsed off. The menthol in this unusually creamy cleanser makes it too irritating for all skin types.

☺ **Continuous Control Acne Wash, Oil-Free** *($4.99 for 6 ounces)* lists 2% salicylic acid as its active ingredient, but any benefit it might have is rinsed down the drain, making this ineffective against acne. It is recommended as a standard, water-soluble cleanser for oily to very oily skin.

☺ **Foaming Facial Cleanser, Oil Free** *($4.39 for 8 ounces)* is recommended if you prefer a water-soluble cleanser with copious foaming action. The foam has no cleansing ability, but the impression it gives is one some consumers prefer, and in the case of this product is not irritating or drying. The antibacterial agent triclosan is listed as an active ingredient, but its effect in cleansing products that are quickly rinsed from skin is negligible.

✓☺ **Foaming Facial Cleanser, Sensitive Skin** *($4.39 for 8 ounces)* is not only Clean & Clear's best cleanser, thanks to its gentle yet very effective water-soluble formula, but is also one of the best beauty buys at the drugstore. It would be even better without fragrance, but that's a minor concern. This cleanser removes makeup easily and is suitable for all skin types except very dry.

☹ **Instant Dissolving Cleansing Sheets** *($4.99 for 24 sheets)* contain sodium lauryl sulfate as the main cleansing agent, making these portable cleansing sheets too drying and irritating for all skin types. They also contain sulfuric acid, a caustic ingredient rarely seen in skin-care products (though fortunately the amount used is tiny).

☺ **Makeup Removing Cleanser** *($4.99 for 6 ounces)* is an almost-gentle, water-soluble cleanser that is made slightly problematic (but not prohibitively so) by the inclusion of drying sodium C14-16 olefin sulfonate as a secondary cleansing agent. This is still an option for those with normal to oily skin. As for its makeup-removing prowess, this cleanser can tackle most water-based foundations, but to remove heavy or silicone-based makeup you will need to use a washcloth with it.

😐 **Warming Daily Face Scrub** *($5.99 for 4 ounces)* contains zeolite, a type of mineral that elicits a warming sensation when mixed with water. It feels nice, but doesn't make this scrub a must-have or more effective than any other. The warmth does not remove "all pore-clogging residue."

☹ **Cooling Daily Pore Toner** *($4.59 for 8 ounces)* lists alcohol as the second ingredient and also contains a form of menthol for a cooling (and irritating) effect on skin. The glycolic and salicylic acids won't exfoliate skin due to the too-high pH of this toner.

☹ **Dual Action Moisturizer, Oil-Free** *($5.99 for 4 ounces)* has a pH that allows its 0.5% salicylic acid to exfoliate skin, but half a percent won't be effective and the menthyl lactate in this moisturizer causes undue irritation.

😐 **Shine Control Moisturizer, Oil-Free** *($5.99 for 4 ounces)* is an exceptionally basic moisturizer that leaves a slight matte finish, but lacks ingredients capable of absorbing oil. Actually, it also lacks any ingredients necessary to create a state-of-the-art moisturizer!

😐 **Invisible Blemish Treatment** *($4.49 for 0.75 ounce)* contains 2% salicylic acid at an effective pH of 3.5. The amount of alcohol (28%) is a problem for irritation and keeps this otherwise well-formulated BHA product from getting a better rating.

✓☺ **Persa-Gel 10, Maximum Strength** *($4.99 for 1 ounce)* remains a very potent, fragrance-free topical disinfectant for blemishes. It contains 10% benzoyl peroxide, the maximum amount approved for over-the-counter sales. Although this amount can be drying and potentially irritating, this is an option for stubborn cases of acne.

☺ **Oil-Absorbing Sheets** *($4.99 for 50 sheets)* are an interesting twist on the standard oil-absorbing papers. These are more like soft plastic sheets with a slight rubbery feel. They work well enough, but it takes several of them to make a difference, just as it does with any of the more standard oil-absorbing papers.

CLEARASIL (SKIN CARE ONLY)

CLEARASIL AT-A-GLANCE

Strengths: Inexpensive; effective topical disinfectants with 10% benzoyl peroxide; a good BHA option for those who prefer pads; a decent selection of water-soluble cleansers and topical scrubs.

Weaknesses: As is true for most anti-acne lines, irritating ingredients with no benefit for skin take precedence; only one sunscreen and it's part of a lackluster three-step kit; no lower-strength benzoyl peroxide products (10% has a higher chance of causing irritation than 2.5% and 5% versions).

For more information about Clearasil, call (866) 252-5327 or visit www.clearasil.com or www.Beautypedia.com.

CLEARASIL BLACKHEAD CONTROL PRODUCTS

☹ **Blackhead Control Treatment Gel** *($7.99 for 0.65 ounce)* lists 2% salicylic acid and has a pH low enough for it to exfoliate and help dissolve blackheads, but the amount of alcohol makes it a problem for all skin types.

☺ **Daily Blackhead Control Scrub with Natural Sea Salt** *($7.99 for 5 ounces)* is a topical scrub with 1% salicylic acid, but its pH is too high for it to have an impact on blackheads. Keep in mind that you can't scrub blackheads away. A topical scrub will help remove dead skin cells on the surface and minimally effect blackheads, but a leave-on BHA (salicylic acid) product gets to the root of the problem because it can penetrate the pore lining where blackheads develop. The sea salt is just a gimmick; it is not the solution for stubborn blackheads. This is an overall good scrub for normal to oily skin.

☹ **Daily Blackhead Control Astringent with Natural Sea Salt** *($8.49 for 6.78 ounces)* lists alcohol as the second ingredient and has enough sea salt to cause dryness, which won't help blackheads but will cause undue irritation.

✓☺ **Daily Blackhead Control Pads with Natural Sea Salt** *($7.99 for 80 pads)*. These alcohol-free pads have 1% salicylic acid and a pH of 3.5, so exfoliation will occur. The sea salt doesn't serve much purpose in this product, and isn't an ingredient that should be on the short list for those dealing with blackheads. However, these pads are an excellent way to enjoy the benefits of a well-formulated BHA product.

CLEARASIL DAILY OIL CONTROL PRODUCTS

☹ **Daily Oil Control Cleansing Wipes with Green Tea & Peppermint** *($8.59 for 25 wipes)* contain, as the name states, peppermint. They also contain witch hazel, and some of the thickening agents chosen won't control oil very well. All told, these wipes are more irritating than helpful for oily skin.

☹ **Daily Oil Control Cream Cleanser with Green Tea & Peppermint** *($7.99 for 5 ounces)* contains peppermint and a lot of fragrance and is not recommended for any skin type.

☹ **Daily Oil Control Gel Wash with Green Tea & Peppermint** *($7.99 for 6.78 ounces)* contains peppermint and a lot of fragrance and is not recommended for any skin type. It is far from being "gentle enough for everyday use."

CLEARASIL ULTRA PRODUCTS

☹ **Ultra Acne Clearing Gel Wash** *($6.99 for 6.78 ounces)* contains 2% salicylic acid, but the pH of this cleanser (and its brief time on skin) won't permit it to work as intended. Further, the inclusion of menthol makes it too irritating for all skin types.

☹ **Ultra Acne Fighting Cleansing Wipes** *($6.99 for 32 wipes)* contain 2% salicylic acid and have a pH of 3.6, so these will exfoliate. However, the hydrogen peroxide and menthol make these cleansing wipes a poor choice for any skin type. As a topical disinfectant hydrogen peroxide is an option, but it generates free-radical damage and that is harmful for skin. It is absolutely not preferable to the more stable and incredibly well-researched disinfectant benzoyl peroxide. Without the hydrogen peroxide and menthol, these wipes, whose solution is not rinsed from the skin, would have been a reliable product.

☹ **Ultra Acne Solution System** *($24.99 for the kit)* comprises four items in a kit designed to address the causes of and help combat facial acne. The **Stay Clear Daily Face Wash** is similar to the Ultra Acne Clearing Gel Wash above, but adds polyethylene beads to the mix so it's a cleanser/scrub. It is still too irritating due to the menthol, so we're not off to a good start. Step 2 involves the **StayClear Daily Toner**, but with alcohol as the second ingredient it's also a problem for all skin types. Things begin looking up with the **StayClear Daily Lotion**, a 0.5% BHA lotion with a pH of 2.3. The pH allows the salicylic acid to exfoliate skin, but is considerably more irritating than a pH of 3–4, which is a safe pH range for skin and salicylic acid. The only product that deserves consideration is the **Quick Start Treatment Cream**. This is a simply formulated 10% benzoyl peroxide lotion that has a slightly absorbent matte finish. Ten percent benzoyl peroxide is a potent disinfectant for blemishes, and in general it is best to start with lower strengths to see if those work for you without pronounced side effects such as dryness or flaking. All told, with three out of four products in this system faltering, the only conclusion is to ignore this kit and keep in mind that separate benzoyl peroxide products are available from Clearasil, Neutrogena, and other drugstore lines.

😐 **Ultra Daily Face Wash** *($6.99 for 6.78 ounces)* contains 2% salicylic acid, but any potential benefit is wasted in a cleanser because it is not left on the skin long enough to work.

And that's not to mention the drawbacks of avoiding the eye area during use and the fact that the pH of this cleanser is too high for the salicylic acid to work as an exfoliant. This is otherwise a standard, water-soluble foaming cleanser that is an option for normal to oily skin—so long as you don't expect it to provide "clearer skin in just 3 days."

☹ **Ultra Deep Pore Cleansing Pads** *($6.99 for 90 pads)* have a pH-correct formula with 2% salicylic acid, but hydrogen peroxide is added to the mix. That isn't excessively irritating, but it is a source of free-radical damage and an impediment to the skin's healing process, both of which are problems that someone already battling acne (or with skin of any type, for that matter) doesn't need.

😐 **Ultra Acne Clearing Scrub** *($6.99 for 5 ounces)* contains 2% salicylic acid (BHA), but the real exfoliating benefit comes from the polyethylene beads because this scrub, just like any other scrub, won't be left on the skin long enough for the BHA to have an effect, even though its pH of 3.6 is low enough for exfoliation to occur. It's a decent scrub option, but the sodium lauryl sulfate makes it less enticing than similar options from Neutrogena or Olay. Leaving it on the skin is an option, but not one I would encourage, given that there are better ways to get the benefits of BHA.

☹ **Ultra Acne Eliminating Astringent** *($7.69 for 6.78 ounces)* lists alcohol as the second ingredient, which makes this too irritating for all skin types. That's a shame, because sans alcohol, the pH of 3 makes the 2% salicylic acid an effective exfoliant.

Ultra Acne Scar Care System *($24.99 for set of 3 products)* is a system designed to reduce the appearance of scars from acne, and by scars they are referring to the flat, reddened, or (depending on your skin color) brown marks left after a blemish heals. These marks are not true scars, nor are they usually permanent, even though it can seem that way if you're staring at them every time you look in the mirror! The Scar Care System includes the following items:

☹ **Exfoliating Acne Wash** *(5 ounces)* contains 2% salicylic acid in a pH-correct cleansing-lotion base. As I have mentioned repeatedly in the past, salicylic acid's benefits are wasted in a cleanser because it is rinsed from the skin before it has a chance to work. This cleanser is made problematic for skin because it contains menthol and because it is so highly fragranced that you could skip applying your regular perfume.

After cleansing, you're directed to apply the 😐 **Protecting Day Lotion with SPF 15** *(1.67 ounces)*. This in-part avobenzone sunscreen won't prevent new acne scars (hyperpigmentation) from forming, but its protective benefit for skin will enhance the natural fading of these marks. The effective yet boring formula lacks antioxidants, significant skin-identical ingredients, and anti-irritants, but it does have a light lotion texture those with normal to slightly dry or slightly oily skin will appreciate. After the sun goes down, Clearasil directs you to apply their Night Repair Lotion.

😐 **Night Repair Lotion** *(1 ounce)* claims to improve the appearance of scars. How it goes about doing that is a mystery because the formula contains nothing that can positively affect the discoloration left behind after a blemish heals. A tiny amount of the plant *Mimosa tenuiflora* is included, an ingredient traditionally used to heal burns and wounds. However, evidence as to whether this plant is really effective for such purposes is conflicting and, given its high tannin content, it is likely to be irritating (Sources: *Revista de Investigacion Clinica*, July–September 1991, pages 205–210; and *Revista de Biologica Tropical*, December 2000, pages 939–954). I have seen no research that shows it to be effective for healing post-inflammatory hyperpigmentation. This is merely an OK lightweight moisturizer for normal to slightly dry skin.

😐 **Ultra Vanishing Acne Treatment Cream** *($9.99 for 1 ounce)* combines 10% benzoyl peroxide with enough glycolic acid to exfoliate skin, which this product's pH of 3.6 allows. However, according to a cosmetics chemist I interviewed, benzoyl peroxide's stability can be negatively affected at this pH level, causing it to break down into benzoic acid (which has no effect on acne). This product's combination of actives sounds intriguing, but their effectiveness may be inhibited by the unknowns about what happens when they are combined. Further, glycolic acid isn't preferred to salicylic acid for acne.

😐 **Ultra Tinted Acne Treatment Cream** *($9.49 for 1 ounce)* is nearly identical to the Ultra Vanishing Acne Treatment Cream above, except this version has a sheer peach tint. It's too peach to use on its own during the day, but can look convincing if a neutral foundation is applied afterward.

OTHER CLEARASIL PRODUCTS

☹ **3 in 1 Acne Defense Cleanser** *($5.99 for 6.78 ounces)* lists 2% salicylic acid as its active ingredient, but it's ineffective because this product is rinsed from the skin so quickly. This would have been a recommended cleanser/scrub hybrid for normal to oily skin, but the menthol makes it too irritating to consider.

☹ **Acne Control Deep Cleansing Scrub** *($4.79 for 5 ounces)* is a topical scrub that's medicated with 2% salicylic acid, but its brief contact with skin and the product's pH keep it from working to fight blemishes. The menthol in this scrub does not make it preferred over other options, and the amount of sodium lauryl sulfate is potentially drying.

☺ **Acne Fighting Cleansing Wipes** *($5.09 for 32 wipes)* cleanse skin and remove makeup while depositing 2% salicylic acid. The pH of 2.9 permits exfoliation, making these wipes a worthwhile option for those battling blemishes. The only caution is to avoid using them around the eye area.

☺ **Acne Fighting Foaming Cleanser** *($4.99 for 5.9 ounces)* claims to prevent breakouts with its 2% salicylic acid. However, in a cleanser this ingredient does not have enough time to work before it is rinsed. This is still a good, water-soluble cleanser for oily skin, but not for use around the eyes.

😐 **Daily Face Wash** *($4.99 for 6.5 ounces)* is a somewhat harsh, water-soluble foaming cleanser because of the inclusion of alkaline potassium stearate and other cleansing agents that aren't the best for skin unless it is very oily. The 0.3% triclosan won't work as an antibacterial agent because its contact with the skin is too brief.

😐 **Daily Face Wash, Sensitive Skin** *($4.99 for 6.5 ounces)* is nearly identical to the Daily Face Wash above, minus the triclosan, but the same basic comments apply. It is too drying for someone with sensitive skin, though it is fragrance-free.

☹ **Icewash Acne Gel Cleanser** *($4.79 for 6.78 ounces)* contains menthol and menthyl lactate, along with drying sodium lauryl sulfate as the main detergent cleansing agent, making this a cleanser to avoid.

☺ **Oil Control Acne Wash** *($4.49 for 6.78 ounces)* is a good, basic, water-soluble cleanser for normal to oily skin. However, the salicylic acid it contains will be rinsed down the drain before it can impact blemish- or blackhead-prone skin. The small amount of isopropyl alcohol is unlikely to cause irritation.

☹ **Pore Cleansing Pads** *($4.99 for 90 pads)* list alcohol as the main ingredient, making these 2% salicylic acid pads too irritating and drying for all skin types—plus the pH is too high for the BHA to function as an exfoliant.

😐 **Adult Care Acne Treatment Cream** *($5.99 for 1 ounce)* contains 2% resorcinol along with 8% sulfur, both topical disinfectants that can be effective against acne-causing bacteria. The tradeoffs are that resorcinol can be exceedingly irritating and drying to skin (Source: *Contact Dermatitis*, April 2007, pages 196–200), and sulfur, while less irritating, can cause superficial dryness. Still, this may be a worthwhile option for someone with acne whose blemishes have not responded to benzoyl peroxide or salicylic acid or to prescription options.

✓☺ **Tinted Acne Treatment Cream** *($5.99 for 1 ounce)* provides 10% benzoyl peroxide in an absorbent base with a sheer peach tint and matte finish. This provides minor camouflage, but the peach tinge can draw more attention to the blemish than you want. Still, this is a potent disinfectant that puts the kibosh on acne-causing bacteria.

✓☺ **Vanishing Acne Treatment Cream** *($5.99 for 1 ounce)* is identical to the Tinted Acne Treatment Cream above, minus the tint. That makes this option more versatile for daytime use with makeup, though this much benzoyl peroxide is best reserved for blemishes that have been unresponsive to lower strengths.

CLINIQUE

CLINIQUE AT-A-GLANCE

Strengths: Less expensive than most department-store lines; one of the best selections of state-of-the-art moisturizers and serums loaded with ingredients that research has shown are of great benefit to skin; excellent sunscreens; good selection of self-tanning products; some very good cleansers and eye makeup removers; some unique mattifying products; a large but wholly impressive selection of foundations, many with reliable sun protection (and shades for darker skin tones); good concealers; some remarkable mascaras; much-improved eyeshadows; loose powder; all of the blush products; some brilliant lipsticks, lip gloss, and the Quickliner for lips; gel eyeliner; well-organized,clearly labeled, and accessible tester units.

Weaknesses: The three-step skin-care routine, because of the bar soaps and irritant-laden Clarifying Lotions; jar packaging downgrades several otherwise top-notch moisturizers; incomplete routines for those prone to acne; skin-lightening products with either unproven or insufficient levels of lightening agents; the pressed-powder bronzer, liquid eyeliner, and brow pencil disappoint; lip plumper; one truly awful mascara.

For more information about Clinique, call (800) 419-4041 or visit www.clinique.com or www.Beautypedia.com. Note: All Clinique products are fragrance-free unless noted otherwise.

CLINIQUE SKIN CARE

CLINIQUE ACNE SOLUTIONS PRODUCTS

☹ **Acne Solutions Antibacterial Facial Soap** *($10 for 5.2 ounces)* has a minimal amount of triclosan, an antibacterial agent with minimal research proving its benefit for acne and no research showing that's it's useful in a rinse-off product. Beyond the useless active ingredient is the fact that this old-fashioned soap is a poor choice for anyone, blemishes or not. It contains menthol, which irritates already inflamed skin.

☹ **Acne Solutions Cleansing Foam** *($17.50 for 4.2 ounces)* would have been an excellent liquid-to-foam cleanser for normal to oily skin, but the peppermint is a problem and salicylic acid's benefit in a cleanser is minimal at best because it is rinsed from skin before it can penetrate into the pore lining. This cleanser does contain some very good (and some unique) water-binding agents, but again, their impact on skin won't be great and the peppermint remains a problem.

☹ **Acne Solutions Clarifying Lotion** *($13.50 for 6.7 ounces)* doesn't improve on Clinique's long-standing Clarifying Lotions (reviewed below). This version still contains a lot of alcohol and a lesser but still potentially problematic amount of witch hazel. Without those, it would be an excellent toner for all skin types, though the 1.5% salicylic acid cannot exfoliate due to the pH of this toner.

☺ **Acne Solutions Clearing Moisturizer, Oil-Free** *($16 for 1.7 ounces)* is one of the most state-of-the-art benzoyl peroxide lotions available today. It contains 2.5% of this topical disinfectant, an excellent amount to apply all over acne-prone skin. The lightweight lotion base feels silky and contains oodles of good-for-skin ingredients, including green tea, acetyl glucosamine, and many soothing plant extracts. The only misstep (one that prevents this product from earning a Paula's Pick rating) is the addition of peppermint extract. The amount is so small as to very likely be a non-issue for skin, but why include it at all when it has no benefit for acne-prone skin?

☹ **Acne Solutions Daytime Shield** *($16 for 1.7 ounces)* is a lightweight, silicone-based moisturizer that could have been a great soothing option for dry skin, except that it contains peppermint, and that adds unnecessary irritation. Also, the lack of sun protection in this product is not what a daytime product is all about.

✓☺ **Acne Solutions Emergency Gel Lotion** *($13.50 for 0.5 ounce)* remains an outstanding topical disinfectant for blemish-prone skin with 5% benzoyl peroxide and a good group of anti-inflammatory agents.

☹ **Acne Solutions Night Treatment Gel** *($16 for 1.7 ounces)* contains 2% salicylic acid, but the pH of this gel makes exfoliation debatable. Moreover, it contains enough alcohol to be irritating, while even the lower amount of peppermint makes for strange bedfellows with the anti-irritants in this product.

😐 **Acne Solutions Post-Blemish Formula** *($13.50 for 0.07 ounce)* claims to gently fade the appearance of post-inflammatory hyperpigmentation—those pesky red or brown marks left over for a period of time after a blemish has healed. However, other than the smattering of anti-irritants, nothing in this lightweight lotion (dispensed through a click-pen precision applicator) will hasten the fading of these unsightly marks. That's because the main "ingredient" necessary to fade post-blemish marks is time. The typically red or pink pigmentation you're seeing is a remnant of your skin's healthy immune response to the blemish, and for most skin types and skin colors it tends to linger long after the blemish is gone. The marks will fade, but it can often take 12 months or longer. If you don't have that kind of patience (and who does?), a better option for speeding up the fading of this type of discoloration is to use a topical exfoliant (a pH-effective AHA or BHA product works well) or a tretinoin product (available by prescription). It is also critical that you wear sunscreen daily to prevent more damage that will impede the skin's healing process.

Finally, when new blemishes appear, take steps to treat skin gently while using effective blemish-battling products, and, whatever happens, do not pick at them and make scabs—that is a surefire way to damage skin further, resulting in darker and longer-lasting post-inflammatory hyperpigmentation. Bottom line: This Clinique product won't make matters worse, but it won't help things either, and as such is relegated to "why bother?" status.

☹ **Acne Solutions Spot Healing Gel** *($12.50 for 0.5 ounce)* lists alcohol as the main ingredient, and although it contains 1% salicylic acid, the pH is too high for it to function as an exfoliant, leaving your skin irritated and still blemished.

☹ **Acne Solutions Body Treatment Spray** *($19.50 for 3.4 ounces)* is a spray-on BHA product that lists 2% salicylic acid as the active ingredient. The pH of this spray won't permit exfoliation to occur, while the amount of alcohol can cause dryness and irritation.

CLINIQUE CX PRODUCTS

☺ **$$$ CX Soothing Cleanser** *($35 for 4.2 ounces)* doesn't provide much cleanser for the money, but it is indeed gentle and does contain soothing ingredients. Completely without detergent cleansing agents, it instead uses a blend of emollients, plant oils, and silicones to dissolve makeup. It does not contain any irritants (not even fragrant plant extracts), so it should be fine for dry to very dry skin that is also sensitive, easily irritated, or dealing with rosacea. The oils do not make this easy to rinse completely, so you may need a washcloth. A lighter, but still gentle, and considerably less-expensive alternative to this cleanser is Clinique's Comforting Cream Cleanser ($17.50 for 5 ounces).

☺ **$$$ CX Protective Base SPF 40** *($45 for 1.69 ounces)* claims to be exceptionally gentle, but two of the four active sunscreen ingredients don't fit that description. Not that they're a problem, it's just that a sunscreen designed for sensitive skin should only contain the mineral sunscreens titanium dioxide and/or zinc oxide. This product contains those actives too, in a moisturizing base suitable for normal to dry skin. It contains some very good soothing agents, but fewer antioxidants than many other Clinique moisturizers. Two types of lecithin are on hand for their cell-communicating abilities, while the iron oxide and mica mineral pigments bring a radiant glow to skin.

😐 **$$$ CX Soothing Moisturizer** *($55 for 1.7 ounces)*. Unfortunately this very nicely formulated moisturizer comes packaged in a jar, which means that the really helpful antioxidant ingredients won't last very long once you open and start using it. The other ingredients make it a decent choice for dry to very dry skin that needs a rich, protective moisturizer, and it is completely fragrance-free. Were it not for the non-airtight packaging that compromises the effectiveness of the antioxidants, this product would have merited a Paula's Pick rating.

✓☺ **$$$ CX Antioxidant Rescue Serum** *($125 for 1 ounce)* is a water- and aloe-based lightweight serum that contains some formidable antioxidants, cell-communicating ingredients, skin-identical substances, and soothing agents. It is ideal for all skin types and can definitely minimize visible signs of irritation and help skin repair a compromised barrier. Despite this praise, you should know that the Lauder companies have several other serums with similar formulas and benefits, none of which cost this much money. In fact, Clinique's own Repairwear Deep Wrinkle Concentrate for Face and Eye ($55 for 1.4 ounces) is just as good in terms of state-of-the-art ingredients.

✓☺ **$$$ CX Rapid Recovery Cream** *($75 for 1.7 ounces)* is Clinique's most expensive moisturizer. The price and exclusivity are designed to make you think you're getting a product that's a considerable step above those sold in Clinique's main line, but that is not the case. Although this is a beautifully formulated, stably packaged moisturizer that covers all the bases when it comes to giving dry skin what it needs to look and feel better, it is not a superior choice when compared with Clinique's less-expensive options. You are assuredly getting a great moisturizer if you buy CX Rapid Recovery Cream, but logically there is no need to spend the extra money. The "unique" selling point of this moisturizer is that it can help skin recover faster from sources of distress, including cosmetic procedures such as laser or microdermabrasion. The claim is valid, but the fact remains that any well-formulated moisturizer can help damaged skin look and feel more normal, and it doesn't mean you need to step up your spending or rearrange your skin-care budget. This product is fragrance-free, but it does contain coloring agents. It is best for dry to very dry skin.

😐 **$$$ CX Redness Relief Cream** *($75 for 1.7 ounces)* is similar to the CX Rapid Recovery Cream above, except this has a less emollient texture and features jar packaging, which won't keep the many antioxidants stable. Specific to this product is the addition of more anti-irritants (good news for those with reddened, rosacea-prone skin) along with the mineral pigment mica, which adds a luminous finish. The salicylic acid does not function as an exfoliant because the pH is too high, but it can still exert anti-inflammatory properties. The selling points for this product will undoubtedly tempt those dealing with rosacea, but this is not a slam-dunk solution for minimizing redness, nor can it significantly reduce the incidence of flare-ups, and it cannot stop rosacea. The external and internal factors that trigger rosacea flare-ups cannot be controlled by nonprescription topical products. Despite the clinical name and medicinal claims, CX Redness Relief Cream is a cosmetic, not an over-the-counter drug that had to prove its claims before it could be sold. The same basic formula and price comparison comments made for the CX Rapid Recovery Cream apply here, too, and this one is also fragrance-free.

☹ **CX Stretch Mark Cream** *($95 for 6.7 ounces)* claims its patent-pending formula stimulates collagen to reduce the appearance of stretch marks. A well-formulated moisturizer can indeed stimulate collagen, but not to the extent of making a visible improvement in stretch marks. Further, the physical signs of stretch marks are actually broken bands of elastin fibers, not collagen. Stimulating collagen won't simultaneously repair elastin fibers, so the most you can expect from this cream in terms of positive benefits is softer, smoother skin. However, the bigger issue is irritation from the menthol and peppermint in this product. They irritate skin, causing it to swell, which can temporarily make stretch marks appear diminished, but the effect is fleeting and in the long run damaging, as the irritation these two ingredients create causes collagen and elastin to break down.

CLINIQUE DERMA WHITE PRODUCTS

☹ **Derma White Moisture Bar, for Very Dry to Dry Combination Skin** *($15 for a 3.5-ounce bar)* is a glycerin- and plant oil–based soap, but that doesn't mean it's a safe choice for those trying to avoid the dryness and poor rinsing characteristics of bar soaps. This cleanser can still be quite drying and the residue it leaves on the skin is not helpful.

☹ **Derma White Purifying Bar, for Combination Oily to Oily Skin** *($15 for a 3.5-ounce bar)* is a sucrose- (sugar) enriched bar soap that contains the irritating menthol derivative menthoxypropanediol as well as menthyl lactate. It is not recommended.

☹ **Derma White C10 Anti-Aging Clarity Formula** *($80 for six 0.24-ounce vials)* is basically a way to see if vitamin C (ascorbic acid) can help banish skin discolorations. Each vial (enough for a one-week supply) contains quite a bit of this antioxidant vitamin, but it's disappointing that alcohol is listed as the third ingredient. Among its many beneficial traits, vitamin C, when stably packaged—as it is in this product—can have a positive effect on hyperpigmentation (Sources: *Dermatologic Surgery*, July 2005, pages 814–817; and *International Journal of Dermatology*, August 2004, pages 604–607). However, other products also contain ascorbic acid and they don't subject skin to irritation from alcohol. This serum-type product also contains angelica extract, which research has shown contains compounds that can cause phototoxicity—making it a poor choice in a product meant to diminish sun- and hormone-induced skin discolorations (Source: www.naturaldatabase.com).

☹ **Derma White Clarifying Brightening Lotion, for Combination Oily to Oily Skin** *($30 for 6.7 ounces)* lists alcohol as the second ingredient, which makes this antioxidant-packed liquid too irritating for all skin types. The angelica extract is also bad news because it can cause a phototoxic reaction when skin is exposed to sun.

☹ **Derma White Clarifying Brightening Lotion, for Very Dry to Dry Combination Skin** *($30 for 6.7 ounces)* doesn't make sense for very dry to dry skin because alcohol is the second ingredient. What a shame, because if it weren't for that and the angelica extract this would have been an extraordinary moisturizing toner with several skin-beneficial ingredients.

☺ **$$$ Derma White Eye Moisture SPF 15** *($32.50 for 0.5 ounce)* has an in-part zinc oxide sunscreen that can offset the potential for the angelica extract (the main plant extract in this product) to cause a phototoxic reaction. Still, this is overall not as impressive as several other eye-area moisturizers from Clinique, since most of the intriguing ingredients appear near the end of the ingredient list. And the sunscreen ingredient octinoxate is not the best for use around the eye, though there isn't much of it in here.

☺ **$$$ Derma White Intense Brightening Complex** *($60 for 1 ounce)* is about as intensive as pulling up a chair to watch a yoga class! Clinique claims this serum-type moisturizer achieves high-intensity brightening, but what does that mean? You may equate "brightening" to "lightening," but they are not the same. Most products claiming to brighten skin lack ingredients (such as hydroquinone or arbutin) that can actually fade coloration or disrupt melanin production. That's important when you remember that skin gets its coloring and most of its discolorations from this skin pigment. What brightening products like this one can do is improve the skin's appearance, but they accomplish that by smoothing the skin with ingredients such as glycerin and silicones, and, in many cases, by adding mica (which provides a soft, shimmering glow), all of which happen to be in this product. Smooth, even-textured, or shimmer-enhanced skin is better able to reflect light, and that is what the "brightening" term really means. However, none of that can change one bit of skin discoloration or overall skin color in any way. This product also contains several antioxidants, tried-and-true skin-identical ingredients, and a token amount of anti-irritant, all adding up to create a lightweight moisturizer for normal to slightly oily skin. This product is best used at night, because the angelica extract it contains can cause a phototoxic reaction. It contains fragrance in the form of gardenia extract.

😐 **$$$ Derma White Moisture Cream** *($34 for 1 ounce)* does not contain ingredients that have a proven whitening effect on skin, and the antioxidants, which are in short supply here, are compromised by jar packaging. This ends up being an OK moisturizer for normal to dry skin. The angelica extract can cause a phototoxic reaction, and the fragrance results from gardenia extract.

☺ **$$$ Derma White Moisture Milk** *($34 for 1 ounce)* misses the mark for a Paula's Pick rating because it contains angelica extract, which can be problematic when worn during the day. This has merit as a nighttime moisturizer for normal to slightly oily skin, though it has no impact on skin discolorations. It does contain some excellent cell-communicating ingredients and antioxidants.

☺ **$$$ Derma White Super City Block SPF 40** *($22.50 for 1.4 ounces)* contains titanium dioxide and zinc oxide for UVA protection, along with a couple of synthetic sunscreen ingredients. The potential for angelica extract to cause a phototoxic reaction is inhibited both by the amount present here, and by the sunscreens. Most of the really interesting ingredients are present in minor amounts, making this less impressive than Clinique's Super City Block Oil-Free Daily Face Protector SPF 25 ($16.50 for 1.4 ounces), reviewed below. The SPF 40 rating is one it appears the FDA will concede as they finalize the revised sunscreen monograph (Source: www.fda.gov).

☹ **Derma White Intense Brightening Mask** *($50 for the set)* is a two-part treatment that is said to speedily brighten skin thanks to something Clinique calls Black-Out Yeast extract. There is no research pertaining to this ingredient's ability to lighten or brighten skin, although yeast can theoretically function as an antioxidant. However, both phases of this duo (**Gel Treatment** and **Activating Spray**) contain enough alcohol to make them more irritating than helpful for skin.

CLINIQUE PORE MINIMIZER PRODUCTS

☺ **$$$ Pore Minimizer Thermal-Active Skin Refiner** *($27.50 for 2.5 ounces)* is Clinique's version of their parent company Estee Lauder's Idealist Micro-D Deep Thermal Refinisher ($46 for 2.5 ounces). The two products are remarkably similar and both claim to open pores to free clogging debris; however, pores cannot be opened or closed like window blinds. Lauder's product has more of a microdermabrasion-at-home marketing slant, whereas the Clinique version positions itself as a "mini-spa for pores." Both products contain the scrub ingredient polyethylene (ground-up plastic) as the exfoliating agent, along with the inorganic salt calcium chloride, which is where the "thermal" part comes in. When calcium chloride is mixed with water (Clinique's directions state that you should use this product on damp skin) it causes an exothermic reaction. Simply put, that's a chemical reaction—in this case, between water and calcium chloride—that generates heat. This is merely a nifty science project, however, and has no benefit for skin.

Heat of any kind does not help minimize pores. In reality, the warm sensation is there just to give the impression that the product is doing something. It is actually the action of massaging scrub particles over the skin that loosens debris (dead skin cells and oil) from the surface of your pores, allowing it to be rinsed away. That will make skin feel smoother and look more even-toned, and can temporarily make pores smaller—but only because the buildup of dead skin cells and oil has been reduced. Almost any topical scrub or even just a washcloth, does this; I no longer recommend baking soda as a scrub. In contrast, chemical exfoliants such as glycolic and salicylic acids surpass topical scrubs because they exfoliate more evenly and thoroughly and with no abrasion. Nevertheless, Pore Minimizer Thermal-Active Skin Refiner will produce smoother, more even-toned skin with consistent use. You don't need to spend this much money to get such results, but there is nothing in this product that is harmful to skin. The pH of 5 prevents the salicylic acid in this product from functioning as an exfoliant.

✓☺ **Pore Minimizer Instant Perfector** *($16.50 for 0.5 ounce)* comes in two shades (light and dark), but the color itself barely registers on the skin. Rather, this product is designed to mattify the skin and create a silky-smooth surface by filling in large pores and absorbing excess oil. This irritant-free formula does just that, and beautifully, too. No, it does not have a long-lasting effect on reducing pore size or holding back every drop of excess oil, but it is a smart product to add to your routine if oil control is an issue. When paired with an ultra-matte foundation (preferably one that has a built-in SPF 15), this can be a formidable option for keeping skin matte most of the day. Pore Minimizer Instant Perfector can also be applied (carefully) over makeup to absorb oil rather than dusting on more powder.

☹ **Pore Minimizer T-Zone Shine Control** *($13.50 for 0.5 ounce)* contains several dry-finish ingredients (such as silicones) that can indeed leave a lasting matte finish on the skin. Unfortunately, they are joined by irritants such as denatured alcohol, witch hazel, and clove extract, and that means this product is not recommended for any skin type.

😐 **Pore Minimizer Refining Lotion** *($18 for 1.4 ounces)* is a water- and silicone-based fluid lotion that also contains a good deal of film-forming agent (which can temporarily make pores look smaller) along with alcohol and the absorbents silica and talc. Clinique claims that, with ongoing use, this product makes the pore walls stronger, but nothing in this formula supports that claim. If anything, daily exposure to the high amount of film-forming agent and alcohol can cause chronic irritation, and that won't strengthen pores in the least. This is best used as a temporary mattifying product, though products like Clinique's Pore Minimizer Instant Perfector above or Smashbox's Anti-Shine Foundation ($26) are more effective options.

☺ **Pore Minimizer Oil Blotting Sheets, for Combination Oily to Oily Skin** *($13.50 for 50 sheets)* are standard, powder-free blotting papers that work as well as most to soak up excess oil and perspiration. Reducing surface oil will make pores appear smaller, but that benefit isn't unique to this product.

CLINIQUE REPAIRWEAR PRODUCTS

😐 **$$$ Repairwear Day SPF 15 Intensive Cream** *($47.50 for 1.7 ounces)* is an excellent, in-part zinc oxide sunscreen in a moisturizing base that's characteristic of the best moisturizers from Clinique, but it also has jar packaging. That means the many light- and air-sensitive ingredients in this product will be compromised once you begin using it.

Some of the plant extracts can be problematic, but they are present in small amounts and the beneficial plant extracts and cell-communicating ingredients have them outnumbered. Clinique maintains that Repairwear "helps block and mend the look of lines and wrinkles," though that's true only to the extent that an effective sunscreen, which this product contains, can prevent further skin damage. As well-formulated as this product is, please don't be fooled into thinking it can repair your skin and eliminate wrinkles, or you're bound to be disappointed. The fact that this is described as an intensive cream may make you think it is for very dry skin, but it's actually best for normal to dry skin.

😐 **$$$ Repairwear Day SPF 15 Intensive Cream Very Dry Skin Formula** *($47.50 for 1.7 ounces)* is a more emollient, dry-to-very-dry-skin-appropriate version of the Repairwear Day SPF 15 Intensive Cream above, and the same basic comments apply, including those about the poor choice of jar packaging.

✓☺ **$$$ Repairwear Day SPF15 Intensive Lotion** *($47.50 for 1.7 ounces)* shares the same in-part zinc oxide sunscreen as the Repairwear Day SPF 15 Intensive Cream product above, but this product comes in a lighter-weight lotion base. That makes it preferred for normal to slightly dry or slightly oily skin types. Otherwise, the same formulary and price comments made above apply here, too. A major advantage this product has over both Repairwear Intensive SPF 15 Creams above is its packaging. The Intensive Lotion is housed in an opaque bottle with a pump applicator, which nicely helps preserve the antioxidants.

✓☺ **$$$ Repairwear Deep Wrinkle Concentrate for Face and Eyes** *($55 for 1.4 ounces)* lists 72 ingredients, so it's reasonable to suppose that at least a few of them might be helpful for your skin—yet how much of any one ingredient is actually in here in a level that is beneficial for skin is questionable. After all, the contents can only add up to 100%.

Claiming to deal with "wrinkles at their base" and to "jump-start natural collagen production," this anti-aging product is one many baby-boomer consumers will take seriously. Despite the somewhat misleading claims (shared by dozens of other products), this product is as state-of-the-art as it gets. What is remarkable is the elegant formula. Just as advanced as most of Clinique's Repairwear products that aren't packaged in jars, its formula includes effective and abundant antioxidants, skin-identical ingredients, cell-communicating ingredients, potent anti-irritants, fatty acids, plant oil, and smoothing film-forming agents. It really is a brilliant formula that has the potential to significantly improve the health and appearance of skin. Will it vanquish wrinkles? No, at least not those related to years of unprotected sun exposure. But it will help skin help itself to an improved, smoothed appearance, thus making earlier damage less apparent. That is reason enough to highly recommend this fragrance-free product. One more comment: The serum texture makes this a suitable product for oily skin looking to benefit from topical antioxidants without making skin feel slick or too moist.

☹ **$$$ Repairwear Intensive Eye Cream** *($38.50 for 0.5 ounce)* has a lot going for it in terms of its plentiful antioxidant content—that's why the choice of jar packaging was a bad one, because these ingredients won't remain potent once the product is opened and used repeatedly. It's a good emollient eye cream for dry skin, but opaque tube packaging would have made it a slam-dunk.

☹ **$$$ Repairwear Intensive Night Cream** *($47.50 for 1.7 ounces)* supposedly "works all night to help block and mend the look of lines and wrinkles" and "rebuilds stores of firming natural collagen." But one could argue that mending the appearance of wrinkles is what any moisturizer can do, making this only another meaningless, albeit on the surface enticing, cosmetics claim. It would be splendid if that were true, but there is no way this moisturizer can accomplish these tasks. As is the case with many other Clinique moisturizers, this is an elegant formulation that covers all the bases when it comes to a modern combination of emollients, skin-identical ingredients, antioxidants, and cell-communicating ingredients—yet the effectiveness of several of those ingredients is compromised due to the jar packaging. This does contain a jasmine oil–derived fragrance in the form of methyldihydrojasmonate, which refutes Clinique's 100% fragrance-free assertion.

☹ **$$$ Repairwear Intensive Night Cream Very Dry Skin Formula** *($47.50 for 1.7 ounces)* is a richer, creamier version of the Repairwear Intensive Night Cream above, and the same basic comments apply. This product's jar packaging won't allow "24-hour antioxidant protection" as claimed. And besides, I wonder how they determined that, given that we don't know with certainty how long topically applied antioxidants can protect skin.

✓☺ **$$$ Repairwear Intensive Night Lotion** *($47.50 for 1.7 ounces)* is a lighter version of the Repairwear Intensive Night Cream above. This water- and silicone-based formula contains a minimal amount of thickening agents, so it's preferred for normal to slightly oily skin. The numerous antioxidants are well-served by this product's packaging, and although it's pricier than some Clinique moisturizers with similar formulas, it beats several department-store moisturizers that cost two to three times as much. It does contain fragrance in the form of methyldihydrojasmonate.

☹ **$$$ Zero Gravity Repairwear Lift Firming Cream, for Combination Oily to Oily Skin** *($52.50 for 1.7 ounces)* promises an instant firming sensation but a sensation isn't the same as an actual result, and about all this moisturizer will do instantly is make skin feel smoother and softer. That won't help skin stand up to gravity's downward assault, but then again, no skin-care product can do that. As is true for most of Clinique moisturizers, this is loaded with antioxidants, cell-communicating ingredients (including retinol), and ingredients that mimic the structure and function of healthy skin. The problem with this product it twofold: jar packaging won't keep the buzz-worthy ingredient stable during use and the inclusion of alcohol (it's the sixth ingredient) prior to any antioxidant is a letdown because alcohol causes free-radical damage. Considering the price and aforementioned detriments, this moisturizer is a tough sell. The mineral pigments in this product lend a soft glow to skin.

☹ **$$$ Zero Gravity Repairwear Lift Firming Cream, for Dry Combination Skin** *($52.50 for 1.7 ounces)* makes the same claims as the Zero Gravity Repairwear Lift Firming Cream, for Combination Oily to Oily Skin above, but omits the alcohol and contains several thickeners to create a creamier texture suitable for normal to dry skin (not combination skin, assuming part of this combination includes oily areas). It's still unfortunate that so many light- and air-sensitive ingredients are prone to breaking down quickly once this jar-packaged moisturizer is opened.

☹ **$$$ Zero Gravity Repairwear Lift Firming Cream, for Very Dry to Dry Skin** *($52.50 for 1.7 ounces)* has a surprisingly lighter texture than the Zero Gravity Repairwear Lift Firming Cream, for Dry Combination Skin above, despite being labeled for very dry skin. The glycerin, plant oil, and emollient thickeners are certainly capable of making any degree of dry skin look and feel better, but the state-of-the-art efficacious ingredients (numerous antioxidants and several cell-communicating ingredients, including retinol) won't last for long once this jar-packaged moisturizer is opened. It is doubtful their presence in this product will stimulate collagen production even a little; in stable packaging, that would be another story.

☹ **$$$ Repairwear Intensive Lip Treatment** *($25 for 0.14 ounce)* functions as a soft spackle for lines on and around the lips. The very thick, lipstick-style balm has several emollients to condition lips, and also contains film-forming agents and waxes that temporarily fill in lines. The addition of peppermint may make you think the product is doing something special, but it's just especially irritating, which isn't great for routine use. Smaller amounts of antioxidants and cell-communicating ingredients are included, but not enough to justify the cost or make this a revolutionary treatment for lip lines.

OTHER CLINIQUE PRODUCTS

☺ **$$$ Comforting Cream Cleanser** *($17.50 for 5 ounces)* is an excellent, lotion-type cleanser for normal to dry skin that is close to being water-soluble, but still requires the use of a washcloth for complete removal. This would be an option for normal to dry or sensitive skin, and it is truly fragrance and irritant-free. Clinique claims you can tissue this off, but is anyone still using tissues to remove their cleanser? If they are, they should stop!

☹ **Extremely Gentle Cleansing Cream** *($26 for 10 ounces)* is standard-issue cold cream and is recommended only for very dry skin not prone to breakouts. It removes makeup easily but also leaves skin feeling greasy and coated.

☹ **Facial Soap Extra Mild** *($11.50 for a 5.2-ounce bar with dish; $10.50 refill)* may be mild, but it's still standard bar soap and as such can be needlessly drying and irritating to skin.

If you prefer bar cleansers, Dove's original Beauty Bar ($8.99 for 6 bars) is actually a better formulation.

☹ **Facial Soap Mild** *($11.50 for a 5.2-ounce bar with dish; $10.50 refill)* is a less emollient version of the Facial Soap Extra Mild above, and the same review applies.

☹ **Facial Soap Oily** *($11.50 for a 5.2-ounce bar with dish; $10.50 refill)* contains a high amount of menthol and sodium borate, both of which are irritating to skin.

☹ **Foaming Mousse Cleanser** *($19.50 for 4.2 ounces)* is a liquid-to-foam cleanser containing potassium-based cleansing agents that give this seemingly benign cleanser a pH of 9, which is way too alkaline for any skin type because it can cause unnecessary dryness and a tight feeling, similar to what you get from bar soap. What a shame, because this simple formulation leaves out many of the irritants (such as lemon and pine) found in other Clinique cleansers.

✓ ☺ **Liquid Facial Soap Extra Mild** *($14.50 for 6.7 ounces)* is not necessarily water-soluble due to its oil content, but it is an excellent option for someone with dry to very dry skin. A true lotion cleanser, it does not contain any detergent cleansing agents, and so is actually a smart choice for someone with sensitive or easily irritated skin (and infinitely better for skin than any of Clinique's bar soaps). The oil content helps dissolve makeup, including mascara, but you'll need a washcloth for complete removal. One nice touch is the anti-irritants, although they are not as beneficial here as they are in leave-on products.

✓ ☺ **Liquid Facial Soap Mild Formula** *($14.50 for 6.7 ounces)* is a standard, but good, water-soluble cleanser for normal to slightly dry or slightly oily skin. Despite its name, it is completely soap-free, and contains gentle but effective detergent cleansing agents and skin-smoothing skin-identical ingredients to prevent skin from feeling dry or tight. It is also completely fragrance-free and does a good job removing makeup.

☹ **Liquid Facial Soap Oily Skin Formula** *($14.50 for 6.7 ounces)* is similar to the Liquid Facial Soap Mild Formula above, but loses points for the senseless inclusion of menthol. This irritant has no benefit for skin, oily or not. What a shame, because without the menthol this would have been a slam-dunk recommendation for normal to oily skin.

☹ **Rinse-Off Foaming Cleanser** *($17.50 for 5 ounces)* produces copious, creamy foam, but the potassium-based cleansing agents can be drying for most skin types, and the inclusion of eucalyptus, pine, lemon, and lavender make this too irritating for everyone and unsuitable for use around the eyes.

☺ **$$$ Take the Day Off Cleansing Balm** *($26 for 3.8 ounces)* is a modern-day version of a classic cleansing cream. It contains emollients and plant oil to dissolve makeup, and is capable of removing stubborn or waterproof formulas. This is best for dry to very dry skin or sensitive skin not prone to breakouts.

☺ **$$$ Take the Day Off Cleansing Milk** *($24 for 6.7 ounces)* is a silky, lightweight cleansing lotion whose solvent does dissolve makeup quickly and easily. This doesn't rinse completely without the aid of a washcloth, but is nevertheless a very gentle option for those with normal to dry, sensitive skin. It is truly fragrance-free.

☹ **Wash Away Gel Cleanser** *($17.50 for 5 ounces)* would be recommended as a very good water-soluble cleanser if it didn't contain eucalyptus, lavender, lemon, and pine—none of which have a single benefit for skin, but all of which can cause irritation.

✓ ☺ **$$$ Take the Day Off Makeup Remover for Lids, Lashes & Lips** *($16.50 for 4.2 ounces)* is a very good, silicone-in-water, dual-phase remover that makes quick work of even the most stubborn foundations, lipsticks, and waterproof mascaras. It is Clinique's most efficient makeup remover and may be used before or after cleansing.

☺ **Rinse-Off Makeup Solvent** *($14.50 for 4.2 ounces)* is a basic, no-frills eye-makeup remover that contains mild detergent cleansing agents to dissolve makeup. It does not contain extraneous ingredients that may irritate the eye.

☺ **$$$ Naturally Gentle Eye Makeup Remover** *($15.50 for 2.5 ounces)* is indeed gentle, but also oily enough to make it difficult to rinse from the eye area or eyelashes. It is an option, but Clinique's Take the Day Off Makeup Remover for Lids, Lashes & Lips above, is less messy, easier to rinse, and effectively removes all types of eye makeup. An interesting side note on this product is that it contains sialyllactose, a complex carbohydrate that is derived from human milk and urine. It's not formally listed as a cosmetic ingredient, but according to a blurb on this product in the March 2002 issue of *Allure*, sialyllactose is a sugar-based emulsifier that is a component of human tears. The idea was to add ingredients to this eye makeup remover that mimic human tears. Ironically, the sesame oil in the formula, while gentle, is assuredly not a component of natural human tears, and like any oil it can cause temporary blurred vision if it gets into the eye.

😐 **$$$ 7 Day Scrub Cream** *($16.50 for 3.5 ounces)* is an oil-based topical scrub for dry to very dry skin. It does not rinse well without the aid of a washcloth, which provides some exfoliation on its own. Still, this is a gentle option with a minimally abrasive formula that contains polyethylene beads to polish skin.

☺ **$$$ 7 Day Scrub Cream Rinse-Off Formula** *($16.50 for 3.4 ounces)* rinses better than the original 7 Day Scrub Cream above, but may still require use of a washcloth for complete removal. It also contains polyethylene as the scrub agent, and is an option for normal to slightly dry skin not prone to blemishes.

☹ **Exfoliating Scrub** *($16.50 for 3.4 ounces)* is Clinique's most abrasive topical scrub and also its most irritating, thanks to menthol.

☹ **Clarifying Lotion 1** *($11 for 6.7 ounces)* lists alcohol as the second ingredient, and that makes this toner too irritating for all skin types.

☹ **Clarifying Lotion 2** *($11 for 6.7 ounces)* is an alcohol-based toner that also contains witch hazel and menthol. The Clinique salespeople may claim that the alcohol is "cosmetics-grade," which sounds nice but doesn't make this product any less irritating.

☹ **Clarifying Lotion 3** *($11 for 6.7 ounces)* is similar to Clarifying Lotion 2, but with less alcohol and no menthol. It's still way too irritating and drying, even for oily skin.

☹ **Clarifying Lotion 4** *($11 for 6.7 ounces)* is nearly identical to Clarifying Lotion 3, and the same review applies.

☺ **Mild Clarifying Lotion** *($11 for 6.7 ounces)* puts all of Clinique's other Clarifying Lotions to shame with its alcohol-free formula that contains 0.5% salicylic acid at an effective pH of 2.9. Although a higher concentration of salicylic acid would be more effective for someone battling blemishes and blackheads, this is a step in the right direction and contains some very good skin-identical ingredients.

☺ **$$$ Moisture Surge Face Spray Thirsty Skin Relief** *($19.50 for 4.2 ounces)* is a very good spray-on, alcohol-free toner. This is a good choice for all skin types, including oily or blemish-prone skin that has minor dry patches.

😐 **$$$ Total Turnaround Visible Skin Renewer** *($32.50 for 1.7 ounces)* cannot exfoliate skin because the amount of salicylic acid is too small and the pH of the product is too high. It's an option for someone with normal to slightly oily skin looking for a silky, lightweight moisturizer. It's unfortunate the antioxidants are diminished by jar packaging, but the cell-communicating ingredients will fare better. The mica and titanium dioxide lend a radiant finish to this moisturizer; but be sure you like this before applying it over shine-prone areas.

✓☺ **$$$ Turnaround Concentrate Visible Skin Renewer** *($36.50 for 1 ounce)* contains what Clinique refers to as "an advanced cocktail of exfoliants," but the only ingredient that has substantiated research behind it to support that claim is salicylic acid. Although present in this silky-smooth lotion at approximately 1%, the pH of 5 limits its ability to exfoliate. Clinique has taken a cue from parent company Estee Lauder and included acetyl glucosamine, which they believe is an effective non-acid exfoliating agent, although there is still no substantiated research proving this ingredient's effectiveness as an alternative to AHA or BHA exfoliants. It does have excellent water-binding properties for skin, and complements the other skin-beneficial ingredients in this product quite well. Although this product won't "renew" skin, it is an outstanding, well-packaged, lightweight moisturizer that contains several antioxidants, vitamins, cell-communicating ingredients, and anti-irritants. It is fragrance-free and best suited for those with normal to oily skin. Fans of Estee Lauder's Idealist ($46.50 for 1 ounce) take note: Turnaround Concentrate Visible Skin Renewer is incredibly similar, right down to its light texture and silky finish.

✓☺ **$$$ Advanced Stop Signs** *($38.50 for 1.7 ounces)* is a very good, antioxidant-rich, stably packaged serum for all skin types. It isn't quite as impressive as the Repairwear Deep Wrinkle Concentrate for Face and Eyes above, but is still worthy of a Paula's Pick rating. Clinique maintains this serum contains a "cluster-buster" complex to break apart and discourage the emergence of dark spots, but there aren't enough such ingredients in this product to make that promise a reality. This does contain coloring agents and the mica casts a subtle glow.

☺ **$$$ Advanced Stop Signs Eye Preventive Cream SPF 15** *($32.50 for 0.5 ounce)* is a creamy, initially greasy-feeling moisturizer that contains zinc oxide as its primary sunscreen agent, a gentle choice for use around the sensitive eye area. There is a synthetic sunscreen agent also, but the small amount should not be a problem for use near the eyes. While the zinc oxide leaves a slight whitish cast on the skin, this can be considered a benefit because it creates a brightening effect under the eye that can soften the appearance of dark circles.

Beyond the sunscreen, the moisturizing base for this elegant formula contains several emollients and skin-identical ingredients. There's also a range of antioxidants (in greater amounts than in the original version of this eye cream), but the jar packaging won't keep them stable once the product is opened. This is still a good option for those with normal to dry skin, or someone with oily skin experiencing dryness around the eyes. Although it is not necessary to purchase a separate sunscreen for the eye area, if your favorite sunscreen tends to cause stinging or burning when applied near the eye area, a product like this one may be the solution. Despite the claims made for this product, Advanced Stop Signs Eye SPF 15 won't make an existing wrinkle revert back to smooth, unlined skin, but it absolutely can reduce the risk of future wrinkles (to some extent) and shield skin from further environmental damage.

☺ **$$$ All About Eyes** *($27.50 for 0.5 ounce)* is one of Clinique's most popular items, and its silicone-based formula leaves skin very smooth and silky. It contains some outstanding ingredients to fortify skin and allow it to repair itself, but many of these are compromised by packaging that exposes them to light and air. Clever cosmetic pigment technology changes the way light is reflected off shadowed areas, temporarily improving the appearance of dark circles (sort of like a concealer but without coverage).

☺ **$$$ All About Eyes Rich** *($27.50 for 0.5 ounce)* is an emollient version of the All About Eyes above, but unlike that product, whose silkiness is largely due to its silicone base, All About

Eyes Rich contains several emollients, chiefly shea butter. It is indeed a moisture-rich product and is preferred for dry to very dry skin around the eyes or elsewhere on the face. It cannot diminish dark circles or puffy eyes as claimed. The usual roster of antioxidants, anti-irritants, and ingredients that mimic the structure and function of healthy skin are present, but the antioxidants won't remain potent for long given the jar packaging. The packaging keeps it from earning a higher rating, but this is still an unquestionably emollient moisturizer, even though its base formula doesn't contain anything that's exclusively "all about eyes."

😐 **$$$ Anti-Gravity Firming Eye Lift Cream** *($32.50 for 0.5 ounce)* is a good emollient moisturizer for dry skin anywhere on the face, but its formula isn't as elegant as that of All About Eyes Rich above. Jar packaging brings this product's score down considerably, and to boot the overall formula has fewer antioxidants than many Clinique moisturizers. None of the ingredients in this product has a special ability to firm or lift eye-area skin, though the product's name implies otherwise.

😐 **$$$ Anti-Gravity Firming Lift Cream** *($39.50 for 1.7 ounces)* purports to lift and firm skin instantly and over time. (Why would it need to do that over time if it does so right away?) It can't do that, of course, but it is a reliable moisturizer for normal to dry skin. It contains several cell-communicating ingredients as well as antioxidants, but their effectiveness is limited by jar packaging.

☺ **$$$ City Block Sheer Oil-Free Daily Face Protector SPF 15** *($15.50 for 1.4 ounces)* is worth a look by those with sensitive or rosacea-afflicted skin that's normal to slightly dry. This lightweight moisturizer contains a blend of titanium dioxide and zinc oxide for sun protection, and has a sheer tint that's cosmetically pleasing. It also contains some good cell-communicating ingredients and antioxidants, but not as much as the Super City Block SPF 25 (reviewed below).

☺ **$$$ City Block Sheer Oil-Free Daily Face Protector SPF 25** *($16.50 for 1.4 ounces)* is similar to the City Block Sheer Oil-Free Daily Face Protector SPF 15 above, with the major difference being that this one contains higher amounts of titanium dioxide and zinc oxide to achieve its SPF rating. Otherwise, the same comments made for the SPF 15 version apply here, too.

CLINIQUE CONTINUOUS RESCUE ANTIOXIDANT MOISTURIZERS

All of the moisturizers below claim to provide consistent protection from free-radical damage. Although each product contains an impressive array of antioxidants, they don't eliminate free-radical damage, they just reduce the problem in a limited but needed manner. Topical application of antioxidants is a major part of taking the best possible care of your skin, but at most they work to minimize, not eradicate, free-radical damage. Perhaps this proves that Clinique is finally taking the issue of stable packaging seriously. Almost all of their moisturizers contain lots of antioxidants, but most of them are packaged in jars that compromise their effectiveness once the product is opened. All of the Continuous Rescue moisturizers are packaged in opaque tubes, which is excellent.

✓☺ **$$$ Continuous Rescue Antioxidant Moisturizer Combination/Oily to Oily** *($39.50 for 1.7 ounces)*. This version is suitable for combination skin, but is too heavy for oily skin or oily areas. It contains some great emollients, silicone, slip agents, Vaseline, several antioxidants, cell-communicating ingredients, and soothing plant extracts. The only frustrating element is that half of the really intriguing ingredients are listed after one of the preservatives, meaning they're basically window dressing rather than being efficacious. However, even without dustings of those ingredients, this fragrance-free moisturizer can still be considered antioxidant-packed, and it is recommended for normal to slightly dry or slightly oily skin.

✓☺ **$$$ Continuous Rescue Antioxidant Moisturizer Dry/Combination** *($39.50 for 1.7 ounces)* is well suited for dry skin or combination skin with dry areas, but is too emollient for use over oily or breakout-prone areas. It is an outstanding blend of water, silicone, thickeners, shea butter, fatty acids, glycerin, antioxidants (in greater quantity than the version for Combination/Oily Skin above), cell-communicating ingredients, and skin-identical ingredients. In short, this fragrance-free moisturizer takes advantage of what solid research has shown is necessary to create a truly state-of-the-art moisturizer. Well done, Clinique!

✓☺ **$$$ Continuous Rescue Antioxidant Moisturizer Very Dry to Dry** *($39.50 for 1.7 ounces)* is the richest of the three Continuous Rescue Antioxidant Moisturizers, and is appropriate for dry to very dry skin. Interestingly, this version contains greater amounts of antioxidants known for their potent anti-inflammatory effect. That attention to detail can help dry skin repair itself because the less inflammation skin endures, the better able it is to strengthen itself and repair damage. Some of the intriguing ingredients aren't present in amounts large enough for skin to take advantage of, but there are enough bells and whistles in this moisturizer to compensate for that.

The Reviews C

☺ **Dramatically Different Moisturizing Gel in Tube** *($11.50 for 1.7 ounces)*. Talk about a long time coming! Well past the time when Clinique clearly knew Dramatically Different Moisturizing Lotion wasn't dramatically different in the least, they still recommended their poorly formulated lotion as an essential skin-care step in their famous three-step routine. Although the original lotion remains a mundane, not-as-good-as-Lubriderm option for normal to dry skin, it is and always has been ill-suited for those dealing with oiliness or breakouts. Therefore, for those loyal to Clinique's basic regimen and for those looking for a more affordable department-store moisturizer, Dramatically Different Moisturizing Gel is a welcome addition. The formula is more a lotion than a gel, but does feel quite light and silky on the skin. It does not contain any oils or heavy thickening agents, and this fragrance-free moisturizer is appropriate for normal to slightly dry or slightly oily skin. The only issue I have with the product is its meager antioxidant content (though it has some great anti-irritants). Most of Clinique's moisturizers are brimming with state-of-the-art ingredients, but this one, though certainly effective for its intended skin types, is plain by comparison—yet dramatically better than their original and still incredibly popular lotion (reviewed below).

😐 **Dramatically Different Moisturizing Lotion** *($11.50 for 1.7 ounces)* is the same as it always was: a basic, mundane, out-of-date, yellow-toned moisturizer built around mineral and sesame oils. It's an option for dry skin and is fragrance-free, but, other than its cheap price tag, there is nothing else attractive or beneficial about this product.

😐 **$$$ Exceptionally Soothing Cream for Upset Skin** *($32.50 for 1.7 ounces)* used to contain an over-the-counter amount of hydrocortisone. Perhaps Clinique reformulated it because customers weren't willing to pay so much for an active they could get at the drugstore for around $5, or maybe it was because repeated use of cortisone thins skin and breaks down collagen. This jar-packaged moisturizer contains some very good soothing agents and skin-friendly emollients to ease dryness, but the antioxidants are exposed to air on first use, leaving them ineffective shortly thereafter. Looking past that, this cream is an option for normal to dry skin.

✓☺ **$$$ Moisture In-Control Oil-Free Lotion** *($35 for 1.7 ounces)* makes the tempting claim of being able to control shine in oily areas while depositing moisturizing ingredients over your dry zones. There is no way a moisturizer can "sense" where skin is oily and where it's dry and then adjust the deposit of ingredients accordingly. Where this product excels is in its blend of lightweight slip agents and dry-finish ingredients that won't feel or look greasy. It also contains some exceptional cell-communicating ingredients and lesser but still impressive amounts of antioxidants. Consider it a winner for normal to oily skin or for use over slightly dry areas on breakout-prone skin.

😐 **$$$ Moisture On-Call** *($35 for 1.6 ounces)* contains mostly water, plant oil, thickener, slip agent, shea butter, silicone, antioxidants, cholesterol, cell-communicating ingredients, anti-irritant, film-forming agent, more thickeners, preservatives, and coloring agents. It's a well-formulated moisturizer for normal to dry skin not prone to breakouts, but the jar packaging spells certain doom for the light- and air-sensitive ingredients, diminishing if not completely eliminating their benefit for skin.

😐 **$$$ Moisture On-Line** *($35 for 1.7 ounces)* has a silkier, less oily, but more substantial feel than Moisture On-Call above, but lacks the same complement of cell-communicating ingredients and antioxidants. That's not a big loss because the jar packaging won't keep most of these ingredients stable. This is an OK option for normal to dry skin. By the way, this product's claim to trigger skin's ability to build and hold moisture can be attributed to any well-formulated moisturizer.

✓☺ **$$$ Moisture Surge Extra Refreshing Eye Gel** *($26 for 0.5 ounce)* is a silky, extremely well-formulated gel moisturizer for slightly dry skin around the eyes or elsewhere. It contains a hefty array of antioxidants, a couple of cell-communicating ingredients, and proven skin-identical ingredients. This would also be a brilliant option for moisturizing dry patches on acne-prone skin because the product's texture makes it unlikely to clog pores.

😐 **$$$ Moisture Surge Extra Thirsty Skin Relief** *($32 for 1.7 ounces)* has a beautifully silky texture and smooth finish, but jar packaging renders most of the state-of-the-art ingredients ineffective after the product is opened. It is best for normal to slightly oily skin.

☺ **Skin Texture Lotion Oil-Free Formula** *($22.50 for 1.25 ounces)* is one of Clinique's older moisturizers, but it still has potential for normal to slightly dry or slightly oily skin. While not brimming with state-of-the-art ingredients, it does have its fair share of antioxidants, a nice blend of anti-irritants, and good skin-identical ingredients, all in stable packaging.

✓☺ **Super City Block Oil-Free Daily Face Protector SPF 25** *($16.50 for 1.4 ounces)* combines an all–titanium dioxide sunscreen with a creamy moisturizing base that's chock-full of antioxidants and that also includes a cell-communicating ingredient. This gentle formula is ideal for those with sensitive skin, including those with rosacea. It is too rich for those prone to blemishes, but can be used by any skin type as an eye-area sunscreen. Super City Block has a sheer tint that goes on translucent, thus preventing the titanium dioxide from creating a whitish coloration on skin.

☺ **Super City Block Oil-Free Daily Face Protector SPF 40** *($16.50 for 1.4 ounces)* is nearly identical to the Derma White Super City Block SPF 40 above, and the same review applies. Why the Derma White version costs several dollars more is a good question.

😐 **$$$ Superdefense Triple Action Moisturizer SPF 25, for Normal to Oily Skin** *($39.50 for 1.7 ounces)* has a great name and is sold with the tagline "makes SPF alone seem almost primitive." I assume what Clinique means is that today we know so much about how skin functions and the role sun damage plays in hurting healthy skin that we recognize it takes more than just standard active ingredients to protect and restore skin. If this was their intention, then I agree!

That's because, given what we now know about antioxidants, anti-inflammatory agents, and barrier-repair ingredients, and the way their presence in sunscreens can make them even more effective on skin, it's a good idea to examine sunscreens beyond what's in their active ingredient list. This particular product is another winner for sunscreen, featuring an in-part avobenzone sunscreen in a light, silky feeling lotion base suitable for normal to oily skin.

According to information in the September 30, 2004, issue of the cosmetics industry newsletter *The Rose Sheet*, the sunscreens in all of Clinique's Superdefense moisturizers are "contained in a floating polymer matrix" to prevent skin irritation. This technology, which is relatively new, potentially can prevent active ingredients from penetrating the skin, which can lead to irritation. Studies of products that combine UVA-protecting actives, such as avobenzone and octinoxate (both used in Clinique's Superdefense products), with various silicone ingredients showed mixed results. In some trials, the silicones slowed the penetration of the actives (thus reducing the potential for a sensitizing reaction), but other trials noted accelerated penetration of the actives, indicating that the specific type of silicone emulsion included must be carefully coordinated with the specific active ingredients (Source: *Journal of Cosmetic Science*, November–December 2004, pages 509–518).

Whether or not Clinique has succeeded in their efforts to create a gentler sunscreen remains to be seen. Further, this technology cannot guarantee that you won't react negatively to one or more of the active ingredients—or potentially to other ingredients in the product—because there are so many other factors that come into play, such as what your skin is sensitive to. Although Clinique deserves commendation for combining effective sunscreen and several antioxidants in a cosmetically elegant product, their choice of jar packaging renders them ineffective shortly after the product is opened, and keeps this from earning a higher rating.

😐 **$$$ Superdefense Triple Action Moisturizer SPF 25, for Normal to Dry Skin** *($39.50 for 1.7 ounces)* shares all of the positive traits (and has the same packaging issue) as the Superdefense Triple Action Moisturizer SPF 25, for Normal to Oily Skin above, except the base formula is an emollient blend appropriate for normal to dry skin. The silicone and petrolatum mix is a great way to get the benefits of both ingredients because the silicone's drier finish helps offset the greasy feel of the petrolatum. Both are excellent for protecting the skin's barrier and preventing moisture loss due to environmental conditions.

😐 **$$$ Superdefense Triple Action Moisturizer SPF 25, for Very Dry Skin** *($39.50 for 1.7 ounces)* shares all of the positive traits (and has the same packaging issue) as the Superdefense Triple Action Moisturizer SPF 25, for Normal to Oily Skin above, except its base formula is preferred for normal to very dry skin. This is slightly more emollient than the Superdefense for Normal to Dry Skin moisturizer above.

☺ **Anti-Gravity Firming Lift Mask** *($22.50 for 3.4 ounces)*. Can a facial mask stop gravity or create firmer, lifted skin? Not even Clinique appears to think so, because the claims for this product make no direct reference to defying gravity or lifting sagging skin other than in the name. Clinique does maintain that regular use of this mask will "erase the look of lines," but any well-formulated moisturizer can (temporarily) do that. After all, we're only talking about the "look of lines," not the lines themselves, which will still be there regardless of how often you use this product. Anti-Gravity Firming Lift Mask is a creamy concoction that contains mostly water, emollient, slip agent, plant oil, several thickeners, antioxidants, anti-irritants, and preservatives, plus mica for a "glow" effect on the skin. This also contains sandalwood extract, which definitely imparts fragrance but has no other significant benefit.

☹ **Deep Cleansing Emergency Mask** *($19.50 for 3.4 ounces)* is a standard clay mask that also contains absorbent cornstarch and an ineffective amount of salicylic acid. The menthol doesn't help and makes this not worth considering over several other clay masks.

😐 **$$$ Turnaround 15-Minute Facial** *($34.50 for 2.5 ounces)* has a formula that's remarkably similar to the Turnaround Concentrate Visible Skin Renewer above. Both contain several forms of silicones, which add significantly to each product's texture and application. Both products also contain acetyl glucosamine, though as mentioned above it shouldn't be relied on for exfoliation, and both products contain salicylic acid. Turnaround 15-Minute Facial is said to deliver the "radiance and smoothness of microdermabrasion with significantly less irritation and stress." This viscous gel-cream does indeed make skin look smooth and radiant, but the way it accomplishes that is as far removed from microdermabrasion as salmon is from a chocolate chip cookie. The silicones and skin-identical ingredients in this product do smooth and plump skin, and the smoother skin is, the better it reflects light, thus appearing more radiant. Nothing in this "facial," however, approximates what happens during a microdermabrasion procedure, where skin is mechanically "polished" using different materials and a controlled device. The amount of salicylic acid is too low (less than 0.5%) to exfoliate skin, though the product's pH of 4 would have allowed that to occur if more salicylic acid were used. Consider this product if you are looking for a uniquely textured mask to treat normal to dry skin. The neutral face rating applies because this antioxidant-rich product is packaged in a jar, which will make the air-sensitive ingredients ineffective shortly after you open it.

☺ **$$$ All About Lips** *($20 for 0.41 ounce)* theoretically smooths and fills in superficial lip lines and lines around the mouth with silicones and film-former, but I would test this out before spending the money. Even if it does have an impact, which is merely temporary and quickly undone if you follow with lipstick or gloss (the product's performance largely depends on leaving it undisturbed), it will be convincing only for the most superficial of lines. This also contains salicylic acid, but not in an amount that will exfoliate skin around the mouth—and it is too drying for use on lips. Still, kudos to Clinique for creating a product like this without adding menthol or other irritants.

☺ **$$$ Moisture Stick** *($14.50 for 0.14 ounce)* is a castor oil–based clear lipstick that nicely takes care of dry, chapped lips. You don't have to spend this much to relieve chapped lips, but this does the job without fragrance or flavoring.

CLINIQUE SUN & SELF-TANNING PRODUCTS

☹ **After-Sun Rescue Balm** *($17.50 for 5 ounces)* contains eucalyptus and peppermint, which make this lightweight moisturizer too irritating for all skin types, and especially for skin that has spent too much time in the sun. What a shame, because there are several good antioxidants in this product.

☺ **Sun-Care Body Gel SPF 15 Sunscreen** *($17.50 for 5 ounces)* has an in-part avobenzone sunscreen in a lightweight, alcohol-free gel base. The formula includes several antioxidants, though not as much of them as in most of Clinique's facial moisturizers with sunscreen. Still, this is a very good option for normal to oily skin, and it is water-resistant.

☺ **Sun-Care Body SPF 25 Sun Block** *($17.50 for 3.4 ounces)* contains only titanium dioxide and zinc oxide as the active ingredients, making it suitable for sensitive or rosacea-prone skin that is normal to dry and not prone to breakouts. The amount of antioxidants isn't wholly impressive, but some is better than none! This sunscreen is water-resistant.

☹ **Sun-Care Body Spray SPF 15 Sun Block** *($17.50 for 5 ounces)* includes avobenzone for UVA protection, but its base formula is mainly alcohol, and the ingredient methyl hydrogenated rosin can cause contact dermatitis.

☹ **Sun-Care Body Spray SPF 30 Sun Block** *($17.50 for 5 ounces)* is similar to the Sun-Care Body Spray SPF 15 Sun Block above, save for the higher percentage of active ingredients needed to make an SPF 30 claim. Otherwise, the same review applies.

☺ **$$$ Sun-Care Lip/Eye SPF 30 Sun Block** *($16.50 for 0.21 ounce)* contains titanium dioxide and zinc oxide along with several synthetic sunscreen agents to create a water-resistant, moisturizing sunscreen stick. The amount of active ingredients makes this a potentially risky product to use near the eyes, but it's a great "spot sunscreen" for exposed scalp, tops of ears, and lips. Two forms of vitamin E serve as antioxidants.

☺ **Sun-Care UV-Response Body Cream SPF 30** *($17.50 for 5 ounces)* features an in-part avobenzone sunscreen in a silky, silicone-enhanced base that's water-resistant. Several antioxidants are included, but none in significant amounts. This is a good option for normal to dry skin from the neck down.

✓☺ **Sun-Care UV-Response Face Cream SPF 30** *($17.50 for 1.7 ounces)* is the face version of the Sun-Care UV-Response Body Cream SPF 30 above. It has a slightly lighter texture and greater amount of antioxidants for the always-exposed face, and is a great option for normal to slightly oily skin. This formula is water-resistant.

☺ **Sun-Care UV-Response Body Cream SPF 50** *($18.50 for 5 ounces)* contains avobenzone for sufficient UVA protection and almost 28% active ingredients to achieve its high SPF rating. That makes this sunscreen potentially irritating but still worth considering for longer days in the sun, assuming you reapply after swimming, perspiring, or toweling off. The base formula contains some very good skin-identical ingredients, antioxidants, and a cell-communicating ingredient. And it looks as though the FDA is becoming amenable to sunscreens rated above SPF 50, though keep in mind the higher SPF ratings are about longer, not better, protection.

✓☺ **Sun-Care UV-Response Face Cream SPF 50** *($15.50 for 1.7 ounces)* is similar to the Sun-Care UV-Response Body Cream SPF 50 above, but this facial version contains more cell-communicating ingredients and a greater array of antioxidants. It is best for normal to slightly oily skin.

✓☺ **Self-Sun Body Quick Bronze Self-Tanner** *($17 for 4.2 ounces)* maintains the status Quo of self-tanning products, containing the same ingredient found in almost all of them, dihydroxyacetone. However, with its silky lotion base this one goes beyond standard by including some good water-binding and soothing agents, making it a cut above most others.

☹ **Self-Sun Body Quick Bronze Tinted Self-Tanner Mousse** *($17.50 for 5 ounces)* contains dihydroxyacetone to turn skin color over time, and is caramel-tinted for instant gratification (and so you'll notice missed spots). It also contains black walnut leaf extract, a plant whose high tannin content can have constricting properties on skin (Source: www.naturaldatabase.com), which makes this a self-tanner to skip.

☹ **Self-Sun Body Self-Tanning Lotion** *($17 for 4.2 ounces)* contains irritating fragrant extracts of coriander, lavender, sage, and cardamom, making this otherwise good self-tanner not worth using over countless others.

✓☺ **Self-Sun Face Quick Bronze Tinted Self-Tanner** *($17 for 1.7 ounces)* is nearly identical to the Self-Sun Body Quick Bronze Self-Tanner above, and the same review applies. There is no reason the body version cannot be used on the face.

☹ **Self-Sun Face Self-Tanning Formula** *($17 for 1.7 ounces)* isn't worth considering over other self-tanners from Clinique or other lines; several turn skin bronze without the potential irritation from the fragrant extracts (including cell-damaging lavender) that are present in this product.

☹ **Self-Sun Radiant Bronze Face & Body Tinted Self-Tanner SPF 15** *($17.50 for 4.2 ounces)* lacks the UVA-protecting ingredients of titanium dioxide, zinc oxide, avobenzone, Tinosorb, or Mexoryl SX, and is not recommended. Used indoors as a self-tanner, this product contains the same ingredient found in almost all self-tanners: dihydroxyacetone.

CLINIQUE MAKEUP

FOUNDATION: ✓ ☺ $$$ Perfectly Real Makeup *($22.50)* is a near-perfect choice for those who want a smooth, lightweight foundation that fulfills its promise of looking as natural as possible. This foundation has a slightly creamy texture that quickly morphs into a soft matte finish once it's blended. Clinique states that Perfectly Real Makeup "feels like nothing at all." It isn't quite that light—you will notice it's there—but your skin will look improved without appearing made-up. It provides sheer to light coverage, so you still need a concealer for red spots or dark circles. The matte finish makes this product preferable for normal to oily skin. It can definitely exaggerate any dry spots, so it's important for your skin to be completely smooth before application. There are 20 shades, and almost all are gorgeous, neutral options with no strong overtones of peach, pink, ash, or rose. The only shades to consider avoiding are 28, 34, and 36, each of which can be too peach for their intended skin tones. There are options for very light skin, as well as some beautiful darker shades, but watch out for shades 46 and 50, which have a slight tendency to turn ashy on the skin.

✓ ☺ **$$$ Perfectly Real Compact Makeup** *($22.50)* is a talc-based pressed-powder foundation with wow-factor silkiness. It glides over skin and doesn't look the least bit heavy, even when applied with the included sponge. Those with normal to slightly dry or oily skin will enjoy the smooth matte finish and light, buildable coverage. Much like the Perfectly Real Makeup above, the range of 20 shades is brilliant. Those with fair to medium skin will find neutral option after neutral option. The only potential problem shades are 116 (too yellow), 120 (slightly peach), and the darkest shade, 148, which looks slightly ash for the depth of its intended skin tone. Your skin won't look "believably perfect," but will look even and polished. A caveat: Those with melasma or rosacea will likely want more coverage than this foundation provides, but its texture is so light it could be brushed over a medium- to full-coverage liquid foundation without detriment.

✓☺ **$$$ Superbalanced Compact Makeup SPF 20** *($26.50; $19.50 for refills)* is a beautiful cream-to-powder foundation with a brilliant in-part zinc oxide sunscreen. As with all cream-to-powders, this is best for someone with normal to slightly oily skin. The matte, slightly powdery finish of Superbalanced Compact Makeup SPF 20 will magnify any dry areas, so if that's an issue be sure to moisturize before application. This foundation blends easily and builds from sheer to medium coverage that does not appear heavy. Its soft, creamy texture sets quickly and feels very light on skin. There are 18 mostly stellar shades, including options for fair and dark (but not very dark) skin. The only shades to use caution with are Cream (can be too yellow), Warm Buff, Sunny (both slightly peach), Honeycomb (can turn orange), and Cream Chamois (slightly peach). Although it cannot make good on its claim to control oil and hydrate dry areas, this is still an exceptional choice if you prefer cream-to-powder makeup with sunscreen.

✓☺ $$$ **Dewy Smooth Antiaging Makeup SPF 15** *($21.50)* is definitely smooth, with a silky, silicone-based texture that feels amazing and blends without a hitch. Titanium dioxide is not only the sunscreen agent, but also lends an opacity that allows this makeup to provide medium to almost full coverage with a satin matte finish that feels slightly moist. This does not make skin look dewy or drenched in moisture, but it is still a great option for normal to dry skin. Beyond the sunscreen, there is nothing anti-aging about the formula. Ignore the marketing hype and you'll be left with a superior foundation that comes in nine mostly gorgeous colors for very light to dark skin. Use caution with Beige Petal, which is slightly peach. By the way, although Repairwear Anti-Aging Makeup SPF 15, reviewed below, has more bells and whistles, Dewy Smooth is much easier to blend and doesn't look as heavy, which makes it a better option.

✓☺ **Almost Makeup SPF 15** *($19.50)* is a very sheer foundation with a broad-spectrum titanium dioxide sunscreen, making it ideal for sensitive skin. It is definitely not akin to traditional foundation, and is available in four great shades, although it lacks a color for dark skin. The product's moist finish is best for normal to dry skin.

✓☺ **Superfit Makeup** *($19.50)* was originally launched as Clinique's contribution to the growing crop of ultra-matte foundations. The fact that it's still around can be attributed to its beautifully silky, weightless texture and its long-wearing, dimensional matte finish. It provides medium coverage, blends on easily, and isn't a chore to remove, though it isn't as oil-resistant as the ultra-matte finish foundations from years past. Still, the tradeoff is minor and this remains a top foundation for oily to very oily skin. Of the 16 shades, 5 are too yellow, peach, or orange for most skin tones. Avoid Vanilla, Golden Beige, Nutty, Deep Caramel, and Toffee Bronze. Shell is slightly pink, but may work for some light skin tones.

☺ $$$ **Moisture Sheer Tint SPF 15** *($26)* has a satin-smooth texture and slightly creamy application that sets to a minimally moist finish. This product is aptly named, as it provides sheer, almost nonexistent coverage. Its sunscreen is in-part titanium dioxide, but it's at a level of only 1%, which may be too low to provide sufficient UVA protection for long days outdoors. Four shades are available, and the best among them are Fair and Neutral. Beige is good but may be too yellow for medium skin tones, while Deep is marginal and has a tendency to turn orange on dark skin. All told, Moisture Sheer Tint is a good option for someone with normal to slightly dry skin seeking sheer coverage.

☺ $$$ **Repairwear Anti-Aging Makeup SPF 15** *($28.50)* continues Clinique's Repairwear lineup as the company's first makeup to feature their so-called line-blocking, line-mending technology. Lines (wrinkles) will indeed be forestalled thanks to this foundation's titanium dioxide sunscreen, but the "mending" part is open to interpretation. This makeup does contain many of the same antioxidants and skin-beneficial ingredients as Clinique's Repairwear skin-care products, but just how much such ingredients will improve wrinkles is not established. As for the makeup itself, it is incorrectly described as "luxuriously moisturizing." It has an initially creamy texture that smooths over skin, blending to a satin matte finish, but it won't thrill those with extremely dry skin, and ends up being far better for normal to moderately dry skin. Coverage is substantial, but with this level of camouflage the tradeoff is a makeup that looks (but doesn't feel) heavier on skin. It would be an excellent choice for those battling redness from rosacea. Not only are such mineral-based sunscreens extra-gentle, but also the amount of coverage they offer (when combined with pigments) will tone down excess redness—assuming you choose your shades carefully.

Clinique hit a stumbling block in regard to shades, however. Although there are some great choices among the 12 options, Porcelain Beige, Warm Golden, Sand, and Nutty are too pink, rose, peach, or yellow to recommend, so choose carefully. This foundation does not include shades for dark skin, although Alabaster is an option for fair skin.

☺ **$$$ Clarifying Powder Makeup** *($21)* is a wonderfully smooth-textured, talc-based powder foundation, especially if you have normal to oily skin. This applies impeccably and leaves a natural matte finish that looks smooth and even, rather than dry or powdery. The five shades are soft and neutral, but best for fair to medium skin only.

☺ **$$$ City Base Compact Foundation SPF 15** *($22.50)* isn't as elegant as Clinique's Superbalanced Compact Makeup SPF 20, but is a consideration for those with normal to slightly dry skin. It's a classic cream-to-powder makeup with an initially creamy application and soft powder finish that doesn't hold up well over oily areas. Except for Porcelain Beige and Almond Beige, the ten shades are excellent and would work for a wide range of skin tones, from light to dark, but not for someone with very light or very dark skin. The SPF 15 sunscreen contains titanium dioxide as the only active ingredient.

😐 **Balanced Makeup Base** *($19.50)* is Clinique's oldest foundation, and the three shades that remain are likely there to placate the consumers who just aren't ready to give this up. It is best for those with dry to very dry skin. The mineral oil–based consistency is emollient and creamy, and it applies well, leaving a natural finish. The coverage is light to medium, but I encourage you to explore Clinique's other liquid foundation options before this.

☺ **Soft Finish Makeup** *($19.50)* is quite similar to Clinique's Balanced Makeup Base above in terms of consistency and coverage, but this one has a silicone-enhanced slip and is slightly sheerer than the Balanced. It's a good foundation for normal to very dry skin but does not have a special ability to make lines and wrinkles less obvious. Of the eight shades, most are beautifully neutral. Soft Bisque is slightly peach, while Soft Porcelain is too pink, and Soft Honey should be considered with care.

☺ **Stay-True Makeup Oil-Free Formula** *($18.50)* now ranks as one of Clinique's oldest foundations, and remains a satisfactory option for those with normal to very oily skin who want an oil-absorbing matte finish. It has a slightly thick texture that blends well despite its lack of slip and it provides medium coverage. Definitely a traditional but worthwhile matte makeup, it is available in nine shades. Among those, avoid Stay Neutral, Stay Porcelain, Stay Golden, and True Bronze due to their overtones of pink or peach.

😐 **$$$ Superbalanced Makeup** *($19.50)* is Clinique's top-selling foundation worldwide (Source: www.elcompanies.com), in no small part because it claims to provide moisture and absorb oil when and where needed—a skin-care dream many women share. However, this ends up doing neither job very well. There is no way a product can differentiate between the oily parts of your face and the dry parts. The absorbent ingredients in it will soak up any oil they come in contact with (including the moisturizing ingredients in this product or in the one you applied to your skin) and the moisturizing ingredients will get deposited over areas you don't want to be moisturized. With Superbalanced Makeup, you get a silicone-in-water liquid that provides light to medium coverage with a smooth, matte-finish foundation that is best for someone with normal to slightly dry or slightly oily skin. Someone with any amount of excess oil would not be happy with the finish or with how it wears during the day. The 21 shades have been refined a bit since this foundation was last reviewed, and a few of the poor colors are gone. Still, compared to several other Clinique foundations, the palette isn't as neutral. The following colors are best avoided by most skin tones: Light, Cream Chamois, Ivory, Linen, Neutral, Vanilla, Porcelain Beige, Sunny, and Honeyed Beige. Alabaster and Breeze are the best neutral shades if you have fair skin, while Amber and Clove are attractive dark shades.

☹ **Work-Out Makeup All-Day Wear** *($19.50)* is a creamy, water-resistant foundation that provides medium coverage and a rather heavy application, though it does hold up well. The problem is that three of the four shades are too pink or rose to look natural. Cloud is the sole recommended shade, but this is not one of Clinique's better foundations.

☹ **Clarifying Makeup Clear Skin Formula** *($19.50)* was once recommended, but upon reviewing it again, there are too many drawbacks to make it a foundation for those with blemished, oily skin. Alcohol is the third ingredient, followed closely by witch hazel and, further down the list, clove extract. None of these ingredients is helpful for skin, and when you consider that the formula tends to separate as well as ball up on skin that has any sort of lightweight moisturizer or serum applied, it's a no-brainer to avoid.

CONCEALER: ✓ ☺ $$$ All About Eyes Concealer *($15.50)* is a state-of-the-art concealer formula thanks to the inclusion of pentapeptides, antioxidants, and elegant skin-identical ingredients. It has a smooth, creamy texture and concentrated pigmentation. A little goes a long way and provides good coverage with minimal slip. The seven shades present mostly true skin-color options, though Light Neutral (the palest shade) is too yellow for most fair skin and Medium Beige is too bright yellow. The others are superb and include options for darker skin. Clinique claims this is recommended for disguising dark circles, and it does indeed work very well for that purpose, without looking thick or cakey.

☺ **$$$ CX Soothing Concealer Duo SPF 15** *($35)* comes in a sleek compact and includes a creamy concealer, pressed powder, and a dual-sided brush composed of synthetic hair. The concealer is available in three shades, all of which are good, though Medium is slightly peach and can be trickier to work with. Concealer application is smooth and even, providing medium coverage with a slight chance of creasing. Lightly brushing on the pale, neutral yellowish powder nicely sets the concealer (you get the same color of powder regardless of the concealer shade). The gentlest part of this product is the sunscreen (in the concealer only), which is all titanium dioxide. It is otherwise no more soothing than any of Clinique's concealers. Keep in mind that if camouflaging diffuse areas or spots of redness is your goal, the All About Eyes Concealer bests this one for coverage.

☺ **$$$ Airbrush Concealer** *($18.50)* is housed in a pen-style applicator; you rotate the base to feed concealer onto the built-in brush tip. It offers a smooth (though too sheer to provide any amount of concealing) application that has an airy, silky texture and sets to a natural matte finish. The two shades are the main issue here, because Fair is too pink and Medium is undeniably peach. However, they are both so sheer that the misguided colors get toned down. By the way, the finished effect on the skin is not akin to airbrushing a photo, where flaws are eliminated. If anything, even minor flaws will still be visible with this concealer, but, to Clinique's credit, they do describe this as being sheer, so it still deserves a happy face rating for those looking more for a highlighter/enhancer than for significant coverage.

☺ **Acne Solutions Concealing Stick** *($13.50)* is packaged as an automatic pencil, and is nonretractable, so don't wind up more than you need. It contains 2% salicylic acid for exfoliation, but because you cannot establish (let alone hold) an acidic pH in a nonaqueous product, its exfoliating properties are at best dubious. However, it is a lightweight concealer in three viable shades that do a good job camouflaging blemish-induced redness. The ingredients that keep it in stick form aren't the best for use directly on a blemish, but this is worth considering to cover the red marks blemishes often leave behind (you know, the ones that take months and months to fade).

☺ **Advanced Concealer** *($13.50)* comes in a squeeze tube and goes on like a thick cream, but quickly dries to a powder. Coverage is very good without looking heavy. This comes in two excellent shades, Matte Light and Matte Medium. The fine print: This concealer works only if the skin under your eyes is smooth; any dry or rough skin will look worse because of this product's powdery finish.

☺ **Line Smoothing Concealer** *($13.50)* promises an instantly firmer look and is said to contain ingredients to bridge wrinkles, making them less apparent. Neither claim becomes reality, but this is still a very good liquid concealer with a smooth, even application, the right amount of coverage for most flaws, and a semi-matte finish that leaves a bit of a glow. I suppose it's that glow that helps reflect light away from wrinkles, but the visual trickery is minor, at least if you have the kind of lines that don't disappear when your face is motionless. Of the seven mostly neutral shades, only Medium Honey (which is bright peach) and Deep Honey (an unattractive ochre hue) should be avoided.

😐 **Quick Corrector** *($13.50)* comes in a tube with a wand applicator and has a fluid, slightly moist application. It smooths on easily and covers well, though the unstable, minimally matte finish can translate into creasing around the eyes. Avoid Medium, which is too pink.

😐 **City Cover Compact Concealer SPF 15** *($13.50)* is one of the few concealers that has a reliable SPF 15 with UVA protection. The two colors are quite workable for fair to light skin and capable of almost full coverage. The problem is that this has a creamy consistency that will crease before you're out the door. If the sun protection appeals to you, make sure you try this at the counter first and see how it wears over time.

POWDER: ✓ ☺ $$$ Blended Face Powder & Brush *($18.50)* is one of the best talc-based loose powders available, and is available in an attractive array of colors. This has a light, supple finish that clings well without caking and doesn't look dry or dull skin's natural glow. Of the seven shades, use caution with Transparency 2 (pale pink but goes on sheer) and Transparency Bronze (nice color, but too shiny, though it's an option for evening sparkle). The finish this powder leaves is best for normal to dry skin. One more point: Toss the brush; it doesn't apply powder well, feels scratchy, and sheds too much.

☺ **$$$ Stay Matte Sheer Pressed Powder Oil-Free** *($18.50)* is a good, talc-based powder with a slightly dry, powdery, sheer finish. The absorbency of this powder is ideal for oilier skin types, but it isn't as refined as the pressed powders from Bobbi Brown, M.A.C., Stila, or even Clinique's own Clarifying Powder Makeup above. The eight shades are beautiful and there are some good options for light and dark skin tones.

☺ **$$$ Soft Finish Pressed Powder** *($18.50)* is intended by Clinique to be used for drier skin, and that makes sense, as this talc-based formula has a creamier, silky feel and smooth, even coverage. The light-diffusing claims are bogus, and this is down to two shades, so your choices are limited. ☺ **$$$ Superpowder Double Face Powder** *($18.50)* is a standard, talc-based pressed powder with a smooth, soft texture. It can be used alone or as a regular finishing powder. There are eight very sheer shades, all terrific. Interestingly, Clinique is now advising against using this product wet—a wise direction!

😐 **$$$ Gentle Light Powder and Brush** *($21)* is a talc-based loose powder that is exceptionally light and soft, yet infused with enough shine to make a chorus of Las Vegas showgirls sparkle with envy. The five shades are beautiful, but this shiny powder clings poorly to skin.

☹ **True Bronze Pressed Powder Bronzer** *($23.50)* has a dry, grainy texture and somewhat spotty, sheer application with shine. It isn't nearly as impressive as it should be, and is not worth considering even though the three tan shades are a balanced mix without too much red or copper.

BLUSH: The color products (blushes, eyeshadows, and lipsticks) are arranged into four groups: Nudes (which are not all that nude), Tawnies, Pinks, and Violets. This is definitely a helpful way to organize a large color collection and the designations mostly make sense.

☺ **$$$ Blushing Blush Powder Blusher** *($18.50)* has the smoothst texture and best color deposit of all of Clinique's powder blushes, but each shade is laden with shine (on most shades, the shine is metallic-looking rather than a soft shimmer). This powder blush is otherwise very workable and easy to blend, but this much shine is best reserved for nighttime glamour.

☺ **$$$ Touch Blush** *($16.50)* is nearly identical to Stila's Rouge Pots ($20). Touch Blush shares the same outstanding traits: an air-whipped texture that's a modern interpretation of cream-to-powder blush, translucent colors that give skin a healthy flush rather than a layer of stronger color, and seamless application. Clinique's packaging makes it easier to use than Stila's version (where the jar opening makes it tricky to grab just a dab of product), but unlike most of Stila's Rouge Pots shades, all but one of Clinique's colors are shiny. Plush Plum has a hint of shine, while the others are imbued with flecks of glitter that are not what I would call subtle. The overdone shine keeps this product from earning a Paula's Pick rating, but this blush is otherwise recommended, especially if your idea of evening makeup includes glittery cheeks.

☺ **Gel Blush** *($12.50)* is worth trying! This traditional gel blush is available in three realistic, sheer colors that blend easily and offer a long-lasting transparent finish. As with all cheek stains, these work best on smooth, flawless skin and must be blended quickly if they are to look convincing. Gel Blush may be applied to lips for a sheer stained effect.

😐 **$$$ Soft Pressed Powder Blusher** *($18.50)* is decently silky but almost too sheer. Color deposit is minimal and requires successive layers to register on most skin tones (and forget about it showing up at all on dark skin). All of the shades are shiny and the shine tends to flake, making this less enticing than the powder blushes from M.A.C., Stila, or Clarins. 😐 **$$$ Blushwear** *($16.50)* is a cream-to-powder blush that is only available in two understated shades. It applies slightly heavy and can be tricky to blend out evenly, but the result is a satin matte finish that feels slightly moist. Unless you're already sold on this product, consider Clinique's Touch Blush or Stila's Rouge Pots instead.

EYESHADOW: Clinique's Colour Surge Eye Shadows come in various formulas, but are organized on the tester unit by color, which makes zeroing in on the one you want difficult without some assistance.

✓☺ **Colour Surge Eye Shadow Velvet** *($13.50)* marks the first time Clinique's eyeshadows have what they've been missing for years: good color concentration and an enviably smooth texture that applies and blends expertly. Their former shadows (still available in the Pair of Shades Eyeshadow Duo product reviewed below) tended to go on very sheer and had a texture that was too flyaway and powdery, hindering application. Colour Surge solves those problems and offers an attractive palette of shades, including a few matte and almost-matte (meaning negligible shine) options; check out Buttermilk, Bewitched, and Crushed Plum.

✓☺ **Colour Surge Eye Shadow Soft Shimmer** *($13.50)* has the same texture and application traits as the Colour Surge Eye Shadow Velvet above, except that each shade of this version has shine. These sublimely silky colors blend beautifully, and although the shine (shimmer) isn't what I consider "soft," the finish is appropriate for daytime makeup if you have unwrinkled eyelids and a smooth underbrow area. The small shade selection is impressive, with only a few pastel tones that you should consider carefully. These also have a slightly softer color intensity than the Colour Surge Eye Shadow Velvet shadows.

✓☺ **Colour Surge Eye Shadow Duo** *($17.50)* has the same ultra-smooth texture and application as the Colour Surge Eye Shadow Soft Shimmer above. If you want to avoid shine, you're out of luck because each Duo contains two shiny colors, albeit in mostly workable combinations. The deeper shades apply smoothly and are an option for creating a shiny, smoky, evening eye makeup. There are some blue-toned duos to watch out for, but the odd pairing of purple with pale gold (in the Beach Plum duo) is actually quite attractive.

✓☺ **$$$ Colour Surge Eye Shadow Quad** *($25)* has the same velvety texture and swift-blending application as Clinique's single and duo Colour Surge Eye Shadows, which is good news! Quads make sense if the shades are well-coordinated, and that is indeed the case with two of the four sets available. Teddy Bear is a beautiful group of nude and earth tones, while Spicy combines bronzes, gold, and taupe-rose shimmer for those who can pull off shiny eyeshadow (though the effect is more shimmery than glittery). The other quads are more difficult to work with because they're slightly mismatched, not to mention that the blue tones won't serve to shape and shade the eye, which is the purpose of eyeshadow. Ignore the applicators that come with this set and stick with full-sized professional eyeshadow brushes for best results.

☺ **Colour Surge Eye Shadow Super Shimmer** *($13.50).* These are nearly identical to the Colour Surge Eye Shadow Soft Shimmer above, except they have more shine, and are best reserved for evening or special occasion makeup. Blue Lagoon and Cornflower Blue should be avoided unless you just cannot do without blue eyeshadow. The shine in these shadows has a greater tendency to flake, which is why these are not rated as a Paula's Pick. However, the flakiness is minimal compared to that of most other eyeshadows with this much shine.

☺ **Touch Base for Eyes** *($13.50)* is one of the better cream-to-powder eyeshadows. This comes in a compact that must be kept closed tightly or the product will dry out and be useless. However, it might dry out even if you follow that guideline, so recommending this is risky. Test this at the counter, but be forewarned that every shade (even the flesh-toned Canvas, Canvas Light, and Canvas Deep) is shiny. This no longer fills the bill for a truly matte eyeshadow base.

😐 **$$$ Pair of Shades Eyeshadow Duo** *($17.50)* represents Clinique's older eyeshadow formula, with a slightly powdery application and sheer colors that aren't for anyone who wants to use eyeshadow to shape and shade the eye. Only eight duos remain, and all but one (No-Show Taupes) have glaring shine. They remain an OK option for sheer eyeshadow if you have fair to light skin.

😐 **$$$ Touch Tint for Eyes** *($14.50)* consists of tubes of semi-sheer, cream-to-powder eyeshadows. These have a creamy, slightly slick texture that makes controlling the color trickier than usual, but they eventually dry down to a soft powder (in feel) finish. The Cream shades are semi-matte, while the Shimmer formula lays on the shine, and go easy on the color. The slick nature of Touch Tint for Eyes makes it prone to creasing unless paired with a powder eyeshadow.

EYE AND BROW SHAPER: ✓☺ **Brush-On Cream Liner** *($14.50)* deserves consideration if you're a fan of Lauder-owned Bobbi Brown's Long Wear Gel Eyeliner ($18) or M.A.C.'s Fluidline ($14.50). Clinique's me-too version is essentially the same thing: a densely pigmented cream-gel eyeliner packaged in a glass jar. The formula applies easily (similar to liquid eyeliner) and sets to a long-wearing finish that won't smear, smudge, or flake even if oily eyelids are a problem. It may seem like a bonus that Clinique included a brush, but unless you want a thick line, you'll want to experiment with fine-tipped options. Among the four shades, Black Honey is shiny and the remainder are classic black, brown, and gray. As with all products of this nature, it must be recapped tightly after each use to prevent the product from drying out.

☺ **Brow Shaper** *($14.50)* is a powder brow color that comes in four excellent shades, though now each of them has shine, which is a bit over the top. The texture is slightly heavy, but these blend onto the brow quite well, even though the brush that comes packaged with them is too stiff and scratchy. For the money, a matte, brow-toned eyeshadow would work just as well and could also double as an eyeshadow; Brow Shaper is too heavy for eyeshadow. ☺ **Superfine Liner for Brows** *($12.50)* is an automatic, nonretractable, very thin brow pencil that works well to softly accent and fill in brows for those who prefer pencils to powder. It applies without dragging or feeling thick, and has a slightly tacky powder finish that lasts with minimal fading and no smearing. The five shades are excellent, and include options for blondes and redheads.

😐 **Quickliner for Eyes** *($14.50)* is a standard automatic pencil that provides a smooth, no-tugging application and is very easy to smudge before it sets. Because this stays creamy, its wear-time is compromised and every shade goes on too soft for quick definition. In addition, each shade also leaves a low-glow sheen; nonshiny options would have been preferred for variety. 😐 **$$$ Kohl Shaper for Eyes** *($15.50)* is a standard pencil that needs sharpening (though a cleverly concealed built-in sharpener is included), but Kohl Shaper for Eyes has a great smooth application that doesn't skip, so drawing one continuous line is a breeze. Once it sets, the creaminess is gone, and it barely moves or smudges. As usual, a classic black shade is available, but all of the other shades have a black base, which makes the blue-toned options acceptable because they come across as deep navy, appearing almost black. 😐 **$$$ Cream Shaper for Eyes** *($13.50)* is a very soft-textured eye pencil. The saleswomen who demonstrated this for me commented that caution is warranted because the tip breaks so easily. The good news is that you need only minimal pressure to get a smooth line of color, though it may take some practice before you get the hang of it. This needs-sharpening pencil goes on creamy and stays creamy, yet (this is the best part) barely smudges. Each shade is infused with shimmer, which should raise a red flag if your eyelids are wrinkled. Otherwise, the glow these pencils provide can be subtly effective. It is best for defining eyes and then smudging the effect for a smoky look, and is not recommended as a lower-lid liner if you have allergies or watery eyes, both of which promote smearing with a creamy pencil like this.

☹ **Eye Defining Liquid Liner** *($13.50)* has an uneven application, takes too long to dry (which encourages smearing), and its brush isn't the best for precise application. ☹ **Brow Keeper** *($14.50)* is a substandard brow pencil that comes in only two colors. It has a slick texture and slightly creamy, sticky finish that prompts smudging and fading.

LIPSTICK, LIP GLOSS, AND LIPLINER: ✓☺ **Colour Surge Lipstick** *($14)* does indeed provide a surge of color, and in a very attractive range of rich, full-coverage shades! This creamy lipstick feels wonderfully light and moist, and leaves a moderately glossy finish. Best of all, the colors really last—even when the creaminess has worn away, a smooth, vibrant stain of color remains, and that means fewer touch-ups! Colour Surge is definitely Clinique's most pigmented lipstick, not to mention its best cream option. Also available is ☺ **Colour Surge Lipstick Metallic Finish** *($14)*, a collection of a half dozen shades that share the same formula as the original Colour Surge Lipstick but with a smooth shimmer (rather than metallic) finish. ✓☺ **Long Last**

Soft Matte Lipstick *($14)* may not be around too much longer based on the dwindling shade selection (all are beautiful), and that would be a shame. This smooth-textured lipstick feels great, provides opaque coverage, and has a satin matte finish that holds true to the "long last" part of this lipstick's name. ✓☺ **Long Last Soft Shine Lipstick** *($14)* has a luscious feel and smooth, even application with opaque coverage. It is nicely creamy without being greasy or too glossy. The color selection is extensive, with equally impressive pale and deep shades.

✓☺ **Colour Surge Impossibly Glossy** *($14.50)* is a pigment-rich tube gloss that daringly offers near-full coverage and a shimmer-infused glossy finish that's moist rather than sticky. The decadent colors are beautiful (actually, they're sexy) and work well alone or paired with a lipstick for added drama.

✓☺ **Quickliner for Lips** *($13.50)* is an automatic, nonretractable pencil that must have been improved (the Clinique salespeople weren't sure) because it now has a super-smooth, just-right creamy application that doesn't feel thick or waxy but does a great job of keeping lipstick from feathering into lines around the mouth. The shade range is gorgeous and easy to coordinate with just about any Clinique lipstick. Just keep in mind that their greasier and glossy formulas aren't for those prone to lipstick feathering. ✓☺ **Superbalm Moisturizing Gloss** *($13.50)* comes in a squeeze tube and is an emollient, balm-like lip gloss that moisturizes while imparting sheer, juicy color and a minimally sticky feel. It's a good way to condition lips while adding a hint of color, and some of the shades have a slight shimmer for a glistening effect.

☺ **Colour Surge Bare Brilliance Lipstick** *($14)* has a sheer, slick texture that, in contrast to many other sheer options, is a bit less slippery and greasy. It has a moist, smooth feel, with a wet-looking finish from each of its eye-catching shades, all of which go on translucent but can be layered for more intensity. ☺ **Colour Surge Butter Shine Lipstick** *($14)* goes on quite thick and feels considerably more greasy than creamy. It has a glossy finish and comes in an attractive selection of shades seemingly based on best-sellers from Clinique's vast lipstick library—but this will bleed into lines around the mouth almost as soon as you apply it, and its longevity is cut short by the extra-emollient formula. It isn't a bad lipstick by any means, just one to approach with caution if you're prone to lipstick feathering and/or want long-lasting color. Those without this problem but with chapped lips should stop by the Clinique counter to explore this lipstick!

☺ **Different Lipstick** *($14)* comes in a classic range of colors with some pretty neutrals and pastel brights, but isn't different from most standard, lightly creamy lipsticks that provide medium coverage. This is not as long-lasting as any of Clinique's lipsticks rated as Paula's Picks. ☺ **Glosswear for Lips** *($13.50)* is a semi-thick, wand-applicator lip gloss that's standard fare. It features some good sheer colors and has a minimally sticky finish. ☺ **Glosswear for Lips Sheer Shimmers** *($13.50)* has a texture that's similar to the regular Glosswear for Lips, but it's slightly less sticky and, of course, the colors leave a shimmer finish. ☺ **Glosswear for Lips Intense Sparkle** *($13.50)* is nearly identical to the original Glosswear for Lips, but with a non-grainy, very sparkly finish.

😐 **$$$ Cream Shaper for Lips** *($15.50)* is a standard lip pencil with a creamy application that goes on smoothly but won't do much to keep lipstick in place. The built-in brush is a nice touch, but not enough to make this worth considering over Quickliner for Lips. 😐 **Sheer Shaper for Lips** *($13.50)* capitalizes on the popularity of the "sheer" makeup looks many consumers are requesting. This is a standard, needs-sharpening lip pencil whose low-impact colors go on very softly and, as a result, tend not to last nearly as long as a regular Lipliner. The pencil has a smooth, slightly creamy application but is basically the Lipliner equivalent of a sheer lipstick, and that means it's too fleeting to keep lips defined and help anchor your lipstick.

☹ **Full Potential Lips Plump and Shine** *($17.50)* is said to have a triple-plumping action and promises to keep the plumpness going for hours. The trio of plumping agents are all of the irritating kind, and include peppermint, capsicum (pepper), and ginger root oils. None of them are good news for lips, especially if this is a product you intend to use routinely. It's otherwise a standard, slightly thick lip gloss with a sticky finish and an attractive selection of sparkle-infused colors. Despite Clinique's gentle reputation (which, at least in the case of their classic three-step skin-care routine, isn't true), this lip-plumping product ends up being more irritating than similar options.

MASCARA: ✓☺ **Lash Doubling Mascara** *($13.50)* does a very good job of living up to its name, as this quickly builds lots of length and a fair amount of thickness with ease. The formula sweeps on with no clumps or smearing—each lash is well defined—so unless you're looking for all-out drama, this is an outstanding choice. ✓☺ **High Impact Mascara** *($13.50)* is simply fantastic and is on my short list of favorite mascaras. If you're looking for mascara that quickly builds substantial length and substantial thickness while defining lashes without clumping, this is a must-try. It wears well throughout the day and is easily removed with a water-soluble cleanser, qualities that make it even more ideal.

☺ **Long Pretty Lashes Mascara** *($13.50)* has an accurate name, as this mascara produces lots of length and does so without clumping, smearing, or flaking. The clean, quick application does not produce any thickness, so it's not as all-out impressive as High Impact Mascara. Still, if length is what you're after, this is well worth trying!

☺ **Gentle Waterproof Mascara** *($13.50)* is a bit of a misnomer, as waterproof mascara in general is hard on lashes for both wear and removal. It is best for creating moderately long, well-defined lashes; thickness is slow going and peters out before reaching anything too dramatic.

😐 **Naturally Glossy Mascara** *($13.50)* is a basic mascara that builds some length and minimal thickness, though it leaves lashes feeling dry and stiff due to the film-forming agents and the amount of PVP (an ingredient used in many hairstyling gels) it contains.

😐 **Lash Building Primer** *($12.50)* is nothing to get excited about. This will only impress you if it is used with a mediocre to poor mascara. In that case, you could expect to see increased length and thickness that would not be possible using the inferior mascara alone. However, when paired with a superior mascara, such as any rated a Paula's Pick, you won't notice much, if any, difference between using the primer and mascara together or simply applying two coats of the mascara.

☹ **High Definition Lashes Brush Then Comb Mascara** *($13.50)* is really bad, and that's not something I see too often with new mascaras. The dual-sided brush features comblike teeth on one side and standard mascara bristles on the other. You're directed to use the bristled portion first to build thickness, then comb through lashes for length and added drama. Neither side works well, though at least the brush side doesn't leave lashes clumped together and spiky-looking. This is one of the few mascaras that requires more effort to apply and neaten than the results merit.

BRUSHES: ☺ **The Brush Collection** *($16.50–$32.50)*. Better late than never! After years and years of having their consultants apply makeup on customers with cotton balls and swabs (not an easy or beautiful task), Clinique finally has its own collection of brushes. Was the wait worth it? Although the company breaks no new ground, most of the brushes are full, well-shaped, and functional for their intended purpose. The prices are similar to most other brushes at the department store. All feature elegant handles that are neither too long nor too short, though no brush cases are currently available. The best options are the ☺ **Blush Brush** *($25)*, ☺ **Concealer Brush** *($16.50)*, ☺ **Eye Shadow Brush** *($18.50)*, ☺ **Eye Contour Brush** *($18.50)*, and ☺ **Eye Definer Brush** *($16.50)*, which is preferred for defining brows rather than eyelining. The 😐 **Eye Shader Brush** *($20)* is very soft and full, making it too large for most eyes, and best for applying a wash of color to the entire eye area. The 😐 **Powder Brush** *($30)* is also quite soft and full, but a bit more density would make it easier to control. The ☺ **Bronzer/Blender Brush** *($32.50)* is incredibly full and a bit unwieldy, but an option for applying powder to large areas of skin.

Adding a unique marketing element to their new brushes is Clinique's assertion that the brush hairs are treated with a long-lasting antibacterial agent to keep them hygienic. That could very well be possible, but it seems Clinique doesn't quite believe it either because they still advise you to clean your brush monthly for hygienic purposes, and the makeup artists clean the brushes with alcohol after each use. It's also important to keep in mind that the kind of bacteria that grow on brushes aren't the kind associated with breakouts, so the antibacterial claim won't help that aspect of your skin's appearance.

FACE AND BODY ILLUMINATING/SHIMMER PRODUCTS: ☺ **$$$ Up-Lighting Liquid Illuminator** *($22.50)* may seem like the latest and greatest when it comes to shimmer, but the four sheer shades in this lightweight lotion don't break any new ground for radiant shine. Each applies smoothly and imparts a hint of color and shine that can be layered for more intensity. Flesh and bronze tones are sold alongside a peach and rosy pink shade, the latter two best used as blush rather than applied all over. The good news is that the shine clings well and the color lasts—though keep in mind the effect of both is subtle. This isn't the best if you want something more noticeable, say, for special occasion evening glamour.

SPECIALTY PRODUCTS: 😐 **Makeup Brush Cleaner** *($12.50)* will remove excess oil and pigment, but washing your brushes with a standard shampoo would work better than using this formulation. Makeup Brush Cleaner is primarily water, alcohol, and detergent cleansing agent, designed to be misted on and tissued off. There is no question this fast-drying formula works in between routine brush cleansing (especially if you need to use the same brushes on multiple people or you want to use one brush to apply two contrasting colors), but most women will find it an unnecessary addition to their makeup accessories. Also, the alcohol can be drying and degrade the brush hair over time.

😐 **CX Color Corrector** *($30)* is a fluid, concealer-like product housed in a pen applicator complete with a built-in synthetic brush. The texture is creamy with a soft powder finish and moderate coverage, though the colors (one sheer green, the other a noticeable peach) aren't the best for camouflaging discolorations. They tend to draw attention to what you're trying to hide, and don't replace a regular, neutral-toned concealer.

COPPERTONE (SUN CARE ONLY)

COPPERTONE AT-A-GLANCE

Strengths: A few effective, basic sunscreens with various but typically lightweight textures (especially the Ultra Sheer); all recommended sunscreens are also water-resistant; inexpensive, which should encourage liberal application and reapplication; reliable self-tanners tailored to various skin tones.

Weaknesses: The majority of their sunscreens lack sufficient UVA-protecting ingredients, even though Coppertone clearly knows about this and routinely reformulates.

For more information about Coppertone, call (800) 842-4090 or visit www.coppertone.com or www.Beautypedia.com.

GENERAL PROTECTION: THE ORIGINAL COPPERTONE PRODUCTS

☹ **Continuous Spray Sunscreen SPF 15** *($9.99 for 6 ounces)* may spray continuously, but lacks the UVA-protecting ingredients of titanium dioxide, zinc oxide, avobenzone, Tinosorb, or Mexoryl SX and also contains 80% alcohol. This sunscreen is not recommended.

☹ **Continuous Spray Sunscreen SPF 30** *($9.99 for 6 ounces)* is nearly identical to the Continuous Spray Sunscreen SPF 15 above, save for a higher percentage of active ingredients. Otherwise, the same comments apply.

☺ **Spectra3 UVA/UVB Sunscreen Lotion SPF 50** *($11.09 for 6 ounces)* is a very good, in-part zinc oxide sunscreen in a lightweight, water-resistant, fragrance-free lotion base. Small amounts of vitamins A, C, and E are included for antioxidant protection, but I suspect the percentage, while not paltry, offers only a "something is better than nothing" benefit.

☹ **Sunblock Lotion SPF 15** *($8.99 for 8 ounces)* lacks the UVA-protecting ingredients of titanium dioxide, zinc oxide, avobenzone, Tinosorb, or Mexoryl SX, and is not recommended.

☺ **Sunblock Lotion SPF 30** *($9.99 for 8 ounces)* has an in-part avobenzone sunscreen to ensure sufficient UVA protection and comes in a smooth, water-resistant lotion base suitable for normal to slightly oily skin. The tiny amount of vitamin E is likely ineffective at providing much, if any, antioxidant protection.

☺ **Sunscreen Lotion SPF 50** *($9.99 for 8 ounces)* is similar to the Sunblock Lotion SPF 30 above, save for the higher percentage of active ingredients needed to create SPF 50. Otherwise, the same review applies.

☹ **Bug and Sun Sunscreen with Insect Repellent SPF 30** *($11.99 for 8 ounces)* repels insects with the chemical DEET (N,N-diethyl-m-toluamide), but leaves skin vulnerable to UVA damage because it lacks the UVA-protecting ingredients of titanium dioxide, zinc oxide, avobenzone, Tinosorb, or Mexoryl SX.

COPPERTONE KIDS PRODUCTS

☹ **Kids Continuous Spray Sunscreen SPF 50** *($9.99 for 6 ounces)* differs from the "adult" version reviewed above and includes avobenzone for UVA protection. However, the alcohol content is still extremely high, and makes this sunscreen too irritating for children's skin.

☹ **Kids Sunblock Lotion Spray SPF 45** *($9.99 for 8 ounces)* lacks the UVA-protecting ingredients of titanium dioxide, zinc oxide, avobenzone, Tinosorb, or Mexoryl SX, and is not recommended.

☹ **Kids Sunblock Stick SPF 30** *($5.99 for 0.6 ounce)* lacks the UVA-protecting ingredients of titanium dioxide, zinc oxide, avobenzone, Tinosorb, or Mexoryl SX, and is not recommended.

☹ **Kids Sunblock Trigger Spray SPF 30** *($10.19 for 6 ounces)* lacks the UVA-protecting ingredients of titanium dioxide, zinc oxide, avobenzone, Tinosorb, or Mexoryl SX, and is not recommended.

☺ **Kids Sunscreen Lotion SPF 50** *($9.99 for 8 ounces)* is identical in every respect to the Sunscreen Lotion SPF 50 above, and the same comments apply. The amount of synthetic active ingredient is not exactly kid-friendly, but there's no reason adults cannot use this sunscreen.

☹ **Kids Lip Balm with Sunscreen SPF 30** *($2.49 for 0.15 ounce)* lacks the UVA-protecting ingredients of titanium dioxide, zinc oxide, avobenzone, Tinosorb, or Mexoryl SX, and is not recommended. Further, the cherry flavor encourages lip-licking, and several ingredients in this product aren't meant to be ingested.

COPPERTONE OIL-FREE PRODUCTS

☺ **Oil Free Faces, Hydrating UVA/UVB Sunblock SPF 30** *($8.99 for 3 ounces)* is oil-free but its absorbent base isn't hydrating. This is a great choice for oily to very oily skin. Avobenzone provides UVA protection, and the fragrance-free, water-resistant lotion feels light and applies easily.

☹ **Oil Free Sunblock Lotion SPF 15** *($9.99 for 8 ounces)* lacks the UVA-protecting ingredients of titanium dioxide, zinc oxide, avobenzone, Tinosorb, or Mexoryl SX, and is not recommended.

☺ **Oil Free Sunblock Lotion SPF 30** *($9.99 for 8 ounces)* includes not a single bell or whistle for extra skin-care benefits, but is a good, basic sunscreen that's water-resistant, and it includes avobenzone for UVA protection.

☺ **Oil Free Sunblock Lotion SPF 45** *($10.99 for 8 ounces)* is similar to the Oil Free Sunblock Lotion SPF 30 above, except its lightweight lotion base feels tackier on skin. This is still a worthwhile option for normal to oily skin from the neck down.

COPPERTONE SPORT PRODUCTS

☹ **Sport Continuous Spray Sunscreen SPF 15** *($9.99 for 6 ounces)* is nearly identical to the Continuous Spray Sunscreen SPF 15 above, and the same review applies.

☹ **Sport Continuous Spray Sunscreen SPF 30** *($9.99 for 6 ounces)* is nearly identical to the Continuous Spray Sunscreen SPF 30 above, and the same review applies.

☹ **Sport Continuous Spray Sunscreen SPF 50** *($10.99 for 6 ounces)* includes avobenzone for sufficient UVA protection, but its alcohol-based formula is too drying for all skin types and increases the chance of irritation from the amount of active ingredients needed to create an SPF 50 sunscreen.

☹ **Sport Sunblock Lotion SPF 15** *($9.99 for 8 ounces)*, ☹ **Sport Sunblock Lotion SPF 30** *($9.99 for 8 ounces)*, ☹ **Sport Sunblock Lotion SPF 50** *($9.99 for 8 ounces)*, ☹ **Sport Sunblock Spray SPF 30** *($9.99 for 7 ounces)*, ☹ **Sport Sunblock Stick SPF 30** *($5.49 for 0.6 ounce)*, ☹ **Sport Trigger Spray SPF 30** *($9.99 for 6 ounces)*, and ☹ **Sport Lip Guard with Sunscreen SPF 15** *($2.49 for 0.15 ounce)* all lack the UVA-protecting ingredients of titanium dioxide, zinc oxide, avobenzone, Tinosorb, or Mexoryl SX, and are not recommended for any type of outdoor activity, not even a quick walk to the mailbox.

COPPERTONE SUNLESS TANNING PRODUCTS

☺ **Endless Summer Sunless Tanning Lotion** *($12.49 for 3.7 ounces)* is a basic, silky-textured self-tanning lotion that uses dihydroxyacetone (DHA) to turn skin color. It is available in versions for light to medium and medium to deep skin tones.

☺ **Gradual Tan, Sunless Tanning Moisturizing Lotion** *($9.49 for 9 ounces)* contains a small amount of dihydroxyacetone to gradually change skin color. This is a good option for face or body, and sets to a soft matte finish. It does contain fragrance.

☺ **Gradual Tan Faces, Sunless Tanning Moisturizing Lotion** *($7.99 for 2.5 ounces)* is nearly identical to the Gradual Tan, Sunless Tanning Moisturizing Lotion above, and the same review applies. Budget-wise, go for the larger size; nothing about this version is specifically suited for facial use.

☺ **Oil Free Sunless Tanning Lotion** *($8.89 for 8 ounces)* is a caramel-tinted self-tanning lotion that provides immediate color so you'll notice missed spots quickly. This contains dihydroxyacetone, as do most self-tanning products; moreover, the solvent ethoxydiglycol enhances penetration and on prepped skin should result in a deeper tan whether you choose the Light/Medium or Dark version.

COPPERTONE TANNING/LOW SPF SUNSCREEN PRODUCTS

☹ **Dry Oil Continuous Spray Sunscreen SPF 10** *($9.99 for 6 ounces)* lacks the UVA-protecting ingredients of titanium dioxide, zinc oxide, avobenzone, Tinosorb, or Mexoryl SX, and contains 80% alcohol, making it very irritating.

☹ **Dry Oil Sunscreen Spray SPF 4** *($8.59 for 6 ounces)* lacks sufficient UVA protection and has a dangerously low SPF rating, along with almost 40% alcohol.

☹ **Dry Oil Sunscreen Spray SPF 8** *($9.69 for 6 ounces)* is the spray-on lotion version of the Dry Oil Sunscreen Spray SPF 4 above, and has the same drawbacks with a marginally higher but still disappointing SPF rating.

☹ **Dry Oil Sunscreen Spray SPF 15** *($9.69 for 6 ounces)* is nearly identical to the Dry Oil Continuous Spray Sunscreen SPF 10 above except for its higher SPF rating. Otherwise the same comments apply.

☹ **Sunscreen Lotion SPF 4** *($8.59 for 8 ounces)* feels like a sunscreen holdover from decades ago, and leaves skin vulnerable to UVA damage.

☹ **Sunscreen Lotion SPF 8** *($6.19 for 4 ounces)* deserves the same review as written for the Sunscreen Lotion SPF 4 above.

COPPERTONE ULTRA SHEER PRODUCTS

✓☺ **Ultra Sheer Faces Sunscreen Lotion SPF 30** *($9.69 for 3 ounces)* not only gets the UVA protection issue right (it includes avobenzone), but this silky, fragrance-free, dry-finish formula also contains several antioxidants and comes in stable packaging. This is one of Coppertone's most elegant water-resistant sunscreen formulas, and is best for normal to very oily skin.

☺ **Ultra Sheer Sunscreen Lotion SPF 30** *($11.89 for 6 ounces)* isn't quite as nice as the Ultra Sheer Faces Sunscreen Lotion SPF 30 above due to a limited presence of antioxidants and the addition of fragrance, but it's still worth considering for its in-part avobenzone sunscreen, water resistance, and a matte finish that doesn't leave skin feeling coated.

COPPERTONE WATER BABIES PRODUCTS

☹ **Water Babies Continuous Spray Sunscreen SPF 50** *($10.99 for 6 ounces)* is one of Coppertone's two alcohol-free, spray-on sunscreens, but the propellant (dimethyl ether) is irritating to skin and can be toxic if too much is inhaled, making it a poor choice for use on children.

☹ **Water Babies Sunblock Stick SPF 30** *($5.79 for 0.6 ounce)* is identical to the Kids Sunblock Stick SPF 30 above, and the same review applies.

☺ **Water Babies Sunscreen Lotion SPF 50** *($9.99 for 8 ounces)* is a good, basic, fragrance-free sunscreen lotion with an in-part avobenzone sunscreen. The combination of synthetic actives is ill-advised for kids, especially babies (it's all too easy for them to get this product in their eyes when they rub them), but is just fine for adults. This sunscreen is water-resistant.

☺ **Water Babies Sunscreen Lotion Spray SPF 50** *($11.09 for 8 ounces)* wins points for its in-part avobenzone sunscreen, alcohol-free, spray-on formula, and lightweight finish that's also water-resistant. Again, the active ingredients aren't the best for use on babies, but this is highly recommended for adults and bests every option from Coppertone's Sport line.

☺ **Water Babies Spectra3 UVA/UVB Sunscreen Lotion SPF 50** *($10.79 for 6 ounces)* is very similar to the Spectra3 UVA/UVB Sunscreen Lotion SPF 50 above, and the same review applies. This water-resistant formula is better for teens and adults than babies.

COSMEDICINE (SKIN CARE ONLY)

COSMEDICINE AT-A-GLANCE

Strengths: Some fragrance-free options; state-of-the-art serums and moisturizers; every sunscreen includes avobenzone for reliable UVA protection.

Weaknesses: Expensive; no products to address acne or skin discolorations—an odd omission from a line whose name and marketing speaks of its medicinal qualities; jar packaging that reduces the effectiveness of several of the included state-of-the-art ingredients; no more medicinal or cosmeceutical than countless other lines.

For more information about Cosmedicine, call (866) 247-4157 or visit www.cosmedicine.com or www.Beautypedia.com. Note: Many of Cosmedicine's moisturizers and serums contain dromiceius oil. More commonly known as emu oil, it is no more beneficial for skin than most other nonvolatile plant oils. There is minimal research showing it to have anti-inflammatory action and that it may speed wound healing, but what heals wounds is not related to wrinkles or other visible signs of the skin's aging (Sources: *Plastic and Reconstructive Surgery*, December 1998, pages 2404–2407; and *The Australasian Journal of Dermatology*, August 1996, pages 159–161).

☺ **$$$ Healthy Cleanse Foaming Cleanser & Toner in One** *($35 for 5 ounces)* is a whole lot of money for what ends up being an incredibly standard, detergent-based, fragrance-free, water-soluble cleanser. It is an option for normal to dry skin, but the cost is anything but healthy.

☺ **$$$ Healthy Cleanse for Oily Skin, Clarifying Cleanser & Toner In One** *($35 for 5 ounces)* is a good water-soluble cleanser for normal to oily skin. The clarifying part is supposed to come from the salicylic acid and tea tree oil in here. Neither is present in an amount that significantly impacts blemishes or blackheads, and both are rinsed from skin before they can provide much, if any, benefit. But in terms of cleansing ability and makeup removal, this works well.

😐 **$$$ Medi-morphosis Self Adjuster Exfoliator** *($42 for 4.2 ounces)* is mostly witch hazel water (which includes alcohol), more water, scrub particles, slip agents, plant extracts, a teeny amount of sodium hyaluronate (a helpful skin reinforcer), and preservatives. There is nothing medical or self-adjusting about this. (Ask yourself, How could this product know what type of skin it is being applied to?) This is nothing more than a topical scrub with particles that dissolve with enough rubbing and/or water. The claim that it reduces the appearance of pores immediately is true for any scrub because it temporarily swells the skin, giving the temporary appearance of smaller pores.

Even more misleading is the declaration that 217 subjects didn't experience irritation. This is not a usage claim, but a repeat insult patch test (RIPT) claim. This type of test involves putting a product on someone's arm or back, placing a piece of tape over it, and checking it several times over a period of weeks. If no irritation is noted, then a company may make the claim that it is not irritating to skin. However, that is misleading because it doesn't relate to the way the product is actually used or to the way it reacts in combination with other products, not to mention that some skin conditions, such as rosacea, don't occur on the forearm or back. This contains a formaldehyde-releasing preservative.

☹ **$$$ Hydra Healer Maximum Strength Moisture Cream** *($75 for 1 ounce)* is a well-formulated emollient moisturizer of mostly water, silicone, and Vaseline along with a nice blend of antioxidants, anti-irritants, and a teeny amount of an ingredient that mimics the skin structure. It does contain some peptides, but there is no research showing they can ever reach developing skin cells when applied topically. While this could have been a decent moisturizer, the jar packaging won't keep the many air-sensitive ingredients stable, which means they quickly deteriorate after opening.

☹ **$$$ Private Nurse Recovery & Repair Cream PM** *($75 for 1 ounce)* is similar to the Hydra Healer above, minus the petrolatum (Vaseline). Again, the jar packaging makes it just as undesirable at this price.

☺ **$$$ Medi-Matte Oil Control Lotion SPF 20** *($42 for 1.35 ounces)* is a well-formulated, though overpriced, sunscreen for normal to oily skin. It does contain avobenzone for UVA protection. However, because you need to apply sunscreen liberally, keep in mind that the product's high price may discourage you from doing that, which would put your skin at risk. Accompanying the sunscreen is a nice blend of beneficial antioxidants, but there is nothing in here that will normalize oil production. The acrylates and silicone polymer it contains do have some oil-absorbing properties, but that's about it.

☹ **$$$ Medi-Matte, Oil Control Spray** *($35 for 2 ounces)* is a fragrance-free blend of dry-finish silicones with preservatives and a thickener. Misting this on skin leaves a weightless matte finish, but using this over finished makeup isn't a good idea because it can disrupt an otherwise smooth, even application. Besides, if your makeup routine includes an absorbent powder and/or a matte finish primer or serum, a product such as this isn't needed. If you decide to try it, it is best used before makeup.

✓☺ **$$$ Primary Care Multi-Tasking Moisturizer SPF 20** *($48 for 1.35 ounces)* is similar to the Medi-Matte Oil Control Lotion SPF 20 above, but with a few more bells and whistles and plant oils, making it a good option for normal to dry skin. This will work great for daily sun protection with antioxidants if you are willing to apply it generously.

✓☺ **$$$ MegaDose PM Skin Fortifying Serum** *($85 for 1 ounce)* is a beautifully formulated, silicone-based serum with a notable array of state-of-the-art ingredients, though the small amount of retinol means it's hardly worth mentioning. While the claims are a bit over the top, this is a worthwhile moisturizer for normal to dry skin. For less money and a similar formulary, Lauder's Perfectionist CP+ ($50 for 1 ounce) is an equally impressive option.

✓☺ **$$$ MegaDose Skin Fortifying Serum** *($80 for 1 ounce)* is almost identical to the PM version above except this contains a few more antioxidants, and the same basic comments apply.

✓☺ **$$$ Opti-mologist Eye Cream with Light Diffusers** *($45 for 0.5 ounce)* doesn't contain anything unique for the eye area. The amount of caffeine present is negligible, and the rosemary oil is not eye-area friendly (it's the last ingredient listed). Still, this is an excellent, silicone-based moisturizer complete with antioxidants and other beneficial ingredients for skin.

✓☺ **$$$ Opti-mologist PM Intensive Eye Cream** *($48 for 0.5 ounce)* is similar to the Eye Cream above, and the same basic comments apply.

😐 **$$$ Physical Conditioning Body Skin Therapy Lotion** *($40 for 4.2 ounces)* is a strange formula because, while it does contain a good amount of sunscreen ingredients, it doesn't have an SPF rating. It is a decently formulated moisturizer for normal to dry skin, and the silicone oils will feel nice on your skin, yet when compared to the latest body lotions from Dove or Olay, this isn't worth the splurge.

☺ **$$$ Global Health SPF 30 Face** *($40 for 1.35 ounces)* is a fairly basic, though well-formulated, sunscreen with avobenzone for UVA protection. The claim that this won't irritate skin is an impossibility. The synthetic sunscreen agents, including avobenzone as well as homosalate, octinoxate, and octisalate, have long track records of being potentially sensitizing (Sources: *Journal of Family Practice*, May 2005, pages 437–440; *Cutis*, March 2005, pages 17–21; and *Contact Dermatitis*, November 1997, pages 221–232). That doesn't mean you shouldn't consider using this, it's just that you shouldn't rely on the claim. Token amounts of antioxidants are included, but not enough to justify the price, especially when you consider the need to apply sunscreen liberally.

😐 **$$$ Global Health SPF 30 Body** *($35 for 4.2 ounces)* is less impressive than the Global Health SPF 30 Face above, primarily because it lacks significant amounts of antioxidants and contains enough alcohol to be potentially irritating. It does feature avobenzone for sufficient UVA protection.

☺ **$$$ Full Benefits Lip Plumper Hydrator & Exfoliator** *($28 for 2.34 ounces)* claims that "In clinical studies, [it]… demonstrated a statistically significant 56% decrease in dry, flaky surface skin." Of course, the study does not tell you if you would have gotten the same results from a different lip balm or from using plain Vaseline, which is the major ingredient in this product. This is a good emollient for dry lips, but the low amount of salicylic acid present means it won't exfoliate your lips. The teeny amounts of antioxidants and collagen aren't going to affect your lips, so don't start looking in the mirror for increased fullness.

☺ **$$$ Honest Face Skin Tint & Treatment SPF 20** *($35 for 1.35 ounces)* is a decent tinted moisturizer for normal to dry skin. It contains avobenzone for UVA protection and a few skin-friendly ingredients that make it more interesting than some. However, for the money and formulation, Neutrogena Healthy Skin Enhancer SPF 20 ($11.99 for 1 ounce) is just as well-formulated, has more color choices, and is available at a price that will make you more inclined to apply it liberally.

COVER GIRL (MAKEUP ONLY)

COVER GIRL AT-A-GLANCE

Strengths: Inexpensive and widely available; a hugely improved selection of foundations, several with reliable sunscreen; good concealers; enviable pressed powders; some fantastic mascaras; mostly great eyelining options; a vast selection of lip color options, from the long-wearing Outlast to sheer lip glosses; well-designed, easy-to-navigate Web site.

Weaknesses: The older foundations are seriously lacking; the newer Advanced Radiance foundations have great textures but disappointing SPF ratings; Professional Loose Powder;

powder blush and eyeshadows; terrible makeup brushes; all of the "Clean" products contain irritating ingredients.

For more information about Cover Girl, call (800) 426-8374 or visit www.covergirl.com or www.Beautypedia.com.

FOUNDATION: Cover Girl would win even higher marks if they would provide adequate testers for all of their products. None of the displays I visited had testers, even for the newest items. Occasionally you'll find mini trial packs of new foundations, but for the most part, you'll be left guessing which shade is best. Note: Almost without exception, Cover Girl's three darkest foundation shades are not sold in Canada.

✓☺ **TruBlend Whipped Foundation** *($7.89)* has a delicately whipped, slightly creamy texture that floats onto skin and feels gossamer-light. Blending progresses very well and it sets to a natural matte finish with a hint of luminosity (not the sparkling or shiny kind). As with Cover Girl's original TruBlend Foundation, most of this version's shades are versatile, meaning you will likely find that, because of the pigment technology they use, you can wear two or three shades without looking unnatural. Among the 15 colors are excellent options for fair to dark skin tones. The only shades to avoid due to overtones of pink, peach, or copper are Natural Ivory, Creamy Beige, Toasted Almond, and Natural Beige (after all, whose skin resembles these shades?). This silicone-in-water foundation is best for normal to slightly dry or slightly oily skin. It's workable for those with dry skin provided you apply a moisturizing sunscreen first.

✓☺ **TruBlend Liquid Makeup** *($9.49)* is identical in almost every respect to Max Factor's Colour Adapt Foundation ($11.99), which isn't surprising given that both companies are owned by Procter & Gamble. Cover Girl's version also has a pump dispenser, as well as a somewhat thick and opaque texture. Yet once you apply it to your skin, it softens immediately and blends effortlessly. Few foundations feel so incredibly light and silky on the skin, and there is no question you will be amazed at how TruBlend conceals minor flaws without camouflaging your underlying skin tone, all while providing a truly natural matte finish.

Like Max Factor's Colour Adapt Foundation, TruBlend has a couple of drawbacks. The tradeoff for such a remarkably natural-looking foundation is that the more pronounced flaws will still be apparent, even when this foundation is layered. Of course, you can use a separate concealer to remedy this, but if you want a foundation to provide adequate coverage for flaws, such as red spots, dark under-eye circles, or brown discolorations (like freckles), this is not the best choice.

Those not concerned with concealing, but who instead want a smooth foundation to even their skin tone, will be most pleased with TruBlend. It's also worth mentioning that this foundation can crease on the eyelids if not set with powder, although when used on its own (meaning no powder), it does a better-than-average job of keeping skin shine-free, and it does not break up on the skin, as some silicone-based foundations can. These traits make TruBlend Foundation an option for all but very dry skin. Fifteen shades are available, and, thanks to the pigment technology in this foundation, you may find more than one shade to match your skin quite well, if not exactly. This foundation has Cover Girl's best palette of soft, neutral shades. There are some excellent options for light to dark (but not very dark) skin, with the best choices being Ivory, Classic Ivory, Creamy Natural, Buff Beige, Classic Beige, Medium Light, Warm Beige, Soft Honey, Classic Tan, Tawny, and Soft Sable. Avoid Natural Ivory (too pink), Natural Beige (too rose), and Creamy Beige (too peach); Toasted Almond is questionable in terms of its rosy undertone, but may be an option for medium skin tones.

✓☺ **TruBlend Powder Foundation SPF 15** *($9.49)* has a mica- and talc-based texture that's buttery, silky, and slightly powdery all at once. That's an admittedly strange description, but it accurately describes this great pressed-powder foundation that features an in-part titanium dioxide sunscreen. It blends beautifully, providing light coverage that leaves skin looking naturally polished rather than thick and powdered. Cover Girl's shade improvements continue with this product. Among the 15 options, almost all are suitable, and they represent a wide range of natural skin tones. The only shades to avoid because they are too pink, peach, or rose are Medium Light, Warm Beige, and Natural Beige. The following questionable shades are OK because this product blends so well, but you should approach them with caution: Classic Beige, Natural Ivory, and Creamy Natural. Classic Ivory is an excellent shade for fair skin; Buff Beige is an ideal neutral for lighter skin tones. This product joins the small group of pressed powders that offer sufficient sun protection. However, keep in mind that products like this are best used in combination with a facial sunscreen or foundation with sunscreen because you're not likely to apply this liberally enough to get the advertised level of sun protection.

✓☺ **AquaSmooth Makeup SPF 15** *($8.50)* is an ultralight, silicone-to-powder compact makeup that smooths easily onto the skin and dries to a soft, powdery matte finish. As with similar foundations, quick, deft blending is key—these formulas dry fast, and are not easy to move once they do. The sunscreen is all titanium dioxide, so even sensitive skin should be able to wear this, though the formula and finish are best for normal to slightly oily skin—dry skin will only look more noticeable with this type of foundation. Although the formula contains waxes, the amount is small enough that it's unlikely to be a problem for blemish-prone skin. The 15 shades offer light to medium coverage. The ones to avoid due to overtones of pink or peach are Natural Ivory, Medium Light, Warm Beige, Natural Beige, Creamy Beige, and Toasted Almond. The remaining shades feature some excellent options for light and dark skin tones.

☺ **Advanced Radiance Age-Defying Sheer Moisturizing Makeup SPF 15** *($7.99)* and ☺ **CG Smoothers SPF 15 Tinted Moisture** *($7.59)* have identical formulas, and both are exceptionally sheer moisturizers that impart the smallest amount of color to the skin. The four shades from each product are also identical, and all worth considering, but keep in mind these are very sheer, so dark circles or red discolorations will require a concealer. Both products are fragrance-free, with a lightweight lotion texture and minimally moist finish. The sunscreen is in-part zinc oxide, making this product appropriate for normal to slightly dry or slightly oily skin. I called Cover Girl to ask if the Advanced Radiance version was going to replace the CG Smoothers version, and was told that was not the case. It seems Cover Girl wants to keep two versions of the same product, with the CG Smoothers product marketed to younger women and the Advanced Radiance targeted toward women over the age of 40. The formula could certainly be more state-of-the-art, especially for older women, but it's recommended as a reliable tinted moisturizer with broad-spectrum sunscreen.

☺ **Advanced Radiance Age-Defying Compact Foundation** *($11.49)* is a silicone-based cream-to-powder foundation with a superior smooth texture that applies almost like a liquid makeup. It feels wonderfully light, blends well, and provides light to medium coverage with a satin matte finish. The 14 shades include some outstanding neutral tones, but 6 of them have undesirable overtones of peach, pink, or rose. The following shades should be avoided: Natural Ivory (fair skin doesn't need this much pink to look good), Medium Light, Warm Beige, Creamy Beige, Classic Beige, and Ivory. Classic Ivory and Buff Beige are great for lighter skin tones, while Soft Sable and Classic Tan are winners for dark skin. If you're wondering about the "Age-Defying" part of this makeup's name, it comes from the inclusion of niacinamide and vitamin E, the same Vita-Niacin complex in many Olay products (Procter & Gamble is the parent company of Cover Girl and Olay). Niacinamide and vitamin E have merit for skin, but the tiny amounts included in this foundation won't offer much benefit. If anything, this foundation's finish can make pronounced wrinkles more apparent, so it isn't the best choice for "mature" skin. Advanced Radiance Age-Defying Compact Foundation is best for normal to slightly oily or slightly dry skin. Any dry areas should be prepped with a moisturizer because this foundation's finish will exaggerate dry spots.

☺ **Fresh Complexion Pocket Powder** *($6.49)* maintains that it will provide "fresh coverage that lasts," but they should have inserted the adjective "sheer" because this talc-based, pressed-powder foundation barely registers on the skin in terms of coverage. It does have a velvety texture that never looks dry or powdery, but the finish almost leaves a glow on the skin—not something those with oily skin have on their makeup checklist. It's best for normal to dry skin that doesn't need to hide anything, but you won't net any lasting shine control with this product. The 15 shades present some visibly pink and peach colors, but the sheerness makes the color almost irrelevant. The ones to use with caution are Buff Beige, Natural Beige, Medium Light, and Classic Beige. Fair to light skin tones have the best chance of finding a perfect shade, while dark skin tones should look elsewhere.

☺ **CG Smoothers All Day Hydrating Makeup** *($7.59)* isn't all that hydrating. In fact, the talc content (it's the fourth ingredient) gives this sheer-to-medium-coverage foundation a soft matte, slightly powdery finish suitable for someone with normal to oily or combination skin. The range of 15 shades is impressive, and the packaging now permits you to see the color, although it's still best to test it on your skin. The following colors are too pink, rose, or peach for most skin tones: Natural Ivory (just slightly pink), Natural Beige, Medium Light, Warm Beige, Creamy Beige, and Toasted Almond. Soft Sable is a beautiful color for dark skin tones. This is fragrance-free.

☺ **Outlast All-Day Liquid Makeup SPF 14** *($11.49)* is a two-part, two-step product that includes a Sunscreen Primer with an in-part zinc oxide sunscreen and a transfer-resistant foundation (All Day Color). The Primer is an elegant, silky lotion that blends easily and dries quickly, although it's a bit too white in color; it would be hard to apply this product liberally, which is a must for sunscreen protection. Even though it isn't an essential step in terms of how the foundation applies or wears, it is necessary if you're not using a separate sunscreen because the Primer contains the SPF part of this foundation. Still, the amount of product you get isn't much, given that it is basically split in two (with only 0.7 ounce of Primer and 0.7 ounce of makeup in each bottle).

The medium-coverage foundation is a water- and silicone-based formula that is a pleasure to blend, setting to a natural matte finish that is excellent for normal to very oily skin. It wears well with minimal fading all day, although your oiliest areas will likely require a touch-up with powder. Cover Girl's selection of 15 shades is impressive, and most of them are true to life and suitable for fair to very dark skin tones. The usual offenders—Classic Beige, Natural Beige, Creamy Beige, and Medium Light—are egregiously pink (whose skin is close to these colors?) and Toasted Almond has a reddish tone that will work for a limited range of darker skin (such as someone of Polynesian descent or some Native American skin tones). Soft Sable is a beautiful dark shade, while Ivory is suitable for fair skin.

One caveat: The whiteness of the Sunscreen Primer can make the darker shades turn slightly ash, so experiment with and without the Primer to see which method works best for your skin color. This foundation requires a silicone- or oil-based cleanser for complete removal. Does this foundation last ten hours, as claimed? As always, that depends entirely on how oily your skin is—but this does hold up better than most, and would have been rated higher if the SPF number hadn't stopped at 14.

😐 **Advanced Radiance Age-Defying Liquid Makeup SPF 10** *($11.99)* gets its sunscreen rating partially from titanium dioxide, so it's sad that the SPF number is too low to rely on for daytime protection. Even more disturbing is Cover Girl's "restores youthful appearance" claims, which would have resonated better with an SPF 15 sunscreen. There is no question you'll be impressed with the airy-yet-creamy texture of this smooth-blending foundation. It blends on easily, providing sheer to light coverage and a radiant finish that enlivens the skin's appearance. Despite the creamy feel, this isn't the best formula for someone with dry skin because the base of silicone and glycerin combined with talc won't be enough to make dryness look or feel better. However, this is an option if you pair it with a moisturizing sunscreen rated SPF 15 or higher. Cover Girl's selection of 14 shades is mostly impressive and includes choices for fair to dark (but not very dark) skin tones.

The following shades are best avoided due to overtones of peach, pink, and red: Natural Ivory (which has enough pink to qualify as a blush), Classic Beige, Natural Beige, Creamy Beige, and Toasted Almond. This foundation does contain the Olay ingredients (remember, Cover Girl and Olay are owned by Procter & Gamble) niacinamide and palmitoyl pentapeptide-3, which is a nice touch, but what a shame the SPF rating falls short of the desired SPF 15.

😐 **Advanced Radiance Restorative Cream Foundation SPF 10** *($10.99)* has an in-part titanium dioxide sunscreen but an SPF rating that's too low to provide sufficient daytime protection (especially if this is your only source of sunscreen). That's a shame, because just about every other aspect of this foundation is top-notch. It has a delicate, whipped texture that feels wonderfully silky and is a pleasure to blend. Coverage goes from sheer to medium and the finish is seamlessly smooth and radiant, thanks to the silicone base. The formula even contains some typical skin-care extras, including antioxidant green tea, peptides, and niacinamide. Five of the eight shades are soft and neutral, suitable for fair to light skin tones. The shades to avoid due to prominent overtones of pink or peach are Natural Ivory, Creamy Beige, and Medium Light. Despite the cream part of the name, this foundation is best for normal to slightly dry skin. It can look too glow-y over oily areas.

😐 **Clean Makeup Fragrance Free** *($4.99)* mercifully omits the sickly sweet scent that is present in the original Clean Makeup formula (reviewed below), as well as the irritating extracts. Unfortunately, most of the 15 shades are just too strongly peach, pink, or rose for most skin tones. The only four shades worth considering are Ivory, Classic Ivory, Soft Honey, and Classic Tan.

😐 **Clean Makeup Oil Control** *($4.99)* is an oil- and fragrance-free liquid foundation that I suppose was Cover Girl's attempt to modernize their original Clean Makeup. It's nice that the irritants and overpowering fragrance were omitted, but the shades still suffer from a preponderance of rose, pink, peach, and orange tones. The foundation itself isn't as silky-smooth as it could have been, and its matte, slightly powdery finish tends to look a bit chalky in the lighter shades. It's an OK light-coverage option for normal to oily skin, but the only worthwhile shades are Ivory, Classic Ivory, Buff Beige, and Creamy Natural.

😐 **Ultimate Finish Liquid Powder Makeup** *($7.49)* is a below-standard, very dated cream-to-powder foundation. It smooths on OK but the high amount of aluminum starch octenylsuccinate causes it to dry almost instantly, and it can feel uncomfortably matte. Ultimately, this is workable only for those with oily skin not prone to blemishes, because the waxlike thickeners in this product certainly won't promote clear skin. The 15 shades are packaged so you can see the color, but remain a mixed bag; 8 of them are too glaringly peach, pink, or rose for most skin tones, so you should avoid Natural Ivory, Creamy Natural, Classic Beige, Medium Light, Warm Beige, Creamy Beige, Natural Beige, and Toasted Almond. Soft Sable and Tawny are worthwhile shades for darker skin tones, but Cover Girl's AquaSmooth Makeup SPF 15 or their Advanced Radiance Age-Defying Compact Foundation are assuredly preferred to this.

☹ **Clean Makeup** *($4.99)* is the original Cover Girl foundation (launched in 1961) that hasn't yet been discontinued despite the fact that it has a dated, basic formula that contains clove, menthol, camphor, and eucalyptus, which are extremely irritating for skin, comes in colors that are largely unusable for any skin tone, and has fragrance that is intrusive. This must be selling well, however, or why would they keep it for so many years? Yet all that means is that there are thousands of women wearing an irritating foundation whose colors haven't kept pace with the vast majority of foundations available, including those from Cover Girl.

☹ **Simply Powder Foundation** *($7.49)* claims it "covers like a liquid," and it may seem convenient to get that benefit from a powder. Don't bother. This talc-based pressed-powder foundation goes on unevenly, looks chalky, and isn't nearly as silky as Cover Girl's superior TruBlend Powder Foundation SPF 15 above. The shades are also mostly problematic, because with the texture and finish this has, even the neutral options just don't look convincing on skin.

CONCEALER: ☺ **Advanced Radiance Age-Defying Correcting Concealer** *($7.49)* is meant to lighten dark areas under the eyes, and the angled felt-tip applicator makes it easier to apply there. This liquid concealer has a thin, silky texture and takes a bit longer than it should to set to a soft matte finish. It's not much for coverage, but it looks natural, highlights well, and won't crease. Four very good shades are available, but there are no options for medium to dark skin. The Under-Eye Disguise shade has a noticeable yellow tinge that appears more neutral on skin. By the way, although it may seem like an endorsement that this product is "Olay recommended," both they and Cover Girl are owned by Procter & Gamble.

☺ **Fresh Complexion Concealer** *($5.49)* is the only Cover Girl concealer to seriously consider. It has a wonderful, lightly creamy texture and a soft application that provides almost too much slip. Although blending this concealer takes a bit more time, the natural matte finish and smooth coverage are worth it. This wouldn't be my top choice if your main concern is great coverage, but those with minor imperfections should check it out. Of the four colors, only Natural Beige is too pink to purchase, but be careful with the slightly pink Creamy Beige, too.

😐 **CG Smoothers Concealer** *($5.99)* is a standard, lipstick-style concealer that doesn't go on as greasy as it appears and provides good coverage with minimal creasing. However, four of the six shades are on the peach side, and the coverage is opaque enough for that to be a problem for some skin tones. Neutralizer is OK, but Illuminator is too whitish pink for even very light skin. This concealer is not recommended for use over blemishes or blemish-prone areas.

😐 **Invisible Concealer** *($4.49)* has a formula and mostly poor colors that have caused it to fall out of favor as a recommended concealer. It provides adequate coverage but has a somewhat tacky finish that isn't as elegant as today's best liquid, wand-applicator concealers. Among the five shades, only the darker ones (Honey and Tawny) are workable.

POWDER: ✓☺ **TruBlend Pressed Powder** *($7.49)* carries on the remarkable pigment technology introduced with Cover Girl's TruBlend Foundation. This talc-based powder has a silky smooth, slightly thick texture that meshes so well with skin you won't know you're wearing powder. Instead, the skin looks refined and finished rather than pasty or dry, an effect that is flattering on all skin types. Six shades are available, and here's where Cover Girl's "matches 97% of skin tones" comes into play. All of the shades are beautiful; in fact, I found I could wear four of the six convincingly. Somehow, the pigments in this powder simply enhance skin without changing its natural color. This is good news, because it means you're not likely to make a mistake choosing a shade—just pick something that looks close to your skin tone and try it on. Chances are, you'll be pleasantly surprised with the results. ✓☺ **Advanced Radiance Age-Defying Pressed Powder** *($6.99)* has a formula, texture, and finish that are identical to those of the TruBlend Pressed Powder above, so the same basic comments apply. Six shades are available, and there's not a bad one in the bunch. Both this and the TruBlend Pressed Powder are wonderful for all but very oily skin—because that will need more shine control than these powders are capable of providing.

☺ **TruBlend Naturally Luminous Loose Powder** *($7.49)* gets its luminosity from the finely milled sparkles it contains, though they don't cling well to skin so the luminous finish is short-lived. This is otherwise an airy, dry-textured, talc-based loose powder that imparts very sheer color from its four shades (most of which look brazenly peach to orange in the container but not on skin). Its soft finish looks fairly natural on skin, too, and it's a good option if you need a sheer loose powder but don't require lots of oil absorption. ☺ **TruBlend Naturally Luminous Bronzer** *($7.49)* has the exact same formula as the TruBlend Naturally Luminous Loose Powder above, except this version comes in two sheer, bronze-toned shades, both suitable for fair to medium skin tones. The shine is more apparent with this powder when compared with the two above, and it has the same problem of not clinging well. However, the sheer hint of tan can be attractive and the shine isn't so distracting as to make this an evening-only product.

☺ **CG Smoothers Pressed Powder** *($5.99)* comes in six suitably neutral colors that leave a subtle, shiny finish on skin. The talc- and mineral oil–based formula is best for normal to dry skin. It leaves a satin finish yet isn't quite as silky as the two Cover Girl pressed powders above.

☺ **Outlast Pressed Powder** *($7.49)* has a noticeably smooth texture and glides over skin with ease. However, this fragrance-free, talc-based powder's finish isn't as natural looking as others, which is why a Paula's Pick rating was not assigned. Six shades are available, and although some (such as Translucent Medium and Translucent Beige) look too peachy pink in the compact, each goes on fairly neutral and sheer. That makes getting the color exactly right less of an issue, and most skin tones will find they can wear two or more of these shades. ☺ **Clean Pressed Powder Fragrance-Free** *($5.49)* isn't "cleaner" than any of the other pressed powders in the Cover Girl line. It's a standard, talc-based powder with a smooth application and soft, slightly dry finish suitable for normal to oily skin. The 15 shades fare much better than those for the Clean Makeup above, with the only missteps being Classic Beige, Warm Beige, Creamy Beige, and the borderline-peach Soft Honey.

😐 **Fresh Look Pressed Powder** *($5.99)* deserves a compliment for its smooth texture and lightweight matte finish, but tends to look dry on skin, creating a flatness that doesn't translate to a fresh complexion. It's best dusted on sheer, and is a reasonably good option for those with oily skin, plus all six colors are soft and neutral. 😐 **Tanfastic Bronzer** *($4.99)* is a pressed, talc-based bronzing powder that comes in two sheer tan shades best for fair to light skin. The dry texture isn't as elegant as many others, likely due to the calcium silicate (the second ingredient) that compromises chances for attaining a silkier feel. It's an OK option, but the bronzing powders from Wet 'N' Wild are nicer and cost less (though Cover Girl's price is nothing to scoff at).

☹ **Clean Pressed Powder for Normal Skin** *($4.99)* is almost identical to its fragrance-free counterpart, but this one includes eucalyptus oil and camphor, both of which are very irritating even in small amounts. It also has a medicinal-sweet fragrance that'll enter a room before you do. ☹ **Professional Loose Powder** *($5.49)* comes in six mostly well-conceived shades and has a fine texture, but that is cancelled out by the pointless inclusion of eucalyptus, camphor, clove oil, and menthol—four potent irritants—and the sickly sweet fragrance.

BLUSH: All but one of Cover Girl's powder blushes contain menthol, camphor, eucalyptus oil, and clove oil—irritants that have no business being in makeup and serve no positive purpose for the skin. ☺ **TruBlend Naturally Luminous Blush** *($7.49)* has the exact same formula as the TruBlend Naturally Luminous Loose Powder above, except this version comes in two sheer blush shades, neither of which does much to impart noticeable cheek color. This is best used as a highlighting powder paired with a standard powder blush, though the two shades are limited to those with fair to light skin.

☹ **Instant Cheekbones** *($5.49)* has three colors in one compact—a blush tone, a contour color, and a shiny highlighter. The colors for these and for the single blush version, ☹ **Cheekers** *($3.99)*, finally are an updated palette of contemporary shades, but have a terribly dry, flaky texture that sweeps on unevenly, creating a blotchy look. ☹ **Classic Color Blush** *($5.69)* is a powder blush that comes in four shades that, although vivid, blend on sheer. These are fairly powdery, and the color intensity is too soft for darker skin tones.

EYESHADOW: ☺ **PowderExact Powder Eyeshadow in a Stick** *($5.99)* does come in a stick, and is more or less a novel approach to standard pressed-powder ey shadow. The twist-up, nonretractable stick goes on smoothly and powder-dry, and thus cannot be blended much. All of the shades have shine, and it's strong enough to call attention to wrinkles. I think this has more youth appeal. It definitely doesn't replace standard powder eyeshadows, but it's a clever departure if you want to shake up your routine. ☺ **CG Eyeslicks Gel Eyecolor** *($5.49)* consists of chubby pencils that go on somewhat wet, which means they glide on easily, and then the color dries to a matte (in feel) finish that doesn't budge or smear all day. Because of the wider pencil head, you can't draw a thin line. In addition, all of the shades are shiny, so these are best used on smooth, taut eyelids for a shadowy effect or on the under-brow area to highlight. Oddly, despite budgeproof wear, this comes off immediately with just water, so don't get caught in the rain!

😐 **Shadow Squease** *($5.49)* may seem like a kicky new way to experiment with eyeshadow, but this liquid-cream product, packaged in a squeeze tube with a built-in sponge applicator, has too much slip for precise blending, and the large shiny particles tend to migrate and flake, though not excessively. Almost all of the colors are soft, so blending shades together is fine, but the effort isn't worth it considering what you can easily attain with powder eyeshadows (although not Cover Girl's).

☹ **Eye Enhancers 1-Kit Shadows** *($3.49)* have a nonsense name because one color (or one of anything) does not a kit make. Each shade has a smooth, unusually dry texture that imparts sheer color, but not without some flaking and skipping during application. Again, these apply very sheer—even the black shade goes on almost translucent. Compared to powder eyeshadows from L'Oreal, Sonia Kashuk, and Jane, these really aren't worth considering. ☹ **Eye Enhancers 3-Kit Shadows** *($5.49)* and ☹ **Eye Enhancers 4-Kit Shadows** *($5.49)* have some potentially workable color combinations (and some real duds), but also have the same formula and application issues as the Eye Enhancers 1-Kit Shadows above.

EYE AND BROW SHAPER: ✓☺ **Liquid Pencil Felt Tip Eyeliner** *($5.69)* is an excellent, gel-based liquid eyeliner that applies easily and stays on without fading or chipping off. It is also very easy to wash off, so if you're a fan of this type of eyeliner, this is a strong contender—and the four shades are all contenders, too. ✓☺ **Outlast Smoothwear All-Day Eyeliner** *($6.99)* is an automatic, silicone-based retractable pencil that features a built-in sharpener, a nice option when you need to sharpen the point to allow you to draw on a thinner line. I was very impressed with how well this pencil goes on and how, once set, it wears fairly well without a trace of smudging or smearing. Some fading does occur, especially by the end of the day, but for the most part this is a slam-dunk recommendation as one of the best eye pencils available at the drugstore. One caution: Removing this requires more than a water-soluble cleanser. OK, two cautions: Avoid Sage, because this shade of green eyeliner isn't pretty on anyone, especially if you want to be taken seriously.

☺ **Perfect Point Plus** *($4.99)* is an automatic eye pencil that glides on easily without being greasy, and it maintains a consistent, sharp point. Chestnut is a great shade as an auburn eyeliner, but Midnight Blue is best avoided. Avoid using the smudge tip—it's not well made and can change your eye makeup look from smoky to messy.

😐 **Perfect Blend Eye Pencil** *($4.49)* hasn't changed since it was last reviewed. It remains a standard but good pencil that goes on slightly drier than most others and has decent staying power. There are six shades, and all come with a sponge tip to ease blending. Avoid Cobalt Blue.

☹ **CG Smoothers Eyeliner** *($5.49)* needs sharpening but is indeed smooth. You won't have any trouble applying this pencil eyeliner, but how long it lasts is questionable given that it sheers out quickly and can look spotted, with patches of color being stronger in one area than another. Stick with Cover Girl's Outlast Smoothwear All-Day Eyeliner instead of this.

☹ **Brow and Eye Makers** *($2.99)* feature two short pencils that are the same color. You're supposed to use one for eyes and one for brows, but the dry, waxy texture makes both of them more appropriate for use as a brow pencil, albeit not a very good one. That's because application can be painful and the finish is tacky enough to be bothersome.

LIPSTICK, LIP GLOSS, AND LIPLINER: ✓☺ **Outlast All-Day Lipcolor** *($9.99)* is identical in every respect to Max Factor's Lipfinity. Both products feature a liquid color you apply to lips (make sure they're clean, dry, and free of any flakes), let set for a moment or two, then apply a glossy top coat for comfortable wear and shine. Outlast wears about the same as Lipfinity, which is to say extraordinarily well. As long as you can commit to regularly applying the moisturizing top coat, you'll be rewarded with feel-good color that lasts through most meals (oily salad dressings or fried foods are this lip color's undoing), and it doesn't come off on cups or people (so go ahead and kiss the ones you love freely). The only minor areas where Cover Girl's Outlast bests Max Factor's Lipfinity are price (Outlast typically costs $1–$2 less) and shade selection.

✓☺ **Outlast Smoothwear All-Day Lipcolor** *($9.99)* is similar to Cover Girl's regular Outlast All-Day Lipcolor, but with less pigment and the tradeoff of a shorter wear time, although Cover Girl claims both products last ten hours. This has the same formula and technology as original Outlast—the only difference is the level of pigment in each color. If you thought the first round of Outlast colors was too bold or intense, consider this sheer option so you can experience one of the best long-wearing lipsticks available. Yes, you need to reapply the Conditioning

Moisturecoat at regular intervals to avoid lips that feel desert dry, but the color itself really does stay put, and that is what makes this type of long-wearing lip color so unique.

☺ **TruShine Lipcolor** *($6.49)* is a moderate-coverage, smooth cream lipstick with a soft gloss finish. The selling point is Cover Girl's claim that the shade range matches 97% of skin tones. That's not surprising, nor is it a marvel of chemistry, because the selection of warm and cool tones coordinates well with a multitude of skin tones and colors. Basically, the shade range is a can't-go-wrong mix of classic neutrals, reds, pinks, plums, and coral hues, most offset by a slight shimmer finish. The deeper shades have more staying power thanks to their pigmentation, while the pastel shades tend to fade quickly. The slippery finish of this lipstick ensures movement into lines around the mouth, but if that's not an issue for you, this is yet another cream lipstick to consider.

☺ **Outlast Double LipShine** *($8.19)* is a sheerer, glossier version of Cover Girl's Outlast Smoothwear All Day Lipcolor. The same application steps are called for, meaning you apply a coat of color, wait for it to set, then brush on the glossy top coat for shine and comfortable wear. The big claim here is that this product lasts longer than the leading lip gloss (whatever product that is wasn't identified), with up to ten hours of wear. Although the color does last for hours (with regular touchups to the top coat to keep lips from feeling parched), it doesn't last evenly for more than a couple of hours. You'll likely notice some fading, especially toward the inner portion of the lips, while the border retains stronger color, sort of like when your lipstick wears off before the Lipliner. It's not a deal-breaker, and there's no question this product wears longer than a regular lip gloss, but it isn't failsafe and does require maintenance to keep up appearances.

☺ **IncrediFULL Lip Color** *($6.49)* follows a trend in the cosmetics industry in which makeup products are positioned as going beyond what is typically expected for their category. This lipstick is a great example. Rather than just positioning it as a creamy, "all-day moisturizing" lipstick with rich color, Cover Girl's angle is to address the needs of women concerned with lips that become thinner with age. IncrediFULL is said to plump lips and add volume, and they even go so far as to proclaim it enhances the natural lip line! The ingredients allegedly responsible for such effects are vitamin E and various B vitamins, including niacinamide. This lipstick also contains an appreciable amount of glycerin, which helps attract moisture to the lips and keep it there, temporarily making them appear fuller. The amount of vitamins in this lipstick is negligible relative to the other standard ingredients, and vitamins won't add volume to lips, at least not in any way close to what collagen or hyaluronic acid dermal injections can accomplish. But that doesn't mean this isn't a worthwhile lipstick. It has a wonderfully creamy feel and imparts opaque color that doesn't feel thick or greasy, although the formula is slick enough to feather into lines around the mouth. The shade selection favors pinks and reds, so unless you're looking for soft, sheer colors, most of the options are attractive.

☺ **Continuous Color Lipstick** *($5.49)* is available in a Creme or Shimmer finish, with the Creme version being preferred for its smoother texture and the fact that the shimmer in the Shimmer version tends to feel grainy as the lipstick's creaminess wears off. Both formulas feel emollient and last decently without feathering into lines around the mouth. ☺ **LipSlicks Lipgloss** *($3.99)* is a basic, emollient, castor oil–based sheer lipstick with some very shiny shades, all in packaging that makes getting it on the lips very tricky for anyone with thin lips. ☺ **Outlast Smoothwear All-Day Lipliner** *($6.49)* is a very good automatic, retractable lip pencil. It glides on with a creaminess that is smooth but easy to control, and does its job of staying put, defining the lip line without migrating into creases or fading before your lipstick does. The shade selection isn't as extensive as Cover Girl's, but most of the colors are versatile.

☺ **CG Wetslicks** *($4.97)* is an improvement on Cover Girl's longstanding lip gloss option, Lipslicks. Lipslicks had a wide, swivel-up applicator, which was tricky to use unless you had naturally full lips. Wetslicks is a conventionally packaged tube-type lip gloss with an angled sponge-tip applicator. Formula-wise, it doesn't set any new standards; it is merely a lightweight, non-sticky lip gloss whose sheer colors are infused with heavy shimmer. The shade selection is sparkling and attractive, with the only drawback being its potent, sweet fragrance. ☺ **Wetslicks Crystals Lip Gloss** *($5.50)* is a gloss to consider if you're a fan of ultra-sparkly lip gloss and prefer a smooth, non-goopy texture that doesn't make lips feel like they're coated in caramel. The shades are more about high shine than about making an impact with color, but if you apply them over lipstick, that's a non-issue. ☺ **Wetslicks Fruit Spritzers** *($5.79)* smell and taste like fruit, and all of the sheer, shimmer-infused shades coat lips with a juicy shine and non-sticky, thick-but-smooth texture. This tube lip gloss is an option if you're looking for soft, sparkling colors; however, the flavor may make you lick your lips more often, which means more frequent touch-ups (not to mention that ingesting extra lip gloss isn't necessarily the best idea).

☺ **Smoothwear Lip Tints** *($6.49)* is a reliable, smooth-textured, squeeze-tube gloss with sheer colors that de-emphasize pigment in favor of shimmer. It is substantially glossy without a trace of stickiness, and yet isn't so slick it immediately moves into lines around the mouth. That will happen eventually (as it does with any lip gloss), but if your lips are prone to feathering, lip gloss shouldn't be the first item you reach for anyway!

😐 **CG Smoothers Lipliner** *($5.79)* is as standard a Lipliner as they come, and the fact that it needs sharpening doesn't make it worth considering over Cover Girl's Outlast Smoothwear All-Day Lipliner, reviewed above.

MASCARA: ☺ **Lash Exact Mascara** *($6.99)* has a unique brush that appears spiky, almost resembling cactus bristles, yet it turns out that the brush does an amazing job of making lashes thick with minimal effort. It's not much for creating length, but if thickness without clumps is what you're after, this is highly recommended and a welcome addition to Cover Girl's gradually getting-better mascara lineup.

☺ **Lash Exact Waterproof Mascara** *($7.99)* has the same rubber-bristled brush as the original (non-waterproof) Lash Exact Mascara above. Cover Girl claims that this special brush has the advantage of allowing you to easily reach every lash, but lots of mascara brushes have that capability. It's more about the size of the brush than what the bristles are made of. In any event, this is an admirable waterproof mascara that builds long lashes quickly along with moderate thickness. You'll notice some minor clumping, especially with lashes at corners of the eye, but that's easily remedied with the brush. This wears all day without a flake or smear, and must be taken off with a silicone- or oil-based remover.

☺ **Volume Exact Mascara** *($6.99)* is riding the success of Cover Girl's popular Lash Exact Mascara, and compared to the progenitor, this formula (also with a rubber-bristled brush) thickens lashes even more and keeps them well-defined with only minor clumping. Successive coats smooth things out, but, oddly, don't make lashes much longer. Some length is attainable, but this is really best as a thickening mascara, and it wears beautifully. ☺ **Volume Exact Waterproof Mascara** *($6.49)* isn't as impressive as the non-waterproof version of Volume Exact, but it works if what you're after is a clean application, soft definition, and a trusty waterproof formula. Lashes never look too coated or too heavy, regardless of how many coats you apply.

The downside is that lashes never get beyond moderately long, and thickness is on the mild side. Depending on what you want out of a mascara, those can be good or bad traits. ☺ **Super Thick Lash Mascara** *($4.99)* does well as a lengthening mascara, easily elongating lashes without clumps. Despite the name, it builds modest thickness, but is best as a lengthening mascara that leaves lashes softly fringed.

☺ **Professional Mascara Classic Look Curved Brush** *($4.99)* makes lashes longer but not the least bit thick. It separates and defines without clumping, though it takes a bit of practice with the curved brush to get an even application. ☺ **Multiplying Mascara** *($4.99)* promises to provide the "look of twice the lashes," and follows this statement with an asterisk. On the back of the package, you'll notice that Cover Girl actually means twice the lashes versus *bare* lashes, which is hardly an impressive feat because most of the mascaras in the world accomplish this with ease. Even so, it is a worthwhile lengthening mascara that nicely separates lashes without clumping and removes easily. ☺ **Curved Brush Fantastic Lash Mascara** *($6.49)* marks one of the few times where I noticed the curved brush makes a difference for the better. With some effort, you can build long, reasonably thick lashes with minor, easily fixed clumping. It also leaves lashes softly curled, and wears well, making it Cover Girl's overall best mascara.

☺ **Multiplying Waterproof Mascara** *($5.99)* allows you to build average length with little thickness. Lashes are well (but not dramatically) defined with a few sweeps and no clumps. This is very waterproof, whether you're anticipating tears or plan to take a dip in the pool. Where things get tricky is trying to remove this extremely tenacious formula! You will need a separate oil- or silicone-based makeup remover on hand to make sure you've completely washed this off. ☺ **Professional Waterproof Mascara** *($4.99)* has a formula that applies easily and with some effort builds noticeable length and minimal thickness. Best of all, it really does hold up when wet yet is easy to remove, coming off almost completely with just a water-soluble cleanser. ☺ **Remarkable Washable Waterproof Mascara** *($4.99)* applies evenly and builds good length with minimal thickness. It isn't as waterproof as others, withstanding only a little water (such as a light rain) and breaking down under water—so swimmers and criers will have to look elsewhere. True to its name, it does wash off easily—but that's the tradeoff for a formula that isn't as waterproof as most others.

😐 **Professional Mascara Classic Look Straight Brush** *($4.99)* has an easier-to-wield wand than the curved version (though I suspect some women like curved brushes, whereas I find them awkward), but this version builds lengthy lashes unevenly and needs more fine-tuning than it should. 😐 **Marathon Waterproof Mascara** *($5.49)* is Cover Girl's most impressive waterproof mascara in terms of how tenaciously waterproof it is, but the lengthened, wet look it creates isn't for everyone, and there's some clumping along the way. This is extremely difficult to remove, even with an oil- or silicone-based remover. It definitely turns your nightly cleansing routine into a marathon of its own.

😐 **Fantastic Lash Mascara** *($6.49)* claims to provide five times the volume of ordinary lashes, which would really be fantastic, but it doesn't deliver. Instead, it excels at creating long (but not impressively long), separated lashes. If you want truly fantastic mascara, you'll have to look to L'Oreal or Maybelline, because Cover Girl's options fall short of fantastic. 😐 **Professional Natural Lash Mascara** *($4.99)* is just a clear, boring mascara that does incredibly little to enhance lashes, and is best used as a soft-finish brow gel. Cover Girl claims this mascara is smudgeproof, but this claim is meaningless—the product is clear, so what difference does it make if some smudging occurs?

☹ **Fantastic Lash Waterproof Mascara** *($6.49)* is fantastically mediocre for length and thickness, although it is waterproof. Still, there are plenty of waterproof mascaras (including others from Cover Girl) that do not flake and smear the way this one does, making Fantastic Lash Waterproof Mascara one to ignore.

BRUSHES: ☹ **Large Blush Brush** *($4.99)* is a poorly constructed brush that is not recommended because the bristles are too soft and too sparse, making color placement and control an issue. The ☹ **Powder Brush** *($5.69)* is cut straight across rather than domed or tapered, a shape that tends to work against the natural contours of the face and makes it easy to over-powder. The ☺ **Eyeshadow Brush** *($4.19)* isn't the most versatile due to its thickness, and if you're only going to offer one eyeshadow brush, it should be flatter and a bit more pointed for better control and blending. This remains an OK option for applying all-over or soft crease color.

SPECIALTY PRODUCTS: 😐 **Clean Makeup Remover for Eyes and Lips** *($4.29 for 2 ounces)* is mineral oil–based and yet this fluid, greasy lotion doesn't remove long-wearing makeup nearly as well as a silicone-based remover. It's an OK option for standard lipsticks that may leave a stain, but is far too greasy to use around the eyes or to remove mascara.

DARPHIN PARIS (SKIN CARE ONLY)

DARPHIN PARIS AT-A-GLANCE

Strengths: Lauder's influence on this line has resulted in only a few improved products; there are some good cleansers; some worthwhile serums and moisturizers.

Weaknesses: Very expensive; no products to address acne or pigmentation issues; only one sunscreen and it has problems; jar packaging for products that contain air- and light-sensitive ingredients.

For more information about Darphin Paris, owned by Estee Lauder, call (866) 880-455-4559 or visit www.darphhin.com or www.Beautypedia.com.

DARPHIN PARIS AROVITA PRODUCTS

😐 **$$$ Arovita C Cream** *($150 for 1.7 ounces)* includes compelling ingredients for creating healthy, radiant skin (including retinol), but they won't be around for long once this jar-packaged moisturizer is opened. Minus the antioxidants, it's a standard emollient option for normal to dry skin. The orange coloring agent is supposed to align with the vitamin C theme of Darphin's Arovita products.

☹ **Arovita Eye and Lip Contour Gel** *($85 for 1 ounce)* contains several fragrance components that can be irritating to skin, but especially so when used around the eyes. This water- and jojoba oil–based gel is not recommended.

😐 **$$$ Arovita Fluid** *($95 for 1 ounce)* is a standard lightweight moisturizing lotion that contains retinol, but in packaging that won't keep this extremely light-sensitive ingredient stable. The amount of vitamin C isn't anything to write home about, and the bitter orange oil can be a skin irritant. In nearly every respect, there isn't any reason to consider this product, and nothing in the formula will reduce excess oil.

😐 **$$$ Arovita C Energic Firming Cream** *($110 for 1.7 ounces)* is an emollient moisturizer for dry skin that contains some very good skin-identical ingredients, but the vitamin C and other antioxidants won't last long after this jar-packaged product is opened. As expected, this will not firm skin. One of the main plant extracts is morinda (listed as *Morinda citrifolia*).

You may be more familiar with this plant's common name of noni (it is sold as a juice and in supplement form with dozens of unsubstantiated health-related claims). There is no research proving morinda can help aging skin in any way, but it does't appear to be a cause for concern either, at least when it comes to topical application.

☹ **$$$ Arovita C Line Response Cream** *($110 for 1.7 ounces)* is actually a much more exciting formula than the Arovita C Energic Firming Cream above, so it's that much more disappointing that jar packaging limits the effectiveness of the light- and air-sensitive powerhouse ingredients that are in here. Given the poor packaging choice, this ends up being a needlessly pricey moisturizer for normal to dry skin.

☺ **$$$ Arovita C Line Response Firming Serum** *($125 for 1 ounce)* is a serum version of the Arovita C Line Response Cream above. It contains some noteworthy antioxidants, skin-identical ingredients, and cell-communicating ingredients, but its translucent glass bottle packaging means the vitamin C and other antioxidants are subject to deterioration unless this is kept stored in a dark place and away from sources of natural light. It is suitable for normal to slightly dry skin not prone to breakouts.

☺ **$$$ Arovita C Line Response Fluid** *($110 for 1.7 ounces)* is very similar to the Arovita C Line Response Firming Serum above, and the same review applies.

DARPHIN PARIS HYDRASKIN PRODUCTS

☹ **$$$ Hydraskin Intensive Moisturizing Serum** *($90 for 1 ounce)* contains mostly water, slip agents, plant oil, glycerin, gemstone extract, antioxidants, water-binding agents, preservative, vitamin E, film-forming agents, fragrance, and potentially irritating fragrance components. It's an OK lightweight moisturizer for normal to oily skin, but for the money not nearly as elegant as the serum-type moisturizers from Estee Lauder or Clinique.

☹ **$$$ Hydraskin Light** *($85 for 1.7 ounces)* is a good lightweight, silicone-enhanced moisturizer for normal to slightly oily skin, but the jar packaging won't keep the plant-based antioxidants stable once the product is opened. This does contain potentially irritating fragrance components.

☹ **Hydraskin Night** *($90 for 1.7 ounces)* contains irritating horsetail extract (listed by its Latin name of *Equisetum arvense*) as well as irritating fragrance components of eugenol, isoeugenol, linalool, and geraniol, among others.

☹ **$$$ Hydraskin Rich** *($85 for 1.7 ounces)* works well for dry to very dry skin but so do many other moisturizers that not only cost less but use packaging that will keep the antioxidants stable while excluding potentially irritating fragrance components.

DARPHIN PARIS INTRAL PRODUCTS

☺ **$$$ Intral Cleansing Milk** *($50 for 6.7 ounces)* is a lighter version of the Cleansing Aromatic Emulsion reviewed below, and better suited for those with normal to slightly dry skin not prone to breakouts. This still ends up being a lot of money for a standard, detergent-free cleansing lotion.

☹ **$$$ Intral Toner** *($50 for 6.7 ounces)* is a basic, alcohol- and fragrance-free toner that contains some good water-binding and soothing agents. It is recommended for normal to dry skin, but so is Neutrogena Alcohol-Free Toner ($6.99 for 8.5 ounces).

☹ **$$$ Intral Balm** *($105 for 1.7 ounces)* is one of the better balms from Darphin because it eschews irritating fragrant oils (though it still contains potentially irritating fragrance components such as limonene and geraniol). This balm is mostly vegetable oil with thickeners, wax, and plant oil. For a lot less money and zero risk of skin irritation, you can treat your very dry skin to plain, extra virgin olive oil or plain jojoba oil instead.

😐 **$$$ Intral Complex** *($110 for 1 ounce)* contains some effective plant-based soothing agents, but that alone doesn't justify this water-based serum's price. Further, the translucent glass packaging demands careful storage so the antioxidants aren't exposed to light (which diminishes their effectiveness). This contains minimal fragrance and is an OK option for oily to slightly oily skin, assuming the price doesn't give you stress breakouts.

😐 **$$$ Intral Cream** *($90 for 1.7 ounces)* is another emollient moisturizer from Darphin whose banal blend of water, thickeners, slip agent, shea butter, and several more thickeners along with tiny amounts of plant extracts isn't all that impressive. This is an OK option for dry to very dry skin, but it does contain some potentially problematic fragrant plant extracts and lesser amounts of potentially irritating fragrance components.

DARPHIN PARIS PREDERMINE PRODUCTS

☹ **Predermine Cream** *($175 for 1.7 ounces)* has the most rudimentary base formula that ends up being an overpriced showcase for tiny amounts of skin-identical ingredients and some problematic plant extracts, along with 14 volatile fragrance component ingredients that add up to trouble for most skin types.

☹ **Predermine Serum** *($310 for 1 ounce)* doesn't contain a single ingredient that even remotely justifies its price, nor can anything in this product boost natural collagen production better than other products. It's an average water-based serum that contains problematic horsetail, jasmine, and iris extracts along with over a dozen fragrance components, most of which are considered skin sensitizers. I don't know who to recommend this to except those who like spending a lot for a potentially troublesome return on their investment.

☺ **$$$ Predermine Wrinkle Corrective Serum** *($195 for 1 ounce)* is one of the best formulations in Darphin's lineup, with ingredients that mimic the structure and function of healthy skin. Although this product deserves its rating because of the plethora of state-of-the-art ingredients it contains, you should know that nearly identical products are available from Clinique's Repairwear line, from Estee Lauder's Perfectionist line, and in Prescriptives Super Line Preventor+ 24 Hour Environmental Skincare ($47.50 for 1 ounce). Along with Darphin, these are all Lauder-owned lines. Whichever product you purchase will produce good results, but won't eliminate wrinkles. If anything, Darphin's option ends up being less impressive because of the volatile fragrance components it contains (a factor that also keeps it from earning a Paula's Pick rating).

☹ **Predermine Mask** *($85 for 1.7 ounces)* is a below-standard, ridiculously expensive clay mask that irritates skin by including iris and horsetail extracts.

DARPHIN PARIS STIMULSKIN PRODUCTS

😐 **$$$ Stimulskin Plus Eye Contour Cream** *($130 for 0.5 ounce)* has some wonderful ingredients for dry to very dry skin around the eyes or elsewhere on the face, but the antioxidants are compromised by jar packaging. Similarly rich moisturizers are widely available for much less money.

😐 **$$$ Stimulskin Plus Firming Smoothing Cream, for Dry Skin** *($230 for 1.7 ounces)* is loaded with state-of-the-art skin-care ingredients, but the potency of most of them (including retinol) is significantly diminished because of the jar packaging. Even if the packaging were better, however, the fragrant oils are potentially irritating, making this a less desirable option at any price.

☹ **$$$ Stimulskin Plus Firming Smoothing Cream** *($230 for 1.7 ounces)* is similar to, but with fewer bells and whistles than, the Stimulskin Plus Firming Smoothing Cream, for Dry Skin above, and the same basic comments apply. For over $200, the least you should expect is packaging that will keep the retinol stable.

☹ **$$$ Stimulskin Plus Intensive Face Lifting Complex** *($350 for 1 ounce)* may sound like a face-lift in a bottle, but doesn't come even a little bit close. This serum contains mostly water, slip agents, castor oil, silicone thickener, skin-identical ingredients, fragrant plant extracts (none capable of lifting or firming skin), antioxidants, alcohol, preservatives, and fragrance. Several of the fragrance components are potentially irritating to skin, and keep this product from earning a better rating. Even without them, this serum pales in comparison to any offered by other Lauder-owned companies.

☹ **$$$ Stimulskin Plus Rejuvenating Lifting Serum** *($295 for 1 ounce)* is very similar to the Stimulskin Plus Intensive Face Lifting Complex above, except with a lower price and more skin-identical ingredients. Otherwise, the same review applies.

OTHER DARPHIN PARIS PRODUCTS

☹ **Azahar Cleansing Micellar Water, All-In-One French Cleanser** *($50 for 6.7 ounces)* may have a French lineage, but who's to say they know how to make great cleansers (wines are another story, but that's not what this book is about). This is merely water with slip agents, fragrant orange oil (which is irritating), a soothing agent (which won't outpace the irritation the orange oil causes), and preservatives. It isn't worth anyone's time or money, and won't help skin in the least.

☺ **$$$ Cleansing Aromatic Emulsion** *($50 for 4.2 ounces)* contains tiny amounts of plant extracts, but is overall a very standard water- and mineral oil–based cleanser for normal to dry skin. The aromatic element of this cleanser is what you're paying for, but that's not what's removing makeup or cleansing the skin. This rinses without the need for a washcloth.

☺ **$$$ Purifying Foam Gel, for Combination Oily Skin** *($50 for 4.2 ounces)* contains tiny amounts of plant extracts, none of them problematic. Nothing about this standard water-soluble cleanser is more purifying than most others; it's just an effective, albeit overpriced, option for normal to oily skin.

☺ **$$$ Refreshing Cleansing Milk** *($50 for 6.7 ounces)* is nearly identical to the Intral Cleansing Milk above, save for a change in plant extracts, which have no bearing on skin but add fragrance to this cleansing lotion. Otherwise, the same review applies.

☺ **$$$ Rich Cleansing Milk** *($50 for 6.7 ounces)* is actually lighter than the two Darphin Cleansing Milks above, although its oil content makes it unsuitable for breakout-prone skin. There are some intriguing antioxidants in this cleanser, but their benefit is quickly rinsed down the drain. It's an otherwise standard cleansing lotion that requires the use of a washcloth for complete removal and is best for normal to slightly dry skin. And the rich price tag? Sheer nonsense!

☹ **Gentle Eye Make-Up Remover** *($45 for 5.1 ounces)* contains fragrant plant extracts with no established benefit for skin and fragrance components, including eugenol and geraniol, neither of which is gentle or suitable for use in the eye area.

☺ **$$$ Exfoliating Foam Gel** *($50 for 4.2 ounces)* is a very standard cleanser/scrub hybrid that contains polyethylene (plastic) beads as the abrasive agent. Although this is workable for normal to oily skin, there is no reason to choose this over topical scrubs from the drugstore unless you steadfastly believe Darphin has all the answers.

☹ **Purifying Toner** *($50 for 6.7 ounces)* lists alcohol as the second ingredient, which is a shame because this is otherwise a well-formulated toner for all skin types.

☹ **Refreshing Toner** *($50 for 6.7 ounces)* contains a high concentration of fig fruit extract, which is known to cause contact dermatitis due to its psoralens content. Psoralens may also cause reactions when skin is exposed to sunlight.

☺ **$$$ Rich Toner** *($50 for 6.7 ounces)* contains a hefty amount of antioxidant black tea ferment, but the translucent packaging won't keep it potent unless it is kept away from light sources. That's the most exciting aspect of this standard but good (and overpriced) toner for normal to dry skin.

😐 **$$$ Skin Mat Balancing Serum** *($85 for 1 ounce)* is a water-based serum that contains about 1% salicylic acid, but the pH of 4.7 prevents it from working optimally as an exfoliant, and at this price that's the least you should expect. Although there are some good anti-irritants in this product, it lacks ingredients capable of making good on its claim of absorbing excess oil. The plant extracts it contains do nothing to reduce the appearance of pores, making this lightly moisturizing serum an expensive letdown.

☹ **Aromatic Purifying Balm** *($75 for 0.5 ounce)* is a rich blend of hazel seed and vegetable oil along with beeswax and several irritating fragrant oils, including sage, thyme, and lavender. It smells divine, but the fragrant oils are very irritating to skin and won't reduce the appearance of skin imperfections as claimed. If anything, they can make matters worse.

☹ **Chamomile Aromatic Care** *($75 for 0.5 ounce)* contains several irritating fragrant oils and fragrance components (such as eugenol) that make this a poor choice for all skin types, especially the product's targeted audience of consumers with blotchy, irritated skin.

☹ **Energic Cream** *($110 for 1.7 ounces)* contains several volatile fragrance components that can be irritating to skin and cause problems when skin is exposed to sunlight. It isn't even a very interesting moisturizer, and the few antioxidants will quickly become powerless due to jar packaging.

☹ **Fibrogene Complex** *($165 for 1 ounce)* lists *Equisetum arvense* (horsetail) as the fourth ingredient, making this product too irritating for all skin types. Horsetail has antioxidant properties, but its high tannin content is constricting and it can irritate skin (Source: www.herbmed.org). Oddly, Darphin claims this product will reduce the tight feeling those with very dry skin may experience!

☹ **Fibrogene Creme** *($150 for 1.7 ounces)* is an exceedingly boring, incredibly overpriced moisturizer that contains enough problematic plant extracts and fragrance components to make it not worth considering for any skin type. Almost any moisturizer from Dove or Neutrogena beats this formula, and without the potentially irritating ingredients.

☹ **Fibrogene Intensive** *($150 for 1.7 ounces)* is similar to the Fibrogene Creme above, and the same basic comments apply.

☹ **Firming Vitaserum 70** *($145 for 1 ounce)* contains irritating horsetail extract (listed by its Latin name *Equisetum arvense*) as well as irritating fragrance components of eugenol, linalool, and geraniol. If you're interested in seeing what a product with soy protein can do for your skin, consider those from Aveeno's Positively Radiant products instead. Aveeno packages those products to keep the antioxidants stable and they also exclude the potentially irritating fragrance components.

☹ **Instant Lumiere Brightening Cream** *($110 for 1.7 ounces)* lists citrus unshiu peel extract as the second ingredient. Although this extract has research showing its inhibitory effect on tyrosine (the amino acid in skin that initiates the production of the skin pigment melanin) and as such has validity as a skin-lightening agent, it also contains a high amount of the volatile fragrance component limonene, which is known to cause contact dermatitis (Sources: www.naturaldatabase.com; and *Journal of Occupational Health*, November 2006, pages 480–486). Therefore, it is not recommended over other skin-lightening agents that do not pose this problematic side effect.

☹ **Instant Lumiere Brightening Serum** *($130 for 1 ounce)* is the serum version of the Instant Lumiere Brightening Cream above. It contains less citrus unshiu peel extract, but is still likely to be problematic for most, and for the money, it's not worth choosing over a skin-lightening product with more reliable depigmenting agents.

😐 **$$$ Instantly Radiant** *($65 for 0.05 ounce)* is an off-putting amount of money for what amounts to primarily water, silicone, thickeners, and talc. The talc, titanium dioxide, and zinc oxide combine to cosmetically brighten the eye area, but this effect is attainable from careful use of any good concealer.

☹ **Intralderm Soothing Gel, for Sensitized Skin** *($50 for 2.6 ounces)* is an affordably priced product for Darphin and contains some state-of-the-art soothing agents ideally suited for sensitive skin. Why they had to ruin a good thing by adding an appreciable amount of skin-sensitizing lavender oil is anyone's guess, but it makes this gel moisturizer impossible to recommend.

☹ **Jasmine Aromatic Care** *($100 for 0.5 ounce)* contains several irritating ingredients for any skin type, including limonene, orange oil, and rosewood oil. Rather than risk irritation why not just treat your dry skin to pure sweet almond oil, which is the main ingredient in this fragrant moisturizer?

☺ **$$$ Lifting and Firming Eye Serum** *($75 for 0.5 ounce)* is an interesting blend of water, slip agents, tree pulp extract (likely functioning as a thickener because there is nothing but anecdotal evidence to support its usefulness for skin care), and some very good skin-identical ingredients and antioxidants. Darphin even left out fragrance components, which is a breath of fresh air given that almost every other product in the line literally stinks with fragrance. This is a worthwhile product for all skin types looking for a lightweight serum. It is not recommended for dry skin around the eyes (you'll want something emollient).

☹ **Myrrh Aromatic Care** *($75 for 0.5 ounce)* follows the same path as most of Darphin's Aromatic Care products and assaults the skin with several irritating volatile oils, including lavender, myrrh, and balsam. This sunflower oil–based moisturizer is not recommended.

☹ **Niaouli Aromatic Care** *($75 for 0.5 ounce)* has the same base as the Myrrh Aromatic Care above, but irritates skin with a potent blend of rosemary, bitter orange, and lavender oil, among other problematic ingredients. Plain sunflower seed oil is distinctly preferred to this product.

☹ **Rose Aromatic Care** *($75 for 0.5 ounce)* contains irritating volatile fragrant oils, including bay, as well as fragrance components that are not helpful for skin. Using plain sunflower or almond oil to moisturize very dry skin is preferred.

☹ **Tangerine Aromatic Care** *($75 for 0.5 ounce)* contains a trio of irritating plant oils, including orange, orange peel, and grapefruit peel. Skip the irritation and the potential for phototoxic reactions and use plain sunflower or jojoba oil if your skin is very dry.

😐 **$$$ Skin Mat Matifying Fluid** *($85 for 1.7 ounces)* is a fairly standard, lightweight moisturizer that helps create a matte finish due to the silicone it contains. The slip agents and thickeners won't keep skin matte for long, but will hydrate slightly dry skin. Although there are some good skin-identical ingredients in this product, it's an overall unimpressive formula for the money and absolutely will not reduce excess oil.

☹ **$$$ Vitaserum Eye Contour 40** *($70 for 0.5 ounce)* contains a good amount of soothing cornflower extract (listed as *Centaurea cyanus*), but is otherwise a basic gel moisturizer that contains a tiny amount of the film-forming agent PVP (think hairspray) to make eye-area skin feel a bit tighter. The oak root extract may be irritating to skin, and overall this product omits many ingredients that could have made it a prime choice for skin.

😐 **$$$ Dark Circles Relief and De-Puffing Eye Serum** *($75 for 0.5 ounce)* would be a good way to see if a product with peptides will work for you, although there is no research proving peptides' mettle for vanquishing dark circles or puffy eyes. The prominence of passionflower extract in this water-based serum looks impressive—if only it had documented benefit for skin. Research surrounding passionflower's potential benefit for skin did not involve the type Darphin uses, nor did that research have to do with eye-area cosmetic woes. The volatile fragrance components in this gel keep it from earning a higher rating, and may be a problem when this is applied near the eyes.

😐 **$$$ Hydrating Kiwi Mask** *($60 for 1.7 ounces)* is a very good, though needlessly expensive, moisturizing mask for normal to dry skin. The packaging will help keep the plant-based antioxidants stable, but it would be better if this product did not contain so many volatile fragrance components.

☹ **Mild Aroma Peeling** *($55 for 1.7 ounces)* is a paraffin-based mechanical scrub that is a poor option for all skin types because it contains irritating sandalwood oil.

☹ **Purifying Aromatic Clay Mask** *($50 for 1.7 ounces)* has far too many irritating fragrant oils to make it an option for any skin type. Bergamot, lavender, lemon, orange, and cypress present far more problems than benefits for skin.

☺ **$$$ Soothing Eye Contour Mask** *($75 for 1 ounce)* would warrant a Paula's Pick rating if it did not contain potentially problematic fragrance components. It's a lightweight gel mask that contains some helpful and truly soothing ingredients as well as antioxidants, plus the cell-communicating ingredient niacinamide. It's an option for all skin types needing mild hydration around the eyes or elsewhere on the face.

☺ **$$$ Vitabalm** *($25 for 0.12 ounce)* ends up being one of the most expensive castor oil–based, lipstick-style lip balms around—but it certainly takes good care of dry, chapped lips. Vitabalm does contain fragrance.

DARPHIN PARIS SUN PRODUCTS

☺ **$$$ Skin Bronze Self-Tanning Face & Body Cream** *($50 for 4.2 ounces)* is a standard, water- and silicone-based self-tanning lotion that contains dihydroxyacetone to turn skin brown. It works as well as any if you decide to overspend in this category.

☹ **Skin Bronze Self-Tanning Face & Body Tinted Cream** *($50 for 4.2 ounces)* contains the volatile fragrance components eugenol, linalool, and others. The potential for irritation makes this otherwise standard self-tanning lotion not worth considering over hundreds of others, most selling for under $20.

☹ **Skin Bronze Self-Tanning Face Tinted Gel** *($50 for 1.6 ounces)* contains the volatile fragrance components eugenol, linalool, and others, plus alcohol. The potential for irritation makes this otherwise standard self-tanning gel not worth considering over hundreds of others, most selling for under $20.

☹ **Soleil Plaisir, Protective Face Cream SPF 30** *($50 for 2.6 ounces)* provides broad-spectrum sun protection and includes avobenzone for UVA protection, but the formula lacks ingredients of interest to justify the price, although it does have a silky-smooth texture. A larger problem is the inclusion of many potent fragrance components, including eugenol. Plenty of sunscreens avoid these irritants, leaving this one not worth considering.

DDF
DOCTOR'S DERMATOLOGIC FORMULA
(SKIN CARE ONLY)

DDF AT-A-GLANCE

Strengths: Several good water-soluble cleansers; every sunscreen includes sufficient UVA-protecting ingredients; some truly state-of-the-art moisturizers and serums; a few good AHA and skin-lightening options; a good benzoyl peroxide topical disinfectant.

Weaknesses: Expensive; products designed for sensitive skin tend to contain one or more known problematic ingredients; several irritating products based on alcohol, menthol, or problematic plant extracts; more than a handful of average moisturizers, many in jar packaging.

For more information about DDF, owned by Procter & Gamble, call (800) 437-7546 or visit www.ddfskin.com or www.Beautypedia.com.

☺ **$$$ Blemish Foaming Cleanser** *($30 for 6.6 ounces)* is a standard, liquid-to-foam cleanser that contains mostly water, detergent cleansing agents, lather agent, and pH-adjusting agents. Salicylic acid is listed an an active, but its contact with skin is too brief for it to affect blemishes. The token amount of azelaic acid won't impact blemishes even a little. The same can be said for the plant extracts, some soothing and some irritating—but none present in an amount great enough to be a problem or to exert a benefit. This is a good, though pricey, option for normal to oily skin.

☺ **$$$ Brightening Cleanser** *($32 for 8.45 ounces)* is similar to the Blemish Foaming Cleanser above, except the azelaic acid is replaced by glycolic acid and the plant extracts are those known (at least in vitro) to have a skin-lightening effect. However, none of these ingredients will be helpful in a cleanser because it's rinsed from the skin before the ingredients can affect pigmentation. This won't lighten, brighten, or exfoliate skin, but it's a good water-soluble cleanser for normal to oily skin.

☺ **$$$ Cellular Cleansing Complex** *($46 for 6 ounces)* is a very expensive version of the original Cetaphil Gentle Skin Cleanser ($6.99 for 8 ounces). The big deal claim is that this is formulated with enzymatic exfoliators. Although enzymes are present (listed as papain), they are unstable ingredients that don't exfoliate skin as efficiently as an AHA or BHA product does. Even if they were equal, the exfoliating benefit wouldn't occur unless you left this cleanser on skin for several minutes or longer, and that's not how most people wash their faces. This is a good lotion-style cleanser for normal to dry skin, but assuredly not worth the extra money compared to Cetaphil.

☺ **$$$ Non-Drying Gentle Cleanser** *($30 for 8.5 ounces)* is billed as ultra-mild, and for the most part, it is. The detergent cleansing agent is one typically seen in "no more tears" baby shampoos and it is fragrance-free. What's not mild is the problematic horsetail and comfrey extracts. Both have their share of problems for skin, but they are unlikely to be an issue in a cleanser (and in the small amounts used in this product). This is a semi-water-soluble cleanser most suitable for normal to slightly dry skin.

☹ **$$$ Sensitive Skin Cleansing Gel** *($30 for 8.5 ounces)* is a standard, detergent-based water-soluble cleanser for normal to oily skin. It is not a slam-dunk for sensitive skin (including rosacea) because of the potentially irritating plant extracts and preservatives it contains.

☺ **$$$ Wash Off Cleanser** *($30 for 8.5 ounces)* contains a tiny amount of coltsfoot extract, which can be problematic in leave-on products due to its alkaloid content. Because this is a rinse-off, water-soluble cleanser it shouldn't be a problem for most skin types. Still, for the money this isn't worth choosing over Clean & Clear Foaming Facial Cleanser, Sensitive Skin ($4.39 for 8 ounces).

☹ **$$$ Clarifying Enzyme Complex** *($32 for 2 ounces)* is a thick, water- and wax-based facial scrub with polyethylene beads that act as the abrasive agent. The tiny amount of papain (enzyme) won't exfoliate skin, but the mechanical process of massaging the polyethylene beads over skin will. There is only one study demonstrating papain as an effective exfoliant, but it used only a pure concentration (Source: *Archives of Dermatological Research*, November 2001, pages 500–507). This formula is only for dry to very dry skin and is not the easiest to rinse.

☹ **$$$ Pumice Acne Scrub** *($32 for 8.5 ounces)* doesn't contain actual pumice, which is great because that would make this polyethylene-based (plastic bead) scrub way too abrasive. Benzoyl peroxide is listed as an active ingredient, but its effect will be limited because this product is rinsed from skin shortly after being applied. This cleansing scrub is best for oily to very oily skin.

☹ **Aloe Toning Complex** *($30 for 8.5 ounces)* contains an amount of comfrey extract that makes it potentially problematic for all skin types. Please refer to Chapter Seven, *Cosmetic Ingredient Dictionary*, for detailed information on why comfrey is a problem for skin.

☹ **$$$ Glycolic 5% Daily Cleansing Pads** *($30 for 56 pads)* have potential as a pH-correct, 5% AHA product in pad form, but the amount of alcohol makes them a less desirable option when compared with most others. They are an OK option for oily skin, and do contain fragrance.

☹ **Glycolic Exfoliating Wash 7%** *($32 for 8.5 ounces)* contains peppermint oil, making it too irritating for all skin types. The amount of glycolic acid is impressive, but the pH of this cleanser and its brief contact with the skin won't permit exfoliation.

☹ **$$$ Salicylic Wash 2%** *($32 for 8.5 ounces)* omits the peppermint oil present in the Glycolic Exfoliating Wash above, and contains 2% salicylic acid instead of an AHA. However, both its brief contact with skin and the pH of the base still prevent exfoliation. This is otherwise a very standard, water-soluble cleanser for normal to oily skin. It should be kept away from the eye area.

☹ **Glycolic 10% Toning Complex** *($32 for 8.5 ounces)* contains alcohol and menthol, and is not recommended for any skin type. What a shame, because this is otherwise a well-formulated 10% glycolic acid toner.

☺ **$$$ Glycolic 10% Exfoliating Moisturizer** *($46 for 1.7 ounces)* contains 10% glycolic acid at a pH of 3.6, making it an effective exfoliant. The lightweight, silicone-enhanced lotion base is suitable for normal to slightly dry skin. Although it contains some great antioxidants and the packaging will keep them stable, the amount of each is so small as to be almost nonexistent.

☹ **$$$ Glycolic 10% Exfoliating Oil Control Gel** *($46 for 1. 7 ounces)* has a pH of 4.1, which limits the effectiveness of the 2% salicylic acid and 10% glycolic acid it contains.

There isn't any other reason to consider this gel, and for the money it doesn't best options from Neutrogena, Alpha Hydrox, or Paula's Choice.

7-Day Radiance Peel Kit *($100 for the kit)* is a four-part, at-home glycolic and salicylic acid peel that is meant to be used as a five-minute exfoliating and post-peel treatment routine for seven days. The ☹ **Radiance Solution** is housed in a glass bottle and contains glycolic acid as the main exfoliant. The percentage of glycolic acid is not listed on the label, and DDF would not divulge this information. However, it appears to be at least a 10% concentration and the base has a pH of 3, so exfoliation will occur.

My concern with this product is the addition of alcohol, lemon peel oil, and grapefruit peel oil. These ingredients are listed before the antioxidants, which are held in powder form in the Radiance Solution's cap. The idea is to pour the powder into the Solution just prior to use to keep the antioxidants "fresh." There is no reason to tolerate the extra irritants when other products can give you the same results without any mixing or excess irritation. The Radiance Solution is applied with cotton swabs (supplied in the Kit) and left on for five minutes, after which you are instructed to apply the 😐 **Neutralizer Pads**. These pads have an alkaline pH of 10, and instantly stop the peel from working because the alkali neutralizes the acid of the Radiance Solution. But a pH of 10 is over the top for skin (meaning really irritating), and unnecessary to neutralize this product. The residue that remains is rinsed off, and then you are advised to apply and leave on the ☹ **Arginine Beta Gentle Resurfacing Serum**, which is a water- and alcohol-based solution that contains salicylic acid (the amount is not revealed, but it appears to be 1%) in a pH of 3. It is definitely problematic that after treating your skin to the alkaline Neutralizer Pads you are then asked to apply another acidic exfoliating product that also contains too much alcohol (you can clearly smell it, which is never a good sign).

The one bright spot in the Kit is DDF's wonderful ✓☺ **Organic Sunblock SPF 30**. The instructions for the Peel wisely recommend practicing "serious sun care," and this titanium dioxide and zinc oxide lotion provides just that, albeit with a slight, unavoidable white cast left on the skin (a characteristic of these mineral-based sunscreens). This antioxidant-rich sunscreen is a fine choice for those with sensitive skin (including those with rosacea).

The prospect of do-it-yourself peels is no doubt intriguing to many consumers, especially when these at-home kits are compared to peels you would receive in a dermatologist's office. Although this Kit will definitely exfoliate the skin, the additional irritants are problematic for all skin types, and the concentration of glycolic acid is not anywhere close to what you would get from an in-office peel, where concentrations of up to 70% glycolic acid and 13% salicylic acid are allowed. Spas and aestheticians can perform peels with up to 40% AHA (typically glycolic or lactic acid); salicylic acid peels are not available as nonmedical treatments. Most in-office peels involve concentrations ranging from 20% to 30%, and are administered as a series of treatments spaced six weeks apart. If you are looking for more striking results from an AHA or BHA peel, I advise you to seek these treatments from a dermatologist rather than wasting money on at-home kits that cannot deliver the same results—especially since the results of at-home peels are also attainable with regular use of pH-correct AHA or BHA products from numerous lines for a lot less money and rigmarole.

😐 **$$$ Bio-Molecular Firming Eye Serum** *($82 for 0.5 ounce)* is a lightweight, water- and aloe-based serum that contains several antioxidants (most in tiny amounts) whose effectiveness is compromised by clear packaging. The peptides and other cell-communicating ingredients have merit and somewhat justify this product's price, but they're not enough to make this worth the investment unless you don't mind overspending for an eye-area product that's best for slightly dry skin.

✓☺ **$$$ C3 Plus Serum** *($62 for 0.5 ounce)* is an excellent product if you're looking for a fragrance-free serum that combines the antioxidant benefits of vitamin C with the skin-enhancing benefits of peptides. Packaged in an airtight opaque bottle to keep the antioxidants stable, C3 Plus Serum also contains a nice complement of skin-identical ingredients, making it worthwhile for someone with oily or blemish-prone skin who wants an antioxidant-rich product. Traditionally, ascorbic acid (the form of vitamin C in this product) has been considered difficult to stabilize. However, new placebo-controlled research shows that a 3% concentration of ascorbic acid (which this product contains) in an emulsion can produce positive results in skin within a short period of time. This means that although the ascorbic acid will break down faster than more stable forms of vitamin C, some immediate efficacy is obtained when the formulation is correct (Source: *Skin Pharmacology and Physiology*, July–August 2004, pages 200–206). Assuming that your skin-care routine includes an effective sunscreen—and without it all the antioxidants in the world will have minimal positive impact on your skin—this is a good product to consider, especially if you'd like to see what the vitamin C and peptides combination can do for your skin.

😐 **$$$ Cellular Revitalization Age Renewal** *($125 for 1.7 ounces)* makes all manner of cellular repair claims tied to the company's proprietary complex of proteins and peptides. However, there isn't much of those high-tech ingredients in this emollient moisturizer for dry to very dry skin, and several of the beneficial ingredients will be compromised by jar packaging. The phytoestrogen ingredients in this product cannot control skin symptoms associated with menopause. If you were intending to explore the potential antiwrinkle benefits of copper, this product contains barely a dusting of it.

😐 **$$$ Daily Matte SPF 15** *($36 for 1.7 ounces)* is a good, fragrance-free, basic, matte-finish sunscreen for normal to oily skin. It includes an in-part titanium dioxide sunscreen and leaves a silky finish. Several antioxidants are part of the formula, but in amounts so small it's unlikely they'll have much impact on skin.

☺ **$$$ Daily Organic SPF 15** *($36 for 1. 7 ounces)* claims the 11 antioxidants it contains provide complete protection from free radicals, but that's impossible because there is no way any amount of antioxidants can shield skin from all sources of oxidative damage. (For example, how do you block oxygen without dying? And there is no sunscreen ingredient that can block every ray of the sun.) This is a good, fragrance-free "mineral" sunscreen whose actives are titanium dioxide and zinc oxide. It is recommended for sensitive skin that is normal to dry or struggling with rosacea.

✓☺ **$$$ Daily Protective Moisturizer SPF 15** *($36 for 1.7 ounces)* combines zinc oxide with other sunscreen actives, including 0.5% avobenzone (which is interesting because, as of this writing, these actives are not permitted for combined use by the FDA, although they are routinely combined in sunscreens sold outside the United States and a proposal is pending that may grant such a combination stateside). In contrast to the other DDF sunscreens above, this superior option has a larger concentration of antioxidants. The base formula is best for normal to slightly dry skin, and this sunscreen is fragrance-free.

😐 **$$$ Dramatic Radiance TRF Cream** *($98 for 1.7 ounces)* is a fairly standard moisturizer whose formula is quite mundane for the price. It contains mostly water, glycerin, emollients, slip agents, silicones, shea butter, film-forming agent, several more thickeners, antioxidants, plant oil, preservatives, and fragrance. It purports to change the way skin utilizes oxygen in an effort to restore "youthful suppleness and elasticity," but does not accomplish that goal. How can a product change the way skin handles oxygen? And does that increase free-radical damage? The claims are the only mildly interesting part of this product, and the only dramatic element of this moisturizer for normal to dry skin is the price.

☺ **$$$ Enhancing Sun Protection SPF 30** *($30 for 4 ounces)* provides broad-spectrum sun protection with its titanium dioxide and zinc oxide sunscreen ingredients, and comes in a tinted moisturizing base for normal to dry skin. Although this is a very good sunscreen, it's disappointing that the antioxidants are barely present and that the formula isn't too exciting when compared to options from Clinique or Estee Lauder. This product is fragrance-free.

😐 **$$$ EPF Moisturizer C3 SPF 15** *($82 for 1.7 ounces)* provides potentially inadequate UVA protection because it contains only 1% titanium dioxide along with UVA-deficient active ingredients. There is a significant amount of vitamins C and E in this product, but their potency is quickly diminished once this jar-packaged product is open. Although vastly overpriced, it's an OK option for normal skin with slight signs of dryness.

😐 **$$$ Erase Eye Gel** *($45 for 0.5 ounce)* is mostly water with film-forming agent, wax, and skin-identical ingredients. It also contains vitamin K, which DDF claims is encapsulated and able to treat dark circles under the eyes. There is no substantiated research proving topical application of vitamin K has any effect on dark circles (something the good doctor would be completely aware of). This can be a decent serum whose film-forming agent will make skin appear temporarily smoother.

✓☺ **$$$ Mesojection Healthy Cell Serum** *($80 for 1 ounce)* is sold as a topical substitute for a procedure known as mesotherapy. This treatment, which is not medically sound but is most commonly used to dissolve fat and improve cellulite, is based on receiving injections that are either homeopathic or pharmaceutical. Strangely, there isn't necessarily any consistency, and the cocktail of ingredients can vary from practitioner to practitioner, which makes this treatment very hard to evaluate (and just because something is popular in Europe doesn't mean it's the global standard. After all, many Europeans still relish sunbathing). The most typically used substance is phosphatidylcholine, but it can also be combined with deoxycholate. A handful of studies have shown that this can successfully reduce fat when injected into the skin, with one study demonstrating this for the under-eye area. Theoretically, the reduction of subcutaneous fat may be caused by inflammatory-mediated cell death and resorption. What does any of this have to do with skin? DDF is hoping the association with injecting potentially helpful substances will correlate with topical application of this water-based serum. They state that this product's technology allows for 85% more potent antioxidant activity to be delivered to the deepest layers of skin's surface (which really isn't that deep, but sounds impressive, doesn't it?). There is no published research to confirm that this antioxidant serum delivers great benefits, but the good news is that it does contain impressive amounts of several antioxidants, in a base that is suitable for normal to dry skin. The second ingredient, methylpropanediol, is a glycol that also functions as a penetration enhancer. That also has nothing to do with mesotherapy, but it's likely this will help the antioxidants travel farther into skin than they would in, say, an alcohol or oil base. The amount of salicylic acid is below efficacious, although this serum has a pH that would allow it to exfoliate if more was used. Interestingly, several antioxidants appear after the preservative, so they don't count for much. But what precedes them further up on the list is more than enough to make this a worthy contender for those looking for a well-formulated (despite wacky claims) antioxidant serum.

✓☺ **$$$ Nourishing Eye Cream** *($45 for 0.5 ounce)* is an outstanding fragrance-free moisturizer for slightly dry skin around the eyes or anywhere on the face. It contains a thoughtful blend of emollients, skin-identical ingredients, silicone, antioxidants, and plant oil.

😐 **$$$ Protective Eye Cream SPF 15 Plus, with CoQ-10** *($46 for 0.5 ounce)* has a great SPF number backed up by an in-part zinc oxide sunscreen, although the creamy base formula is lackluster and unimpressive. This product includes some intriguing ingredients, but they are present in such minute amounts as to be almost inconsequential for skin. There are less expensive, more impressive sunscreens available from Neutrogena, Clinique, and Olay, to name a few. By the way, there is nothing about this product that makes it better for the eye area.

✓☺ **$$$ Retinol Energizing Moisturizer** *($85 for 1.7 ounces)* presents retinol along with several antioxidants in a slightly emollient lotion base suitable for normal to dry skin. This well-packaged product contains some beneficial fatty acids and nonvolatile plant oils that go beyond merely moisturizing skin. If you're going to splurge on a moisturizer, this product won't prove to be a letdown (provided you keep your expectations in check about it making you look years younger).

✓☺ **$$$ Silky C Serum** *($72 for 1 ounce)* is a very good non-aqueous serum that silkens skin with silicones while treating it to stabilized vitamins C and E and soy, while also providing the cell-communicating ingredient retinol. The antioxidant content of this serum isn't quite as prodigious as DDF's C3 Plus Serum above.

😐 **$$$ Ultra-Lite Oil-Free Moisturizing Dew** *($36 for 1. 7 ounces)* contains some ingredients that support the name, but the amount of wax and thickeners doesn't make this a slam-dunk solution for those battling blemishes. This is one of the less-impressive DDF moisturizers whose antioxidant content is almost too minor to matter. It's an OK option for normal to slightly oily skin.

😐 **$$$ Wrinkle Relax** *($82 for 0.5 ounce)* used to be sold as FauxTox, but DDF abandoned that cute if inaccurate name in favor of Wrinkle Relax to avoid legal complications from the real Botox owners. Is there any mistaking what this product is supposed to do? DDF touts its combination of two "non-toxic anti-aging peptides" as being able to prevent lines formed from facial expressions. One of the peptides is palmitoyl pentapeptide-3, which has no research proving it works in any capacity similar to Botox (it's a good ingredient, just incapable of relaxing expression lines). The main peptide is acetyl hexapeptide-3, which I have written about extensively because it shows up in so many products claiming to work like Botox. Please refer to Chapter Seven, *Cosmetic Ingredient Dictionary*, for detailed information about acetyl hexapeptide-3. In the end, this serum's peptides have water-binding properties and can function as cell-communicating ingredients (assuming enzymes in the skin don't break them down before they reach their target), but this product is overpriced for what you get—and not even Botox works like Botox when applied topically, rather than being injected into the skin.

☺ **Matte Finish Photo-Age Protection SPF 30** *($28 for 4 ounces)* is a good, in-part avobenzone sunscreen for normal to slightly oily skin, though the main thickening agent keeps it from being matte for long. More important than the short-lived matte finish is the fact that this sunscreen has a nice array of antioxidants and a soothing agent. This is a good example of a sunscreen that goes beyond the basics.

✓☺ **Moisturizing Photo-Age Protection SPF 30** *($28 for 4 ounces)* is similar to the Matte Finish Photo-Age Protection SPF 30 above, except this version is preferred for slightly dry skin and contains more antioxidants and at higher concentrations. The lightweight moisturizing base will work well under makeup, and this product is fragrance-free.

☺ **Organic Sun Protection SPF 30** *($28 for 4 ounces)* is an antioxidant letdown compared to the other DDF sunscreens above, though this titanium dioxide and zinc oxide sunscreen has merit for normal to dry skin. It's not the best for sensitive or rosacea-affected skin because it is fragranced, and it's a shame that the many antioxidants are present in such minuscule amounts.

☺ **$$$ Benzoyl Peroxide Gel 5%, with Tea Tree Oil** *($24 for 2 ounces)* is a simply formulated but effective topical disinfectant for blemish-prone skin. The amount of tea tree oil is not enough to function as a disinfectant (it just adds fragrance), but the benzoyl peroxide takes care of that on its own.

☺ **$$$ Fade Cream 15** *($40 for 1.7 ounces)* is an effective skin-lightening product that contains 2% hydroquinone. However, you should ignore the claim that it "protects as if you were wearing an SPF 15 because it contains a sunscreen." There are sunscreen ingredients in this product, but they're not listed as actives, and these ingredients won't keep skin shielded from the full spectrum of UVA rays. In particular, the product does not have an SPF rating, and you have to wonder if the FDA knows about this—because making this claim about sun protection without an SPF rating would not make any regulatory board in the world very happy. There isn't anything else to extol beyond the hydroquinone, which makes this a pricier option while offering no incentives to justify the cost.

☹ **Fade Gel 4** *($52 for 0.5 ounce)* contains alcohol, lemon oil, and lime oil, all of which are very irritating to skin, especially when combined with active ingredients (hydroquinone in this case) that may make skin more sensitive.

☺ **$$$ Intensive Holistic Corrector Swabs** *($42 for 28 swabs)* packs a gel-like solution into a long plastic swab with a sponge-tip applicator on one end. Pushing the sliding plastic parts of the swab together feeds the solution onto the applicator, with the idea being a targeted application to trouble spots. This contains a hefty amount (likely 10–12%) of glycolic acid, but the pH of 4.1 prevents it from working fully as an exfoliant. The plant extracts (none of which are truly "holistic") include mulberry and licorice root, which have limited research concerning their ability to affect hyperpigmentation. This ends up being a gimmicky, excessively packaged kit for the money, and it is no match for an effective skin-lightening product with hydroquinone or even an effective concentration of stabilized vitamin C.

☺ **$$$ Intensive Holistic Lightener** *($50 for 0.5 ounce)* is similar to the Intensive Holistic Corrector Swabs above, but in a more sensible package and with a pH-correct formula that permits the glycolic acid to function as an exfoliant. This product contains DDF's DermaWhite complex, which consists of amino acids along with kojic acid. Kojic acid has merit as a skin-lightening agent, but its efficacy, safety, and formulary quirks (it's a very unstable ingredient) have kept it from eclipsing the gold standard status of hydroquinone (Source: *Journal of the American Academy of Dermatology*, December 2006, pages 1048–1065). Further, the amount of salicylic acid and azelaic acid (other agents that can help pigmented areas look better) is too small to impart a benefit. That makes Intensive Holistic Lightener an effective AHA product with dubious skin-lightening ability.

☺ **$$$ Intensive Hydration Mask** *($32 for 2 ounces)* is a wonderfully rich mask for dry to very dry skin and it is fragrance-free, but you can get a similar benefit from applying plain safflower or sesame oils (the main ingredients after water in this mask) to dry skin and then washing it off after several minutes.

☺ **$$$ Nutrient K Plus** *($54 for 1 ounce)* is supposed to be the answer for those dealing with broken capillaries because it contains vitamin K (phytonadione). There is lots of research pertaining to vitamin K's circulation-enhancing benefit when it's consumed orally, but this has not been demonstrated for topical application (Source: www.naturaldatabase.com). There is no reason to believe this lackluster moisturizer will have a visible effect on broken capillaries.

☹ **Redness Relief** *($48 for 1 ounce)* positions itself as a botanically based treatment to soothe reddened or hypersensitive skin. I'm always suspicious of such claims because so many botanical ingredients tend to be problematic for skin, and that turns out to be the case here, too. Although DDF included some very good anti-irritants (all plant-based), they also added *Ranunculus ficaria* extract. This weed may have antibacterial and antifungal properties, but applied topically it can cause irritation and possibly photodermatitis (Source: www.naturaldatabase.com).

unrated **RMX Essential** *($200 for 56 .067-ounce packets)* caused quite a stir when it launched in Sephora stores in 2006, mostly because of its regimented usage instructions and lofty price. The original RMX lineup included the Essential version as well as RMX Intense ($550) and RMX Maximum ($1,000). The latter two were discontinued because, according to a Sephora insider, they were "ahead of their time." That's funny, because most cosmetics companies are trying to outdo the competition with ahead-of-time products. I'm fairly certain the real reason the Intense and Maximum versions disappeared is because, quite simply, consumers weren't buying into the absurd price and accompanying inane claims. So that leaves RMX Essential at a comparatively cheap $200. After delving into this product's formulation, it leaves far more questions than answers, which is why it didn't get a rating. Do not make the mistake of thinking this is medicine or the high cost is equal to proof or evidence that it is the best formulation out there—it isn't. There is no published research to prove that this product will change your skin so it will never be the same again, but who really knows? You have to take Dr. Sobel's word for it because, other than that there are no studies to rely on.

From an ingredient standpoint, there's a little bit of everything in RMX Essential. It contains several popular peptides (cell-communicating ingredients), ingredients that mimic the structure of skin, and antioxidants. Lots of these ingredients are clearly intriguing, but they are by no means unique to this formula. If the amount of these substances is meant to be the strong suit, there's no indication of how much of any ingredient you are actually putting on your skin; you just have to take the company's word for it that these ingredients are "concentrated." As far as cell-communicating ingredients, this product contains basically palmitoyl oligopeptide, acetyl hexapeptide, and palmitoyl pentapeptide-3, all described in my Web site's Cosmetic Ingredient Dictionary and in Chapter Seven, *Cosmetic Ingredient Dictionary*. Most of the research that cosmetics companies rely on for their "belief" in the value of peptides is performed by the manufacturers of the ingredients. Independent research about how peptides affect wrinkles when applied topically is practically nonexistent (Source: *International Journal of Cosmetic Science*, June 2005, page 155). Whether peptides ever get to the skin cell and have an impact there is just not known. Many researchers feel that they don't (peptides are notoriously unstable and easily broken down by enzymes in the skin), but obviously there are those researchers who do. One thing that is known, at least, is that they are beneficial as skin-identical ingredients. All in all, $200 for two month's worth of RMX Essential packets is a lot of money for guessing.

The second ingredient in RMX Essential is colostrum, which is the thick yellowish fluid secreted by the mammary glands during the last weeks of pregnancy and the first days after a baby is born, before actual milk is produced by the breast. (The source of colostrum used in supplements and skin-care products is primarily bovine.) Colostrum is a highly nutritious substance, loaded with proteins, immune-building substances, and growth factors. Primarily, colostrum is about antibodies and growth factors to help the infant fight viruses and bacteria and to jump-start the growth of muscle, bone, and tissue. A small amount of research shows that colostrum can have benefit when applied topically for wound healing, but there is also research that shows it is not helpful.

Either way, wrinkles and aging skin are not wounds (getting cut by a knife isn't related in any way to the slow process of how skin comes to be wrinkled and look older), so the little research that has been done does not relate to anything claimed on the label of this product (Sources: *Indian Journal of Pediatrics*, July 2005, pages 579–581; *Cells Tissues Organs*, January 2000, pages 92–100; *Australasian Biotechnology*, July–August 1997, pages 223–228; and *Journal of Dermatologic Surgery Oncology*, June 1985, pages 617–622).

Further, if you're supposed to believe that colostrum's growth hormone content can impact your skin, then you would also have to believe that other constituents of colostrum would also have an effect. A major component of colostrum is a laxative to help newborns, whose digestive tracts are not fully formed. Anyone for a laxative while they fight wrinkles?

Farther down on the ingredient list is something called glycoproteins-Y28. It is nowhere to be found, whether in a search of medical journals, in *The International Nomenclature of Cosmetic Ingredients* (INCI, a compendium of cosmetic ingredients), or in an Internet search. Glycoproteins are fairly well understood, but exactly what the Y28 designation stands for is unknown. Most likely it's a specific receptor site on the cell that this ingredient is destined for, but that's just a guess because there is no way to know (Source: *Archives of Biochemistry and Biophysics*, June 1998, pages 232–238).

In general, glycoproteins are cell-to-cell communicating ingredients created when a protein links with a carbohydrate. In the body, glycoproteins play a critical role in the way various systems recover from internal and external stresses; they also are fundamentally involved in cellular repair, among other functions. Beyond that, studies on whether they can affect skin as a cell-communicating ingredient when applied topically just aren't anywhere to be found in science (Sources: www.glycoscience.com; www.anatomyatlases.org; and *Journal of Immunology*, November 1, 2000, pages 5295–5303, and September 1991, pages 1614–1620).

What we do know is that glycoproteins function very well as ingredients that mimic the structure of skin. When combined with saccharides, glycoproteins form polysaccharides and glycosaminoglycans (hyaluronic acid) that help keep skin cells and the skin's framework intact.

As high-tech as this RMX formula is, it contains retinyl palmitate instead of retinol or retinaldehyde. Here, the research is fairly clear: in the skin retinyl palmitate does not convert to retinoic acid—the active, beneficial form of vitamin A—as readily as retinol or retinaldehyde. That's important, because retinoic acid is the substance that can communicate with a skin cell to tell it to function normally (Sources: *Skin Pharmacology and Physiology*, May–June 2004, pages 124–128; *European Journal of Pharmaceutics and Biopharmaceutics*, May 2000, pages 211–218; and *Journal of Investigative Dermatology*, September 1997, pages 301–305).

One more ingredient that stands out is prasterone (dehydroepiandrosterone, DHEA), a naturally occurring pro-hormone that in the body is converted primarily to androgens (male steroids) and to a lesser degree estrogens. As an oral supplement, DHEA is controversial because long-term use has been associated with women developing secondary masculine traits, liver damage, disrupted menstrual cycles, and defects in fetuses, and, for men, with decreased sperm count. More superficial risks include hair loss, acne, and weight gain. When applied topically, it is possible that DHEA can increase collagen production and prevent collagen destruction by decreasing matrix metalloproteinases (MMP), but the research about this is extremely limited and the studies that do exist were done on only a handful of people (Sources: *Drug Delivery*, September–October 2005, pages 275–280; *Journal of Endocrinology*, November 2005, pages 169–196; *Journal of Investigative Dermatology*, November 2005, pages 1053–1062, and February 2004, pages 315–323; *Gynecological Endocrinology*, December 2002, pages 431–441; www.fda.gov; and www.mayoclinic.com/health/dhea/NS_patient-dhea).

By now you probably see what I mean about this being a hard product to review. For example, I still can't decide with any certainty whether it is worth any amount of money. And I can't give you an answer because there is simply no way to know. The ingredients appear to be helpful for skin, but how much more helpful than other combinations, or in exactly what capacity, remains a mystery. As skin-care formulations get more technical, it would be nice if they came with more than just the formulator's word on their reliability. Without research to point the way (and in the cosmetics industry, products launch well before research has proven their effectiveness, as was the case with this one), it is all speculation and conjecture. Still, this product does have some state-of-the-art ingredients and may be worth a try by those with unlimited skin-care budgets.

☹ **Sulfur Therapeutic Mask** *($34 for 4 ounces)* is a standard clay mask that also contains 10% sulfur. Sulfur is a topical disinfectant that is very irritating and highly alkaline, and can cause problems for skin.

😐 **$$$ Ultra-Lite Peel, with Elm Extract** *($40 for 1 ounce)* is designed as a leave-on peel product for sensitive skin, and the chief exfoliant is arginine. Arginine is an amino acid that functions as an antioxidant and may have wound-healing properties, but there is no research showing it to be an exfoliant (Sources: *Journal of Surgical Research*, June 2002, pages 35–42; *Nitric Oxide*, May 2002, pages 313–318; *European Surgical Research*, January-April 2002, pages 53–60; and www.naturaldatabase.com). The exfoliant in this product is approximately 1% salicylic acid, and the pH is low enough for it to function in that manner. However, alcohol precedes it on the list and makes this a less-appealing BHA option due to the kickback from irritation. Elm extract has no research establishing its benefit for skin when applied topically.

☹ **Glossy Lip Therapy SPF 15** *($18 for 0.25 ounce)* includes an in-part titanium dioxide sunscreen in a rich, lanolin-based lip balm loaded with other emollient ingredients. What a shame it also contains peppermint oil, which makes it too irritating for routine use.

DECLEOR PARIS (SKIN CARE ONLY)

DECLEOR PARIS AT-A-GLANCE

Strengths: None of note.

Weaknesses: Expensive; 85% of Decleor Paris's products contain volatile essential oils that have limited to no benefit for skin and are known irritants; almost all the sunscreens lack the right UVA-protecting ingredients; no product to address acne or skin discolorations; inappropriate jar packaging.

For more information about Decleor Paris, owned in-part by Shiseido, call (888) 414-4471 or www.decleor.com or www.Beautypedia.com.

DECLEOR PARIS AROMESSENCE PRODUCTS

☹ **Aromessence Angelique Night Balm** *($66.50 for 1 ounce)* has an oil-based, emollient texture that those with very dry skin will love, but your skin won't appreciate the irritation from the rosemary, geranium, and angelica oils (the latter is phototoxic, so it's good this is recommended for nighttime use).

☹ **Aromessence Angelique Nourishing Concentrate** *($63.50 for 0.5 ounce)* is mostly hazel seed, wheat germ, and avocado oils, all of which are available separately at health food stores and are a far better choice than this overpriced "concentrate" and its irritating fragrant oils of rosemary, geranium, and angelica.

☹ **Aromessence Essential Balm** *($66.50 for 1 ounce)* contains irritating basil, bitter orange, and neroli oils and is not recommended. This very fragranced balm would make a much better candle than skin-care product! Basil oil has mutagenic properties and its active constituents (concentrated in the oil) are bad news for skin (Source: *Natural Medicines Comprehensive Database*, 2006).

☹ **Aromessence Iris Night Balm** *($71 for 1 ounce)* contains fragrant geranium oil as well as lavender oil, and the latter is capable of causing skin-cell death when applied topically (Source: *Cell Proliferation*, June 2004, pages 221–229).

☹ **Aromessence Iris TimeCare Concentrate** *($80 for 0.5 ounce)* claims to redefine features, but you can take that to mean causing visible irritation and possibly contact dermatitis from the litany of problematic fragrant volatile oils it contains.

☹ **Aromessence Neroli Comforting Concentrate** *($63.50 for 0.5 ounce)* is similar to the Aromessence Iris TimeCare Concentrate above, only with a different blend of problematic oils.

☹ **Aromessence Rose D'Orient Soothing Concentrate** *($63.50 for 0.5 ounce)* is similar to the Aromessence Iris TimeCare Concentrate above, only with a different blend of problematic oils.

☹ **Aromessence Rose D'Orient Night Balm** *($66.50 for 1 ounce)* absolutely won't reduce signs of irritation given the number of volatile plant oils it contains. Routine use of this product is likely to cause irritation and inflammation.

☹ **Aromessence Ylang-Ylang Purifying Concentrate** *($63.50 for 0.5 ounce)* smells divine, but the blend of ylang ylang, geranium, rosemary, and bay oils won't do your skin one bit of good, and none of these oils can control sebaceous (oil) gland secretions.

☹ **Aromessence Ylang-Ylang Night Balm** *($66.50 for 1 ounce)* is not recommended because it contains irritating ylang ylang and basil oils.

☹ **Aromessence Lip Balm** *($23 for 0.4 ounce)* won't nourish lips as claimed because the nourishing ingredients are impeded by the irritants lemon, orange, and cinnamon oils.

DECLEOR PARIS AROMA PURETE PRODUCTS

☹ **Aroma Purete Matt Finish Skin Fluid** *($38.50 for 1.69 ounces)* is a silicone-enriched moisturizer that has mattifying properties, but irritates skin with *Cananga odorata* flower oil. Also known as ylang ylang, this oil has research demonstrating its relaxing quality when inhaled, but that's how most essential oils are best enjoyed (Source: *Phytotherapy Research*, September 2006, pages 758–763).

☹ **Aroma Purete Instant Purifying Mask** *($40 for 1.69 ounces)* contains a high amount of ylang ylang oil, which can be irritating to skin (Source: www.naturaldatabase.com). This is otherwise a very standard clay mask that is easily replaced by many others that not only omit problematic ingredients but also cost much less.

☹ **Aroma Purete Matifying Powdered Blotting Papers** *($25 for 48 sheets)* are talc-imbued papers that also contain cornstarch, pigment, and lots of fragrance, including ylang ylang oil. Considering the potential for irritation and the exorbitant price, these are not recommended.

DECLEOR PARIS AROMA WHITE PRODUCTS

☺ **$$$ Aroma White Brightening Make Off Cream, Face and Eyes** *($34 for 5 ounces)* won't help unevenly pigmented skin in terms of lightening discolorations, but this is a good, irritant-free cleansing cream for dry to very dry skin. It requires a washcloth for complete removal, but does remove makeup well.

😐 **$$$ Aroma White Brightening Treatment Lotion** *($34 for 8.4 ounces)* is a fairly basic gel-textured toner that contains more fragrant orange and kiwi water than mulberry extract. The latter is the only ingredient in this product that can have an effect on melanin production, but there isn't enough of it here to bring a benefit for hyperpigmented skin.

☹ **Aroma White Brightening Matifying Fluid SPF 15** *($50.50 for 1.69 ounces)* lacks the UVA-protecting ingredients of titanium dioxide, zinc oxide, avobenzone, Tinosorb, or Mexoryl SX. and is not recommended.

😐 **$$$ Aroma White Brightening Night Cream** *($62 for 1.69 ounces)* is a good emollient moisturizer for dry to very dry skin, though its jar packaging compromises the stability of the few antioxidants present. The tiny amount of mulberry extract won't lighten skin one iota, so this is not the moisturizer to choose if you're looking to fade sun- or hormone-induced discolorations.

😐 **$$$ Aroma White Brightening C+ Essence** *($75 for 3 0.33-ounce vials)* only contains vitamin C in the sense that some of the plant extracts in this serum are a natural source of it. However, it's doubtful the vitamin C content is still viable once the extract has been processed, which makes pure, stabilized forms of vitamin C preferred. There's no compelling reason to consider this treatment kit, particularly since the antioxidants are compromised by non-opaque bottles, making it more a waste of money than anything else.

☹ **Aromessence White Brightening Concentrate** *($75 for 0.5 ounce)* contains fragrant rose and orange oils along with lemon peel, all of which are irritating to skin and all of which have no positive effect on pigmentation.

😐 **$$$ Aroma White Brightening Purifying Mask** *($44 for 1.69 ounces)* is a standard clay mask dressed up with claims of preventing dark spots and featuring a list of plant oil and extracts that are no match for an over-the-counter skin-lightening product that contains hydroquinone. Not only that, but a mask is designed for occasional use and is rinsed off, and not even proven skin-lightening agents would work if you were following that routine.

😐 **$$$ Aroma White Brightening Spot Corrector** *($31 for 0.5 ounce)* lists active ingredients that aren't regulated as such, including roman chamomile. There is no evidence that any of Decleor Paris's self-proclaimed "actives" will correct dark spots and pigment imperfections, or help prevent new spots from forming. This is basically clay, thickeners, and cornstarch along with a form of vitamin C not known to be effective on discolorations, and the plant extracts this product contains aren't helpful for that either.

DECLEOR PARIS EXPERIENCE DE L'AGE PRODUCTS

😐 **$$$ Experience De L'Age Triple Action Eye and Lip Cream** *($60 for 0.5 ounce)* is said to be specially formulated for the eye and lip area, but the ingredients don't support that. For example, if Decleor Paris believes these areas are "delicate," then why did they include problematic iris extract and herbs such as *Bupleurum falcatum* root, which do not have established safety records for topical application (Source: www.naturaldatabase.com). This creamy moisturizer has some beneficial ingredients for dry skin, but it's not an antiwrinkle product with "corrective action" and is very overpriced for what you get. The fragrance components it contains are best kept away from the eyes and mouth.

☺ **$$$ Experience De L'Age Triple Action Light Cream** *($95 for 1.69 ounces)* has a lighter texture than the Experience De L'Age Triple Action Eye and Lip Cream above, but makes similar claims and contains the same problematic and questionable plant extracts. The base formula is an OK moisturizer for normal to slightly dry or slightly oily skin.

☺ **$$$ Experience De L'Age Triple Action Rich Cream** *($95 for 1.69 ounces)* is a more emollient (but not "rich") version of the Experience De L'Age Triple Action Light Cream above, but makes the same claims and has the same problematic plant extracts. It's an option for normal to dry skin, but the jar packaging won't keep the antioxidants stable.

☹ **Experience De L'Age Triple Action Gel Cream Mask** *($45 for 1.69 ounces)* is a silky-textured mask that would be better without the problematic iris extract and irritating menthol derivative.

DECLEOR PARIS HARMONIE PRODUCTS

☹ **Harmonie Delicate Soothing Emulsion** *($65.50 for 1.69 ounces)* begins as one of Decleor Paris's more intriguing moisturizer formulas, but quickly heads in the wrong direction due to the inclusion of irritating (not calming, as claimed) lavender, thyme, bitter orange, rose, and marjoram oils. This is one to steer clear of if you have sensitized, reddened skin—unless you want to make matters worse.

☹ **Harmonie Essentielle Ultra Soothing Cream** *($65.50 for 1.69 ounces)* contains the same potent cocktail of irritating essential oils as the Harmonie Delicate Soothing Emulsion above, and the same review applies.

☹ **Harmonie Gentle Soothing Cream** *($65.50 for 1.69 ounces)* contains the same potent cocktail of irritating essential oils as the Harmonie Delicate Soothing Emulsion above, and the same review applies.

☺ **$$$ Harmonie Soothing Eye Contour Gel** *($34.50 for 0.5 ounce)* has a lotion texture and is actually an impressive formula for normal to dry skin. It contains rose oil and a couple of problematic plant extracts, but in amounts unlikely to cause problems. You should still keep this away from the eye area.

☹ **Harmonie Gentle Soothing Mask** *($42 for 1.69 ounces)* contains the same group of irritating essential oils as the Harmonie Delicate Soothing Emulsion above, and is equally problematic for all skin types, particularly "reactive skin," for which Decleor Paris specifically designed this product.

DECLEOR PARIS HYDRA FLORAL ANTI-POLLUTION

☹ **Hydra Floral Anti-Pollution "Flower Dew" Moisturising Gel-Cream for Eyes** *($38 for 0.5 ounce)* has a delicate, gel-cream texture, but its main ingredients are orange fruit and peppermint leaf water, which, though diluted, are still far too irritating to use around the eyes. (Decleor Paris claims these plant ingredients make up 10% of the product, which is really depressing news if true.) Farther down the list are fragrant neroli oil and other fragrant components, such as amyl cinnamal, linalool, and limonene—all problematic ingredients for skin, and incapable of diminishing dark circles and puffiness. If anything, the irritating ingredients in this moisturizer will create, not ease, puffy eyes.

☹ **Hydra Floral Anti-Pollution "Flower Nectar" Moisturising Cream** *($54 for 1.69 ounces)* lists orange fruit and peppermint leaf water as the main ingredients, as well as the other irritants mentioned above for the Hydra Floral Anti-Pollution "Flower Dew" Moisturising Gel-Cream for Eyes. This product is absolutely not recommended for any skin type.

☹ **Hydra Floral Anti-Pollution "Fresh Flower" Moisturising Emulsion** *($54 for 1.69 ounces)* contains the same irritating ingredients mentioned above for Decleor Paris's other Hydra Floral Anti-Pollution products, and is not recommended. Even without the irritants and the many fragrant components, this is an incredibly boring moisturizer formula for the money.

☹ **Hydra Floral Anti-Pollution "Flower Essence" Moisturising Mask** *($38 for 1.69 ounces)* doesn't improve in any way on the other Hydra Floral Anti-Pollution products reviewed above because it contains the same group of irritating ingredients, albeit in a more emollient base. How any of these products is supposed to protect skin from pollution is beyond me, so don't count on that or any other significant benefit.

☹ **Hydra Floral Anti-Pollution "Flower Petals" Eye and Lip Moisturising Mask** *($39 for 1 ounce)* rounds out the Hydra Floral Anti-Pollution collection and completes the progression of irritation that will result from combined or continued use of this line of products. Putting this much peppermint, orange, and neroli on your lips is almost as bad as using it near your eyes, and none of these ingredients (or any other ingredient in the product) can alleviate dark circles or puffiness—if anything, irritating ingredients make matters worse.

DECLEOR PARIS NUTRI-DELICE PRODUCTS

☹ **Nutri-Delice Delicious Ultra-Nourishing Cream** *($54 for 1.69 ounces)* is a very emollient, water- and oil-based moisturizer that would be much better for dry skin if the ceramide content were increased and the irritating angelica oil eliminated. This oil contains chemical constituents that can be phototoxic, including bergapten, imperatorin, and xanthotoxin. Although some of the components of angelica oil have antioxidant ability, it is a risky ingredient to use on skin if you are going to expose your skin to sunlight (Sources: www.naturaldatabase.com; and *Journal of Agricultural and Food Chemistry*, March 2007, pages 1737–1742). That news is neither nourishing nor delicious.

☹ **Nutri-Delice Delightful Extreme Protection Cream** *($61 for 1.69 ounces)* is similar to the Nutri-Delice Delicious Ultra-Nourishing Cream above, and the same review applies.

☹ **Nutri-Delice Meltingly Soft Nourishing Cream** *($54 for 1.69 ounces)* is similar to the Nutri-Delice Delicious Ultra-Nourishing Cream above, and the same review applies.

😐 **$$$ Nutri-Delice Nourishing Cereal Mask** *($38 for 1.69 ounces)* includes cereal grains such as oatmeal and wheat germ in a water-and-oil base suitable for dry to very dry skin. The tiny amount of angelica oil is unlikely to be a problem, provided you rinse this mask from your skin and don't wear it in the presence of sunlight. This is a decent mask but it's more a do-nothing than anything resembling nourishment for skin.

OTHER DECLEOR PARIS PRODUCTS

☹ **Cleansing Gel** *($31 for 8.4 ounces)* contains peppermint leaf water as a main ingredient as well as irritating (but delicious-smelling) ylang ylang oil, making it a poor choice for all skin types.

☹ **Cleansing Cream** *($33 for 8.4 ounces)* is a cold cream–style cleanser that contains irritating angelica and geranium oils. That's not as much of an issue in a rinse-off product, but given the number of cleansers for normal to dry skin that don't contain potentially problematic ingredients, why choose this one?

☹ **Cleansing Milk** *($31 for 8.4 ounces)* contains lavender and bitter orange oils, both of which are irritating and only serve to add fragrance.

☹ **Cleansing Oil** *($32 for 8.4 ounces)* contains irritating lavender, lemon peel, and bitter orange oils and is not recommended. If you prefer cleansing with oil, try plain olive oil or sunflower seed oil and save your skin from irritation.

☹ **Cleansing Water** *($32 for 8.4 ounces)* contains several irritating fragrant oils and has a formula that ranks below average for overall cleansing ability.

☹ **Foaming Cleanser** *($33 for 6.7 ounces)* has merit as a water-soluble cleanser, but the irritating lavender and bitter orange oils serve only to damage the skin's hydrolipidic film, which this cleanser is supposed to protect.

☹ **Eye Make-Up Remover Lotion** *($24.50 for 5 ounces)* is very standard in that it contains the same cleansing agents as most non-silicone eye-makeup removers. It falls below standard due to the fragrant rose flower oil it contains, which should not be used near the eyes or tear ducts.

☹ **Purete Exfoliante Natural Micro-Smoothing Cream** *($35 for 1.69 ounces)* contains black pepper oil and menthol, which makes no sense from any skin-care point of view and is just really bizarre. It also uses coconut shell powder as the abrasive agent, which, while natural, has uneven surfaces that can cause micro-tears in skin.

☹ **Fresh Hydrating Mist** *($20.50 for 5.07 ounces)* irritates skin with lavender and bitter orange oils and is otherwise a very boring, overpriced spray-on toner.

☹ **Matifying Lotion** *($30 for 8.4 ounces)* lists peppermint leaf water as the second ingredient and also contains fragrant ylang ylang oil and extracts of cinnamon and ginger. This is a recipe for potpourri, not a skin-care product to tackle oiliness.

☹ **Tonifying Lotion** *($31 for 8.4 ounces)* won't rebalance skin, but it will irritate it thanks to the amount of lavender and bitter orange oil.

☹ **Alpha Morning Alpha Hydrating Cream SPF 12** *($52 for 1.69 ounces)* does not contain the UVA-protecting ingredients of titanium dioxide, zinc oxide, avobenzone, Tinosorb, or Mexoryl SX, and is not recommended. That's a shame, because the pH of 4 allows the glycolic and lactic acids to function as exfoliants—yet you definitely do not want to wear this during daylight hours.

😐 **$$$ Hydrotenseur Eye Contour Firming Serum** *($45 for 0.5 ounce)*. Other than some standard skin-identical ingredients, there isn't much to write about this water-based serum. It's OK for a quick fix, but shortchanges the eye area by omitting antioxidants.

😐 **$$$ Instant de Beaute Radiant Lifting Fluid** *($48 for 1.69 ounces)* is a decent, lightweight, "primer"-type moisturizer to apply before makeup if you have normal to oily skin. It contains mostly water, wheat protein, emulsifier, slip agent, plant oil, film-forming agent, vitamin E, and preservatives. It is, amazingly, fragrance-free.

☹ **Prolagene Energising Gel** *($33.50 for 1.69 ounces)* claims to be a complete skin-care treatment, working to smooth imperfections that are both natural and accidental. It cannot do that, and is a very basic, watery gel formula that contains irritating osmanthus oil.

☹ **Soin Du Soir Night Repair Cream** *($47 for 1.69 ounces)* is a below-standard emollient moisturizer because it contains irritating bitter orange oil and bitter orange wax. Nothing in this moisturizer is capable of repairing skin, day or night.

☹ **Source D'Eclat Instant Radiance Moisturiser** *($49 for 1.69 ounces)* contains several problematic ingredients for skin, including citrus oils, oak root, and volatile fragrance components. The radiance comes from the mineral pigments mica and titanium dioxide, but you can get that effect from many other products that don't subject skin to irritation.

☹ **Vitalite Nourishing Firming Cream** *($66 for 1.69 ounces)* has several very good non-volatile plant oils for dry to very dry skin, but it contains enough geranium oil to cause irritation while providing minimal benefit, and that's never the goal.

☹ **Vitaroma Wrinkle Prevention and Radiance Face Emulsion** *($63 for 1.69 ounces)* continues Decleor Paris's pattern of emollient moisturizers infused with irritating essential oils. This product's offending ingredients include citronella and rose moschata oils.

☹ **Vitaroma Wrinkle Prevention Eye Contour Cream** *($42 for 0.5 ounce)* lists several of its most intriguing ingredients (vitamin E, retinol, lecithin) well after problematic ones such as geranium and citronella oils, neither of which is appropriate for skin around the eyes (or anywhere else on the face).

☹ **Clay and Herbal Cleansing Mask** *($38.50 for 1.69 ounces)* doesn't break any new ground in terms of clay masks, but will irritate skin with arnica and horsetail extracts.

☹ **Phytopeel** *($40.50 for 1.69 ounces)* contains lemon peel, lavender, thyme, and marjoram oils, all of which would serve much better in a salad dressing than as something to apply to skin.

☹ **Source D'Eclat 10-Day Radiance Powder Cure** *($32 for 0.33 ounce)* is a two-part product where you mix a vitamin C powder (pure ascorbic acid) with a glycol-based serum, apply it, and then your complexion becomes radiant. Vitamin C is mentioned as a skin stimulator, but the real stimulation (and irritation) comes from the citrus oils in the serum, and volatile fragrance components such as eugenol and limonene don't make matters any better.

☹ **Source D'Eclat Radiance Revealing Peel-Off Mask** *($40 for 1.69 ounces)* contains two types of drying alcohol as the main ingredients, along with irritating citrus oils and other problematic plant extracts.

☹ **Nourishing Lip Treatment** *($20 for 0.14 ounce)* contains cinnamon oil as well as problematic fragrance components, including eugenol and linalool. Plain Vaseline would be a much better, and much less expensive, lip moisturizer.

DECLEOR PARIS SUN PRODUCTS

☹ **Aroma Sun Anti-Sunburn Refreshing Gel-Cream, for Face & Body** *($35 for 4.17 ounces)* should not be applied to skin anywhere on the body because of the number of irritating volatile oils it contains. This is far from a refreshing experience for your skin, but your nose will be pleased with the scent.

☹ **Aroma Sun Express Hydrating Self-Tan Spray, for Body** *($35 for 5 ounces)* is a spray-on self-tanner that lists alcohol as the second ingredient and also contains a significant amount of irritating volatile plant oils.

☹ **Aroma Sun High Protection Sun Stick SPF 25, for Lips & Sensitive Areas** *($20 for 0.26 ounce)* lacks the UVA-protecting ingredients of titanium dioxide, zinc oxide, avobenzone, Tinosorb, or Mexoryl SX, and is not recommended. Even if it had sufficient UVA sunscreen ingredients, this contains problematic fragrant oils that would make it hard to recommend.

☹ **Aroma Sun Protective Anti-Wrinkle Cream SPF 15, for Face** *($35 for 1.69 ounces)* lacks the UVA-protecting ingredients of titanium dioxide, zinc oxide, avobenzone, Tinosorb, or Mexoryl SX, and is not recommended.

☹ **Aroma Sun Protective Anti-Wrinkle Cream SPF 30, for Face** *($35.50 for 1.69 ounces)* lacks the UVA-protecting ingredients of titanium dioxide, zinc oxide, avobenzone, Tinosorb, or Mexoryl SX, and is not recommended. Not to mention that the antiwrinkle claim is bogus.

☹ **Aroma Sun Protective Beautifying Mist SPF 8, for Face & Body** *($35 for 5 ounces)* lacks the UVA-protecting ingredients of titanium dioxide, zinc oxide, avobenzone, Tinosorb, or Mexoryl SX, and is not recommended. Moreover, the SPF rating is too low for daytime protection.

☹ **Aroma Sun Protective Hydrating Spray SPF 20, for Face & Body** *($35 for 5 ounces)* lacks the UVA-protecting ingredients of titanium dioxide, zinc oxide, avobenzone, Tinosorb, or Mexoryl SX, and is not recommended.

☹ **Aroma Sun Protective Hydrating Spray SPF 30, for Face & Body** *($35 for 5 ounces)* lacks the UVA-protecting ingredients of titanium dioxide, zinc oxide, avobenzone, Tinosorb, or Mexoryl SX, and is not recommended.

☹ **Aroma Sun Protective Hydrating Sun Milk SPF 15, for Face & Body** *($35 for 4.2 ounces)* lacks the UVA-protecting ingredients of titanium dioxide, zinc oxide, avobenzone, Tinosorb, or Mexoryl SX, and is not recommended.

☹ **Aroma Sun Protective Satiny Oil SPF 8, for Body & Hair** *($35 for 5 ounces)* does not list any active sunscreen ingredients, and is mostly triglyceride, thickener, emollient, and fragrance. The geranium and rose oils are volatile substances that can irritate skin and may cause further problems to skin when exposed to sunlight.

☹ **Aroma Sun SPF 8 Hydrating Self-Tanning Milk, for Face & Body** *($35.50 for 4.2 ounces)* is one of two Decleor Paris sunscreens that get the issue of UVA protection right, thanks to its in-part avobenzone sunscreen. Unfortunately, this self-tanner's sunscreen rating is too low and you're not likely to apply such a product daily or liberally. Plus the fragrant oils can cause irritation.

☹ **Aroma Sun SPF 10 Hydrating Tinted Self-Tanning Gel-Cream, for Face** *($35 for 1.69 ounces)* contains avobenzone like the Aroma Sun SPF 8 Hydrating Self-Tanning Milk, for Face & Body, above, but it also contains volatile fragrant oils to irritate skin and a pepper resin that makes matter worse, especially if applied around the eyes.

☹ **Aromessence Repairing After-Sun Balm, for Body** *($47 for 1.69 ounces)* is an oil- and wax-based balm that contains some excellent ingredients for dry, parched, weather-beaten skin. But it also contains several irritating fragrant oils, including skin-damaging lavender oil.

☹ **Aromessence Repairing After-Sun Balm, for Face** *($37 for 0.5 ounce)* is similar to the Aromaessence Repairing After-Sun Balm, for Body above, and the same review applies.

☹ **Aromessence Solaire Protection Booster, for Face** *($62 for 0.5 ounce)* contains what Decleor Paris refers to as a "cocktail of essential oils that work in synergy to increase cells' natural defenses against sun damage," but that's completely false. Sunflower, rice bran, and wheat germ oil will keep skin from drying out in the sun, but won't prevent sun damage. Further, the volatile components geranium and rose oils are irritating to skin.

☹ **Aromessence Solaire Protection Booster, for Body** *($65 for 3.3 ounces)* makes the same invalid claim as the Aromessence Solaire Protection Booster, for Face above, and the same review applies.

DERMABLEND

The only reason to consider this line is if you have complexion issues that demand serious coverage.

DERMABLEND AT-A-GLANCE

Strengths: None of note.

Weaknesses: Please refer to the individual product reviews below because almost every one has its own problems and distinct weaknesses; the makeup provides substantial coverage but the tradeoffs may not be worth it.

For more information about Dermablend, owned by L'Oreal, call (877) 900-6700 or visit www.dermablend.com or www.Beautypedia.com.

DERMABLEND SKIN CARE

☹ **Acne Results Cleansing Gel** *($9 for 2 ounces)* contains 2% salicylic acid as an active ingredient, but its brief contact with skin ensures it won't work as an exfoliant. A bigger problem for this cleanser is the inclusion of menthol, which makes it too irritating for all skin types.

☹ **Remover** *($15 for 6.3 ounces)* will help remove the thick, long-wearing Dermablend makeup because it contains TEA-lauryl sulfate as the main detergent cleansing agent. Unfortunately, that makes this water-soluble cleanser too drying for all skin types. An oil- or silicone-based makeup remover will do a better job without drying skin.

😐 **$$$ Hydrating Complex Creme with Vitamins A, C & E** *($30 for 3.75 ounces)* is an emollient moisturizer built around petrolatum (Vaseline) and several thickeners. It also contains some good antioxidants—retinol and soybean oil—but the jar packaging will quickly render their active properties ineffective. This will take care of dry skin, but in basic rather than advanced fashion.

😐 **$$$ Wrinkle Fix** *($15 for 0.12 ounce)* has been part of the Dermablend lineup for years, and is nothing more than a mineral oil–based, lipstick-style moisturizer. It's fine for spot-treating very dry skin, and the fragrance-free formula is suitable for use around the eyes, but so is plain Vaseline, for pennies. This balm will make wrinkles look better, but it won't "fix" them.

☹ **Acne Results Spot Gel** *($12 for 0.5 ounce)* is an ineffective 2% BHA product because the pH is too high for the salicylic acid to exfoliate skin; plus the formula's alcohol content is potentially irritating.

☹ **Chromatone Fade Creme** *($18.25 for 3.75 ounces)* lists 2% hydroquinone as the active ingredient, but the jar packaging will render it ineffective shortly after the product is opened. The other active is sunscreen agent octyl methoxycinnamate, which by itself does not provide sufficient UVA protection.

DERMABLEND MAKEUP

Dermablend does not disappoint if you have something to hide, but in public (especially in daylight), it will be no secret to others that you're wearing heavy-duty makeup. The concept is well-meaning, but from a reviewer's standpoint, rating these products is a tough call; whether or not to use makeup to camouflage rather than to enhance skin is a personal decision. The need for this type of makeup is intertwined with potentially delicate self-esteem issues. However, if using such cosmetics to conceal what bothers you about your skin increases your self-esteem,

I'm all for it. When it came to rating Dermablend's products, I compared them directly to similar niche products rather than using the makeup-at-large approach I take with mainstream cosmetic lines. Dermablend is worth exploring if you can tolerate the unavoidable tradeoffs in exchange for concealing what's bothersome about your skin.

FOUNDATION: 😐 **$$$ Cover Creme SPF 30** *($27.50)* is Dermablend's original foundation. It offers completely opaque coverage via a thick-textured, slightly greasy cream. The SPF 30 rating is now official (previously it was claimed, but no active ingredient was listed) and it is pure titanium dioxide. This foundation is recommended for all skin types. However, there's no doubt that those with oily, blemish-prone skin will find its texture and finish unappealing, even when used with powder. There are 20 shades, though many of them have decidedly unnatural overtones of peach, pink, rose, orange, and copper. The best neutral to passable shades are Pale Ivory, Warm Ivory, Rose Beige, Sand Beige, Yellow Beige, Almond Beige, Golden Beige, Caramel Beige, Olive Brown, Toasted Brown, Chocolate Brown, and, for very dark skin, Deep Brown. One caution: Not every shade of Cover Creme lists SPF 30 and an active ingredient. If you decide to try this, be sure to purchase only the shades that indicate an active ingredient to support the SPF 30 claim. The formula is waterproof, but will rub off on clothing or furniture, even when set with powder.

Cover Creme is also available as 😐 **$$$ Compact Cover Creme** *($20)*, which features seven shades, each with a name that corresponds to its matching Cover Creme SPF 30 foundation above. The ones to avoid include True Beige, Medium Beige, and Honey Beige. This is identical in every respect to the original Cover Creme, except for the packaging. 😐 **$$$ Smooth Indulgence Foundation** *($25)* is seemingly designed to be a modern interpretation of the full coverage attainable from Dermablend's original Cover Creme. This water- and silicone-based liquid foundation has a very smooth texture with nice slip—it's definitely easier to blend than the Cover Creme. It also provides almost as much coverage, but with a much lighter feel. The problem? It still appears heavy on skin and its powdery matte finish looks like makeup, no two ways about it. Estee Lauder, Prescriptives, M.A.C., and Lancome all offer foundations that provide significant coverage while looking more natural on skin, making this a less-enticing option. Among the seven mostly good shades, only Soft Beige and Caramel Beige are too peach to recommend.

☹ **Leg and Body Cover Creme** *($18)* provides the most significant, immediate coverage of any foundation I have ever seen, but the result is a dry, ashen finish that does not look natural or skinlike in the least. Dermablend advertises it as a new, silky formula and it is silky, but none of the other problematic elements were corrected, including this foundation's tendency to separate and continually change color as it is blended (something I rarely witness). Exuviance by Neostrata's Corrective Leg & Body Makeup ($16.50) is better in every respect, and includes a titanium dioxide and zinc oxide SPF 18.

CONCEALER: 😐 **$$$ Smooth Indulgence Concealer** *($18)* shares the same traits as the Smooth Indulgence Foundation above, only with greater coverage. The tradeoff for nearly complete camouflage of dark circles, blemishes, or redness is a finish that feels light and silky but looks heavy. Making matters worse is the fact that three of the four shades are noticeably peach to orange. Nude is the only workable option, but there are better full-coverage concealers available. 😐 **$$$ Quick-Fix** *($17)* is an oil-based, lipstick-style concealer with minimal slip. It provides intense coverage but will crease into lines around the eyes. Dermablend recommends this as a cover-up for acne, but using this thick, wax-based concoction over a blemish only proves that misery loves company. There are ten shades, and most are a far cry from realistic skin tones. Light, Beige, Ivory, Caramel, and Deep are the only shades worth considering, and then only if you have dry skin and need complete coverage.

☹ **Smooth Indulgence Redness Concealer** *($17)* has a slightly lighter, more fluid texture than the regular Smooth Indulgence Concealer, but its sheer green tint doesn't do a great job of minimizing redness and it can be tricky to blend with a flesh-toned foundation color. ☹ **Cover Duet Custom Corrector** *($21.50)* is a dual-sided liquid concealer that has a liquid-like texture and soft matte finish. Although this provides good coverage, all of the duos have at least one shade that's too peach or yellow to recommend.

POWDER: 😐 **$$$ Loose Setting Powder** *($19)* is nothing more than talc and a preservative—not the critical product it's made out to be if you're considering Dermablend. The instructions for Cover Creme indicate this is "the key to the wearability and smudge-resistance of Dermablend," but any talc-based powder will do the same thing, and then you can ignore the mediocre colors offered here, especially Original, which is pure white. 😐 **$$$ Matte & Shimmer Bronzer** *($18)* is labeled as such on Dermablend's Web site, but on the product itself it reads **Brush-On Bronzer**. This talc-based pressed-powder bronzer duo features a matte peachy bronze shade paired with a sparkling copper color. There are better and less expensive bronzing powders to consider before this one, but it's an OK option for medium skin tones.

☹ **Solid Setting Powder** *($17)* is a talc-based, pale white pressed powder that has a soft, smooth application, but the color is too difficult to work with, especially if you have medium to dark skin.

DERMALOGICA (SKIN CARE ONLY)

DERMALOGICA AT-A-GLANCE

Strengths: Good eye-makeup remover; a combination AHA/BHA product; a couple of commendable moisturizers.

Weaknesses: Expensive; almost every category has one or more products that contain irritating ingredients with no established benefit for skin; poor sunscreens; no products to comprehensively address the needs of acne-prone or hyperpigmented skin; unusually suspicious about any requests for ingredient information. My research assistant repeatedly contacted Dermalogica (as a consumer) and was told that questioning their ingredients was strange and "a very odd request" by every person she spoke to.

For more information about Dermalogica, call (800) 831-5150 or visit www.dermalogica.com or www.Beautypedia.com.

☹ **Anti-Bac Skin Wash** *($29.50 for 8.4 ounces)* is a standard, detergent-based cleanser that also contains mint, menthol, and camphor, none of which serve any purpose for skin other than to cause irritation and inflammation. This does contain triclosan, an antibacterial ingredient that has no research showing it to be effective for acne, despite the fact that there is controversy as to whether daily use may be problematic in regard to generating bacterial resistance.

☹ **Clearing Skin Wash** *($32 for 8.4 ounces)* contains a small amount of salicylic acid that is rinsed from skin before it can impact blemishes, while the main detergent cleansing agent is the drying, irritating sodium C14-16 olefin sulfonate. This also contains several irritating plant extracts rather high up on the ingredient list, making it an all-around bad choice.

☹ **Dermal Clay Cleanser** *($29.50 for 8.4 ounces)* is an odd mixture of plant oil, clay, detergent cleansing agents, thickeners, and several irritating plant extracts. This concoction won't help oily or "congested" skin, but could very well make matters worse, mostly because it doesn't rinse well.

😐 **$$$ Essential Cleansing Solution** *($29.50 for 8.4 ounces)* is a cold cream–style cleanser that is an option for dry to very dry skin, but it's not so enticing owing to the inclusion of a few potentially irritating plant extracts.

☹ **Precleanse** *($32 for 5.1 ounces)* is marketed as "the professional's deep cleansing weapon," but is nothing more than a mix of trigylceride with several nonvolatile plant oils. Also included are two forms of lavender and forms of citrus that serve to fragrance the product and irritate skin. For the money, irritant-free jojoba or olive oil is preferred.

☹ **Skin Purifying Wipes** *($15 for 6 wipes)* contain balm mint (*Melissa*), witch hazel, and camphor, all of which are irritating to skin. The amount of salicylic acid isn't sufficient for exfoliation, and the pH wouldn't allow that to happen even if it contained a decent amount.

☹ **Special Cleansing Gel** *($29.50 for 8.4 ounces)* contains irritating essential oils of lavender and balm mint (*Melissa*) and is neither recommended nor the least bit special.

☹ **The Bar** *($17.50 for a 5-ounce bar)* is a soap-free bar cleanser that contains some tea tree oil and lesser amounts of some irritating plant extracts and essential oils. Its base formula is similar to Dove's Beauty Bars, so if you prefer this type of cleanser, stick with Dove and avoid the irritation this bar can cause.

☹ **Ultracalming Cleanser, for Face and Eyes** *($29.50 for 8.4 ounces)* contains lavender as a chief ingredient, which prevents this otherwise well-formulated cleansing lotion from being ultra-calming or recommended.

☺ **$$$ Soothing Eye Makeup Remover** *($21.50 for 4 ounces)* is a standard, but good, detergent-based eye-makeup remover that is free of fragrance and the irritating plant extracts Dermalogica puts in their facial cleansers.

😐 **$$$ Daily Microfoliant** *($47.50 for 2.7 ounces)* costs a lot for what amounts to cellulose, talc (the exfoliants in this cleansing scrub), detergent cleansing agents, plant extracts, and irritating essential oil of grapefruit peel. There is no reason to choose this over a standard topical scrub, or just using a washcloth with your water-soluble cleanser.

😐 **$$$ Skin Prep Scrub** *($28 for 2.5 ounces)* is a detergent-based, water-soluble cleanser that contains cornmeal as the scrub agent. It would probably be better to just use cornmeal from the grocery store if you want a cornmeal scrub, because then at least you wouldn't be applying some of the irritating plant extracts that are present in this product, including arnica and ivy. Although these ingredients are probably present in such small amounts that they don't have much effect on skin, why are they in here at all?

☹ **Multi-Active Toner** *($27.50 for 8.4 ounces)* is multi-irritating because it contains lavender, balm mint, pellitory, arnica, and ivy. None of these ingredients are humectants (as Dermalogica asserts) and they certainly are not "skin-repairing."

☹ **Soothing Protection Spray** *($30 for 8.4 ounces)* is supposed to protect skin from reactive ozone, which is impossible. Perhaps they made that claim to skirt the fact that this toner irritates, not soothes, skin with lavender oil and the menthol derivative menthoxypropanediol.

☹ **Daily Resurfacer** *($65 for 35 individually wrapped applications, 0.51 ounce total)* is an extremely expensive, somewhat gimmicky way to exfoliate skin, and its exfoliating benefit is dubious. Enclosed in a jar are almost three dozen packets of a liquid solution and a pre-soaked sponge designed to fit on your index finger. You're directed to massage this in circular motions over skin, with no need to rinse. The solution has in its base a bitter-orange extract, which is a fragrant extract and a skin irritant, so things aren't off to a good start. Salicylic acid (BHA) is included, at about a 1% concentration, but the AHAs touted on the label are sugarcane and apple extracts, neither of which are true AHAs that can exfoliate skin, or at least not with any supporting research. Either way, the pH of this solution is too high for exfoliation to occur, so you're left hoping the sponge applicator will be abrasive enough to do the job. (It isn't, but that's a good thing.) Making matters worse, especially because the product remains on the skin, is grapefruit peel oil. This citrus oil can cause contact dermatitis and phototoxic reactions due to its volatile chemical constituents (Source: www.naturaldatabase.com).

☹ **Gentle Cream Exfoliant** *($33.50 for 2.5 ounces)* ends up being Dermalogica's idea of gentle, but that includes irritants such as sulfur and lavender oil. Who's formulating these products and marketing them so disingenuously?

☹ **Medicated Clearing Gel** *($35 for 1.7 ounces)* clears the way for blemished skin to become irritated and inflamed due to the many fragrant oils it contains, including sage, rosemary, and ginger. The 2% salicylic acid is useless due to this gel's pH, which is above 4.

☺ **$$$ Skin Renewal Booster** *($45 for 1 ounce)* is a 10% AHA and 0.5% BHA product whose pH of 3.6 is great for exfoliation. The aloe base is excellent for all skin types, though this does contain some thickeners that may be a problem for blemish-prone skin. Skin Renewal Booster contains a few fragrant plant extracts, but in amounts unlikely to cause a problem. Finally, the packaging of this product will help keep the retinol stable.

☹ **Active Moist** *($34 for 1.7 ounces)* contains lavender and arnica, both problematic ingredients for skin. This is otherwise a very bland, lightweight moisturizer lacking any state-of-the-art ingredients to justify its price.

😐 **$$$ Barrier Repair** *($35 for 1 ounce)* is a silicone-based moisturizer that also contains some vitamin E, plant oils, vitamin C, and anti-irritants. The silicone feels silky on skin and this would be an option for someone with normal to dry skin. It is not rated higher because the antioxidants are in such short supply.

☹ **Climate Control** *($29.50 for 0.75 ounce)* cannot shield skin from environmental pollutants or protect it from reactive ozone (ozone is bad to breathe, too, so how does this moisturizer protect us from that?). Its an oil- and wax-based formula that would have been recommended for dry to very dry skin if it did not contain geranium oil and lavender.

☹ **Day Bright SPF 15** *($46.50 for 1 ounce)* lacks the UVA-protecting ingredients of titanium dioxide, zinc oxide, avobenzone, Tinosorb, or Mexoryl SX, and is not recommended. Even with sufficient UVA protection, the balm mint and orange oil are irritating to skin.

☹ **Extra Firming Booster** *($45 for 1 ounce)* has an irritating bitter orange flower base and only makes skin feel firmer because of the PVP (a hairstyling film-forming agent) it contains. The ylang ylang oil can cause contact dermatitis and itchy skin, which isn't what you want from any product.

☹ **Gentle Soothing Booster** *($45 for 1 ounce)* could have earned highly recommended status due to its roster of genuinely soothing plant extracts. However, the St. John's wort (*Hypericum*) extract can cause severe phototoxic reactions on sun-exposed skin, and that's hardly gentle (Source: www.naturaldatabase.com).

😐 **$$$ Intensive Eye Repair** *($43 for 0.5 ounce)* should not be used around the eyes because the first ingredient is fragrant rose extract. It is an OK moisturizer for normal to dry skin elsewhere on the face, though the arnica extract is present in an amount that may prove irritating to sensitive or reactive skin.

☺ **$$$ Intensive Moisture Balance** *($37 for 1.7 ounces)* lists rose extract as the first ingredient, which makes this a very fragranced moisturizer whose blend of thickeners, silicone, aloe, and antioxidants is fairly good. Without the rose extract this would have rated a Paula's Pick; it includes the cell-communicating ingredient lecithin and does not contain any irritating plant extracts or oils. Those with normal to dry skin may want to consider it.

☹ **Multivitamin Power Concentrate** *($52 for 45 capsules, 0.65 ounce total)* has antioxidant finesse and a non-aqueous formula, but it's sabotaged by irritating citrus oils of lime, orange, and grapefruit. This is a dangerous product to apply to skin if it will be exposed to sunlight.

☺ **$$$ Multivitamin Power Firm, for Eye and Lip Area** *($47 for 0.5 ounce)* contains mostly silicones, thickeners, vitamin E, vitamin A, antioxidants, anti-irritant, plant oils, plant extracts, and vitamin C. It's a good antioxidant serum for all skin types, but has no special benefit (and is not emollient enough) for the lips. Although this is a very good formulary, it's not as impressive as the top serum options from Lauder-owned lines.

☹ **Night Bright** *($48.50 for 0.75 ounce)* contains balm mint (*Melissa*) as the main ingredient, along with lesser amounts of problematic lemon and lime. The plant extracts in this serum have some proven skin-lightening ability, but the irritants make this one to skip.

☹ **Oil Control Lotion** *($34 for 2 ounces)* contains 1% salicylic acid at an effective pH of 3.6, but is not recommended because it irritates skin with balm mint, camphor, and menthol. What a shame, and none of the plant extracts in this lotion can have any effect on skin's oil production.

☹ **Power Rich** *($175 for 5 0.3-ounce tubes; 1.5 ounces total)* promises a pharmaceutical-strength formula that will show a difference after just one week. This rose flower– and silicone-based serum isn't powerful or rich, and it doesn't contain ingredients that have a pharmaceutical quality. It does irritate skin with essential oils of jasmine, ginger, and grapefruit.

☹ **Sheer Moisture SPF 15** *($37 for 1.3 ounces)* includes zinc oxide for UVA protection, but has a lavender base and contains lavender oil. This sunscreen also contains English walnut oil (listed as *Juglans regia*), which, when applied topically, can cause yellow to brown skin discolorations and contact dermatitis (Source: www.naturaldatabase.com).

☹ **Sheer Tint Redness Relief SPF 15** *($39 for 1.3 ounces)* does not provide skin with sufficient UVA protection, and in addition it's a problem that a sheer, moisturizing tint designed to reduce redness contains sensitizing lavender oil as well as the fragrance components limonene and linalool.

☹ **Skin Hydrating Booster** *($53 for 1 ounce)* lists balm mint (*Melissa*) as the main ingredient and also contains lavender oil, making this far too irritating for all skin types.

☹ **Skin Smoothing Cream** *($36 for 1.7 ounces)* contains a potentially irritating amount of arnica as well as sensitizing ylang ylang oil. Even if you wanted to tolerate these ingredients, the moisturizer is an overall boring formula with a paltry amount of antioxidants.

😐 **$$$ Super Rich Repair** *($75 for 1.7 ounces)* is sold as the company's "most intense, super-concentrated cream." Super Rich Repair is indeed an emollient, oil-rich moisturizer, even if it is packaged so that the effective ingredients won't stay stable. Plus the antioxidants in here are present only in very small amounts. (In fact, there's more preservative than state-of-the-art ingredients, a ratio that isn't good news, considering the premium price of this moisturizer.) So much for being super.

Another issue is the inclusion of several essential oils, including sandalwood, eucalyptus, cedarwood, and geranium, which all work in opposition to the anti-irritants, and that means the two types of ingredients cancel each other out. All in all, this moisturizer will certainly make dry to very dry skin feel better, but for the money and because of the needless inclusion of fragrant irritants, you'd be better off considering state-of-the-art (and non-jar packaged) formulas from Clinique, Skinceuticals, or Prescriptives.

☺ **$$$ Total Eye Care SPF 15** *($37.50 for 0.5 ounce)* lists only titanium dioxide as the active ingredient, making this a gentle sunscreen to use around the eyes. Iron oxides, talc, and mica provide a brightening effect to shadowed areas, while lightweight emollients moisturize. The formula lacks significant amounts of antioxidants and interesting skin-identical ingredients, but is an option for normal to dry skin.

☹ **Anti-Bac Cooling Masque** *($33.50 for 2.5 ounces)* contains several irritating ingredients, almost too many to list, including balm mint, rose oil, rosewood oil, and balsam.

☺ **$$$ Intensive Moisture Masque** *($36.50 for 2.5 ounces)* has some good ingredients for dry to very dry skin, and includes antioxidant vitamins. However, the antioxidants are best left on skin and the titanium dioxide (the second ingredient) creates a strong whitening effect that isn't what you'd want to wear all day. Not to mention that the orange oil can cause irritation.

☹ **Multivitamin Power Recovery Masque** *($40 for 2.5 ounces)* includes some very good plant oils and antioxidants, but those are countered by irritating plant extracts as well as the potent menthol derivative menthoxypropanediol, making this impossible to recommend for any skin type.

☹ **Sebum Clearing Masque** *($39 for 2.5 ounces)* is a clay mask that contains several menthol derivatives as well as menthol itself, which makes it too irritating for all skin types. Menthol has no effect on oil production or absorption; the pH of 4.5 prevents the salicylic acid from clearing "congested follicles" (though that term is classic spa-talk).

☹ **Skin Hydrating Masque** *($33.50 for 2.5 ounces)* is based around irritating bitter orange flower extract and also contains irritating ivy, pellitory, and arnica extract, all of which cancel out the effect of the anti-irritant plant extracts in this well-intentioned but problematic mask.

☹ **Skin Refining Masque** *($32.50 for 2.5 ounces)* contains the same irritating plant extracts as the Skin Hydrating Masque above, but makes matters worse by adding menthol and sage to the mix. There are many clay masks that absorb oil and refine skin's texture without causing undue irritation.

☹ **Special Clearing Booster** *($41 for 1 ounce)* is a needlessly expensive topical disinfectant with 5% benzoyl peroxide as the active ingredient. This water-based solution is not recommended because it contains St. John's wort, sage, lemon, and ivy.

☹ **Overnight Clearing Gel** *($40 for 1.7 ounces)* has a pH of 4, which is borderline for its 2% salicylic acid to exfoliate skin. While some exfoliation is assured, this product contains several irritating plant extracts and oils, including sage, rosemary, and citronella. Camphor is also in the mix. What a shame, because without the copious irritants this would have been an above average BHA option for all skin types.

☹ **Clearing Mattifier** *($40 for 1.3 ounces)* contains 2% salicylic acid, but the pH of 4.7 doesn't allow it to function as an exfoliant. The silicones in this product leave a soft matte finish, but the amount of cinnamon bark extract is cause for concern and makes this unhelpful BHA product a poor option (not to mention expensive, considering several products can provide a matte finish like this does).

☹ **Concealing Spot Treatment** *($30 for 0.5 ounce)* contains 5% sulfur, a potent disinfectant that can be unusually drying and irritating for skin. This also contains a large amount of witch hazel and irritants including camphor and cinnamon bark.

DERMALOGICA SUN PRODUCTS

☹ **After Sun Repair** *($30 for 3.4 ounces)* contains far too many irritating plant extracts and essential oils to be even slightly capable of repairing sun-exposed skin. If anything, the irritant potential of the essential oils will further damage skin and negatively affect the healing process.

☹ **Extra Rich Faceblock SPF 30** *($48 for 1.7 ounces)* would have been an excellent, in-part zinc oxide moisturizing sunscreen for normal to dry skin, but it contains irritating essential oils of sandalwood, eucalyptus, and geranium. Without these troublesome ingredients, this would be highly recommended due to its antioxidant and cell-communicating ingredient content.

☹ **Full Spectrum Wipes SPF 15** *($22 for 15 wipes)* not only lack the correct UVA-protecting ingredients, but also contain balm mint and several irritating essential oils, including spearmint.

☹ **Multivitamin Bodyblock SPF 20** *($35 for 4.2 ounces)* contains avobenzone for sufficient UVA protection, but also has lavender oil, which can irritate skin and cause skin-cell death (Source: *Cell Proliferation*, June 2004, pages 221–229).

☹ **Oil-Free Matte Block SPF 20** *($45 for 1.7 ounces)* includes titanium dioxide for UVA protection and comes in a lotion base that contains some good antioxidants. Unfortunately, it also contains enough grapefruit peel oil to be irritating and possibly cause a sensitizing reaction on sun-exposed skin.

☹ **Solar Defense Booster SPF 30** *($33 for 1 ounce)* contains avobenzone, so this one has good UVA protection! However, it also contains balm mint and lemon extracts plus lavender oil, all skin irritants.

☹ **Solar Shield SPF 15** *($10 for a 0.28-ounce stick)* is an emollient sunscreen in stick form that lacks the UVA-protecting ingredients of titanium dioxide, zinc oxide, avobenzone, Tinosorb, or Mexoryl SX. Making matters even worse is the inclusion of menthol and grapefruit oil.

☹ **Super Sensitive Faceblock SPF 30** *($45 for 1.7 ounces)* contains lavender oil, which is completely unsuitable for "super sensitive" skin. It's good that the active ingredients are only titanium dioxide and zinc oxide, and the formula has some well-researched antioxidants and soothing agents, but the lavender oil trumps them all.

☹ **Ultra Sensitive Faceblock SPF 25** *($26 for 1.7 ounces)* lists balm mint as the first ingredient, which may make skin ultra-sensitive and irritated. This completely titanium dioxide sunscreen also assaults skin with several ouch-inducing essential oils, including thyme, rosewood, and orange.

☹ **Waterblock Solar Spray SPF 30** *($38 for 4.2 ounces)* leaves skin vulnerable to UVA damage because it lacks titanium dioxide, zinc oxide, avobenzone, Tinosorb, or Mexoryl SX. It also contains irritating balm mint extract and grapefruit peel oil.

DIOR

DIOR AT-A-GLANCE

Strengths: Every sunscreen offers sufficient UVA protection; a handful of outstanding cleansers and makeup removers; some extraordinary foundations, some of which include sunscreen; the liquid concealer; very good loose powder, powder blush, and powder eyeshadows; some great mascaras; brow gel; elegant creamy lipsticks and several good lip glosses; Dior's makeup tester units are much more accessible and user-friendly. I also found their counter staff to be more accommodating and definitely less condescending than several other European-bred lines.

Weaknesses: Expensive; lackluster moisturizers and serums that contain more fragrance and preservatives than elegant ingredients; irritating toners and self-tanners; ordinary masks; lack of products to address the needs of those with blemishes or skin discolorations; some foundations with SPF ratings that are too low; the cream concealer; mostly average makeup brushes.

For more information about Dior, call (212) 931-2200 or visit www.dior.com or www.Beautypedia.com.

DIOR SKIN CARE

DIOR CAPTURE PRODUCTS

😐 **$$$ Capture Levres Lip Contour Wrinkle Creme** *($35 for 0.52 ounce)* temporarily smooths lines around the mouth due to the amount of acrylate-based film-forming agent it contains. How long the effect lasts depends on how deep your lip lines are and how much you move your mouth. All told, this isn't really an exciting formula and the most intriguing ingredients are barely present.

😐 **$$$ Capture R-Lisse Smooth-Away Wrinkle Treatment** *($42 for 1.7 ounces)* is a very boring moisturizer that makes skin look smoother thanks to polyvinyl alcohol. Although this can be an irritating ingredient, the amount in this product is unlikely to cause a problem. Still, this is severely lacking in significant amounts of state-of-the-art ingredients, and contains fragrance components that can be sensitizing.

😐 **$$$ Capture R60/80 Filler Intense Deep Wrinkle Filler** *($67 for 0.67 ounce)*. So what do the numbers R60/80 mean? According to Dior's Web site, the R60 stands for 60% reduction in wrinkles after just one hour following application and 80 represents the claim that "After 1 month: 80% of women surveyed noticed a visibly younger-looking appearance." In addition, all of Dior's Capture R60/80 products contain their patented C.U.R.E. complex; the letters stand for Cutaneous Ultra-Revitalizing Extract. Dior does not reveal what specific ingredients make up this complex, but the ones on the label are not exactly earthshaking or even vaguely as unique as the name attributed to them. Further, in every Capture R60/80 product, the beneficial ingredients are listed well after the fragrance and preservatives, meaning that the amounts present are most likely not enough to deliver much, or at least no more than any other supposed antiwrinkle product. This water- and silicone-based serum makes skin feel silky and contains film-forming agents to smooth superficial wrinkles, but that's about it.

😐 **$$$ Capture R60/80 First Wrinkles Smoothing Eye Creme** *($49 for 0.5 ounce)* is a lighter version of the Capture Levres Lip Contour Wrinkle Creme above, and the same basic comments apply. The amount of film-forming agent in this product may prove irritating for use around the eyes.

😐 **$$$ Capture R60/80 Nuit Enriched Wrinkle Night Creme** *($80 for 1.7 ounces)* is a standard, jar-packaged emollient moisturizer for dry skin. Its creamy texture shortchanges skin of many essential ingredients it needs, and it contains more fragrance and preservatives than antioxidants or skin-identical substances.

😐 **$$$ Capture R60/80 Nuit Intense Wrinkle Night Fluid** *($64 for 1 ounce)* is hardly a "miracle fluid." For all the exaggerated promises and claims, this is just a good, but relatively uninspired, moisturizer, and the price doesn't add up when the formula is primarily water, thickeners, film-forming agent, slip agents, preservatives, fragrance, and tiny amounts of a few antioxidants. It contains palmitoyl pentapeptide-3, but in a concentration of less than 0.1%. Considering that the company that sells that ingredient recommends at least a 3% concentration, the amount here falls into the "less-than-useful" category. This product also contains retinol and the packaging will keep it stable, but there are other products with retinol that cost far less than this one. Dior's marketing campaign definitely earns a merit badge for doing everything it can to make the ordinary sound compellingly extraordinary.

😐 **$$$ Capture R60/80 Ultimate Wrinkle Creme, Light & Fresh Texture** *($76 for 1.7 ounces)* is just as lackluster a product as the Intense Night Wrinkle Fluid above, only this one is said to "contain a biological complex of marine origin for gentle exfoliating action." The only ingredient it contains that comes close to matching that description is glucosamine, and the amount of it in this product is minuscule, not to mention that glucosamine does not exfoliate the skin (though it is often positioned as a gentle alternative to AHA or BHA products). Dior's naming this product Ultimate Wrinkle Creme can only mean they are completely out of the loop when it comes to what ingredients it takes to create a good moisturizer with significant amounts of antioxidants and other skin-beneficial substances. This product contains mostly water, sunscreen agents (not listed as active ingredients, so they cannot be relied on for sun protection), slip agents, film-forming agents, preservatives, and fragrance. The few antioxidants and skin-identical ingredients (similar to those in all the R60/80 products) show up too close to the end of the ingredient list to matter, and the jar packaging hinders what little benefit they offer.

😐 **$$$ Capture R60/80 Ultimate Wrinkle Creme, Rich Texture** *($76 for 1.7 ounces)* is nearly identical to the Ultimate Wrinkle Creme, Light & Fresh Texture above, except that this one contains an emollient thickener and some silicone, which makes it better for normal to dry skin. Otherwise, the same basic comments apply.

😐 **$$$ Capture R60/80 Yeux Wrinkle Eye Creme** *($54 for 0.51 ounce)* is basically a hybrid of the two Ultimate Wrinkle Creams above, with a silky texture that's in between a cream and a lotion. Although this feels quite nice, the formulation lacks worthwhile amounts of antioxidants, skin-identical ingredients, and anti-irritants, and there is little reason to consider this a special formulation for the eye area. It contains mostly water, film-forming agent, emollient, slip agent, a long list of thickeners, preservatives, fragrance, plant extracts, and the tiniest amount of vitamin C and glycosaminoglycans (water-binding agent) imaginable.

😐 **$$$ Capture R-Flash Instant Ultra-Smoothing Fluid** *($57 for 0.5 ounce)* is sold as the "magical" skin care, but for Dior the main thing here is to convince you this generic, water-based serum is worth the splurge. The sorbitol and algin can create a slight tightening effect, but the after-feel is somewhat tacky and the effect is strictly cosmetic. Meanwhile, skin is shortchanged of ingredients that, while not tightening, actually have benefit.

☹ **Capture Sculpt 10 Contouring Gel-Emulsion, Focus Chin-Throat** *($100 for 1 ounce)* sounds like a face-lift in a bottle with all its claims of targeting skin that's begun to sag or expand (as with a double chin). But then the second ingredient is alcohol, and nothing that follows can reshape skin or redefine its contours. The notion that a cosmetic product can do that is as ridiculous as this product's formula.

☹ **$$$ Capture Sculpt 10 Lifting Firming Creme** *($80 for 1.7 ounce)* is another lackluster Dior moisturizer claiming to lift, tighten, support, and deeply strengthen skin. The claims are Park Avenue elite, while the formula borders on Skid Row in terms of leaving skin wanting much more, especially at this price.

☹ **$$$ Capture Sculpt 10 Lifting Firming Fluid** *($80 for 1.7 ounces)* is the lotion version of the Capture Sculpt 10 Lifting Firming Creme above, and other than this containing more alcohol, the same review applies.

☹ **$$$ Capture Sculpt 10 Re-Plumping Emulsion, Focus Cheeks-Lips** *($75 for 0.5 ounce)* claims to target sunken cheeks and make them appear more plump and toned. It is completely incapable of this feat and ends up being an exceedingly boring, potentially irritating moisturizer that is a barely passable option for normal to oily skin.

☹ **$$$ Capture Totale Multi-Perfection Concentrated Serum** *($125 for 1 ounce)* is an average water- and silicone-based serum that contains enough film-forming agent to make skin look smoother temporarily. For the money, it is not preferred to the truly state-of-the-art serums from Olay, Paula's Choice, Estee Lauder, or Neutrogena.

☹ **$$$ Capture Totale Multi-Perfection Creme** *($115 for 1.7 ounces)* claims to correct all the visible signs of aging, but since there's no sunscreen here you can forget about making your wrinkles or dark spots look any better. It's a standard, emollient moisturizer for normal to dry skin that contains far more fragrance than legitimate bells and whistles (and the jar packaging won't help keep the tiny amount of antioxidants stable once this is opened).

☹ **$$$ Capture Totale Multi-Perfection Eye Treatment** *($75 for 0.5 ounce)* attributes its Multi-Perfection name to its alleged ability to correct wrinkles, discolorations, and dark under-eye circles. Considering the price, it would be rewarding if this product really were a "totale" treatment for eyes, but it's not. As with most Dior moisturizers, including those meant for the eye area, it is inadequately formulated—all of the interesting ingredients are listed well after the preservative and fragrance, which means they are barely present. Interesting or not, none of the ingredients in this product will prolong skin's youthful appearance, nor is it soothing, as claimed. It's just a lightweight, water- and silicone-based moisturizer with enough film-forming agent to make the eye area look temporarily smoother.

☹ **$$$ Capture XR60/80 Extra Vital Restoring Serum** *($82 for 1.7 ounces)* contains mostly water, film-forming agent, slip agents, glycerin, the cell-communicating ingredient lecithin, and skin-identical ingredients. The peptides are present in meaningless amounts, being surpassed by the amount of fragrance and preservatives in this unexciting, non-vital serum.

☹ **Capture Anti-Taches D-30 Age Spot Correction Intensive Concentrate** *($45 for 0.06 ounce)* lists alcohol as the second ingredient, which makes this intensely irritating. The mineral pigments add a reflective glow to skin that can cosmetically blur the appearance of dark spots—but your money is better spent on a product with ingredients that have greater impact on skin discolorations without causing undue irritation.

☹ **$$$ Capture Totale Rituel Nuit, Multi-Perfection Intensive Night Restorative** *($125 for 1.8 ounces)* takes a cue from competitor Chanel's ultra-pricey Sublimage Essential Regenerating Cream (reviewed above), claiming that its rare, revitalizing plant, longoza, is "grown only in Madagascar" and, therefore, must have phenomenal benefits for aging skin. Why is it that such ingredients never seem to show up in Peoria or Houston? Why only in exotic locales? Are exotic plants automatically better for skin? The mystique makes it sound like you're buying something unique or special. The marketing myths about plants or rare species of seaweed, from remote countries or islands where they're gathered by tribal harvesting practices, and on and on, seem never-ending. Speaking of marketing nonsense, Longoza is actually a city in Madagascar, and the plant of that name appears to be a form of wild ginger. Yet it's not present anywhere in this product. That's OK, though, because there's no evidence that any species of ginger can "turn back the clock" for your skin. This ends up being a silky-textured but basic moisturizer that contains mostly water, glycerin, silicone, slip agent, film-forming agent, emollients, alcohol, more film-forming agent, salt, preservative, and fragrance. It's a mediocre option for normal to slightly dry skin.

☹ **Capture Totale Rituel Nuit, Multi-Perfection Nighttime Soft Peel** *($75 for 3.4 ounces)* lists alcohol as the second ingredient, which makes this product too irritating for all skin types. The amount of salicylic acid is way too small and the pH is way too high for it to be effective as an exfoliant, making this a complete waste of time and money.

☺ **$$$ Capture Anti-Taches D-30 Age Spot Correction Hand Cream SPF 15** *($45 for 2.6 ounces)* features avobenzone for sufficient UVA protection and has a lightweight but substantial-feeling base formula. As is the case with most Dior products, the most intriguing ingredients are barely present, being overshadowed by fragrance and preservatives. Still, the sunscreen element alone is enough to earn a happy face rating.

Dior Prestige Products

😐 **$$$ Dior Prestige Exquisite Cleansing Creme** *($55 for 6.9 ounces)* is a basic, lotion-style cleanser that will need a washcloth to remove all the makeup. There are no words for how ordinary this is. Lines from Nivea to Pond's all have options that surpass this one. The tiny amounts of antioxidants and anti-irritants in this product are barely worth mentioning.

😐 **$$$ Dior Prestige Exquisite Cleansing Foam** *($45 for 0.5 ounce)* is a glycerin-based, water-soluble cleanser whose cushiony lather feels luxurious, just like many other foaming cleansers that wouldn't dare charge this much. The amount of potassium hydroxide can be drying, making this cleanser's use limited to those with oily skin (and a freewheeling budget).

☹ **Dior Prestige Exquisite Lotion** *($55 for 6.7 ounces)* lists alcohol as the second ingredient, which at this price is just insulting. Even if the company's talked-up rare flower nectar had some benefit for skin, the alcohol would cancel it. Any, and I mean any, drugstore toner beats this product.

😐 **$$$ Dior Prestige 20 + 1 Nutri-Restoring Creme** *($250 for 1.7 ounces)* pledges to give skin a second youth due to the 20 rare ingredients it contains, in addition to the rare flower nectar present in all of the Prestige products. In many ways, this moisturizer is actually less impressive than most others from Dior. It contains sunscreen ingredients but doesn't list an SPF rating, has far more fragrance than beneficial extras, and none of the "rare" ingredients have research proving they're anti-aging miracle workers for skin. Topping all of this disappointment is jar packaging, which means the plant extracts' antioxidant capability will be compromised as soon as you open the product. Your money is better spent on a series of AHA or BHA peels, or saving up for dermal fillers, all procedures that really do make aging skin look better.

😐 **$$$ Dior Prestige 20 + 1 Nutri-Restoring Fluid** *($250 for 1.7 ounces)* is the lotion version of the Dior Prestige 20 + 1 Nutri-Restoring Creme above, and aside from its better packaging, the same review applies. Even with stable packaging, however, this is an absurdly overpriced product unless you have unwavering faith in Dior's flower nectar.

☺ **$$$ Dior Prestige Revitalizing Creme** *($155 for 1.7 ounces)* claims to shower skin with pleasure, but the only pleasure is the one Dior receives from selling such a needlessly expensive moisturizer that isn't worth a fraction of the cost. It contains some very helpful ingredients for dry skin, but none that don't show up in hundreds of other products. Further, the amount of antioxidants is paltry and the jar packaging won't keep them stable.

☺ **$$$ Dior Prestige Revitalizing Essence** *($180 for 1 ounce)* is said to contain an ultra-concentration of Dior's precious flower nectar, but there's more of this ingredient in the Prestige moisturizers above. Regardless of the amount, there is no evidence anywhere that it's the key to restoring youthfulness. This is a pricey, water- and silicone-based serum with a tiny amount of plant oil and more fragrance than antioxidants. It is best for normal to slightly dry skin, but spending this much is not warranted.

☺ **$$$ Dior Prestige Revitalizing Eye Creme** *($78 for 0.5 ounce)* lists the third ingredient as aluminum starch octenylsuccinate, an absorbent that is about as far from moisturizing as you can get. This contains a small amount of skin-identical ingredients, antioxidants, and anti-irritants, but for this kind of money, that's an insult. The fragrance components in this product should be kept away from the eye area.

☺ **$$$ Dior Prestige Intensive Cure** *($280 for 3 0.3-ounce bottles)* promises to gradually transform skin and bring it to its highest level of revitalization (how they quantified that wasn't explained, but it sure sounds good). The system is separated into three "cures." **Cure 1** and **Cure 2** are nearly identical and consist primarily of water, glycerin, the Prestige flower nectar, glucose, slip agents, skin-identical ingredients, and preservative. **Cure 3** adds a triglyceride for more moisture and has a greater amount of vitamin E than Cures 1 or 2. Yet none of these is a restorative potion for aging skin, nor is it necessary to follow Dior's week-by-week successive regimen. This is basically an assembly of products made out to be a super-potent elixir, just waiting for women with money to burn to plunk down their credit cards. You'll get softer, smoother skin, but any hopes beyond that will undoubtedly be dashed—and there are lots of less-expensive ways to be disappointed (such as sitting through Halle Berry in *Catwoman*).

☺ **$$$ Dior Prestige Massage Mask** *($110 for 1.7 ounces)* is a good emollient mask for normal to dry skin, but is made less impressive by its prohibitive price and the potentially irritating fragrance components. Besides, the backbone ingredients in this formula, while effective, can be found in countless other moisturizing masks.

☺ **$$$ Dior Prestige Revitalizing Mask** *($110 for 10 0.67-ounce masks)* is a silkier, lighter version of the Dior Prestige Massage Mask above. Best for normal to oily skin, its formula is similar to many silicone-enriched serums. For the money, you'd be better off using an Olay Regenerist or Total Effects serum (as a mask or leave-on product) than this concoction.

DIORSNOW PRODUCTS

☹ **DiorSnow Pure Whitening Foaming Cleanser** *($31 for 3.6 ounces)* won't whiten skin one iota, and ends up being a foaming cleanser that's potentially drying due to the amount of alkaline potassium hydroxide it contains. It also contains the irritating menthol derivative menthoxypropanediol, and is not recommended.

☹ **DiorSnow Pure Whitening Aqua Lotion** *($46 for 6.7 ounces)* lists alcohol as the second ingredient, making this neither refreshing nor whitening. In fact, nothing in this poorly formulated toner has the ability to lighten skin discolorations.

☺ **$$$ DiorSnow Pure UV Ultra-Protective Whitening UV Base SPF 50 – PA +++** *($45 for 1 ounce)* is an in-part titanium dioxide sunscreen with a fluid texture and soft matte finish suitable for normal to oily skin. The additional titanium dioxide and mineral pigments mica and iron oxides create a subtle whitening and brightening effect. This product contains no ingredients capable of lightening skin discolorations other than the protection the sunscreen offers them, which is true for any well-formulated sunscreen that is used religiously.

😐 **$$$ DiorSnow Pure Whitening Moisturizing Creme** *($65 for 1 ounce)* pales in comparison to the best moisturizers from Estee Lauder, Clinique, and Prescriptives. The amount of vitamin C is encouraging, but the jar packaging won't keep it or the couple of other antioxidants in the product stable. Once again, nothing in this moisturizer will impact skin discolorations.

☺ **$$$ DiorSnow Pure UV Ultra-Whitening Spot Corrector SPF 50 – PA+++** *($42 for 0.63 ounce)* contains almost 20% titanium dioxide, along with other sunscreen actives, which assures you of significant broad-spectrum sun protection. Sold as a spot treatment, this whitens skin cosmetically (the titanium dioxide and iron oxides provide concealer-like coverage) and is best paired with a skin tone–correct foundation. This is an OK, though very expensive, option for normal to oily skin not prone to blemishes. With its fragrance components, this product should be kept away from the eye area.

☹ **DiorSnow Pure Whitening Skin Repairing Essence** *($85 for 1.7 ounces)* lists alcohol as the second ingredient, which makes it too irritating for all skin types. Immediately after the alcohol is the stable vitamin C derivative magnesium ascorbyl phosphate. Research into magnesium ascorbyl phosphate's ability to lighten skin via inhibition of melanin is scientifically promising (Sources: *Phytotherapy Research*, November 2006, pages 921–934; *Skin Research and Technology*, May 2002, page 73; and *Journal of the American Academy of Dermatology*, January 1996, pages 29–33). These studies used 3% and 10% concentrations, respectively—and although this Dior product may meet that criterion, the alcohol makes this potentially effective skin-lightening product an irritating proposition.

Dior HydrAction Products

Most of the HydrAction products below claim to be infused with Dior's exclusive Aquacept Complex, which uses aquaporin technology. You may recall that aquaporins are a series of ten different proteins that form water channels in living things to regulate the water content of skin and other organs. Aquaporin-3 is the one that's abundant in skin, and is a major way that glycerol (glycerin) and its derivatives are transported through the top layers of skin. So what Dior is really stating is that the products listed below contain glycerin, which helps the skin retain water in between cells. That's great—but hundreds (possibly thousands) of skin-care products contain glycerin, and preventing water loss is only one part of keeping skin healthy and maintaining proper moisture balance.

😐 **$$$ HydrAction Deep Hydration Refreshing Spray** *($30 for 3.36 ounces)* is a basic spray-on toner that contains glycerin and some novel skin-identical ingredients, but the latter are present in a meager amount. This is an ordinary toner for normal to dry skin with an extraordinary price.

😐 **$$$ HydrAction Deep Hydration Defense Fluid SPF 15** *($46 for 1.7 ounces)* is a very standard moisturizing sunscreen that contains avobenzone for UVA protection. Although this is a good option for normal to dry skin, it should be brimming with ingredients that further boost skin's environmental defenses (such as antioxidants), and it isn't.

☹ **HydrAction Deep Hydration Radical Serum** *($67 for 1.7 ounces)* contains too much alcohol to be hydrating or capable of giving skin an "extra moisture boost." It also contains fragrance components that can irritate skin, and that won't help it look radiant or healthy.

😐 **$$$ HydrAction Deep Hydration Rich Creme** *($46 for 1.7 ounces)* is a moisturizer whose formula is almost identical to Dior's Prestige Massage Mask (reviewed above, and which, despite the directions for the mask, can be left on skin like a moisturizer). Why this one costs $64 less is a mystery. In either case, both products are acceptable for normal to dry skin, but both are also easily replaced by less-expensive and better-formulated products.

😐 **$$$ HydrAction Deep Hydration Sorbet Creme** *($33 for 1 ounce)* is a lightweight, refreshing, cream-gel moisturizer that's an OK option for normal to oily skin. It contains a dusting of antioxidants, but the jar packaging won't keep them stable.

😐 **$$$ HydrAction Deep Hydration Sorbet Gel** *($46 for 1.7 ounces)* is nearly identical to the HydrAction Deep Hydration Sorbet Creme above, and the same review applies.

😐 **$$$ HydrAction Deep Hydration Intensive Mask** *($32 for 2.5 ounces)* is a standard moisturizing mask for normal to dry skin. Almost any moisturizer at the drugstore can take this product's place, as it pretty much covers the basics (though it does so with lots of fragrance).

😐 **$$$ HydrAction Deep Hydration Pore Reducing Treatment** *($33 for 0.67 ounce)* smooths skin's texture with its mixture of glycerin and silicones. However, since alcohol is the second ingredient, this will also irritate, and the fragrance components compound this side effect.

OTHER DIOR PRODUCTS

😐 **$$$ Cleansing Gelee, for Face, Lips and Eyes** *($32 for 6.7 ounces)* is a fluid cleanser that contains cleansing agents typically found in eye-makeup removers. This product removes makeup quite well, but the fragrance components can be problematic for use around the eyes, which limits its appeal.

☺ **$$$ Cleansing Milk, for Face and Eyes** *($29 for 6.7 ounces)* shouldn't be used around the eyes because of the volatile fragrance components it contains, but is otherwise an innocuous lotion cleanser for normal to dry skin. You'll need a washcloth for complete makeup removal.

☺ **$$$ Cleansing Water, for Face and Eyes** *($29 for 6.7 ounces)* is a standard but effective water-based makeup remover. It is not adept at removing long-wearing or waterproof makeup, but is a fine water-soluble option for removing other types of makeup.

😐 **$$$ Rinse-Off Cleansing Foam** *($29 for 5.3 ounces)* has merit if you prefer foaming cleansers, but the amount of potassium hydroxide is potentially drying and makes this Foam best for oily skin. Needless to say, Neutrogena and L'Oreal sell similar cleansers for considerably less money.

✓☺ **$$$ Self-Foaming Cleanser** *($28 for 5 ounces)* is a very good all-around cleanser for all skin types. Gentle but effective cleansing agents combine with skin-softening ingredients to remove makeup and leave skin satin-smooth. If you're going to splurge on a Dior cleanser, make it this one.

✓☺ **$$$ Duo-Phase Eye Make-Up Remover** *($25 for 4.2 ounces)* is an excellent, fragrance-free, silicone-enhanced makeup remover that may be used around the eyes or anywhere on the face. The price should give you pause (Almay and Neutrogena sell similar products for under $6), but this is still recommended.

☺ **$$$ Exfoliating Face Scrub** *($31 for 2.5 ounces)* is a rich, creamy topical scrub that contains polyethylene as the abrasive agent. It is suitable for dry to very dry skin, and its only drawback (well, aside from the fragrance) is that it doesn't rinse easily.

☹ **Energizing Toner** *($28 for 6.7 ounces)* lists alcohol as the second ingredient and contains insignificant amounts of helpful ingredients for any skin type.

☹ **Matifying Toner** *($29 for 6.7 ounces)* contains too much alcohol and also irritates skin with camphor and menthol. The inclusion of castor oil is odd for a toner that claims to mattify skin and minimize pores.

😐 **$$$ Soothing Toner, Alcohol-Free** *($29 for 6.7 ounces)* contains a tiny amount of soothing ingredients and ends up being a truly ho-hum, overpriced toner for normal to dry skin.

😐 **$$$ Masque Magique, Purifying Radiance Mask** *($30 for 2.5 ounces)* contains lightweight hydrating ingredients along with lesser amounts of alcohol and silicone. It's an OK mask for normal to slightly dry skin, but there's nothing magical about it and the amount of antioxidants is insignificant.

☺ **$$$ Blotting Papers** *($21 for 150 sheets)* are standard, powder-free oil-blotting papers. They come in attractive, chic packaging, and that's what you're really paying for. What's inside can be easily replaced by countless less-expensive options.

☹ **Lip Beautyfier** *($26 for 0.27 ounce)* contains camphor, menthol, and a pepper extract, all of which serve to irritate, not beautify, lips.

DIOR SUN PRODUCTS

😐 **$$$ Dior Bronze Beautifying Moisturizer** *($32 for 4.7 ounces)* is a floral- and coconut-scented body and hair moisturizer that contains a good blend of glycerin, slip agents, oil, and silicones. It has a beach-y appeal, but contains some fragrance components that can be a problem for skin if it is exposed to sun without protection.

☹ **Dior Bronze Self-Tanner Natural Glow, Body** *($27 for 4.4 ounces)* lists alcohol as the second ingredient, and contains the same ingredient (dihydroxyacetone) found in most self-tanning products. Knowing this, why subject your skin to irritation from this much alcohol?

☹ **Dior Bronze Self-Tanner Natural Glow, Face** *($26 for 1.8 ounces)* contains far too many potentially irritating fragrance components to make it worth choosing over countless other self-tanning products, not to mention the needlessly high price for a very basic formula.

☹ **Dior Bronze Self-Tanner Shimmering Glow, Body** *($27 for 4.5 ounces)* is similar to the Dior Bronze Self-Tanner Natural Glow, Face above, and the same review applies.

DIOR MAKEUP

FOUNDATION: ✓☺ $$$ DiorSkin Compact SPF 20 *($41)* has an ultra-silky, talc-based texture and smooth, seamless application that matches similar products from Lancome, Estee Lauder, Chanel, and Laura Mercier. However, Dior's version has a drier finish and feels less creamy than my favorites in this category, though theirs includes an in-part titanium dioxide sunscreen, which is a big plus. As a touch-up over foundation or moisturizer with a well-formulated sunscreen, this can be a nice adjunct to your makeup routine. Each of the nine shades is beautiful and recommended. One caveat: This does contain shiny particles that are visible on the skin in daylight, so be careful if this is not the look you are after.

☺ **$$$ DiorSkin Pure Light Sheer Skin-Lighting Makeup SPF 15** *($41)* has a beautifully fluid, sheer, elegant texture with a flawless application that leaves a slightly moist, radiant finish that those with normal to slightly dry skin will appreciate. The in-part titanium dioxide sunscreen makes this sheer-coverage foundation an ideal all-in-one product as the weather heats up, but to ensure adequate sun protection it must be applied liberally and evenly (and don't forget to apply regular sunscreen to your neck and chest area). Of the eight shades, only two (shades 202 and 400) are poor options because of strong overtones of peach; the rest are a mostly neutral lot suitable for fair to medium skin tones.

☺ **$$$ DiorSkin Eclat Satin** *($41)* is Dior's foundation for those with dry skin, and it delivers—with a creamy, moisturizer-like texture that has a natural affinity for skin. It provides medium to almost full coverage, yet does so without looking thick or cakey and leaves an attractive dewy finish. Six shades are available, but watch out for the slightly peach #400 and avoid #402, which is glaringly rose. The fact that this foundation is highly fragranced keeps it from earning a Paula's Pick rating.

☺ **$$$ DiorSkin AirFlash Mist Makeup** *($60)* is an aerosol foundation that can be tricky to use, but with a little patience the results are rewarding. The coverage you get depends on your application. Spraying it in your hand at close range and then applying to the face will net medium to full coverage that looks surprisingly natural, and is far less messy than holding it 12 inches or more from your face (as the Dior makeup artist I spoke to recommended). Either way it provides a sheer veil of color and coverage. Once sprayed on, AirFlash dries, well, in a flash—so blending must be quick. Luckily, this blends evenly and sets to a long-wearing, silky matte finish that will require more than a water-soluble cleanser to remove. Only four shades are available, with options for fair to medium skin, but each one is excellent. Although this is pricey, it is a unique twist on liquid foundations (even those that are silicone-based) and does indeed feel weightless, which is ideal for oily to very oily skin. By the way, since this foundation can get on your clothing or hairline as you spray it (especially given that you should keep your eyes closed when doing so), it is best applied before dressing, with your hairline protected by a towel or headband, because if you aren't careful it can get all over. The mist this produces is ultra-fine, but some spotting can occur when spraying from the distance that Dior recommends, and do make sure the opening doesn't clog or a mess will ensue.

😐 **$$$ DiorBronze Sun Glowing Moisturizer SPF 10** *($35)* features an in-part titanium dioxide sunscreen, but SPF 10 is frustratingly low for daytime. Although not recommended as your sole source of sunscreen, this lightweight tinted moisturizer blends easily, provides sheer coverage, and has a soft, natural matte finish. The formula is best for normal to oily skin, and comes in three workable shades.

😐 **$$$ DiorSkin Icone Photo Perfect Creme-to-Powder Makeup SPF 10** *($41)* isn't the perfect choice when you know you're going to be photographed. This is a cream-to-powder makeup in a tube, similar to Chanel's superior Double Perfection Creme Powder Makeup SPF 15 ($42). With Chanel's version you get an effective sunscreen that meets the minimum standard for daytime protection. Dior's version includes an in-part titanium dioxide sunscreen, but the SPF rating falls short. The texture is initially thick but softens quickly and blends well, setting to a powder finish. Unless you're careful during application, the finish can look heavy and too powdery. This is not a foundation for someone with any degree of dry skin, which further limits its appeal. It is best for normal to slightly oily skin and provides medium coverage. The range of eight shades is impressively neutral; only shades 032 and 042 are too peach to consider. Shade 001 is a colorless primer that makes skin feel very silky, but it isn't essential if you are using a silicone-based moisturizer or serum as part of your skin-care routine.

😐 **$$$ DiorSkin Sculpt Line-Smoothing Lifting Makeup SPF 20** *($52)*. There is nothing in this foundation that will make lines look smoother, at least not any more so than any other foundation, but that cosmetic effect is a poor substitute for wrinkle prevention, which is where an effective sunscreen comes in. Unfortunately, this anti-aging makeup misses the mark by not including the UVA-protecting ingredients of titanium dioxide, zinc oxide, avobenzone, Tinosorb, or Mexoryl SX. That's truly a shame, because it has a creamy-smooth texture and a beautiful application perfect for those with normal to dry skin who prefer a slightly moist finish and medium to full coverage. Six of the nine shades are excellent, with Ivory 010 being a prime choice for very fair skin. Rosy Beige 032 is too peach, Honey Beige 040 is slightly rose, and Dark Beige 050 is noticeably rose. In terms of sculpting or lifting, don't count on such benefits, especially with insufficient sun protection. This does contain a tiny amount of peptides, but they're listed after the preservative, meaning their benefit to skin will be minimal at best. There are enough positives to make this worth considering, but not over similar foundations that get the critical issue of sun protection right.

☺ **$$$ DiorSkin Fluide Foundation SPF 12** *($41)* has a lot going for it, but its too-low SPF 12, though in-part titanium dioxide, keeps it from earning a higher rating. If sunscreen in foundation isn't a concern, this is worth considering for its modern texture and beautiful application. This liquid foundation is housed in a pump bottle, and its pump works more effectively than most when it comes to controlling how much product is dispensed. It has one of the silkiest textures around, and is supremely easy to blend, setting to a satin matte finish and providing light to medium coverage. Fourteen shades are available (Dior's broadest palette), including options for very light and dark skin tones. Just watch out for the following colors, because all are too peach, pink, or orange to recommend: 202 (slightly pink, an option for some light skin tones), 203, 300, 302, 303, and 400.

CONCEALER: ✓☺ **$$$ DiorSkin Sculpt Lifting Smoothing Concealer** *($29)* has a price that should give you pause, but there's no denying that this is a formidable concealer that is worthy of your attention. The silky, silicone-enhanced formula begins slightly thick, but blends very well. It has minimal slip, so it does a great job of staying precisely where you place it, drying to a satin matte finish that provides significant coverage. Dark circles and redness are easily erased, but this concealer never looks too thick and it creases only minimally. It comes in three superb shades, though only for fair to medium skin tones. Forget about the sculpting and lifting claims because they are mere fantasy, but the rest is as real as it gets.

☹ **Hydrating Concealer** *($25)* is a creamy, medium- to full-coverage concealer that has a pervasive sweet fragrance. Blending this is frustrating because it never sets, and it tends to crease unless heavily set with powder, which isn't a good look. Add the 4 mostly poor shades to that and this is an easy one to ignore.

POWDER: ☺ **$$$ DiorSkin Loose Powder** *($42.50)* is a talc-based powder with a silky, finely milled texture and satin matte finish suitable for normal to dry skin. All three shades go on almost translucent, so there's no need to worry about getting the color exactly right. This does come with a worthwhile brush instead of the more typical powder puff.

☺ **$$$ DiorSkin Pressed Powder** *($35)* is also talc-based and has an expectedly heavier (but still natural-looking) application when compared with its loose counterpart. It isn't the most absorbent powder, so those with very oily skin will not be satisfied, but for all other skin types this is recommended, and all three shades are very good.

☺ **$$$ Dior Essential Bronzing Powder** *($39)* is a monumental improvement over Dior's former pressed bronzing powder. Not only have the texture and application been improved, but also the range of four colors now resembles golden, tan, and bronze tones rather than the former version's peachy orange hues. The only drawback is the shine. Each shade is imbued with large sparkling particles that tend to flake off. It's not a huge drawback, but a bronzing powder at this price should be as close to perfect as possible.

BLUSH: You will not be disappointed with the sublime texture and application of ✓☺ **$$$ DiorBlush** *($32.50)*. In a word, it is superlative, and most of the available colors are excellent, with several soft choices that apply evenly. Each shade is infused with shine, but it's not too intrusive. This blush, like Estee Lauder's Tender Blush ($25) has that extra something that pushes it above and beyond the best, and, comparing French lines, Dior's powder blush puts Lancome's to shame.

✓☺ **$$$ Pro Cheeks Ultra-Radiant Blush** *($30)* has a spongy texture that turns into an airy cream-to-powder blush that's a cinch to apply and blend. In fact, if you're new to this type of blush this is almost foolproof, and the translucent colors look remarkably natural. (It's still blush, though, so "natural" is a relative term.) Among the four shades, the only non-blush tone is Limelight, which is opalescent, very pale pink, and best for highlighting, if you use it at all.

☺ **$$$ Sunshine Blush** *($41)* is a pressed-powder blush/bronzer that includes four shades (two for blush, one bronze tone, and one highlighter) in a compact. Dior has offered this type of product for years, and some women will indeed find it convenient. You have the option of using each color individually (a tricky feat given there are no dividers between the stripes of color) or sweeping a brush over the whole powder cake for one uniform color. Either way you'll get decent pigmentation and noticeable shine, which makes this best for evening wear.

EYESHADOW: ✓☺ **$$$ 5-Color Eyeshadow Compact** *($52)* represents Dior's classic eyeshadow offering and has been around almost from this line's inception. The texture of these is like powdered sugar and although the formula puts emollience before absorbent ingredients like talc, it doesn't crease. Each shade applies very smoothly, doesn't flake, and provides more coverage (and definitely has a stronger color payoff) than most powder eyeshadows. The ongoing problem is Dior's often contrasting or overly trendy color combinations. Sadly, these tend to outnumber the workable sets, though the following are worth considering: Beige Massai, Incognito, Night Dust, Sweet Illusion, and Tender Chic. All of these are predominantly shiny, but if that's your thing the shine goes on softer than in the past and clings beautifully. It's still too shiny for wrinkled or drooping eyelids, but younger women with the means to afford these eyeshadow sets will be impressed.

✓☺ **$$$ 1-Colour Eyeshadow** *($23.50)* has a formula different from that of the 5-Colour Eyeshadow Compact reviewed above, but it's still enviably silky, almost creamy. The application is excellent, as is the color saturation, making these single shadows a pleasure to work with. The drawback for those with wrinkles is the amount of shine. If wrinkles aren't a concern and you want shine, there are some attractive brown, gray, and off-white shades to consider (and the requisite blue and green shades to ignore).

✓☺ **$$$ 2-Colour Eyeshadow** *($32)* carries on the tradition Dior established long ago of offering powder eyeshadows with an ultra-fine, supremely silky texture that feels almost creamy and blends superbly. The vast majority of Dior's eyeshadows are replete with shine, and that carries on here, too. Each duo features a light and dark complementary or tone-on-tone blend, so as long as you avoid the blue, bright pink, and lime green duos the combinations are all pretty much can't-go-wrong. However, unless your eye area is perfectly smooth and unwrinkled, these are too shiny for daytime wear. Younger women who are not yet dealing with visible signs of aging on their eyelids (such as the models Dior tends to use in their eye-makeup ads) can use these shadows with abandon. The best pairings are Diorchic, Diorgraphic, and Diorwild. The talc-free formula can be used wet or dry, with wet application intensifying the color (often to a flattering effect).

☺ **$$$ DiorShow Eyecolor** *($30)* is packaged in a click pen with a built-in synthetic brush applicator. The formula is creamy-slick, but blends to a finish that feels matte and looks shiny. In fact, shine is the name of the game here because you'll see more of that than color. Use caution when dispensing, as this tends to get slightly chunky if you don't clean the brush between uses. Overall this is more novelty than practical, and doesn't surpass Dior's shiny powder eyeshadows.

😐 **$$$ Eye Show** *($30)* has the same formula and texture characteristics as the Pro Cheeks Ultra-Radiant Blush above, but it doesn't translate as well to eyeshadow. The trend-driven colors are difficult to work with and all are infused with chunky shine that looks more flashy than classy. Used as directed, these tend to crease quickly and, unlike the blush, the colors fade easily, leaving behind bits of sparkles. This is minimally waterproof.

EYE AND BROW PRODUCTS: ✓☺ $$$ Brow Gel *($17)* is a standard, lightweight brow fixative. The brush is excellent, with both long and very short bristles, so every hair will be tamed, and this has a minimally sticky finish that's a step above similar brow-taming products.

☺ **$$$ Style Liner** *($30)* is an inkwell-style liquid eyeliner that applies better and dries faster than Dior's Liquid Eyeliner below. The thin, flexible brush is the perfect length for controlled application, and you'll find this doesn't chip or smear once dry. If only the colors were better! Still, a classic black option is available and is the only shade I recommend unless you want a space-age iridescent finish. ☺ **$$$ Liquid Eyeliner** *($30)* is a long-lasting liquid liner that comes with a good brush that makes even application easy. The bottom of the pen houses the liquid and you have to click the base to feed the brush. If Dior sold refills, this would be an option; since they don't, this is absurdly overpriced for what you get, though still deserving of a happy face rating.

😐 **$$$ Crayon Eyeliner** *($24)* is a standard though quite creamy pencil that makes smearing almost a certainty. Perhaps that's why a smudge tip was included, as this only works for smoky eyes, preferably when set with a coordinating powder eyeshadow. 😐 **$$$ Crayon Eyeliner Waterproof** *($24)* needs routine sharpening, but does have a soft, creamy application. The finish, though waterproof, feels tacky, so consider this a special occasion pencil and know that it's not recommended over automatic pencils that stay put, such as Cover Girl's Outlast version.

☺ **$$$ Powder Brow Pencil** *($24)*. Although an automatic, twist-up brow pencil or a powder eyeshadow with a thin brush is easier to use to create realistic eyebrow definition, this remains one of the better standard brow pencils. It has a soft powder texture that fills in and defines brows without looking heavy (no Joan Crawford arches here!) and comes in three beautiful shades suitable for blonde to medium brown brows. The mascara brush at the opposite end of the pencil is a nice touch for softening the result.

😐 **$$$ DiorShow Brow** *($17)* puts the spotlight on your brows thanks to its glitter-infused tinted gel formula. The dual-sided brush is great at allowing you to create a softer or more defined effect, and the shine tends to cling to brow hairs rather than flake onto the eyelid. Although this is worth considering if you want glossy-looking, glitter-infused brows, the finish feels somewhat dry and stiff, though it does keep unruly hairs in place. The two shades include sheer blonde and brunette.

LIPSTICK AND LIPLINER: ☺ $$$ Rouge Dior Replenishing Lipcolor *($26)* makes all sorts of claims in terms of long wear and amplified color technology, but for all the hype this is nothing more than a standard, but good, creamy lipstick. It offers enticing shades with medium opacity and a soft glossy finish. The pigments in this lipstick are more concentrated than usual, which means the colors last longer. However, you'll likely be ready for a touch-up before then because the glossy finish is short-lived.

☺ **$$$ Dior Addict Lipstick** *($24.50)* has a soft, creamy texture and a slightly greasy-feeling finish. That may feel great, but it doesn't help in the longevity department. The majority of the colors are fine, with most having an iridescent or soft shimmer finish.

☺ **$$$ Dior Addict Pearl Shine Lipstick** *($23)* is identical to the Dior Addict Lipstick, but with a pearlized finish that makes each shade more light reflective.

☺ **$$$ Dior Addict Ultra-Gloss** *($23.50)* has an emollient, lanolin-based formula that is great for dry lips and provides a smooth, glossy finish that isn't sticky. The sheer- to light-coverage colors are a tantalizing mix, with options for the color-shy and for those with a flair for the dramatic. It's not the ultimate gloss, but at least those prone to over-spending won't be disappointed!

☺ **$$$ DiorKiss** *($19)* is one decadent lip gloss! Its thick, syrupy texture feels semi-sticky on lips and each of its bold yet sheered-down colors has a rich, vinyl-like shine. This tube gloss with a built-in angled applicator is a splurge, but if you love lip gloss and enjoy having several variations from which to choose, this is a new option worth seeking out—and it lasts longer than most. ☺ **$$$ Dior Addict Plastic Gloss** *($24.50)* has a reflective, plastic-like finish, hence the name. The colors are applied with a sponge-tip wand, and each goes on feeling thick and sticky, though this (and the strong pigmentation) does keep the gloss around longer than slick formulas.

☺ **$$$ DiorShow Gloss Show Spectacular Sparkling Lip Gloss** *($27)* is a soft-textured, fancifully packaged pot-type lip gloss that features a handful of sheer, versatile colors laced with large particles of glitter. The finish is indeed sparkling and this is a good choice for gloss fans looking to put the spotlight on their lips. It is completely non-sticky, but as the emollience wears away the glitter may begin to feel grainy—not as noticeably as with similar glosses, but still something to keep in mind.

😐 **$$$ Dior Addict Ultra Shine Sheer Lipcolor** *($24.50)* is a standard, slightly greasy sheer lipstick with a sparkling, glossy finish that feels slippery. The shade range offers choices from the softest nude to bright, vibrant pinks and corals. However, this lipstick is more style than substance (the attractive holographic packaging alone costs vastly more than the lipstick), and it doesn't really offer anything special or unique for your lips. As with all sheer lipsticks, these won't last long before you need a touch-up. Note also that the glitter particles tend to stick around long after the color has faded, so it would be best to cover the entire lip area with a Lipliner beforehand.

☺ **$$$ RougeLiner Automatic Lipliner** *($23)* is an automatic, retractable lip pencil made to coordinate with the Rouge Dior Replenishing Lipcolor above. The application is a step above most pencils, being silky with just the right amount of creaminess. It sets to a nearly smudgeproof finish and is an easy recommendation for those who prefer to spend their cosmetics dollars at the department store. One disappointment: The shade selection is unusually small, and favors brown tones. They're workable, but not for those who prefer Dior's (or anyone else's) brighter hues or reds.

😐 **$$$ Lipliner Pencil** *($24)* is a standard, creamy-finish Lipliner that comes in a dwindling array of colors (almost all of which are brown-based) and has a lipstick brush at one end. It's exceptionally overpriced for what you get, but it does the job.

MASCARA: ✓☺ **$$$ DiorShow Waterproof Mascara** *($23)* is Dior's best waterproof mascara to date. Although the brush is enormous and can be difficult to work with, you will find it produces copious length and respectable thickness without clumps or smears. The formula is tenaciously waterproof, but easier than most to remove, making this highly recommended if your mascara budget extends to Dior's price point.

☺ **$$$ MaximEyes** *($23)* claims to add lush length and intense depth to even the puniest lashes with just one coat. Unless your definitions of "lush" and "intense" are fairly lenient, you're bound to be disappointed with this mascara if you stop at one coat. Like most mascaras, it takes several coats to produce beguiling lashes, and MaximEyes is no exception. Actually, with several coats this turns out to be quite impressive! It lengthens and provides slight thickness without a clump or smear in sight, and wears well all day.

☺ **$$$ DiorShow Mascara** *($23)* has one of the largest brushes I've ever seen on a mascara wand, which makes it a bit tricky to work with, and nearly impossible to reach the small lashes near the eye's inner and outer corners, but with patience and practice every lash can be covered. The payoff is extraordinarily long, thick lashes with minimal to no clumping, and beautiful separation. Beyond the cumbersome brush, the only caveat with this mascara is its potent fragrance. There is no reason for mascara to contain fragrance, but then again, this is Dior.

☺ **$$$ DiorShow Black Out Spectacular Volume Intense Black-Kohl Mascara** *($23)* has a large brush that is similar to but more spiral-shaped than the DiorShow Mascara above. It can be difficult to control and apply evenly, but with patience this builds dramatically thick, full lashes. This is also one of the blackest mascaras I've tried; the color really makes an impact. You'll appreciate how soft this keeps lashes, plus it wears beautifully yet removes easily with a water-soluble cleanser. A less cumbersome brush would have earned this a higher rating.

😐 **$$$ UltimEyes Mascara** *($23)* promises a look of "sculpted, defined, seemingly endless lashes," but it doesn't deliver. This isn't a mascara to dismiss altogether, but a product this pricey should make lashes long enough to make the investment worth it. At best, UltimEyes Mascara separates lashes well while building modest length and some thickness (without major clumps). 😐 **$$$ DiorShow Unlimited Ultra-Lengthening Curving Mascara** *($23)* actually thickens better than it lengthens, and nothing about its performance deserves "ultra" status. Application tends to be a bit uneven and slightly wet, so you'll get some smearing unless you're meticulous (or wipe down the wand beforehand). It wears well and does leave lashes softly curled, but all in all, if Dior mascaras are your thing, consider their superior MaximEyes mascara before this.

FACE AND BODY ILLUMINATING/SHIMMER PRODUCTS: ☺ **$$$ DiorSkin Moisturizing Radiance Makeup Base** *($39)* has a fluid consistency that isn't moisturizing in the least. Rather than add color to skin, it has a brightening effect thanks to the mica and titanium dioxide it contains. Skin is left with a soft, pearlescent shimmer that works alone or can be mixed with foundation to create a radiant glow. ☺ **$$$ DiorShow Powder** *($40)* is a sparkling loose powder packaged in a jar with an attached synthetic sponge. Powder is dispensed onto the sponge when the container is inverted, and you "buff" it onto your skin. Although more for shine than color, the talc-based formula is airy and sheer, and the shiny particles stay put surprisingly well, making this a pricey but worthwhile shimmer powder.

☺ **$$$ Skinflash Radiance Booster Pen** *($33)* promises "professional lightworks in a flash." What this really ends up being is merely a click-pen applicator set up so that you need to twist the base of the component to feed product onto the attached synthetic brush. This produces a flesh-toned liquid that at first appears to be a concealer. Yet once it's applied to skin it practically vanishes into it, providing minimal coverage as it sets to a natural matte (in feel) finish. Basically, this is a sheer highlighter with a touch of shimmer to help light reflect more evenly off skin. To some extent, this can soften minor flaws and subtle discolorations. It is best for creating soft highlights under the eye, on the brow bone, and down the bridge of the nose, and the fact that this blends so well into skin makes it a pleasure to work with, especially if you're attempting a complex highlighting/contouring makeup application. Three shades are available, and though each is initially pink or peach, they "neutralize" once blended. The effect this product provides can be created with less-expensive concealers (just make sure the color you select is at least one shade lighter than your skin tone or the highlighting effect won't work).

☹ **$$$ DiorGlam** *($55)* provides a pressed-powder eyeshadow and highlighting powder in one chic silver compact with an attached brush. It's the sort of product you'd expect to fall out of Paris Hilton's evening bag, and the concept is shine, shine, shine. Because Dior knows how to produce extremely silky powders, these apply smoothly and cling well, but the shine is too much for anyone concerned about downplaying wrinkles or uneven skin texture.

BRUSHES: The small collection of **Brushes** *($25–$40)* is respectable but by no means perfect or worthy of must-have status. Given Dior's vast selection of makeup, it's surprising their brush choices (especially for eye makeup) are so limited. The brushes to consider include the ☺ **$$$ DiorShow Blush Brush** *($35)*, which is better than the flimsy ☹ **$$$ DiorShow Powder Brush** *($40)*. Also good are the ☺ **$$$ DiorShow Eyeshadow Brush** *($25)*, and the synthetic hair ☺ **$$$ DiorShow Foundation Brush** *($30)*, which is not as large as many others, making it easier to reach tight spaces.

SPECIALTY PRODUCTS: ☺ **$$$ DiorSkin Control Colors** *($24)* is Dior's contribution to the concept of color-correcting cosmetics, similar to what Estee Lauder did with their Prime FX line. Unlike standard color correctors, the fluid formula imparts sheer color and leaves a sparkling shine with a matte feel. Actual color correction is almost zilch, but that's good because the concept, though well-meaning, rarely looks convincing in natural light. Think of the three shades as highlighters with shine and try blending this with your foundation for a touch of evening glamour.

☺ **$$$ Blotting Papers** *($21 for 150 sheets)* are standard, nonpowdered blotting papers that absorb excess shine, but so do many other versions that wouldn't dare charge this much for what amounts to tissue paper. What you're paying for is the elegant Dior-embossed carrying case that includes a built-in mirror. It's definitely a chic way to blot, but what a shame Dior doesn't sell refill packs so you only have to pay for the extravagance once. These serve their purpose, but whether or not to spend this much for elegant packaging is up to you.

DOVE (SKIN CARE ONLY)

DOVE AT-A-GLANCE

Strengths: Inexpensive; some state-of-the-art water-soluble cleansers and moisturizers; available in every major drugstore and mass-market store; Dove's latest ad campaigns emphasizing the natural beauty of real women are a refreshing and long-overdue change of pace; the company offers several programs and inspiring articles that encourage women to embrace themselves as they are and build their self-esteem.

Weaknesses: A few products with low SPF ratings; problematic ingredients in some products designed for sensitive skin; many bar cleansers; the Pro-Age line is overall disappointing.

For more information about Dove, call (800) 761-3683 or visit www.dove.com or www.Beautypedia.com. Note: All Dove products contain fragrance unless otherwise noted.

DOVE COOL MOISTURE PRODUCTS

☹ **Cool Moisture Beauty Bar** *($2.99 for 2 4.25-ounce bars)* is a standard bar cleanser that contains a combination of detergent cleansing agents and ingredients found in traditional soap. This makes for a drying experience that doesn't rinse well, and it is not recommended.

✓☺ **Cool Moisture Facial Cleansing Cloths** *($5.99 for 30 cloths)* are a convenient way to cleanse skin, especially when you're on the go. The sturdy cloths are steeped in a gentle water-soluble cleansing solution that's suitable for all but very oily skin. The amount of cucumber and green tea isn't significant, and what counts most is how well these work to refresh skin and remove makeup.

✓☺ **Cool Moisture Foaming Facial Cleanser** *($5.99 for 6.76 ounces)* is an excellent water-soluble cleanser for all skin types except very dry. It produces a soft lather, removes makeup well, and rinses easily.

DOVE DEEP MOISTURE PRODUCTS

☺ **Deep Moisture Creamy Facial Cleanser** *($5.99 for 6.76 ounces)* feels creamy and sounds suitable for dry skin, but the detergent cleansing agents present are best for normal to oily skin. This is a very good, water-soluble cleanser that contains some absorbent ingredients to leave skin feeling clean and looking matte; it is not deeply moisturizing.

😐 **Deep Moisture Day Cream SPF 15** *($7.49 for 1.69 ounces)* protects skin from UVA rays with its in-part avobenzone sunscreen. It is formulated in a lightweight, smooth-finish cream base suitable for normal to slightly dry or slightly oily skin. It contains a smattering of ingredients that mimic the structure and function of healthy skin, though the jar packaging isn't preferred.

☺ **Deep Moisture Facial Lotion SPF 15** *($7.49 for 4.05 ounces)* is similar to but with a thinner texture than the Deep Moisture Day Cream SPF 15 above, and the same basic comments apply. This option has better packaging, but the lack of antioxidants is disappointing.

DOVE ENERGY GLOW PRODUCTS

☹ **Energy Glow Beauty Bar** *($8.99 for 6 4.25-ounce bars)* is a standard bar soap cleanser, and the dulling residue it leaves won't promote a healthy glow, as claimed. This can be too drying for all skin types.

😐 **Energy Glow Brightening Facial Cleansing Pillows** *($4.49 for 14 pillows)* are small pillows that contain a powdered mixture of citric acid and baking soda (sodium bicarbonate) that causes a fizzy, foamy effect when they're moistened, as you're d rected to do before cleansing. Neither side of the pillow is too abrasive, and each is easy to maneuver around the face, but the amount of citric acid may make it irritating, and this is definitely not to be used around the eyes. Of concern is the drying detergent cleansing agent sodium C14-16 olefin sulfonate. However, the amount of it in these pillows is likely too low to cause problems. I wouldn't choose this over a good water-soluble liquid cleanser, and these certainly aren't economical (if you use two pillows per day you'll be out of them in a week), but they're an OK option if you're feeling experimental and will make sure not to use them around the eyes.

☺ **Energy Glow Skin Brightening Facial Cleanser** *($4.99 for 5 ounces)* is a foaming, water-soluble cleanser that's laced with exfoliating beads (the gentle plastic kind, made of polyethylene). It's a good option for a cleansing scrub, but won't make skin any brighter than other similar scrubs, or simply using a washcloth with your facial cleanser. The exfoliating beads make this cleanser a problem for use around the eyes; however, this is just fine as a morning cleanser to awaken skin without irritation.

😐 **Energy Glow Brightening Eye Cream SPF 8** *($10.99 for 0.5 ounce)* has an SPF number that's embarrassingly low, even though the sunscreen includes zinc oxide for UVA protection. Nothing about this formula makes it specific to the needs of the eye area (it can be used anywhere on the face), although this thick but soft cream's high silicone content and its texture allow it to function as a soft spackle for eye-area wrinkles. The effect is temporary, and it does work, but how long it lasts will depend on how expressive you are. Still, this is a disappointing product for daytime use unless you're willing to pair it with another product with SPF 15 or higher. What a shame, because the packaging Dove chose will keep the antioxidants stable, and the product is fragrance-free.

✓☺ **Energy Glow Brightening Moisturizer SPF 15** *($10.99 for 1.7 ounce)* is a well-formulated moisturizer, and it features an in-part zinc oxide sunscreen. The creamy formula moisturizes without feeling greasy, and includes antioxidants as well as ingredients that mimic the structure of healthy skin. The mica, zinc oxide, and titanium dioxide blend adds a subtle whitening effect that's translucent, so the result is indeed more a skin-brightening than the pasty, pale look that you can get from some other products. This fragranced daytime moisturizer is best for someone with normal to slightly dry or slightly oily skin that's not prone to blemishes.

😐 **Energy Glow Brightening Night Cream** *($10.99 for 1.69 ounce)* has a luxuriously silky yet lightweight cream texture and contains some good antioxidants, although the jar packaging won't help keep them stable. It also contains several good skin-identical ingredients. The "brightening" effect is courtesy of zinc oxide, and Dove put in enough of it to create a soft white cast on the skin, which, coupled with mica, creates a brightening glow. The effect is strictly cosmetic, and not much use at night (do you really care if your skin glows while you sleep?), but it is harmless.

😐 **Energy Glow Daily Face Moisturizer with a Touch of Self-Tanner** *($6.99 for 1.7 ounces)* omits all of the bells and whistles (most of which are truly beneficial for skin) seen in most of Dove's other moisturizers. Instead, the two formulas available for this product (one for Fair to Medium Skin, the other for Medium to Dark Skin) include the self-tanning ingredients dihydroxyacetone and erythrulose. Both provide a subtle sunless tan, but it's a shame these lightweight lotions end up being one-note products when Dove's other options provide a symphony.

😐 **Energy Glow Daily Moisturizer with Subtle Self-Tanners** *($7.99 for 8.5 ounces)* is the "for the neck down" body moisturizer version of the Energy Glow Daily Face Moisturizer with a Touch of Self-Tanner above, and the same review applies. The facial and body versions are nearly identical formula-wise, so if you're curious to try this, it's obvious which one to choose.

DOVE PRO-AGE PRODUCTS

This subcategory from Dove doesn't break any new ground with its formulas (and several products are outright disappointments), but it's getting attention for its use of real, unmodel-like women in print and television ads. The company's goal was to break with tradition and stereotypes in an effort to create an "affirmative and hope-driven" marketing campaign. I admire Dove for presenting such a realistic picture of women rather than more images of airbrushed perfection. I only wish their formulas for mature skin (to use that nebulous term that doesn't accurately reflect the needs of skin as it ages) were truly different and took advantage of well-researched, state-of-the-art ingredients. They missed the boat on that, but at least some of what's on board has benefit for normal to dry skin, as well as normal to fine or thin hair of any age.

☹ **Pro-Age Beauty Bar** *($3.49 for 2 8.5-ounce bars)* is a standard bar cleanser that is soap-free, but the ingredients necessary to keep it in bar form can still clog pores and impede rinsing. The "fine exfoliants" in this beauty bar are no match for the superior combination of a water-soluble body wash and washcloth, or a standard body scrub.

☺ **Pro-Age Foaming Facial Cleanser** *($5.99 for 5 ounces)* is a very good, water-soluble cleanser for normal to dry skin, but nothing in it is capable of "optimizing surface cell turnover," a process that slows down as skin ages. This product will leave skin feeling clean, soft, and smooth, but supplying moisture via a cleanser is not a tremendous anti-aging benefit or something that's unique to this product.

😐 **Pro-Age Day Moisturizer SPF 15** *($11.99 for 1.7 ounces)* is actually a disappointing product from Dove, although it does not leave your skin vulnerable to UVA damage. An in-part zinc oxide sunscreen is included, and the base formula has a lightweight texture and silky finish. The letdown is that Dove's other facial moisturizers are full of ingredients that mimic the structure and function of healthy skin as well as several antioxidants. Those ingredients are in short supply here, and that's not a plus for aging skin. This is a worthwhile daytime moisturizer for normal to slightly dry skin, provided you don't mind a soft shimmer finish, but its positioning for skin of "advancing age" isn't reflected in the formulation here.

😐 **Pro-Age Eye Treatment SPF 8** *($11.99 for 0.5 ounce)* includes an in-part zinc oxide sunscreen, but the SPF rating is woefully low. In addition, the only antioxidant is a tiny amount of olive oil, making this inappropriate for anyone concerned with forestalling the signs of aging.

😐 **Pro-Age Neck & Chest Beauty Serum** *($8.99 for 3.4 ounces)* is a water- and silicone-based serum with a good amount of antioxidant olive oil. It will leave skin anywhere on the body feeling silky-smooth. However, in terms of being a boost for improving the appearance of aging skin it would be better if Dove included ceramides, retinol, some anti-irritants, and more antioxidants. Admittedly the price is a bargain, but this isn't a state-of-the-art product for skin showing signs of aging. Also, don't forget that the neck and chest area need sun protection as much as the face, and no amount of anti-aging ingredients can take the place of that.

😐 **Pro-Age Rich Night Cream** *($11.99 for 1.69 ounces)* doesn't contain significantly rich ingredients, but instead has a lightweight cream texture built around silicones and glycerin. The amount of olive oil is decent but its effectiveness is compromised by jar packaging. The inclusion of the cell-communicating ingredient linolenic acid is a nice touch, but once again this formula should have had more stacked in its favor to address the needs of aging skin.

DOVE SENSITIVE SKIN PRODUCTS

☹ **Sensitive Skin Beauty Bar** *($10.69 for 8 4.25-ounce bars)* is similar to Dove's other Beauty Bars and is not recommended. This option is particularly troublesome for anyone with sensitive skin because it contains fragrant rosewood, cedarwood, and rose oils.

✓☺ **Sensitive Skin Foaming Facial Cleanser** *($5.99 for 6.76 ounces)* is a very well-formulated, water-soluble cleanser that removes all types of makeup and rinses easily. The only caveat is that this fragrance-free cleanser's cleansing agents may be too drying for someone with sensitive skin. It is best for those with normal to oily or blemish-prone skin.

☺ **Sensitive Skin Day Cream** *($7.49 for 1.69 ounces)* is a beautifully formulated, silky-textured moisturizer—though without sunscreen it's best for nighttime use unless paired with a product rated SPF 15 or greater. The problem here is jar packaging, which compromises the stability of the many light- and air-sensitive ingredients in this product. It contains fragrance in the form of coriander seed oil.

☺ **Sensitive Skin Facial Lotion** *($7.49 for 4.05 ounces)* has some terrific ingredients to create and maintain healthy skin, including ceramides, anti-irritants, antioxidants, and linolenic acid. However, it is not suitable for sensitive skin because it contains fragrant coriander oil. This oil's linalool content can cause contact dermatitis (Source: www.naturaldatabase.com), and although there's not much of it in this product it's enough to keep it from earning a higher rating.

OTHER DOVE PRODUCTS

☹ **Calming Night Beauty Bar** *($8.99 for 6 4.25-ounce bars)* differs from Dove's other Beauty Bars only in its fragrance and the inclusion of token amounts of "looks good on the label" ingredients such as honey extract. It's still bar soap and can be too drying for all skin types.

☹ **Nutrium Nourishing Bar** *($10.69 for 8 4.25-ounce bars)* is similar to the Calming Night Beauty Bar above, save for the addition of plant oil. Otherwise, the same basic review applies.

☹ **Beauty Bar, Pink** *($2.79 for 2 4.25-ounce bars)* is standard-issue, no-frills bar soap. Yes, it does contain a detergent cleansing agent and moisturizing stearic acid, but the overall effect on skin is still drying, and it doesn't rinse easily.

☹ **Beauty Bar, Unscented** *($2.79 for 2 4.25-ounce bars)* is similar to the Beauty Bar, Pink above minus the coloring agents. It contains masking fragrance.

☹ **Beauty Bar, White** *($2.79 for 2 4.75-ounce bars)* is nearly identical to the Beauty Bar, Unscented above, and the same review applies.

✓☺ **Daily Hydrating Cleansing Cloths** *($6.99 for 30 cloths)* are nearly identical to the Cool Moisture Facial Cleansing Cloths above, and the same review applies. The tiny amount of corn oil is unlikely to be a problem for blemish-prone skin.

☹ **Gentle Exfoliating Beauty Bar** *($10.69 for 8 4.2-ounce bars)* is a standard bar cleanser that contains a very small amount of the abrasive agent polyethylene. You won't notice much exfoliating benefit, and the eventual buildup from the soap will prevent skin from sloughing on its own.

☺ **Gentle Exfoliating Daily Facial Cleanser** *($5.99 for 6.76 ounces)* is recommended for those with normal to oily or combination skin looking for a water-soluble cleanser/scrub hybrid.

☺ **Gentle Exfoliating Daily Facial Cleansing Pillows** *($4.99 for 14 pillows)* are nearly identical to the Energy Glow Brightening Facial Cleansing Pillows above, and the same review applies.

☺ **Essential Nutrients Day Cream SPF 15** *($6.89 for 1.69 ounces)* is an OK moisturizer with sunscreen for normal to slightly dry skin. It includes avobenzone for UVA protection, but the jar packaging won't keep the antioxidants in this stable.

✓☺ **Essential Nutrients Day Lotion** *($6.59 for 4.05 ounces)* includes an in-part avobenzone sunscreen as part of its lightweight, hydrating base, which is best for normal to oily skin. This wins additional accolades for including several antioxidants and ingredients that mimic the structure and function of healthy skin, all in stable packaging.

☹ **Skin Vitalizer Facial Cleansing Massager** *($11.99 with 6 Exfoliating Pillows)* is a battery-operated, hand-held cleansing tool designed for use with Dove's Cleansing Pillows. It provides a "powered" cleansing and exfoliation that I suppose goes beyond what manual cleansing can do, but all in all this isn't a must-have if you're using another exfoliating product (such as a topical scrub, washcloth, or, better yet, a well-formulated AHA or BHA product, something Dove doesn't offer).

DR. BRANDT (SKIN CARE ONLY)

DR. BRANDT AT-A-GLANCE

Strengths: Provides complete ingredient lists on the company Web site; an outstanding makeup remover; sunscreens with built-in bronzing effect; a novel skin-lightening product.

Weaknesses: Expensive; overwhelming number of products that contain irritating ingredients with no established benefit for skin; no products to comprehensively address acne or oily skin; every Poreless product is a disappointment; jar packaging; the "prescription-strength" tag line is completely without substantiation.

For more information about Dr. Brandt's products, call (800) 234-1066 or visit www.drbrandtskincare.com or www.Beautypedia.com.

DR. BRANDT LINELESS PRODUCTS

☹ **$$$ Lineless Gel Cleanser, for All Skin Types** *($40 for 8 ounces)* is an OK, water-soluble cleanser for normal to oily skin, but it is not without drawbacks. The inclusion of sodium lauryl sulfate, the standard for measuring irritation, as a secondary cleansing agent isn't the best, nor is the arnica extract. Still, this is better than the previous version, which contained problematic lavender oil.

☹ **Lineless Tone, for All Skin Types** *($40 for 8 ounces)* lists witch hazel as the second ingredient, which negates the effect of the anti-irritants that follow, as does the inclusion of lavender oil.

☹ **Lineless Anti-Glycation Serum** *($90 for 1.5 ounces)* claims to address the effects of glycation on skin cells. Advanced glycation end-products (AGEs) are abnormal, cross-linked, and oxidized proteins that might play a role in the aging process. That oxidation process also involves sugars, particularly in the form of glucose, which is one of the primary ways the body gets its fuel for producing energy and "get up and go" power.

This is because glucose can also, through an enzymatic trigger, attach itself to proteins anywhere in the body and form "glycated" substances that damage tissue by making it stiff and inflexible. AGEs directly affect the surface layers of skin as well as structures beneath the surface, such as collagen and elastin. What is still unknown, despite ongoing research, is whether topical application of ingredients known to disrupt the internal process AGEs go through to damage normal proteins (including collagen) can have any effect on skin. Brandt's serum is claiming to prevent the effects of glycation while strengthening the collagen and elastin fibers, but for now, that claim is still wishful thinking.

A couple of ingredients do stand out for their potential role in mitigating the effects of AGEs: carnosine and prolinamidoethyl imidazole. Both of these ingredients have demonstrated potent antioxidant ability, but there is no conclusive research pertaining to their use in cosmetic formulations meant to combat AGEs, so whether or not they'll really work for that purpose is a leap of faith (Sources: *Life Sciences*, April 2006, pages 2343–2357; and *Pathologie-biologie*, September 2006, pages 396–404).

Even if this serum could put a stop to AGEs and therefore slow the skin's aging process, this product contains lavender oil, which has been proven to cause skin-cell death (Source: *Cell Proliferation*, June 2004, pages 221–229). That error alone makes this pricey serum not worth considering, as any potential AGE-mitigating benefit from the aforementioned ingredients isn't worth the irritation the lavender oil can cause.

☹ **Lineless Cream, Age-Inhibitor Complex, for Normal to Dry Skin** *($100 for 1.7 ounces)* contains irritating lavender oil (which doesn't inhibit one second of aging), and lists most of its antioxidants well after the preservatives, meaning they're barely present. Even if there were greater amounts, Brandt's choice of jar packaging will quickly render them ineffective.

☺ **$$$ Lineless Eye Cream, for All Skin Types** *($60 for 0.5 ounce)* is a very good moisturizer for dry skin around the eyes, or anywhere on the face. It contains mostly water, emollients, plant oil, green tea, silicones, anti-irritant plant extracts, aloe, more plant oil, skin-identical ingredients, and preservatives. The inclusion of geranium oil isn't ideal, but the amount is unlikely to be a problem.

😐 **$$$ Lineless Gel** *($100 for 1.5 ounces)* is a very light, gel-type moisturizer that contains appreciable levels of antioxidants, yet it also includes a significant amount of drying ethyl alcohol, which isn't helpful for skin. This is packaged to keep the antioxidants stable, and may be an OK option for very oily skin.

☹ **Lineless Soothing Mask** *($40 for 1.7 ounces)* is a thin-textured, extremely standard gel mask that irritates skin with fragrant geranium and lavender oils. It is not recommended.

DR. BRANDT PORELESS PRODUCTS

☹ **Poreless Cleanser, for Oily/Combination Skin** *($35 for 8 ounces)* contains irritating sodium lauryl sulfate along with lavender and rosemary oils, making this cleanser a problem for any skin type.

☹ **Poreless Tone, for Oily/Combination Skin** *($35 for 8 ounces)* lists alcohol as the second ingredient, followed by witch hazel. Adding insult to injury are the irritating oils of rosemary and lavender, making this toner a no-go regardless of pore size.

☹ **Poreless Gel, for Oily/Combination Skin** *($55 for 1.7 ounces)* lists witch hazel as the second ingredient, and also contains potentially irritating levels of film-forming agents as well as the menthol derivative menthyl lactate. The fact that such a poor concoction is from a dermatologist is just embarrassing.

☹ **Pore Effect, for Oily/Combination Skin** *($55 for 1.7 ounces)* is said to stimulate cellular turnover, but it doesn't contain ingredients capable of doing that. It will, however, irritate skin because it contains lavender and rosemary oils.

☹ **Poreless Moisture, for Oily/Combination Skin** *($42 for 3.5 ounces)* contains lavender and rosemary oils, both volatile substances with more detriments than benefits for skin.

☹ **Pores No More, for Oily/Combination Skin** *($45 for 1 ounce)* is a very expensive blend of silicones and silicone polymers that mattify skin and absorb excess oil. It works quite well, but it isn't good news that it also contains lavender oil. Given the potential irritation and the price, why not consider the superior options from Clinique's Pore Minimizer line over this faulty option?

☹ **Poreless Purifying Mask** *($40 for 3.5 ounces)* has an insulting price for what amounts to a below-standard clay mask that has the potential to needlessly irritate skin with menthyl lactate. It is not recommended.

OTHER DR. BRANDT PRODUCTS

☹ **Anti-Irritant Cleanser, for Dry/Sensitive Skin** *($40 for 6.7 ounces)* is anti-irritant in name only. This relatively standard, lotion-style, creamy cleanser could have been an exceptionally gentle option for dry, delicate skin if not for the inclusion of irritating geranium oil. Dr. Brandt recommends that women use this cleanser after a peel or laser treatment, but the last thing that already-sensitized skin that is trying to heal needs is a dose of irritation!

☺ **$$$ Laser Lightning Foaming Cleanser, for All Skin Types** *($45 for 8 ounces)* is a good though very expensive cleanser for normal to dry skin. Slightly lathering but not completely water-soluble because of the amount of castor oil, this will cushion dry skin and remove makeup easily. The tiny amount of mandarin orange peel oil is not likely to cause problems. By the way, nothing in this cleanser will help fade freckles or dark spots, nor does it have anything to do with lasers.

✓☺ **$$$ D-Face Makeup Remover** *($35 for 4 ounces)* is a very good, detergent-based makeup remover for all but very oily skin. The rice bran oil helps dissolve stubborn makeup while the licorice extract provides an anti-irritant benefit.

☹ **Microdermabrasion In A Jar** *($75 for 1.7 ounces)* doesn't deserve consideration over the multitude of other topical scrubs claiming to mimic the effects of microdermabrasion because they use the same crystals. Brandt's version is quite abrasive, and further irritates skin because it contains orange and lemon oils. Even without those troublesome ingredients, Neutrogena's version is very effective and one-third the price.

😐 **$$$ "A" Cream, Night Cream** *($65 for 1.7 ounces)* is a very good emollient moisturizer those with dry skin will appreciate, but it's packaged in a clear jar, which means the antioxidants (including a good amount of grape seed oil) and retinol won't remain stable once the jar is open and the product is exposed to air. If you're looking for the benefits of retinol, consider the superior, less-expensive options from Aveeno, Neutrogena, and RoC, which are packaged so the retinol remains stable.

😐 **$$$ "C" Cream, for Dry/Dehydrated Skin** *($58 for 1.7 ounces)* promises a smoother, more radiant complexion with fewer lines and wrinkles, but that claim can be attributed to any good, standard moisturizer, and that is exactly what "C" Cream is. Despite the spotlight-on-the-vitamin name, the stability of the vitamin C and other antioxidants in this product is definitely at risk because they're packaged in a jar. This is still an option for normal to dry skin, but for the money, better packaging should have been chosen.

☹ **"C" Gel** *($90 for 1 ounce)* is a silicone-based antioxidant serum that contains grape seed oil and vitamins C and E, although the forms used are not identified. (In fact, Brandt's listing violates FDA guidelines for ingredient disclosure because liposomes are not an ingredient but rather a delivery system.) Although the antioxidants are assuredly helpful for skin, the lavender, grapefruit, and geranium oils are not, making this one to ignore.

☹ **Contour Effect** *($185 for 1.7 ounces)* not only has a ridiculous price tag, but also shortchanges skin by including only meager amounts of exciting ingredients and then further reducing their efficacy with jar packaging. Contour Effect is supposed to restore volume and plumpness to aging skin while boosting cells' energy (which declines with age and years of sun exposure). Although this moisturizer has an elegant, silky texture based largely on silicone technology, its unique ingredient, *Bacopa monniera* (also known as brahmi), has zero research pertaining to its benefit for skin. There's quite a bit of research examining oral consumption of this herb, but even that doesn't have anything to do with its ability to restore the diminishing substances (such as fat pads and collagen) whose loss causes skin to slacken and droop. Further, the inclusion of lavender oil causes skin cell death; how is that supposed to rev up cellular energy? Your money is much better spent on dermal fillers that really do restore volume and plumpness to aging skin (an alternative Brandt would likely not admit, even though he offers such procedures in his practice).

☹ **Crease Release, with GABA Complex** *($150 for 1 ounce)* is a basic emollient moisturizer that claims to rapidly reduce wrinkles with gamma amino butyric acid (GABA). Please refer to Chapter Seven, *Cosmetic Ingredient Dictionary*, in this edition for detailed information on this ingredient. GABA cannot and does not work as Dr. Brandt claims, and this moisturizer irritates skin because it contains the allergenic fragrance component eugenol. Eugenol is a standard substance used to test for skin allergies, and has a deleterious effect on skin's immune cells (Sources: *Molecular Immunology*, March 2007, ePublication; and *Biological Chemistry*, September 2006, pages 1201–1207).

☹ **Infinite Moisture, for Dry/Dehydrated Skin** *($65 for 1.7 ounces)* is a mixed bag of what to include and what not to include when formulating a skin-beneficial moisturizer. This product begins well, with an emollient and several good skin-identical ingredients, but begins to unravel with the addition of guarana and kola nut extracts, each in higher-than-usual amounts. Guarana is an herb that contains two and a half times more caffeine than coffee, has constricting properties on skin, and is a skin irritant. Kola nut has plenty of caffeine as well, but of greater concern is its amine content, which can form nitrosamines—potential carcinogens that are not something you want to routinely (if ever) apply to your skin (Source: *Food and Chemical Toxicology*, August 1995, pages 625–630). This product also contains irritating geranium and ylang ylang oils, which have no place in a moisturizer except to add fragrance. What a shame, because this is otherwise an excellent, well-packaged moisturizer for normal to slightly dry skin.

☹ **Liquid Skin, for All Skin Types** *($70 for 1.7 ounces)* is said to mimic skin's structure in an effort to provide a better canvas for your night cream. First, skin does not need to be prepared for nighttime moisture—not if you're using a state-of-the-art product loaded with antioxidants and ingredients that help support skin's intercellular matrix. Second, Liquid Skin's silicone-heavy formula lacks several essential components that comprise skin's structure, including lipids (such as cholesterol), hyaluronic acid, and even good old-fashioned glycerin. Instead, Brandt included tiny amounts of amino acids and even smaller amounts of ceramides and soybean sterols. They look good on the label, but will have minimal impact on skin in the amounts used. Moreover, the mandarin orange peel oil can cause irritation, and has nothing to do with encouraging skin to replenish itself. Estee Lauder, Clinique, Prescriptives, Olay, Neutrogena, and Paula's Choice all offer less-expensive serums that truly contain ingredients that mimic skin's support structure.

☺ **$$$ r3p Cream** *($125 for 1.7 ounces)* makes me sigh heavily, but not because it's a bad product. Rather, the price is astonishing for what amounts to a relatively standard but effective moisturizer for normal to slightly dry skin. It cannot make good on its claims for exfoliation because it contains no ingredients that would make that happen. Coming from a dermatologist, this is a moisturizer you should expect to be brimming with state-of-the-art ingredients such as antioxidants and those that mimic the skin's intercellular matrix; alas, that isn't the case. These ingredients are present in this product, but barely, serving as little more than window dressing. This cream does contain acetyl hexapeptide-3, an ingredient that is present in many products claiming to topically reduce muscle contractions, and that use phrases like "similar to Botox." Such claims are not made here, but you should be aware that this ingredient is incapable of exerting any muscle-relaxing effect on skin, nor is it exclusive to high-end doctors' lines. The other two peptides serve as skin-identical ingredients, but they are present in amounts so small that any benefit to skin is likely negligible. This product contains fragrance in the form of lavender oil, but contains less of it than other Brandt products.

☹ **r3p Eye, for All Skin Types** *($80 for 0.5 ounce)* has a lush, emollient texture and contains several ingredients that are brilliant for dry to very dry skin. The antioxidants won't last for long once this jar-packaged eye cream is opened, while the lavender oil is toxic to skin cells and definitely not an ingredient that should be applied near the eye.

😐 **$$$ V-Zone Neck Cream** *($60 for 1.7 ounces)* is sold as a specialty product for addressing sun-damaged skin on the neck and décolleté area, but there is nothing in this product to prevent you from using it anywhere on the body, including the face. This emollient cream contains about 5% glycolic acid at a pH that allows for exfoliation. It's not very impressive when it comes to antioxidants, but is an OK (though overpriced) option as an AHA cream for dry skin.

☺ **$$$ Daily UV Protection SPF 30, Face, Light Bronze** *($30 for 1.7 ounces)* combines an in-part avobenzone sunscreen with creamy moisturizers and potent cell-communicating ingredients. The formula is enhanced by its sheer bronze tint, allowing for sun protection with instant color gratification. This is not rated higher because it contains potentially sensitizing orange oil, but it is still recommended, and is best for normal to dry skin.

☺ **$$$ Daily UV Protection SPF 30, Face, Medium Bronze** *($30 for 1.7 ounces)* is identical to the Daily UV Protective SPF 30, Face, Light Bronze above, except this version provides a darker color and is preferred for medium to tan skin tones. Otherwise, the same comments apply.

😐 **$$$ Laser A-Peel Peeling System, for All Skin Types** *($100 for the kit)* marks Brandt's contribution to the peel-at-home kits made popular by Lancome, L'Oreal, and a handful of other cosmetics companies. The difference here is that Brandt goes over the top by claiming that his three-step kit is a treatment that "mimics the results of laser technology." That is no more an accurate statement than it is to suggest that taking an aspirin is akin to open-heart surgery.

Step 1 in this kit is to apply the **Prepping Solution** *(2 ounces)*. This toner-like product is supposed to be applied after cleansing to remove impurities and to prepare skin to be treated with the next step. It's an antiquated formula that is mostly water and alcohol, and so it will increase the risk of irritation and dryness and should not be used, not to mention that alcohol causes cell death and free-radical damage. A water-soluble cleanser and a gentle toner would remove all impurities and are all the prep you need before using any AHA product, which leads us to Step 2, the **Peeling Solution** *(1.7 ounces)*. This lotion contains a blend of glycolic and lactic acids at a concentration of 10% (5% glycolic, 5% lactic, as confirmed by Dr. Brandt's customer service team) and at an effective pH of 3.6. A few bells and whistles are also included in this product, but in such tiny amounts your skin won't notice them. You're instructed to leave the Peeling Solution on the skin for five minutes, and then rinse with water. That's actually not enough time for the AHAs to penetrate and work as effectively as they would if you left this solution on longer, and I see no reason why you couldn't do just that. Several companies sell effective 10% AHA lotions quite similar to this, and leaving their products on the skin works great with no problem, with the results supported by research published in medical journals!

Dr. Brandt's instructions are to rinse the Peeling Solution and then apply Step 3, the **Soothing Gel** *(1 ounce)*. This is a very well-formulated, well-packaged moisturizer with a gel texture. It contains several beneficial ingredients for skin, including lecithin, glycerin, grape seed oil, and green tea extract. Although recommended for all skin types, someone with dry to very dry skin will want something more emollient. At least this final step isn't a throwaway product, as is the case with similar kits from other companies!

In terms of the "works like laser technology" claim, there haven't been any studies done to compare the effects of cosmetic levels of AHAs (less than 20% concentrations) to the effects of laser treatments. Think of it this way: If the claim were true, then any product containing 10% AHA would easily replace laser resurfacing. So you needn't waste $100 on Brandt's product to find out if his claim is real.

To be clear about the difference, the exfoliation from chemical peels performed at a doctor's office using concentrations of more than 40% has been compared to laser resurfacing, and each method has its pros and cons. But cosmetic products are not related to those procedures. Comparing Dr. Brandt's "Laser in a Bottle" to a laser procedure is like comparing a canoe to a speedboat.

If you want to consider an 8% to 10% AHA product you don't need this kit. All that's necessary is one effective (meaning pH-correct) AHA product with 10% glycolic acid, lactic acid, or gluconolactone (an AHA option researched by Neostrata). Alpha Hydrox, Neutrogena, M.D. Formulations, and Pond's all have great options in this regard, and all cost far less than this version.

***unrated* Laser Lightening Serum, for All Skin Types** *($110 for 1 ounce)* has a water-based serum texture and bases its lightening ability around the ingredient fullerene. A fullerene is defined as a cagelike, hollow molecule composed of hexagonal and pentagonal groups of atoms. Their major element is carbon, and fullerenes constitute the third form of carbon after diamond and graphite.

Various fullerene molecules exist. There is one study that compared a fullerene derivative (C60-fullerene) to arbutin and vitamin C (L-ascorbic acid). It revealed that C60-fullerene has an inhibitory effect on melanin in the presence of UVA radiation. Therefore, over time and with diligent use of sunscreen, its ongoing use should fade sun-induced skin discolorations and prevent new discolorations from appearing. The study also demonstrated that this fullerene derivative was better at inhibiting melanin formation than arbutin or L-ascorbic acid, though the concentrations used in the study were not revealed (Source: *Archives of Dermatological Research*, February 28, 2007, ePublication). Whether or not Brandt used this fullerene derivative is not known, and one study isn't much to go on (especially when the tried-and-true skin-lightening agent hydroquinone has volumes of research attesting to its efficacy). It is also important to point out that there is research showing fullerenes to be extremely risky (Source: *Environmental Health Perspectives*, July 2004, pages 1058–1062). With so many questions about this ingredient left unanswered, this serum is best left on the shelf. You need not be a guinea pig for anyone.

☺ $$$ Laser in a Bottle Laser Relief *($85 for 1.7 ounces)*. The notion that skin-care products can mimic the effects of laser treatments on skin is nothing less than ridiculous, but when such products are created and endorsed by a dermatologist it becomes downright ludicrous. Dr. Brandt has had success with other products he sells that claim to work like microdermabrasion and Botox injections, so why not add another one that misleads consumers on faux-laser treatments too?

The big to-do about Laser in a Bottle is something called QuSomes. This delivery system is said to transport potent ingredients deeper into the skin, presumably to the same depth laser treatments reach. Supposedly, delivering such ingredients deeper into the skin mimics the elastin- and collagen-stimulating effects of lasers. But there is no research to support any of this, or at least nothing that was not sponsored by BioZone, the company that developed and sells QuSomes. Even so, the information on the company's Web site isn't all that impressive, and definitely not to the extent that Dr. Brandt's claims promote it.

Another issue is the fact that just delivering "potent" ingredients to skin cannot have the same effect, in any way, shape, or form, as what lasers do. By "potent," I assume Dr. Brandt means antioxidants, because nothing else in his product is notable. But that's like saying a kite works the same way as a jet airplane! Skin likes making collagen, and will continue to do so at a healthy rate if it is protected from environmental damage (notably, sun exposure) and the resulting destructive inflammation it causes. Antioxidants assist in this process by helping reduce inflammation by reducing free-radical damage, and thereby stimulating collagen synthesis (Sources: *Dermatologic Surgery*, July 31, 2005, pages 814–817; *Experimental Dermatology*, June 2003, pages 2374–2384; and *BMC Dermatology*, September 28, 2004, page 13). But antioxidants do not work in the same manner as non-ablative and ablative lasers. The various wavelengths of laser light generate variable amounts of heat, triggering a response that stimulates collagen and potentially healthy, new skin-cell production. There is not a shred of research that favorably compares the effects of topically applied antioxidants (regardless of the delivery system) with the proven positive effects of laser treatments.

This product deserves a happy face rating not for its outlandish claims, but because it is an antioxidant-rich, fragrance-free moisturizing lotion for normal to dry skin with packaging designed to keep the antioxidants stable during use. It's pricey, but it will make skin softer and smoother while exerting an anti-inflammatory effect that may help reduce redness. The tiny amount of menthone glycerin acetal, derived from mint, is used primarily as a flavoring agent and for fragrance; it is unlikely to be problematic for skin when present in such small amounts.

☹ **Laser in A Bottle Laser Tight** *($110 for 1.7 ounces)* is similar to the Laser in a Bottle Laser Relief above, and the same comments about Dr. Brandt's claims and what is actually possible apply here as well. There is no reason why this product should cost more than its Laser in a Bottle counterpart above, but the bigger problem is the inclusion of such a large amount of lavender oil. Even in amounts as low as 0.25%, lavender oil has proven to be cytotoxic to skin cells (Source: *Cell Proliferation*, June 2004, pages 221–229). Its benefits to skin are controversial and mostly anecdotal, and, based on its potential to damage skin cells, I do not recommend products that contain it.

☹ **Vitamin Moisture Mask, for Dry/Sensitive Skin** *($25 for 1.7 ounces)* is an odd mix of film-forming agent, clay, and emollients, which is bound to confuse dry skin, and the lavender oil is a problem for sensitive skin. In case you're wondering, vitamins are in short supply.

DR. DENESE NEW YORK

DR. DENESE AT-A-GLANCE

Strengths: Several well-formulated serums and moisturizers that are reasonably priced; a very good matte-finish, tinted sunscreen with zinc oxide; uses well-researched, proven ingredients that truly benefit skin, and uses them in higher concentrations than most skin-care lines.

The Reviews D

Weaknesses: Some problem cleansers and toners; inclusion of unnecessary irritants such as lavender oil and menthol; limited options for sun protection; a few gimmicky, multistep kits that are easily replaced by other products in her line; Dr. Denese's book contains several erroneous claims about what skin needs and how to take care of it, and some of this information is contradicted by her own products!

For more information about Dr. Denese New York, call QVC at (800) 345-1515 or visit www.qvc.com or www.Beautypedia.com. Note: All Dr. Denese products contain fragrance unless otherwise noted.

☺ **$$$ Hydrating Cleanser** *($22 for 6 ounces)* is a simply formulated, detergent-based cleanser that contains borage oil to soften skin and facilitate makeup removal. The big-deal ingredients that supposedly justify the price are coenzyme Q10, vitamin A, and vitamin E. The vitamins are barely present in this cleanser and the CoQ10 is completely absent, which is strange. However, even if it were present, neither the CoQ10 nor the other vitamins can have a positive effect on the skin because when they are included in a cleanser they are rinsed off before they have a chance to have any impact. So, paying extra for such bells and whistles isn't necessary. Regardless, this is still a good cleanser for normal to slightly dry skin.

☹ **DermaClean Gentle BHA Cleanser** *($19 for 8 ounces)* does contain BHA (salicylic acid), but the amount is not specified, although the pH of 3.2 will permit exfoliation. The inherent problem with including BHA in a cleanser is that it is not left on the skin long enough to have an optimal effect because it is quickly rinsed off your skin and down the drain. The main problem with this otherwise well-formulated cleanser is the high amount of lavender oil, which is irritating to skin and should not get anywhere near the eyes or mucous membranes (Source: *Cell Proliferation*, June 2004, page 221). Contrary to claim, the vitamins in this cleanser do not exfoliate.

😐 **$$$ Doctor's Microdermabrasion Cream** *($34.90 for 4 ounces)*. Unlike most microdermabrasion scrubs, which contain aluminum oxide crystals, Dr. Denese opted to use pumice, one of the more abrasive scrub agents available. The base formula has sufficient oil and emollients to prevent the pumice from being too rough on skin, but between this and the various AHA peels in this line, we're talking potential exfoliation overload. This product also contains small amounts of several irritating plant extracts. If you're looking for a topical scrub, the microdermabrasion-in-a-jar versions from Neutrogena, Susan Lucci's Youthful Essence, Clinique, and Olay Regenerist are better and less expensive. But remember, simply using a washcloth with your cleanser can easily net the same results.

☹ **Pore Refining Toner** *($19 for 8 ounces)* is a water- and aloe-based toner that would have been much better for skin if it didn't include irritating witch hazel, lavender oil, and several citrus extracts. This toner does contain AHAs, but the pH of 6 prevents them from functioning as exfoliants. This product is not recommended.

😐 **$$$ Triple AHA/BHA Two Step Weekly Facial Peel** *($39 for the kit)* is a two-part system. The **Doctor's Triple AHA/BHA Peel** contains glycolic, salicylic, and lactic acids and has a pH of 3.6, so exfoliation will occur (unlike the Pore Refining Toner above). The percentage of glycolic acid is not revealed, but it is likely in the 8% to 10% range, while the lactic and salicylic acids are likely present in concentrations below 1%. The peel contains enough alcohol to cause undue irritation, and the addition of grapefruit peel oil doesn't help matters. After leaving the peel on the skin for no more than five minutes, you're supposed to stop it with the **Neutralizing Mineral Powder**, which is composed of alkaline mineral powders. This powder will indeed stop the peeling action, but so would generously rinsing your skin with tap water, so this second product isn't necessary. Overall, although this will produce results, they're not going to be comparable to those you'd get from a stronger AHA or BHA peel administered by a physician. Moreover, you can achieve better results with less irritation by applying a well-formulated AHA gel, cream, or lotion (which should specify the amount of AHA it contains) and leaving it on the face. In that sense, this two-part peel, though effective, isn't preferred to a leave-on, alcohol-free AHA or BHA product.

☹ **Firming Facial Pads** *($35 for 60 pads)* have a pH of 3.8 and contain 10% glycolic acid in a water-based solution that is delivered to the skin when you wipe the pad over your face. These pads will exfoliate skin, but they tend to leave a sticky finish, and the inclusion of irritating menthol is senseless. Given the poor aesthetics, the menthol, the price, and the fact that many effective AHA products have superior formulas, you needn't add this to your cart.

☹ **Cellular Firming Serum** *($64 for 1 ounce)* is one of several serums in the Dr. Denese line. This formula is nothing if not intriguing, because it contains a blend of AHAs and BHA as well as the skin-lightening ingredients arbutin and kojic acid. It also contains hydroquinone PCA, although that isn't the same as hydroquinone because it does not have the ability to lighten skin. Dr. Denese claims this product tingles when applied to skin, and attributes this tingling to the alpha lipoic (thioctic) acid. However, it's more likely that the combination of alcohol with glycolic and lactic acids is what causes the sensation, and that isn't great for skin. It is true that at the appropriate pH, AHA or BHA products may cause slight tingling or stinging due to the manner in which they work on skin. But you want to avoid the additives, such as alcohol, that add to this irritation. This serum has a lot going for it, but it fails to successfully combine the benefits of exfoliation and skin lightening without causing excess irritation.

😐 **Baggage Lost Puff Reducing Gel** *($25 for 1 ounce)* is a lightweight moisturizer that doesn't contain anything that can noticeably reduce puffiness or dark circles under the eye. Classic "deflating" ingredients such as cucumber show up, but no topical ingredient or blend can address the cause of age-related puffy eyes. The second ingredient, sweet almond seed extract, has soothing properties—nice but not a cure-all for under-eye woes.

😐 **Doctor's Night Recovery Cream** *($39.50 for 2 ounces)* is an excellent formula for those with dry to very dry skin. It includes fatty acids, ingredients that mimic the structure and function of healthy skin, plant oils, anti-irritants, many antioxidants, and cell-communicating ingredients, including retinol. Unfortunately, the jar packaging means that many of these ingredients (especially the retinol) won't remain stable once the container is open and exposed to air. With improved packaging, this would be one of the best moisturizer formulas money can buy.

☹ **Doctor's Skin Recovery Serum** *($49 for 1 ounce)* has so much going for it, especially if you have normal to dry skin and are seeking an antioxidant-rich serum with retinol. It's unfortunate that several irritating plant extracts were included, because they ruin an otherwise stellar product. Balm mint, coltsfoot, horsetail, and St. John's wort are the biggest offenders.

✓☺ **$$$ HydroShield Eye Serum** *($44 for 0.5 ounce)* contains silicone, antioxidants, ceramides, retinol, several fatty acids, and preservatives. This fragrance-free serum is an outstanding formulation that is recommended for all skin types. It may be used around the eyes or anywhere on the face. Its lightweight texture and matte finish make it well-suited for those with oily skin looking for the benefits of antioxidants and retinol without heaviness. This is a product any dermatologist would be proud of!

✓☺ **$$$ HydroShield Ultra Moisturizing Face Serum** *($49 for 0.5 ounce)* is nearly identical to the HydroShield Eye Serum above, and the same review applies.

☹ **Instant Wrinkle Press** *($65 for 0.5 ounce)* has a great name, but can't press wrinkles flat. It is a slightly opaque, thick cream that contains a considerable amount of gamma aminobutyric acid (also known as GABA). GABA is an amino acid that acts as a neurotransmitter inhibitor and is associated with reducing seizures and depression. When taken as a supplement, it affects the way nerves fire. Some cosmetics lines, including Dr. Denese's, want consumers to associate this internal effect with wrinkle reduction. The theory is that if GABA can stop nerves from firing in the brain, it should be able to control the nerve impulses that affect facial muscles—the kind that lead to expression lines. There is no research proving GABA is a revolutionary (let alone effective) antiwrinkle ingredient, but we do know that in the body GABA does not work alone. Keeping nerves from being triggered requires a lot of other components. Even Botox doesn't affect muscle movement when rubbed on skin. Don't fall for the hype, and don't use this product, primarily because it promises to be "intensely cooling." What provides this sensation? An appreciable amount of menthyl lactate, a derivative of menthol that should not get near the eye—yet that's exactly where the directions for this product indicate users should apply it.

✓☺ **$$$ Neck Saver Serum** *($34 for 1 ounce)* is a brilliantly formulated serum that can be used on the face or from the neck down. It contains a blend of silicones, antioxidants, retinol, ceramides, several cell-communicating ingredients, plant extracts (a couple with undetermined benefit for skin), and preservatives. The clover extract in this serum adds fragrance.

☹ **Pore Reducing Serum** *($49 for 1 ounce)* ends up being an expensive way to irritate skin while not reducing pore size beyond the visual trick of using irritation to swell skin, which makes pores less noticeable. There are lots of very good ingredients in this serum, but they're eclipsed by the amount of isopropyl alcohol it contains.

😐 **$$$ RestorEyes Eye Cream** *($45 for 0.5 ounce)* is an even better formulation than the HydroShield Eye Serum above, so why the neutral rating? Jar packaging. Thanks to that poor choice, the many antioxidants in this product (plus its retinol) will be useless shortly after the product is opened. This is still a good option for a silky-textured, normal-to-dry-skin moisturizer anywhere on the face.

☹ **Skin Recovery Serum** *($49 for 1 ounce)* is similar to the HydroShield Eye Serum and HydroShield Ultra Moisturizing Face Serum above, but suffers by comparison because it contains several problematic ingredients that have no established benefit for skin, including balm mint, coltsfoot, St. John's wort, and horsetail extracts. There is no reason to consider this serum over the two mentioned above, or similar products from other lines, including Clinique, Olay, and Neutrogena.

😐 **$$$ Skin So Tight Instant Anti-Wrinkle Gel** *($38 for 1 ounce)* contains the absorbents silica and sodium magnesium silicate in a water base. Applying this serum to skin results in a temporary tightening effect, but the lack of moisture in this product may make wrinkles look worse, especially if skin is dry. This is not as impressive as several other Dr. Denese products.

😐 **$$$ SPF 30 Defense Day Cream** *($49 for 2 ounces)* features an in-part zinc oxide sunscreen and is slightly tinted to offset the white cast this ingredient can leave on skin. The product is described as being able to "intensely hydrate" the skin, but the inactive ingredients don't support this claim because they are primarily dry-finish silicones, aloe, and talc. The jar packaging won't keep the antioxidants in the formula stable during use, and why Denese switched back to the jar from the former opaque tube is a mystery. This fragrance-free sunscreen is best for normal to slightly oily skin not prone to blemishes.

☹ **Triple Strength Neck Wrinkle Smoother** *($36.36 for 2 ounces)* has an odd price, but that's what's listed on Denese's Web site, so there you have it. This moisturizer, which isn't specific to the neck, contains mostly water, chelating agent, glycerin, plant oils, and emollients suitable for dry to very dry skin. The jar packaging means that the many antioxidants and retinol won't remain stable during use, though most of them are present only in meager amounts anyway.

✓☺ **$$$ Triple Strength Wrinkle Smoother** *($54 for 2 ounces)* won't help reduce lines resulting from facial expressions, but it is an elegant moisturizer for normal to dry skin. It contains mostly water, film-forming/"opacifying" agent, thickener, several peptides, shea butter, skin-identical ingredients, retinol, anti-irritant, antioxidants, preservatives, and fragrance. The opaque tube packaging helps keep the light- and air-sensitive ingredients stable. The level of acrylate film-forming agent in this moisturizer does lend a slight tightening and "firming" effect to skin, but this tactile benefit is temporary and incapable of keeping expression lines at bay. Dr. Denese states in her book that this product has "three times the Oligopeptide of the industry standard." That sounds impressive, but is less so when you consider that there is no industry standard for this ingredient, nor any independent research showing it has antiwrinkle efficacy on skin. Nevertheless, this moisturizer does have a higher amount of peptides than many competing products and they can, in theory, function as cell-communicating ingredients.

☺ **$$$ Triple Strength Eye Wrinkle Smoother** *($60 for 0.5 ounce)* is similar to but more emollient and less exciting than the Triple Strength Wrinkle Smoother above. Peptides are present in lesser quantities than its partner product, and the group of ingredients said to reduce dark circles (including hesperidin methyl chalcone and vitamin K) don't have substantiated research proving they work for this purpose. This is still a worthwhile product for use around the eye or elsewhere on the face, and is best for normal to dry skin.

☹ **$$$ Vitamin C Line Filling Radiance Cream** *($38 for 0.5 ounce)* contains hardly any vitamin C, but even if it were present in abundance it wouldn't remain potent for long once the jar is opened. This silicone-based, fragrance-free moisturizer has a beautifully silky finish and contains an impressive range of antioxidants (including retinol) and skin-identical ingredients. It's an option for normal to slightly dry skin, but what a shame the packaging isn't better.

☹ **$$$ Wrinkle-Less Line Reducing Serum** *($69 for 1 ounce)* is a simple serum of water, water-binding agent, the "works-like-Botox" (but there is no research to prove this) acetyl hexapeptide-3, wheat-based thickener, slip agent, and preservative. Describing this product as "rich" and "all natural" is a joke, because it is not emollient in the least—and when was the last time you saw butylene glycol in your grocer's produce department? It won't reduce wrinkles, but will lightly hydrate normal to slightly oily skin. For this amount of money, though, you should expect a serum loaded with antioxidants, cell-communicating ingredients, and the like. Their absence makes this serum a tough sell and it's not recommended over others in the Denese line.

☺ **$$$ Wrinkle Rest Expression Line Peptide Concentrate** *($100 for 1.7 ounces)* is a silicone- and glycerin-based serum that primarily claims to moisturize skin by infusing the top layers with lipids (fats). However, it doesn't contain any lipids, and the peptides aren't as concentrated as they are in other Denese products. This contains an ingredient listed as pinacolyl-trans retinoate, which the company making it says is a retinol derivative. The only information about this ingredient (trade name RETexture Granactive RD-101) comes from the manufacturer, which is about as reliable as McDonald's saying hamburgers are nutritional powerhouses. It likely has antioxidant ability similar to other forms of vitamin A, but there's no proof it is as efficacious as tretinoin (Retin-A) without the irritation. This serum won't put wrinkles to rest, but is a good option for normal to slightly dry skin.

☺ **$$$ Hyaluronic Wrinkle Filler Serum and Cream** *($59 for the kit)* is a two-part system—but for the life of me I can't figure out why these products needed to be separated. The decision seems to be more marketing caprice than necessity. Step 1 is a serum, which consists solely of water, vitamin B5, slip agent, preservative, skin-identical ingredients, and more preservatives. Step 2 is a silicone-based cream whose formulary is nearly identical to the Vitamin C Line Filling Radiance Cream above, except this product is packaged in an opaque tube, which is preferred to a jar. The products are said to work in tandem to reduce creases, but since the ingredients in the serum could have easily been added to the cream, why bother splitting them up? The system does constitute an effective moisturizer for normal to slightly dry or slightly oily skin, but compared to other Denese products it's disappointingly short on antioxidants. The skin-identical ingredients can temporarily plump skin, reducing the appearance of creases, but neither these ingredients nor the effect are unique to this product.

✓☺ **HydroSeal Hand & Decollete Serum** *($35 for 3 ounces)* is just as nice as the other recommended serums in this line, containing an impressive mix of silicones, plant oil, skin-identical ingredients, retinol, antioxidants, cell-communicating ingredients, and several ingredients that mimic the structure and function of healthy skin. Notice the larger size and lower price compared to the other Dr. Denese serums? That's a plus, because your skin will benefit from its use whether on the hands or face! The amount of plant oil in this fragranced serum makes it suitable for normal to dry skin.

✓☺/☹ **Two-Step Peel and Seal Neck Saver System** *($46 for the kit)* includes the **Doctor's Neck Saver Serum** (also available separately and reviewed above) along with **Neck Saver Firming Pads**. The Serum is excellent but best purchased on its own because the Firming Pads are problematic. Although they contain approximately 8% glycolic acid and 1% salicylic acid, the pH of 4.1 makes them marginal for exfoliation. However, any assumptions that care was taken to avoid irritating the neck are unfounded because the pads also contain the irritants menthol and lavender oil, and these are not recommended.

😐 **$$$ Damage Reversal Pads** *($45 for 60 pads)* contain a solution of 2% hydroquinone in a water base with an effective amount of glycolic acid. However, because these pads are packaged in a jar, the hydroquinone will quickly become inactive, as will the arbutin and antioxidants; what a shame. At best, this is a pricey way to exfoliate skin with AHA.

☺ **$$$ Damage Reversal Treatment Stick** *($28 for 0.16 ounce)* is the only concealer I know of that contains hydroquinone as an active ingredient. Denese opted for a 1.5% concentration, which won't be as effective as traditional 2% versions, but is still worth considering as a skin lightening and concealing product in one. The dual-sided component includes two shades of lipstick-style cream concealer. Both shades are neutral and work well on light skin tones used separately or blended together. The texture is thick and this doesn't have much slip, but it covers well and stays in place. It is fragrance-free.

✓☺ **$$$ Perfect Pucker Line Filler with Pro-Peptide Factor** *($36.50 for 0.3 ounce)* has an incredibly long ingredient list, and once you get past the silicones and thickeners, it reads like a "who's who" of antioxidants. Peptides are present, too, but although they are helpful they do not have the ability to fill in vertical lines above the lip. What does help with that are the silicones in this thick cream. Applied "generously," as the label indicates, this will serve as a spackle for lip-area lines. It temporarily creates a smoother surface that reflects light better, which further improves the appearance of this trouble spot. This product would also work to "fill in" lines around the eyes, but how long it works depends on how expressive you are. The more the skin in this area moves, the less time the effect lasts, and you may not be that impressed to begin with. Still, there is no reason not to see if this product does minimize the appearance of lines for you, and it is packed with beneficial ingredients, as well as being fragrance-free.

✓☺ **$$$ Pro-Peptide Makeup Primer** *($39 for 1 ounce)* surpasses most primers due to the sheer variety of good-for-skin ingredients it contains. The silicone-based gel makes skin feel supremely silky and supplies it with some very good skin-identical ingredients, antioxidants, and cell-communicating ingredients. It is a shame that half the bells and whistles (including retinol) are listed after the preservative, but this can still be considered a state-of-the-art "primer" for all skin types or a lightweight moisturizer for normal to oily skin.

☺ **$$$ Triple Strength Lip Smoother** *($29 for 0.3 ounce)* is a minimally emollient moisturizer that contains a lot of film-forming agent and a smattering of state-of-the-art ingredients, including retinol, several peptides, and hyaluronic acid. It is designed to be used for lines around the mouth and on the lips, and does have a temporary tightening and smoothing effect. Use on lips demands a follow-up application of a lipstick, balm, or gloss because it can make them feel uncomfortably dry.

☹ **Lip Firm Gloss SPF 15** *($11 for 0.3 ounce)* lacks the UVA-protecting ingredients of titanium dioxide, zinc oxide, avobenzone, Tinosorb, or Mexoryl SX, and is not recommended.

☺ **$$$ Glow Younger Clear Self Tanner for Face & Body** *($25 for 3 ounces)* contains a glycol that aids in penetration of the self-tanning agent dihydroxyacetone. Another point of difference for this self-tanner is the inclusion of peptides, turning what could have been just a self-tanner into something more special. The water-based, fragrance-free formula is suitable for all skin types.

☺ **$$$ SunShield Powder Brush SPF 20 UVA/UVB** *($29.50)* is a talc-based loose powder packaged in a component that houses the powder in a central chamber. Pushing a button on the bottom shoots powder onto the attached brush. The component also includes a numeric dial which allows you to control how much powder is dispensed. Sun protection is assured from actives of titanium dioxide and zinc oxide. The amount of these minerals lends a dry matte finish to this silky powder, and also provides light to medium coverage, depending on how much is applied (a sheer application is best to avoid a heavy, powdered look). The drawbacks are that replacing the cap over the brush isn't easy and causes the bristles to splay unless you're very careful, and there is only one shade (best for fair to light skin tones only). Still, this is recommended if you have normal to oily skin and you want a portable powder with effective sunscreen.

😐 **$$$ Smart Concealer for Face** *($24)* is also known as **Smart Concealer Duo Compact for Face and Eyes**. Housed in a sleek compact are two creamy concealers, each with its own formula. The Eye Concealer has a smoother texture and applies easier, though is slightly prone to creasing into lines under the eye; the Face Concealer has a thicker, drier texture that can feel heavy and doesn't provide what most would consider natural-looking coverage. The full-size brush that's included is useful, though synthetic bristles would've made it even better. Unfortunately, the shades for each of the three sets aren't the easiest to work with. Light and Medium are slightly peach while Tan is slightly rose-toned.

E.L.F. COSMETICS (MAKEUP ONLY)

E.L.F. COSMETICS AT-A-GLANCE

Strengths: Inexpensive; lip gloss with broad-spectrum sunscreen; praiseworthy powder blush and eyeshadows; brow gel/clear mascara; oil-blotting papers are a steal.

Weaknesses: Mostly average formulas in smaller packaging than what's typical; terrible concealer; limited options for foundation; average to not-worth-it-at-any-price brushes.

For more information about E.L.F. Cosmetics, call (800) 231–4732 or visit www.eyeslipsface.com or www.Beautypedia.com. Note: E.L.F. Cosmetics is sold in many dollar stores and at select Target stores. However, the best way to experience the entire collection is to visit their Web site.

FOUNDATION: ☹ **All Over Cover Stick** *($1)* is a very tiny stick foundation with an unattractively thick, greasy texture that blends decently but still looks heavy on skin (sort of like theatrical greasepaint). The waxlike thickening agents put acne-prone skin on the fast track for more blemishes, and two of the three shades are very peach. It does not contain a single "active natural" ingredient, and is in no way preferred to any other stick foundation.

😐 **Shielding Hydrotint SPF 15** *($1)* does not list active ingredients on the carton or product itself, so this cannot be relied on for sun protection. It has a strong fragrance, and a sheer texture that gives minimal coverage, providing a satin matte finish that is best for those with normal to dry skin. Among the four shades, only Tone 3 should be avoided. However, this product is not recommended for its sunscreen.

CONCEALER: ☹ **Tone Correcting Concealer** *($1)* has a silky, moist texture that never sets, so this liquid concealer is prone to fading and creasing. That's not good news, especially when combined with its spotty coverage and three fairly peach colors.

POWDER: ☺ **Clarifying Pressed Powder** *($1)* claims to help treat and prevent breakouts, but it contains absolutely nothing that is capable of doing that. This is a very good, talc-based pressed powder with enough mineral oil and petrolatum to create a satin-smooth texture that's best for normal to dry skin. It applies sheer, all four colors are great, and it leaves a satin matte finish that doesn't look the least bit powdery. The Tone 3 and Tone 4 shades function as bronzing powders for light to medium skin tones.

😐 **Healthy Glow Bronzing Powder** *($1)* is a talc-based pressed bronzing powder that has an initially smooth texture, but that can apply unevenly because it tends to grab onto your skin. Its dry finish (enhanced by clay) also makes it difficult to blend. The Sunkissed shade is a rosy bronze tone with shimmer that can work for light to medium skin tones, while Warm Tan is more versatile. The Luminance shade isn't bronze-toned at all, and is best for highlighting with a shimmer finish, assuming you have the patience to deal with this product's application and blending issues.

BLUSH: ☺ **Natural Radiance Blusher** *($1)* is a pressed-powder blush with a smooth, slightly thick texture that applies evenly and imparts sheer color with a soft glow for a soft shine finish. The pigmentation of the shades is best for fair to medium skin tones; layering produces a slightly greater color payoff.

😐 **All Over Color Stick** *($1)* is a tiny, twist-up color stick meant for use anywhere on the face. The sheer, shimmer-infused colors are best for highlighting features, such as the brow bone or top of the cheekbone, and the fragrance-free formula is best for normal to dry skin. This product is not emollient enough to use on your lips (nor are the colors well-suited for lips) and applying it to your eyelid or crease area guarantees creasing due to the moist finish.

EYESHADOW: ☺ **Brightening Eye Color** *($1)* presents a selection of eyeshadow quads packaged with sponge-tip applicators, which should be tossed out. These quads are an amazing value for the money, especially if you prefer sheer colors and don't mind shine (every quad has some amount of shine, but none are outright glittery). They have a reasonably smooth texture and apply evenly, and every set has at least one shade that can serve as powder eyeliner. The best sets include Matte Mauve (it's almost matte), Butternut, Drama, and Nouveau (the olive-green shade in this one goes on khaki and blends well with the other colors). You can find eyeshadows that last longer and have a texture that's more elegant, but you'll pay a lot more for the privilege.

☺ **Custom Eyes** *($1 per shade; $1 for refillable 4-pan compact)* are powder eyeshadows sold singly so that you can customize a quad set of your own. The compact holds four colors, and it can also hold the Custom Lips and Custom Face shades below. These eyeshadows have a different formula than the Brightening Eye Color above. They're powder-free and based on oil and waxes, which result in a smooth, creamy-feeling texture that applies like a powder, but unfortunately are also prone to creasing and fading, especially if your eyelids are oily. These are still worth testing because they blend well and go on sheer. The best shades (all with some amount of shine) are Pink Ice, Wisteria, Mocha, Ivory, Dusk, and Moondust.

EYE AND BROW SHAPER: 😐 **Brightening Eye Liner** *($1)* is a basic, creamy eye pencil that needs routine sharpening. It applies smoothly and remains creamy enough to smudge slightly, so it's best for smoky eye designs where you intend to soften the line rather than keep it solid. Classic shades are available; the Gilded shade has a metallic shine.

😐 **Professional Eye Widener** *($1)* is a creamy, standard pencil with a sharpener built into the cap. You're instructed to stroke the pencil along the upper lash line and on the inside rim of the lower lash line to create the illusion of larger eyes. This is a theatrical makeup technique that tends to look obvious in person (and in daylight), not to mention the risk of putting a cosmetic product so close to the eye itself. This is an OK option as a soft white shimmer pencil for the upper lash line.

LIPSTICK, LIP GLOSS, AND LIPLINER: ✓☺ **Super Glossy Lip Shine SPF 15** *($1)* wins as the best product from E.L.F. Cosmetics because nowhere else will you find a supremely smooth, non-sticky lip gloss with gorgeous sheer colors and excellent sun protection courtesy of its in-part titanium dioxide sunscreen. Pink Kiss, Candlelight, Goddess, and Mauve Luxe have a soft metallic finish, while Angel is a colorless shade with flecks of glitter (definitely not a sophisticated look). The remaining colors have a soft shimmer and all of them have a fruity scent and taste. At this price, why not buy all the shades?

☺ **Moisture Care Lip Color** *($1)* is a castor oil–based lip gloss packaged in a click pen with a built-in angled sponge-tip applicator. It takes dozens of rotations to feed the color onto the applicator, but once the flow is primed, successive applications are a cinch. This has a thick, emollient texture and glossy, non-sticky finish. Every shade applies sheer, including the deeper-looking reds and plums. ☺ **Hypershine Lip Gloss** *($1)* has a combination of thickness and slickness that's unusual, but it applies smoothly and leaves a non-sticky, moderately (not hyper) glossy finish. The click pen with brush applicator works well and though this gloss offers only a small selection of shades they go on nearly transparent, making these a safe bet to apply over any color of lipstick.

☺ **Hypershine Mini Cell Phone Lip Gloss Charms** *($5)* are sold as mini versions of the Hypershine Lip Gloss above. They have a different formula that's more emollient but not glossier. The set presents eight glosses with an overcap that can be attached to any shade so it can be worn as a charm (or added to a key ring). This is primarily a teen-appeal product, but is an option for adults who want a tiny gloss to tuck into an evening bag.

☺ **Soothing Lip Gloss** *($1)* isn't too soothing because it is flavored with mint, but that's not as detrimental to lips as adding pure menthol or one of its derivatives. This is a good, basic lip gloss with a slightly thick texture and a non-sticky gloss finish. The red and orange hues apply almost as strong as they look, while the other shades go on sheer.

☺ **Custom Lips** *($1 per shade; $1 for refillable 4-pan compact)* are pans of lip color that you add to a compact. You can add up to four shades, or you can mix and match with E.L.F. Cosmetics's Custom Eyes and Custom Face shades. These have a thick texture with a slight slip and minimally emollient finish. Every color, even the deep reds and plums, applies very sheer. The only issue with a product like this is that it requires finger application unless you're willing to tote a lip brush.

😐 **Therapeutic Conditioning Lip Balm** *($1)* is an emollient, oil-based stick lip balm that comes in assorted fruit flavors. It's very basic, doesn't impart much gloss, and the fruity element of each shade can be cloying. 😐 **Feather Proof Moisturizing Lipliner** *($1)* has a formula that's way too greasy to prevent feathering, and it needs routine sharpening. This is an OK lip pencil that comes in a mostly pink-tinged range of shades, but spending a bit more at the drugstore will open the door to several superior lip pencils.

☹ **Plumping Lip Glaze** *($1)* is a waxy-feeling, dual-sided lip gloss that contains a lot of menthol, which plumps lips by virtue of irritation but ends up being too irritating for frequent use (and touch-ups with this very sheer gloss would definitely be frequent).

MASCARA: ☺ **Earth & Water Mascara Duo** *($1)* has a New Age-y name that doesn't really explain the fact that this is a dual-sided mascara. One side is regular mascara, the other is waterproof. The regular mascara is surpassingly good, allowing quick and dramatic lengthening of lashes with minimal clumps and delivering a long-lasting finish. In contrast, the waterproof version (which has the same brush as the regular mascara) goes on thin, doesn't build much length, doesn't thicken, and is only mildly waterproof. Although not equally impressive, for the price, even half of this mascara is a beauty steal.

✓☺ **Wet Gloss Lash & Brow Clear Mascara** *($1)* houses the same clear gel formula in a dual-sided, dual-brush component. One end is for eyebrows (and the brush is suitable for brow application) and the other for lashes (with an equally suitable brush). The gel applies smoothly, is non-sticky, and does a great job of grooming brows or providing slight lash enhancement while leaving a subtle glossy finish. All this for $1? Sold!

FACE AND BODY ILLUMINATING/SHIMMER PRODUCTS: ☺ **Shimmering Facial Whip** *($1)* comes in a tiny tube and dispenses as a lotion that tends to drag a bit during application. It sets to a slightly moist finish that imparts gleaming shimmer that's too strong for daytime unless blended very well. Most of the sheer shades are best for the cheeks or for highlighting lips; Toasted and Citrus are good options for eyeshadow, but be sure to set this with a powder eyeshadow to avoid creasing.

BRUSHES: All of E.L.F. Cosmetics's brushes are sold individually for $1 each. As you may have expected, the quality isn't top of the line. What's missing from many of them is soft, dense hair that allows precision application of color and expert blending. Still, some of these are surprisingly good for the money (they beat any pre-assembled brush set from major drugstore lines). The ones to consider are the ☺ **Eyelash and Brow Wand**, ☺ **Brow Comb and Brush**, ☺ **Defining Eye Brush** (best for shadow, not for applying powder eyeliner), and the synthetic ☺ **Eyeliner Brush**.

😐 **Professional Complete Set** *($9)* includes nine brushes that cover all the basics from powder to lashes and eyelining options, all packaged in a tri-fold case. Most of the brushes are below average and no match for pricier options, but this can work if you need a second set for casual makeup. The 😐 **Professional 5-Piece Brush Collection** *($10)* includes basic brushes for powder, blush, and eyeshadow, but none of them are good enough to make this your primary brush set, even though the price is right.

😐 **Professional 9-Piece Master Set** *($15)* includes the Total Face Brush, Blushing/Bronzing/Blending Brush, Foundation Brush, Defining Eye Brush, Blending Eye Brush, Smudge Eye Sponge, Eyelash/Brow Wand, Brow Comb/Brush, and Lip Defining Brush, all packaged in a deluxe roll-up case. A couple of the tools are great, but the rest are average to poor, making this a sketchy set to consider.

☺ **Mechanical Eyelash Curler** *($1)* is so named because the handle is spring-loaded and must be kept together with the included plastic clasp. This is a standard, workable eyelash curler and is worth a try, but only if your lashes don't curl well on their own from use of an outstanding mascara. Still, this costs next to nothing and can be nice to have around if you ever decide to try a lash curler.

SPECIALTY PRODUCTS: ☺ **Custom Face** *($1 per shade; $1 for refillable compact)* is a group of smooth-textured powder colors meant for use anywhere on the face. However, the small shade range makes it ideally suited for use as a blush. Dusting pink, peach, or rose tones all over your face would look odd, and only one of these shades (Bronzed) is appropriate as eyeshadow. All of them have some amount of shine, with Coy being almost matte. The color saturation is stronger than that of the Custom Eyes or Custom Lips products, but it can be applied sheer.

😐 **The Collection** *($10)* includes two brushes (only the Eye Shadow Brush is recommended), two eyeshadow quads (both tricky colors to work with), two shades of Super Glossy Lip Shine SPF 15, a Healthy Finish Bronzing Powder, All Over Cover Stick, All Over Color Stick, and E.L.F. Cosmetics's dual-sided mascara. This collection presents some of the best and worst of what E.L.F. Cosmetics offers, and although not every product is five-star you're still getting a lot for your money.

☺ **The Ultimate Kit** *($15)* allows you to sample the range of E.L.F. Cosmetics's lip glosses, including the Super Glossy Lip Shine SPF 15, along with two workable eyeshadow quads and an All Over Color Stick. You'll definitely get your money's worth, because there's not a bad product in the bunch, save for the menthol-laden Plumping Lip Glaze.

☺ **Natural Lash Kit** *($1)* and **Dramatic Lash Kit** *($1)* are a good, inexpensive way to experiment with false eyelashes. Both kits present a full set and include a tiny tube of adhesive, which is convenient. The kits are aptly named based on the results they provide, although getting false eyelashes to look natural isn't an easy feat.

☺ **Eye Makeup Remover Pads** *($1 for 18 pads)* offer a very gentle, fragrance-free formula infused onto small round pads. They produce a slight lather and should be rinsed from the skin (or used before cleansing), but they work well to remove non-waterproof makeup.

✓☺ **Professional Shine Eraser** *($1 for 50 sheets)* is the best value around for oil-blotting papers. These powder-free sheets work quickly to mop up excess shine before touching up with powder. They are supposedly infused with green tea extract, which the company says will retexture skin to mask facial imperfections, but, of course, these do no such thing.

Note: The E.L.F. Cosmetics selection also includes minor, nonessential tools that some may find suitable, but for the most part these sponges, sponge-tip applicators, and puffs are poorly made and do not enhance an artful makeup application.

ELIZABETH ARDEN

ELIZABETH ARDEN AT-A-GLANCE

Strengths: Moderately priced; some excellent serums (including the ceramide capsules) and moisturizers; good cleansers for normal to dry skin; good makeup remover; good concealer, pressed powder, eyeshadow, lipsticks, and mascara; well-organized tester units.

Weaknesses: No products for those battling blemishes; no skin-lightening products; no AHA or BHA products or topical scrubs; several products whose sunscreen lacks sufficient UVA protection; none of the foundations with sunscreen provide sufficient UVA protection; lackluster eye and brow pencils; some problematic lip color products; mediocre brushes; jar packaging.

For more information about Elizabeth Arden, call (800) 326-7337 or visit www.elizabetharden.com or www.Beautypedia.com.

ELIZABETH ARDEN SKIN CARE

ELIZABETH ARDEN CERAMIDE PRODUCTS

😐 **$$$ Purifying Cream Cleanser** *($26 for 4.2 ounces)* is a basic, water- and mineral oil–based cleansing lotion that contains barely any ceramides. The tiny amount of sandalwood oil isn't great for skin or for use in the eye area, but is not likely a cause for concern. This will require a washcloth for complete removal and is suitable for normal to dry skin.

☹ **Purifying Toner** *($26 for 6.7 ounces)* lists alcohol as the second ingredient and also contains some potentially irritating plant extracts, all of which undermine the effectiveness of the ceramides and other skin-identical ingredients in this misguided toner.

✓☺ **$$$ Ceramide Advanced Time Complex Capsules Intensive Treatment for Face and Throat** *($65 for 60 capsules; 0.95 ounce)* have been a hallmark of Arden's Ceramide line for years, and they remain a good choice if you're looking for a silky, silicone-based serum that contains some beneficial ingredients for normal to very dry skin types not prone to breakouts. The silicone is joined by emollients, lipids, ceramides, plant oil, and antioxidant vitamins, all packaged to ensure potency before use. The drawback to these capsules is that you must use all the contents each time, because leaving them open is not only potentially messy, but will also allow the antioxidants to quickly degrade.

☺ **$$$ Ceramide Eyes Time Complex Capsules** *($47 for 60 capsules; 0.35 ounce)* are not quite as exciting or helpful for skin as the Ceramide Advanced Time Complex Capsules above. These contain witch hazel and nettle extract, both of which may prove irritating for some skin types when used around the eye area. Kept away from the eyes, these are an option for normal to slightly oily skin; they contain some good antioxidants and, of course, ceramide.

☹ **Ceramide EyeWish Eye Cream SPF 10** *($43 for 0.5 ounce)* not only has an SPF rating that's too low for daytime protection, but also leaves skin vulnerable to UVA damage. UVA rays cause wrinkles, so this product's shortage of protection in that regard isn't what's needed to keep eye-area wrinkles at bay.

✓☺ **$$$ Ceramide Gold Ultra Restorative Capsules** *($68 for 60 capsules; 0.95 ounce)* are an interesting way to provide normal to very dry skin with a short but very effective roster of ingredients that can restore a healthy skin-barrier function, all while supplying elements that skin needs to look and feel its best. Unlike Arden's other Ceramide capsules reviewed above, this formula eliminates the silicone and squalane and gets right down to business with a ceramide-based formula. Cell-communicating ingredients follow, and Arden also included two forms of antioxidant vitamin A as well as some vitamin E. As claimed, these capsules are fragrance- and preservative-free. They are definitely a consideration for those dealing with eczema or rosacea (assuming your rosacea-prone skin is not also oily).

😐 **$$$ Ceramide Moisture Network Night Cream** *($56 for 1.7 ounces)* takes the "everything but the kitchen sink" concept, and, well, includes the sink! With over 90 ingredients, this moisturizer doesn't leave any stone unturned when it comes to providing dry skin with emollients, oils, skin-identical ingredients, antioxidants, ceramides, plant extracts, and even a few anti-irritants. But is that better for skin? It definitely isn't from the standpoint of allergic reactions, because it stands to reason that the more ingredients a product contains, the greater the likelihood that your skin will react to one or more of them. The other downside to packing so many ingredients into a moisturizer is that, aside from the ingredients that create the product's texture and finish, you're only getting tiny amounts of them (the ingredients can only add up to a 100% total content). It is unknown whether tiny amounts of several ingredients (such as antioxidants or anti-irritants) are better for skin than larger amounts of just a few. And even the antioxidants in this moisturizer are subject to quick deterioration due to jar packaging. This Arden product isn't without its flaws because it does contain balm mint extract and some fragrant components (linalool, hexyl cinnamal) that can spell trouble for skin, but the amounts used are likely too small to be cause for concern.

☹ **Ceramide Plump Perfect Eye Moisture Cream SPF 15** *($46 for 0.5 ounce)* lacks the UVA-protecting ingredients of avobenzone, titanium dioxide, zinc oxide, Tinosorb, or Mexoryl SX, and is not recommended. None of the ingredients in this eye cream can combat puffiness. If anything, applying the synthetic sunscreen agents in this product too close to the eyes can cause puffiness (and irritation).

☹ **Ceramide Plump Perfect Lip Moisture Cream SPF 30** *($27.50 for 0.5 ounce)* has a lot going for it, starting with an effective, in-part avobenzone sunscreen in an emollient base that includes ceramides and shea butter, and packaging that keeps light- and air-sensitive ingredients stable. In order to plump up your lips, though, peppermint, balm mint, and menthol were added, even though they merely cause irritation and do not make lips perfect, just chapped, dry, and inflamed. What a shame, because this is otherwise a great sunscreen option for lips.

😐 **$$$ Ceramide Plump Perfect Moisture Cream SPF 30** *($62 for 1.7 ounces)* doesn't disappoint with its in-part avobenzone sunscreen and SPF rating, but for the money the base formulation is disappointing. It contains mostly water, slip agent, emollient, silicones, glycerin, and preservative. Not a bad ordinary roster for taking care of normal to dry skin and offering great sun protection. But considering the price tag, the exciting state-of-the-art ingredients (ceramides, antioxidants, anti-irritant plant extracts, and skin-identical ingredients) should be present in more than just a dusting. This is still a good option for a daytime moisturizer for normal to dry skin, but it's not as enticing as other options with stable packaging and a larger amount of skin-beneficial substances.

☺ **$$$ Ceramide Plump Perfect Targeted Line Concentrate** *($65 for 0.5 ounce)* has a lot of wonderful things going for it, including a supremely silky texture and nearly weightless finish suitable for all skin types. The pump-dispensed serum is packed with antioxidants and ingredients that mimic the structure and function of healthy skin, as well as lesser amounts of a couple of cell-communicating ingredients. The only drawback keeping it from earning a Paula's Pick is the volatile fragrance components, which can be irritating. Their presence is minimal, but they ding this product relative to similarly well-formulated serums from Estee Lauder, Prescriptives, and Clinique.

😐 **$$$ Ceramide Time Complex Moisture Cream** *($49 for 1.7 ounces)* should have better packaging to keep its antioxidants stable. There are several state-of-the-art ingredients in this product, but with sodium chloride (salt) as the fourth ingredient, they won't impact skin in the manner they should.

☹ **Ceramide Time Complex Moisture Cream SPF 15** *($49 for 1.7 ounces)* lacks the UVA-protecting ingredients of titanium dioxide, zinc oxide, avobenzone, Tinosorb, or Mexoryl SX, and is not recommended.

☺ **$$$ Ceramide Plump Perfect Firming Facial Mask** *($58 for 4 0.5-ounce masks)* are cloth masks steeped in a moisturizing solution that includes lightweight hydrating agents, several ceramides, a peptide, cell-communicating ingredients, stabilizers, and preservatives. Although this fragrance-free product has some impressive attributes, you're not getting much for your money considering that only four single-use masks are included.

Elizabeth Arden Intervene Products

☺ **$$$ Intervene 3-in-1 Daily Cleanser Exfoliator Primer** *($20 for 5 ounces)* sports a name that sounds like a time-saver if there ever was one. However, the only truth in the name is the "cleanser" part, as that's essentially all this pricey product is. The tiny amount of polyethylene beads included creates a mild exfoliating action, but it's not akin to the results from using a standard facial scrub, or even a washcloth for that matter. Still, it's a well-formulated cleanser for normal to slightly dry or slightly oily skin, and it removes makeup easily while rinsing cleanly. However, keep in mind that there are countless water-soluble cleansers available for a fraction of the price that leave skin feeling just like this product does.

😐 **$$$ Intervene Pause & Effect Moisture Cream SPF 15** *($55 for 1.7 ounces)* deserves credit only for its innovative name and its in-part avobenzone sunscreen. The Intervene portion of the name is meant to describe how it can interrupt the aging process and the wrinkles associated with that process. Arden goes beyond basic anti-aging claims and states that this product also "helps minimize imbalances in the look of skin caused by fluctuating hormonal and protein levels." They don't explain what these imbalances are or how their product corrects these problems, so it may be as simple as addressing the dryness that can accompany postmenopausal skin, benefits that aren't specific to this product but rather are common to all moisturizers. Although this is an effective sunscreen in a lightweight moisturizing cream base, it contains a fair amount of narcissus bulb, which may cause contact dermatitis, while having no established benefit for skin. Red clover is present to minimize skin symptoms of menopause, but its benefit when applied topically has not been proven (Sources: www.naturaldatabase.com; and *Contact Dermatitis*, August 1997, pages 70–77). Although some worthwhile ingredients appear farther down on the ingredient list, many of them will be compromised by this product's jar packaging. In the end, this is a costly sunscreen, not a wrinkle intervention.

😐 **$$$ Intervene Pause & Effect Moisture Lotion SPF 15** *($55 for 1.7 ounces)* is similar to the Intervene Pause & Effect Moisture Cream SPF 15 above, and also includes an in-part avobenzone sunscreen. The primary differences are in texture (with this one being a thin but substantial lotion) and packaging (with this product featuring an opaque bottle that will keep its antioxidants stable). Although the latter feature is positive, the presence of problematic narcissus bulb is too great to ignore, and makes this an iffy proposition for skin, even though the sunscreen portion is right-on.

OTHER ELIZABETH ARDEN PRODUCTS

😊 **$$$ 2-in-1 Cleanser, for All Skin Types** *($18 for 5 ounces)* is a standard, water-soluble foaming cleanser that's a good option for normal to slightly dry or oily skin. It contains a couple of problematic plant extracts, so keep it away from the eye area and rinse it promptly.

😊 **$$$ Hydra-Gentle Cream Cleanser, for Dry/Sensitive Skin** *($18 for 5 ounces)* would be better for its targeted sensitive-skin customer if it did not contain fragrance; however, this is a very good, silky cleansing lotion that removes makeup and does not contain detergent cleansing agents.

✓😊 **$$$ All Gone Eye and Lip Makeup Remover** *($16 for 3.4 ounces)* is an impressive, fast-acting, water- and silicone-based makeup remover. The lack of fragrance and the inclusion of an anti-irritant make this a cut above many others.

😊 **$$$ Hydra-Splash Alcohol-Free Toner, for All Skin Types** *($18 for 6.8 ounces)* contains mostly water, slip agent, algae, soothing agent, witch hazel, skin-identical ingredients, plant oil, and emollients. It's a good option for normal to dry skin and would rate a Paula's Pick without the witch hazel.

☹ **Bye Lines Anti-Wrinkle Serum** *($42 for 1 ounce)* contains a significant amount of coriander oil, so it's not so much "bye lines" as "hello irritation." The main fragrance component of this oil is linalool, which can cause allergic reactions and make skin more sensitive to sunlight (Source: *Herbal Drugs and Pharmaceuticals*, Medpharm GmbH Scientific Publishers, 1994).

☹ **Daily Moisture Lotion SPF 15** *($35 for 1.7 ounces)* lacks the UVA-protecting ingredients of titanium dioxide, zinc oxide, avobenzone, Tinosorb, or Mexoryl SX, and is not recommended.

😐 **Eight Hour Cream Skin Protectant** *($16 for 1.7 ounces)* lands on many fashion magazines' "best of beauty" lists for its long-standing history and versatility. However, it's just a blend of emollients with fragrance, salicylic acid (incapable of exfoliating in this product), plant oil, vitamin E, and preservatives. (So much for the validity of the "best" lists in fashion magazines!) Plain Vaseline, which makes up the bulk of this formula, would work just as well.

✓😊 **$$$ Extreme Conditioning Cream SPF 15** *($36 for 1.7 ounces)* provides UVA protection with its in-part avobenzone sunscreen and comes in an emollient, silky, antioxidant-enriched base. The opaque pump bottle will keep the light- and air-sensitive ingredients stable, so this is an all-around exceptional daytime moisturizer for normal to dry skin.

😐 **$$$ First Defense Advanced Anti-Oxidant Lotion SPF 15** *($39 for 1.7 ounces)* is a good, though standard, sunscreen lotion that contains avobenzone for UVA protection. The water- and silicone-based lotion leaves skin feeling silky and moist, but all of the interesting skin-identical ingredients and, most important, the antioxidants, are minimally present. Actually, the more than 40 ingredients show up in short supply here, which means that you essentially get a whole lot of nothing. Arden claims that the carnosine and wolfberry plant extract are proven to outperform vitamins A, C, and E at neutralizing skin-damaging free radicals. Yet if that's true, there is no substantiated research to support it. Carnosine has a good amount of promising research concerning its antioxidant benefit when taken orally, but compared to the piles of research on topical use of the three aforementioned vitamins, information on topical use of carnosine is scarce. As for the wolfberry, there isn't much of it in here to extol, and there is insufficient reliable information about its effectiveness whether it's used topically or consumed (Source: www.naturaldatabase.com).

☹ **First Defense Advanced Anti-Oxidant Cream SPF 15** *($39 for 1.7 ounces)* is a more emollient version of the First Defense Advanced Anti-Oxidant Lotion SPF 15 above, and also includes an in-part avobenzone sunscreen. The same formulary issues (that is, the intriguing ingredients are listed after the preservative) apply here, too, though this formula adds irritating grapefruit juice, which serves no purpose in a sunscreen other than to cause irritation and possibly a photosensitizing reaction.

😐 **$$$ Good Morning Skin Serum** *($31 for 0.5 ounce)* is a silicone-based serum that contains several plant extracts, some of which can have antioxidant properties for skin and some that can be skin irritants. The teeny amount of mulberry is not enough to inhibit melanin production. What this product lacks is a significant quantity of skin-identical ingredients, which would have made this a far better way to say good morning for skin.

😐 **$$$ Good Night's Sleep Restoring Cream** *($36 for 1.7 ounces)* is designed to be used at night, yet contains three sunscreen ingredients, which is unnecessary and can cause irritation. This rich-textured cream contains a frustrating blend of problematic and helpful plant extracts. The helpful plants have antioxidant properties, but won't remain stable once this jar-packaged product is opened. The amount of lavender extract is unlikely to cause problems, but if you're interested in this plant's sleep-inducing effect, a far better method would be to inhale lavender essential oil or potpourri before bedtime.

☹ **Matte Moisture Lotion, Oil Free** *($34 for 1.7 ounces)* has a matte finish thanks to the amount of alcohol and talc it contains. There are less irritating ways to keep skin shine-free than with an alcohol-laden moisturizer, and this also contains some potentially irritating plant extracts.

☺ **$$$ Overnight Success Cellular Renewal Serum** *($47 for 1 ounce)* promises to resurface and regenerate skin's appearance, giving your skin enhanced clarity and a less blotchy appearance. Yet the best thing this serum has going for it is that its silicone base will leave skin feeling exceptionally silky. In terms of enhanced clarity, there is nothing in the product that can make skin clearer. However, because silicones can even out your skin's texture you may perceive more clarity. This is because of how silicone functions on skin: smooth-textured skin is better able to reflect light, which does improve its appearance, but that's a cosmetic effect, not an anti-aging breakthrough.

Arden wisely filled this serum with several very good skin-identical ingredients and antioxidants, ingredients you should expect to see in any serum (or moisturizer), especially in this price range. Even better, packaging for this product will ensure that the antioxidants remain stable during use. The inclusion of the Australian flower extract *Centipedia cunninghamii* (also known by its less appealing garden name, old man weed) is curious, because it is commonly used as a medicinal remedy for colds and chest pain (Source: *Natural Medicines Comprehensive Database*, 8th Edition, 2006). Reliable, substantiated information about this extract's effect on skin doesn't seem to exist. The extract does not appear to be harmful or irritating, but there are no proven studies pertaining to its usefulness as an antiwrinkle ingredient. My one complaint about this product is its intense fragrance. I don't often comment on a specific skin-care product's scent, but this serum's perfumey scent lingers on the skin long after it has been absorbed. Both Clinique and my line have similar products that are fragrance-free and less expensive, but this product is definitely an option for all but sensitive skin types seeking either a lightweight moisturizer or antioxidant product.

😐 **$$$ Perpetual Moisture 24 Cream** *($38.50 for 1.7 ounces)* is another moisturizer in which the effectiveness of the many antioxidants is compromised by jar packaging. However, a larger offense is Arden's decision to include balm mint extract, which poses a risk of irritation for skin. The amount is likely too small to be a problem, but this otherwise nicely done moisturizer for normal to dry skin would be better without it.

😊 **$$$ Perpetual Moisture 24 Lotion** *($38.50 for 1.7 ounces)* is a lighter-weight version of the Perpetual Moisture 24 Cream above, and is packaged in an opaque pump bottle, which better preserves the effectiveness of its antioxidants. This is a mostly outstanding moisturizer for normal to slightly dry or slightly oily skin. It would earn a Paula's Pick rating if not for the balm mint extract. Regarding Arden's claims that this product "pre-empts moisture loss at its source," that is merely a standard for any well-formulated moisturizer; it should indeed contain ingredients that keep moisture in skin (preventing moisture loss) and draw moisture to the skin's surface. This Arden product contains essential ingredients that do just that.

😊 **$$$ Prevage Anti-Aging Treatment** *($150 for 1.7 ounces)* continues the carefully orchestrated launch of Prevage ($115 for 1 ounce), which was first marketed to physicians and is now available in what is termed an "over-the-counter" version, marketed under the Elizabeth Arden name. Arden partnered with Allergan, the company that makes Prevage, to create a product that contains the "powerful" antioxidant idebenone (listed on the ingredient list as hydroxydecyl ubiquinone). What is the difference, you ask, between the dermatologic version and the one sold at the Arden counter? The original Prevage formula is billed as "physician-strength" and contains 1% idebenone, while Arden's cosmetics-counter version contains 0.5% idebenone. The physician-strength angle is bogus because idebenone is not a drug of any kind, nor is it regulated or akin to any type of prescription treatment. There is no reason it can't be sold in any retail channel. Such positioning and exclusivity is clever marketing on Allergan's part (the company also distributes Botox and markets the M.D. Forte skin-care line).

The intense curiosity about this product has been nothing short of amazing, with most women asking me if idebenone really is *the* best antioxidant available. The study that showed idebenone has the antioxidant muscle to surpass others involved only 30 subjects, and compared idebenone to vitamins C and E, alpha lipoic acid, coenzyme Q10, and kinetin. The study did not, however, compare the effects of idebenone to many of the hundreds of other potent antioxidants that commonly appear in other skin-care products, nor did it compare the effects of idebenone with the effects of a combination of antioxidants. Perhaps a cocktail of antioxidants would far surpass idebenone—we don't know. Interestingly, a study comparing the protective effect of idebenone on sun-exposed skin found it ineffective compared to topical application of vitamins C and E with ferulic acid, but this study was conducted in part by Dr. Sheldon Pinnell, whose Skinceuticals line sells an antioxidant serum with those very ingredients (Source: *The Journal of Investigative Dermatology*, May 2006, pages 1185–1187).

The world of antioxidants is far more complex than the mere handful that Allergan compared to idebenone. To date, there are still no published, peer-reviewed studies that support idebenone's alleged superiority. This does not mean idebenone is not a valid antioxidant for skin. Given what we know about how ubiquinone performs in the body, it is definitely not a throwaway ingredient. What is fairly certain, however, is that it is neither the best nor most potent antioxidant around. Comparing Allergan's original Prevage formula to Arden's is like comparing night and day. Arden's water-in-silicone version is silky-smooth, and with a formula that's nearly identical to that of Allergan's "medically positioned" (however inaccurate that is) Prevage MD ($150 for 1 ounce). Both Prevage products are water-in-silicone serums that contain several skin-friendly ingredients, including glycerin, phospholipids, green tea, sodium hyaluronate, and algae.

Which Prevage product to choose isn't a tough decision, given that efficacy levels for idebenone have not been established. The fact that Arden's product contains 50% less than the original Prevage is inconsequential, and there is no research proving that 1% idebenone is preferred to Arden's 0.5%. Is Arden's readily available version worth the money? Despite its elegant formula, the answer is "no." Considering that idebenone is not the definitive antioxidant and that many companies are producing antioxidant serums and lotions that contain a cocktail of antioxidants, Arden's price point is undeservedly high. The product is a worthwhile option, and the formula is suitable for all skin types—unless you're sensitive to fragrance. But money-wise, lots of companies have antioxidant-loaded products that cost less (in some cases, much less) and, due to their blend of antioxidants, potentially offer skin a greater complement of benefits. One last note: The mica in both Prevage products lends a slight shimmer to skin, which the companies describe as enhancing skin's radiance; it's just a glitter-effect, nothing more.

✓☺ **$$$ Prevage Eye Anti-Aging Moisturizing Treatment** *($95 for 0.5 ounce)* provides less product that the original Prevage product reviewed above, yet the price ends up being much higher on an ounce-per-ounce comparison basis. Good thing it is a more impressive formula! Claiming to be "anti-everything" that you don't like about the skin around your eyes, it is mostly a blend of silicones with sea water and algae. Lesser amounts of several antioxidants (including idebenone, listed as hydroxydecyl ubiquinone) and cell-communicating ingredients are included, but the good news is that the small amount of each adds up to a significantly beneficial product for slightly dry skin anywhere on the face. Don't count on this serum-type product to banish dark circles or deflate puffiness, but do count on it to provide skin with an array of excellent ingredients to help it look its best. The mica and titanium dioxide pigments add a soft shine to skin, but the effect on dark circles pales in comparsion to the camouflage a good concealer can provide.

😐 **Velva Moisture Film** *($39.50 for 6.7 ounces)* is a very dated moisturizer recommended for combination or oily skin. The thickeners and lanolin make it inappropriate for these skin types, particularly if breakouts are a concern. Actually, this formula makes Clinique's boring Dramatically Different Moisturizing Lotion look like a state-of-the-art product, which isn't saying much.

😐 **$$$ Visible Difference Refining Moisture Cream Complex** *($49.50 for 2.5 ounces)* has been in the Arden line for years, which means customers are still buying it. It's a jar-packaged, very standard moisturizer for normal to dry skin that contains a tiny amount of antioxidants and doesn't compete favorably with today's state-of-the-art moisturizers.

☹ **Peel & Reveal Revitalizing Treatment** *($30 for 1.7 ounces)* contains two forms of drying, irritating alcohol as the main ingredients and the jar packaging will make the many antioxidants unstable shortly after the product is opened. Finally, several of the plant extracts (horsetail, orange, and lemon among them) are irritating to skin.

☹ **Eight Hour Cream Lip Protectant Stick SPF 15** *($16 for 0.13 ounce)* lacks the UVA-protecting ingredients of titanium dioxide, zinc oxide, avobenzone, Tinosorb, or Mexoryl SX, and is not recommended. Neutrogena, Cover Girl, and Paula's Choice all have sheer lipsticks or balms with reliable sun protection.

ELIZABETH ARDEN MAKEUP

FOUNDATION: ☺ **$$$ Flawless Finish Mousse Makeup** *($32)* is the original mousse foundation. It's packaged in a metal can that uses a propellant to distribute an airy, bubbly, flesh-toned foam, which blends on better than you might expect, though you might end up wasting some product until you get used to the dispensing method. Coverage is sheer, and the texture has enough slip to allow for adequate blending. This dries to a soft matte finish and is an option for normal to slightly oily or dry skin. If you're prone to breakouts, you will appreciate the absence of potentially pore-clogging thickening agents in this formula. Thirteen shades are on hand, including some great colors for fair skin tones, but avoid Melba, Bisque, and Natural. Champagne and Ginger are slightly pink, and should be considered carefully.

😐 **$$$ Ceramide Plump Perfect Makeup SPF 15** *($39.50)* has many positive attributes, but for a foundation purporting to reduce the appearance of wrinkles, its cardinal error was not including a sunscreen that offers UVA-protecting ingredients. This is otherwise a modern formula that does include ceramides, though it takes more than that to create radiant, healthy-looking skin. The silky texture blends easily, providing medium coverage and leaving a soft matte finish. Ten shades are available, with some enticing options for light to medium skin tones. Avoid Honey, Cameo, Mocha II, and Bisque, and avoid this altogether if you're looking for a foundation with reliable sunscreen.

😐 **$$$ Flawless Finish Sponge-On Cream Makeup** *($32)* has been part of Arden's makeup lineup for years, but that's not necessarily a good thing. This fairly thick and somewhat greasy petrolatum- and mineral oil–based compact makeup is only for someone with dry skin. It starts out very thick and moist, providing medium to full coverage with a creamy, opaque finish. It blends well enough, but most women don't need this much coverage, and the fragrance is quite strong. Those who are loyal to this makeup may want to reconsider what they want from a foundation. Of the 11 shades, the following are too pink, orange, or peach: Vanilla, Softly Beige, Porcelain Beige, Toasty Beige, Gentle Beige, and Toasty Rose.

😐 **$$$ Flawless Finish Dual Perfection Makeup SPF 8** *($32)* is a talc-based pressed-powder foundation with a silky feel and a very smooth finish. The SPF rating is embarrassingly low—by itself this is a no-no for daytime—but it is part titanium dioxide, so if you pair it with an effective SPF 15 sunscreen it would add some extra protection. The formula works best for someone with normal to slightly dry or slightly oily skin, and most of the 12 colors are excellent. The only ones that should be avoided due to their peach casts are Buff and Cameo.

😐 **$$$ Flawless Finish Bare Perfection Makeup SPF 8** *($29)*, other than having a way too low SPF without adequate UVA protection, is actually an impressive foundation suitable for normal to dry skin. With a smooth, moist texture and satin finish capable of delivering sheer to light coverage, it's worth a look, but it's not recommended over foundations that go the distance to protect skin with SPF 15. There are 15 shades to consider, including a couple of good options for darker skin tones. The shades that should be avoided due to overtones of peach, orange, or pink are Bisque, Cameo, Honey, Mocha II, and Fawn. Buff is slightly peach but may work for some light skin tones.

☹ **$$$ Flawless Finish Radiant Moisture Makeup SPF 8** *($29)* is an elegant, moisturizing foundation for those with normal to very dry skin. What a shame the sunscreen lacks adequate UVA-protecting ingredients and that the SPF rating is pitifully low. This somewhat thick, creamy makeup provides medium coverage and a moist finish that can look thick if not blended carefully. The 11 shades include some notable neutral options; the ones to avoid due to peach or pink tones are Bisque, Cameo, Honey, Mocha II, and Fawn.

CONCEALER: ✓☺ Flawless Finish Concealer *($16)* remains an excellent wand-applicator type concealer with a lightweight, smooth texture and an opaque, soft matte finish that poses almost no risk of creasing. The three colors are superbly neutral, and best for fair to medium skin. Surveying Arden's entire makeup collection, this is one of a handful of items that is really worth your attention (and money).

POWDER: ☺ $$$ Flawless Finish Pressed Powder *($22)* appears to have been improved, because it now competes nicely with other talc-based pressed powders that leave a silky, sheer, real-skin finish rather than looking dry or chalky. It comes in five shades, though each is so sheer the color is almost a non-issue. One more thing: This deposits so minimally on skin that someone with very oily areas will be disappointed and need to find a more absorbent powder.

☹ **$$$ Flawless Finish Loose Powder** *($22.50)* has a silky but drier-than-usual texture and doesn't compete with the stellar choices from Lauder-owned lines or French-themed lines, including Lancome and Chanel. It serves its purpose, but tends to look like powder rather than polished, perfected skin. The five sheer shades are nonintrusive and suitable for fair to tan skin.

☹ **Bronzing Powder Duo** *($29.50)* is a talc-based, pressed-powder bronzer that features two shiny colors in one compact. Each shade has a dry, slightly grainy texture but sheer application. The overall performance doesn't come close to matching the price, and this makes it not worth considering over countless other bronzing powders.

BLUSH: ☹ $$$ Color Intrigue Cheekcolor *($21)* is a collection of pressed-powder blushes, each with a slightly dry, grainy texture and sheer, blendable application. Every shade has some amount of shine, but the truly underwhelming texture doesn't make this worth considering over blushes rated with a happy face or greater.

EYESHADOW: ✓☺ Color Intrigue Eyeshadow *($14.50)* is ideal. Each shade has a wonderful, satin matte, nonpowdery finish and a texture that blends and layers beautifully. Every shade has at least a touch of shine, but the good news is the shiniest shades leave more of a sheen than glitter or sparkles, and these shadows don't flake. The almost-matte options include Teak, Urban, Vanilla, and Wheat. ☺ **Color Intrigue Palette Eyeshadow Quad** *($30)* share the same formulary and application traits as the single Eyeshadow above, but here you get four shades in one compact. I wish the color combinations were more thoughtful; the quads I saw weren't the easiest shades to work with, and every one was very shiny. The shades tend to change seasonally, so keep your eyes open for an attractive grouping where you can realistically use more than two colors!

EYE AND BROW SHAPER: ☹ Color Intrigue Eyeliner *($16)* wins points for being an automatic, retractable pencil with an easy-glide application, but because it stays creamy you'll find that it fades and smears easily. All of the shades have a slight to strong metallic finish, which can be a fun departure, though perhaps too distracting for day-to-day wear. If you decide to try this, it works best to create a smoky eye, rather than a long-lasting line.

☺ **Smoky Eyes Powder Pencil** *($16)* is definitely powdery, and best used to draw a thick line that you then smudge for a smoky appearance; otherwise this will smudge on its own. It needs routine sharpening but applies without pulling or tugging—always a plus.

☹ **Dual Perfection Brow Shaper and Eyeliner** *($17)* has a dry, grainy texture and is meant to be used wet, yet once dry the powder tends to flake. There are much easier, longer-lasting ways to shape and define the eyebrow and line the eye.

LIPSTICK, LIP GLOSS, AND LIPLINER: ✓☺ $$$ Color Intrigue Lipstick *($18.50)* comes in almost two dozen shades, each with beguiling names such as Seduction, Entrapment, and Drama. The color selection favors bolder, shimmer-infused colors, and includes some decadent reds and rich browns. As for the lipstick itself, it is creamy-smooth without feeling a bit slick or greasy. This is one of the few creamier lipsticks that won't immediately creep into lines around the mouth, and it sets to a semi-matte finish that allows for reasonably long wear (it helps that these lipsticks have lots of pigment, too!).

✓☺ **$$$ Ceramide Plump Perfect Lipstick** *($21.50)* contains a tiny amount of palmitoyl pentapeptide, not enough to plump lips (though even a large amout of this peptide lacks reliable research confirming its plumping prowess). Despite that letdown, there's no denying that this is a remarkable cream lipstick. The colors are riveting, the texture sublime, and the non-greasy, non-slippery finish lasts longer than many other creamy lipsticks. As an added bonus, the formula is rich in ceramides and antioxidants—a rarity in lipstick formulas at any price.

☺ **$$$ Exceptional Lipstick** *($18.50)* is a great name for what is a standard, but good, creamy lipstick. These all tend to have a slight to strong glossy finish and enough stain to allow for longer wear. The color range is smaller than ever due to the newer (and better) Color Intrigue Lipstick above.

☺ **High Shine Lip Gloss** *($15)* doesn't distinguish itself as a "must-have" lip gloss, but it's a workable option with a medium-thick texture and slightly sticky finish. The sheer shades are infused with sparkles, and luckily they don't make lips feel grainy as the moisturizing effect wears off.

☺ **Lip Definer** *($15)* is an automatic, nonretractable pencil that goes on smoothly and sets to a semi-matte finish that does a reasonable job of keeping lipstick from feathering into lines around the mouth.

☺ **Smooth Line Lip Pencil** *($15)* is a standard, needs-sharpening pencil that slides over lips without tugging or skipping. It is more creamy than greasy, and would have been rated higher if routine sharpening weren't required. Arden included a lip brush on the opposite end of the pencil, and it's surprisingly good.

☹ **Eight Hour Cream Lip Protectant Stick SPF 15** *($16)* won't protect lips from the sun's UVA rays because it lacks any of the UVA-protecting ingredients of titanium dioxide, zinc oxide, avobenzone, Tinosorb, or Mexoryl SX. In addition, the sheer colors can't provide the physical-type block that opaque lipsticks offer, so this product is not recommended. ☹ **Crystal Clear Lip Gloss** *($14)* is a very thick, sticky gloss that is flavored with spearmint, which tastes nice but can be irritating for the lips.

MASCARA: ✓☺ $$$ Defining Mascara *($17)* applies cleanly and makes lashes dramatically long, but it takes a while to build the lashes. Clumping is minimal, and if thickness isn't your major goal, this is highly recommended.

☺ **$$$ Double Density Maximum Volume Mascara** *($18)* is a mascara whose name conflicts with the actual results you'll notice. This isn't a poor mascara—far from it. But if your definition of "dramatically" thickened lashes is textbook, you'll see that this mascara is primarily about clump-free lengthening. You will get some thickness, with effort, but not an effect most people would call dramatic. This mascara is worth trying if your expectations are not as lofty as Arden's claims.

☹ **$$$ Two-Brush Mascara** *($17)* must be for those who can't decide what type of mascara brush they prefer. This dual-ended mascara features a regular-size spiral brush that allows for some average lengthening (but little else), and a small, short-bristled brush that allows you to reach every lash while building considerable length and some thickness. Guess which side I preferred! Most women will prefer one side to the other, which means you're paying top dollar for half a mascara—and who wants to do that?

☹ **Lash Optimizer Primer with Conditioners** *($14)* contains hydrated silica as a main ingredient. That's not a bad thing, but since this is absorbent by nature, it negates any conditioniong benefit stated in the product name. This ends up being another superfluous lash primer; it makes very little difference if you are already using an outstanding mascara (and if you aren't, why not?) and a slightly discernible difference with average mascaras. The concept of lash primers (or anything primer-related) appeals to many women; if a lash primer is what you want, consider Smashbox's Layer Lash Primer ($16), which produces good results and really is conditioning.

FACE AND BODY ILLUMINATING/SHIMMER PRODUCTS: ☺ **$$$ Sheer Lights Illuminating Pen** *($22)* is sort of a concealer/shimmer hybrid. Housed in a click pen with a built-in brush applicator is a smooth-textured liquid that blends well (it has enough slip for movement but not so much that you can't control where the shine goes) and dries to a matte (in feel only) finish with subtle shine. Three shades are available, with the yellow-toned Natural and pink-toned Soft being preferred over the orange-toned Warm. It's a practical way to softly illuminate or highlight certain features.

☹ **$$$ Sheer Lights Illuminating Tinted Moisturizer SPF 15** *($27)* leaves your skin vulnerable to UVA damage because it does not contain the UVA-protecting ingredients of titanium dioxide, zinc oxide, avobenzone, Tinosorb, or Mexoryl SX. That's a shame, too, because this sheer, tinted moisturizer with soft shimmer comes in stable packaging and has an antioxidant-rich formula that's ideal for normal to dry skin. Each of the four shades veers toward being too pink or peach, but the sheerness negates this fact.

BRUSHES: Professional application tools aren't this line's strong point, which may explain why their brushes are neither displayed nor advertised. The ☹ **Eye Brush #1** *($35)* and ☹ **Multipurpose Brush #3** *($20)* are decent options, but not worth considering over the impressive (if for nothing more than the number of choices) from M.A.C.

SPECIALTY PRODUCTS: ☹ **$$$ Lip-Fix Creme** *($19.50)* is supposed to prevent lipstick from feathering. Packaged in a tube, it goes on like a moisturizer and must dry before you put on your lipstick, which is not convenient for touch-ups during the day. Anti-feathering products that come in lipstick or lip-liner forms mean there's no waiting between applications, and you don't need to remove what you have on to reapply more—and those options make Arden's version less enticing. ☹ **Eye-Fix Primer** *($19)* is supposed to be a sheer cream for the eyelid to prevent makeup creasing; it's basically water, silicone, talc, and wax. Forget this boring, superfluous product and just use the Flawless Finish Concealer above, which would work as well, if not better, than this product.

ERNO LASZLO

ERNO LASZLO AT-A-GLANCE

Strengths: One good toner; some good moisturizers; pH-correct AHA product; tinted moisturizer with sunscreen; workable concealer, powders, and powder blush.

Weaknesses: Expensive; the majority of products contain one or more considerably irritating ingredients; basic skin-care regimen revolves around using drying bar soap and alcohol-laden toners; how one splashes their face with water has nothing to do with good skin care; the TranspHuse line; jar packaging.

For more information about Erno Laszlo, call (888) 352-7956 or visit www.ernolaszlo.com or www.Beautypedia.com.

ERNO LASZLO SKIN CARE

ERNO LASZLO TRANSPHUSE PRODUCTS

☺ **$$$ TranspHuse Eye** *($70 for 0.5 ounce)* contains some potent antioxidants for skin, but their benefit is diminished because of the jar packaging chosen for this moisturizer. It's an option for dry skin around the eye or anywhere on the face, but for the money, this product should have packaging that keeps its pricier light- and air-sensitive ingredients stable.

☹ **TranspHuse Night Serum** *($165 for 1 ounce)* is mostly water and film-forming agent, and doesn't impress by including far more preservatives than beneficial ingredients for skin, all of which are in short supply, while they should be front and center in a product costing so much. This product also contains lavender oil, which is irritating to skin and can cause cell death, and a preservative (methylisothiazolinone) that is contraindicated for use in leave-on products because of its irritation potential.

☹ **TranspHuse Topical** *($128 for 1 ounce)* is one of the cornerstone products of what Laszlo refers to as their "Surgiceuticals" line of products. However, nothing in any of the TranspHuse products replaces or even mildly approximates the results possible from in-office procedures such as Botox or dermal fillers. TranspHuse Topical is a water- and silicone-based lotion that contains some good (and a few unique) antioxidants, but the clear bottle packaging demands protection from light to keep them stable. Of more concern is the inclusion of the irritating menthol derivative menthoxypropanediol. Its tingle may make you think something wrinkle-relaxing is happening, but it's just trickery without a benefit.

☹ **TranspHuse Lip pHixative** *($48 for 0.12 ounce)* contains the irritating menthol derivative ethyl menthane carboxamide, and is not recommended. If you want to plump lips with such ingredients, you can do so without having to spend this much money (sucking on a peppermint has the same effect), just keep in mind that the effect is temporary—meaning minutes not hours—and doesn't approach what medically performed lip injections can accomplish.

☹ **TranspHuse pHixation** *($72 for 0.06 ounce)* contains some very good ingredients to support skin and help it appear smoother. Things go south not only because of overblown claims of targeting deep lines and wrinkles, but also owing to the inclusion of two potent menthol derivatives. How these irritants are supposed to be the equivalent of cosmetic corrective procedures is a good question, but this gives you some idea of what a waste of time and money these products are.

OTHER ERNO LASZLO PRODUCTS

☹ **Active pHelityl Oil, Pre-Cleansing Treatment for Dry to Slightly Oily Skin** *($36 for 6.8 ounces)* is absolutely the wrong product for someone with slightly oily skin. It's a blend of mineral and plant oils, most of which are beneficial for dry to very dry skin, and all of them are capable of dissolving makeup. The inclusion of irritating chaulmoogra oil is disappointing and makes using plain mineral oil or olive oil preferred, but only if your skin is dry to very dry.

☺ **$$$ Active pHelityl Two-In-One Cleanser, for Dry and Slightly Dry Skin** *($39 for 3.3 ounces)* claims to be the ultimate cleanser for dry to slightly dry skin, but the only thing ultimate is the price. Considering both size and price, this ranks as one of the most expensive cleansers in this book. However, it is a good water-soluble option for all skin types except very dry. The talked-up botanicals and fruit extracts are present in microscopic amounts, and don't justify the cost.

☹ **Active pHelityl Soap, for Dry and Slightly Dry Skin** *($32 for a 6-ounce bar)* is a standard, tallow-based bar soap that contains sulfated castor oil, which makes it even more drying.

☹ **Beta Wash, for Blemish-Prone Skin** *($34 for 6.8 ounces)* lists sodium C14-16 olefin sulfonate as the main detergent cleansing agent, which makes it too drying for all skin types. Even with a gentler cleansing base, the peppermint oil and menthol in here are overly irritating for any skin type.

☹ **HydrapHel Cleansing Bar, for Extremely Dry Skin** *($32 for a 6-ounce bar)* is an incredibly standard, shockingly priced bar soap that is too drying for all skin types. Someone with extremely dry skin will find this soap distinctly problematic.

☹ **Sea Mud Soap, for Normal, Slightly Oily and Oily Skin** *($32 for a 6-ounce bar)* contains mud in the form of silt, but that doesn't help oily skin when it's combined with standard-issue bar soap ingredients and fragrant irritants such as eugenol.

☹ **Special Skin Soap, for Oily and Extremely Oily Skin** *($32 for a 6-ounce bar)* combines drying soap ingredients, and adds insult to injury by including the extremely irritating detergent cleansing agent sodium lauryl sulfate. This is double trouble for any skin type, including extremely oily skin.

☹ **Multi-pHase Makeup Remover, for All Skin Types** *($32 for 4 ounces)* contains several irritating ingredients, including a significant amount of arnica, ivy, and horsetail. Performance-wise, water- and silicone-based makeup removers from drugstore lines work just as efficiently without the irritants.

☹ **Conditioning Preparation, for Oily to Extremely Oily Skin** *($32 for 6.8 ounces)* is mostly alcohol and resorcinol, a very drying topical disinfectant that is rarely used for acne treatment anymore. Plus, suspending it in alcohol, as it is here, makes it devastating for any skin type. If you want red and irritated skin, this is the product to choose.

☹ **Controlling Lotion, PM Oil Control for Slightly Dry and Normal Skin** *($45 for 4 ounces)* contains glycolic, lactic, and salicylic acids and has a pH of 2.6, which is a bit low and can result in irritation. That wouldn't be terrible except that the irritation comes without the benefit of the AHAs and BHA, since there is barely enough of them in here to have any effect on skin.

☹ **Extra Controlling Lotion, PM Oil Control for Slightly Oily to Extremely Oily Skin** *($45 for 4 ounces)* is similar to but more silicone-laden than the Controlling Lotion, PM Oil Control product above, and the same review applies. Both the regular and Extra Controlling Lotions contain rosemary oil, which is irritating and won't make skin less oily.

☹ **Heavy Controlling Lotion, PM Oil Control for Slightly Oily to Extremely Oily Skin** *($34 for 6.8 ounces)* is mostly water, alcohol, silica, and absorbent minerals. It will promote a powdery, matte finish but at the expense of drying and irritating skin.

😐 **$$$ HydrapHel Skin Supplement, Freshener for Extremely Dry and Dry Skin** *($32 for 6.8 ounces)* is the only Laszlo toner someone with dry skin should consider. This alcohol- and irritant-free toner is a good change of pace from the pathetic assortment of irritating toners in this line, but it's still a boring formulation that lacks any state-of-the-art ingredients for dry skin.

☹ **Light Controlling Lotion, Toner for Slightly Dry to Oily Skin** *($32 for 6.8 ounces)* lists alcohol as the second ingredient, which makes it a problem for any skin type.

☹ **Regular Controlling Lotion, PM Oil Control for Slightly Dry and Normal Skin** *($34 for 6.8 ounces)* will regularly irritate skin thanks to the amount of alcohol. Also, the mix of absorbent ingredients and glycerin is strange, because the absorbents prevent the glycerin from moisturizing the skin.

☹ **Sea Mud Two-In-One Cleanser, for Normal to Oily Skin** *($39 for 3.3 ounces)* is a below-standard scrub because it contains the irritating menthol derivative menthyl lactate. Sea mud (present in this product as silt) is not the answer for normal to oily skin, though it can have absorbent properties when left on skin for a brief period.

☺ **$$$ Advanced Retexturizing Complex** *($97 for 1.7 ounces)* is an effective option for an AHA product, and the pH of 3.4 permits exfoliation to occur. The chief AHA in here is gluconolactone, but it's present only at about 3% and it isn't as effective as many other AHA products that don't come with such a prohibitive price tag. Still, this is an option for all skin types and contains some good antioxidants.

😐 **$$$ Active pHelityl Cream, PM Moisturizer for Slightly Dry Skin** *($44 for 1.75 ounces)* is a very basic, jar-packaged emollient moisturizer for dry skin. Considering the price, there really isn't anything worth getting excited about.

😐 **$$$ Antioxidant Complex for Eyes** *($48 for 0.5 ounce)* is a gel-textured moisturizer that cannot make good on its claims that botanical extracts can lighten dark circles or reduce puffiness under the eyes. It's fine if your eye area needs lightweight hydration, but the effectiveness of the few antioxidants will be compromised by clear packaging.

☹ **Antioxidant Mattifying Complex SPF 15, for Normal to Extremely Oily Skin** *($59 for 3 ounces)* provides UVA protection via an in-part avobenzone sunscreen, but the base formula contains enough witch hazel to be irritating for skin. Further, the thickening agents and lack of absorbent ingredients means oily skin won't stay matte for long.

☹ **Antioxidant Moisture Complex SPF 15, for All Skin Types** *($62 for 3 ounces)* lacks the UVA-protecting ingredients of titanium dioxide, zinc oxide, avobenzone, Tinosorb, or Mexoryl SX, and is not recommended.

😐 **$$$ C10** *($66 for 1 ounce)* claims to contain 10% vitamin C, but I doubt the amount is that high (it's more likely 5% to 7%). Even with more vitamin C (which isn't necessarily better), the jar packaging won't keep it or the other antioxidants in this moisturizer stable once it's opened.

😐 **$$$ HydrapHel Emulsion SPF 15, for Extremely Dry and Dry Skin** *($56 for 2.1 ounces)* has an in-part avobenzone sunscreen going for it, but is otherwise an unremarkable formula whose antioxidants will lose their potency due to the jar packaging.

😐 **$$$ HydrapHel Intensive, for Extremely Dry and Dry Skin** *($62 for 2.1 ounces)* is loaded with substantial emollients for its intended skin type, but what a shame the vitamin E and other antioxidants are compromised by jar packaging.

😐 **$$$ Intensive Decollete Cream SPF 20** *($84 for 2.1 ounces)* contains an in-part avobenzone sunscreen in a nonaqueous, silicone base. It claims to lighten sun spots and hyperpigmentation, but the amount of kojic acid that could help with that is minuscule and the jar packaging won't keep this air- and light-sensitive ingredient stable.

☹ **Moisture Firming Throat Cream** *($49 for 2 ounces)* contains fragrant geranium and cypress oils in amounts very likely to be irritating. Angelica extract is also a problem for skin, and none of this is the least bit firming.

😐 **$$$ Ocu-pHel Emollient, Nourishing Eye Treatment** *($68 for 0.53 ounce)* has, despite a strange name, a basic but good emollient formula for slightly dry to dry skin anywhere on the face. It is unfortunate that, once again, jar packaging limits the effectiveness of the antioxidants.

☺ **$$$ pHelitone Eye Treatment** *($57 for 0.5 ounce)* is a very good moisturizer for normal to dry skin anywhere on the face. The plant extracts are non-irritating, though it would be better if the antioxidant content were higher. This does contain coloring agents.

☹ **pHelityl Cream, PM Moisturizer for Normal Skin** *($62 for 2.1 ounces)* is a mundane moisturizer that is overpriced for what you get, especially considering that many of its fragrance components (including eugenol and coumarin) are sensitizing.

☹ **pHelityl Lotion, for Slightly Dry to Slightly Oily Skin** *($54 for 3 ounces)* contains chaulmoogra oil and comfrey extract, both of which are problem ingredients for skin that lack evidence of any topical benefits (Source: www.naturaldatabase.com). This product supposedly increases skin's oxygen uptake, but all that would mean is more free-radical damage (and why include antioxidants in a product meant to help skin retain more oxygen?).

☹ **pHelityl Lotion SPF 15** *($57 for 3 ounces)* lists avobenzone for sufficient UVA protection, but contains chaulmoogra oil (listed as taraktogenos kurzi seed oil), which makes this too potentially irritating for all skin types.

😐 **$$$ pHormula No. 3-9** *($95 for 1 ounce)* is said to be Erno Laszlo's prescription for perfect skin. Perfection sounds great, but this ends up being similar to most of the other ordinary emollient moisturizers this line offers. It contains mostly water, Vaseline, silicone, emu oil, silicone polymer, slip agent, wax, and vitamin E. The healing ingredient alluded to is *Calophyllum tacamahaca* seed oil. Also known as tamanu, this oil comes from the nut of the laurelwood tree. There is no substantiated research proving this oil can heal wounded skin (and, lest we forget, wrinkles are not wounds), though there is research showing that topical application can cause contact dermatitis (Source: *Contact Dermatitis*, October 2004, pages 216–217).

😐 **$$$ R.E.M. Intensive Night Therapy, for Slightly Dry Skin** *($97 for 2.1 ounces)* is a moisturizer whose jar packaging won't allow its many antioxidant ingredients to repair, energize, and moisturize skin (that's what the R.E.M. stands for). However, not all antioxidants are moisturizing by themselves, and none of them will remain stable on exposure to air. This otherwise is a ho-hum moisturizer for dry skin.

☹ **R.E.M. SPF 30 Intensive Day Therapy, for All Dry Skins** *($74 for 3 ounces)* features avobenzone for UVA protection (listed by its chemical name butyl methoxydibenzoylmethane), but contains enough chaulmoogra oil to make it too irritating for all skin types.

☹ **Timeless Skin Age Preventative Treatment, for All Skin Types** *($78 for 1 ounce)* has some state-of-the-art ingredients, but ends up being a very expensive way to irritate skin because it contains tangerine, mandarin orange, and basil oils.

😐 **$$$ Total Skin Revitalizer Facial Hydration Enhancer, for All Skin Types** *($60 for 1 ounce)* is a lightweight moisturizer that contains some good skin-identical ingredients, but several of the fragrance components can be sensitizing, making this a less effective option.

☺ $$$ **Total Skin Revitalizer for Eyes** *($52 for 0.5 ounce)* is a good emollient moisturizer for dry skin anywhere on the face. The non-irritating plant extracts outnumber the potentially problematic ones, and it contains a nice complement of antioxidants and soothing agents.

😐 **$$$ Hydra-Therapy Skin Vitality Treatment, Two Phase Moisture Mask for All Skin Types** *($38 for 4 applications of each phase)* is a two-part mask. Phase 1 consists of water, film-forming agent, skin-identical ingredients, and preservatives, while Phase 2 is just absorbent minerals and pigment. It's a gimmicky product with minimal benefit, but can be an OK mask for oily or breakout-prone skin, since it doesn't contain any ingredients that aggravate blemishes or clog pores.

☹ **Sea Mud Exfoliating Mask** *($42 for 3.5 ounces)* contains a lot of alcohol along with lesser, but still offensive, amounts of peppermint oil and the fragrance component farnesol, making this too irritating for all skin types.

☹ **Targeted Blemish Treatment** *($27 for 0.5 ounce)* hits the target when it comes to causing irritation and making inflamed blemishes look worse because it contains several irritating ingredients. Alcohol, witch hazel, peppermint oil, camphor, and cinnamon do not make for clear, happy skin.

☹ **Timeless Concentrate Mask** *($54 for 1 ounce)* lists alcohol and polyvinyl alcohol as the second and third ingredients and also contains several irritating citrus oils, making it a problem for all skin types. Without those ingredients, this could have been a very good mask for dry skin.

☹ **Total Blemish Treatment** *($82 for 2 ounces)* is a ridiculously priced BHA product whose 1% salicylic acid content cannot exfoliate because the pH is too high. It's also not good news that cinnamon bark and arnica are on hand to cause irritation, while not being helpful for blemish-prone skin.

☹ **Total Face & Body Protection SPF 30** *($42 for 7 ounces)* includes avobenzone for UVA protection but also contains menthol, which only serves to irritate skin.

ERNO LASZLO MAKEUP

FOUNDATION: ☺ **$$$ Tinted Treatment SPF 15** *($38)* contains a minimum of treatment ingredients, so it's not as state-of-the-art as the word treatment implies. However, the in-part avobenzone sunscreen is great and this has a light yet creamy texture appropriate for normal to dry skin. It blends well and provides sheer coverage and a natural, slightly moist finish. The six shades are mostly neutral—only Tan and Dark stand out for their slightly peach and orange tones.

😐 **$$$ Absolute Finish Mousse Foundation SPF 15** *($47)* lacks the UVA-protecting ingredients of avobenzone, titanium dioxide, zinc oxide, Tinosorb, or Mexoryl SX, which is really disappointing because it would otherwise be a superb foundation. The silicone-based formula is mousse-like but not as airy as the name implies. It glides over skin and sets to a silky matte finish capable of light to medium coverage. The range of ten shades is outstanding—not a bad option in the bunch. The only weak point is the insufficient sunscreen; this is otherwise recommended for those with normal to oily skin willing to pair it with a separate product to provide the necessary UVA protection.

☹ **Regular Normalizer Shake-It** *($40)* is Laszlo's long-standing foundation for controlling oily skin, but the strong (and irritating) alcohol base means it is difficult to apply, can streak, provides minimal coverage, and dries out the skin. There are dozens of better foundations for someone with very oily skin concerned with shine control.

CONCEALER: ☺ $$$ Perfect Concealer for Face & Eyes *($34)* is almost perfect. Its beautifully creamy texture provides remarkable coverage without looking heavy or thick, but the cream finish means creasing into lines under the eye is inevitable. If you're willing to tolerate that and do touch-ups during the day, this is recommended. The three shades are great, with Shade 1 being just slightly pink. This type of concealer is not recommended for use over blemishes, but is ideal for concealing redness from rosacea.

POWDER: ☺ $$$ Controlling Face Powder Loose *($38)* and **☺ $$$ Controlling Face Powder Pressed** *($34)* are both talc-based, and have supremely soft textures and a natural finish on the skin. Each comes in three very good neutral shades. Laszlo used to recommend these powders for oily skin, but they are now correctly indicated for use by those with dry skin. **☺ $$$ Duo-pHase Face Powder Loose** *($38)* and **☺ $$$ Duo-pHase Face Powder Pressed** *($34)* have lighter, drier, talc-based textures and a stronger matte finish than the Controlling powders above, making them preferred for normal to oily skin. Each version comes in three soft, neutral shades that do not have a trace of shine. **☺ $$$ Multi-pHase Bronzer** *($38)* combines several bronze, gold, and tan tones in one mosaic pressed-powder compact. Sweeping a brush over the powder allows it to come off as one color (a warm golden tan) on skin. It's silky-smooth rather than dusty, and provides a satinlike finish with subtle shine. Not a bad option for fair to medium skin, but also one that's overpriced for what you get.

BLUSH: ☺ $$$ Multi-pHase Blusher *($38)* has the same multiple color and mosaic pattern as the Multi-pHase Bronzer above, only this product comes in one blush tone that mixes pale to medium pinks with a touch of peach and rose. The result on cheeks is a soft, warm rose color that applies evenly. Whether or not to spend this much money on powder blush really comes down to how much you like the color, but it's one you've seen before in almost every cosmetics line, price notwithstanding.

ESTEE LAUDER

ESTEE LAUDER AT-A-GLANCE

Strengths: Lots of Paula's Picks; some of the most state-of-the-art moisturizers and serums around; excellent sunscreens and self-tanning products; some good cleansers, toners, and makeup removers; excellent retinol product; several above-standard self-tanning lotions; several categories of makeup excel, including some extraordinary foundations (that include shades for darker skin tones), concealers, powders, blush, and eyeshadows; a mostly good selection of eye, brow, and lip pencils; their long-wearing lip color and some of the lipsticks are supremely good; well-organized tester units and, usually, well-trained counter personnel.

Weaknesses: Several items are highly fragranced; incomplete and/or problematic products for anyone battling blemishes; no effective AHA or BHA products; many of the Re-Nutriv products are priced too high given similar, less-expensive options from Lauder; some of the sunscreens and foundations with sunscreen lack sufficient UVA protection; the mascaras; the brushes aren't on par with those from other Lauder-owned lines, such as Bobbi Brown or M.A.C.; some superfluous specialty products and problem pencils; jar packaging.

For more information about Estee Lauder, call (877) 311-3883 or visit www.esteelauder.com or www.Beautypedia.com.

ESTEE LAUDER SKIN CARE

ESTEE LAUDER ADVANCED NIGHT REPAIR PRODUCTS

✓☺ **$$$ Advanced Night Repair Concentrate Recovery Boosting Treatment** *($85 for 1 ounce)* serves as a partner product to Lauder's enduring Advanced Night Repair serum. This concentrated version (supposedly with five times the amount of patented recovery complex than the original Advanced Night Repair) is meant to be used for three weeks, after which you revert to your usual routine of applying original Advanced Night Repair. Considering that the price for the Concentrate is double that of the original Advanced Night Repair, you may wonder if this allegedly more potent version is worth the upgrade. It turns out that the formulas are similar in some ways, but the differences are notable enough to definitely make Advanced Night Repair Concentrate the superior product, and not only for three weeks. Its silicone content gives the Concentrate a silkier texture than the original, but the big difference is in the larger amount of antioxidants Lauder packed into the Concentrate version. This is enough of a difference to consider the original antiquated. Whether or not the extras are worth the money is up to you. Clinique's Repairwear Deep Wrinkle Concentrate for Face and Eye ($55 for 1.4 ounces) is just as well-formulated, as is Estee Lauder's Perfectionist CP+ ($55 for 1 ounce), reviewed below.

A major ingredient in the Advanced Night Repair Concentrate and in the original Advanced Night Repair is bifida ferment lysate. The bifida portion refers to bifidobacteria, a strain of bacteria found in the human body and believed to provide immune protection and prevent gastrointestinal problems (in other words, it's a friendly strain of bacteria). How does it relate to skin care? Claims made for this ingredient are that it can do for the face what it does for the body, enhance the immune system and decrease bad bacteria. There is no published information establishing that to be true. Oral consumption of this bacteria (it is often present in yogurt and can be purchased in supplement form) has a couple of studies that show it can be of benefit in helping with infant eczema, but that's about it when it comes to skin (Source: www.naturaldatabase.com).

😐 **$$$ Advanced Night Repair Eye Recovery Complex** *($48 for 0.5 ounce)*. The kicker with this moisturizer is that it claims to address pretty much every eye-area skin-care woe you can think of, from puffiness to dark circles, wrinkles, and environmental damage. It sounds like the ultimate choice for eyes, but we've all heard this song before with countless other Lauder eye products, from Uncircle to Unline to Eyezone, along with a vast selection from the ten other lines under Lauder's ownership. Still, skin-repairing claims aside, this is indeed a very good, silicone-based moisturizer that would take good care of dry skin anywhere on the face. It contains mostly water, silicones, emollients, thickeners, anti-irritants, antioxidants, skin-identical ingredients, vitamins, film former, and preservatives. Unfortunately, the antioxidants lose potency once this jar-packaged product is opened.

😐 **$$$ Advanced Night Repair Protective Recovery Complex** *($46.50 for 1 ounce)* is the original Night Repair product, and although this water-based serum has some very good ingredients for all skin types, it just isn't as exciting as Lauder's superior Advanced Night Repair Concentrate Recovery Boosting Treatment or their Perfectionist CP+. Lauder recommends it as an essential for all skin types, but it isn't—at least not anymore.

ESTEE LAUDER CLEAR DIFFERENCE PRODUCTS

☺ **$$$ Clear Difference Deep Pore Purifying Facial** *($21 for 2.5 ounces)* is a standard, overpriced clay mask that differs little from almost any other clay-based mask. It is worth considering because it does not contain irritants and will absorb excess oil while smoothing skin, but the price for this benefit (when dozens of less-expensive products offer the same thing) makes this needlessly costly despite the positives.

☹ **Clear Difference Targeted Blemish Gel** *($16 for 0.5 ounce)*. Sigh! Here is another anti-blemish product that breaks no new ground and instead is the same old, same old combination of alcohol and irritants. This product features 0.5% salicylic acid as its active ingredient, but that concentration is only minimally effective against blemishes. And along with that issue, the pH of the gel is too high for it to work as an exfoliant. Lauder somewhat distinguishes this product from the general run-of-the-mill blemish products by including some skin-soothing agents, but with the base of alcohol and witch hazel here their benefit to skin is lost.

☹ **Clear Difference Advanced Oil-Control Hydrator** *($32.50 for 1.7 ounces)* lists alcohol as the second ingredient, and that makes this otherwise fine moisturizer a problem for all skin types. This product does not contain ingredients that can keep skin "hydrated inside, perfectly matte outside." Rather, the predominance of alcohol keeps the moisturizing ingredients from doing their job. How unfortunate, because the price is downright affordable (for a Lauder moisturizer, anyway) and this contains some excellent skin-identical ingredients (though few antioxidants). Clinique's Moisture In Control Oil-Free Lotion ($32.50 for 1.7 ounces) costs more, but offers a superior formula with a similar lightweight texture that those with normal to oily or combination skin would appreciate.

ESTEE LAUDER DAYWEAR PRODUCTS

😐 **$$$ DayWear Plus Multi Protection Anti-Oxidant Creme SPF 15, for Normal/Combination Skin** *($38 for 1.7 ounces)* leaves out the petrolatum found in the DayWear Plus for Dry Skin below and instead uses silicones for a lighter-feeling, creamy emulsion. This formula is indeed suitable for normal to combination skin, and contains an in-part avobenzone sunscreen. Unfortunately, it is packaged in a clear jar, which will quickly negate the benefits of including such an inspired variety of antioxidants. This does contain fragrance.

😐 **$$$ DayWear Plus Multi Protection Anti-Oxidant Creme SPF 15, for Dry Skin** *($38 for 1.7 ounces)* also has an in-part avobenzone sunscreen that would be an excellent choice as a daytime moisturizer for dry skin were it not for jar packaging that limits the long-term effectiveness of the antioxidants. It does contain some good skin-identical ingredients and the familiar DayWear cucumber fragrance, but what a shame the antioxidants won't last long.

✓☺ **$$$ DayWear Plus Multi Protection Anti-Oxidant Lotion SPF 15, for Oily Skin** *($38 for 1.7 ounces)* has a fluid, non-greasy texture and a lightweight feel on the skin. This is not a matte-finish sunscreen, and there's no way to guarantee it won't cause breakouts (this is true of all sunscreens), but it is worth auditioning if you have oily skin and have not been able to find a foundation with sunscreen that works for you. The packaging will definitely keep the many antioxidants stable much longer than the two DayWear Creams above, and this also contains some intriguing cell-communicating ingredients.

✓☺ **$$$ DayWear Plus Multi Protection Anti-Oxidant Moisturizer Sheer Tint Release Formula SPF 15, for All Skin Types** *($38 for 1.7 ounces)* has an in-part avobenzone sunscreen, which makes for great UVA protection from this lightly emollient lotion. The soft tan tint looks great over a variety of skin tones, and is a believable color for those with fair skin if they want to pull off a slightly tan look. Coverage is sparse, and, like the other DayWear Plus products, this includes a nice array of antioxidants and some cell-communicating ingredients. Lauder's opaque tube packaging for this product ensures that the antioxidants remain stable. Although the sunscreen is the same, the base formulation is different from those of the other DayWear Plus products, and is best for normal to slightly dry or slightly oily skin.

☺ **$$$ DayWear Plus Multi-Protection Anti-Oxidant Lotion SPF 30, for Normal/ Combination Skin** *($38 for 1.7 ounces)* is another well-formulated, well-packaged sunscreen from Estee Lauder. The active ingredients include titanium dioxide and zinc oxide for UVA protection, and the lightweight lotion texture slips on without a trace of the white cast typical of mineral sunscreens (the formula includes synthetic sunscreens, too). This product is loaded with antioxidants, cell-communicating ingredients, and ingredients that mimic the structure and function of healthy skin. The only drawback is the fragrance, which is stronger than it needs to be. For a daytime moisturizer available at the department store, this runs circles around what Lancome, Clarins, and Chanel have to offer in the way of sunscreens, and Lauder's price point offers better protection for your budget as well. Another job well done, and it is indeed appropriate for normal to combination skin types.

ESTEE LAUDER FUTURE PERFECT PRODUCTS

😐 **$$$ Future Perfect Anti-Wrinkle Radiance Creme SPF 15, for Dry Skin** *($45 for 1 ounce)* is being marketed as Lauder's high-tech answer to the dilemma of aging skin. Take a look at these claims: "Estee Lauder Research cracks the code of visible aging to dramatically change the destiny of your skin.... Helps re-ignite skin's natural age-fighting ability.... The look of lines and wrinkles is significantly reduced." Does this mean Lauder can empty its counter and discontinue all their other products that have yet to "crack the code of visible aging"? Obviously not, because they continually launch new ones, and the old ones are rarely discontinued.

This supposedly "futuristic" moisturizer uses what Lauder refers to as cell vector technology. Supposedly, these vectors (guides) can recognize and immediately respond to skin and "the visible effects of its inherent deficiencies" to make "lines and wrinkles visibly retreat." Yet for all of this technical talk, what Lauder has produced is, in simple terms, an excellent in-part avobenzone sunscreen whose base formula is excellent for dry to very dry skin. A well-formulated, broad-spectrum sunscreen is the only true antiwrinkle product we have at our disposal. This is because sunscreens act on the skin to deflect or absorb ultraviolet light before it can damage skin, and that means all well-formulated sunscreens have cracked the code, not just Lauder's. What sunscreens cannot do is make lines and wrinkles go away, an idea that is certainly implied in the ad copy for this product.

It turns out that cell vector technology is less an intriguing formulary advantage and more a marketing concept to convince consumers that this is *the* anti-aging product to buy. Although the claims are a bit outlandish, the formula has some excellent attributes, but the antioxidants and other light-sensitive ingredients suffer from jar packaging. This contains a small amount of mica that leaves a soft shimmer on skin. If you decide to try this anyway, it's best for dry to very dry skin.

😐 **$$$ Future Perfect Anti-Wrinkle Radiance Creme SPF 15, for Normal/Combination Skin** *($45 for 1 ounce)* is a less emollient, lighter version of the Future Perfect Antiwrinkle Radiance Creme SPF 15, for Dry Skin, above, and the same basic comments apply. This is indeed appropriate for those with normal to combination skin, though someone with a very oily T-zone will likely find this product too rich. Another negative is the price, which makes it less likely that someone will use it liberally enough to provide effective sun protection. Plus, the jar packaging is disappointing given the number of antioxidants in this daytime moisturizer.

😐 **$$$ Future Perfect Anti-Wrinkle Radiance Eye Creme** *($42 for 0.5 ounce)* is a wonderfully rich, elegantly formulated eye cream whose only downfall is jar packaging that compromises the potency of the many antioxidants and other light- and air-sensitive ingredients. The mica and titanium dioxide provide a cosmetic brightening effect to soften the appearance of dark circles under the eye.

✓ 😊 **$$$ Future Perfect Anti-Wrinkle Radiance Lotion SPF 15, for Normal/Combination Skin** *($65 for 1.7 ounces)* is the lotion version of the Future Perfect Anti-Wrinkle Radiance Creme SPF 15, for Normal Combination Skin, above, and the same basic comments apply. Again, it's appropriate for normal to combination skin, but perhaps too rich (and the mica too shimmery) for someone with a very oily T-zone. And the price may make it less likely that someone will use it liberally enough to provide sufficient sun protection. Still, the packaging in this case will keep the state-of-the-art formula's antioxidants stable, and it is loaded with other skin-beneficial ingredients.

ESTEE LAUDER HYDRA COMPLETE PRODUCTS

😐 **$$$ Hydra Complete Multi-Level Moisture Creme, for Dry Skin** *($40 for 1.7 ounces)* purports to quench skin's deepest thirst thanks to its mineral-rich bio-water. That's the hook, but if you'll pardon the pun, it doesn't hold water—and if the bio-water is so good, why isn't it used in all the Lauder products?. Minerals aren't a must-have in skin-care items (they're far more beneficial for skin when consumed as part of a healthy diet), which leaves you with … water. It takes far more than water to treat "thirsty" skin; luckily, this moisturizer also has what it takes to make normal to dry skin look and feel better. The drawback is jar packaging, which hinders the effectiveness of the many antioxidants. It does contain some good cell-communicating ingredients.

😐 **$$$ Hydra Complete Multi-Level Moisture Eye Gel Creme** *($38.50 for 0.5 ounce)* is a silky, lightly hydrating, fragrance-free moisturizer that is suitable for normal to slightly dry skin anywhere on the face. It contains Lauder's usual assortment of antioxidants, soothing plant extracts, and plentiful skin-identical ingredients, but would be more worthy of its elite status without jar packaging. Contrary to claim, the algae extract in this product, while a good water-binding agent, cannot alleviate puffy eyes.

😐 **$$$ Hydra Complete Multi-Level Moisture Gel Creme, for Normal/Combination Skin** *($34 for 1.7 ounces)* has a supremely silky texture and is loaded with antioxidants—what a shame the jar packaging won't keep them stable once this product is opened! This is still worth considering by those with normal to oily skin because it contains some intriguing cell-communicating ingredients and impressive skin-identical ingredients (the neutral rating pertains to the problematic packaging).

✓ 😊 **$$$ Hydra Complete Multi-Level Moisture Lotion, for Normal/Combination Skin** *($40 for 1.7 ounces)* is similar to the Hydra Complete Multi-Level Moisture Gel Creme, for Normal/Combination Skin, above, except this has a lighter texture and packaging that will keep the air- and light-sensitive ingredients stable. Antioxidants are in good supply, as are cell-communicating ingredients, skin-identical ingredients, and ingredients that mimic the structure and function of healthy skin.

ESTEE LAUDER IDEALIST PRODUCTS

✓☺ **$$$ Idealist Refinishing Eye Serum** *($48 for 0.5 ounce)* is the complement to Lauder's top-selling Idealist Skin Refinisher reviewed below. The Eye Serum is similar to the original Idealist product, but the formula is updated to capitalize on the latest skin-care ingredients. Included in this water- and silicone-based gel-cream are long-proven emollients (petrolatum), several antioxidants (the packaging will keep them stable), state-of-the-art skin-identical ingredients, and anti-irritants. It won't minimize puffiness or significantly brighten the eye area, but it will protect skin and help it function more normally. This would be even better without the fragrance, but that's a minor complaint for such a thoughtfully formulated product. By the way, this can be used anywhere on the face—there is nothing in this product that makes it unique for the eye area.

☺ **$$$ Idealist Pore Minimizing Skin Refinisher** *($46.50 for 1 ounce)* is Lauder's all-in-one solution to problems such as large pores, flaky skin, redness, and, of course, fine lines. It launched in summer 2007 as a replacement for the company's original (and very popular) Idealist Skin Refinisher. What's the difference? Well, Lauder is now claiming that this product makes pores appear one-third smaller, instantly, and that this version contains three times more acetyl glucosamine than the original formula. It does indeed contain more acetyl glucosamine, but is that an advantage? Derived from sugar, acetyl glucosamine doesn't have known exfoliating properties (Lauder claims it helps unglue the bonds that hold dead skin cells to the surface, something a well-formulated AHA or BHA product accomplishes). Acetyl glucosamine's primary constituents are mucopolysaccharides and hyaluronic acid. Found in all parts of the skin, it has value as a water-binding agent and is effective (in high concentrations) for wound healing. There is also research (*Cellular-Molecular-Life-Science*, 53(2), February 1997, pages 131–140) showing that chitins (also known as chitosan, which is composed of acetyl glucosamine) can help in the complex process of wound healing. However, that is a few generations removed from acetyl glucosamine being included in a skin-care product. Procter & Gamble has published research on the skin-lightening effect of acetyl glucosamine when used at concentrations of 2% or more in combination with niacinamide (such as in their Olay Definity moisturizers), but although Lauder is likely using that amount, they left out niacinamide (Source: *Journal of Cosmetic Dermatology*, March 2007, pages 20–26).

There are some notable ingredients in Idealist Pore Minimizing Skin Refinisher, but in terms of making skin look better and pores appear smaller, it does so mostly by cosmetic trickery. For example, the strong silicone base instantly makes skin look smoother, so it reflects light better, and it can temporarily fill in large pores and superficial lines. Cosmetic pigments (iron oxides, mica, and titanium dioxide) provide a brightening effect, imparting a "glow" to your skin. Beyond the light show, plant-based anti-inflammatory ingredients help minimize minor redness and antioxidants such as green tea help keep skin protected from free-radical damage. What's not good news is the inclusion of lavender and orange along with the fragrance components limonene and linalool. They're present in a greater amount than in the original Idealist, and may be potentially irritating, which keeps this product from earning a Paula's Pick. If you decide to give this a go, it is best for normal to oily skin.

☺ **$$$ Idealist Micro-D Deep Thermal Refinisher** *($46 for 2.5 ounces)* is Estee Lauder's contribution to the category of topical scrubs that are alleged to mimic the effect of microdermabrasion. Many similar scrubs (including the Dermapolish Treatment Cream scrub from Lauder-owned Prescriptives) contain the conventional ingredient polyethylene (ground-up plastic) as the exfoliating agent, and so does this one. But this one also includes the inorganic salt calcium chloride, which is where the thermal part comes in. Lauder claims that the calcium chloride delivers a "detoxifying thermal action," which is "activated when Micro-D is applied to the skin. The process allows pores to open, preparing skin for detoxifying and refreshing action." Sidestepping the issue that pores cannot open (or close) like doors or windows, how can this simple salt detoxify them? What toxins are lurking in pores, anyway? No one has ever explained the never-ending myth that the skin or pores need to be purged of toxins. I'd like to learn the name of just one toxin!

The truth is our pores are not harboring toxins that require a product like this to expel them. What happens when calcium chloride is mixed with water (Lauder recommends using this product on damp skin) is called an exothermic reaction. That means a chemical reaction (in this case, between water and calcium chloride) that generates heat. However, other than a brief sensation of warmth, this process brings no benefit to the skin. It certainly does not detoxify the skin or aid in minimizing pores, any more than a warm day does. If it does anything, the warm sensation just leaves the impression that the product is "working." Instead, it is the scrub particles being massaged over the skin that loosen debris (dead skin cells and oil) from the surface of your pores, allowing it to be rinsed away. That will make skin feel smoother and look more even-toned, and can temporarily make pores smaller—but only because the buildup of dead skin cells and oil has been removed. Almost any topical scrub, including plain cornmeal, or even a washcloth can do this, while chemical exfoliants (such as glycolic and salicylic acids) surpass topical scrubs because they exfoliate more evenly and thoroughly without the mechanical abrasion.

Lauder has buffered the abrasive agents with silicones, and although this makes them more gentle on the skin, it can present some difficulty when you rinse the product. A small amount of jade powder is included, too, but these exotic additions don't add much to the results of Idealist Micro-D. It can add to the abrasiveness of the polyethylene and calcium chloride, but that isn't really necessary and can approach overkill if you use this scrub too often or too aggressively.

Overall, this is a pricey way to exfoliate, although if used with caution it can indeed produce silky-smooth skin. Idealist Micro-D would work best for normal to oily skin or slightly dry skin. Those with very dry skin would do better with a creamier scrub that does not contain calcium chloride, which can be a bit drying.

ESTEE LAUDER PERFECTIONIST PRODUCTS

☺ **$$$ Perfectionist Correcting Concentrate for Deeper Facial Lines/Wrinkles** *($42 for 0.11 ounce)* is packaged in a pen-style applicator with an angled tip that supposedly allows you to zero in on your most troublesome expression lines and wrinkles. You're likely wondering if what gets dispensed can really relax lines and reduce the look of wrinkles. Forget about the relaxing part, because nothing in this product is capable of that feat. Lauder uses acetyl hexapeptide-3, also known as argireline, for this alleged effect, but it has never been proven to work as claimed. Even Botox doesn't relax wrinkles when applied topically, as opposed to being injected.

This water- and silicone-based formula will help temporarily to smooth and fill in lines and wrinkles, making them look less apparent. It's a cosmetic effect, similar to what you get with lots of moisturizers. What's most exciting about this product is that it is jam-packed with ingredients that are beneficial to skin, including several antioxidants, cell-communicating ingredients, anti-irritants, and a plethora of ingredients that mimic the structure and function of healthy skin. So how come this Perfectionist product was not rated a Paula's Pick? In a word, alcohol.

Although not present in an amount significant enough to cause irritation, it's listed before the many state-of-the-art ingredients, an unwelcome blemish on an otherwise spotless formulation. Perfectionist Correcting Concentrate is best for normal to dry skin, and is fragrance-free.

☺ **$$$ Perfectionist Correcting Concentrate for Lip Lines** *($35 for 0.08 ounce)* is meant to be the product to correct any flaws around your lips. The claims are literally mouth-watering: "In as fast as 1 week, the fine lip lines around your mouth look remarkably reduced as our exclusive BioSync Complex™ quickly strengthens skin's suspension and amplifies natural collagen levels. By Month 1 and beyond, deep vertical lip lines look lifted away, helping redefine the contours around your lips so they appear fuller, softer, more sensual." A great story, but it's just mumbo jumbo—it never says anything substantive. Lauder is careful never to state that the vertical lines around the lips will be eliminated, removed, gone forever, or done away with. Rather, they will only *look* lifted away, an optical illusion at best and one that doesn't have to be structural. What does "amplifies natural collagen levels" mean anyway? Any moisturizer can help skin build collagen, so that isn't unique to this concoction. Like any moisturizer the effect is hardly unique and is bound to be short-lived unless you make a concerted effort to keep your mouth perfectly still all day long, which isn't realistic. The happy face rating pertains to this product's overall formulation as an aid to making skin around the lips look better, not to Lauder's claims.

✓☺ **$$$ Perfectionist [CP+] with Poly-Collagen Peptides Correcting Serum for Line/Wrinkles/Age Spots** *($55 for 1 ounce)* is another one of Lauder's "works like Botox" products, complete with the same absurd claim everyone else selling such products is using. "Now, triumph over wrinkles without toxins, lasers or injections. Estee Lauder Research boldly advances the fight against wrinkles—and now age spots—with our most comprehensive treatment ever." Before I discuss the formula, I want to mention that this product is not a substitute in any way, shape, or form for Botox, lasers, or any type of dermal filler. No topical cosmetic product is capable of attaining anywhere near the results obtainable from those medical corrective procedures.

Clearly, the desire for such a product is strong, or companies such as Lauder, L'Oreal, Lancome, Revlon, and a host of others wouldn't keep consumers' hopes alive with such claims as "it virtually immobilizes lines and wrinkles without affecting your natural facial expressions" or that their product can intercept "the cycle of irritation that can increase the depth and length of a wrinkle." These suggestions (which is what advertising of this nature always is: impression, not fact) are just that, and nothing more. If your lines were immobilized, your facial expressions would definitely be affected. Furthermore, deep wrinkles are not inherently caused by simple irritation, but rather by deep inflammation from cumulative unprotected sun exposure and myriad other factors that include things like hormone loss and cell senescence, to name a few.

So what's in this product that can allegedly smooth wrinkles without (eek!) resorting to needles or other medical procedures? The "CP" in the product's name stands for collagen peptides. According to information from Lauder, patent-pending "triple enzyme technology rushes" this collagen peptide complex to "even the most prominent wrinkles." Yet a patent has nothing to do with proof of efficacy, it is only about who else can use an ingredient or combination of ingredients related to a particular claim.

While there is much hope that peptides may help skin, they are easily broken down by enzymes, and that doesn't help get them to the cell. It all adds up to another dubious "treatment" product that isn't any more perfecting than those in Lauder's original, now-defunct Perfectionist incarnation.

Aside from the correcting claims, this silky formulation has numerous skin-identical ingredients and, further down the lengthy ingredient list, antioxidants that will help improve the way skin looks and feels (though these would have been more useful if they were present in larger amounts).

If you were hoping Lauder's showcased CP+ peptide solution was the answer, you should know that the amount of peptides in this product is not unique, nor is it more than in other peptide-containing products from Olay's Regenerist, Neutrogena's Active Copper, or even, dare I say, StriVectin. Perfectionist [CP+] contains acetyl hexapeptide-3, an ingredient that is common in many products claiming to "work like Botox." As I have written before, there is no substantiated research proving that this peptide is capable of affecting muscle contractions to the point of smoothing a wrinkle, and if it could work topically (as claimed), why wouldn't it affect other areas it contacts, such as your fingers?

☹ **$$$ Perfectionist Peel, 2-Step Enzyme Activating Treatment** *($85 for the kit)* begs you to "peel away the years and reveal refined, radiant skin." It claims results said to be similar to those from a professional glycolic acid peel (30% strength), so it's no wonder why curiosity about this product has been so intense. Step 1 of this duo is the **Thermal Facial Peel** (meant to remind you of Thermage, the radio-frequency medical procedure). It is a nonaqueous, silicone-based cream you apply to damp skin and leave on for 15 minutes. The second ingredient, magnesium sulfate, produces a warming sensation when mixed with water, so you feel like something is happening even when it really isn't. It would be nice if this form of magnesium had something to do with exfoliation, but it doesn't, nor does the small amount of acetyl glucosamine in this product (an ingredient Lauder claims is a gentle AHA alternative, despite a lack of published research supporting the claim). Salicylic acid is on hand, too, but in an amount that's too small (and with a pH that's too high) for it to function as an exfoliant.

Step 2 involves removing the Thermal Facial Peel with **Calming Neutralizer Pads**. These water-based, jar-packaged pads contain mostly yeast extract along with green tea and Japanese knotweed, both effective antioxidants, although they won't remain effective for long given the packaging. The Neutralizer Pads help balance the slightly alkaline Thermal Facial Peel, but this is essentially a toner formula, and you can get the same neutralizing effect by simply rinsing the Peel with water. All told, this is a pricey product whose results don't come close to those of a professional peel and whose primary attribute is a warming sensation that has no rejuvenating effect on skin. The only benefit I can imagine is if you somehow get a boost from the 15 minutes of relaxation after using this basically do-nothing product.

☹ **$$$ Perfectionist Power Correcting Patch for Deeper Eye Lines/Wrinkles** *($50 for 3 pairs)* purports to make your eye area look ten years younger in 20 minutes, all without the hassle of a doctor's visit or the pain of a needle. These patches are meant to fit the eye contour area and contain a solution of water, film-forming agent, potassium chloride (can be an eye irritant, so use caution), acetyl hexapeptide-3, slip agent, and preservative. Lauder is banking on acetyl hexapeptide-3 being capable of working just like Botox to take the years away, but it doesn't—not even Botox works like Botox when applied topically rather than injected. Further, this is a pricey way to deliver any type of skin care, a benefit that in this case is limited given the nature of the formulation and the amount of hairspray-type ingredient it contains.

ESTEE LAUDER RE-NUTRIV PRODUCTS

☺ $$$ **Re-Nutriv Intensive Hydrating Creme Cleanser** *($39 for 4.2 ounces)* is an emollient, creamy cleanser for dry to very dry skin. It's pricey for what you get, but will hydrate and remove makeup efficiently (though not without the aid of a washcloth).

✓☺ $$$ **Re-Nutriv Intensive Softening Lotion** *($40 for 8.4 ounces)* is an incredibly well-formulated toner that's chock-full of helpful ingredients for all skin types, including antioxidants and cell-communicating ingredients. If you're going to spend a lot of money on a toner, this option has visible rewards! One caution: Lauder included gold in this product, likely to reinforce their marketing of Re-Nutriv as luxury skin care. If you have metal allergies (such as to nickel), this may be a problem; research has shown those with nickel allergies often have a similar though less-intense response to skin contact with other metals, including gold (Source: *Clinical and Experimental Immunology*, December 2006, pages 417–426).

😐 $$$ **Re-Nutriv Creme** *($85 for 1.7 ounces)* is a very emollient, mineral oil–based moisturizer for dry skin. It does contain some good skin-identical ingredients and antioxidants, but jar packaging won't keep the antioxidants stable.

😐 $$$ **Re-Nutriv Intensive Lifting Creme** *($158 for 1.7 ounces)*. While this is a good moisturizer with lots of good skin-identical ingredients, antioxidants, and anti-irritants, there is nothing in it that will lift skin anywhere, and the price is nothing less than obscene given the ingredient list and jar packaging. Estee Lauder charges a lot less for other moisturizers that have a similar ingredient list and are appropriately packaged to keep the light- and air-sensitive ingredients stable during use.

😐 $$$ **Re-Nutriv Intensive Lifting Eye Creme** *($78 for 0.5 ounce)* is a very emollient eye cream for dry to very dry skin, but it won't lift skin or reduce dark circles. It comes up comparably short in antioxidants, but even if they were there in abundance, jar packaging wouldn't keep them stable once the product is opened.

😐 $$$ **Re-Nutriv Intensive Lifting Creme for Throat and Decolletage** *($100 for 1.7 ounces)* is a good emollient moisturizer for dry skin that contains a good mix of plant oils, skin-identical ingredients, and a small amount of antioxidants. There is nothing in this formulation that makes it better for the throat and chest area than for the face, and the jar packaging is disappointing.

✓☺ $$$ **Re-Nutriv Intensive Lifting Serum** *($175 for 1 ounce)* boasts it is Lauder's "ultimate" anti-aging/repair formula, which you'd think would leave the hundred-plus other anti-aging/repair products the Lauder company sells unnecessary and superfluous. But aside from that realization, does this live up to that lofty assertion? It isn't all that ultimate in the least. Without question, there are some extraordinary ingredients in this product that can make a difference in the health, resilience, and appearance of skin. The packaging is such that the many antioxidants and the cell-communicating ingredient retinol will remain stable during use, but you don't need to spend this much to get the advantageous ingredients that make this product a winner. Lauder's Perfectionist CP+ serum and their Advanced Night Repair Concentrate Recovery Boosting Treatment offer similar benefits (albeit with different textures), and Clinique has equally impressive options in their Repairwear line. The base formula of this Re-Nutriv serum is preferred for normal to dry skin.

✓☺ $$$ **Re-Nutriv Intensive Protective Base SPF 30** *($65 for 1.7 ounces)* is a brilliant though pricey option for a daytime moisturizer if you have normal to slightly oily skin. The in-part avobenzone sunscreen protects from UVA rays, while the formula is brimming with antioxidants and cell-communicating ingredients to boost skin's environmental defenses. A less-expensive but not quite as impressive version of this product is Lauder's DayWear Plus Multi-Protection Anti-Oxidant Lotion SPF 30, for Normal/Combination Skin ($38 for 1.7 ounces). The mica and titanium dioxide in this product cast a soft glow on skin—something we lose naturally as we age (and as years of sun damage begin to show)—but that is hardly unique to this product.

☹ **$$$ Re-Nutriv Lightweight Creme** *($85 for 1.7 ounces)* is an emollient but overall lackluster formula compared to most other Lauder moisturizers, including those selling for half this price. The "Lightweight" portion of the name is misleading due to this moisturizer's oil content.

☹ **$$$ Re-Nutriv Re-Creation Day Creme SPF 15 and Re-Creation Night Creme** *($900 for the set; 1.7 ounces of each product)* tries to justify its astonishingly high price by not only being a two-piece set, but also by showcasing the fact that these products are "endowed with tomorrow's science, including eight U.S. and international patents pending." Lauder's idea of tomorrow's science includes using "a wealth of rare plants and minerals known to create life, respond to natural stresses, and promote longevity." That point deserves additional explanation, because it sounds amazingly helpful. It is true that countless plants have internal support systems that allow them to survive and, in many cases, thrive, despite constant exposure to the elements and sunlight, but that doesn't translate to humans. The natural systems that a growing plant uses to sustain itself are built around antioxidants and other cellular ingredients responsible for defending a plant from environmental aggressors. Yet that process in a living plant doesn't explain what happens when a portion of it is uprooted, extracted, and chemically treated to be mixed into a cosmetic product. The plant extracts used in the products below have antioxidant capability, but they cannot transfer their own life-sustaining benefits to your skin, so please don't think that this Re-Nutriv duo is the antiwrinkle answer we've all been waiting for. Further, patents have nothing to do with proof of efficacy. Patent law is about establishing a unique ingredient or group of ingredients that can't be used by anyone else. That doesn't mean the ingredients work or have any purpose whatsoever; in a cosmetic, it is all marketing hype and legalese that has nothing to do with the well-being of your skin.

Turning to the products, ☹ **$$$ Re-Nutriv Re-Creation Day Creme SPF 15** includes avobenzone for UVA protection and has a silky, lightweight cream texture suitable for normal to slightly dry skin. However, jar packaging spells an unstable future for the many antioxidants in this product (one more example of how antioxidants from plants are subject to deterioration when removed from their living source), which is a major misstep from a product costing $450. All you'll be getting is an elegantly textured daytime moisturizer with sunscreen—and how liberally are you going to apply this product knowing its cost is equivalent to a monthly automobile payment? ☹ **$$$ Re-Creation Night Creme** is not only disappointing due to jar packaging, but also, for the money, it lacks many of the state-of-the-art ingredients found in dozens of other Lauder moisturizers. Talk about insulting a consumer's intelligence! Yes, there are some unusual species of seaweed in this moisturizer, but the other antioxidants and cell-communicating ingredients are also found in other products that wouldn't dare charge this much (and seaweed is not a cure-all for aging skin, nor is it an expensive ingredient to include in a product). In summation, this duo is more dour than dynamic, and won't give skin of any age a new lease on life.

☹ **$$$ Re-Nutriv Revitalizing Comfort Creme** *($115 for 1.7 ounces)* is another Lauder moisturizer for dry skin that contains dozens of light- and air-sensitive ingredients subject to deterioration once this jar-packaged product is opened. This has merit, but why would you want to spend so much for ingredients that won't remain stable?

☹ **$$$ Re-Nutriv Revitalizing Comfort Eye Creme** *($60 for 0.5 ounce)* is similar to the Re-Nutriv Intensive Lifting Eye Creme above, and the same review applies. In some respects this is a better formula, but it doesn't deserve more than a neutral face rating because of jar packaging.

☹ **$$$ Re-Nutriv Ultimate Lifting Creme** *($250 for 1.7 ounces)* wants to endow your skin with amazing powers, but this isn't a Superhero secret—it's just another well-formulated moisturizer for normal to dry skin that includes many antioxidants (though not as many as some less-expensive Lauder moisturizers), which won't last long once this jar-packaged product is opened. The radiance and "next generation optical effects" come from the pearl powder, mica, and titanium dioxide in the formula. This isn't futuristic, it's a commonplace way to manipulate the way light reflects off skin and is found in many other products, including Lauder's antioxidant-rich, well-packaged Spotlight Skin Tone Perfector ($32 for 1.7 ounces). What would really make this the ultimate moisturizer is opaque, pump-bottle packaging and even greater amounts of antioxidants.

☹ **$$$ Re-Nutriv Ultimate Lifting Eye Creme** *($100 for 0.5 ounce)* promises to be "the most extravagant eye care you've ever experienced." Well, along with ignoring that, you can also ignore this product's claims of reducing the appearance of dark circles and puffiness—even today's best skin-care formulations cannot effectively remedy these common complaints. This product is remarkably similar to Lauder's Re-Nutriv Intensive Lifting Eye Creme above, and once again jar packaging makes this a less desirable option. The texture feels extravagant, but it won't perform as claimed. This product is fragrance-free.

✓☺ **$$$ Re-Nutriv Ultimate Lifting Serum** *($200 for 1.7 ounces)* claims to be the ultimate repair product, which is odd because so do several other Lauder products. You have to wonder, if they are all advertised as ultimate, how do you know which one really is the best? It's not this option, but only because of its prohibitive price. There is much to applaud about this formula, whose chief antioxidant is pomegranate. Another major ingredient is a species of mushroom known as *Inonotus obliquus*, which has no research pertaining to its benefit for skin. However, one study demonstrated its anti-tumor capability when one if its triterpenoid extracts was applied to mouse skin (Source: *Bioorganic and Medicinal Chemistry*, January 2007, pages 257–264). Other antioxidants and cell-communicating ingredients are present, along with some plant extracts that have no established benefit for skin, but nevertheless provide the "everything but the kitchen sink" image to make you think it is jam-packed with good-for-skin ingredients. Although this is an impressive product, it isn't worth considering over Lauder's Advanced Night Repair Concentrate, Perfectionist CP+, or Lauder-owned Clinique's Repairwear Deep Wrinkle Concentrate for Face and Eyes. If you choose to splurge on this option, at least you can do so knowing you're getting a well-formulated product.

✓☺ **$$$ Re-Nutriv Intensive Lifting Hand Creme SPF 15** *($45 for 3.4 ounces)* has an in-part avobenzone sunscreen and an elegant formula that will take very good care of dry skin on the hands (or elsewhere). The opaque tube will help keep the antioxidants in this product stable, and it moisturizes without leaving hands feeling super-slick or greasy. Pricey, but well done, and definitely an option for on-the-go sun protection for always-exposed hands.

☺ **$$$ Re-Nutriv Intensive Lifting Mask** *($70 for 1.7 ounces)* is a very good moisturizing mask for normal to dry skin, but for the money, the formula cannot compete with Lauder's superior, less expensive Resilience Lift Extreme Ultra Firming Mask ($40 for 2.5 ounces) reviewed below.

ESTEE LAUDER RESILIENCE LIFT PRODUCTS

😐 **$$$ Resilience Lift Extreme Overnight Ultra Firming Creme** *($75 for 1.7 ounces)* is supposed to use exclusive nighttime technology to lift and firm skin by "taking advantage of skin's own restorative rhythms," but if that's true, then the same claim can be applied to most of Lauder's moisturizers. This formula doesn't distinguish itself from the pack, and includes a similar complement of antioxidants, cell-communicating ingredients, emollients, and ingredients that mimic the structure and function of healthy skin. It's a shame an otherwise superior moisturizer for normal to dry skin has jar packaging to hinder the effectiveness of its antioxidants.

☹ **Resilience Lift Extreme Ultra Firming Creme SPF 15, for Dry Skin** *($70 for 1.7 ounces)* lacks the UVA-protecting ingredients of titanium dioxide, zinc oxide, avobenzone, Tinosorb, or Mexoryl SX, and is not recommended.

😐 **$$$ Resilience Lift Extreme Ultra Firming Creme SPF 15, for Very Dry Skin** *($70 for 1.7 ounces)* provides the UVA protection missing in the Resilience Lift Extreme Ultra Firming Creme SPF 15, for Dry Skin, above, but the amount of titanium dioxide (0.9%) may still leave skin vulnerable to UVA damage. This is otherwise an exceptionally emollient formula whose many antioxidants are at risk for quick deterioration due to jar packaging.

😐 **$$$ Resilience Lift Extreme Ultra Firming Eye Creme** *($49.50 for 0.5 ounce)* is similar to, but has a lighter texture and fewer bells and whistles than, the Re-Nutriv Intensive Lifting Eye Creme above, and the same basic comments (including jar packaging) apply. The "luminizing optics" are just cosmetic pigments that reflect light from skin, cosmetically minimizing shadowed areas around the eye.

✓☺ **$$$ Resilience Lift Extreme Ultra Firming Lotion SPF 15, for Normal/Combination Skin** *($70 for 1.7 ounces)* bests the other Resilience Lift Extreme moisturizers with sunscreen above, not only because it contains more titanium dioxide for UVA protection, but also because it has much better packaging. As a result, this is a winning option for normal to dry skin (it's not the best for use over oily areas, so isn't appealing for combination skin) provided you aren't hooked by the lifting and firming claims, which won't materialize. What this does do is provide reliable sun protection in an elegant moisturizing base that contains a state-of-the-art mix of antioxidants and cell-communicating ingredients. Liberal application is necessary to ensure protection, so you have to be OK with replacing this fairly often to avoid putting your skin at risk for sun damage, but other than that caveat, go for it.

😐 **$$$ Resilience Lift Eye Creme** *($48 for 0.5 ounce)* is another emollient eye cream for dry skin that does contain "intense hydrators" such as shea butter, but its antioxidant blend won't hold up once this jar-packaged product is opened, and that's a letdown considering the price.

✓☺ **$$$ Resilience Lift Extreme Ultra Firming Mask** *($40 for 2.5 ounces)* takes an everything-but-the-kitchen-sink approach to skin care, and includes almost every major emollient, antioxidant, water-binding agent, skin-identical substance, and cell-communicating ingredient I've ever heard of. It's certainly a powerhouse formula for dry to very dry skin and is best left on as a moisturizer rather than used occasionally as a mask to be rinsed off. This mask is supposed to revitalize skin with advanced lifting and firming technology, but it can't do that. It doesn't even contain ingredients to create a temporary tightening effect, and that are often used in products to convince you that your skin really is being firmed and lifted. However, as long as you're not banking on this product being a face-lift in a tube, it is without question a formidable moisturizer that treats dry skin to a bevy of ingredients that will improve its feel and appearance.

ESTEE LAUDER VERITE PRODUCTS

☺ **$$$ Verite LightLotion Cleanser** *($23.50 for 6.7 ounces)* is an emollient, cold cream–style cleanser that is an option for someone with dry, sensitive, or reddened skin not prone to breakouts.

😐 **$$$ Verite Soothing Spray Toner** *($23.50 for 6.7 ounces)* is an OK toner that consists mostly of water and slip agents. The plant extracts have soothing properties, and this is fragrance-free for those with sensitive skin.

😐 **$$$ Verite Calming Fluid** *($60 for 1.7 ounces)* is a fragrance-free, lightweight moisturizing lotion that's sort of a stripped-down version of other Lauder moisturizers. It contains significantly fewer antioxidants, and the soothing agents should have been more prominent. Still, it's an option for normal to slightly oily skin and leaves a silky finish.

😐 **$$$ Verite Moisture Relief Creme** *($50 for 1.7 ounces)* is a standard, slightly emollient moisturizer for normal to slightly dry skin. The jar packaging won't keep the minor amount of antioxidants stable once opened, but it is fragrance-free.

✓☺ **$$$ Verite Special EyeCare** *($37.50 for 0.5 ounce)* is a very emollient, water-based moisturizer that contains a good mix of skin-identical ingredients, antioxidants, and cell-communicating ingredients. Like all Verite products, this is fragrance-free.

OTHER ESTEE LAUDER PRODUCTS

☺ **$$$ Perfectly Clean Light Lotion Cleanser** *($23 for 6.7 ounces)* is a water-based emollient cleansing lotion that does not contain detergent cleansing agents, so it is a good option for dry to very dry skin. This product can do a reasonably good job of removing makeup, but you may need to pair it with a washcloth or wipe it off altogether to ensure complete removal.

😐 **$$$ Perfectly Clean Splash Away Foaming Cleanser** *($19 for 4.2 ounces)* lists alkaline and drying potassium myristate as the main cleansing agent, so this will be a problem cleanser for all skin types except very oily. It does remove makeup completely, but is nearly akin to washing with standard bar soap.

☺ **$$$ Soft Clean Moisture Rich Foaming Cleanser** *($19 for 4.2 ounces)* is a creamy, cushiony cleanser whose potassium-derived cleansing base can produce a copious foam, although that has little to do with a product's cleansing abilities. This can be a good, water-soluble cleanser for normal to slightly dry or slightly oily skin. It contains more fragrance than Lauder's other cleansers.

☺ **$$$ Soft Clean Tender Creme Cleanser** *($19 for 4.2 ounces)* is a standard cleansing cream for normal to dry skin. It does not contain detergent cleansing agents, but it can remove most types of makeup without the aid of a washcloth. Used around the eyes (to remove eye makeup or mascara), it can leave a greasy film that is not preferred, especially when compared with a silicone-based makeup remover or water-soluble cleanser. For the money, you may want to try Dove Pro-Age Foaming Facial Cleanser ($5.99 for 5 ounces) over this pricier option.

☹ **Sparkling Clean Oil-Control Foaming Gel Cleanser** *($23 for 6.7 ounces)* is a somewhat drying water-soluble cleanser that would have been an option for oily skin, but the inclusion of irritating menthyl lactate makes it a less than sparkling option.

☹ **Sparkling Clean Purifying Mud Foam Cleanser** *($19 for 4.2 ounces)* is a water-soluble foaming cleanser that contains soap-based potassium myristate as its main cleansing agent. It can be drying for all but very oily skin, especially with the "mud" (clay) thrown in. The deal-breaker is the addition of irritating menthyl lactate, which won't purify skin in the least.

☺ **$$$ Gentle Eye Makeup Remover** *($15.50 for 3.4 ounces)* is a very standard, but effective, fragrance-free, detergent-based eye-makeup remover. Several less-expensive versions at the drugstore easily replace this, but it's an option if you want to spend more.

☺ **$$$ Take It Away LongWear Makeup Remover Towelettes** *($17.50 for 45 towelettes)* feature a formula that is remarkably similar to that of the Gentle Eye Makeup Remover above, only steeped into disposable towelettes. This product is not adept at removing long-wearing or waterproof makeup and ideally should be rinsed from skin because, left on, the detergent cleansing agent can be drying.

☺ **Take It Away Total Makeup Remover** *($22 for 6.7 ounces)* is a water-and-wax concoction with a lotion texture that does an efficient job of removing most makeup without irritating skin.

☺ **$$$ So Polished Exfoliating Scrub** *($22 for 3.4 ounces)* could also be named "So Expensive Exfoliating Scrub" because, although it's an effective topical scrub option for normal to oily skin, it differs little from those available in the drugstore for one-third the price.

😐 **$$$ Perfectly Clean Fresh Balancing Lotion** *($19.50 for 6.7 ounces)* is a very standard toner that lists alcohol as the second ingredient, and that makes this too drying and irritating for all skin types. It cannot "balance" skin, and the exotic plant extracts are a mix of irritants and anti-irritants, which means that basically they cancel each other out.

☺ **$$$ Soft Clean Silky Hydrating Lotion** *($19.50 for 6.7 ounces)* is one of the most original and skin-beneficial toners in the Estee Lauder line, and would be a great option for normal to dry skin. It is alcohol-free, and contains mostly water, silicone, thickener, slip agent, plant extracts (including fragrant floral extracts), skin-identical ingredients, emollient, anti-irritant, Vaseline, film-forming agent, fragrance, and preservatives. The tiny amount of caffeine is unlikely to be a problem, but this toner is a bit too fragrant for someone with very sensitive skin.

☹ **Sparkling Clean Mattifying Oil-Control Lotion** *($19.50 for 6.7 ounces)* lists alcohol as the second ingredient, which is drying and irritating for skin, and also contains the alkaline ingredient barium sulfate, which is a potential skin irritant. Keep in mind that you can't "dry up" oil because it isn't wet. Drying ingredients also negatively affect skin cells, and that doesn't help skin in the least. Many better mattifying options are available, with one of the more interesting versions being Smashbox's Anti-Shine ($26).

✓☺ **$$$ Fruition Extra Multi-Action Complex** *($46.50 for 1 ounce)* contains a blend of synthetic hydroxy acids along with salicylic acid (BHA), but the total amount is very likely less than 1%, and the pH of 4.1 is just above the acceptable range for exfoliation to occur. So why the excellent rating? Although this won't exfoliate skin to the same degree that a well-formulated AHA or BHA product will, the silky lotion formula has a potent amount of antioxidant green tea and contains several other well-researched antioxidants as well as soothing agents, plus a cell-communicating ingredient. It is an excellent moisturizer for slightly oily to oily skin (I know, I know, Lauder positions this as a treatment product, but at its heart it is just a well-formulated moisturizer).

😐 **$$$ Age-Controlling Creme** *($63.50 for 1.7 ounces)* has jar packaging and is one of Lauder's longest selling moisturizers. Antioxidants are in short supply, but my goodness is this emollient! It would be very effective for someone with painfully dry skin.

☺ **$$$ Estoderme Emulsion** *($30 for 4 ounces)* is an emollient moisturizer for dry skin that contains some good skin-identical ingredients and antioxidants, though not to the extent of several other options from Lauder.

☹ **Eyzone Repair Gel** *($38.50 for 0.5 ounce)* contains the preservatives methylisothiazolinone and methylchloroisothiazolinone (Kathon CG), which are contraindicated for use in leave-on products due to their sensitizing potential (Sources: *Contact Dermatitis*, November 2001, pages 257–264; and *European Journal of Dermatology*, March 1999, pages 144–160).

😐 **$$$ Skin Perfecting Creme Firming Nourisher** *($38 for 1.7 ounces)* is an OK moisturizing cream for normal to slightly dry skin. There is no reason to consider this one over hundreds of other more modern formulas (with better packaging).

☹ **Swiss Performing Extract** *($42 for 3.4 ounces)* is another longtime moisturizer from Lauder, and although it is based around emollient, antioxidant grape seed oil and comes in stable packaging, the fragrance components (including eugenol), which are not present in many other moisturizers in this line, are irritating.

✓☺ **$$$ Diminish Anti-Wrinkle Retinol Treatment** *($80 for 1.7 ounces)* contains about the same amount of retinol (roughly 0.25%) as most products, but it's loaded with antioxidants, sophisticated skin-identical ingredients, and cell-communicating ingredients, all in stable packaging. Lauder has tempered its claims for this "treatment" since it first came on the scene several years ago, but it remains an incredibly well-formulated product for normal to dry skin types who want to try a moisturizing retinol product.

✓☺ **$$$ So Clean Deep Pore Mask** *($22 for 3.4 ounces)* begins as a standard clay mask, but the twist here is the inclusion of some very good soothing agents, cell-communicating ingredients, and skin-identical ingredients. The hydrating ingredients don't hold up that well against the absorbent clay, but they do make this mask more cosmetically elegant, aid rinsing, and leave skin looking smoother. In terms of penetration, this mask doesn't go any deeper than most others; it just has a formula that's a cut above.

😐 **$$$ So Moist Hydrating Facial** *($22 for 3.4 ounces)* is a good moisturizing mask for dry to very dry skin, but isn't as elegant as many other Lauder moisturizers.

😐 **$$$ Spotlight Skin Tone Perfector** *($32 for 1.7 ounces)* provides a soft, radiant glow thanks to the cosmetic pigments it contains. They won't make skin look perfect in every light, but can enliven dull, sallow skin, and the silicone-enriched moisturizing base contains some reliable antioxidants and soothing agents.

😐 **$$$ Stress Relief Eye Mask** *($29.50 for 10 0.4-ounce packettes)* won't relieve stress by itself, but you may feel more relaxed if you take the time to lie down as the fluid solution on these eye-shaped pads hydrates skin. The formula is mostly water with slip agents, skin-identical ingredients, and a tiny amount of cucumber, which won't reduce puffiness.

ESTEE LAUDER SUNLESS TANNING PRODUCTS

✓☺ **$$$ Body Performance Naturally Radiant Moisturizer** *($35 for 6.7 ounces)* is an emollient self-tanning lotion for the body that browns skin with dihydroxyacetone, as with most self-tanning products. The difference? This option includes several skin-beneficial ingredients that are missing from most self-tanners, and that elevates its status.

☺ **Body Smoother Exfoliating Creme** *($20 for 5 ounces)* is a standard, easy-to-rinse body scrub that contains polyethylene (plastic) as the abrasive agent. It's an option for all skin types except very dry.

☹ **Fast Tan Quick-Dry Sunless Spray SPF 15** *($29 for 4.2 ounces)* lacks the UVA-protecting ingredients of titanium dioxide, zinc oxide, avobenzone, Tinosorb, or Mexoryl SX, and is not recommended.

☺ **$$$ Go Bronze Plus Tinted Self-Tanner for Body** *($28.50 for 5 ounces)* doesn't have the same complement of skin-identical ingredients as the Body Performance Naturally Radiant Moisturizer above, but has a silkier texture and comparably weightless finish. This self-tanning lotion contains dihydroxyacetone to turn skin color, and cosmetic pigments (including shimmer pigments) for an instant bronze glow.

✓☺ **$$$ Go Bronze Plus Tinted Self-Tanner for Face** *($22.50 for 1.7 ounces)* has a formula that's similar to that of the Go Bronze Plus Tinted Self-Tanner for Body above, but also contains some great antioxidants and a cell-communicating ingredient, making it an overall better formula tailored for facial use. Otherwise, the same comments apply.

☹ **Go Bronze Plus Tinted Self-Tanner for Face SPF 15** *($24 for 1.7 ounces)* has a base formula that's nearly identical to the Go Bronze Plus Tinted Self-Tanner for Face above, but for some inexcusable reason it lacks the UVA-protecting ingredients of avobenzone, titanium dioxide, zinc oxide, Tinosorb, or Mexoryl SX, and is not recommended.

😐 **$$$ Go Tan Sunless Towelettes** *($28 for 10 towelettes)* proves convenience has a price, as these toss-away towelettes are steeped in a water-based solution that includes the self-tanning ingredient dihydroxyacetone and little else of note. They do turn skin tan, but application isn't just swipe on and forget about it—this must be blended thoroughly and evenly over smooth skin for best results.

😐 **$$$ Go Tan Sunless Towelettes for Face and Decolletage** *($23 for 10 towelettes)* are nearly identical to the Go Tan Sunless Towelettes above, and the same review applies.

☺ **$$$ Sunless SuperTan, for Body** *($26.50 for 4.2 ounces)* is available in Medium and Dark versions, both of which contain dihydroxyacetone to color the skin. The water- and silicone-based formula is silky-smooth and does indeed dry quickly, but I'd still be careful for an hour or so before getting dressed or coming into contact with fabrics you don't want to stain.

✓☺ **$$$ Sunless SuperTan, for Face** *($22.50 for 1.7 ounces)* comes in Medium and Dark shades; the Dark option simply has more of the self-tanning ingredient dihydroxyacetone. Both versions have a silky silicone base and contain antioxidants, skin-identical ingredients, and other helpful ingredients that make them more than just standard self-tanning lotions.

ESTEE LAUDER SUNSCREEN/AFTER-SUN PRODUCTS

😐 **$$$ After Sun Rehydrator for Body** *($18.50 for 5 ounces)* is a decent lightweight body moisturizer, but comes up short by including too few antioxidants and skin-identical substances to replenish what's lost when skin is weather-beaten.

☹ **Body Shimmer Sunscreen SPF 15** *($22.50 for 5 ounces)* lacks the UVA-protecting ingredients of titanium dioxide, zinc oxide, avobenzone, Tinosorb, or Mexoryl SX, and is not recommended.

✓☺ **Multi-Protection Sun Lotion for Body SPF 30** *($22 for 5 ounces)* frustratingly encourages tanning by claiming its Anti-Spot Protection "helps prevent sun spots and patchiness to create a tan that looks more even, more radiant...." This in-part avobenzone sunscreen for normal to slightly dry skin contains some outstanding antioxidants and cell-communicating ingredients, but avoiding sun spots demands liberal application, reapplication when necessary, and a willingness to seek shade whenever possible, not to mention the need for protective accessories such as hats and sunglasses. The Paula's Pick rating pertains to the formula itself, not to the disingenuous, dangerous endorsement of creating the perfect tan from the sun.

✓☺ **Multi-Protection Sun Lotion for Face SPF 30** *($22 for 1.7 ounces)* is similar to the Multi-Protection Sun Lotion for Body SPF 30 above, and the same review applies. The Body version may be used on the face; there's no need to purchase both products.

☹ **Multi-Protection Sun Towelettes for Body SPF 15** *($25 for 10 packs)* lack sufficient UVA protection and have a base formula that's primarily alcohol, making this a double-whammy problem for all skin types.

☹ **Multi-Protection Sun Spray SPF 15, Oil-Free** *($22 for 4.2 ounces)* has the same formulary concerns as the Multi-Protection Sun Towelettes for Body SPF 15 above, and the same review applies.

ESTEE LAUDER MAKEUP

FOUNDATION: Estee Lauder's foundations offer something for everyone in terms of texture and formulation, not to mention a better-than-ever shade range that includes options for darker skin tones. Foundation samples are readily available for almost all of the formulas reviewed below, so don't hesitate to ask for these if you're uncertain about shade or formula. I found that salespeople at all the Lauder counters I visited more than happy to provide complimentary foundation samples, no purchase required.

✓☺ **$$$ Individualist Natural Finish Makeup** *($32.50)* is one of the silkiest, most blendable, and natural-looking foundations Estee Lauder has ever produced. Its soft cream texture has just enough slip on skin for controlled application, yet it sets to a natural (meaning not powdery or flat-looking) matte finish suitable for normal to slightly dry or slightly oily skin. As natural as this looks, it provides medium coverage. This is accomplished by specially treated reflective pigments (what Lauder refers to as Ideal Match technology) that somehow blur imperfections while allowing your skin tone to show through. However they want to explain it, the process works—I only wish this had a sunscreen, too, for those with oilier skin who don't need to layer products. A staggering 24 shades are available, and I am pleased to report that all but 2 are outstanding, true-to-life, real-skin colors, including some remarkable pale tones and non-ashy options for dark to very dark skin tones. Avoid the too rose Fresco and too peach Cocoa (also labeled as "Rich Cocoa").

✓☺ **$$$ DayWear Plus Multi Protection Tinted Moisturizer SPF 15** *($35)* combines an in-part avobenzone sunscreen with an antioxidant-rich lotion that's beautifully suited for normal to dry skin. Coverage is sheer, just as it is for most tinted moisturizers, while the finish is satinlike. What makes this Lauder moisturizer different is the very good assortment of skin-friendly ingredients that take it above and beyond what some other tinted moisturizers with sunscreen provide. Among the four neutral-to-yellow shades, the only tricky one is Medium, and even that is still worth trying to see if it works for you.

☺ **$$$ Re-Nutriv Ultimate Lifting Creme Makeup SPF 15** *($80)* is Lauder's most expensive foundation, and your first question may be, "Is it worth the money?" Although this creamy foundation has a lot going for it, the answer is "no." It has a titanium dioxide–based sunscreen, which is great for protecting skin, but so do countless other foundations that cost significantly less. Lauder goes on and on about the skin-care technology behind this foundation, but it won't lift skin in the least. The base formula isn't nearly as exciting as many of their well-formulated moisturizers, plus the jar packaging won't keep the antioxidants in here stable. Texture-wise, this is extra rich, almost to the point of being greasy. It slides over skin and is easy to blend, but doesn't ever set, so you're left with a creamy finish that must be set with powder. You'll get medium coverage without much effort, and it's hard to get less than that, even if you apply a sheer layer (but don't do that because you'll cheat your skin of the sun protection it needs). Ten shades are available, and most of them are very good. Avoid the too-rose Outdoor Beige and Auburn. Based on the emollience of this foundation, I recommend it only for someone with dry to very dry skin, assuming you're willing to pay the exorbitant price.

☺ **$$$ Re-Nutriv Intensive Lifting Makeup SPF 15** *($65)* is elegantly packaged in a frosted-glass jar complete with golden cap and trim, and includes a titanium dioxide sunscreen. In contrast to the pricier Re-Nutriv Intensive Lifting Creme Makeup SPF 15 above, this has a silkier, silicone-based formula that blends down to a satin matte finish that is not at all emollient—nor something those with dry skin would enjoy. It's best for those with normal to slightly dry or slightly oily skin seeking medium coverage and a whatever-it-may-cost makeup. The ten shades are impressively neutral, with the exceptions being Outdoor Beige and Auburn, both of which are too rose to look convincing. Like its companion product, this foundation is not capable of lifting the skin, but it will lift lots of money from your bank account.

☺ **$$$ Minute Makeup Creme Stick Foundation SPF 15** *($32.50)* is a stick foundation that was once discontinued, but there was such a clamor from customers to bring it back that Lauder did, albeit in fewer shades than it originally had. The "Minute" part of the name is inaccurate because this takes just as long to apply as most other foundations, but it does have a smooth, cream-to-powder texture that blends well. This is best for someone with normal skin and minimal to no oiliness. Minute Makeup's powder finish is minimal and doesn't hold up over oily areas very long. I disagree with Lauder's claim that it's non-acnegenic because there are several ingredients that could trigger breakouts, not the least of which is the active sunscreen ingredient, titanium dioxide, which is great for UVA protection but can be problematic for acne-prone skin. All six shades are superb, but only for fair to medium skin tones. A more modern interpretation of this foundation with a broader shade palette is M.A.C.'s Studio Stick SPF 15 ($27.50).

😐 **$$$ Ideal Matte Refinishing Makeup SPF 8** *($32.50)* uses something called AeroPowder technology to create a modern-day powdery matte finish. I must say this silicone cream is a unique foundation. Ideal Matte dispenses as thick as toothpaste but softens immediately upon blending, producing skin that looks smooth and even-textured. The finish is best described as flexible satin matte, meaning that once dry, it leaves a matte finish but without the flat look that is characteristic of traditional matte foundations. Ideal Matte's finish doesn't last as long as you might hope (shine in your oiliest areas will be visible shortly after application), but the result is so realistic and skinlike you may decide to tolerate less oil control for a more natural look. It is best for someone with normal to slightly oily skin. Coverage is billed as medium, but it's really sheer to light. The dismal SPF 8 is lamentable, though it is titanium dioxide–based. Fifteen shades are available, with options for fair to deep skin tones. Almost all of the shades are beautiful; the only poor options are Henna (seemingly a great neutral, but can turn ashy on medium skin tones), Outdoor Beige (slightly peach), Pale Almond (slightly pink, but may be OK for some fair skin tones), and Warm Gold (slightly too yellow, but may be worth trying).

😐 **$$$ Resilience Lift Extreme Ultra-Firming Makeup SPF 15** *($33.50)* doesn't provide an ultra- or even a mildly firming benefit. If anything, the lack of sufficient UVA-protecting ingredients leaves skin vulnerable to sun damage, which encourages loss of firmness. As with most new foundations, this has a lush, silky texture that slips on like a second skin and blends very well. It has a radiant satin finish that makes normal to dry skin look much better, which makes the lack of UVA protection even more disappointing. If you are willing to wear an effective sunscreen underneath this foundation, there are some excellent options among the 15 shades, including colors for dark (but not very dark) and fair skin. The following colors are too pink, peach, or copper for most skin tones: Outdoor Beige, Pale Almond, and Rich Cocoa. Ivory Beige is slightly pink but may work for some fair skin tones; ditto for Shell Beige, although it has a slightly peach cast.

☹ **$$$ Equalizer Smart Makeup for Combination Skin SPF 10** *($32.50)* is similar in concept to Lauder-owned Origins' Stay Tuned Balancing Face Makeup ($17.50) and Clinique's Superbalanced Makeup ($22.50). All of these foundations make the same improbable claim of being able to moisturize dry areas while absorbing oil from oily areas. How a product could hold back its moisturizing ingredient from one area while absorbing oil or moisture from another is a mystery, and in fact it doesn't work—which you will be able to tell immediately after your first application. All claims aside, Equalizer leapfrogs over Stay Tuned and Superbalanced by adding an all titanium dioxide–based sunscreen. The SPF 10 is a shame because it's not enough for daytime protection, and brings this foundation's rating down compared to the similar versions previously mentioned. Equalizer has a very silky, light texture, offering sheer to medium coverage with a soft, slightly powdery finish that is best for those with normal to slightly oily skin. The powder finish will exaggerate any dry spots, so address those before application. There are 21 shades, and the majority of them are wonderful. Pearl is a gorgeous shade for very fair skin, while Nutmeg, Truffle, and Mocha are beautiful, non-ashy dark shades. Avoid the Vanilla, Rich Fawn, and Copper due to overtones of peach or rose.

☹ **$$$ Futurist Age-Resisting Makeup SPF 15** *($33.50)* leaves out the most important anti-aging weapon anyone can have: a sunscreen with sufficient UVA-protecting ingredients! How disappointing that a foundation with such a superlative texture and luminous finish has this as its major flaw. Almost as upsetting is that the base formula was modified to include several state-of-the-art ingredients (if ever there was a foundation that functions like skin care, this is it), yet Lauder didn't improve the deficient sunscreen element. Sigh! If you have normal to dry skin and are prepared to wear a sunscreen underneath, you will get a great medium-coverage foundation. Unusual for Lauder is that half of the 16 available shades are too rose, orange, or copper for most skin tones: Fawn, Pale Almond (slightly pink), Tender Cream, Cool Sand, Golden Petal, Cameo, Sunlit Topaz, and Bare Beige are best avoided, or at the very least auditioned carefully.

☺ **$$$ Double Wear Stay-in-Place Makeup SPF 10** *($32.50)* is great—at least when it comes to a terrific matte finish that doesn't move. If you have normal to oily skin, you'll be impressed with the application and the way it holds up over a long day, and the texture isn't as thick and hard to move as it once was. The SPF is too low for it to be your sole source of daytime protection, but it is pure titanium dioxide. If you have oily skin and want to give this a try, pair it with one of Neutrogena's matte-finish sunscreens with UVA protection. There are now 21 shades offered, more than ever before. Shell and Ecru are excellent for fair skin, and darker skin tones are well-served, too. The shades to steer clear of due to pink, orange, or peach tones are Suede, Rich Cocoa, and Rich Ginger (though this may be a workable option for dark skin tones).

☹ **$$$ Double Wear Stay-in-Place Powder Makeup SPF 10** *($32.50)* lists titanium dioxide as its sole active ingredient, but the SPF rating is below the benchmark, making this talc-based pressed-powder foundation best as an adjunct to another product (foundation or moisturizer) rated SPF 15 or greater. It has a very smooth but thick texture that blends well and provides light to medium buildable coverage. The strong matte finish has a bit of chalkiness to it that primarily affects the darker shades, which tend to go on or turn ash. Among the 18 shades are some great neutral options for fair to medium skin, but avoid Spice, Soft Tan, and Rich Cocoa due to their ashen finish. The absorbency and matte finish of this pressed-powder foundation make it best for oily to very oily skin.

😐 **$$$ Fresh Air Makeup Base** *($23.50)* is an old-fashioned liquid foundation exclusively for oily skin. It blends on lighter than you might expect and sets quickly to a strong, clay-based matte finish, similar to Clinique's Stay True Makeup Oil-Free Formula ($18.50), which is actually the better foundation, especially considering Fresh Air's uninspired shades.

😐 **$$$ Maximum Cover Camouflage Makeup for Face & Body SPF 15** *($28.50)* has a more fluid texture, with enough slip to make controlling the application tricky. It doesn't provide as much coverage as the name indicates (this isn't Dermablend), but it does cover well, provides a titanium dioxide sunscreen, and blends to a solid matte finish. The range of four shades is limited but commendable, with only Creamy Tan being a bit too peach. A Green Corrector shade is also offered, but it's intensely green and will make it extremely obvious that you are wearing an odd shade of makeup, even when mixed with a flesh-toned shade.

☹ **Lucidity Light-Diffusing Makeup SPF 8** *($32.50)* does not include the UVA-protecting ingredients of titanium dioxide, zinc oxide, avobenzone, Tinosorb, or Mexoryl SX and its SPF is much too low for adequate daytime protection. In addition, this has become a dated liquid foundation with few redeeming qualities. It was once recommended, but given its shortcomings it doesn't deserve serious consideration over many other foundations with better textures that get the sunscreen issue right.

☹ **Country Mist Liquid Makeup** *($23.50)* is a holdover from several years ago, and is a standard, no-frills, emollient foundation for normal to dry skin that comes in disappointing colors and is not worth considering. Even the Lauder salespeople I spoke with were embarrassed this foundation was still around, and were reluctant to even show it to me.

☹ **Impeccable Protective Compact Makeup SPF 20** *($32)* is a substandard cream-to-powder makeup whose sunscreen does not afford sufficient UVA protection. The four shades are average, and this is absolutely not worth considering over the stellar cream-to-powder foundations from Clinique, Prescriptives, Clarins, and Cover Girl.

☹ **Double Matte Oil Control Makeup SPF 15** *($32.50)* does not offer the UVA-protecting ingredients of titanium dioxide, zinc oxide, avobenzone, Tinosorb, or Mexoryl SX, and also has other undesirable traits (including the irritant balm mint and a preponderance of peachy shades), which make it a poor choice for all skin types. Revlon's ColorStay foundations are much better for someone with oily skin that needs a long-wearing matte finish and excellent sun protection.

CONCEALER: ☺ **$$$ Ideal Light Brush-On Illuminator** *($24.50)* is sold as a concealer and radiance-reviving product in one. The click-pen applicator feeds product onto a synthetic brush tip. This makes spot application easy, but it is possible to dispense too much product, and there's no way to put it back. This concealer works better as a highlighter due to its sheer texture. Coverage is not sufficient enough to hide darkness under the eyes, camouflage redness, or blur sun-induced discolorations. It layers well for areas that do need more coverage, but why bother when a standard concealer does that with considerably less product? As a highlighter, this product adds a soft-focus effect to skin, sets to a satin matte finish, and actually works better when paired with a regular concealer (applied afterward). You can dab it on to highlight under the eyes, the brow bone, or bridge of the nose. Seven shades are offered, and the only one to be careful with is Medium Deep, which is slightly peach. Soft Pink has a name that may raise concerns, but although it is pink-based, it applies so sheer that it's not a bad choice for fair skin.

☺ **$$$ Smoothing Creme Concealer** *($19.50)* comes in a squeeze tube, so be cautious of dispensing too much. It has a soft, creamy texture and a natural finish that allows for medium coverage with minimal chance of creasing. This can easily look too thick and heavy if not blended well; with practice, you'll find it a workable option. Among the six shades, Smooth Ivory is only for very fair skin, and Smooth Medium may be too peach for some skin tones. The remaining shades are great, including Smooth Extra Deep for dark skin tones.

😐 **$$$ Double Wear Stay-in-Place Concealer SPF 10** *($19.50)* is a liquidy, ultra-matte concealer that provides nearly opaque coverage and includes a titanium dioxide sunscreen. I am a bit surprised the SPF stopped at 10 (which is why this did not earn a happy face rating) because the active ingredient list has titanium dioxide at 17%. That should be equal to more than an SPF 15, but perhaps Lauder thought a higher SPF would be off-putting for use around the eyes. That's not the case from my perspective, though—I'd welcome it. This formula has minimal slip and dries quickly to a matte finish that won't budge, so blending must be precise. Three very good shades are available, with no options for tan to dark skin.

☹ **Re-Nutriv Intensive Concealing Duo** *($38)*. They have to be kidding about this being "the ultimate" concealer! This is one of the thickest, greasiest concealers around, and although it provides sufficient coverage, it looks heavy and creases endlessly. You get two colors in one very elegant-looking mirrored compact, the idea being to use the lighter shade to disguise dark circles and the darker shade to conceal other flaws. Mixing the shades is an option, and one that works best given the peachy pink tone present in two of the three available duos. The Light/Medium Duo has the best shades, but this is not a creamy concealer I'd encourage you to try.

POWDER: ✓☺ $$$ AeroMatte Ultralucent Pressed Powder *($26)* directs you to "finish flawlessly" because "AeroMatte is so soft and air-light sheer, all you see is skin." And that's really true with this amazing, talc-based powder. AeroMatte has a supremely silky, cashmere-like texture that is a pleasure to work with because it never leaves skin looking too powdered or dry. It is available in eight neutral-toned shades, including options for darker skin (these options also work well as bronzing powder on light to medium skin tones). Lauder recommends this powder for all skin types, a point with which I almost concur. Someone with very oily skin will want a powder more absorbent than this, and the cornstarch in this formula may present a problem for those battling blemishes. Otherwise, it is highly recommended, although it's a good idea to apply it with a powder brush rather than the included applicator.

☺ **$$$ Re-Nutriv Intensive Smoothing Powder** *($50)* has a supremely silky, almost creamy-feeling, talc-based texture. It meshes perfectly with skin and leaves a polished finish complete with a noticeable amount of shine. I suppose that part is what Lauder hopes will distract you from noticing that your wrinkles aren't really smoothed, but at least it's not blatant sparkles. If you're going to spend too much money on a loose powder, this is definitely one of the better ones to consider. All four shades are soft and neutral, imparting just a hint of color.

☺ **$$$ Re-Nutriv Intensive Comfort Pressed Powder** *($50)* is also talc-based and shares the same level of silkiness as the Re-Nutriv Intensive Smoothing Powder above. Because this version is pressed, it offers more coverage and a longer-lasting matte (in feel) finish. The shine is toned down compared to the loose version, but still visible. All told, this is a very good, though pricey, powder for normal to very dry skin. It doesn't look the least bit powdery, and comes in four excellent shades.

☺ **$$$ Lucidity Translucent Loose Powder** *($29.50)* is now talc-free and has an intriguing texture that's difficult to describe because Lauder opted not to use talc alternatives such as mica and cornstarch. The texture is very light and feels weightless and smooth on skin. It leaves a soft, radiant shine, which is supposed to downplay wrinkles but doesn't really have that effect. Still, this is recommended for normal to dry skin and it comes in six beautiful shades, including options for dark (but not very dark) skin.

☺ **$$$ Bronze Goddess Soft Matte Bronzer** *($29.50)* may not make you feel worthy of goddess status, but if it will keep you from tanning, it's worth the investment! This pressed-powder bronzer doesn't have the smoothst texture around, but it's still worthwhile and does apply evenly, leaving a soft shine. The single shade is a realistic tan color that's neither too red nor too orange, but it's best for light to medium skin only.

😐 **$$$ Lucidity Translucent Pressed Powder** *($25)* has a talc-based formula that goes on smoothly but quite dry. It leaves skin looking powdered and doesn't do a thing to soften the appearance of lines, but that's not a realistic quality to look for in powder anyway. The six sheer shades tend to be a bit peach or pink, but that's not really noticeable on skin. I wouldn't choose this over the superior AeroMatte Ultralucent Pressed Powder above.

😐 **$$$ Double-Matte Oil-Control Pressed Powder** *($25)* has a talc- and silica-based formula. The texture is similar to that of the Lucidity Translucent Pressed Powder above, but with an even drier, slightly chalky finish. Although that can be a problem for some skin tones, a powder this dry is a boon for those with very oily skin. All seven shades are good, and include options for dark skin.

BLUSH: ✓☺ $$$ Tender Blush *($25)* has a sumptuously silky texture and super-smooth application that doesn't streak or skip. The color intensity is neither too sheer nor too strong, making it an excellent choice for classic blush with a modern formula that goes the distance. The shade range is very attractive, and presents several almost matte options, including Petal, Nude Rose, True Sand, Pink Kiss, and Rosewood. Wild Rose is too shiny for daytime wear; the amount of shine in the remaining shades is soft but definitely noticeable.

☺ **$$$ BlushLights Creamy CheekColor** *($25)* is a silky-smooth cream-to-powder blush that offers eight sheer, attractive colors, but must be applied with a deft hand because it dries almost immediately to a soft powder finish. The semi-translucent colors feel so light they seem to float over the skin, but the formula lasts (though not as well as a powder blush). Most of the shades have a hint of shine; only Honey Shimmer and Pink Shimmer are too shiny for daytime wear.

😐 **$$$ Blush All Day Natural CheekColor** *($24.50)* has a soft, dry texture that feels slightly grainy and doesn't apply as smoothly as Lauder's preferred Tender Blush. The shades apply color-true, and there are options for very light to medium skin tones. Each blush color has some shine, with the most obvious being Potpourri, Raspberry, Rose Marble, and Pink Sand.

😐 **$$$ Tender Blush Sheer Stick** *($25)* is a twist-up blush/highlighting stick that disappoints more than it excites. The texture isn't quite cream-to-powder, but it's not that silky either. Application doesn't have the same pleasant glide you find in many similar products (Avon's long-standing Split Second Blush Stick, priced at $8, comes to mind). All of the colors are so sheer they're nearly see-through, and each has a slight to moderate shine. Once blended, this does feel silkier, but the color payoff is weak and the non-powder finish encourages fading. This isn't a terrible product, just one to test at the counter to be sure you like the application and wear.

EYESHADOW: ✓☺ Pure Color EyeShadow *($17.50)* has been reformulated and, although the previous version was amazingly silky and applied beautifully and color-true, this one is even better. It has an enviable silkiness and ultra-smooth texture that meshes with skin rather than looking like powder sitting on top of it. Another refinement is the departure of the chunky, Lucite containers. Now each shade is packaged in a flat compact that includes a built-in mirror and throwaway sponge-tip applicator. None of the shades sold singly are truly matte, but the almost-matte options (which have a slight reflective quality suitable for daytime wear) include Sand Box, Chocolate, Mink, Taupe, Ivory Box, Plum Pop, and Slate. Sticking to its pure color name, the rest of the shades include traditional and trendy options, with the following shades being either too difficult to work with or too clownish for anything but high-fashion or theatrical makeup: Ivy, Cherry, Aqua, and Lagoon. Pumpkin is a deep orange shade that is tricky to work with, but, if blended with a deeper brown, is an attractive pairing for darker skin tones.

☺ **$$$ Pure Color EyeShadow Duo** *($30)* has a texture similar to the Pure Color EyeShadow above, but the application is softer. Both shades in each duo are shiny, so these aren't for wrinkled or drooping eyelids. More than half of the duos are contrasting colors that are difficult to work with; the best pairings are Saturn, Jupiter, Solar Orbit, and Moon Dust.

☺ **$$$ Graphic Color EyeShadow Quad** *($37)* leaves me torn, because I really wanted to rate this a Paula's Pick. These powder eyeshadows have a wonderfully smooth texture and seamless, even application. They deposit more color than Lauder's Pure Color EyeShadows above, making them great for formal makeup or for use on darker skin tones. I don't even mind that there are no matte quads to consider, because the biggest problem is the colors themselves. Either the shade combinations are difficult to work with or the tone-on-tone gradations are too bright or pastel to achieve the purpose of eyeshadow (which is to shape and shade the eye area). It's no coincidence that the most workable quad, Sizzling Coral, is often sold out at Lauder counters and on their Web site. If the color combinations were thoughtfully coordinated, this would be a slam-dunk recommendation. For now, a happy face rating will have to do.

EYE AND BROW SHAPER: ☺ $$$ Automatic Eye Pencil Duo *($23.50, $11.50 for refill)* is a standard, twist-up, retractable pencil in an elegant container that features a pointed sponge tip for softening and blending. Although pricey, the refills are a bargain and then you have the sexy container. The formula sports a drier finish than in the past, making these less prone to smearing or fading. The Plumwood shade is an attractive alternative to traditional black or brown liner.

☺ **$$$ Automatic Brow Pencil Duo** *($23.50, $11.50 for refill)* comes in the same elegant, refillable packaging as the Automatic Eye Pencil Duo above, but instead of the sponge tip you get an angled brow brush. The pencil has a dry but smooth texture that applies evenly without being too thick or greasy, nor does it deposit too much color at once. The shade selection includes options for blondes and redheads, but the brow brush is too stiff and scratchy for consistent, comfortable use.

😐 **$$$ Artist's Eye Pencil** *($18.50)* is a standard pencil with a smooth and slightly creamy application that sets to a relatively solid finish that goes the distance. The pencil includes a sponge tip for softening the line, and the "artist" portion comes into play with the movable rubber gripper. This accessory is designed to provide more control during application, but isn't really needed and it can be a problem if it slides as you're drawing a line. Ten shades are available, and two of them (Copper Writer and Plum Writer) have shimmer. Blue Iris (a deep royal blue) is the only misstep, though some women will undoubtedly find this shade irresistible.

☹ **$$$ Artist's Brow Mobile Essentials** *($25)* isn't all that essential or particularly mobile. It's packaged in a container just slightly wider than (and reminiscent of) a mascara tube. Inside you'll find a dual-ended pencil (for eyelining and brow defining), a pair of tweezers, a brow brush, and a clear brow gel. It sounds convenient, but the products themselves are mediocre. The pencils, housed in the middle of the unit, are too short (probably to conserve space) and are standard fare: neither too creamy nor too dry. The brow gel works well, but can feel slightly sticky. Once you get to the tools, you feel shortchanged, and not because each piece is so incredibly tiny. The tweezers have a decent point, but feel flimsy and, well, cheap. And the brow brush, though compact, has incredibly stiff and scratchy bristles—not something you'd want to endure with every makeup application. As clever as this packaging may seem, it is more gimmicky than practical.

☹ **$$$ Two-in-One Eyeliner/Browcolor Compact** *($26)* goes on wet or dry, but works best when used wet. It comes in one compact with two colors: brown and black. Although it does fill in brows or line the eye, the color selection is limited and almost any matte eyeshadow can perform the identical function. The supplied tools are too small to be useful, and the brow brush is too stiff and scratchy.

☹ **Artist's Mechanical Eye Pencil** *($23.50)* may seem convenient because you get an automatic, retractable eyeliner pencil and coordinating eyeshadow in one component. However, the pencil is too creamy and prone to smearing because it never sets, and the twist-up, retractable cream eyeshadow does the same thing. There's also the issue of pairing green and blue eye pencil shades with similar shadow colors, but this isn't worth trying anyway, at least not if you want your eye makeup to last. ☹ **Natural Brow Filler** *($17)* is a chunky one-color eyebrow pencil that needs sharpening and isn't by any means a one-size-fits-all product. The broad tip makes it hard to control the color through the brow, the creamy texture ensures eventual fading, and the color isn't in the least natural if you have very light or dark brows. ☹ **Pure Color EyeLiner** *($22.50)* is lavishly packaged, yet the liquid liner housed inside a gorgeous Lucite bottle is sketchy at best. There are traditional and extreme shades, each imbued with subtle to obvious iridescence (the black shade has the least amount). Application has been improved so you get a solid line of color from beginning to end of the lash line. The frustrations begin with this liner's slow dry time and the fact that it tends to flake during the day. For this much money, forget the pretty packaging—I'd settle for improvements in the product itself.

LIPSTICK, LIP GLOSS, AND LIPLINER: ✓☺ $$$ Double Wear Stay-in-Place Lip Duo *($24)* has a formula, application process, and performance identical to that of (Lauder-owned) M.A.C.'s Pro Longwear Lipcolour ($19.50). There is a slight price difference, and it's worth mentioning that Lauder's version has the limitation of not offering additional variations of the glossy top coat. Otherwise, this and M.A.C.'s version take first place as the best long-wearing lip colors on the market, although, for this category of lip products, the term "best" is relative. We've tested every major contender in this group, from the original Max Factor Lipfinity to copycat versions from Cover Girl, L'Oreal, Lancome, Maybelline, Revlon, and Smashbox. Most of them have similar positive attributes and all of them wear longer than traditional lipsticks (even those with a matte finish). Lauder and M.A.C.'s versions excel because they have the smoothst textures and the most even wear. When the color starts to fade (and exactly when that occurs depends greatly on the type of food—greasy or messy—you eat), it does so without chipping or flaking. In addition, the glossy top coat feels light and is completely non-sticky, while others run the gamut from thick and syrupy to super-slick. There are drawbacks to be sure, such as needing to routinely reapply the top coat to ensure comfortable wear, but that's a much simpler task than touching up lipstick, where in most cases you need a mirror (especially if you wear reds or other strong colors). Speaking of color, Lauder's shade selection is smaller than M.A.C.'s, but there's not a bad one in the bunch!

✓☺ **$$$ Electric Intense LipCreme** *($22)* is Lauder's best traditional lipstick, though "traditional" is too boring a word to describe this elegant, creamy lipstick. It glides on and feels light and not too slippery. Each stunning shade is saturated with color that provides longer-than-anticipated wear and has a good stain. If you're going to spend over twenty dollars on a lipstick, this is a great place to start the search! ✓☺ **$$$ Electric Intense Liquid LipCreme** *($22)* is equally great, though the formula doesn't last as long due to its glossy finish. Housed in a pen-style applicator and applied with a built-in synthetic brush, this liquid lipstick feels exceptionally smooth, is completely non-sticky, and comes in a terrific assortment of colors, each providing sheer to light coverage.

☺ **$$$ Pure Color Long-Lasting Lipstick** *($22)* is too creamy to make good on its long-lasting claim, but the colors are richly luxurious and this has a beautifully smooth application that feels creamy without being greasy. It isn't too slick either, which means there's much less chance of it feathering into lines around the mouth, although that will occur if paired with lip gloss. The shade selection is enticing and the component opulent—you'll want to touch up in public with this one! ☺ **$$$ Pure Color Crystal Lipstick** *($22)* promises "sheer electricity, daring shine," but the only thing that will get a charge out of this slick, glossy lipstick is your credit card. The colors are fetching, but fleeting, with a glossy sheen that feels emollient. ☺ **$$$ Pure Color Crystal Lipstick with Neon Glow** *($22)* is nearly identical to the Pure Color Crystal Lipstick above, except that these shades are infused with glitter for an even shinier (not neon) finish. This gets extra points because the glitter doesn't feel grainy as the lipstick wears away. ☺ **$$$ Pure Color Velvet Lipstick** *($22)* is a smooth, comfortably creamy lipstick that comes in a small but enticing selection of colors. The formula isn't all that different from Lauder's original Pure Color Lipstick, and the packaging is every bit as opulent. This feels weightless on the lips and leaves a soft, semi-opaque creamy finish. It has enough movement to slip into lines around the mouth, but is far less greasy than traditional lipsticks. ☺ **$$$ Pure Color Gloss** *($18)* carries over the opulent packaging of its lipstick predecessor, but the formula itself, while good, is nothing spectacular. It feels relatively light and applies smoothly with its sponge tip, leaving a moist, glossy finish. The only significant point of difference is that the colors have more intensity than your average lip gloss. ☺ **$$$ Pure Color Crystal Gloss** *($18)* has the same basic formula as the Pure Color Gloss above, but these colors have more shimmer and the pigmentation is softer. Watch out for the glitter-infused shades because they tend to feel grainy as the gloss wears off. ☺ **$$$ Pure Color Crystal Gloss with Neon Glow** *($20)* is nearly identical to the Pure Color Crystal Gloss above, except that each sheer shade has a brilliant shimmer finish that's slightly metallic (not neon). All of the shades are exquisite. ☺ **$$$ High Gloss** *($16)* is "all you really need to shine," at least if you only want shiny lips. This tube lip gloss has a smooth, slightly thick feel with a minor amount of stickiness. High Gloss is exactly the finish you'll get from each of the sheer shades, including a colorless option and several with shimmer. The only caveat is the strong fragrance; make sure you're OK with that before you purchase!

☺ **$$$ Artist's Mechanical Lip Pencil** *($23.50)* is a dual-sided product that is worth considering. One end is a twist-up, retractable lip pencil that provides a creamy, easy-glide application that stays surprisingly well. The other end houses a coordinating sheer, glossy lipstick that is not much for long wear. However, there's no denying that this is a convenient way to line and color the lips.

😐 **$$$ Electric Sheer LipShine** *($22)* is a smooth, lightweight, cream lipstick that feels great and comes in a beautiful array of sheer colors, some of which are so pale they wash out the lips if used alone (but are fine paired with a Lipliner). Each shade is imbued with crystalline glitter pigment, and although it doesn't feel grainy the particles are large and make lips look speckled—not smooth and soft. 😐 **$$$ All-Day Lipstick** *($17)* is extremely creamy, bordering on greasy, with medium coverage and no stain to speak of. It does not hold a candle to any of the Lauder lipsticks reviewed above, and absolutely does not last all day (actually, it barely makes it through coffee breaks). 😐 **$$$ Automatic Lip Pencil Duo** *($23.50; $11.50 for refill)* is a standard, twist-up, retractable Lipliner, but the tip of the pencil comes out of a wider-than-normal opening, which makes it too thick to be capable of drawing a thin outline around the mouth. That's not a deal-breaker, but what you may not like is that this pencil stays creamy, diminishing its longevity. The built-in lip brush is a nice touch, but not enough to warrant a happy face rating. 😐 **$$$ Artist's Lip Pencil** *($18.50)* has a much better texture and longer-lasting finish than the Automatic Lip Pencil Duo above, but the fact that it needs sharpening and has an inferior built-in lip brush keeps it from earning a better rating. If you're intrigued, the shade range is expansive. Like the Artist's Eye Pencil, it comes with a movable rubber gripper; I don't think it's too useful, but your experience may differ.

☹ **Lip Conditioner SPF 15** *($16)* is basically a lipstick without pigment, but the fact that it does not contain the UVA-protecting ingredients of titanium dioxide, zinc oxide, avobenzone, Tinosorb, or Mexoryl SX makes it not worth considering.

MASCARA: ✓☺ **$$$ Illusionist Waterproof Maximum Curling Mascara** *($21)* is Lauder's best mascara by a considerable margin. Unlike the non-waterproof version of Illusionist (reviewed below), this formula is indeed waterproof and builds substantial length and curvaceous thickness with nary a clump in sight. It may take some time to impress, but with patience you will find this an exemplary waterproof mascara that leaves lashes noticeably full and softly curled. There are less-expensive waterproof mascaras available at the drugstore that perform as well as this, but if purchasing mascara from a department-store line is your cup of tea, this product is a satisfying drink.

☺ **$$$ Projectionist High Definition Volume Mascara** *($19.50)* has a great unconventional name, and it also comes with the benefit of producing pronounced lashes. Although results with this mascara are good overall, getting there can be a messy proposition. Length outshines thickness here, but with successive coats it builds reasonably dramatic, defined lashes. Expect minor clumping and a slightly uneven deposit of mascara that requires careful comb-through and you won't be disappointed.

☺ **$$$ Lash XL Maximum Length Mascara** *($21)* won't become any mascara-lover's new favorite for all-out length, but it does do a respectable job of defining and moderately dramatizing lashes without clumping or flaking. Its lengthening abilities don't qualify as maximum, but this does make lashes perceptibly longer with just a few strokes, and builds some thickness, too.

😐 **$$$ Illusionist Intense Maximum Curling Mascara** *($21)*. The curl your lashes get from this mascara isn't of the maximum variety, but it does quickly make lashes longer without clumps or smearing. Thickness is present, but in a supporting role, and you're left with remarkably long, naturally curled lashes. For truly maximum curl, you'll need to pair this with an eyelash curler, especially if your lashes are straight or tend to grow downward.

☹ **$$$ MagnaScopic Maximum Volume Mascara** *($21)* supposedly makes lashes 300% thicker. Lauder even refers to it as "the fast track to thick lashes." If that's the case, then it must be a poorly traveled track, because thickness was hard to come by even after successive applications—and there were clumps along the way. Where MagnaScopic really excels (beyond its clever name) is for lengthening and long wear. If you're willing to put up with a slightly uneven application and have the patience it takes to separate clumped lashes, this is a good (but not great) option. If thickness and truly maximum volume are your mascara mantra, consider Clinique's High Impact Mascara ($13.50) or L'Oreal's Lash Architect Mascara ($6.99). ☹ **$$$ More Than Mascara** *($21)* is less than adequate, at least if you're expecting a payoff of substantial length with some thickness, because this mascara provides neither. In terms of this being a "moisture-binding" formula, it doesn't contain much that makes it different from countless other mascara formulas, though it does leave lashes feeling soft. ☹ **$$$ Lash Primer Plus** *($18.50)* is sold as a pre-mascara conditioning base for lashes, but that is an unwarranted step given the industrywide availability of superlative one-step mascaras. The formula closely matches that of most mascaras, save for the addition of a tiny amount of nut oils.

BRUSHES: Estee Lauder's **Brushes** *($18.50–$40)* aren't terrible, but the collection as a whole isn't as elegant, functional, or attractive as those from Lauder-owned M.A.C., Bobbi Brown, or Prescriptives. At Lauder's price points, I expected, but didn't observe, higher quality. Still, if you're keen on exploring brushes with the Lauder logo, the best ones to consider are the ☺ **$$$ Foundation Brush 1F** *($30)*, ☺ **$$$ Blush Brush 2F** *($30)*, ☺ **$$$ Bronzer Brush 5F** *($35)*, **Base Contour Brush 8E** *($22)*, ☺ **$$$ Eyeshadow Blending 11E** *($25)* and, if you don't mind the stubby handle, the ☺ **$$$ All-Over Face and Body Brush 14F/B** *($35)*.

SPECIALTY PRODUCTS: ☺ **$$$ Prime FX Face Definer** *($25)* is a two-step product that plays up a basic makeup principle: light brings features forward, dark makes them recede. Packaged in a single unit are a brush-on highlighter (Liquid Light) that offers sheer, pearlized color to brighten features such as the underbrow area or top of the cheekbone, and a cream-based neutral brown tone (Dark Creme) for contouring and creating shadow. The highlighter part is simple enough to use, but the shadow part will take practice and ample checking in daylight to make sure what you intended as soft contouring or sculpting does not look smudged or dirty. If you decide to try this product, ask a Lauder makeup artist for a demonstration, and then practice at home to make sure you can duplicate the results. Even in adept hands, highlighting and contouring is tricky. For regular use this isn't practical, but makeup artists might find this a convenient product.

☹ **$$$ Prime FX Makeup Refresher** *($18)* is nothing more than an overpriced, alcohol-free toner that does little to freshen or set your makeup. If anything, misting skin covered with makeup doesn't get the ingredients to the skin, it just lies on top of the makeup, and that can encourage smearing. This product is an OK option for use after cleansing as a toner, but it's a fairly expensive way to go about it. ☹ **$$$ Makeup Brush Cleanser** *($15)* is a basic, water- and alcohol-based cleanser that does remove makeup and oil buildup from brushes, but it's best for someone who needs to clean their brushes quickly because they are using them on multiple people. For your personal brush collection, occasional washing with a gentle shampoo is all you need to keep them in good shape—it does not require a specialized product.

☹ **Prime FX Lip Amplifying Base** *($20)* fills in lines on and around the lips, thanks to silicone technology and film-forming agents. However, although it can produce localized inflammation that makes lips temporarily fuller, the peppermint oil included is unwise—it is even more irritating to lips than to skin. The question of whether having fuller lips is worth the irritation is one each consumer must answer, but in the long run, I wouldn't recommend assaulting your lips with anything irritating, peppermint oil or otherwise.

EUCERIN (SKIN CARE ONLY)

EUCERIN AT-A-GLANCE

Strengths: Inexpensive and widely distributed; fragrance-free cleansers.

Weaknesses: Sunscreens without UVA-protecting ingredients; anti-redness products that added questionable ingredients instead of increasing the anti-inflammatory agents; nothing for acne-prone skin; jar packaging.

For more information about Eucerin, call (800) 227-4703 or visit www.eucerin.com or www.Beautypedia.com.

EUCERIN REDNESS RELIEF PRODUCTS

✓☺ **Redness Relief Soothing Cleanser** *($8.99 for 6.8 ounces)* is a gentle, fragrance-free, water-soluble cleansing gel whose simple formula is ideal for those with sensitive, easily irritated skin. It contains licorice root extract, a good anti-irritant, but considering the amount of it here and the limited time it's in contact with your skin, it will not lead to "immediate redness relief." The good news is that this cleanser isn't apt to make persistent facial redness worse. It is best for normal to slightly dry or slightly oily skin.

😐 **Redness Relief Daily Perfecting Lotion SPF 15** *($14.99 for 1.7 ounces)* deserves praise for including titanium dioxide for sufficient UVA protection, but there are problems with this formula, especially for those with reddened, easily irritated skin. The active ingredients are two synthetic sunscreens, which, while generally well tolerated, are not the best for someone with sensitive skin. Eucerin would have been wise to use just titanium dioxide and/or zinc oxide as the active(s). Another issue is the inclusion of denatured alcohol. There's not a lot of it in the product, but for someone with red, sensitive skin, it's cause for concern. The alcohol is more prevalent than the played-up licorice extract, which is present in such a small amount its soothing benefit to skin is negligible. Finally, this lotion is tinted mint green in an effort to cancel facial redness. Such color-correction rarely looks convincing, but in this case it's so sheer as to be barely noticeable on skin, so it doesn't matter one way or the other. This moisturizing sunscreen is an OK option for normal to dry skin that is not affected by redness or sensitivity, but it's certainly not what current research indicates is a state-of-the-art formula.

😐 **Redness Relief Soothing Anti-Aging Serum with Coenzyme Q10** *($14.99 for 1 ounce)* is a somewhat basic, fragrance-free serum that could have been much more impressive if it included more soothing agents and antioxidants. Nothing in this serum is known to make reddened, easily sensitized skin less red, but it won't make it worse (unless you happen to be sensitive to one of the ingredients, which is always the risk for someone with sensitive skin). Ubiquinone (coenzyme Q10) cannot reduce fine lines and wrinkles. There is much more research concerning this antioxidant when it is consumed orally than when it's applied topically, though it certainly has merit for skin because it reduces sun-induced inflammation and can inhibit the collagen-weakening protease MMP-1 (Sources: *Journal of Cosmetic Dermatology*, March 2006, pages 30–38; and *Biofactors*, volume 18, 2003, pages 289–297).

☹ **Redness Relief Soothing Moisture Lotion SPF 15** *($14.99 for 1.7 ounces)* is very similar to the Redness Relief Daily Perfecting Lotion SPF 15 above, except this option is not tinted. Otherwise, the same review applies, including the comment about the amount of alcohol.

☹ **Redness Relief Soothing Night Creme** *($14.99 for 1.7 ounces)* doesn't have much to it, though it is fragrance-free, which is great for sensitive skin. Given what we know about what skin needs to look and feel healthy, whether it is sensitive or not, this jar-packaged moisturizer lacks interest. Consisting primarily of water, glycerin, panthenol, and triglycerides, it's an extremely simple, slightly emollient formula for normal to slightly dry skin. What's missing are antioxidants, cell-communicating ingredients, and a more sophisticated mix of ingredients that mimic the structure and function of healthy skin. It does contain licorice extract for its anti-irritant properties, but given the small amount, I am skeptical that someone with persistent redness or rosacea will notice their symptoms abating. Still, if you're curious, this bland formula shouldn't make reddened, sensitive skin worse.

☹ **Redness Relief Tone Perfecting Creme** *($14.99 for 0.08 ounce)* is designed as a spot concealer for particularly troublesome red or blotchy areas. Housed in a click-pen applicator with a built-in sponge tip, this thick, mint green–tinted cream does a poor job of concealing redness and looks painfully obvious on skin. The high amount of titanium dioxide creates an unattractive whitish cast, and the formula tends to settle in pores. Several regular (meaning flesh-toned) concealers from companies such as Revlon, Maybelline, L'Oreal, Dior, and M.A.C. do a much better job concealing redness or blotches, and in a way that looks natural and skinlike rather than green and pasty.

OTHER EUCERIN PRODUCTS

✓☺ **Gentle Hydrating Cleanser** *($6.99 for 8 ounces)* contains the essential ingredients necessary to create a detergent-based, water-soluble cleanser that is suitable for all skin types, except very dry. The fragrance-free formula is truly gentle, removes makeup well, and doesn't leave a residue on skin. What more could you ask for?

☹ **Clear Skin Formula Deep Action Toner** *($5.99 for 6.8 ounces)* puts drying, irritating alcohol and a form of potentially pore-clogging castor oil together in one product meant for breakout-prone skin. If this seems contradictory, you're right; this toner is one to leave on the shelf in favor of better options.

☺ **Extra Protective Moisture Lotion SPF 30** *($9.29 for 4 ounces)* is a good, basic, fragrance-free daytime moisturizer for normal to dry skin not prone to blemishes. The in-part titanium dioxide and zinc oxide sunscreens keep skin well shielded from the sun, while the silicone-enhanced formula doesn't feel too heavy or tacky. What's missing are antioxidants to help boost skin's natural defenses, and that's what keeps this from earning a higher rating.

☹ **Q10 Anti-Wrinkle Sensitive Skin Creme** *($10.99 for 1.7 ounces)* contains some well-documented antioxidants in a light yet creamy base formula. Unfortunately, jar packaging won't keep the antioxidants stable, leaving you with an average choice for normal to dry skin.

☹ **Q10 Anti-Wrinkle Sensitive Skin Lotion SPF 15** *($11.29 for 4 ounces)* does not contain the UVA-protecting ingredients of titanium dioxide, zinc oxide, avobenzone, Tinosorb, or Mexoryl SX, and is not recommended. No antioxidant around can make up for an omission like this, at least if your goal is to keep skin from wrinkling and sagging.

☹ **Skin Renewal Day Lotion SPF 15** *($9.29 for 4 ounces)* lacks the UVA-protecting ingredients of titanium dioxide, zinc oxide, avobenzone, Tinosorb, or Mexoryl SX, and is not recommended. This faulty sunscreen also contains two preservatives not meant for use in leave-on products due to their irritation potential.

EXUVIANCE (SEE NEOSTRATA)

FREEZE 24-7 (SKIN CARE ONLY)

FREEZE 24-7 AT-A-GLANCE

Strengths: The company provides complete ingredient lists on their Web site.

Weaknesses: Expensive; products do not work as claimed; most of these products contain one or more known irritants; a line that bills itself as providing "Age-Less Skincare" should be ashamed of not offering a conventional sunscreen.

For more information about Freeze 24-7, call (877) 373-3934 or visit www.freeze247.com or www.Beautypedia.com.

unrated **Ice Shield Facial Cleanser with Sunscreen SPF 15** *($48 for 4.2 ounces)* claims to be, and actually is, a first. This is a cleanser with active sunscreen ingredients that are supposed to remain on skin after rinsing. The actives include avobenzone for UVA protection and the cleansing base does its job to remove surface oil, dirt, and makeup. So is Freeze 24-7 really on to something? Is applying sunscreen now as simple and convenient as washing your face? Apparently, yes.

According to an article in *Happi* magazine, the company behind this cleanser/sunscreen technology is Aquea Scientific. They market an ingredient mixture known as Wash-On (also known as Aquea SPF). According to the article, this is "a patented technology to encapsulate active ingredients into micron sized particles, which are then positively charged. As a result, encapsulated active ingredients are attracted to negatively charged skin and hair. Active ingredients delivered through the system will remain attracted to the skin and hair throughout the day, even after patting dry." That sounds great, but does it really work?

Aquea Scientific CEO Dave Compton commented, "This isn't super glue, we believe it's the best way right now of attracting actives to skin [in] the presence of surfactants." I was curious if any tests had been done to prove that the sunscreen actives said to adhere to skin after rinsing are enough to protect skin from UV damage. There was no information available on the FDA's Web site, and Aquea Scientific's site simply referred to extensive clinical testing done by independent labs, which doesn't explain anything. I was able to reach Mr. Compton via telephone and he explained to me that because this product is a first (there's never been a cleanser with active sunscreen ingredients that adhere to skin after rinsing), the FDA has no prescribed testing method. Compton stressed that they did due diligence by performing FDA-mandated static testing to determine the product's potential SPF range. However, based on FDA testing protocols, this involved leaving the mixture on skin, not rinsing it off as the consumer is directed to do at home. So it wasn't a huge surprise that the active ingredients left on skin provided a certain amount of sun protection.

Compton went on to explain that they worked with a lab to perform "real-world testing" with human volunteers. This involved applying the compound to wet skin, massaging it in, then washing it off. The cleansed skin was then tested under ultraviolet light and it was determined that the sun protection did, in fact, remain on skin. I also spoke to a cosmetics chemist who specializes in sunscreen formulation about this technology. He was familiar with it and believed it to be effective based on the information he had seen.

However, neither Aquea Scientific nor Freeze 24-7 was willing to share the clinical test results with the public, and the information is not published. Granted, it doesn't have to be published or shared, but you'd think a company on to something so exciting would be a bit more forthcoming. Still, speaking with Mr. Compton was interesting and he commented that several mass-market brands are working on products that use this technology. For now, Ice Shield Cleanser is the only way to take advantage of it and it's considerably expensive. It's good news to know that we may see less-expensive products that promise a quick, convenient way to apply sunscreen.

What remains unclear is what happens when additional skin-care products are applied over these sunscreen actives. Does the sunscreen diminish if you apply an exfoliant, moisturizer, and/or makeup on top of the actives adhering to your skin? I suspect it would, as did the sunscreen chemist I spoke with, because simply charging ingredients so they adhere to skin doesn't mean they're impervious to rub-off once other products are applied afterward (or with a towel when you get out of the shower). I phoned Mr. Compton again, leaving a message expressing this concern in detail, and asked him to return my call. As this book goes to press, he has not gotten back to me. Therefore, I am cautiously recommending this product as a good sunscreen option provided you do not apply other products over it, unless those products also include broad-spectrum sun protection.

😐 **$$$ Skin Glace Daily Detoxifying Cleanser and Mask** *($65 for 3.3 ounces)* is said to restore vital oxygen to skin thanks to its self-foaming technology. A couple of the main ingredients in this cleanser are solvents that have an oxygenating effect when mixed with water. However, despite the copious foam many consumers love, supplying oxygen to intact, otherwise healthy skin, isn't good news! Increasing the amount of oxygen skin absorbs only leads to more free-radical damage. I doubt this cleanser/mask hybrid's oxygenating effect is long-lasting or stable enough to impact skin, but if it is, that's a hindrance, not a benefit. This is otherwise an odd mix of detergent cleansing agents, silicone, clay, slip agents, and thickeners. It is needlessly expensive but an OK cleanser for normal to oily skin not anticipating "treatment" results.

☹ **IceCrystals Anti-Aging Prep and Polish** *($65 for 2.6 ounces)* is a very abrasive scrub that is also exceptionally irritating to skin because it contains basil, peppermint, and lemon peel oils. This is absolutely not recommended and is easily replaced by any topical scrub at the drugstore.

☹ **Freeze 24-7 Anti-Aging Eye Serum** *($105 for 0.5 ounce)* is a water- and glycerin-based serum that contains a high amount of the irritating fragrance component eugenol, and is not recommended. Even without eugenol, nothing in this serum can eliminate dark circles or puffy eyes.

☹ **Freeze 24-7 Anti-Wrinkle Cream** *($115 for 1 ounce)* is sold as a pre-moisturizer step to quickly and dramatically (no skin-care products ever claim to work slowly and methodically, do they?) diminish lines and wrinkles as well as stretch marks on the body, not to mention any other skin flaw you can imagine. It comes in a moisturizing base and does contain GABA, but none of this is helpful for wrinkles or stretch marks (stretch marks don't go away with Botox injections either), so this is even more ridiculous. Because it also contains the fragrance component eugenol, it is a skin irritant. The resulting irritation may cause you to think the product is working, but I assure you this reaction is problematic, both for the short- and long-term health of your skin.

☹ **IceCream Anti-Aging Moisturizer** *($80 for 1.7 ounces)* is supposed to be used with the Freeze 24-7 Anti-Wrinkle Cream above to further reduce lines and wrinkles. So much for the other products being wrinkle-banishing superstars in their own right—now you need another product to get the best results, and, of course, both of them are expensive. Just as with the Anti-Aging Eye Serum and Freeze 24-7 Anti-Wrinkle Cream, this contains GABA, although it comes with no substantiated proof that it works in a manner similar to Botox injections. IceCream also contains acetyl hexapeptide-3, a synthetic peptide that is sold as another alternative to Botox. It has its share of precautions, too, assuming it works the way the manufacturers claim. Fortunately it doesn't, and that's good news for consumers who may be impressionable enough to consider the snake oil–like claims asserted for these products. The eugenol included is a skin irritant, and the antioxidants don't stand a chance once this jar-packaged moisturizer is opened.

😐 **$$$ IceCream Double Scoop Intensive Anti-Aging Moisturizer** *($95 for 1.7 ounces)* leaves out all of the works-like-Botox peptides and GABA and is just a moisturizer. Of course, the claims are tempting and speak of the long-term firming and toning benefits, but all this will do is refine the texture of normal to slightly dry skin. Jar packaging won't keep the few antioxidants in this product stable after it is opened.

😐 **$$$ PlumpLips Lip Plumper** *($40 for 0.28 ounce)* contains enough niacin (nicotinic acid) to produce a brief warming sensation on the lips, which is counteracted by the cool tingle you'll feel from the menthol in this glosslike product with a selection of sheer shades. It doesn't plump lips so much as irritate them by encouraging excess blood flow to the lips that can temporarily make them swell. You won't go from thin lips to a full-on Julia Roberts' pucker, but you will see a difference. The unfortunate element is that the difference comes at the expense of irritating your lips. In the long run this will do more harm than good, though occasional use is acceptable. By the way, the clear tube packaging won't keep the retinol in this formula stable.

GARNIER NUTRITIONISTE (SKIN CARE ONLY)

GARNIER NUTRITIONISTE AT-A-GLANCE

Strengths: Inexpensive; well-formulated moisturizers (those in non-jar packaging); an intriguing serum.

Weaknesses: Lack of sufficient UVA protection from the sunscreens; mostly irritating cleansers; no products for blemish-prone skin; no products to address uneven skin tone or skin discolorations; ineffective BHA products; jar packaging; their marketing angle of merging nutrition and skin-care science as about as unique as wearing a white wedding dress.

For more information about Garnier Nutritioniste, call (800) 370-1925 or visit www.garniernutritioniste.com or www.Beautypedia.com.

GARNIER NUTRITIONISTE NUTRI-PURE PRODUCTS

☺ **Nutri-Pure Detoxifying Cream Cleanser, Oil-Free** *($5.99 for 6.7 ounces)* is a water-soluble cleanser with a slightly creamy texture. Adding nutrients (antioxidants) to a cleanser is somewhat of a waste because they are rinsed from skin before they can exert a benefit. In this case, there's more fragrance than nutrients. Although this won't detoxify skin (nor does skin need to be detoxified), it is an effective option for normal to slightly dry or slightly oily skin. The tiny amount of peppermint extract is unlikely to cause irritation.

☹ **Nutri-Pure Detoxifying Gel Cleanser** *($5.99 for 6.7 ounces)* is a very fragrant water-soluble cleanser that contains enough peppermint extract to cause irritation. This is paired with the potent menthol derivative menthoxypropandediol, which only compounds the irritation and is problematic for use around the eyes. The dermatologists behind this line should've known better, but perhaps the cooling effect was created so consumers think the product is working to detoxify their skin, but that's not what's happening.

☹ **Nutri-Pure Detoxifying Wet Cleansing Towelettes, Oil-Free** *($5.99 for 25 wet towelettes)* have minimal cleansing ability (they don't remove mascara, as claimed) and end up being irritating to skin thanks to the amount of peppermint steeped in each cloth. If you're a fan of cleansing cloths or wipes, Olay, Dove, and Pond's have much better options for around the same price.

😐 **Nutri-Pure Microbead Cream Scrub, Oil-Free** *($5.99 for 5 ounces)* is a creamy facial scrub that contains polyethylene as the abrasive agent. The exfoliating granules are larger and, as such, can be a bit rough on skin even in the creamy base of this scrub. The amount of peppermint isn't terrible, but the tingling sensation it causes is concerning, and doesn't make this scrub preferred to most others.

GARNIER NUTRITIONISTE SKIN RENEW PRODUCTS

☺ **Skin Renew Daily Anti-Fatigue Eye Cream** *($12.99 for 0.5 ounce)* claims to boost surface cell regeneration to diminish dark circles and puffiness. This lightweight moisturizer not contain ingredients capable of doing that, and even if it did boost skin-cell turnover (regeneration), that isn't going to help dark circles or puffiness in any way. The amount of salicylic acid in this product isn't enough to exfoliate skin. It's a good option for slightly dry skin anywhere on the face and includes more than token amounts of antioxidants. Used around the eyes, the mica and titanium dioxide will cosmetically blur the appearance of dark circles by reflecting light from shadowed areas.

😐 **Skin Renew Daily Regenerating Moisture Cream** *($12.99 for 1.7 ounces)* has a formula that bests most of those from Lancome's moisturizer collection (remember, L'Oreal owns Lancome and Garnier), which makes the choice of jar packaging unfortunate because it won't keep the vitamins and antioxidants stable after the product is open. As is, it's an OK option for normal to slightly dry skin. The salicylic acid is not present in an amount great enough to exfoliate, and the fragrance components at the end of the ingredient list pose a slight risk of irritation.

☺ **Skin Renew Daily Regenerating Moisture Lotion** *($12.99 for 2.5 ounces)* is similar to, but has a thinner texture than, the Skin Renew Daily Regenerating Moisture Cream above, and also has packaging to keep its antioxidants stable during use. The glycerin- and silicone-enriched formula is ideal for normal to slightly oily skin and leaves a soft matte finish. This would rate a Paula's Pick were it not for tiny amounts of the fragrant additives linalool, limonene, and geraniol. One more thing: The pH of this moisturizer is too high for the salicylic acid to function as an exfoliant.

☹ **Skin Renew Daily Regenerating Moisture Lotion, SPF 15 Sunscreen** *($12.99 for 2.5 ounces)* lacks the UVA-protecting ingredients of titanium dioxide, zinc oxide, avobenzone, Tinosorb, or Mexoryl SX, and is not recommended. Even with sufficient UVA protection, the base formula is a step down from the Skin Renew Daily Regenerating Moisture Lotion above.

☺ **Skin Renew Daily Regenerating Serum** *($12.99 for 1.7 ounces)* makes skin feel very silky thanks to the amount of silicone it contains. Also on hand are appreciable levels of antioxidants and some interesting skin-identical ingredients. This serum's main drawback is its potentially irritating fragrance components (linalool, limonene), and for that and some minor formulary reasons, it is not preferred to serums from Olay Regenerist or Neutrogena Healthy Skin. Once again, the amount of salicylic acid and the pH of this product won't permit exfoliation to occur.

😐/☹ **Skin Renew Regenerating Micro-Polish Kit** *($16.99 for the kit)* is a two-step process, but the only one to take seriously is the **Polishing Exfoliator with Aluminum Oxide Crystals**. This microdermabrasion-in-a-jar scrub uses alumina as the abrasive agent, which can still be rough on skin despite the inclusion of emollient mineral oil and shea butter. It can be a good topical scrub if used carefully (meaning not too much pressure), though it takes longer than usual to rinse and may require a washcloth for complete removal. The second part is the faulty **Post-Treatment Regenerating Moisturizer SPF 15**, which lacks sufficient UVA-protecting ingredients and isn't a very interesting formula to begin with, making it not worth considering on any level. Routinely exfoliating skin with a topical scrub or AHA or BHA product demands careful adherence to daily sun protection, and that's where this kit falls short and puts your skin at risk.

GARNIER NUTRITIONISTE ULTRA-LIFT PRODUCTS

☺ **Ultra-Lift Anti-Wrinkle Firming Eye Cream** *($14.99 for 0.5 ounce)* doesn't (surprise!) contain any ingredients capable of lifting or noticeably firming skin, but it's an elegant formula with a silky cream texture and a good amount of antioxidant vitamin A (as retinyl palmitate). The other intriguing ingredients are present in lesser amounts, but include some effective skin-identical ingredients and passion fruit oil, which supplies skin with several essential fatty acids and adds a soft fragrance to this moisturizer that's best for normal to dry skin anywhere on the face.

☺ **Ultra-Lift Anti-Wrinkle Firming Moisture Cream** *($14.99 for 1.6 ounces)* is similar to the Ultra-Lift Anti-Wrinkle Firming Eye Cream above, except this version has a thicker texture and less silky finish. It is minimally fragranced and overall a worthwhile moisturizer for normal to dry skin. Its fortifying action on surface skin cells will not result in a deep-lifting action, as claimed. Such lifting and tightening of slackened skin is the essence of an artful, medically precise, surgeon-performed face-lift—nothing a moisturizer can match.

☹ **Ultra-Lift Anti-Wrinkle Firming Moisture Cream, SPF 15 Sunscreen** *($14.99 for 1.6 ounces)* continues L'Oreal's (parent company of Garnier) frustrating predilection for launching sunscreens that lack sufficient UVA-protecting ingredients. They know better, and have for years, so products like this are in no way deserving of a purchase or even a second glance.

😐 **Ultra-Lift Anti-Wrinkle Firming Night Cream** *($14.99 for 1.7 ounces)* contains several ingredients that are necessary to make dry to very dry skin look and feel better, including glycerin and shea butter. Although those and the thickening agents in this moisturizer serve dry skin well, the product's jar packaging compromises the effectiveness of the antioxidants, and that's ultra-disappointing.

☹ **Ultra-Lift Anti-Wrinkle Firming Serum** *($14.99 for 1.7 ounces)* lists alcohol as the third ingredient, which is detrimental for skin and cancels out the beneficial effect the antioxidants in this serum may have had. If you want a serum from Garnier, their Skin Renew Daily Regenerating Serum above is the one to choose.

GIORGIO ARMANI

GIORGIO ARMANI AT-A-GLANCE

Strengths: For skin-care products there are none. The makeup is a very different story: outstanding foundations, superb powder textures, a brilliant shimmer fluid, and a neutral palette make this line a must-see, and several products have a gorgeous finish.

Weaknesses: Expensive; lack of options to address most consumers' skin-care needs; foundations with sunscreen that do not provide sufficient UVA protection; the cream blush; mascaras that aren't as impressive as they should be.

For more information about L'Oreal-owned Giorgio Armani makeup, call (877) ARMANI-3 or visit www.giorgioarmanicosmetics.com or www.Beautypedia.com. Note: Although not fully distributed across the United States, Armani cosmetics has a presence in most major cities and the products may be purchased from Armani's Web site.

GIORGIO ARMANI SKIN CARE

😐 **$$$ Luminous Cleansing Milk** *($32 for 6.76 ounces)* is an absurdly priced but very standard, mineral oil–based cleansing lotion. It's fine for normal to dry skin and will remove makeup, but so will plain baby oil or any good cleansing lotion from the drugstore.

☹ **Luminous Clarifying Lotion** *($32 for 6.76 ounces)* lists alcohol as the second ingredient and also contains the irritating menthol derivative menthoxypropanediol. This won't make skin luminous, just irritated and dry.

😐 **$$$ Luminous Hydrating Lotion** *($32 for 6.76 ounces)* is nothing more than water, glycerin, film-forming agent, preservative, a tiny amount of honey, and coloring agents. This is very basic, but lightweight, and no match for hundreds of other moisturizers or "primers" designed to be worn under makeup.

😐 **$$$ Crema Nera** *($225 for 1.76 ounces).* In an attempt to justify the outrageous price for this product, Armani's marketing team has concocted a story of heroic proportions. This "cell regenerating cream" was supposedly inspired by Giorgio Armani's trips to Pantellaria, an Italian island between Sicily and Tunisia. Somehow Armani discovered that the petrified lava from this island's volcanoes contains everything needed to "nearly perfectly recapture the earth's rejuvenating secrets." (Ah, so the fountain of youth is really in Italy). So basically what they're asking you to swallow is that fossilized lava can somehow generate new skin cells and restore radiance to aging skin. According to an article in the August 2007 issue of fashion magazine *W*, L'Oreal (Armani's owner) researchers studied obsidian (volcanic rock) on this island and worked with experts on volcanoes at Naples's Vesuvian Observatory. The minerals sodium, potassium, silica, and iron are claimed to be collectively responsible for oxygenating skin (which by the way generates free-radicals) and helping skin to absorb water (something the top dead layers do exceptionally well all on their own if there is enough moisture in the environment). In short, those minerals or any lava are useless topically on skin and absorbing water is only a small part of what makes skin healthy.

This water- and silicone-based moisturizer does contain all of those minerals, but none of them are capable of achieving skin-perfecting results, including regenerating cells. There is a tiny amount of salicylic acid, but certainly not enough to prompt exfoliation (now that would have been really helpful for skin).

Beyond all of the nonsense claims and useless input from volcanic experts, this is a shockingly boring formula whose only redeeming value is a silky, elegant texture. The fifth ingredient is paraffin, as in paraffin wax, and the other thickening agents that make up the bulk of this product are as inexpensive as it gets. There are a few token antioxidants in here, but whatever slight benefit they may have provided is lost because of jar packaging. Armani stated that his goal was "to have one cream for a lifetime … I want one product that does everything." Lots of women feel that way, too, but there is no product that can fill that bill (who knows what new discoveries lay around the corner?) and this product doesn't even come close to making a valid attempt.

Crema Nera falls drastically short of being an all-encompassing product for anyone's skin: it does not contain sunscreen, is inappropriate for blemish-prone skin, won't be emollient enough for very dry skin, and lacks ingredients that reinforce skin's structural components. On top of all that, the fragrance and fragrance components can be problematic for sensitive skin. When all is said and done, Crema Nera is the skin-care version of a red carpet fashion faux pas.

GIORGIO ARMANI MAKEUP

FOUNDATION: ✓☺ $$$ Designer Shaping Cream Foundation SPF 20 *($65)* earns a place on the ever-growing list of über-pricey foundations, but at least there is a lot to love about this particular option. Its higher-than-usual sunscreen is in-part titanium dioxide, and this is one of the creamiest yet lightweight foundations for dry to very dry skin you're likely to find. Its emollient texture feels decadently silky and blends very well, though it takes time to set to a soft satin finish. Dry skin is left with a radiant glow, while coverage stays in the medium range. The range of 12 shades is, by and large, quite neutral. The only shades to be careful with are the slightly peach #6 and slightly orange #9.5. Shade #2 is gorgeous for fair skin, and those with light to just-medium skin have several excellent choices. The silk fibers and oil in this foundation do not contour skin, so don't mistake this for a face-lift in a jar (though that's likely how the lofty price was determined). It is a rich yet not heavy-feeling cream foundation with a superb blend of ingredients to replenish dry skin while leaving a soft glow.

✓☺ $$$ Luminous Silk Foundation *($55)* is the foundation every Armani makeup artist I spoke to raves about. It's not hard to see why, because this liquid foundation has a fluid, ultra-smooth texture that floats over the skin and dries to a natural, slightly matte finish with a faint hint of shine. For light coverage and an unbelievably skinlike result that comes in 15 mostly gorgeous colors for fair to dark skin, this foundation is tough to beat. The only misstep is shade 0, which is pure white and tends to look ashen. Luminous Silk Foundation is best for normal to slightly dry or slightly oily skin.

✓☺ $$$ Silk Foundation Powder *($48)* is a wet/dry talc-based powder foundation that has a buttercream-smooth texture, excellent application, and natural matte (in feel) finish. The shade range has been cut in half, but the six remaining options are beautifully neutral, with each providing a hint of shine. This provides light to medium coverage and may be worth the splurge if you prefer powder foundations, although, exceptional as this is, equally impressive versions are available for less money from Laura Mercier, M.A.C., and Estee Lauder.

☺ $$$ Matte Silk Foundation *($55)* has a thicker texture and less slip than the Luminous Silk Foundation above, but still blends well. It dries down to a soft, satin matte finish that is minimally absorbent, so this is not a winner if you have oily areas and want shine control. Coverage is medium and the formula comes in just six shades, of which two (#4 and #7) are slightly to noticeably peach. This is worth considering if you have normal to slightly dry skin.

☹ **$$$ Hydra Glow Foundation SPF 15** *($57)* continues Armani's trend of creating foundations with exceptional textures and a shade range that almost perfectly defines neutral. The bad news is that the sunscreen does not contain the UVA-protecting ingredients of titanium dioxide, zinc oxide, avobenzone, Tinosorb, or Mexoryl SX. Considering the high price, that oversight is particularly egregious, because protecting your skin from the detrimental effects of UVA radiation is just too important to ignore. If you have normal to dry skin and are willing to pair this foundation with an effective sunscreen, it has a fluid, slightly creamy application that provides medium coverage and a slightly moist finish, which lends a subtle, non-sparkling glow to skin. The amount of coverage it provides isn't what I would call natural, so you can ignore Armani's claims that this foundation looks like "a second skin." Estee Lauder did a better job making that claim a reality with their excellent Individualist Natural Finish Makeup ($32.50). Hydra Glow Foundation SPF 15 is available in ten shades and, with one exception (shade 6.5 is a yellow tone that can turn a bit too olive), they are beautifully neutral.

CONCEALER: ☺ **$$$ Skin Retouch** *($33)* has an initially thick texture that melts into skin and blends well, but it's also crease-prone unless a generous amount of powder accompanies it. The four shades are mostly great, with 5.5 being too orange for most medium to dark skin tones. Coverage-wise, this adequately disguises redness and dark circles.

☹ **$$$ High Precision Retouch** *($34)* is a liquid concealer applied with the type of long, thin brush usually reserved for liquid eyeliners. You can indeed be precise with the brush, but it's not the best for covering large areas, such as darkness under the eye. Its fluid texture provides medium coverage and blends decently, but because it never really sets, it won't last long before fading and creasing. The four shades are mostly very good, though 4.5 is slightly bright for medium skin tones.

POWDER: ✓☺ **$$$ Sheer Powder** *($44)* is a very smooth, suitably dry, talc-based pressed powder that has a sheer, almost imperceptible finish on the skin (save for the hint of shine it leaves) and comes in four stunning neutral colors. ✓☺ **$$$ Micro-fil Loose Powder** *($47)* has an airy, ultra-fine texture and a seamless finish that is incapable of looking too dry or powdery on skin. The three colors are excellent, though each one leaves a very soft sparkle—something those with oily skin will not be thrilled with, but that those with dry skin will find attractive.

☺ **$$$ Sheer Bronzer** *($42)* is a collection of three pressed bronzing powders, each with a silky but dry texture that is tightly pressed, so the application is sheer. These brush on evenly and leave a soft, shimmering finish. It's not as natural as a true tan (which doesn't glisten), but the believable colors compensate for that. Shade #1 is tricky because it tends to look a bit too brown, but it works as a soft contour color.

BLUSH: ☹ **$$$ Sheer Blush** *($40)* is a good powder blush with a silky, dry texture and smooth application that imparts minimal color. For this amount of money, you should expect (and get) a bigger color payoff. As is, the palette of nude and soft pastel tones provides a bit too much shine for daytime wear.

☹ **Sheer Cream Blush** *($40)* isn't that creamy or sheer, so the name is misleading. This blush has more of a powder texture that's slightly moist. The texture is unique but the application is a problem because it can go on chunky and deposit color unevenly. The shades have more pigment than Armani's Sheer Blush, but in trying to be unique they ended up with a disappointing product.

EYESHADOW: The pressed powder ☺ **$$$ Eyeshadow** *($24)* features an impressively smooth texture that is a pleasure to work with. The shades apply sheer and don't allow you to build much color intensity beyond that, though they cling well to skin. All of the shades have some amount of shine (typically a soft shimmer), with the following being almost matte: 6, 7, 12, 21, and 39. Numbers 1, 15, and 27 are too blue, green, or lilac to recommend. ☺ **$$$ Eye Mania, Eye Design Colors** *($55)* represent Armani's quad eyeshadows, and share the same smooth texture, application, and sheerness as the single Eyeshadow above. All four colors in every quad are shiny, but the shine doesn't flake and it's sheer enough to be wearable for daytime (unless you have wrinkled skin around the eyes). The most workable quads are numbers 2 and 4.

😐 **$$$ Cream Eye Shadow** *($26)* is not a true cream (or even a cream-to-powder) eyeshadow. Rather, it's a creamy-feeling pressed-powder shadow that can be a bit too powdery and imparts more shine than color. It's an OK option for evening makeup, but shiny eyeshadows don't need to cost this much, designer label or not.

EYE AND BROW SHAPER: 😐 **$$$ Smooth Silk Eye Pencil** *($24)* is a standard pencil (in that it needs regular sharpening), but otherwise it has a wonderfully silky application that sets to a reasonably solid finish. For the money, this is above average, though it's not preferred to automatic pencils. Unless you're interested in using eye pencil for shock value, avoid numbers 3 and 6. 😐 **$$$ Brow Defining Pencil** *($24)* also needs sharpening, but for those who don't mind the inconvenience, this has a smooth, dry application and soft powder finish that really stays in place. The three shades present no options for dark brown or red/auburn brows, a strange oversight from a line of this nature.

LIPSTICK, LIP GLOSS, AND LIPLINER: ✓☺ **$$$ Lipstick Mania** *($25)* feels lightweight and sufficiently creamy without being slick or too sheer. The medium coverage is akin to classic lipstick, but this lasts longer than most. The shade selection is Armani's largest among their lipsticks, but, oddly, the palette is a mixed bag. Still, that doesn't prevent this excellent creamy lipstick from deserving a Paula's Pick rating.

✓☺ **$$$ Lip Shimmer** *($26)* is a splurge, but one you may not mind making if a fantastic lip gloss tops your list of makeup must-haves. This elegant, lightweight, and completely non-sticky lip gloss is applied with a brush and comes in a beautiful selection of colors, each with varying degrees of shimmer. ✓☺ **$$$ Midnight Lip Shimmer** *($26)* is similar to the Lip Shimmer, but is applied with a sponge-tip applicator instead of a brush and the colors are bolder with a strong iridescent finish. Otherwise, the same texture comments apply.

☺ **$$$ ArmaniSilk High Color Cream Lipstick** *($25)* is very similar to Lipstick Mania in that it feels light and creamy without being slick, but the colors are a strange mix of sheer and opaque shades, many including large particles of glitter that distract from some otherwise stunning shades. If you're curious, there are some worthwhile colors, but choose carefully. ☺ **$$$ Shine Lipstick** *($25)* is suitably creamy and offers an attractive glossy finish that's a step above Armani's Sheer Lipstick. The color range is remarkably well-edited and includes some stunning reds. The stain these shades leave give this lipstick a longevity boost that is most welcome.

😐 **$$$ Sheer Lipstick** *($25)* has a moisturizing but greasy feel, although it isn't so slick it slides right off your lips. As the name states, the colors are sheer, and since they provide no stain, you're paying top dollar for a lipstick that likely won't make it past the morning commute. 😐 **$$$ Smooth Silk Lip Pencil** *($25)* needs to be sharpened, which isn't the best, but it applies well without being too creamy and the colors stay in place. Although this will last longer than your average creamy lip pencil, the caveat is that the colors sheer out unless you layer during application. 😐 **$$$ Shine Lip Gloss** *($21)* is a thick, viscous, sticky tube-type gloss that is similar to M.A.C.'s LipGlass ($12.50) and, given the price difference and wide availability of M.A.C. (and countless other lip gloss–toting lines), this is one you can safely pass up.

MASCARA: ✓☺ $$$ Soft Lash Mascara *($25)* is an admirable lengthening mascara that does not clump or flake and allows you to define lashes quickly, plus it layers effortlessly. It isn't much for thickness, but remains a superior lengthening mascara.

😐 **$$$ Star Lash Curling Mascara** *($25)* does indeed provide a soft curl to lashes, but don't expect to abandon your trusty eyelash curler if you typically rely on it for lash enhancement. This formula, and its L'Oreal-inspired, slightly curved brush, builds appreciable thickness and adequate length, but not without some clumps along the way. The overall application is uneven, necessitating extra time to comb through lashes for a separated, clean look. If you're up for the challenges this mascara presents, it does wear well and removes easily.

😐 **$$$ Maestro Instant Volume Mascara** *($26)* is another comb mascara. Although it does create instant volume, the best-looking result required more work than a mascara should. The variegated minicombs deposit a lot of mascara on lashes, but their layout doesn't allow for even application. Therefore, brushing through lashes with a clean mascara wand is necessary to make things look clean yet full. If you're curious to try this type of mascara, L'Oreal's Volume Shocking Mascara ($12.95) is half the price and has a much better application. 😐 **$$$ Soft Lash Primer** *($25)* is essentially a mascara without color, and it builds a waxy base coat on which to apply a regular mascara. A product like this is superfluous if you are already using an excellent mascara, and there are plenty of those to be found for significantly less money than this primer.

BRUSHES: Armani's ☺ **$$$ Brushes** *($24–$55)* have been improved, but they weren't that deficient in the first place. Overall, it's a functional, well-assembled brush collection without any glaring omissions, though the price point doesn't make them preferred to less-expensive brushes. The ☺ **$$$ Face Brush** *($55)* and ☺ **$$$ Blush Brush** *($43)* are full, soft, and luxurious (which they should be at this price), while the ☺ **$$$ Large Eye Contour Brush** *($40)* and ☺ **$$$ Blender Brush** *($45)*, which Armani recommends for applying foundation, are also standouts for their versatility. The 😐 **$$$ Lip Brush** *($24)* is too standard for the money, and because it's a nonretractable brush and without a cap, portability is a problem.

The ☺ **$$$ 10-Brush Luxury Pouch** *($125)* doesn't include any brushes, but for those with unlimited budgets, it is an exquisite high-quality leather pouch with Armani-embossed silver closures. It is designed to fit the shorter-than-usual Armani brushes, so if you're considering this for brushes from another line, make sure they'll fit before purchasing. ☺ **$$$ Weekender** *($125)* is a combination brush and travel case, with the exterior being made of supremely soft black leather. The set allows you to pack essential makeup brushes as well as cosmetics, though it isn't roomy enough to hold everything you'll need for full-face makeup application. Still, for the Hamptons' crowd with a minimalist weekend makeup routine, this may prove irresistible.

FACE AND BODY ILLUMINATING/SHIMMER PRODUCTS: ✓☺ $$$ Fluid Sheer *($55)* is similar in texture and application to the Luminous Silk Foundation above, but is meant to "sculpt" and "illuminate" the complexion. For a touch of radiant shine or to softly highlight or shadow your features in the evening, these are fine and they blend well with foundation or moisturizer. The shade range presents potential options for blush, contour, or bronzing—and, of course, highlighting. Best of all, the shine effect doesn't flake and stays in place on all but the oiliest skin.

SPECIALTY PRODUCTS: ☺ **$$$ Fluid Master Primer** *($55)* costs a lot for what amounts to just silicone. That's all that's in this product! Although it has a silky matte finish and can facilitate makeup application, you don't have to spend this much for equal results. If you choose to do so, this product won't disappoint (well, unless you're expecting long-lasting oil control), but the price is strictly about the designer name.

☺ **$$$ Makeup Vanity Case** *($250)* is a leather makeup case that offers plenty of storage options for all manner of cosmetics, many more than the average woman needs. It's best for working makeup artists, though you'd have to be steadily employed to justify the expense for this case over equally functional but less-expensive cases from Sephora. **Vanity Tray** *($225)* is a gorgeous yet simple black lacquered tray to organize and display makeup on your vanity. It is too large for most bathroom countertops and is definitely an indulgent purchase, but it is well made and serves its purpose for at-home use.

😐 **$$$ Master Corrector** *($35)* is a series of color-correcting liquids packaged in slim, shapely components and outfitted with a precision brush applicator. The thin, light texture is easy to blend, but the four colors are too obvious on skin, so you end up substituting one color "flaw" for another. The Green shade is less green than most, but doesn't look convincing unless you blend it with another color. The Yellow option is so yellow it's almost jaundiced; Pink and Orange are workable but only if carefully applied and deftly blended. I suspect most women won't want to bother with this product. I know I wouldn't.

GLYMED PLUS (SKIN CARE ONLY)

GLYMED PLUS AT-A-GLANCE

Strengths: Cleansers; pH-correct AHA products; most of the sunscreens; reliable products to address hyperpigmentation.

Weaknesses: Expensive; often over-the-top claims; the Serious Action acne line is mostly seriously irritating; jar packaging; this is not an all-inclusive line for anyone's skin.

For more information about Glymed Plus, call (800) 676-9667 or visit www.glymedplus.com or www.Beautypedia.com.

GLYMED PLUS AGE MANAGEMENT SKIN CARE SYSTEM PRODUCTS

☺ **$$$ Gentle Facial Wash** *($30 for 8 ounces)* claims to be the most popular product in the Glymed Plus line, which, given its ordinary nature (it's just a standard water-soluble cleanser for all skin types), is nothing to brag about. The amount of glycolic acid is not enough to exfoliate and, even if it were, that benefit is lost in a cleanser because it is rinsed from skin too soon. The price is what is really obnoxious because nothing in here warrants even a portion of the cost.

☹ **Facial Hydrator** *($41 for 4 ounces)* is a water- and alcohol-based toner that's about as hydrating as sandpaper. It also contains several irritating plant extracts, including ivy, arnica, and pellitory, along with lemon, lime, and balm mint oils. Ouch!

☺ **$$$ AHA Accelerator** *($59 for 4 ounces)* claims to contain a 20% combination of AHAs and BHA, but salicylic acid (BHA) is not listed on the ingredient label. The AHAs glycolic and lactic acids are, and at a pH of 3 they will exfoliate. I am skeptical that the concentration is 20%; however, because if that's true then the amount of glycol listed before the AHAs would need to be greater, which would result in a very tacky-feeling product. Still, I'd wager this contains at least 10% AHAs, and the additional water-binding and soothing agents are good (as is this formula) for all skin types.

☹ **Eye and Lip Renewal Complex** *($37 for 0.75 ounce)* has the correct pH range for the glycolic and lactic acids it contains to exfoliate, if only they amounted to more than 2% of the formula! As is, the AHAs function as skin-identical ingredients, but the lotion base lacks interest and the ylang ylang oil is sensitizing (Source: *Medycyna Pracy*, 2006, pages 431–437).

☺ **$$$ Intense Peptide Skin Recovery Complex** *($75 for 1 ounce)* would be a great way to experience a peptide-rich moisturizer if not for the jar packaging. There isn't a lot of research proving peptides have a noticeable impact on wrinkles, but in theory—when they are in stable packaging—peptides may be cell-communicating ingredients and also have benefit as skin-identical ingredients. Glymed claims this moisturizer contains ingredients that "target lines and wrinkles deep within the skin's infrastructure," but it is doubtful those ingredients (peptides) make it beyond the skin's surface layers because naturally present enzymes break down the peptides before they can reach the depth of a wrinkle, much less work to "rebuild" it. Although not intense, this is an OK moisturizer for normal to dry skin.

☺ **$$$ Photo-Age Environmental Protection Gel SPF 15** *($33.50 for 4 ounces)* is a good, in-part titanium dioxide sunscreen gel for normal to oily skin. The glycerin and silicone base glides on without feeling greasy, and the chamomile is soothing. The cascara bark is not an antioxidant; in fact, it has no history of (or reason for) topical use. This bark extract was subject to some controversy in 2002 because of its use in laxative products, and has since been banned by the FDA for use in drug products, though it may still be sold as an over-the-counter supplement (Source: *Federal Register*, May 2002, pages 31, 125–131).

☺ **$$$ Photo-Age Environmental Protection Gel SPF 30** *($45.50 for 4 ounces)* goes above and beyond in attempting to sound medicinal and superior to other sunscreens, but is just a good, in-part titanium dioxide sunscreen for normal to slightly dry skin not prone to breakouts (the formula contains castor oil). The amount of antioxidants isn't as impressive as the claims state, and the price is cause for concern if it in any way discourages you from applying it liberally.

☹ **Photo-Age Protection Cream SPF 15** *($32.50 for 2 ounces)* does not contain the UVA-protecting ingredients of titanium dioxide, zinc oxide, avobenzone, Tinosorb, or Mexoryl SX, and is not recommended.

☺ **$$$ Treatment Cream** *($56 for 2 ounces)* has merit as a 12% glycolic acid moisturizer for normal to dry skin. The pH of 3.2 allows exfoliation to occur, but this would be better if jar packaging hadn't been chosen. As is, the antioxidants in this product won't remain potent once it is opened.

☹ **Vital A Cream** *($41 for 1 ounce)* claims to contain the highest level of retinyl palmitate available without a prescription, but what about the fact that there is no prescription level of this vitamin A derivative? Glymed must be hoping you'll confuse retinyl palmitate with prescription tretinoin (Renova) or the more effective form, retinol.Their claim doesn't jibe with the ingredient statement either, because this product doesn't appear to include more retinyl palmitate than most others in this line. Another issue: This product is not "synthetic-free," as stated. Silicones are definitely synthetic ingredients, as are the preservatives in this product. The amount of horsetail is the icing on this faulty cake, as it is too astringent and irritating for skin, despite having antioxidant ability (Source: www.herbmed.org).

☹ **Anti-Aging Exfoliant Masque** *($40.50 for 4 ounces)* contains fennel oil, which can cause a phototoxic reaction when skin is exposed to sunlight (Source: www.naturaldatabase.com). This mask also contains an insufficient amount of AHAs or BHA to exfoliate skin, and the pH is too high.

☹ **Arnica+ Healing Cream** *($46.50 for 2 ounces)* lists arnica extract as the second ingredient and also contains other problematic plant extracts with no established benefit for skin. The company claims to use "mega-doses" of arnica extract and oil, though arnica oil doesn't appear on the ingredient list. Whether in extract or oil form, arnica can cause contact dermatitis, and its medicinal use is recommended only for short-term application on unbroken skin (Sources: *American Herbal Products Association's Botanical Safety Handbook*, CRC Press, LLC, 1997; and *Contact Dermatitis*, November 2001, pages 269–272, and October 2002, pages 189–198).

☺ **$$$ Comfort Cream** *($32.50 for 2 ounces)* contains hydrocortisone, but does not list it as an active ingredient, which is in violation of FDA labeling for over-the-counter drugs. A call to the company revealed that the product contains 1% hydrocortisone, the same as considerably less-expensive versions sold at the drugstore. This will work, but you don't have to spend the extra money for comparable results. Just do keep in mind that using cortisone on a regular basis thins skin and causes the breakdown of collagen.

✓☺ **$$$ Derma Pigment Bleaching Fluid** *($37 for 2 ounces)* is a very good, water-based fluid with 2% hydroquinone. It claims to contain azelaic acid, too, but the company uses the salt form (dipotassium azelate) instead, which has no reported function for skin. This hydroquinone fluid is best for normal to very oily skin.

☺ **$$$ Derma Pigment Skin Brightener** *($38 for 2 ounces)* contains mostly water, glycerin, AHA (about 5%), plant oil, aloe, antioxidants, kojic acid, thickeners, skin-identical ingredients, and preservatives. This is a good, pH-correct, glycolic acid–based moisturizer for normal to slightly dry skin. Kojic acid has some ability to inhibit melanin production, but it suffers from poor stability and is a relatively unreliable ingredient. Consider this a good AHA (rather than skin-lightening) product with some good elements for normal to dry skin.

✓☺ **$$$ Living Cell Clarifier** *($38.50 for 2 ounces)* contains live yeast cells, sort of like those that make bread dough rise. There is no known benefit to using these on skin, but it won't hurt skin either. This product also contains bearberry, licorice, a form of vitamin C that can be helpful for inhibiting melanin production, other antioxidants, skin-identical ingredients, and anti-irritants. The yeast part is hokey, but overall this is a well-formulated, lightweight moisturizer for normal to slightly dry skin.

☺ **$$$ Quickies Pocket Packs SPF 15** *($39.95 for 30 wipes)* is identical to the Photo-Age Environmental Protection Gel SPF 15 above, only in wipe-on towelette form. They are indeed convenient for reapplication when on the go, but otherwise the same comments apply.

GLYMED PLUS CELL SCIENCE PRODUCTS

☹ **Cell Science Mega-Purifying Cleanser** *($30 for 6.5 ounces)* contains irritating lavender oil and a lot of angelica extract, making this impossible to recommend. The main plant oil in this cleanser is sunflower, and you'd be better off using that instead, assuming your skin is dry to very dry and not prone to blemishes.

☺ **$$$ Cell Science Skin Recovery Mist** *($32 for 4 ounces)* is a basic, spray-on, alcohol- and fragrance-free toner that contains mostly water, algae, and aloe. The additional skin-identical ingredients make this appropriate for normal to dry skin.

☺ **$$$ Cell Science Cell Serum** *($83 for 0.5 ounce)* would be rated higher if not for the mysterious listing of "certified organic herbs" (which is not in compliance with FDA regulations). You don't really know what you may be putting on your skin, and that's a shame, because this water- and silicone-based serum contains some very good antioxidants and ingredients that mimic the structure and function of healthy skin. This serum is best for normal to dry skin.

✓☺ **$$$ Cell Science Eye Calm** *($36 for 0.3 ounce)* is a well-formulated, emollient eye cream that contains several nonvolatile plant oils, antioxidants, and a small but good selection of skin-identical ingredients. It is fragrance-free.

😐 **$$$ Cell Science Superior C Renewal Cream** *($95 for 1 ounce)* is merely silicones with vitamins C, E, and A. The antioxidant vitamins will lose potency once this jar-packaged product is opened, preventing them from working as intended, and in turn making this costly, serum-type moisturizer a disappointment. With a packaging change, this would definitely be an option.

😐 **$$$ Cell Science Photo-Age Protection Cream 30+** *($55 for 2 ounces)* has titanium dioxide for sufficient UVA protection, which is joined by other sunscreen agents in a moisturizing base suitable for normal to slightly dry skin. It is disappointing that the antioxidants and other air-sensitive ingredients are subject to deterioration due to jar packaging.

😐 **$$$ Cell Science Repair Cream** *($74 for 2 ounces)* is a very emollient moisturizer for dry to very dry skin, but its repairing benefits are minimized because the many antioxidants in this product won't remain stable due to jar packaging.

😐 **$$$ Cell Science Ultra Hydro Gel** *($63.50 for 2 ounces)* goes on and on about the hyaluronic acid it contains, yet it actually contains the less-expensive (but still effective) salt-based form, sodium hyaluronate. Otherwise, this is a lightweight, fragrance-free gel moisturizer for oily to very oily or sensitive skin not prone to significant dryness. It would deserve a higher rating if it were more than just a one-note song; that is, it would have been far better with antioxidants and cell-communicating ingredients.

😐 **$$$ Cell Science Vitamin E-Sensual Cell Cream** *($74 for 2 ounces)* is said to fight aging by reducing the lipid peroxidation that destroys skin cells. Lipid peroxidation is a form of free-radical damage, and although this moisturizer for dry to very dry skin contains the antioxidants grape seed oil and vitamin E, the jar packaging won't keep them stable once you open the product, making it less effective for its intended purpose. This moisturizer is fragrance-free.

☹ **Cell Science Capillary Repair** *($61 for 2 ounces)* makes all manner of claims pertaining to repairing broken capillaries and plugging microscopic leaks that lead to capillary inflammation. A major ingredient in this product is horse chestnut extract. There is research showing that oral consumption of standardized horse chestnut extract can reduce symptoms of chronic venous insufficiency, and it may be a plant extract that has promise for reducing the appearance of wrinkles, but nothing supports Glymed's claims that topical application will improve the appearance of damaged capillaries (Sources: www.naturaldatabase.com; *Dermatologic Surgery*, July 2005, pages 873–880; and *Journal of Cosmetic Science*, September/October 2006, pages 369–376). The horse chestnut won't help capillaries, and the lavender and rosemary oils can cause irritation and make inflamed areas of skin appear worse.

😐 **$$$ Cell Science Clarifying Masque** *($41.50 for 2 ounces)* is a standard clay mask weighed down by some problematic plants, including lavender and lemongrass. The addition of plant oils may make this less drying, but also makes it a confused product. Who is supposed to use this when it's too rich for oily, blemish-prone skin and too absorbent for dry skin? It's an option for normal skin not prone to blemishes, but the price is a burn for what you get.

☺ **$$$ Cell Science Hydrating Masque** *($41.50 for 2 ounces)* contains the same problematic plants as the Cell Science Clarifying Masque above, though in their infusion form they are likely too diluted to cause irritation. That leaves you with a moisturizing mask for normal to dry skin whose helpful antioxidants are best left on skin as long as possible.

☹ **$$$ Cell Science Immune Booster Serum** *($95.50 for 1 ounce)* contains enough horsetail infusion to be potentially irritating to skin, and that won't help in terms of boosting its immune function. There aren't any unique ingredients in this water- and silicone-based serum, so I suppose if it really can restore power to the skin's immune cells (Langerhans cells), then so can most of the other Glymed serums, as well as those from many other companies. This fragranced serum is best for normal to dry skin.

unrated **Cell Science Progesterone Cream** *($51.50 for 1.7 ounces)*. The only reason to consider this product is because of the progesterone content. Other than that it is a fairly ordinary moisturizer. Topically applied progesterone has proponents and critics. There is research showing it absorbs poorly into skin, so this would have little, if any, benefit (Source: *Skin Pharmacology and Physiology*, June 2006, pages 336–342), but there is also research showing that a 2% concentration of progesterone can help skin elasticity and firmness (Source: *British Journal of Dermatology*, September 2005, pages 626–634). Other research indicates that creams or lotions penetrate poorly but gels do much better (Source: *Menopause*, March 2005, pages 232–237).

Of course, none of this explains the issue of the risk for endometrial cancer associated with long-term progesterone use (Sources: *British Journal of Obstetrics and Gynecology*, June 2000, pages 722–726; and *Journal of Clinical Pharmacology*, May 2005, pages 614–619). In terms of all the research I've seen, this summary from a retrospective study published in *The Medical Journal of Australia* (May 2005, pages 237–239) is one to consider very carefully: "The claims for transdermal progesterone creams and the hypothesis on which they are based have been founded on anecdotal information rather than on sound scientific research. In a number of small but carefully conducted prospective, double-blind, randomized studies, progesterone cream has been shown to be no different from placebo in its ability to control vasomotor, psychosexual or mood symptoms. It does not induce a positive response in the biochemical markers for bone metabolic activity or plasma lipid levels. Creams containing progesterone in the doses currently available for clinical use do not fulfill the criteria necessary for them to be endorsed as a therapeutic agent to treat menopausal hormone deficiency." Whatever you decide about the use of progesterone creams, be aware that there are far less-expensive versions available at most health food or vitamin supplement stores than this pricey version.

☹ **Cell Science Lip Science** *($36 for 0.3 ounce)* is sold as a "completely natural" alternative to lip injections. First, lip injections can be natural because they often use collagen, hyaluronic acid, or even your own fat. In terms of formulation, nothing in this product can make it come close to emulating the results of lip injections. This water- and oil-based lip moisturizer ends up being a problem because it contains peppermint oil, which swells lips by virtue of irritation.

GLYMED PLUS SERIOUS ACTION: THE ACNE MANAGEMENT SKIN-CARE SYSTEM

☺ **$$$ Serious Action Sal-X Purifying Skin Cleanser** *($32.50 for 8 ounces)* is worth considering as a water-soluble cleanser for normal to oily skin, blemish-prone or not. However, the 2% salicylic acid is best left on skin, not rinsed quickly as it would be with this fragrance-free cleanser.

☺ **$$$ Serious Action Skin Wash** *($32.50 for 8 ounces)* is a gentler version of the Serious Action Sal-X Purifying Skin Cleanser above, with 2.5% benzoyl peroxide as the active ingredient instead of salicylic acid. The same effectiveness comments apply here, too; benzoyl peroxide is best left on skin rather than rinsed shortly after application. Further, it should not be used near the eyes or mucous membranes, meaning that this is a cleanser to use cautiously. Benzoyl peroxide isn't completely wasted in a cleanser—it's just that you have a greater chance of success if you leave it on longer than you would a cleanser.

☹ **Serious Action Sal-X Exfoliating Cleanser** *($32.50 for 8 ounces)* contains grapefruit peel and orange oils, which make it too irritating for all skin types.

☹ **Serious Action Skin Exfoliant Wash** *($32.50 for 8 ounces)* contains lavender oil, making it too irritating for all skin types. Neutrogena makes several medicated scrubs with cleansing potential, if that's what you're after—and keep in mind that acne cannot be scrubbed away.

☹ **Serious Action Skin Astringent No. 2** *($29.50 for 8 ounces)* claims to dry up acne, but the only thing you can dry up is water. Using drying ingredients such as the isopropyl alcohol in this toner may make acne lesions smaller because the skin is dehydrated, but you may end up damaging skin and hurting its healing process, especially when it's paired with the other irritants in this product, including menthol, arnica, and ivy.

☹ **Serious Action Skin Astringent No. 5** *($30.50 for 8 ounces)* contains an amount of salicylic acid not approved for over-the-counter use in terms of treating acne, and the pH of this astringent is too high for it to function as an exfoliant. This ends up being an exceedingly irritating product that has the same roster of unhelpful ingredients as the Serious Action Skin Astringent No. 2 above.

☹ **Serious Action Skin Astringent No. 10** *($33 for 8 ounces)* contains 10% salicylic acid (which is hopefully a mistake on their label), an amount the FDA does not permit for use in anti-acne products sold over the counter—a category this product qualifies for, as it is readily available for consumers to order online. It contains a lot of alcohol along with lesser but still problematic amounts of menthol, St. John's wort, and ivy. This product is a serious problem for a consumer who uses it.

☹ **Serious Action Skin Gel with Tea Tree Oil** *($57 for 4 ounces)* is a very expensive way to irritate skin. The glycolic, salicylic, and lactic acids won't exfoliate skin because the pH of this product is too high, but the camphor, eucalyptus oil, and alcohol will all make acne-prone skin look and feel worse. Oddly, the ingredient list for this product makes no mention of tea tree oil.

☹ **Serious Action Masque** *($41 for 4 ounces)* hurts to write about! This clay mask contains alcohol, so it's more drying than most clay masks, and it irritates skin with camphor, eucalyptol, thymol, and arnica. Further, what is soybean oil doing in a product meant to be used on oily, acne-prone skin?

☹ **Serious Action Nooners Acne Wipes** *($39.95 for 30 wipes)* is full of drying, irritating ingredients that shouldn't be applied to skin at any time of day. The salicylic acid will not exfoliate skin because the pH of these wipes is too high.

☹ **Serious Action Skin Medication No. 5** *($32 for 4 ounces)* would be recommended as a very good topical disinfectant with 5% benzoyl peroxide if it did not contain cell-damaging lavender oil.

☹ **Serious Action Skin Medication No. 10** *($32.50 for 4 ounces)* is nearly identical to the Serious Action Skin Medication No. 5 above, except this contains 10% benzoyl peroxide. Otherwise, the same review applies.

☹ **Serious Action Skin Peeling Lotion** *($33 for 4 ounces)* contains sulfur, salicylic acid, resorcinol, and alcohol, so I would absolutely call this seriously irritating and a misguided concoction for acne if ever there was one. There are far better ways to exfoliate skin and disinfect it at the same time without using these three ingredients at the same time, and lavender oil only makes matters worse. "Skin Peeling" is right, because with a pH of 2.3 this is one very harsh product.

☹ **Serious Action Sulfur Masque** *($35.50 for 4 ounces)* contains 10% sulfur, which is a very potent disinfectant, and has a high pH that can actually encourage the growth of bacteria! Unfortunately, it is also very irritating and the tradeoff may not be worth it, especially considering the grapefruit oil in this clay- and talc-based mask.

GLYMED PLUS SUN PRODUCTS

☺ **$$$ Tan In, Fast-Acting Sunless Tanning Cream** *($40.99 for 6 ounces)* is a self-tanning lotion for normal to dry skin that contains dihydroxyacetone, the same ingredient found in most self-tanning products. This also contains caramel, which provides instant sheer color, and mica, which adds a soft shimmer.

GOOD SKIN

GOOD SKIN AT-A-GLANCE

Strengths: Price; several state-of-the-art moisturizers and serums; superb cleansers; some well-rounded sunscreens that go beyond just protecting skin from sunlight; hand cream with sunscreen; several fragrance-free products; one awesome foundation; powder blush; loose powder; loose shimmer powder; easily accessible tester units.

Weaknesses: A few sunscreens with paltry amounts of UVA-protecting ingredients; some problematic anti-acne products and a lack of topical disinfectant for blemishes; the makeup items with sunscreen lack sufficient UVA-protecting ingredients; the anti-acne foundation and concealer; the mascara; jar packaging; the displays aren't easily understood and sales help is often hard to find.

For more information about Good Skin, owned by Estee Lauder and sold exclusively at Kohl's, call (866) 352-8338 or visit www.goodskindermcare.com or www.Beautypedia.com.

GOOD SKIN SKIN CARE

GOOD SKIN ALL BRIGHT PRODUCTS

✓☺ **All Bright Moisture Cream** *($23.50 for 1.7 ounces)* has a compelling assortment of state-of-the-art ingredients covering every category that could make your skin happy, along with a wonderful silky texture. There's only one misstep, but it's barely worth mentioning. In essence, this is a very good moisturizer for normal to dry skin—just don't count on it to improve skin discolorations. Mulberry extract and glycyrrhetinic acid (a derivative of licorice) have only a small amount of research showing them to have benefit in this regard, and this research included only a handful of participants who applied those ingredients at high concentrations (Sources: *International Journal of Dermatology*, April 2000, pages 299–301; and *Skin Lightening and Depigmenting Agents*, www.emedicine.com/derm/topic528.htm).

✓☺ **All Bright Moisturizing Sunscreen SPF 30** *($12 for 1.7 ounces)*, with 2% avobenzone, can be relied on for sufficient UVA protection. It also has an array of beneficial ingredients for skin, and that all adds up to a decent daily sunscreen. It isn't the best formula for sensitive skin, but a well-formulated sunscreen of any kind is the first line of defense to improve the appearance of skin discolorations—and prevent them in the first place. Yeast is a good water-binding agent, but has zero effect on discolorations.

✓☺ **All Bright Hand Cream SPF 15** *($16 for 1.7 ounces)* features an in-part titanium dioxide sunscreen in an emollient, antioxidant-rich base that's ideal for dry hands (though it does leave a slightly greasy finish that can make your hands feel slippery). Women often ask me if I know of a good, portable sunscreen they can use just for their hands, and here's a great one to try!

☹ **All Bright 2 Step Facial Peel Pads** *($30 for the kit)* is a poorly conceived product. One jar holds the **Peel Pads**, which contain 10% citric acid (better known as the sour salt used in cooking that imparts extreme tartness to food), a buffering agent (to raise the pH), lime, glycerin, and preservatives. Citric acid is rarely used in cosmetics as an exfoliant, so there is no research that demonstrates either its efficacy or potential problems when used for this purpose (Source: www.fda.gov/ohrms/dockets/dailys/03/Feb03/020403/8004d35c.pdf). Whether it would work in a way similar to glycolic acid, lactic acid (AHA), or salicylic acid (BHA) is anyone's guess. The second jar contains **Neutralizer Pads**, which offer little more than water, slip agents, and bicarbonate of soda. These pads are intended to neutralize the acidity of the citric acid, but rinsing really well with water does the same thing. When you add it all up, why go through a two-step exfoliating process for unknown results when a simple, well-formulated AHA or BHA product can do the job better and without all the fuss?

☺ **All Bright Spot Treatment** *($16 for 0.5 ounce)* is supposed to dramatically dissolve dark spots and discolorations because of the yeast ferment and fruit extracts it contains. The amount of fruit extracts is barely worth mentioning, and although there's a considerable amount of yeast extract, there is no research aligning it with any measure of skin-lightening ability. In the end, this is a lightweight, serum-like moisturizer for normal to slightly dry skin.

GOOD SKIN ALL CALM PRODUCTS

✓☺ **All Calm Creamy Cleanser** *($15 for 6.7 ounces)* is indeed creamy and fairly emollient, so you need a washcloth to be sure you remove all of it and get all your makeup off as well. A blend of thickeners, plant oils, and silicones makes this extremely helpful for someone with dry skin, regardless of whether your skin is sensitive or not.

😐 **All Calm Soothing Toner** *($15 for 6.7 ounces)* is a simple blend of water, slip agents, glycerin, skin-identical ingredients, anti-irritants, and an antioxidant. It isn't a particularly exciting formulation, but it has potential for normal to dry skin. The lavender extract keeps it from earning a higher rating.

✓☺ **All Calm Gentle Sunscreen SPF 25** *($12 for 1.7 ounces)* is aptly formulated for someone with sensitive skin. The sunscreen base is purely titanium dioxide and zinc oxide, which means you get excellent sun protection with almost no risk of irritation. It also has a wonderful silky feel with a nice array of impressive, state-of-the-art ingredients. While it does contain coloring agents to lessen the white appearance of the sunscreen ingredients on skin, it is fragrance-free. This one is a winner!

😐 **$$$ All Calm Moisture Cream** *($22.50 for 1.7 ounces)* contains some good soothing agents and antioxidants, but since these ingredients are light- and air-sensitive, their potency is compromised by the jar packaging. This ends up being a decent option for normal to dry skin, but better packaging would have made it so much, well, better!

☺ **All Calm Moisture Lotion** *($22.50 for 1.7 ounces)* is a silky, lotion-textured moisturizer with a smattering of skin-identical ingredients, anti-irritants, and antioxidants. It's not a great moisturizer for someone with normal to dry skin, but it's definitely a good one.

☹ **All Calm Redness Tamer** *($15 for 0.13 ounces)* is merely an emollient, green-tinted concealer that doesn't contain anything that can calm down what might be causing your skin to be red. Besides, green doesn't cover red, and you end up with a noticeably green cast to the area you are trying to cover.

GOOD SKIN ALL FIRM SKIN CARE

☹ **All Firm Moisture Cream SPF 15** *($23.50 for 1.7 ounces)* does contain the UVA-protecting ingredient titanium dioxide, but in a concentration of less than 1%, which is not enough to make it reliable for protecting skin from the full spectrum of the sun's damaging rays. It does have an impressive array of ingredients that would make it noteworthy for skin, but putting these unstable ingredients in jar packaging means that any benefit from them is time-limited due to the way they decompose on contact with air. That, together with the less-than-exciting sunscreen ingredients, means this is a product that can stay on the shelf.

✓☺ **All Firm Rebuilding Serum** *($25 for 1 ounce)* is a good, lightweight moisturizer with a very good mix of interesting state-of-the-art ingredients. This is definitely helpful for skin, and the weightless texture works for many skin types. Just don't expect to see firmer skin anytime soon.

GOOD SKIN ALL RIGHT SKIN CARE

☹ **All Right Medicated Cleanser** *($12 for 4.2 ounces)* contains 1% salicylic acid, but it's in a cleanser, so the exfoliating acid is rinsed down the drain before it has an opportunity to benefit the skin. The inclusion of peppermint wrecks an otherwise good, water-soluble cleanser for normal to oily skin.

☹ **All Right Purifying Toner** *($12 for 6.7 ounces)* has alcohol and witch hazel headlining the ingredient list, so the only thing "all right" about this product is the name. The 1.5% salicylic acid it contains is a good exfoliant, but the risk of irritation, redness, and dryness posed by the other ingredients means it isn't worth the price of admission.

☹ **All Right Mattifying Gel** *($12 for 0.5 ounce)* could have been a contender for helping someone with a minor blemish problem, thanks to its 0.5% salicylic acid content, but the alcohol listed prominently in second place on the ingredient list makes the potential for irritation and dryness more likely, and that doesn't help any skin type.

☺ **All Right Oil-Free Lotion** *($17.50 for 1.7 ounces)* is a 0.5% salicylic acid lotion with a pH of 3.8, so it will provide minor exfoliation (1% salicylic acid is preferred). The small amounts of antioxidants and anti-irritants are a thoughtful touch, and this does have a smooth texture with a decent matte finish for someone with normal to oily skin.

✓☺ **All Right Oil-Free Sunscreen SPF 30** *($12 for 1.7 ounces)* is an exceptionally well-formulated sunscreen, listing avobenzone as one of the active sunscreen ingredients to cover the UVA spectrum, along with antioxidants, cell-communicating ingredients, and ingredients that mimic skin structure. Appropriately, it has a dependable matte finish. Now this really is all right!

☺ **All Right Portable Anti-Acne Swabs** *($6.50 for 12 swabs)* are intended to provide a way to precisely apply salicylic acid (BHA) directly to a blemish without getting it on the surrounding skin. The stem of the cotton swab contains a liquid solution of 2% salicylic acid, and when you break the tip the fluid flows into it, ready to apply to the blemish-prone area. The pH of 3.6 ensures the salicylic acid will work as intended.

Although BHA can help disinfect and reduce inflammation (salicylic acid is both an antibacterial agent and an anti-irritant, since it is closely related to aspirin), it can also work preventively to keep breakouts from happening in the first place. With this product, however, you don't get enough to apply all over, you barely get enough for even a couple of blemishes. This ends up being a fairly pricey way to treat acne, unless you happen to be the lucky person who gets only one or two pimples a month.

☹ **All Right Spot Treatment** *($8.50 for 0.5 ounce)* is a 1% salicylic acid topical exfoliant that would be a slam-dunk recommendation if it didn't contain menthol, which only serves to irritate skin.

OTHER GOOD SKIN PRODUCTS

☺ **Clean Skin Foaming Cleanser** *($10.50 for 6.7 ounces)* is a standard but good detergent-based, water-soluble cleanser for normal to oily skin. It leaves skin feeling clean but not too dry; this would be rated higher if not for the amount of grapefruit extract it contains.

✓☺ **Perfect Balance Gel Cleanser** *($10.50 for 6.7 ounces)*, just as the name says, does have a very good balance going for it. It has an effective assortment of gentle detergent cleansing agents, which makes it a very good water-soluble cleanser for someone with normal to oily or combination skin.

✓☺ **Soft Skin Creamy Cleanser** *($10.50 for 6.7 ounces)* is a very good emollient cleanser for dry skin that contains a nice blend of emollients, plant oils, and silicone. You may need to use a washcloth to be sure it is all rinsed off, but all in all this is an excellent product.

☺ **$$$ Microcrystal Skin Refinisher** *($25 for 1.7 ounces)* is a lotion-style scrub that contains alumina as the abrasive agent. Alumina has a texture akin to salt, which makes this fairly gritty and scratchy, so be extra careful if you decide to give it a try. A handful of antioxidants and anti-irritants are included, but will be rinsed off before they can have any effect. For manual exfoliation, this is a pricey and perhaps overly rough scrub; gentler options are definitely available.

✓☺ **Polished Skin Gentle Exfoliator** *($14 for 3.4 ounces)* comes in a gel formulation that is, indeed, quite gentle, and for exfoliation it works well. Because the base doesn't have other cleansing agents, you wouldn't want to rely on this alone for cleansing; you'd need to use it after using a water-soluble cleanser.

😐 **All Hydrated Moisture Cream** *($22.50 for 1.7 ounces)* has many formulary positives, but the overriding negative is that jar packaging will render several of the most helpful ingredients ineffective shortly after you begin using this. The fragrance-free, silky-finish formula is suitable for normal to dry skin not prone to blemishes.

✓☺ **Clean Skin Oil-Free Lotion SPF 15** *($15 for 1.7 ounces)* is a very good moisturizer for someone with normal to oily skin who needs a reliable sunscreen with UVA-protecting ingredients. With an impressive 3% avobenzone, this one fills the bill for the kind of sun protection skin needs. It is appropriately lightweight, with a slight matte finish (though it won't hold up all day). It has a decent, amount of ingredients that mimic skin structure, a cell-communicating ingredient, antioxidants, and anti-irritants. It is also fragrance-free and coloring agent–free. Now that's what I'm talking about!

😐 **$$$ Instant Lightening Eye Cream** *($21 for 0.5 ounce)* has a fairly matte finish and isn't the best if you have dry skin around your eyes. The "instant lightening" claim relates to the inclusion of mica, which adds a small amount of shine, and titanium dioxide, which adds a teeny amount of whiteness, but that won't fool anyone. None of the other ingredients can instantly or even slowly lighten the eye area. Other than that, this does contain a decent group of state-of-the-art ingredients, but they would have worked so much better for lots of women if the base had a nicer texture.

☺ **$$$ Perfect Balance Moisture Lotion SPF 15** *($15 for 1.7 ounces)* contains 1.2% titanium dioxide for UVA protection, which is going in the right direction, but it's still not a big enough improvement to warrant an all-star rating. All the best state-of-the-art ingredients are present in this product, and it does have a light silky feel that makes it a wonderful option for someone with normal to dry or combination skin.

😐 **$$$ Smoothing Lifting Eye Cream** *($21 for 0.5 ounce)* is far more emollient than the Instant Lightening Eye Cream above, and would be preferred by those who tend to have drier skin in the under-eye area. It also has an impressive range of antioxidants, ingredients that mimic skin structure, cell-communicating ingredients, and anti-irritants, which made this a strong contender as a Paula's Pick. But why, oh, why, did they have to package it in a jar? These smart-to-include ingredients are all air sensitive, and the jar packaging will render them ineffective in a short time. Sigh! Very disappointing!

By the way, the Good Skin Web site poses the following question: "Do I really need to use a separate eye cream, or will my everyday moisturizer do?" The answer they provide is: "The skin around the eyes is more fragile than that of the face, and therefore requires more delicate formulas specifically targeted for the area." My response is: While the skin around the eye does have some differences from the skin on the rest of the face—in thickness and in the number of oil glands present—I've yet to see an eye cream, including this one, that is formulated in any way that makes it "unique" for the eye area only. In reality, skin anywhere on the body requires the same, skin-friendly ingredients to improve cell production, generate healthy collagen, and make skin feel silky-smooth.

☺ **Smooth-365 Intensive Clarity + Smoothing Peptide Serum** *($42.50 for 1.7 ounces)* ranks as the most expensive Good Skin product, but is it worth the investment? Said to perfect "the overall quality of our skin's appearance right now and into the future" gets things off to a questionable start. That's because without a sunscreen, this cannot prevent sun exposure from making your appearance imperfect. This silicone-based serum will make all skin types feel wonderfully silky, and it contains some good antioxidants and mulberry root extract, which can have a positive impact on skin discolorations (though likely not in the amount used in this product). There is only one peptide in this product, and the amount used is rather small. Although this is an option, it is not as well-rounded or state-of-the-art as Good Skin's Tri-Aktiline Instant Deep Wrinkle Filler below.

😐 **Soft Skin Moisture Cream SPF 15** *($15 for 1.7 ounces)* does contain titanium dioxide for UVA sun protection, but not very much. A 1% concentration is disappointing, but not terrible. A higher concentration would have provided far better UVA protection. All in all, this is a reliable, emollient moisturizer for normal to dry skin. The assortment of antioxidants, ingredients that mimic skin structure, and cell-communicating ingredients is impressive, but several of these ingredients will be compromised once this jar-packaged product is opened.

✓☺ **$$$ Tri-Aktiline Instant Deep Wrinkle Filler** *($39.50 for 1 ounce)* is supposed to help eliminate wrinkles, frown lines, brow lines, and lines around the eye, leaving you flawless, lineless, and, presumably, expressionless. Not to worry. This water- and silicone-based serum doesn't come close to achieving its goals (and, of course, Good Skin's "stringent tests" establishing efficacy were neither available for review nor published). Although it won't send wrinkles and expression lines packing, it does provide a dose of antioxidants, sophisticated skin-identical ingredients, and cell-communicating ingredients, and it comes in packaging that will keep them stable. It has what it takes to promote and maintain healthier skin and does so without adding fragrance, a lack that's always a plus. You'll only be disappointed if you believe the wrinkle-eliminating claims. Those with realistic expectations should definitely consider this product, though its texture is best for normal to slightly dry or slightly oily skin.

☺ **$$$ Megabalm Ultra Soothing Lip Treatment** *($9.50 for 0.24 ounce)* is a standard, Vaseline-based lip balm that will take good care of dry, chapped lips. The tiny amount of sage leaf is unlikely to be irritating. This does contain coloring agent.

GOOD SKIN MAKEUP

FOUNDATION: ✓☺ All Firm Makeup *($15)* is the best foundation in Good Skin's makeup collection. The fluid texture blends very well, feels silky, and leaves a gorgeous, natural-looking smooth matte finish. This is meant to soften the appearance of lines and wrinkles, but it cannot do that. It will provide light to medium coverage without looking or feeling heavy, and the formula does contain some intriguing extras such as peptides and several cell-communicating ingredients. There are 12 shades, most of which are suitably neutral and appropriate for fair to dark (but not very dark) skin tones. Consider Level 4 Warm and Level 5 Cool carefully because of their peachy-pink tones, and avoid the obviously pink Level 4 Cool and rosy-copper Level 6 Cool. All Firm Makeup is best for normal to slightly dry or slightly oily skin.

😐 **Sheer Color Makeup SPF 15** *($15)* has a satin-smooth texture that adds a soft, moist finish to skin while providing sheer coverage and a hint of color. The range of 12 shades provides some neutral and not-so-neutral options, though the lesser shades are so sheer that the peach or pink tones aren't bothersome. The problem is that the sunscreen lacks sufficient UVA protection, making this a poor choice for those looking for an all-inclusive daytime moisturizer.

☹ **All Right Makeup** *($15)* doesn't deserve its name because the alcohol-laden formula is far from all right. Other irritants added to this foundation for acne-prone skin include eucalyptus and clove, neither of which are the least bit helpful. The 0.5% amount of salicylic acid is hardly enough to provide exfoliating benefits; there are better BHA products available. This foundation also has an unpleasant texture, separates easily, and has an uncomfortably dry finish.

CONCEALER: 😐 Two Perfect Eye Concealer Duo *($15)* is a dual-sided product in which one end is a liquid concealer and the other is a pale yellow "corrector" for dark circles. Both formulas have enough slip to make blending easy and they provide moderate coverage with a matte finish. The concealer portion doesn't look as flawless as it should; even a slight over-application can create a too-opaque finish that calls attention to itself. Furthermore, half of the six shades are too orange or peach to consider, those being Level 3, Level 4, and Level 5. Level 6 is slightly copper but may work for some dark skin tones, while the yellow "corrector" shade is the same regardless of its partner color (which won't look good on medium to dark skin tones).

☹ **All Right Anti-Acne Concealer** *($12)* lists 0.5% salicylic acid as an active ingredient, which is an amount most won't find effective enough (and it's ineffective in this concealer because of its pH above 4). This tube concealer has a very dry, difficult-to-blend texture and finish that causes the lighter shades to appear chalky, while the darker shades are too peach or orange to consider. The final strike is the inclusion of drying, irritating sulfur.

POWDER: ✓☺ Totally Natural Loose Powder *($16)* has an absolutely beautiful, smooth texture that sets makeup and makes skin look refined rather than dry and powdered. The finish is so skin-like, it's difficult to believe this is a talc-based powder. It is best for normal to dry skin (someone with oily skin won't appreciate the finish), and all four shades are sheer and highly recommended. This powder, like all Good Skin makeup, is fragrance-free.

☺ **Sheer Color Finishing Powder** *($15)* is a very standard talc-free pressed powder. Kaolin (clay) is used instead of talc or mica, and although this results in a drier finish, application remains smooth and even. Best for normal to very oily skin, this powder's six shades are mostly great; only Level 4 suffers from being a bit pink, but is still worth considering.

☺ **All Firm Finishing Powder** *($15)* is said to soften lines and shadows by manipulating light, but all this talc-based pressed powder does is impart a subtle shine to skin. That won't have the line-softening effect advertised, and may actually make lines appear more prominent. Still, this powder's smooth, dry texture and satin matte finish make it an option for all skin types except very oily. Four of the six shades are splendid; Level 5 and Level 6 are neutral dark tones but both have an ashen finish.

BLUSH: ✓☺ **Naturally Cheeky Powder Blush** *($15)* rates as another winner from Good Skin. This pressed-powder blush has an exceptionally smooth texture, applies beautifully, and allows you to build intensity without looking oversaturated. Although the palette of shades is great, each has some amount of shine. The almost-matte options include Pink Lotus, Spring Rose, Tuscan Sun, Golden Ginger, and Plum Crush.

☺ **Cheer Up All-Over Healthy Color** *($16)* is a creamy-feeling pressed powder that applies easily and imparts a sheer, peachy-pink glow to skin. It is too sheer to use as standalone blush (unless you have very fair skin) but works well as a highlighter over blush or on top of the cheekbone.

😐 **Fresh & Cheeky Cream Blush** *($15)* is a thick, oil-based traditional cream blush that is only recommended (with caveats) for those with dry to very dry skin. The greasy texture and strong pigmentation make this tricky to apply without looking clownish, and blending isn't all that smooth. The Golden Light shade is best for highlighting.

EYESHADOW: 😐 **Smooth Color Eyeshadow Duos** *($14.50)* are powder eyeshadows whose texture and application is disappointing compared to the eyeshadow options from Estee Lauder and Clinique (Lauder owns Good Skin). Most of the duos have pairings that are closer to tone-on-tone than complementary colors with one shade being suitable for crease color, which creates shadow and depth. The only pairs worth considering (if you're OK with a less-than-smooth texture) are Nutmeg Spice and Natural Stone.

LIPSTICK AND LIP GLOSS: ☺ **Natural Shine Lipstick** *($12.50)* is a very good lightweight cream lipstick with a slick application and soft gloss finish. This would be rated a Paula's Pick if the colors had more longevity. As is, even the red shades deposit minimal stain and demand more frequent touch-ups. ☺ **Megabalm Tinted Lip Gloss** *($9.50)* is a sheer lip balm in a tube. It has a smooth, emollient feel and provides a wet-looking gloss finish that's only slightly sticky. The shade range is small but good, and each looks darker in the tube than it does when applied to lips.

☹ **Creamcolor Lipstick SPF 15** *($12.50)* has an unusually greasy texture and its sunscreen leaves lips vulnerable to UVA damage because it does not contain titanium dioxide, zinc oxide, avobenzone, Tinosorb, or Mexoryl SX.

MASCARA: 😐 **Lash Lengthening Mascara & Conditioner** *($12.50)* is a dual-sided mascara, with one end being traditional mascara and the other a lash conditioner. The latter is a joke because the amount of alcohol in this clear "primer" will only leave lashes feeling dry.

Applying it before the mascara doesn't enhance its results. The mascara itself does a decent job of making lashes longer and defined, but doesn't hold a candle to superior, less expensive mascaras at the drugstore.

FACE AND BODY ILLUMINATING/SHIMMER PRODUCTS: ☺ **Soft Reflection Illuminating Loose Powder** *($18)* can be messy to apply and feels slightly grainy, but the multi-colored shiny finish is attractive and clings surprisingly well wherever it is applied. Only one shade is offered, and it is versatile enough to be used by all skin colors.

HARD CANDY (MAKEUP ONLY)

HARD CANDY AT-A-GLANCE

Strengths: One nice option each for foundation, powder, and eyeshadow; some very good lip gloss choices; an above average mascara; offers complete product ingredient lists on their Web site.

Weaknesses: Mostly average to below-average formulas, many with glitter; a terrible concealer; no good options for eye or brow shaping; a horrible brush set.

For more information on Hard Candy, call (866) 330-2263, or visit www.hardcandy.com or www.Beautypedia.com.

FOUNDATION: ☺ **Hint Tint** *($16.50)* provides just a hint of sheer colors, and comes in four excellent neutral shades for fair to medium skin tones. The texture is light yet creamy, and it leaves a moist finish best for normal to dry skin. That doesn't describe most teens (who typically are dealing with oily skin and breakouts) but this is a sophisticated-enough formula that it should interest adults (though for daytime you'd need to pair it with a sunscreen containing UVA-protecting ingredients).

CONCEALER: 😐 **Out-Damn Spot! Concealer** *($12.50)* is a needs-sharpening pencil concealer that has a creamy texture and opaque, heavy finish that is difficult to soften. The oil and waxes in the formula make it ill-suited for use on blemishes, and it creases when used under the eye, further limiting its appeal. It does feature two very good colors, though only for fair to light skin tones. I wonder if any teens will get the *Macbeth* reference?

POWDER: ☺ **Complexion Perfection** *($15)* is too sheer to make skin look perfect, but this talc-based pressed powder has a beautiful, silky application and natural matte finish from each of its four soft, neutral colors. The formula contains polyethylene and although it lends a smooth quality to the powder cake, it also makes it feel a bit plastic-like, so this is definitely one to test at the counter before purchasing.

☹ **O-blot-erate** *($16)* is meant to cut oily shine on contact, and the talc- and calcium carbonate-based formula's dry texture and finish will do that. The problem is that the single shade is an unattractive grayish-white that's laced with shine. It applies almost colorless, but adding shine to a powder meant to minimize it is sort of like jogging with a cigarette dangling from your mouth.

BLUSH: 😐 **Sweet Cheeks Liquid Blush** *($13.50)* imparts more shimmer than color, as each of the shades goes on very sheer. The water-based, lotion-like texture makes blending a bit tricky and it has a tacky finish, but this is definitely a way to add a sheer layer of shine to your complexion.

EYESHADOW: ☺ **Eye Candy** *($12.50)* represents a collection of single eyeshadows with a different (and better) formula than the Eye Shadow Quartets below. The pressed powder feels silky-smooth and applies evenly with minimal to no flaking. Even better is that a handful of the shades are versatile, classic choices. Consider Buttered Popcorn, Butterscotch, Caramel, Lollipop, and Taffy, but note that these shades are shiny and not meant for wrinkled eyes. The 1-piece slider component is cute and functional.

The 😐 **$$$ Eye Shadow Quartets** *($28)* have an improved texture that feels and applies much smoother, but the color combinations remain mostly unworkable and best for a shocking, rather than sophisticated, eye design. Every shade is shiny, ranging from a soft shimmer to all-out glitter. The low-glow shades adhere well and stay put, but the glittery ones flake. If you decide to check these out, the best ("best" being a relative term) quads are Old Skool and Moody. And if you like variety, check out the nine-shade **Eye Candy Eye Shadow Palette** *($22)*, which includes pastel shades along with neutrals and one deep shade for lining, all with moderate to intense shine.

☹ **Bling Bling** *($16)* is one of the newer and least impressive Hard Candy products. The product consists of a small jar of loose glitter and two "magnetic" bases, one a flesh tone and the other an inky black. You apply the base and then the glitter, which sticks to it (though not very well). The bases are thick, difficult to blend, and finish sticky while the glitter is grainy and flakes, making a mess of the whole concept.

EYE AND BROW SHAPER: ☹ **Training Brow Kit** *($10)* is a poor substitute for the Brow Kit that Hard Candy used to sell. This dual-sided product includes a standard pencil on one end and a clear brow gel on the other. The pencil is very small and won't last long considering the frequent sharpening it needs, and the dry, waxy texture is disappointing. The brow gel fares better but remains slightly sticky and isn't worth the price of admission. ☹ **Super Slim Eye Pencil** *($8)* is a standard pencil that needs sharpening and although it's slim, that holds no special benefit because it doesn't change the dry texture and the Technicolor shades that teens will love, but for all the wrong reasons.

☹ **Glitter Eye Pencil** *($14.50)* needs sharpening but has a smooth, powdery texture that glides on effortlessly. The problem? The glitter infused into every shade flakes with little provocation, ending up in your eyes or on your face.

LIPSTICK, LIP GLOSS, AND LIPLINER: ✓☺ **Bon Bon Lip Gloss Set** *($18)* comprises three dual lip glosses packaged to resemble bonbons. Each gloss has a silky-smooth, non-sticky texture and imparts sheer to light coverage color with a hint of shimmer, and competes well with the best lip glosses available. You get a lot of lip gloss here for the money (six shades total) which is why this set was not rated with a triple dollar sign.

☺ **10 Years of Gloss** *($10)* commemorates the 10th anniversary of Hard Candy, which occurred in 2005. The oversized faux jewel compact holds a generous amount of sheer, bubblegum pink shimmer gloss that is slick and non-sticky. ☺ **Candy Coating Lip Gloss** *($12)* has the lightest texture of all the Hard Candy lip glosses, and is applied via a click pen with built-in brush. The sheer colors are completely non-sticky and do not smell or taste like their names (Caramel, Jelly Bean, etc.). ☺ **Sweet Spot Lip Gloss** *($11)* is a collection of orange-flavored lip glosses that begs you to keep licking your lips, which only causes them to dry out and makes you reach for the lip gloss again. If you can avoid temptation (or just don't care for the taste of artificial orange), this is a good gloss that sticks around without being overly sticky or thick. Each sheer shade is infused with multidimensional shimmer, which catches light from every direction. It's a sweet indulgence for nighttime glamour, and small enough to fit in any evening bag.

😐 **Lollipop Lip Gloss** *($6)* really does resemble a lollipop, but don't eat it. A round compact lip gloss is attached to a stick, which looks cute but serves no purpose other than kid appeal. Luckily, the emollient gloss itself is pretty good, though you have to put up with fruit- or candy-like fragrance. 😐 **Kiss & Tell** *($12)* combines lip gloss with the fortune-telling properties of the famed Magic 8 Ball. The cap of the gloss contains a cube suspended in mysterious blue fluid. Just like the Magic 8 Ball, you shake the cap and ask a question, waiting for the answer to float into view. It's an extra touch that teens may like, but I doubt you'll be sitting in traffic, asking your lip gloss cap if you should exit now or rip into the bag of potato chips in the back seat. The gloss itself is unremarkably standard, with minimal color deposit and just a hint of stickiness. 😐 **Super Shine Gloss** *($12)* is applied with a synthetic brush and feels thick and syrupy, though it's undeniably glossy. Despite a large color selection, every shade goes on very sheer with varying degrees of shimmer. The stickiness of this gloss isn't pleasant, and prevents it from earning a happy face rating. 😐 **$$$ Stain & Shine** *($15)* offers a liquid lip stain and glittery lip gloss in one sleek dual-sided component. The lip stain applies unevenly and looks spotted unless blended immediately. Two sheer berry shades are available and they're reasonably long-lasting. The gloss ensures comfortable wear without disrupting the stain, though it is slightly sticky. I wouldn't choose this over the sheer options from Cover Girl Outlast or Max Factor Lipfinity Everlites, but it's nonetheless a decent option.

😐 **Key To My Heart Lip Gloss** *($6)* is a very standard sticky, sheer lip gloss housed in a Lucite cube attached to a keychain. I guess this is worthwhile if you always remember your keys but forget your lip gloss, but that's about it. 😐 **Charmed Lip Gloss Bracelet** *($16)* is a rubber, snap-on charm bracelet that looks and feels juvenile. The cuteness quotient is solidified by the charm-sized lip glosses (you get two per bracelet) that have a tiny wand applicator and impart sheer, glossy color. Paris Hilton would have owned this when she was a kid, and I wouldn't be surprised if she considered it now. 😐 **$$$ Midnight Snack** *($18.50)* is a deluxe lip gloss set that contains four food-flavored lip glosses housed in a box that resembles a refrigerator. It's indulgence without the calories, because lip gloss isn't for eating. The glosses are standard fare, and contain ingredients for a wet-look moisturizing shine. 😐 **$$$ Lip Sync Quartet** *($25)* presents small amounts of four lip glosses in one compact with a tiny, almost useless synthetic lip brush. Each gloss has an unpleasant thick texture and sticky finish, with colors ranging from transparent to moderate coverage, almost approaching that of a traditional lipstick. It's an average product but may be worth considering if you like all the colors.

☹ **Lip Sorbet** *($10.50)* comes in a tube and the slightly sticky formula imparts sheer, glossy color not much different from all of the other Hard Candy glosses above, except this formula contains menthol, which makes it too irritating for lips.

MASCARA: ☺ **Lash Freak Mascara** *($11)* surprised me because it turned out to be a terrific all-purpose mascara that applied without a hitch and wears without flaking or smearing. This is definitely one to consider unless you crave extreme length or thickness.

The 😐 **Glitter Lash Freak Mascara** *($14.50)* applies with a comb rather than a brush and leaves shards, rather than particles, of glitter sticking to your lashes. The look is unique for occasional fun, and the glitter pieces cling tenaciously but some flaking can occur by day's end, making this one to consider carefully.

BRUSHES: ☹ **Tools of Attraction II** *($29.50)* is a 5-piece brush set with carrying case that is one of the most shoddy and unprofessional I have seen. These brushes make the ones from Urban Decay look Rembrandt-worthy and are not even recommended for girls to experiment with makeup on their dolls.

FACE AND BODY ILLUMINATING/SHIMMER PRODUCTS: ☺ **Shaker Body Shimmer** *($15)* is packaged to resemble a cylindrical salt shaker, and works well as a talc-based shimmering body powder. The shiny effect is noticeable but not garish, and it has decent cling. Some flaking is inevitable, but for the most part you'll be pleased with this powder and its two versatile shades.

SPECIALTY PRODUCTS: Once the backbone of this line's business, the ***unrated*** **Vintage Nail Polish** *($7)* is now only offered in a few shades, including Sky, the pale blue polish that started it all. The formula is toluene- and dibutyl phthalate–free, and is otherwise a standard, but good, nail polish formula with unconventional colors.

☺ **Princess Palette** *($25)* and ☺ **Punk Palette** *($25)* are themed face-designs in a box, with each set including three eyeshadows, a blush, a shimmer powder, and two lip glosses. The texture, application, and performance of every product are surprisingly good, but using every item on a face of any age is definitely shine overkill. The Princess Palette features soft pink and mauve tones while the Punk Palette includes warmer, earthy colors with a bit more pigmentation. Either set would make a fun gift for a teen, and the interior of the box features sensible, step-by-step application tips.

😐 **Jewel Box Eye & Lip Palette** *($18)* is a kit that contains various Hard Candy products that are also sold separately. Included are the Super Shine Lip Gloss in seven shades and various colors from the Eyeshadow Quartets. The included applicators are below average, but everything else in this set is nicely organized and portable, assuming you like all the colors.

HYDRODERM (SKIN CARE ONLY)

HYDRODERM AT-A-GLANCE

Strengths: Hydroderm provides complete product ingredients on their Web site.

Weaknesses: Expensive; none of the products can make good on the most enticing portion of their claims; yet another antiwrinkle hope-in-a-jar story that won't come true; reports online of women having a terrible time trying to get a refund on these products once they discover that they don't work as claimed.

For more information about Hydroderm call, (800) 840-5576 or visit www.hydroderm.com or www.Beautypedia.com.

☹ **Skin Restoring Facial Wash** *($24.99 for 5 ounces)* will not restore skin, but just irritates and dries it because the main detergent cleansing agent is sodium C14-16 olefin sulfonate. That fact makes the price for what you get very depressing.

😐 **$$$ Microbead Exfoliant** *($45 for 1 ounce)* is a water- and algae-based AHA product that contains a very small amount of glycolic acid that cannot exfoliate, nor is the pH of this product low enough for that to occur. What you're left with is a lightweight, serum-type product with little benefit for skin.

😐 **$$$ Age-Defying Wrinkle Reducer** *($79.95 for 1 ounce)* contains mostly collagen, water, alcohol, glycerin, nut glycerides, thickener, slip agents, peptides, and preservatives. The big claim here is that they're using the whole collagen molecule and have somehow developed a system to transport it directly into the skin. That's not really saying much, because it's reasonable to assume the collagen could penetrate a couple of superficial layers of surface skin anyway—no big deal. The peptides have theoretical cell-communicating benefits, but there is no substantiated research anywhere proving they reduce wrinkles, let alone by 45% as Hydroderm claims. The alcohol content makes this really a waste of time.

☹ **$$$ Fast Acting Wrinkle Reducer** *($79 for 1 ounce)* is the self-proclaimed star product of the Hydroderm line, yet its formulation is so mundane it's laughable. It contains mostly collagen, water, preservatives, protein, amniotic fluid, and vitamin C. Hydroderm's customer service department told me that the amniotic fluid (the liquid surrounding a developing fetus inside the womb) comes from a plant source! I almost dropped the phone. However, the amount of this ingredient is so minute as to be insignificant for skin, much less worthy of discussion. Suffice it to say it doesn't make skin grow younger.

The showcase ingredient for this product is collagen, and that was also a surprise. I thought the collagen fad was truly a thing of the past because it never worked and there is no research showing it ever did. Almost every antiwrinkle product sold in the late '80s and '90s contained collagen, and wrinkles did not go away or slow down then either. Applying collagen on top of the skin cannot affect the collagen in the skin, and the same is true for the product's protein content: it doesn't add to the protein in your skin. Collagen and protein are both good water-binding agents, but that's about it.

This product also contains the acid form of vitamin C, but such a small amount is present that it is barely detectable and, therefore, unable to help skin (Sources: *Experimental Dermatology*, June 2003, pages 237–244; and *Dermatologic Surgery*, March 2002, pages 231–236). By the way, the ingredient synasol on the ingredient label is a trade name for ethyl alcohol. Deceiving, yes, and it doesn't meet the FDA regulation that says the ingredient's actual name must be listed, but the amount in this product is probably not enough to be a problem for skin.

😐 **$$$ Intense Oil-Free Facial Moisturizer** *($69.95 for 1 ounce)* is a lightweight moisturizer for normal to oily skin that contains acetyl hexapeptide-3 as a main ingredient. For more information about this peptide, please refer to Chapter Seven, *Cosmetic Ingredient Dictionary*, in this book. Needless to say, it won't get rid of wrinkles and the jar packaging is far from the best.

😐 **$$$ Triple Effects Eye Serum** *($60 for 1 ounce)* purports to reduce puffiness and dark circles, which it cannot do. Oddly, it also claims to release magnesium chloride (MgCl) into skin because of its vasodilating effect. If the goal is to reduce dark circles, you don't want to increase blood flow to the under-eye area—that would only make dark circles more pronounced (think of what happens when someone gets a black eye—the blood vessels beneath the skin swell in response to the injury, releasing more blood into the area). MgCl doesn't function to reduce dark circles, although it can be drying to skin when used in large amounts (which is not the case here). This is an OK moisturizer for slightly dry skin and an expensive way to see if acetyl hexapeptide-3 does anything amazing.

☺ **$$$ First Impression** *($77 for the kit)* is sold as a three-piece set meant to increase lips' fullness without "stinging, pain, or inconvenience." The set consists of **Daytime Lip Care**, which is just an emollient lip balm with a tiny amount of peptide; **Nighttime Lip Repair**, which is a silicone-enhanced lip moisturizer with some vitamin E and soybean oil (and a lot of fragrance); and **Gentle Lip Scrub**, which is a standard, water-based scrub that contains polyethylene beads as the scrubbing agent and tiny amounts of ingredients you're meant to think are natural AHAs, but that aren't. This scrub will help remove dry, flaky skin from lips, but should be used gently (and would be better in a creamy base). Nothing in this trio will add collagen to lips, and these products don't come close to what is possible from collagen or hyaluronic acid injections. Despite this, at least the products don't contain irritants and can make lips softer and smoother—at a dear price.

HYLEXIN
(SEE BREMENN RESEARCH LABS)

IDEBENOL
(SEE BREMENN RESEARCH LABS)

ILLUMINARE (MAKEUP ONLY)

ILLUMINARE AT-A-GLANCE

Strengths: Excellent foundation, blush, and eyeshadow options, all with broad-spectrum sun protection; great brushes and application pad.

Weaknesses: Tactile issues that may be of concern for some consumers. No sheer coverage foundation options.

For more information on Illuminare, call (866) 999-2033 or visit www.illuminarecosmetics.com or www.Beautypedia.com. Note: Illuminare offers trial sizes of most of their products; refunds are only available for full-size products.

FOUNDATION: This is Illuminare's main focus, and each foundation contains zinc oxide and titanium dioxide as the UVA-protecting sunscreens. Although they claim the shades are the same for each foundation, I found enough differences among them to warrant avoiding a shade in one formula but not another. Each foundation is packaged in a squeeze tube. ✓ ☺ **$$$ Ultimate All Day Foundation/Concealer Matte Finish Sunscreen Makeup SPF 21** *($27)* starts out thick and a bit dry, but blends surprisingly well and has an incredibly smooth, ultra-matte finish that does not budge once it has set. Without a doubt, oily to very oily skin types will love this foundation's inordinately long-wearing formula, and the coverage, though medium to opaque, is relatively natural-looking (this is still makeup, after all). Removing it takes some effort, and is easiest with a silicone-based or mineral oil–based cleanser and a washcloth. The five shades are all excellent and best for very fair to tan skin. Applying this with Illuminare's Fast Application Pad (reviewed below) makes a big difference (for the better) in how this appears on skin. This is far too matte for those with normal to dry skin to contemplate. For that skin type, ☺ **$$$ Fantastic Finish Foundation Moisturizing Sunscreen Makeup SPF 21** *($27)* will work much better. This moist, creamy makeup also begins thick but has improved slip so blending is much easier, with or without moisturizer. You'll get light (if blended on sheer, but keep in mind that will compromise sun protection) to medium coverage with a soft satin finish. Of the five shades, Sienna Sun and Florentine Fair are still a touch too peach for most light to medium skin tones. ☺ **$$$ Extra Coverage Foundation/Concealer Semi-Matte Finish Sunscreen Makeup SPF 21** *($27)* has a thicker texture and heavier, more opaque finish than the Fantastic Finish makeup above, but, true to its name, this offers full coverage and tends to work best as a spot concealer (especially for reddened areas) rather than as a full-face foundation. Still, if you have normal to dry skin and need the coverage, this is a good choice (it beats the pants off anything from Dermablend), and of the five colors, only Florentine Fair is too peach to work for most light skin tones (it is much better suited to medium skin tones). Note that this is not recommended to conceal blemishes because the opaque nature of the mineral sunscreens may make blemishes worse.

BLUSH: ✓☺ **$$$ Perfect Color Blush Ultimate SPF 21** *($18)* has an identical texture, application, sunscreen, and finish as the Ultimate All Day Foundation/Concealer above. This makes it an excellent counterpart to any matte foundation for those who prefer a nontraditional blush option. The concentrated colors are all top-notch and include options for dark skin tones; each wears extremely well without fading or slipping. Definitely a unique blush option, and the sun protection is an added bonus.

☺ **$$$ Perfect Color Blush SPF 21** *($18)* is identical in texture, application, and finish to the Fantastic Finish foundation, except that these are natural blush tones that add a healthy glow to the cheeks. The sunscreen is titanium dioxide and zinc oxide, and the formula is concentrated, so only a tiny dab is needed for soft, sheer color. This leaves a moist finish that is ideal for normal to very dry skin. Those with oily skin or large pores will likely not enjoy this blush's finish and feel on the skin.

EYESHADOW: ✓☺ **$$$ All Day Eye Colors SPF 15** *($18)* are creamy, thick-textured eyeshadows that come in a squeeze tube and can be applied with fingertips, a sponge, or a synthetic brush. You only need a little of this potent formula to get a soft wash of color that blends decently and that, once it sets, lasts all day without fading or creasing. These really do wear amazingly well, and the colors are exceptionally neutral. Perla Bianca and Perla Rossa have a soft shimmer, but this is easy to sidestep if you're so inclined. If you want a change from powder eyeshadows and want one with sunscreen (pure titanium dioxide and zinc oxide), this is one of the best formulas I have come across, and the matte finish is sorely missing among others of its kind. This requires an oil- or silicone-based product to remove. Note that, with the right tools, some of the shades can be used as long-wearing eyeliner or to shape and define eyebrows.

BRUSHES: ✓☺ The selection of synthetic brushes from Illiuminare are all worth considering, especially if you're using their products. The **Foundation Brush** *($25)*, **Eye Color/ Concealer Brush** *($15)*, and **Eye Liner/Brow Brush** *($10)* are all firm yet soft, and well-shaped for their intended purposes. All of them are available in the **Application Tools Kit** *($50)* which also includes the fantastic **Fast Application Pad** *(sold separately for $10; 2 Pads come in the Kit)*. This sponge-like applicator with a flocked fabric cover works beautifully with all of Illumiunare's foundations, and may be used with any liquid or cream makeup. The advantage of using this Pad with Illuminare's foundation is that it provides a smoother, more natural finish and is much more elegant than applying with fingers (as is true for any foundation).

JAN MARINI SKIN RESEARCH, INC.
(SKIN CARE ONLY)

JAN MARINI SKIN RESEARCH AT-A-GLANCE

Strengths: Most of the products are fragrance- and colorant-free; excellent AHA and retinol options, including an AHA combined with sunscreen; Age Intervention Eyelash Conditioner; the water-soluble cleansers.

Weaknesses: Expensive; some categories contain ingredients (growth factors, hormones, and interferon) with unreliable track records or whose long-term risks, if any, remain unknown; sunscreens that lack sufficient UVA-protecting ingredients; jar packaging.

For more information about Jan Marini Skin Research, call (800) 347-2223 or visit www.janmarini.com or www.Beautypedia.com.

JAN MARINI AGE INTERVENTION LINE

What most of the Age Intervention products contain that makes them different from the other products in Marini's line are pregnenolone acetate, progesterone, and estradiol. These are the first cosmetic products I've seen that contain estradiol. However, the other two ingredients are not unique to Marini's line. Revlon sold products for years that contained pregnenolone acetate, and there are many products that contain progesterone.

Pregnenolone acetate is a precursor (trigger to create) other hormones; it is synthesized naturally from cholesterol and can affect levels of progesterone and estrogen in the body when taken orally. When applied to skin it may work as a water-binding agent, but up to now there is no information on whether it can be absorbed through skin, and there is no research showing it can change aging (including menopausal) skin.

Concerning progesterone, a study published in the *American Journal of Obstetrics and Gynecology* (June 1999, pages 1504–1511) states that "In order to obtain the proper (effective) serum levels with use of a progesterone cream, the cream needs to have an adequate amount of progesterone in it [at least 30 milligrams per gram]. Many over the counter creams have little [for example, 5 milligrams per ounce] or none at all." Marini does not provide information about how much progesterone her products contain. A double-blind study involving 40 peri- and postmenopausal women using a cream containing 2% progesterone versus one without had some intriguing results: The progesterone cream showed statistically significant increases in skin firmness and elasticity compared to the control, but wrinkle depth changed little (Source: *The British Journal of Dermatology*, September 2005, pages 626–634). Unfortunately, the Age Intervention products with progesterone do not appear to contain anywhere close to that amount, so the same results are unlikely.

Estradiol is definitely unique to Marini products. The body produces three main forms of estrogen—estrone, estradiol, and estriol—and estradiol is the most physiologically active form. One study revealed that topical application of estradiol has photoprotective properties due to its anti-inflammatory nature, while another small-scale study showed that topical application of 0.01% estradiol had collagen-stimulating effects on postmenopausal skin (Sources: *Proceedings of the National Academy of Sciences of the United States of America*, August 22, 2006, pages 12837–12842; and *European Journal of Obstetrics, Gynecology, and Reproductive Biology*, February 2007, pages 202–205). However, as a component of estrogen, it is not without its risks and unknowns.

Decreased production of estrogen by the ovaries can lead to symptoms such as hot flashes, night sweats, vaginal dryness, urinary tract infections, depression, and irritability. Estrogen replacement can help relieve these symptoms. Although estrogen offers many benefits, it is not indicated for everyone and women should evaluate their individual risks versus benefits with their physician or health-care provider. Whether or not natural estrogens are safer than other forms has not been well-researched, and the FDA considers the claims and safety of cosmetics containing them to not be proven.

Correspondence with representatives from Jan Marini revealed that the ingredients in her Age Intervention Complex (which she does not list individually as required, but rather refers to as the aforementioned "Complex") include interferon, coenzyme Q10, plankton, and MSM (methylsulfonylmethane). Listing a group of ingredients as a complex is not in compliance with FDA or international regulations for cosmetic labeling.

MSM may have some anti-inflammatory benefit for skin, but there is little research supporting its benefit in topical application (Source: www.naturaldatabase.com). Interferon refers to any in a group of soluble glycoproteins known to have antiviral activity. Specific types of interferon include alpha interferon and gamma interferon. It is produced naturally by immune cells when the body is under attack by viruses or bacteria, and can also be delivered topically or via injection. Although interferon and its derivatives have established pharmacological benefit when applied topically, the conditions it is useful for have nothing to do with aging, at least not in terms of making skin firmer, preventing sagging, or changing hormonal levels. Further, when interferon is used via prescription, its dosage and use are scheduled and controlled. There may be risks with applying a skin-care product with an unknown amount of interferon every day.

In summation, applying hormones and interferon topically to skin is something I strongly suggest should not be taken lightly. These are not benign cosmetic ingredients, and there is limited research establishing either benefits or risks for peri- and postmenopausal skin.

😐 **$$$ Age Intervention Eye Cream** *($60 for 0.5 ounce)* is a very emollient eye cream that contains some excellent nonvolatile plant oils and very good water-binding agents. Lots of antioxidants are included, but they won't remain stable for long once this jar-packaged product is opened. This is an option for dry to very dry skin, but the unknowns surrounding long-term use of products with hormones and interferon are a cause for concern.

😐 **$$$ Age Intervention Face Cream** *($60 for 1 ounce)* is very similar to the Age Intervention Eye Cream above, except this has a few more bells and whistles. Otherwise, the same comments apply.

😐 **$$$ Age Intervention Face Serum** *($60 for 1 ounce)* is a water- and oil-based serum that contains some great water-binding agents and lesser amounts of antioxidants. Although it is an option for normal to slightly dry skin, the concerns about long-term application of interferon and hormones remain.

✓ ☺ **$$$ Age Intervention Eyelash Conditioner** *($160 for 0.23 ounce)* is a star product for Marini, and one I did not review favorably in my newsletter because the company was not forthcoming about what was in the product, which caused quite a bit of controversy, at least behind the scenes. That has since changed. Early versions of this product were labeled Age Intervention Eyelash, sold with amazing claims, and listed "eyelash growth factor" (which isn't an ingredient but a made-up name) instead of the chemical compound, leaving users in the dark about what was in it and thus making it impossible for me to accurately review the product. Marini and team eventually changed the claims, packaging, and name of this product, which led to the revelation of what eyelash growth factor really is.

My assistant had an eye-opening discussion with Marini herself about this product, and although most if it was off the record, the bottom line is, despite tempered claims, that this product stands a very good chance of making eyelashes longer and darker. It contains mostly water, water-binding agents, pH adjuster, slip agent, preservative, film-forming agents, and the "active" ingredient, which is listed as 7-(3,5-dihydroxy-2-(3-hydroxy-4-(3-(triflormethyl) phenoxy)-1-butenyl) cyclopentyl), N-ethyl, 1R-(alpha(Z), 2beta (1E,3R), 3alpha, 5alpha)).

What is this nearly indecipherable ingredient? It is similar to a class of ingredients known as prostaglandin analogues. These drugs, including latanoprost, bimatoprost, and travoprost, are used to treat eye health problems such as glaucoma or ocular hypertension. One of the common side effects of ocular administration of eye drops containing prostaglandin analogues is growth and darkening of the eyelashes.

It wasn't much of a stretch (though a novel one) to assume that topical application of a very low dose of these drugs might have a similar effect, and that perhaps a non-drug version could be created for cosmetic purposes to enhance the appearance of eyelashes. Age Intervention Eyelash Conditioner is applied once per day, and goes on just like liquid eyeliner (minus color). Although Marini does not position this product as being able to grow eyelashes, thus avoiding costly drug testing, research on the prostaglandin analogues' effect on eyelash growth is intriguing. The "active" ingredient listed above is, according to Marini, a customized analogue her lab worked on, and is not a drug. It is chemically similar to prescription prostaglandin analogues, which is why it should work for most people, although how well it works may vary, so keep your expectations realistic. It is also important to note that results take several weeks to become visible and ongoing use is required to maintain the results.

(Sources for the above information: *Clinical and Experimental Ophthalmology*, November 2006, pages 755–764; www.nlm.nih.gov/medlineplus/druginfo/medmaster/a602027.html; http://dermatology.cdlib.org/93/commentary/alopecia/wolf.html; www.medscape.com/viewarticle/443657; and *Drugs of Today*, January 2003, pages 61–74).

The company reports that one tube of this product lasts six months, a statement I have personally found to be accurate. If this works for you, it could be argued that approximately $27 per month is a small price to pay for longer, fuller lashes. Despite my enthusiasm for this product, many of today's mascaras can produce prodigiously long, thick lashes without the expense and routine use this product calls for. Still, if it works for you, it's possible you will need less mascara or a less dramatic formula or you might get better results with the mascara you are currently using, which reduces the chance of mascara flaking, clumping, or smearing. Without a doubt, this is one of the most unusual products reviewed in this book.

***unrated* Age Intervention Regeneration Booster** *($225 for 6 0.25 ounce bottles; 1.5 ounces total)* ranks as Marini's most expensive product to date, and is said to be an "extraordinary new skin care compound [that] captures the emerging science of topical Telomerase Enzyme as a realistic science-based option for dramatically younger looking skin." Telomerase is explained in detail in the review for Re Vive's Peau Magnifique Youth Recruit ($1,500 for 4 0.03-ounce vials), reviewed elsewhere in this book. The bottom line is that the telomerase enzyme is not the antiwrinkle answer. There is only one potentially convincing piece of research on the role of telomerase in preventing skin from further aging, and it's not a slam-dunk or without cause for concern. The study examined using telomerase to extend the life span of fibroblasts (cells that contribute to the building of connective fibers, including collagen). The problem is that the study was done in vitro, and concerned adding telomerase to dermal fibroblast cells and then monitoring these cells for behavioral changes. The results showed that telomerase kept fibroblast cells alive, and as such may reverse the manner in which cell reproduction slows down as we age. How this applies to stimulating telomerase activity on intact, healthy skin is an unknown, and assuming it will work just as this study showed is a leap of faith (Source: *Experimental Cell Research*, August 2000, pages 270–278). Moreover, keep in mind that doing or using something that causes telomerase activity to increase in the body (which normally regulates telomerase on its own) may lead to the unchecked growth of cells that won't die—the basis for most types of cancer. Becase these vials contain telomerase enzyme and we don't know how this actually works on skin (for better or potentially worse), it is left unrated.

The water- and oil-based fluid is loaded with peptides, ceramides, plant oil, silicones, and emollients that help restore a healthy barrier to dry skin. The peptides have theoretical cell-communicating ability, while other cell-communicating ingredients and antioxidants play supporting roles (though antioxidants aren't present in amounts that justify this product's price). Despite these positives, the inclusion of telomerase and several growth factors make this Age Intervention product too potentially risky to consider—and you don't want to be any skin care company's guinea pig. For more information on the various growth factors, please refer to Chapter Seven, *Cosmetics Ingredient Dictionary*.

JAN MARINI ANTIOXIDANT LINE

☹ **Antioxidant Daily Face Protectant, SPF 30, Waterproof** *($36 for 2 ounces)* lacks the UVA-protecting ingredients of titanium dioxide, zinc oxide, avobenzone, Tinosorb, or Mexoryl SX, and is not recommended. In terms of antioxidants, this product comes up short, and it takes more than antioxidants to protect skin from sunlight.

☺ **$$$ Antioxidant Daily Face Protectant Tinted, SPF 30, Waterproof** *($50 for 2 ounces)* is a good, slightly moisturizing, water-resistant sunscreen that contains avobenzone for sufficient UVA protection. Despite the name, the only antioxidant is yeast extract (incorrectly listed by its trade name Nayad S). This has a sheer tint and soft shimmer that would work for light to medium skin tones.

😐 **$$$ Recover-E** *($32 for 1 ounce)* contains vitamin E and a few other antioxidants, but they won't remain stable once this jar-packaged, otherwise bland moisturizer, is opened.

😐 **$$$ Skin Silk Protecting Hydrator** *($32 for 1 ounce)* is a standard, slightly emollient moisturizer for normal to dry skin that's not prone to blemishes. The antioxidant plant oils won't retain potency once this jar-packaged product is opened.

☹ **Body Block SPF 30, Waterproof** *($20 for 4 ounces)* lacks the UVA-protecting ingredients of titanium dioxide, zinc oxide, avobenzone, Tinosorb, and Mexoryl SX, and is not recommended. This also does not contain a single notable antioxidant.

JAN MARINI BENZOYL PEROXIDE GROUP

😐 **$$$ Benzoyl Peroxide 2.5% Wash** *($20 for 8 ounces)* is a cleanser, and because a cleanser is washed away, the benzoyl peroxide (the effective ingredient), which should stay on the skin to work, will be rinsed down the drain. This is otherwise a standard, but good, water-soluble cleanser for all but very dry skin.

☹ **Benzoyl Peroxide 5%** *($20 for 4 ounces)* is a topical disinfectant listing 5% benzoyl peroxide as the active ingredient. That's great, but the amount of sodium lauryl sulfate makes an already potentially drying product far more likely to cause problems. This does not compare favorably with leave-on benzoyl peroxide products from the drugstore.

☹ **Benzoyl Peroxide 10%** *($20 for 4 ounces)* is nearly identical to the Benzoyl Peroxide 5% above, except this contains a 10% concentration. The same concerns apply.

JAN MARINI BIOGLYCOLIC LINE

✓☺ **$$$ Bioglycolic Bioclean** *($20 for 8 ounces)* is a good option for a water-soluble cleanser for all skin types. It removes makeup easily, is fragrance-free, and doesn't contain a single potentially problematic ingredient, making it a top choice. This cleanser does not contain any AHAs, and that's just fine because their benefit would be wasted in such a product.

😐 **$$$ Bioglycolic Facial Cleanser** *($20 for 8 ounces)* differs from the Bioglycolic Bioclean above because it contains glycolic acid and has a minimalist cleansing base. Unless you're willing to leave this on skin, it's not the best idea if you want to get the benefits of glycolic acid. It is an OK cleanser for normal to slightly dry or slightly oily skin, but should not be used around the eyes or to remove eye makeup.

😐 **$$$ Bioglycolic Oily Skin Cleansing Gel** *($20 for 8 ounces)* is similar to the Bioglycolic Facial Cleanser above, but with a higher amount of detergent cleansing agent and a lesser amount of glycolic acid. Otherwise, the same basic comments apply.

😐 **$$$ Bioglycolic Cream** *($48 for 2 ounces)* is a pricey but effective option for normal to dry skin that needs an AHA product. Glycolic acid is the second ingredient listed, and the pH of 3.2 allows it to exfoliate. This would be rated higher if it did not contain comfrey extract, which can be problematic for skin once it is absorbed.

😐 **$$$ Bioglycolic Eye Cream** *($28 for 0.5 ounce)* goes beyond just being an eye cream with AHA (it contains glycolic acid at about 10% with a pH of 3) and claims to have an effect on the fat pockets of the lower eyelids. Supposedly, this cream contains ingredients that can induce lipolysis (a process that allows fat cells to be released from areas resistant to fat metabolism) so it also minimizes under-eye bags to "re-contour" the eye area. One of the ingredients in this eye cream, methylsilanol theophyllinacetate alginate (trade name: Theophyllisilane C) shows up in a few anti-cellulite products. However, there is no research anywhere proving it can affect fat cells in skin when applied topically. Consider this an AHA moisturizer, and disregard all the other claims.

☹ **Bioglycolic Facial Lotion** *($36 for 2 ounces)* has a pH of 3 so the sufficient amount of glycolic acid will exfoliate skin. This product doesn't offer much else, and the inclusion of a significant amount of comfrey makes it a problem for all skin, and definitely not preferred to the AHA products from Alpha Hydrox, Pond's, or Neutrogena.

✓☺ **$$$ Bioglycolic Facial Lotion SPF 15** *($36 for 2 ounces)* omits the comfrey found in the Bioglycolic Facial Lotion above and protects skin from sun with a pure titanium dioxide sunscreen. The combination of sun protection and an effective amount of glycolic acid at a pH of 3.2 makes this a winning, triple-duty product for normal to dry skin.

☹ **Bioglycolic Sunless Self-Tanner** *($20 for 4 ounces)* contains approximately 2% glycolic acid, which is too small an amount to exfoliate. The pH of this self-tanner (it contains dihydroxyacetone to darken skin, just like hundreds of other self-tanning products) is 2.6, making it too irritating for all skin types.

☺ **Bioglycolic Lightening Gel** *($28 for 2 ounces)* contains a potentially effective amount of AHAs at a pH of 3.2 to permit exfoliation. The skin-lightening agent is kojic acid, but it is not preferred to other options, such as hydroquinone or stabilized vitamin C. If anything, kojic acid has research pointing to stability issues in skin-care products (Sources: *Bioorganic and Medicinal Chemistry Letters*, June 2004, pages 2843–2846; and *Journal of Cosmetic Science*, March–April 2004, pages 139–148). This is still an option as an AHA product for normal to oily skin.

😐 **$$$ Bioglycolic Bioclear Cream** *($40 for 1 ounce)* contains about 8% to 10% AHA and about 1% BHA in a fairly basic, lightweight moisturizing formula. It would work well for exfoliation for someone with normal to dry skin. BHA can exfoliate both in the pore and on the surface of skin, while AHA concentrates on the surface. In some ways it is redundant to have both, but some people find that better for their skin type.

This also contains azelaic acid (a component of grains such as wheat, rye, and barley), which has been shown to be effective for a number of skin conditions when applied topically in a cream formulation at a 20% concentration (Source: *International Journal of Dermatology*, December

1991, pages 893–895). However, other research suggests that azelaic acid is more irritating than hydroquinone when mixed with glycolic acid or kojic acid (Source: *eMedicine Journal*, www.emedicine.com, November 5, 2001, volume 2, number 11). Regardless, this product contains far less than 20% azelaic acid, so it is hard to say what, if any, effect it would have on skin. The group of potentially irritating plant extracts in this product makes it less desirable.

☺ **$$$ Bioglycolic Bioclear Lotion** *($40 for 1 ounce)* is a stripped-down version of the Bioglycolic Bioclear Cream above, and ends up being a better choice because it eliminates the problematic plant extracts and simply exfoliates skin with a pH-correct combination of 2% salicylic acid and 8–10% glycolic acid, all in a fragrance-free gel base.

☹ **Bioglycolic Acne Gel I** *($28 for 2 ounces)* contains alcohol and lavender oil, which make it too irritating for all skin types.

☹ **Bioglycolic Acne Gel II** *($28 for 2 ounces)* contains alcohol and lavender oil, which make it too irritating for all skin types.

JAN MARINI C-ESTA LINE

☺ **$$$ C-ESTA Cleansing Gel** *($20 for 6 ounces)* is a basic, but good, water-soluble cleanser for all skin types. It does contain fragrance.

😐 **$$$ C-ESTA Cream** *($60 for 1 ounce)* contains a good amount of vitamin C in the form of ascorbyl palmitate, but the jar packaging won't keep this light- and air-sensitive ingredient stable during use, and there isn't much else to extol about this product.

😐 **$$$ C-ESTA Eye Contour Cream** *($32 for 0.5 ounce)* does not contain a single ingredient backed by any evidence to show that it can diminish dark circles via vasodilation. And actually, you don't want to encourage vasodilation, because dilating veins encourages more blood to flow to an area, and it is this expansion of blood vessels and pooling of blood beneath thin under-eye skin that has a darkening effect, resulting in dark circles. So, if anything, you'd want to reduce the blood flow to the area. However, in this case it's moot, because this product doesn't contain ingredients that can cause vasodilation. In fact, there are no topical ingredients that can accomplish that without being problematic for skin. This jar-packaged moisturizer has a lot of vitamin C, but it won't remain stable once the product is opened.

☺ **$$$ C-ESTA Eye Repair Concentrate** *($44 for 0.5 ounce)* contains a good amount of vitamin C in a serum texture and in packaging that will keep the vitamin C stable. Other than that, there's one significant water-binding agent in this product, and the other goodies appear after the preservatives. It is an option for normal to slightly dry skin.

☺ **$$$ C-ESTA Serum** *($60 for 1 ounce)* combines effective water-binding agents with vitamin C and silicone plus a tiny amount of vitamin E. This is a well-designed, well-packaged product if you're curious to try a vitamin C serum.

☺ **$$$ C-ESTA Serum, Oil Control** *($60 for 1 ounce)* lacks any absorbent ingredients needed to control excess surface oil. It also can't regulate oil production, something that is not possible with a topical product, but this is a good lightweight moisturizer with vitamin C and green tea for normal to oily skin.

☺ **$$$ C-ESTA Facial Mask** *($40 for 2 ounces)* promises face-contouring results, but just delivers light moisture, soothing agents, and the antioxidant capability of vitamin C. This is a good mask for normal to dry skin, but to obtain the most benefit, leave it on overnight.

☺ **$$$ C-ESTA Lips** *($32 for 0.5 ounce)* assumes that none of the other C-ESTA products can be used around the mouth, so now you have one just for the lips and skin in that immediate area. This isn't necessary. There are no ingredients in here that are unique or special for the lip area. The formula is almost identical to the C-ESTA products above for skin, and the same comments apply.

JAN MARINI ENZYME LINE

😐 **$$$ Clean Zyme** *($16 for 4 ounces)*, despite all the fancy words about how papaya (source of the enzyme papain) works on skin, there is no research showing it to have exfoliating properties on skin, and definitely none showing it to be preferred over AHAs or BHA. The Web site www.naturaldatabase.com states that there is insufficient reliable information to support the effectiveness of papaya (also known as green papaya, which is how Marini lists it). Note: Persons allergic to latex, kiwi, or figs are very likely to have a negative reaction to papain, the enzyme component of papaya (Source: *Clinical and Experimental Allergy: Journal of the British Society for Allergy and Clinical Immunology*, August 2004, pages 1251–1258).

😐 **$$$ Skin Zyme** *($28 for 2 ounces)* lists green papaya concentrate as the main ingredient, followed by plant oil, thickeners, slip agent, preservative, honey, vitamin E, and fragrance. The enzyme component of papaya is not a reliable way to exfoliate skin, though some people may notice a slight benefit, and the other ingredients in this product will make skin feel smooth.

😐 **$$$ Day Zyme** *($38.99 for 1 ounce)* is similar to the Skin Zyme above, only without the plant oil and in a base that's better for those with oily skin. It contains a citrus fragrance.

😐 **$$$ Night Zyme** *($39.99 for 1 ounce)* is very similar to the Skin Zyme above, only with added ginger, which can be a skin irritant when applied topically, though the amount in this product is unlikely to have that effect.

JAN MARINI FACTOR-A & FACTOR-A PLUS LINE

😐 **$$$ Factor-A Cream** *($36 for 1 ounce)* is an emollient moisturizer for dry to very dry skin. It contains some very effective water-binding agents, but, if you're to believe the ingredient list, no retinol (or any other form of vitamin A). The jar packaging won't keep the antioxidants stable once opened, and some of the plant extracts can be irritating (though there's not much of them in here).

☹ **Factor-A Plus Cream** *($36 for 1 ounce)* features what the company calls Factor A Plus Complex, which should be listed as retinol—and whatever else is in this complex. (One consistent pattern in Marini's line is failing to meet FDA regulatory ingredient labeling guidelines.) The complex may also contain glycolic acid. Marini claims it does contain glycolic acid, but it is not listed separately, and it should be. The product has a pH of 3, but without knowing if glycolic acid is really in the product, I wouldn't bank on this for exfoliation. Further, the retinol will deteriorate because of the jar packaging. Adding a selection of irritating plant extracts doesn't make for delicious icing on this already flavorless cake.

☺ **$$$ Factor-A Lotion** *($32 for 1 ounce)* is a relatively standard but worthwhile moisturizer for normal to dry skin that contains more retinyl palmitate than retinol, but at least the packaging will keep the retinol stable. It also contains vitamins C and E and a tiny amount of niacinamide.

☹ **Factor-A Plus Lotion** *($32 for 1 ounce)* lists alcohol as the second ingredient, making this too irritating for all skin types. The AHAs in this product are not as helpful for acne-prone skin as BHA (salicylic acid) would be.

✓☺ **$$$ Factor-A Eyes for Dark Circles** *($60 for 60 capsules)* are single-use capsules and a great way to get the benefits of retinol, as it can remain very stable in this kind of packaging. The silicone base lends a pleasant application and silky finish, while the antioxidants green tea and vitamin C lend support. Marini claims the vitamin K in this serum addresses the cause of dark circles, but there is no published research to support topical application of vitamin K for that purpose. This is still an excellent retinol/antioxidant product for all skin types.

✓☺ **$$$ Factor-A Plus Mask** *($60 for 2 ounces)* is an intriguing, well-formulated mask for normal to oily skin. The 2% salicylic acid will exfoliate skin thanks to the pH of 3.2, while antioxidants, soothing agents, and cell-communicating ingredients provide benefit. Given the number of bells and whistles in this product, it would be a waste to rinse it after only a few minutes; there is nothing in this fragrance-free product that cannot be left on skin overnight, and that's what you should do to get the most benefit.

JAN MARINI TRANSFORMATION LINE

Jan Marini uses "transforming growth factor" in the group of products below. The transforming growth factor (TGF beta-1) is a complex protein known to bring about changes in connective tissue and is responsible primarily for wound healing. It stimulates collagen production, or a far better description, according to Dr. Bruce A. Mast, M.D., Division of Plastic and Reconstructive Surgery, Department of Surgery, University of Florida, Gainesville, would be that TGF beta-1 "is a proscarring component of healing." Dr. Mast explained that for a wound to heal, the body has to be able to create scar material, or collagen, for skin. But that kind of collagen production is not related to the skin's intrinsic support structure. Dr. Mast's concern in regard to including TGF beta-1 in skin-care products is that if it really works, it could encourage scar formation on the surface of the skin, and that won't improve the appearance of wrinkles.

There is limited research about this substance, with only one small-scale study of note that compared the wrinkle-reducing effects of TGF beta-1 against other topically applied growth factors. According to the study, the visually graded improvement in the appearance of wrinkles among 31 subjects was 21.7%. That's mildly impressive, but keep in mind that the TGF beta-1 was mixed with stabilized vitamin C (also present in the Marini products below) and not measured on its own merit (so it could have been the vitamin C that played an active role in the improvement). Nor was the effect of TGF beta-1 compared with the effect of other ingredients, such as retinol, green tea, or other antioxidants, or cell-communicating ingredients, such as niacinamide for one. Further, the amount of TGF beta-1 and vitamin C used in this study was not revealed, and there is no published research from Marini or anyone else to establish skin-care formulary protocols for this growth factor (Sources: *Dermatologic Surgery*, May 2006, pages 618–625; *The Journal of Biological Chemistry*, May 2005, pages 18163–18170; and *The FASEB Journal*, August 2002, pages 1269–1270).

😐 **$$$ Transformation Cream** *($60 for 1 ounce)*. The big-deal ingredient in this product is transforming growth factor (TGF beta-1). As described above, the claims for the actions of this ingredient are at best exaggerated, and its effectiveness is not established in skin-care products. This also contains some good water-binding agents and a small amount of antioxidants, but jar packaging won't keep them stable. It does contain fragrance and, despite the claims, there are no peptides listed.

😐 **$$$ Transformation Eye Cream** *($44 for 0.5 ounce)* also contains TGF beta-1, and the same comments apply. This one also contains sugarcane extract, but that is not an AHA and, even if it were, the pH is not appropriate for exfoliation. This version does contain a more impressive mix of water-binding agents and antioxidants, but the choice of jar packaging means the ingredients won't stay stable after it's opened.

☹ **Transformation Serum** *($60 for 1 ounce)* contains a high amount of transforming growth factor, but there are so many unknowns about this ingredient that applying so much of it is a potential risk for skin. The effective water-binding agents won't have much benefit on skin due to the presence of several irritating plant extracts, including comfrey, arnica, ivy, and pellitory.

JANE (MAKEUP ONLY)

JANE AT-A-GLANCE

Strengths: Inexpensive; great loose powder, powder blush, and eyeshadows (each with matte-finish options, though less so for the eyeshadow); one outstanding lipstick that rivals those costing much more; the Shimmering Bronzer; some good mascaras.

Weaknesses: The foundations with sunscreen lack sufficient UVA-protecting ingredients; mediocre pencils; one of the worst liquid eyeliners around; average to problematic lip glosses; inexpensive brushes that still aren't worth it.

For more information on Jane, call (800) 820-JANE or visit www.janecosmetics.com or www.Beautypedia.com.

Note: You may notice that just about every Jane product contains plant extracts of juniper, aloe, nettles, and elder flowers. The first letter of each plant extract spells, what else—Jane! That's the most exciting thing about these otherwise standard plants because, with the exception of aloe, none of them have much benefit for skin (and the amount of aloe in each is minuscule—so don't count on that one).

FOUNDATION: No testers are available for Jane's foundations. One thing to note is that some of the colors appear slightly peach or pink in the bottle, but blend on soft and neutral. Luckily, most drugstores selling this line have generous return policies if you discover you've chosen the wrong shade.

☺ **Be Pure Mineral Makeup** *($6.99)* is a mica-based, talc-free loose-powder foundation that's buffed onto skin via the affixed sponge. The powder is dispensed onto the sponge through a controlled sifter, allowing for smooth application, quick blending, and sheer coverage. It's good this powder's component was designed to apply the product sheer because using it without the sponge results in a thick appearance that's difficult to blend and a chalky finish. All five shades are worth considering, and this mineral makeup is less shiny than most others, making it more advantageous for oily (but not very oily) skin. Just like most loose mineral makeup, this version contains a lot of bismuth oxychloride to enhance coverage and create an absorbent finish.

😐 **Oil-Free Face Makeup** *($3.69)* doesn't contain any oil but it does contain thickening agents that have the potential to clog pores—one more reason you can't rely on an "oil-free" claim if blemishes are a concern. Beyond the name, this is now a really dated liquid foundation that provides a long-wearing matte finish but feels somewhat tacky and isn't nearly as silky as many competing foundations, including those from Cover Girl and L'Oreal. Among the six shades, avoid Vanilla (slightly peach) and Soft Beige (too rosy).

😐 **Sheer Protection Formula SPF 15** *($5.49)* has a better, smoother formula than the Oil- Free Face Makeup above, but lacks the UVA-protecting ingredients of titanium dioxide, zinc oxide, avobenzone, Tinosorb, or Mexoryl SX. It is otherwise a good liquid foundation due to its even application, sheer to light coverage, and slightly moist finish suitable for normal to dry skin. Six shades are offered, and the only one to view with caution is the slightly peach Ivory Bisque.

😐 **Be Pure Mineral Foundation** *($5.99)* has nothing to do with minerals unless they're referring to mineral oil, a major ingredient in this old-fashioned liquid foundation. It has a decent lightweight cream texture that blends well and provides medium coverage and a moist finish suitable for normal to dry skin. However, half of the six shades are strongly pink to rose. Avoid True Beige, Creamy Beige, and Beige to Tan. The remaining colors are OK options for fair to light skin tones.

☹ **Nearly Foundation Tinted Moisturizer SPF 30** *($4.99)* would have been a great product for teens or women of any age if only it provided sufficient UVA protection. Because it is lacking in that department, there isn't any reason to consider this sheer tint over the many fine options that get the essential sun protection element right.

CONCEALER: 😐 **No Show Oil-Free Concealer** *($3.79)* and 😐 **No Show One Touch Concealer** *($3.79)* have as many pros as cons, with the pros being a relatively smooth, fluid texture, strong matte finish, and three very good shades for each. The cons include the time these take to blend, the sketchy coverage, and the lack of a silky finish. They're worth considering if you have oily skin, but the matte-finish concealers from Revlon are better.

POWDER: ✓ ☺ **Translucent Loose Staying Powder** *($3.79)* is also known as Staying Powder Loose Powder. Although recommended to control shine (which most powders do), it's actually a great option for adding a polished, smooth finish to makeup for those with normal to dry skin. The talc-based formula feels almost creamy, and has a wonderful affinity with skin. Two of the three shades are excellent options best for fair to light skin; Colorless has a soft yellow cast (so it's not really without color); Sheer Shimmer applies sheer but leaves behind large particles of shine that cling poorly, so it is not recommended.

😐 **Oil-Free Finishing Powder** *($3.79)* is a talc-based pressed powder with a soft, silky-dry texture that applies sheer and even, with a slight powdery finish. Among the six shades, Bisque-to-Creamy, Beige-to-Peachy, and Cocoa-to-Honey are too peach for their intended skin tones. The three lightest shades work best, but note that Colorless is misnamed because it does impart color to skin (a soft, neutral ivory). 😐 **Oil-Free Bronzing Powder** *($3.99)* is a standard, smooth-textured, talc-based pressed bronzing powder. Each shade is laced with sparkles that don't stay put, and two of the three shades are too orange or copper, despite their sheerness. The best shade is Sunkissed Bronze, which is suitable for fair to light skin tones.

☹ **Be Pure Mineral Powder** *($6.99)* is a mess in almost every sense of the word. Although this has a silky, light texture from its talc-free, mica-based formula, the component with a built-in brush (that feels terrible on skin) falls apart easily. This results in spilled powder, and you don't get very much powder to begin with! Even with the component taped together (mine fell apart in three places), the way this powder is dispensed makes it all too easy to overapply, resulting in a heavy-looking finish (from the bismuth oxychloride). The shades are fine, but the component and cap (which cannot be put back on without ruining the brush) are a classic case of caveat emptor!

BLUSH: ✓ ☺ **Blushing Cheeks Blush** *($3.79)* remains a best buy at the drugstore due to its silky-smooth texture and sheer application, which rivals powder blushes costing four times this amount. The shades are very good and include an even mix of matte and soft shine options, but they're too soft for tan to dark skin tones. The matte colors include Blushing Baby Doll, Blushing Blossom, Blushing Wine, and Blushing Petal.

☺ **Blushing Cheeks Cheek Shapers** *($3.99)* include a pressed-powder blush and contour shade in a split-pan compact. One shade in each pairing is very shiny, and the shine doesn't stay in place too well, which isn't the best look. These do apply smoothly and most of the sets are well-coordinated. ☺ **Shimmering Blush** *($5.99)* plays off of Jane's Shimmering Bronzer (reviewed below), and that's preferred because of its superior texture. The blush version presents five stripes of shimmering color, at least two of which are suitable for blush (the others are best for highlighting). This firmly pressed powder imparts much more shine than color and applies very sheer, so you need successive layers if you want much more than a subtle payoff. The good news is the shine clings well and blends evenly to a soft, radiant finish. The supplied brush is not preferred to a full-size blush brush, but works in a pinch.

☺ **Be Pure Mineral Crushed Blush** *($5.99)* has a very silky texture for a loose powder blush that is clay-based. It also applies evenly and softly, imparting radiant (read: shiny) color that clings well and meshes with skin rather than just sitting on top of it. Of course, the clay base tends to feel drier eventually, making this preferred for normal to oily skin. Two of the shades (Honey and Sunbrushed) are better as shiny highlighting powders than as blush.

😐 **Be Pure Mineral Blush** *($4.99)* is listed on Jane's Web site as **Be Pure Pillow Blush** because of the quilted pattern of this pressed-powder blush. By any name, this initially silky blush with a dry finish and noticeable shine tends to apply unevenly. It can be softened afterward, but is definitely a blush to use with restraint or you'll end up with strong, blotchy color. The hidden brush is completely useless, but the built-in mirror is a nice touch. The small selection of shades favors pinks, but the intensity is best for medium skin tones.

EYESHADOW: 😐 **Eye Zing Shadow** *($3.49)* is a standard powder eyeshadow with a reasonably smooth application and a soft, silky texture. The colors have more pigment than you'd expect, and layer well for added intensity. Unfortunately, many of the shades have a glittering shine that tends to flake, or the colors are too striking or pastel to use around the eyes. The matte shades include Dream Cream, Rock Star, Browny Points, and Hip Bone. 😐 **Eye Zing Carry Along** *($4.49)* has the same formula and application traits as the Eye Zing Shadow above, but is packaged as quads made up of shades from the single Eye Zings. Every quad has some shiny shades, but if that doesn't bother you, 02 Browns is the easiest to work with. The other quads tend to be tone-on-tone (such as varying degrees of blue eyeshadow) or mismatched, making for a difficult eye design, while the Metallic quads offer two good groupings, labeled Hollywood and Chicago.

😐 **Eye Zing Mix & Match** *($4.99 for six shades; $6.99 for eight shades)* features a lineup of powder eyeshadows, each containing shades from the single Eye Zing Shadow formula reviewed above. They're packaged in slim palettes, and designed less to be used together than to give the user multiple shadow options to create a variety of looks. City Tones is a good set to consider among the six-shade sets; the eight-shade sets include more contrasting colors, but at least three in each work well together.

EYE AND BROW SHAPER: ☺ **Fan Club Lash & Brow Mascara** *($3.99)* is a lightweight, clear brow gel that also adds very subtle definition to the lashes. It does not contain film-forming agents, so it's non-sticky, but it is not the best choice if you have unruly brows that need to be held in place.

☹ **ColorSticks Eye Color & Liner** *($3.99; $1.99 for sharpener)* are standard, slightly chunky eye pencils that have a super-smooth application and a soft, minimally creamy finish. All of the colors leave a shimmer finish and don't last long enough (nor are they pigmented enough) to use as eyeliner. If you don't mind sharpening these, they're worth considering as a sheer cream eyeshadow or highlighter.

☹ **Gliding Liners Eye Pencil** *($3.49)* is a standard pencil that doesn't glide as much as drag over skin, but it isn't terrible; it just isn't acceptable given other options nearby from other lines, particularly Cover Girl. The formula has a soft powder finish that promises better staying power than most pencils, but it needs regular sharpening, which is a pain. If you decide to try it, be aware that almost all of the shades have a shimmer or metallic finish. Black Magic is a good, basic matte black.

☹ **Going Steady Eye Definer** *($3.49)* is a twist-up, thick-textured cream eyeliner that applies very smoothly but doesn't set, so it smears in no time and fades within hours. It's workable if you set it with powder shadow, but why not just use that to line your eyes rather than as a stopgap for a substandard liner?

☹ **One Liners for Eyes** *($3.49)* are automatic, nonretractable pencils that apply decently, but have a dry, tacky finish that tends to look crinkled rather than smooth. They're OK if smudged out for a smoky eye design. The best shades are Coffeeline, Blackline, and Smokeline.

☹ **Eye Pencil Triplet** *($4.99)* provides three automatic, retractable, mini eye pencils in one case. Each applies well but the creamy texture smears and smudges easily, especially if you have oily eyelids. In most of the sets, two of the three colors are too bright for eyeliner, but if you're in an experimental mood and under the age of 20, these may seem appealing.

☹ **Endless Eye Quick Dry Eye Liner** *($3.49)* is one of the worst liquid eyeliners in the history of makeup (OK, that may be a bit of an exaggeration, but I have tested a lot of these and I don't remember ever reacting this way to an eyeliner). It has a terrible, flimsy brush that splays, the colors (of which none are all that attractive) apply unevenly and look splotchy, and … well … just don't buy it!

LIPSTICK, LIP GLOSS, AND LIPLINER: ✓☺ **Lipkick Rich Color Lipstick** *($4.49)* is also known as **Moisture Rich Color Lipstick**, and although it's marketed to teens, adults would do well to stop and explore this beautifully creamy, opaque lipstick. It has a smooth, even application and feels very light while providing a soft, glossy (not greasy) finish. It can creep into lines around the mouth, but not as quickly as many other creamy lipsticks. The color palette, though small, is sophisticated, and definitely better suited to adults than teens. Great job, Jane—let's hope this lipstick gets noticed because it is one of the top creamy choices at the drugstore. ☺ **LipHuggers Lipstick** *($3.69)* has teen appeal because of the many pale, frosted colors, but there are a handful of gorgeous, opaque shades to explore, and the formula is smooth and creamy without being too slippery or greasy. It has a semi-matte finish that offers longer wear, and isn't flavored or overly fragranced either!

☺ **Megabites Glossy Gloss** *($3.69)* comes in a squeeze tube and is a smooth, lightweight gloss with sheer, sparkling colors and a non-sticky finish. The drawback is that every shade is flavored, though it's not as pervasive as in the Megabites Flavorful Lipstick below. ☺ **Gloss 'N Line** *($4.99)* combines lip gloss and an automatic, retractable lipliner in one component. The gloss portion feels thick and looks very glossy without being sticky, which is great. The liner is very standard, and definitely too creamy to last with the gloss. However, lining and filling in lips with the pencil and topping with gloss (thus mixing the two shades together) is flattering.

☺ **Lipstick Ribbons** *($4.99)* provide five "ribbons" of sheer, glossy lip color in one mirrored compact complete with a workable lip brush. None of the shades are much for color (despite looking intense in the container), but they feel smooth, keep lips moisturized, and leave a soft, glossy sheen. If you prefer sheer lipstick and don't have an issue with it bleeding into lines around your mouth, this is quite a bargain!

😐 **Megabites Flavorful Lipstick** *($3.69)* is a set of standard, but good, cream lipsticks that are either fruit-, drink-, or dessert-flavored, and the taste may seem inviting or repulsive, depending on your mood. Were it not for the pervasive flavor, these would have gotten a higher rating. The formula is slick enough to slide into any lines around the mouth.

😐 **Attitubes! Lipgloss** *($4.39)* is a thick, sticky lip gloss applied with a wand. It's nothing special, and not the most comfortable gloss to wear, but the texture does keep it around longer than usual. 😐 **ColorSticks Lip Color & Liner** *($3.99; $1.99 for sharpener)* is a coconut oil–based, slightly chunky lip pencil that needs sharpening. This is meant as a lipliner and lipstick in one, but works best as a smooth, lightweight cream lipstick with a soft, creamy (not glossy) finish. The color selection is again geared more toward adults. The main drawback is the difficulty keeping this sharpened because of the soft tip.

😐 **Lip Pencil Triplet** *($4.99)* is nearly identical to the Eye Pencil Triplet above, except in this product you get three mini lipliners that go on smoothly but are too creamy to last past mid-morning. The color groupings have nothing to do with one another, but if your lipstick taste runs from soft nudes to hot fuchsia, you'll be covered!

☹ **Lip Plumping Color and Gloss** *($4.49)* offers three greasy lip colors and one slick gloss in a quad-style compact. A dual-sided mini lip brush is also included, but it's a bit too stiff for routine use. Even if it were ideal, the formula contains camphor and other irritants meant to swell lips, and is not recommended. ☹ **Max Lip2 Lip Plumper, Clear** *($5.49)* is a clear lip gloss that's slightly sticky and meant to plump lips "without injections." After trying this, I'd wager the injections are possibly less painful. Jane chose irritating menthol and cinnamon oil to make lips fuller, and the sting is evident immediately. The cinnamon is quite strong, and almost like dabbing your lips with mouthwash or schnapps. This is too irritating even for occasional use.

MASCARA: ☺ **Max Lash^2 for Intense Volume** *($4.99)* is a dual-sided mascara. Step 1 is a white primer, and step 2 a traditional mascara. The primer does nothing to improve the application or results. If anything, the mascara alone is preferred for nicely defined, clump-free length and a touch of thickness, though it takes several coats. I don't recommend the primer step, so you're essentially paying for just the mascara, though the price still makes it a bargain.

☺ **Fan Club Curling Mascara** *($3.99)* builds impressive length and a smidgen of thickness while leaving lashes with a soft curl. If you normally use an eyelash curler for definition, you'll still need it with this, but it remains a good lengthening mascara to consider. ☺ **Fan Club Curling Mascara Water-Resistant** *($3.99)* has a name that you should pay attention to, because there is a difference between "water-resistant" and "waterproof." This mascara holds up through tears and light rain, but not through swimming or showering. It's a good choice for modest length and a bit of thickness, but is best for those who want a natural lash look without clumps. It does not curl lashes.

☺ **Hi-Fiber Mascara** *($3.99)* promises "a true false eyelash effect," but the reality isn't that exciting, at least if you're looking for a mascara to take your lashes from puny to wow. Hi-Fiber Mascara builds length and thickness in nearly equal measure, but isn't as dramatic as it once was. Despite the name, I didn't detect any fibers in this mascara, which is good because they tend to flake into the eyes throughout the day. This actually wears well and removes easily.

☺ **Hi-Fiber Waterproof Mascara** *($3.99)* is a decent waterproof mascara if you need moderate length and aren't too concerned about building thickness. It doesn't clump or smear and lasts all day without chipping, but it requires an oil- or silicone-based cleanser for complete removal.

☹ **Max Lash² for Dramatic Color** *($4.99)* is another dual-sided mascara like the Intense Volume version above, but in this version the colorless primer is replaced by a mascara with an intense tint. You still get a regular black mascara, and that is applied first. Then the "Dramatic Color" portion is added, if desired. The dramatic colors are strong hues, but both formulas contain fibers that flake during wear, making this one to skip.

FACE AND BODY ILLUMINATING/SHIMMER PRODUCTS: ✓☺ **Shimmering Bronzer** *($5.99)* is shine done right, because this smooth-textured, almost creamy-feeling pressed powder applies beautifully and clings well. You get five "stripes" of shimmer powder in one compact, complete with a workable brush and mirror. These are well-coordinated colors, and you can blend them as one shade (to use as bronzer or blush, depending on the set) or use one or more colors for eyeshadow and highlighting. This product bests Bobbi Brown's Shimmer Brick Compact because it is silkier (though Jane copied their concept), and because Brown's versions cost six times what Jane is charging.

☺ **Summer Glow Gel Bronzer** *($4.99)* offers much more than a "summer glow." Wearing this ultra-shiny bronzing lotion (it's not a true gel) will add such a gleam to your skin you might temporarily blind passersby. Two shades are available, but they're very sheer, so think of this as a high-shine lotion with a very soft bronze cast.

☹ **Staying Powder Shimmer Loose Powder** *($3.69)* is a very shiny loose powder that's messy to apply and the shine barely clings to skin. Only one shade is available, but that's OK because this is all about adding shine, not color. Even so, there are many neater ways to obtain shine than from this poorly conceived powder.

BRUSHES: Jane's ☺ **Brushes** *($3.49 each)* aren't awful; they are just the wrong shape and tend to have a poor consistency. The prices are rock bottom, but the performance is not impressive. The exception is the **Brow/Lash Comb**, which is workable but could benefit from more variegated bristles.

JANE IREDALE

JANE IREDALE AT-A-GLANCE

Strengths: Pom Mist toner; lip balm with SPF 15; the makeup is mostly excellent, particularly the powder-based products, which include Iredale's contribution to mineral makeup; mostly great makeup brushes.

Weaknesses: Two problematic toners; many of the claims made for these products are not supported by solid research; the Circle/Delete concealer, poor eye pencils; PureMoist LipColours SPF 18 contain irritating peppermint; some superfluous specialty products; the makeup is not as skin-caring as the claims may lead you to believe, though it is a worthwhile option for those with sensitive skin.

For more information about Jane Iredale, call (800) 762-1132 or www.janeiredale.com or www.Beautypedia.com.

JANE IREDALE SKIN CARE

☹ **Balance Antioxidant Hydration Spray** *($17.50 for 2 ounces)* was formulated "specifically to help balance the skin's oil production and pH," but nothing in this toner can have that effect, plus the skin handles it's own pH fairly well via sweat and oil production. (After all, oil production is regulated internally by hormones, so external factors have only a negligible influence.) Further, this toner contains irritating tangerine extract as a major ingredient, as well as myrrh. Tangerine can be a skin irritant (though the extract is not as potent as the oil), and myrrh can cause contact dermatitis due to its volatile components, though it does have anti-inflammatory benefits (Source: www.naturaldatabase.com). However, myrrh is not worth seeking out over several other plants whose soothing benefits are not offset by the potential for sensitization. ☹ **D2O Hydration Spritz** *($17.50 for 2 ounces)* lists *Cananga odorata* extract (ylang ylang) water as the main ingredient, which isn't hydrating at all, it's fragrant and irritating. The myrrh extract is also a problem, which is a shame because this toner has some very good water-binding agents. The heavy water has no established benefit for skin.

✓☺ **$$$ Pom Mist** *($17.50 for 2 ounces)* is an antioxidant-laden toner that also contains some good water-binding agents and the cell-communicating ingredient lecithin. It is highly recommended for all skin types and is fragrance-free.

✓☺ **Lip Drink SPF 15** *($10.50 for 0.18 ounce)* contains a pure zinc oxide sunscreen and has a plant oil–based formula that is wonderfully conditioning for lips. I disagree with Iredale's claim (and there is no research to prove it) that petrolatum-based lip balms put users on a "continual drying cycle," but that doesn't change the fact that this is a very well-formulated lip balm. The only potential caution is the lemon peel oil, but there's only a tiny amount of it in here and it's unlikely to be a problem.

😐 **$$$ More Lip Lip Plumper** *($18 for 0.25 ounce)* is made for those who have some trepidation about collagen or hyaluronic acid lip injections, and promises to give you "the same full pout without the pain." All this emollient lip balm does is swell lips temporarily with ginger root oil. Ginger root oil can be irritating, so proceed with caution; products like this should be used only occasionally—and the results are not comparable to what's possible with cosmetic lip injections.

JANE IREDALE MAKEUP

FOUNDATION: ☺ **$$$ Amazing Base Loose Minerals SPF 20** *($42)* contains titanium dioxide and zinc oxide as the active sunscreen ingredients and these definitely contribute to the powder's opacity, cling, dry finish, and long-wearing capabilities. This loose-powder foundation is talc-free and has a very smooth texture that tends to get drier in feel and appearance the longer it's worn. You can use it dry or can mix it with a moisturizer to approximate a liquid foundation or to allow for easier application over drier skin. (Keep in mind, however, that mixing it will diminish the powder's sunscreen properties.) Either method can be messy, which is true for any loose-powder application, and that's a definite drawback. Amazing Base provides medium to full coverage. The smooth, dry texture and comparatively lighter finish (though it still looks like powder makeup) with a faint bit of shine is preferable to many other mineral makeups. It is much less shiny than the bareMinerals foundation from bare escentuals. Most of Iredale's 15 shades are superbly neutral, but some go on a bit lighter or darker than they appear, so testing them on your skin is imperative. The only shade to be careful of, due to its slight peach-rose tone, is Honey Bronze. This version lacks any colors for darker skin tones.

☺ **$$$ PurePressed Pressed Minerals SPF 18** *($48)* is a pressed-powder version of the Amazing Base above, except this one is more matte and not as thick, so oilier skin will be less likely to experience a heavy, caked look once the skin's oil and the powders mix. The sunscreen is pure titanium dioxide and zinc oxide. The same basic comments made for Amazing Base apply here as well; however, this offers a considerably more tidy application and a slightly broader range of shades, including some exemplary options for darker skin tones called **Global Shades**. These are richly pigmented and as a result do not look as ash or gray on deeper skin tones like many other powders can. Of the 18 shades, the only ones to consider avoiding are Honey Bronze and Teakwood. The vast majority of skin-true shades here are gorgeous, just as they are for the Amazing Base.

☺ **$$$ Liquid Minerals A Foundation** *($46)* combines "light-diffusing, soft focus" minerals with "ingredients that replenish the cellular layers of the epidermis." That sounds tempting until you realize that lots of ingredients in liquid foundations (such as glycerin and cholesterol) offer this benefit. This non-powder entry from Iredale is a bit tricky to dispense from its pump applicator, but does have a silky, water-light texture and does provide a smooth, sheer-coverage matte finish. The minerals (pigment) are encapsulated and dispense somewhat chunky, which makes blending a bit more difficult. However, once you get the hang of it, this foundation applies well with a sponge or synthetic brush. Among the 18 shades, a few (Golden Glow, Autumn, and Honey Bronze) are a bit too peach for some medium skin tones, but are still worth considering. Warm Sienna is slightly gold, while the rest of the shades are beautifully neutral and appropriate for fair to dark skin. This is a much lighter alternative to either of the powder-based mineral foundations above and although it contains some great water-binding agents, the matte finish makes it best for normal to slightly oily or oily skin.

CONCEALER: ☺ **$$$ Disappear** *($24)* is positioned as "the ultimate in camouflage creams" and is designed to conceal tattoos. It doesn't provide *that* much coverage, but does a great job concealing minor redness and other bothersome discolorations. The semi-liquid consistency has just enough slip to blend well, and once dry its matte finish stays put. The formula contains several antioxidants, but the "blemish control botanicals" are a far cry from tried-and-true anti-blemish actives such as benzoyl peroxide or salicylic acid. Iredale maintains that the green tea extract in this concealer combats acne, but research does not support this assertion when green tea extract is applied topically instead of consumed in the diet. All four shades are outstanding and best for fair to medium/tan skin.

😐 **$$$ Active Light Under-Eye Concealer** *($25)* is a thick liquid concealer dispensed from a click-pen applicator and applied with the built-in synthetic brush. The smooth texture blends readily and provides nearly full coverage with a slightly flat, opaque finish. Creasing is minimal and the formula contains several skin-friendly ingredients—though it includes too many waxes for use over breakouts. The major problem is with the colors, half of which look nothing like skin and, when used over dark circles, essentially trade one discoloration problem for another. Avoid shades 4, 5, and 6, all of which are too pink or peach. Shades 1, 2, and 3 are yellow-toned options, but only for very fair to light skin to tones. This is not preferred to Estee Lauder's Ideal Light Brush-On Illuminator ($24.50).

☹ **Circle/Delete** *($29)* comes in a pot with two colors; one is a lighter tone, the other a medium tone. The texture is quite thick and creamy, and you will get opaque coverage. This will definitely crease, and applying one of the mineral powders over it tends to look heavy and obvious. Last, the three duos have colors that are a far cry from real skin tones, and blending them together is tricky. ☹ **Enlighten Concealer** *($28)* is a creamy concealer available in a single shade that is blatantly orange. Supposedly, this color is the key to erasing the look of dark circles, bruising, and hyperpigmentation (brown spots). The opacity of this concealer will provide coverage of those skin issues, but the resulting color is awful. The tiny amount of arbutin in this product is likely insufficient to lighten discolorations, plus the packaging chosen won't keep it stable during use.

POWDER: ✓☺ **$$$ Amazing Matte Loose Powder** *($31)* comes in one shade, and although it's translucent it still looks best on fair to light skin. This talc-free, mica- and rice starch–based powder looks beautiful on the skin and provides a dry, matte finish that does a good job of keeping excess shine (oil) in check. The mica lends a subtle glow to skin without being at all sparkly, making the strong matte finish look more natural. This is an impressive product for oily to very oily skin; the only caution has to do with using rice starch (a food-based ingredient) over blemishes.

☺ **$$$ So-Bronze** *($41)* is a talc-free, pressed bronzing powder that comes in two shades. The number 1 option is best for fair to light skin and features minimal shine, while number 2 is darker and has a separate, crescent-shaped shiny powder segment that really lays on the sparkles. Both options have a smooth but dry texture and apply evenly (just use them sparingly).

😐 **$$$ PureMatte Finish Powder** *($36)* feels matte and has a light, dry texture oily skin will love, but it contains more shine than both of Iredale's foundation powders above. There is one shade, and it's suitably neutral, although limited to light skin. Rice starch is not an ideal ingredient to use over blemishes.

BLUSH: ✓☺ **$$$ PurePressed Blush** *($26)* has a silky texture that goes on exceedingly smooth. The color range is impressive, offering equally good options for light and dark skin tones, but note that each shade has a touch of shine.

😐 **$$$ In Touch Cream Blush** *($26)* has a smooth, almost slick texture and comes in a portable, twist-up stick. Each blush shade is sheer and leaves skin with a moist-glow finish. The drawbacks are that this won't last the whole day, you get a surprisingly small amount of product for the money, and the artificial chocolate scent and flavor will be off-putting for many. It does not, as the company states, smell "just like your favorite truffle." Wet 'N' Wild and Avon make better twist-up blush sticks for less money; those looking to spend this amount should consider the options from NARS or Bobbi Brown.

EYESHADOW: ✓☺ **$$$ PurePressed Eye Shadows** *($17.50)* are sold as singles and have a formula and application identical to the PurePressed Blush above, which is great. Each shade applies evenly without flaking or skipping, and tends to go on color-true. Note: The eyeshadow shades that still list bismuth oxychloride as the first ingredient feel drier and don't apply as smoothly. Look for the shades that list titanium dioxide and dimethicone as the main ingredients. Each shade has at least a slight amount of shine, but it is downplayed to a soft glow in many. The shiniest shades tend to deposit the least amount of color, and are best for highlighting the brow bone.

✓☺ **$$$ Duo Eye Shadows** *($27)* have the same formula as the PurePressed Eye Shadows above, and the same review applies. All of the pairings are well done, but you will need a deeper shade for eye lining.

😐 **$$$ Triple Eye Shadows** *($27)* suffer from mostly poor or exceedingly shiny color combinations, and most of the colors still use the primarily drier-textured version, which isn't as easy to work with as the latest formula (only available in certain shades, though not clearly identified). The only workable sets are Triple Cognac and Cloud Nine, but two of the three shades in Pink Bliss are good.

☺ **Eye Highlighter Pencil** *($15)* is a standard chunky pencil with a pale pink shade on one end and an opalescent white shade on the other. The shine is intense without being glittery, and the only issue is that the creamy texture doesn't last too long around the eye, so some fading and creasing are unavoidable.

EYE AND BROW SHAPER: ✓☺ $$$ PureBrow Colours *($16)* are soft-tinted brow mascaras that ably enhance the brows. Five superior shades are available, including options for blonde and auburn brows. It does not get sticky or make brows look greasy or too thick, and the brush deposits just the right amount of product (unless your brows are very full or bushy).

☺ **$$$ PureBrow Fix & Mascara** *($20)* is a standard, PVP-based, clear brow gel that works as well as those sold at the drugstore. The only advantage of this is that it comes with two brushes, though most will find one preferable. ☺ **$$$ Liquid Eye Liner** *($20)* goes on slightly wetter than most, but the brush is great, being flexible enough to glide easily along the lash line, yet it lets you maintain control. Dry time is slower than average, but once set the formula stays in place and wears well. I would encourage you to explore the liquid eyeliner options from L'Oreal or Almay first, but this is an option if you want to spend more money. ☺ **$$$ Super-Shape Me Brow Kits** *($62)* is a very expensive way to shape and shade your eyebrows, but I suppose some may find the entire kit practical. Included in a large mirrored compact are two brow powders, a tinted brow wax, a pale yellow lid primer, and small but workable brow brushes and mini tweezers. The talc-free brow powders go on smoothly and have a soft matte finish. Whether you choose the blonde, auburn, or brunette kit, the two brow colors are basically one shade apart, and either one is workable depending on whether you want a soft or stronger (meaning darker) brow. The coordinating, non-sticky brow wax grooms and enhances the powder color, but isn't essential unless your brows are naturally unruly (but a good trim works better than matting them down). As for the primer, its cream-to-powder texture wears decently, but it tends to apply quite opaque and must be softened for best results. On the pro side, it does nicely camouflage redness from tweezing, or any bluish-purple tones on the eyelid. I wish this weren't so costly because for the most part it's a nicely done kit, though you can achieve the same brow-enhancing results with fewer products purchased separately.

☺ **$$$ Cream to Powder Eyeliner** *($26)* includes one matte and two shimmer-finish, cream-to-powder shades in a single compact. Each applies smoothly and sets to a relatively solid powder finish, though it isn't impervious to smudging and smearing. All in all, this doesn't compare to the long-wearing, gel-type eyeliners from Bobbi Brown, M.A.C., or Stila.

☹ **Eye Pencils** *($9)* are creamy, run-of-the-mill pencils that apply a bit too thick and smudge easily. Iredale's Cream to Powder Eyeliner above lasts longer, as do her powder eyeshadows.

LIPSTICK, LIP GLOSS, AND LIPLINER: ☺ Lip Pencils *($9)* have a creamy texture and attractive colors, but are otherwise standard and require routine sharpening.

☹ **PureMoist LipColours SPF 18** *($19)* are one of the few lipsticks with sunscreen that offer UVA protection (Iredale uses zinc oxide), but this plus is sidelined by the irritating peppermint extract that is also included. Granted, these lipsticks don't have the most elegant texture, but the boon of sun protection would have made them worth trying if not for the irritating peppermint. ☹ **PureMoist LipSheres SPF 18** *($19)* are sheerer versions of the PureMoist LipColours above, and share the same pro (excellent broad-spectrum sunscreen) and con (too much peppermint). ☹ **PureGloss for Lips** *($19)* has been reformulated and now comes with a flocked sponge-tip applicator. These sheer, minimally sticky glosses are available in some enticing colors, but the inclusion of ginger root oil produces a tingly-warm sensation that means lips are being irritated, not cared for.

MASCARA: ☹ **$$$ PureLash Lengthening Mascara** *($16)* builds moderate length with a very clean, clump-free application. Thickness is scarce, and this isn't what I would call dramatic mascara, but it does the job and stays on all day. ☹ **$$$ PureLash Mascara** *($16)* offers decent (but unimpressive) length with a soft curl. This doesn't thicken lashes in the least, but it wears well and removes easily. ☹ **$$$ PureLash Conditioner** *($16)* is essentially a basic mascara formula without pigment. Used as a primer, it bulks up lashes prior to mascara application, although it's no better than applying two or three coats of a good mascara. This does contain conditioning agents, but lashes don't need conditioning the same way hair does.

FACE AND BODY ILLUMINATING/SHIMMER PRODUCTS: ☺ **$$$ Moonglow** *($46)* comes with four pressed shimmer powder wedges in one compact. There are no dividers between the colors, but each is big enough to use alone with any number of eyeshadow brushes. Using a blush or powder brush is tricky and will result in one color (a soft golden bronze with a hint of copper—shades having nothing to do with the moon), but the effect is flattering for evening or glamour makeup.

☹ **24-Karat Gold Dust** *($12)* is just mica, iron oxides, and real gold flakes. Combined, they make this simply a shiny loose powder whose glistening effect works nicely for evening glamour.

BRUSHES: The brushes available here are mostly excellent, and the ones to consider for their workable shapes and soft but firm feel are the ✓☺ **Deluxe Eye Shader** *($21.50)*, ☺ **Chisel Powder** *($24.50)*, ☺ **Eye Shader** *($9)*, and ☺ **Eye Contour** *($9.50)*; ☺ **Eye Liner/Brow** *($12)* and ☺ **Camouflage Brush** *($15)* are options as well, and both are synthetic. The ☺ **$$$ Handi Brush** *($39)*, which is recommended for applying Jane Iredale's powder bases, is cut straight across and applies the powder much like a sponge would, and may be worth a test to see how you like the results. It definitely provides a heavier coverage and matte finish. Iredale's ☺ **$$$ Foundation Brush** *($35.80)* is also worth auditioning if you're curious to see if you prefer this type of brush to a makeup sponge. The ☹ **White Fan Brush** *($12)* has little practical purpose and is easily replaced by other brushes.

Several ☺ **Makeup Bags** *($16.50–$38)* round out Iredale's implement collection, with many including room for brushes and additional compartments, pouches for traveling, or space just to keep your most-used cosmetics organized. You may not find these at salons or spas selling Jane Iredale products, but they are available online.

SPECIALTY PRODUCTS: ☺ **$$$ One-4-All** *($56)* is meant for serious Jane Iredale fans. Included in one sleek, mirrored compact are three eyeshadows, two cream-to-powder eyeliners, two shades of lip gloss, a cream-to-powder blush, and brow powder. Three palettes are available, with Neutral being the easiest to work with. The Warm and Cool sets contain either blue or green eyeshadow and liner colors, which won't do much to shape and shade the eye. A brush is included as well, and it's a step above what you'll find in similar kits. Although this is rated highly, keep in mind that kits like this are a value only if you know you will use most, if not all, of the colors.

☺ **$$$ Lid Primer** *($18)* comes with your choice of two cream-to-powder shades, a soft pearlized ivory or a shimmering pink. Both apply easily, have a slight tendency to crease, and offer significant coverage. Despite the shine, these are good choices if you have any discoloration on your eyelid and don't like the look you get using concealer and powder prior to eyeshadow.

☹ **$$$ Absence Oil Control Primer SPF 15** *($35.50)*, according to the claims, seems to be the product those with overactive oily skin have been searching for—yet the formula doesn't give much credibility to the oil-control and regulating claims. Although it's nice that the sunscreen is pure titanium dioxide and zinc oxide, some of the major ingredients (including candelilla wax and fatty acids from macadamia nut oil) in this cream-to-powder primer won't help oily skin. The colorless base of the original Absence slips over skin and sets to a matte finish, but those with truly oily skin will find it doesn't last as long as they'd like. Absence 2 has a sheer peach tint (not tan, as described) that is borderline problematic for medium skin tones. Both versions are an OK option if your foundation doesn't contain sunscreen and you want to prep your skin with a matte-finish product; just don't expect it to regulate your skin's oil production.

☹ **$$$ Botanical Brush Cleaner** *($15 for 4 ounces)* is mostly alcohol and witch hazel (which is partially alcohol) along with citrus oils for fragrance. Alcohols function as solvents and will break down makeup on your brushes, but not without the eventual side effect of making the brush bristles feel dry. This is a decent option if you don't want to dampen your brushes with water, but one you should use only intermittently.

☹ **$$$ Sugar & Butter Lip Exfoliator/Plumper** *($24)* is a dual-sided product that features an oil-based stick with brown sugar crystals to exfoliate lips and a sheer pink shimmer lipstick designed to plump them. The scrub portion definitely takes care of dry, flaky skin on the lips yet can feel too abrasive unless used very gently. Iredale encourages users to eat the sugar crystals rather than rinsing them (nothing in this portion of the product is harmful to ingest), but that enourages lip-licking, which begins the dryness/chapping cycle anew. This is further aggravated when you apply the Lip Plumper, because it contains mint and ginger (listed on the box as "flavor") that cause a cooling, tingling sensation. Lips become inflamed from the irritation, but this type of product isn't the best for routine use due to the irritation it causes. And the amount of product you get is really tiny, which doesn't justify the price.

☹ **$$$ Facial Blotting Papers** *($11 for 100 sheets)* are average blotting papers because they simply don't absorb oil as well as several other options. Perhaps this is because the papers are made from flax seeds, which are themselves somewhat oily, but whatever the reason, standard tissue paper works better, as do the blotting papers composed of polypropylene (a plastic-like substance).

JURLIQUE INTERNATIONAL (SKIN CARE ONLY)

JURLIQUE INTERNATIONAL AT-A-GLANCE

Strengths: A handful of good moisturizers whose plant extracts have established benefit for skin.

Weaknesses: The majority of the products contain plant extracts or oils known to be irritating (in some cases, significantly so) for skin; the only sunscreen has irritating fragrant oils; no AHA, BHA, anti-blemish, or skin-lightening products; the Ultra-Sensitive line puts already delicate skin on the fast track for more problems; no recommended cleansers; mostly irritating toners/toning mists; no reliable preservative system is used.

For more information aboaut Jurlique International, call (800) 854-1110 or visit www.jurlique.com or www.Beautypedia.com. Note: All of Jurlique International's products are highly fragranced.

JURLIQUE INTERNATIONAL ULTRA-SENSITIVE SKIN CARE

All of Jurlique International's Ultra-Sensitive products contain Szechuan peppercorn extract and gromwell extract (Latin name *Lithospermum officinale*). Szechuan peppercorn is a significant skin irritant and gromwell extract can cause cell damage (Source: *American Herbal Products Association* (AHPA), www.ahpa.org). There is one study indicating gromwell can reduce UVB damage to skin, but other ingredients (such as green tea or pomegranate) can do that without putting skin at risk for irritation (Source: *Biological and Pharmaceutical Bulletin*, May 2007, pages 928–934). Most of the Ultra-Sensitive products also contain lavender, which can cause skin-cell death (Source: *Cell Proliferation*, June 2004, pages 221–229). None of these products are recommended for any skin type, much less for sensitive skin.

☹ **Ultra Sensitive Face Wash** *($42 for 6.8 ounces)*. See comments above.

☹ **Ultra-Sensitive Make-Up Remover** *($46 for 3.4 ounces)*. See comments above.

☹ **Ultra-Sensitive Hydrator/Toner Gel** *($31 for 3.4 ounces)*. See comments above.

☹ **Ultra-Sensitive Aromatic Hydrating Concentrate** *($46 for 1.7 ounces)*. See comments above.

☹ **Ultra-Sensitive Day Moisture Lotion** *($75 for 3.4 ounces)*. See comments above.

☹ **Ultra-Sensitive Night Treatment Gel** *($77 for 3.4 ounces)*. See comments above.

☹ **Ultra-Sensitive Nurturing Mask** *($75 for 4.4 ounces)*. See comments above.

OTHER JURLIQUE INTERNATIONAL PRODUCTS

☹ **Cleansing Lotion Makeup Remover** *($29 for 3.4 ounces)* contains too many plant irritants to list, and is completely inappropriate for cleansing, especially around the eyes. The amount of alcohol is also cause for concern.

☹ **Foaming Facial Cleanser** *($35 for 6.8 ounces)* contains a lot of witch hazel and also has lavender oil, which is irritating to skin and a distinct problem in a cleanser if it gets near the eyes.

☹ **OPC Make-up Remover** *($30 for 3.4 ounces)* lists only water and herbal extracts from horsetail (which is too astringent for skin) and lavender (which is irritating and should not be used around the eyes). With no cleansing agents, this product is nothing more than an irritation for skin.

☹ **Face Wash Cream** *($24 for 1.4 ounces)* begins with almond and oat water, but the herbal extract mix that follows contains some problematic ingredients, plus alcohol. The geranium leaf oil is another problem, and is best enjoyed by inhaling it, rather than exposing your skin to it.

☹ **Aromamist-Clarity Blend** *($26 for 1.7 ounces)* lists alcohol as the second ingredient, and contains irritating oils of orange, lavender, pine leaf, and lemon. Ouch! This would make a better furniture polish than skin-care product!

☹ **Aromamist-Pampering Blend** *($26 for 1.7 ounces)* claims to pamper your skin and senses, but only the latter is accurate. The fragrant oils in this toning mist are incredibly irritating for all skin types.

☹ **Aromamist-Romance Blend** *($26 for 1.7 ounces)* is similar to the Aromamist-Pampering Blend above, save for a change in irritating fragrant oils. Otherwise, the same review applies.

☹ **Aromamist-Travel Blend** *($26 for 1.7 ounces)* is similar to the Aromamist-Clarity Blend above, only with fewer irritants. Otherwise, the same review applies.

☹ **Chamomile Floral Water** *($35 for 3.4 ounces)* lists alcohol as the second ingredient, which ruins an otherwise very soothing toner.

☹ **Chamomile-Rose Aromatic Hydrating Concentrate, for Dry to Delicate Skin** *($51 for 1.7 ounces)* claims to be highly concentrated, which makes the alcohol and rose oil in this product that much more irritating to skin. There is no research showing that the natural ingredients in this product have a balancing effect on skin.

😐 **$$$ Day Care Conditioner** *($35 for 3.4 ounces)* is an OK toner for normal to slightly dry skin. The plant extracts are either soothing for skin or have no established benefit (or risk), but they do add fragrance.

☹ **Herbal Recovery Mist AG, for Normal to Dry Skin** *($46 for 1 ounce)* is similar to the Day Care Conditioner above, but is not recommended because it adds lavender and horsetail to the mix.

☺ **$$$ Herbal Recovery Mist DS, for Delicate and Sensitive Skin** *($46 for 1 ounce)* is too fragrant for delicate or sensitive skin (fragrance is always an issue for a sensitizing or allergic reaction), but it can be a good toner for normal to slightly dry skin. With the exception of rose and daisy, all of the extracts and oils have soothing properties for skin.

☹ **Herbal Recovery Mist MD, for Dry and Mature Skin** *($46 for 1 ounce)* shares common ingredients with the Herbal Recovery Mist DS above, but adds problematic lavender and horsetail extracts plus rose oil, making it a problem for any skin type.

☹ **Herbal Recovery Mist OP, for Oily Skin** *($46 for 1 ounce)* is nearly identical to the Herbal Recovery Mist MD above, and the same comments apply. Isn't it interesting how such similar products purport to work for skin types that are polar opposites?

☹ **Lavender Floral Water** *($35 for 3.4 ounces)* contains too much alcohol and lavender oil, and is not recommended for any skin type.

☹ **Lavender-Lavandin Aromatic Hydrating Concentrate, for Normal to Dry Skin** *($44 for 1.7 ounces)* only serves to irritate skin with its volatile oils and alcohol. None of this is harmonizing for skin, as claimed.

☹ **Lemon Lime Aromatic Hydrating Concentrate, for Oily Skin** *($44 for 1.7 ounces)* contains lemon and lime oils, making it more suitable for a cocktail additive than a helpful product for those with oily skin.

☹ **Pine Needles Aromatic Hydrating Concentrate** *($44 for 1.7 ounces)* may make your Christmas tree smell better, but it's a terrible product for skin because it contains a high amount of pine leaf oil and alcohol.

☹ **Pure Rosewater Freshener** *($31 for 3.4 ounces)* is purely irritating thanks to the amount of rose oil and alcohol it contains.

☹ **Rosemary-Sage Aromatic Hydrating Concentrate** *($44 for 1.7 ounces)* contains a lot of rosemary oil as well as several irritating plant extracts and sage oil. Talk about setting skin off on a cascade of inflammation!

☹ **Arnica Cream** *($32 for 1.4 ounces)* contains a prodigious amount of arnica, which may appeal to fans of natural products, but only serves to make this moisturizer an irritating experience for skin.

☹ **Arnica Lotion** *($28 for 1.7 ounces)* is the lotion version of the Arnica Cream above, and aside from a texture change and the addition of alcohol, the same comments apply.

☺ **Calendula Cream** *($32 for 1.4 ounces)* is an emollient moisturizer for normal to dry skin that contains some good plant oils and anti-irritants, along with lesser amounts of natural water-binding agents (honey) and antioxidants.

☹ **Calendula Lotion** *($28 for 1.7 ounces)* contains enough witch hazel and alcohol to be a problem for all skin types, not to mention that these ingredients undermine the effectiveness of the calendula.

☹ **Day Care Face Cream** *($34 for 1.4 ounces)* contains some good and bad plant extracts for skin, but what tips the scales in favor of an unhappy face rating is the inclusion of orange and rose oils. For daytime this product must be worn with a sunscreen, or at least I'd like to see a recommendation on the label to use one and not rely on this alone.

☹ **Day Care Face Lotion** *($36 for 1 ounce)* is the lotion version of the Day Care Face Cream above, and the same review applies.

☹ **Day Care Face Oil** *($39 for 1 ounce)* contains petitgrain oil, a citrus oil that can be irritating to skin. The avocado and macadamia nut oils are not the least bit helpful for someone with oily skin.

☺ **$$$ Elder Cream** *($39 for 1.4 ounces)* contains elderberry extract, from a plant whose flavonoid content makes it an antioxidant-rich option for skin. This cream for normal to dry skin also contains stabilized vitamin C and, surprisingly for Jurlique International, no other plant extracts besides elderberry.

☹ **Eye Gel** *($121 for 1 ounce)* doesn't help make skin soft and supple because it contains arnica as its main ingredient. That's a shame, because almost all of the other plant extracts in this gel are very good antioxidants.

😐 **$$$ Herbal Recovery Gel** *($67 for 1 ounce)* is similar to the Eye Gel above, minus the arnica. The majority of plants in this gel are good for skin, while a few are here just for fragrance. This is an OK option for slightly dry skin, but do not use it near your eyes.

☹ **Neck Serum** *($75 for 1 ounce)* contains jasmine, myrrh, orange, and frankincense oils, all of which are irritating for skin and have no positive "influence" on the delicate neck area.

😐 **$$$ Viola Cream** *($39 for 1.4 ounces)* contains viola extract. Also known as heart's ease, this is a plant with established anti-inflammatory and antioxidant activity. The chickweed and daisy don't add much beyond fragrance, but this is an OK, though fairly basic moisturizer for normal to dry skin.

☹ **Wrinkle Softener Beauty Cream** *($72 for 1.4 ounces)* makes antiwrinkle claims that are neither more exciting nor truer than those made by most other moisturizers. The difference is that this one irritates skin with some problematic plant extracts and fragrant oils of rose and orange.

☹ **Blemish Cream** *($28 for 0.3 ounce)* contains several thickeners that can be a problem for blemishes. Tea tree oil has not been shown to be effective as a topical disinfectant for acne in the amount this product contains. The colloidal sulfur can have disinfecting properties, but is also significantly irritating, and for most acne sufferers, the tradeoff isn't worth it.

☹ **Deep Penetrating Cream Mask** *($39 for 1.7 ounces)* ends up confusing skin because it contains a blend of absorbent clay and emollients, so neither ends up being that effective. This mask is not recommended for anyone because it contains lavender and lemon peel oils.

😐 **$$$ Moor Purifying Mask** *($38 for 1.7 ounces)* contains Moor extract, a trade name for silt extract, which is another way of saying clay, and it has no special properties for skin. The blend of problematic and helpful plant extracts isn't the best, nor is the alcohol content of this mask, but it's an OK option for oily skin.

☹ **Lip Care Balm** *($23 for 0.3 ounce)* has ingredients that soften and smooth dry, chapped lips, but the fragrant ylang ylang and pepper seed oils will cause inflammation and end up making chapped lips worse.

Jurlique International Sun Products

☹ **$$$ Bronzer** *($37 for 1 ounce)* is a sheer, tan-tinted moisturizer that contains some pro and con plant extracts and fragrant ylang ylang oil. It's a decent option for normal to dry skin, but countless tinted moisturizers offer more without any risk of irritation.

☹ **Sun Lotion SPF 30+** *($63 for 3.4 ounces)* deserves praise for its in-part titanium dioxide sunscreen, but the price is astronomical and that definitely won't encourage you to apply this liberally, which is an essential element in making sure you get the stated SPF protection. Further, this is impossible to recommend because it contains irritating pine leaf, bitter orange, lavender, and cypress oils.

Kiehl's (Skin Care Only)

Kiehl's At-A-Glance

Strengths: Provides complete ingredient lists on their Web site; Kiehl's staff is generous when it comes to providing samples and product information; some good cleansers; a worthwhile selection of sunscreens with avobenzone for UVA protection; a reliable lip balm; many fragrance-free items.

Weaknesses: Expensive for what you get; the Blue Herbal products are terrible for acne; no products to successfully address skin discolorations; the toners; the self-tanner; jar packaging; advertised plant extracts typically show up in very short supply.

For more information about L'Oreal-owned Kiehl's, call (800) 543-4572 or visit www.kiehls.com or www.Beautypedia.com.

Kiehl's Abyssine Products

☹ **$$$ Abyssine Cream** *($40 for 1.7 ounce)*. Abyssine's star attraction is alteromonas ferment extract (abyssine). The claim is that this "survival molecule" (it isn't really a molecule, it's a plant extract) thrives under extreme conditions such as volcanic ocean vents. Translated into cosmetic-speak, that must mean it is a wondrous ingredient for staving off the signs of aging. Whenever an exotic-sounding skin-care ingredient is ballyhooed, there is one thing that's rarely discussed in relation to its alleged benefit for skin. And that one thing is: What, if anything, do the characteristics of the plant or ingredient (such as seaweed or plankton) that allow it to thrive and survive in its native environment have to do with how it will perform when harvested and mixed into a product for skin? The story behind the ingredient is often overblown to the point that this fundamental logic gets lost. In this case, the bottom line is that abyssine does not parlay its survival-of-the-fittest benefits to your skin (more specifically, it can't stave off your wrinkles). At best, it functions as a water-binding agent, but there isn't very much abyssine in this product anyway. This is an OK, fragrance-free, jar-packaged moisturizer for normal to dry skin. It contains a simple mix of water, silicone, glycerin, plant oil, petrolatum, and token amounts of innocuous plant extracts.

☹ **$$$ Abyssine Eye Cream** *($30 for 0.5 ounce)* is a fairly standard moisturizer for normal to dry skin anywhere on the face. It contains mostly water, glycerin, silicone, emollient, thickeners, absorbents (which mean the product is not as hydrating as advertised), slip agent, wax, a long list of water-binding agents (all present in such small amounts that they don't amount to much), film-forming agents, and preservatives. Nothing about this eye cream will deter the effects of aging on skin, but, like all moisturizers, it can make fine lines and wrinkles appear smoother.

☹ **Abyssine Lotion SPF 15** *($40 for 2.5 ounces)* lists all of its interesting ingredients after the preservative, a common occurrence in Kiehl's skin-care products. What this means is that they are essentially window dressing to make this in-part titanium dioxide sunscreen seem like more than it really is. That fact and the inclusion of several irritating plant oils (including lavender) make this a no-go for any skin type.

☹ **Abyssine Serum** *($42 for 1.7 ounces)* lists alcohol as the second ingredient, which makes this serum problematic for all skin types. Further, almost all of the showcased ingredients are listed after the preservatives, giving you an idea of how (un)important they are to this Kiehl's product.

KIEHL'S BLUE HERBAL PRODUCTS

☹ **Blue Herbal Gel Cleanser** *($20.50 for 8.4 ounces)* does contain 1.5% salicylic acid, but in a cleanser this ingredient is wasted because it's not left on the skin long enough to have an effect. The real problem with this cleanser is the inclusion of ginger, cinnamon, menthol, and camphor. If you are using this product, believe me, I feel your pain!

☹ **Blue Astringent Herbal Lotion** *($15 for 8.4 ounces)* has been part of the Kiehl's line since 1964. Considering how much more we know about what skin needs to look and feel its best, it's hardly surprising that this alcohol-based toner is outdated; but with menthol, camphor, and aluminum chlorohydrate (an ingredient in many antiperspirants) as well … oy!, this is also incredibly irritating! This isn't a treatment for blemished skin, it's a punishment.

☹ **Blue Herbal Spot Treatment** *($15.50 for 0.5 ounce)* lists alcohol as the second ingredient, and further down the list are a slew of other irritants, including menthol, camphor, witch hazel, cinnamon, and ginger. What was Kiehl's thinking?

KIEHL'S BRIGHT PRODUCTS

☹ **Brightening Botanical Cleansing Cream** *($22.50 for 5 ounces)* contains a large amount of the alkaline ingredient potassium hydroxide, which makes this foaming cleanser too drying for all skin types. A much better, less-expensive version of this cleanser is L'Oreal's Hydra Fresh Foaming Face Wash, for Normal to Dry Skin ($6.26 for 6.5 ounces).

☹ **Brightening Botanical Clarifying Toner** *($34.50 for 8.4 ounces)* lists alcohol as the second ingredient, which makes this an expensive burn for skin. It also contains the potent menthol derivative menthoxypropanediol.

😐 **$$$ Brightening Botanical Moisture Fluid** *($40 for 2.5 ounces)* contains a very small amount of plant extracts with limited research concerning their skin-lightening ability (and what research exists studied much higher concentrations than Kiehl's uses). This is just a water- and silicone-based moisturizer with vitamin C. The vitamin C, as ascorbyl glucoside, has limited research pertaining to its skin-lightening ability. The most current study involved pairing an unknown amount of it with niacinamide and using ultrasound technology to enhance penetration, possibilities that don't come with this product (Source: *Skin Research and Technology*, May 2006, pages 105–113).

KIEHL'S CRYSTE MARINE PRODUCTS

😐 **$$$ Cryste Marine Firming Cream** *($45 for 1.7 ounces)* makes a big deal out of the Mediterranean-sourced flower (*Crithmum maritimum*, or rock samphire) extract it contains. Supposedly, this flower can increase the renewal rate of skin cells, but there is no information to support this claim. Even if it had such an effect, the amount in this product is minuscule (there's more preservative than flower extract). That leaves you with a pricey moisturizer that has some respectable qualities (the glycerin, silicone, and squalane base gets things off to a good start), yet this remains an ordinary choice when compared to similarly priced products from other department-store lines, such as Clinique and Estee Lauder. Nothing in this product is capable of firming skin.

☹ **$$$ Cryste Marine Firming Eye Treatment** *($35 for 0.5 ounce)* is incapable of firming skin and the jar packaging will render the tiny amounts of antioxidants ineffective shortly after you open the product. At best, this will make dry skin anywhere on the face feel softer and smoother. For the money, you should expect more.

☹ **Cryste Marine Firming Serum** *($48 for 1.7 ounces)* is primarily water, glycerin, silicone, alcohol, and slip agents. The rice protein cannot firm skin, although it and a few other ingredients in this serum are good water-binding agents. This would be an OK option if it did not contain the irritating menthol derivative menthoxypropanediol.

☹ **$$$ Cryste Marine "Ultra Riche" Lifting and Firming Cream** *($45 for 1.7 ounces)* makes a claim that conflicts with basic physics. According to Kiehl's, this rather boring but emollient moisturizer for normal to dry skin contains "Hyaluronic Filling Spheres." The sponge-like absorbency of these spheres is said to trap the skin's own water, causing the molecules to expand, which "immediately" lifts skin. Assuming the spheres work as claimed (although the amount of sodium hyaluronate in this product is next to nothing), the effect would not be to lift skin but rather to stretch it or make it puffy. Of course, when you look at it that way, the appeal pretty much vanishes.

KIEHL'S RARE EARTH PRODUCTS

☺ **$$$ Rare-Earth Oatmeal Milk Facial Cleanser #1, for a Normal to Oily Skin Type** *($20.50 for 8.4 ounces)* doesn't contain any earth that is remotely rare, just standard kaolin, better known as clay. But I guess if you want to make something ordinary sound unique, that is one way to do it. All in all, what you're getting in this product are standard detergent cleansing agents and clay. Clay can be slightly tricky to rinse off, but it does leave skin soft and is an option for someone with oily skin.

☺ **$$$ Rare-Earth Facial Cleansing Masque, for Normal to Oily and Oily Skin Types** *($17.50 for 5 ounces)* is a very standard, but effective, clay mask for normal to oily skin. The addition of some soothing plant extracts may be helpful for inflamed or irritated skin.

☹ **Rare-Earth Face Masque (Gently Astringent for Oily-Acne Skin)** *($16 for 4.2 ounces)* is not preferred to the Rare-Earth Facial Cleansing Masque above because it lacks the bells and whistles available in many other masks, and adds irritating sulfur, despite an overall claim of being a gentle product.

KIEHL'S ULTRA FACIAL PRODUCTS

☹ **$$$ Ultra Facial Cream** *($22.50 for 1.7 ounces)* provides another story about two special ingredients extracted from remote locations, also claimed to be valuable for skin because they can survive in harsh climates (lots of plants can survive harsh climates, but rubbing them on your skin is not going to help you with sun damage or with frigid conditions). It also doesn't help that these miracle plants are present in such tiny amounts, and the jar packaging won't keep any of the token amount of antioxidants stable during use. This is definitely more ordinary than ultra for normal to dry skin.

😐 **$$$ Ultra Facial Moisturizer** *($33 for 8.4 ounces)* remains a very popular product for Kiehl's, sort of like the original Dramatically Different Moisturizing Lotion remains a hot seller for Clinique. Both products cover the basic needs of someone with normal to dry skin, but lack anything truly beneficial or state-of-the-art for skin. The tiny amounts of plant oils and vitamins in this moisturizer will have little to no impact, though it is fragrance-free.

☹ **Ultra Facial Moisturizer SPF 15** *($29.50 for 4.2 ounces)* lacks the UVA-protecting ingredients of titanium dioxide, zinc oxide, avobenzone, Tinosorb, or Mexoryl SX, and is not recommended. Even if this had sufficient UVA protection, it is an exceptionally boring moisturizer for the money.

☹ **Ultra Facial Tinted Moisturizer SPF 15** *($24.50 for 2.5 ounces)* comes in three sheer shades and has a much more interesting (though still lackluster) formula than the Ultra Facial Moisturizer SPF 15 above. However, the absence of sufficient UVA protection makes this a poor choice for daytime.

KIEHL'S YERBA MATE TEA PRODUCTS

☺ **$$$ Yerba Mate Tea Cleanser** *($20.50 for 8.4 ounces)* is a very standard, but good, water-soluble cleanser for normal to oily or slightly dry skin. The amount of black tea ferment is too small to matter, but even if it were present in prodigious amounts it would just be rinsed down the drain before it could exert any antioxidant benefit. This cleanser contains fragrance in the form of lemon fruit extract.

☹ **Yerba Mate Tea Toner** *($24.50 for 8.4 ounces)* is mostly water with slip agents, but loses points for including irritating peppermint and ivy stem. The amount of mate (*Ilex paraguariensis*) is minimal and of little benefit for skin.

☺ **$$$ Yerba Mate Tea Lotion** *($35 for 2.5 ounces)* is infused with yerba mate, but this caffeine-containing plant (most often consumed as tea) has no established benefit for skin. It contains several vitamins and minerals, but not in amounts that would allow the skin to derive much benefit, and its volatile components (including tannins and theobromine) cancel out any potential benefits of the other constituents. In the case of this lotion, the amount of yerba mate is minimal. This is a good moisturizer for normal to slightly oily skin. It has a soft matte finish and provides skin with some effective water-binding agents, a tiny amount of antioxidants, and a cell-communicating ingredient.

OTHER KIEHL'S PRODUCTS

☹ **Foaming Non-Detergent Washable Cleanser, for Combination or Oily Skin** *($17.50 for 8.4 ounces)* is not in the least a non-detergent cleanser because the second ingredient listed is sodium C14-16 olefin sulfate, a detergent cleansing agent (technically called a surfactant) that is present in shampoos and known for stripping hair color. By any dictionary definition, this is a standard detergent cleanser that can be drying and irritating for skin.

☺ **Gentle Foaming Facial Cleanser, for Dry to Normal Skin Types** *($17.50 for 8.4 ounces)* is accurately named. This standard, water-soluble cleanser doesn't have much to it, but it's fragrance-free and does the job for its intended skin types.

☺ **Oil-Based Cleanser and Make-Up Remover** *($20.50 for 8.4 ounces)* ends up being an emollient, somewhat greasy way to remove makeup, but it works for dry to very dry skin not prone to blemishes. The small amount of alcohol is not a cause for concern.

☺ **Ultra Moisturizing Cleansing Cream** *($20.50 for 8 ounces)* is a standard, cold cream–style cleanser that is a good option for dry, sensitive skin, including those with rosacea, and is fragrance-free. You may still need to use a washcloth to remove all of your makeup.

☺ **Washable Cleansing Milk, for Dry, Normal to Dry or Sensitive Skin Types** *($17.50 for 8.4 ounces)* is a lotion cleanser that is an option for normal to dry skin, though it isn't all that washable without the help of a washcloth. The trace amounts of milk and vitamins in this product are barely detectable.

☺ **$$$ Supremely Gentle Eye Make-Up Remover** *($16.50 for 4.2 ounces)* has gentle written all over it, but they should have added "greasy," too, because the amount of oil in this remover leaves a discernible film on skin. This is best for dry skin, and best used before a standard, water-soluble cleanser. It will remove makeup with minimal effort.

☺ **$$$ Epidermal Re-Texturizing Micro-Dermabrasion** *($40 for 2.5 ounces)* is your basic microdermabrasion-in-a-jar topical scrub, with alumina as the abrasive agent. The emollients and silicone in this product help protect skin from the alumina, which can be rough on your skin if not used very gently. Although pricey, this is a good, fragrance-free scrub for normal to dry skin.

😐 **$$$ Milk, Honey and Almond Scrub** *($20.50 for 6 ounces)* is a rather inelegant, from-the-kitchen scrub that contains almond-seed meal and grain flours to exfoliate skin. The honey base makes this somewhat sticky while the plant oils impede rinsing, which adds up to a passable but barely worthwhile scrub for normal to dry skin.

😐 **$$$ Pineapple Papaya Facial Scrub, Made with Real Fruit** *($25 for 3.4 ounces)* relies partly on pineapple enzymes to exfoliate skin. Not only are enzymes unreliable exfoliants, but the jar packaging chosen for this product won't keep them stable. The corncob powder is a low-tech exfoliant, but is what saves this scrub for normal to oily skin from being a total waste of time and money.

✓☺ **Ultra Moisturizing Buffing Cream with Scrub Particles** *($14.50 for 4 ounces)* is a very good moisturizing scrub for dry skin. Unlike the other Kiehl's scrubs above, this contains rounded polyethylene (plastic) beads as the abrasive agent. It is fragrance-free.

☹ **Calendula Herbal-Extract Toner, Alcohol-Free, for Normal to Oily Skin Type** *($34.50 for 8.4 ounces)* is such a basic, nearly do-nothing toner that the price is ludicrous. If you're interested in calendula for skin care, buy a bottle of the oil from a health food store or steep the plant in hot water, let it cool, and bottle your own. Either option is an improvement over this product.

☹ **Cucumber Herbal Alcohol-Free Toner, for Dry or Sensitive Skin** *($15 for 8.4 ounces)* contains balm mint, juniper, pine needle, and arnica, making it too irritating for all skin types, especially sensitive skin.

☹ **Herbal Toner with Mixed Berries and Botanical Extracts, for Normal to Oily Skin Types** *($24.50 for 8.4 ounces)* contains berries supposedly placed in each bottle by hand, but aside from looking kind of neat, they have no impact on skin. What will impact skin (negatively) is the peppermint in this poorly formulated toner.

☹ **Rosewater Facial Freshener-Toner, for Normal to Oily Skin** *($15 for 8.4 ounces)* lists alcohol as the second ingredient and contains too little of anything of redeeming value for skin.

☹ **Rosewater Toner #1, for an Oily Skin Type** *($15 for 8.4 ounces)* is even more irritating and drying than the Rosewater Facial Freshener-Toner above because it adds witch hazel and menthol to the mix.

☹ **Tea Tree Oil Toner, for Oily or Normal to Oily Skin Type** *($24.50 for 8.4 ounces)* contains some tea tree oil, but any benefit it has is offset by the irritation caused by the eucalyptus, sage, lavender oil, and other volatile fragrant oils in this toner.

😐 **$$$ Anti-Oxidant Skin Preserver** *($60 for 1.4 ounces)* is an incredibly rich moisturizer for very dry skin, but comes up short with antioxidants, including just a tiny amount of vitamins A, C, and E—none of which will survive for long because of jar packaging.

😐 **Centella Recovery Skin Salve** *($42 for 2.5 ounces)* contains mostly water, silicones, glycerin, slip agents, and preservatives. The tiny amount of plant extracts has negligible benefit for irritated skin, but at least nothing in this fragrance-free moisturizer is likely to cause irritation or bother sensitive skin.

😐 **$$$ Creamy Eye Treatment with Avocado** *($24 for 0.5 ounce)* is good for dry skin anywhere on the face, but the amount of antioxidants is tiny and they won't last long once this jar-packaged product is opened.

😐 **Creme D'Elegance Repairateur, Superb Tissue Repairateur Creme** *($49.50 for 4.2 ounces)* is nothing more than an average emollient moisturizer for dry skin. The name is fancy, but the formula is outdated, and the most intriguing ingredients amount to less than a dusting.

☺ **$$$ High-Potency Skin-Firming Concentrate** *($55 for 1.7 ounces)* is a lightweight, serum-type moisturizer with a fairly modern assortment of helpful ingredients for skin. Of course, none of them are capable of addressing "multiple skin firmness concerns," but they can help skin restore a healthy barrier and prevent moisture loss. This is fragrance-free.

😐 **Imperiale Repairateur, Moisturizing Eye Balm** *($17.50 for 0.5 ounce)* contains some outstanding ingredients to treat and protect very dry skin, so it's unfortunate that the impressive amount of vitamin E won't remain stable for long due to jar packaging. This still has merit as a balm for dry patches.

☺ **Light Nourishing Eye Cream** *($20 for 0.5 ounce)* is a good, emollient moisturizer for dry skin anywhere on the face. The only antioxidant of note is vitamin E, but the formula is fragrance-free and suitable for sensitive skin.

😐 **$$$ Lycopene Facial Moisturizing Cream** *($60 for 1.4 ounces)* talks up its lycopene and beta carotene content, but these vegetable-derived antioxidants are in severely short supply in this product, plus the jar packaging won't keep them stable during use. This ends up being a very expensive emollient moisturizer for dry skin.

😐 **Lycopene Facial Moisturizing Lotion** *($35 for 1.7 ounces)* is the lotion version of the Lycopene Facial Moisturizing Cream above, and although less costly, it's also a less interesting formula, offering little benefit to normal or slightly oily skin.

😐 **Panthenol Protein Moisturizing Face Cream, for Normal to Dry and Dry Skin Types** *($17.50 for 2 ounces)* is an OK emollient moisturizer for its intended skin type. Most of the interesting ingredients are listed well after the preservative, so they don't count for much.

☺ **$$$ Powerful Strength Line Reducing Concentrate** *($55 for 1.7 ounces)* is mostly slip agent, silicone, vitamin C, more silicones, film-forming agent, and the cell-communicating ingredient adenosine. Although this is a one-note product, it's an option if you want a stably packaged vitamin C serum.

😐 **Sodium PCA "Oil-Free" Moisturizer** *($17.50 for 2 ounces)* is oil-free but also very boring, offering little for normal to oily skin other than silicone and thickeners. The tiny amount of antioxidants will deteriorate quickly due to jar packaging.

☹ **Ultra Protection Moisturizing Eye Gel with SPF 15** *($30 for 0.5 ounce)* lacks the UVA-protecting ingredients of titanium dioxide, zinc oxide, avobenzone, Tinosorb, or Mexoryl SX, and is not recommended.

☺ **$$$ Ultra Moisturizing Eye Stick SPF 30** *($20 for 0.18 ounce)* is a rich, balm-like sunscreen stick that contains an in-part avobenzone sunscreen. The amount of synthetic active ingredients may be too high to use around the eyes, but this can be a very good sunscreen for other exposed areas, such as the ears, scalp, or the top of your feet. It is fragrance-free.

😐 **Algae Masque** *($25.50 for 2 ounces)* has algae extract, but it's the very last ingredient on the list! This mask for normal to dry skin would be more accurately named Glycerin Masque, because that's the main ingredient, along with some slip agents and thickeners. Overall, this is a boring option for skin.

😐 **Drawing Paste** *($15.50 for 0.5 ounce)* is supposed to control surface oiliness and maintain "skin integrity," but it contains several plant oils, wax, shea butter, and lanolin oil, which make it completely inappropriate for oily or blemish-prone skin. There are absorbents in this product, but what they can do is counteracted by the waxes and oils. At least Kiehl's didn't put irritating sulfur in this product.

😐 **Imperiale Repairateur Treatment Line Formula "MM" Moisturizing Masque** *($37.50 for 2.5 ounces)* is a very basic moisturizing mask for normal to dry skin. It does not contain anything unique for people who are routinely subjected to dry airplane cabin air, but it can, just like most emollient moisturizers, help prevent moisture loss.

☺ **$$$ Over-Night Biological Peel** *($40 for 1.7 ounces)* is supposed to be as potent as a 10% glycolic acid product, but it contains no alpha hydroxy acids, or beta hydroxy acid for that matter. Instead, this water- and silicone-based fluid contains urea, which is indeed an exfoliant, albeit a far less sexy version than AHAs or BHA because it's derived from urine. Urea definitely has exfoliating and water-binding properties when used on skin, and unlike AHAs and BHA, its efficacy is not pH-dependent. Much as AHAs do, it can cause a stinging sensation on application. Urea can be beneficial for those with dry skin because, although the manner in which it works isn't fully understood, it has proven very effective at reducing moisture loss from the epidermis (Source: *Dry Skin and Moisturizers Chemistry and Function*, Loden & Maibach, 2000, pages 235–236). Kiehl's ingredient list also points to HEPES as an enzyme activator. However, this ingredient (hydroxyethylpiperazine ethane sulfonic acid) functions as a buffering agent, which should help reduce any potential irritation from the urea. Although this peel is pricey and not necessarily superior to an AHA (or BHA) product, it is nevertheless a novel approach to exfoliating skin if you're curious to try something different, or if your skin has not responded favorably to AHA products.

😐 **Soothing Gel Masque** *($17 for 2 ounces)* is a lightweight gel mask suitable for normal to oily skin experiencing dry patches. The green tea has soothing benefits, but the jar packaging won't keep it stable for long.

☺ **Lip Balm #1** *($5.50 for 0.5 ounce)* is a very standard, Vaseline-based lip balm that contains a good blend of emollients to prevent dry, chapped lips. It is fragrance-free.

KIEHL'S SUN PRODUCTS

☺ **All-Sport "Non-Freeze" Face Protector SPF 30** *($18.50 for 1.4 ounces)* features avobenzone for sufficient UVA protection and has a nonaqueous, wax-based formula suitable for very dry skin, particularly in cold climates. This sunscreen is too heavy for day-to-day wear, and is not recommended for use over blemish-prone areas.

☹ **Sun-Free Self-Tanning Formula** *($22.50 for 5 ounces)* doesn't distinguish itself performance-wise from other self-tanners containing dihydroxyacetone. However, it can be irritating to skin because it contains many volatile fragrant oils and extracts.

☹ **Sunscreen Creme SPF 15** *($15.50 for 4.2 ounces)* leaves skin vulnerable to UVA damage because it lacks the UVA-protecting ingredients of titanium dioxide, zinc oxide, avobenzone, Tinosorb, or Mexoryl SX, and it is not recommended.

☹ **Ultra Protection Water Based Sunscreen Lotion SPF 25** *($27 for 4.2 ounces)* doesn't provide ultra protection because it lacks sufficient UVA-protecting ingredients of titanium dioxide, zinc oxide, avobenzone, Tinosorb, or Mexoryl SX. What a shame, because this has a great lightweight texture.

☺ **UV Protective Everyday Facial Moisturizing Sunscreen Cream SPF 15** *($29.50 for 3.4 ounces)* is Kiehl's version of similar sunscreens with Mexoryl SX from L'Oreal-owned Lancome, La Roche-Posay, and L'Oreal's own line (recall that L'Oreal holds the patent for Mexoryl, which is why for the time being only their brands contain it). Although each of these companies' options provides sufficient UVA protection via Mexoryl SX (ecamsule) and avobenzone, each has a boring lotion formula that is void of antioxidants or other state-of-the-art ingredients. This is recommended for normal to oily skin needing a lightweight, effective sunscreen, but for the money this should have provided more.

☺ **UV Protective Suncare Sunscreen Cream, for Face And Body SPF 20** *($32.50 for 3.4 ounces)* is nearly identical to the UV Protective Everyday Facial Moisturizing Sunscreen SPF 15 above except this version adds titanium dioxide to gain its higher SPF rating. Otherwise, the same comments apply; UVA protection is definitely assured with this blend of Mexoryl SX, avobenzone, and titanium dioxide.

☺ **Vital Sun Protection Lotion SPF 15** *($18.50 for 5 ounces)* is a very good, in-part avobenzone sunscreen for UVA protection; it is appropriate for someone with normal to slightly oily skin. It contains a film-forming agent that provides water resistance, which Kiehl's advertises on the product label. My only point of contention with this sunscreen is the claim that "minimal chemical ingredients" are used, which I'm sure they've chosen to say to try to imply that their sunscreen is superior to others, and it just isn't true. It contains 18% active ingredients—all of them synthetic sunscreen agents—and synthetic preservatives and film-forming agents. Kiehl's claim of using a "minimal" amount doesn't add up to anything like a genuine definition and is a completely disingenuous statement. This product is fragrance-free and does contain vitamin E for some antioxidant benefit.

☺ **Vital Sun Protection Lotion SPF 30** *($18.50 for 5 ounces)* is similar to the Vital Sun Protection Lotion SPF 15 above, except this contains a higher concentration of active ingredients to achieve its SPF 30 rating. Otherwise, the same basic comments apply.

☺ **Vital Sun Protection Lotion SPF 40** *($18.50 for 5 ounces)*. Just to be clear, sunscreens with higher SPF ratings do not provide better protection, just the same amount of protection for a longer time (meaning the amount of time you can stay in the sun without getting burned). For example, an SPF 30 and an SPF 40 (as long as they both have UVA-protecting ingredients) both protect skin from the same amount of the sun's rays. As this book goes to press, the FDA is considering raising the SPF labeling allowance, with their proposal concerning moving from the current recommended maximum SPF rating of SPF 30 and raising this to SPF 50. However, that still has to do with longer, not better, protection.

Regardless of the SPF number, liberal application and regular reapplication are keys to staying protected during prolonged periods of sun exposure. This sunscreen is similar to the Vital Protection SPF 15 and SPF 30 products above, except that it contains a higher concentration of active ingredients and a larger amount of film-forming agent for water resistance. Otherwise, the same comments apply regarding formula and skin type.

☹ **Vital Sun Protection Spray SPF 15** *($17.50 for 4.2 ounces)* has an effective, in-part avobenzone sunscreen that is compromised by the alcohol base, which is drying for skin.

☺ **Vital Sun Protection Spray SPF 25** *($17.50 for 4.2 ounces)* is an alcohol-free version of the Vital Sun Protection Spray SPF 15 above, which raises the question of why that product couldn't have also been made without the alcohol. At any rate, this is a very good, in-part avobenzone sunscreen in a moisturizing, water-resistant spray formula.

☹ **Lip Balm SPF 15** *($8.50 for 0.5 ounce)* is an emollient lip balm available in clear or tinted shades, but none of them provide sufficient UVA protection, which leaves lips vulnerable to sun damage.

KINERASE (SKIN CARE ONLY)

KINERASE AT-A-GLANCE

Strengths: Some antioxidant-rich products in stable packaging; every sunscreen offers sufficient UVA protection; mostly fragrance-free products.

Weaknesses: Cleanser; toning mist; some moisturizers and a serum with irritating ingredients; the Clear Skin products; unknowns about topical application of kinetin and zeatin.

For more information about Kinerase, call (800) 826-9755 or visit www.kinerase.com or www.Beautypedia.com. Note: For more information on kinetin, please refer to Chapter Seven, *Cosmetic Ingredient Dictionary.*

The Reviews K

KINERASE PRO+ THERAPY PRODUCTS

☺ **$$$ Pro+ Therapy Skin Smoothing Cleanser** *($39 for 5.1 ounces)* is a basic, water-soluble cleanser that is a good, though pricey, option for normal to oily skin. The AHAs in this cleanser cannot exfoliate skin due to their brief contact with it, though the pH is within range.

☹ **Pro+ Therapy Advanced Repair Serum** *($132 for 0.5 ounce)* lists alcohol as the second ingredient, which makes this a very expensive way to irritate skin, and it just can't repair skin the way they claim it can. In addition to kinetin, this serum contains zeatin, another plant growth hormone responsible for cell differentiation. Suresh I. S. Rattan, the same doctor who published research on kinetin, was responsible for the sole study on zeatin's effects on skin. The study was performed in vitro and had some promising results, including increasing the ability of skin cells to decompose hydrogen peroxide, meaning that zeatin can be considered an antioxidant. Interestingly, Dr. Rattan's study specifically mentions zeatin's ability to help skin cope with ethanol (alcohol) stress (Source: *Rejuvenation Research*, March 2005, pages 46–57). That revelation, however, neither explains nor justifies Kinerase including so much alcohol in this serum, unless they wanted to prove Dr. Rattan right at the expense of irritating their customers' skin!

😐 **$$$ Pro+ Therapy Ultra Rich Day Repair** *($149 for 1.7 ounces)* isn't as rich as the name states, but has some emollient properties for dry skin. Jar packaging compromises the effectiveness of most of this product's intriguing ingredients. If you're interested in seeing how the plant growth hormones kinetin and zeatin may affect aging skin, this may be worth a try. However, we don't know at this point if light and air exposure from jar packaging may negatively affect these ingredients too. In theory, I suspect it would at least diminish their antioxidant potential.

✓☺ **$$$ Pro+ Therapy Ultra Rich Eye Repair** *($85 for 0.5 ounce)* is, aside from the unknowns surrounding ongoing use of the plant growth hormones kinetin and zeatin, a very good moisturizer for dry skin anywhere on the face. It contains some great water-binding agents along with cell-communicating ingredients, antioxidants, and ingredients that reinforce skin's support structure. This product is fragrance-free, too.

😐 **$$$ Pro+ Therapy Ultra Rich Night Repair** *($149 for 1.7 ounces)* contains some impressive ingredients for skin, including several ceramides, a peptide, and a significant amount of the antioxidant ergothioneine. How disappointing that jar packaging won't keep these ingredients stable once this emollient, fragrance-free moisturizer for normal to dry skin is opened.

☺ **$$$ Pro+ Therapy Advanced Radiance Facial Peel** *($85 for 15 packets; 0.5 ounce each)* ends up being an expensive way to experience the benefits of the AHA lactic acid. Each packet contains a sponge-tip applicator steeped in this water- and aloe-based solution. The pH of 3.2 allows the approximately 8% lactic acid to exfoliate as you swab this over skin, but it is overall no more effective than considerably less-expensive AHA lotions or serums. The only reason to consider this product is if you're intrigued by the combination of lactic acid with zeatin, though there is no research to support their combined use.

😐 **$$$ Pro+ Therapy Ultra Hydrating Repair Mask** *($89 for 1.7 ounces)* is a lightweight, but hydrating mask for normal to slightly dry skin. It does not contain significant amounts of ingredients known to repair skin, but will feel soothing. The pH, at above 5, prevents the salicylic acid from functioning as an exfoliant.

OTHER KINERASE PRODUCTS

☹ **Gentle Daily Cleanser** *($30 for 6.6 ounces)* lists sodium lauryl sulfate (SLS) as the main detergent cleansing agent, which makes this water-soluble cleanser far from gentle. It is otherwise indistinguishable from countless options at the drugstore (except for the price and inclusion of SLS). Paying this much money for something so standard and ordinary should be illegal.

☹ **Hydrating Antioxidant Mist** *($35 for 6.6 ounces)* has a lot going for it, including glycerin and hyaluronic acid as water-binding agents; antioxidants such as green tea, ergothioneine, and beta-glucan; and an alcohol-free formula. What a shame all this good stuff is degraded by the inclusion of bergamot oil. This citrus oil has photosensitizing and melanogenic (melanin-producing) properties, and should absolutely not be included in skin-care products (Source: *Journal of the American Academy of Dermatology*, September 2001, pages 458–461).

😐 **$$$ Clear Skin Moisture Light** *($75 for 1.7 ounces)* is an insanely overpriced moisturizer with ludicrous claims. Kinerase maintains that this emollient lotion (a triglyceride and thickeners comprise the bulk of the formula) banishes shine upon application while also reducing blemishes. Don't bet on it; in fact, the thickening agents in this moisturizer that's best for normal to dry skin may make blemishes worse or prompt new ones. And it absolutely won't leave a shine-free finish. This contains an ineffective amount of salicylic acid, though even if more was used, the pH is above 5, which means it cannot work to exfoliate clogged pores.

😐 **$$$ Intensive Eye Cream** *($59 for 0.7 ounce)* contains a very small amount of kinetin (which is fine, because we don't know how much is needed to exert a benefit) and is otherwise a basic, slightly emollient eye cream comparable to several options at the drugstore, including those from Nivea, Dove, and Neutrogena.

☹ **$$$ Kinerase Cream** *($117 for 2.8 ounces)* combines very standard thickening and emollient ingredients with a soybean-based antioxidant, silicone, preservatives, vitamin C, water-binding agents, and a tiny amount of kinetin (N6-furfuryladenine). There is no reason to choose this over several more elegant formulas loaded with antioxidants and cell-communicating ingredients, unless you think kinetin is the ultimate anti-aging ingredient.

☹ **$$$ Kinerase Cream with SPF 15** *($135 for 2.8 ounces)* features an in-part avobenzone sunscreen, and unless you're gung-ho for kinetin, that's the only exciting element in this simple product. Why anyone would want to spend this much money for a bit of sunscreen that will likely not last more than a few weeks (if it's applied liberally to the face and neck as sunscreen should be) is beyond me, but at least those who do will be getting sufficient broad-spectrum protection.

☹ **$$$ Kinerase Cream with SPF 30** *($135 for 2.8 ounces)* provides sufficient UVA protection via its in-part titanium dioxide sunscreen. The base formula is nothing to write home about (or even talk to a stranger about) because the impressive ingredients are present in minute amounts. This is still an option for normal to dry skin, but at this price, are you really going to apply it liberally (so essential in getting the level of sun protection stated on the label)?

☹ **$$$ Kinerase Lotion** *($117 for 2.8 ounces)* is a lighter version of the Kinerase Cream above, and is suitable for normal to slightly oily skin. The tiny amount of antioxidants doesn't justify the price, so be aware you're paying a premium to find out if kinetin is the answer for your wrinkles and other aging skin issues (thus far, research hasn't proven kinetin all that amazing).

☺ **$$$ Kinerase Lotion with SPF 30** *($135 for 2.8 ounces)* is similar to the Kinerase Cream with SPF 30 above, and the same review applies. The amount of kinetin in both products is conservative, to say the least.

☹ **Ultimate Day Moisturizer** *($125 for 2.8 ounces)* is not the ultimate choice for daytime because it does not contain sunscreen. This slightly emollient moisturizer contains some state-of-the-art ingredients to help dry skin look and feel better. However, the latest research on kinetin hasn't proven it to be an antiwrinkle luminary or even a dim light (Source: *Annals of the New York Academy of Sciences*, May 2006, pages 332–342). Despite some positives, this moisturizer is problematic for all skin types because it contains grapefruit peel oil, which can cause contact dermatitis and a phototoxic reaction due to its volatile components (Source: www.naturaldatabase.com).

☹ **Ultimate Night Moisturizer** *($125 for 2.8 ounces)* is similar to the Ultimate Day Moisturizer above, except it contains a higher concentration of irritating grapefruit peel oil. What a shame, because aside from the potential unknowns of topical kinetin, this moisturizer contains some brilliant ingredients for dry skin.

☹ **Under Eye Rescue** *($75 for 0.7 ounce)* would be more truthfully labeled "Under Eye Irritation," thanks to menthyl lactate, a derivative of menthol. Although only a tiny amount is included, any amount is problematic in a product designed for application around the eyes. This is otherwise a respectable formula, though not worth its cost, especially when compared with state-of-the-art products like those in the Clinique Repairwear line.

☺ **$$$ C6 Peptide Intensive Treatment** *($96 for 1 ounce)* expands on kinetin products by adding vitamin C and peptides to the mix, so it would seem kinetin isn't quite the answer to skin-care woes after all. When bragging about kinetin didn't get much attention from the consumer, Kinerase must have decided to jump on the peptide/vitamin bandwagon by creating this product with acetyl hexapeptide-3, the ingredient used in many products claiming to work "better than Botox." I have discussed this ingredient in the past and it appears that I'll have to keep commenting on it because cosmetics companies keep using it—even though there is no substantiated evidence concerning its effectiveness. For a detailed description of this ingredient, please refer to Chapter Seven, *Cosmetics Ingredient Dictionary*, in this book.

In the end, this product is a good moisturizing lotion that contains antioxidant vitamins C and E, and some standard, but effective, water-binding agents. Whether or not to spend almost $100 to see what kinetin and acetyl hexapeptide-3 might do for your skin is up to you, but I don't recommend it. That $100 could achieve a much more reliable benefit for your skin elsewhere.

☹ **Clear Skin Blemish Dissolver** *($39 for 0.12 ounce)* lists alcohol as the second ingredient and also contains a high amount of lemon extract, which only serves to create a very irritating product.

☹ **Clear Skin Regulating Mask** *($55 for 2.8 ounces)* proves Kinerase should stick with kinetin because they clearly know nothing about what blemish-prone skin needs. If they did, they wouldn't have launched this irritant-laden mask. Lime, basil, and spearmint oils are just a sampling of the offenders in this unhelpful product.

☹ **Clear Skin Treatment Serum** *($79 for 1 ounce)* lists alcohol as the second ingredient, which makes this too drying and irritating for all skin types. The amount of salicylic acid is too small to exfoliate skin, and kinetin has no research proving its anti-acne worth.

☺ **$$$ Instant Radiance Facial Peel** *($75 for 15 0.05-ounce pre-moistened applicators).* Let me preface my review by saying that the happy face rating is merely for the very basic but effective exfoliating formula. It is in no way a recommendation that this is preferred over versions from other companies that are far better and far less expensive. Having said that, what you are wasting your money on are premoistened, individually packaged sponge applicators on a stick. Each sponge is about the size of a quarter and is steeped in a solution of primarily aloe, fruit acids, and lactic acid. Kinerase claims that aloe and fruit acids exfoliate, too, but there's no substantiated proof of that, and the amount of aloe and fruit acid in this peel is insignificant anyway. Although the company would not reveal the percentage of lactic acid, it's likely around 5%, and the pH of 3.2 permits exfoliation to occur. This is an incredibly and unnecessarily expensive way to exfoliate skin, but it's an option. In other words, economically speaking, this is not preferred over numerous AHA lotions, gels, or creams that contain at least 5% or more glycolic or lactic acids, or BHA products that contain 2% salicylic acid. Nevertheless, it is an AHA-containing product with an effective pH. It's a bit like paying $75 for a small bottle of aspirin; the aspirin will work, but at the price, it's just a burn.

☺ **$$$ Lip Treatment** *($38 for 0.35 ounce)* ranks as one of the most expensive lip balms around. But to Kinerase's credit, it's not your typical wax-based formula (although there's nothing wrong with those). More a lip cream than a balm, and designed to be used on and around the lips, it contains an intriguing blend of thickeners usually found in moisturizers, such as non-volatile plant oils, potent antioxidants (present in amounts greater than mere window dressing), soothing plant extracts, water-binding agents, kinetin, and peptides. This product won't make lips plump because it doesn't contain ingredients that cause lips to swell, but it will make dry lips feel smooth and soft, and, as with any moisturizer placed over fine, dry lines, it will make them look better, although the effect is not permanent. Lip Treatment would get a Paula's Pick rating if not for the unknowns surrounding topical use of kinetin.

KISS MY FACE (SKIN CARE ONLY)

KISS MY FACE AT-A-GLANCE

Strengths: Inexpensive; generous sizes; some very good sunscreens, including several lip balms with broad-spectrum protection; occasional use of antioxidants without troublesome plant extracts; some fragrance-free products; sold in most health food stores and many large drugstores.

Weaknesses: Nearly all products contain one or more problematic plant extracts or volatile plant oils; the Obsessively Organic line is a dud; no products to treat acne or lighten skin discolorations; several bar soaps; no reliable AHA or BHA products; irritating toners; problematic self-tanner.

For more information about Kiss My Face, call (800) 262-5477 or visit www.kissmyface.com or www.Beautypedia.com.

KISS MY FACE OBSESSIVELY ORGANIC PRODUCTS

☹ **Obsessively Organic Clean for a Day Creamy Face Cleanser** *($13 for 4 ounces)* contains several plant extracts and ingredients that, organic or not, can cause irritation. The tangerine oil makes this a risky cleanser to use anywhere near the eyes. Without the problematic plants, this would have been a very gentle cleanser for normal to dry skin.

☹ **Obsessively Organic Shea Soy Facial Cleansing Bar** *($11 for a 5-ounce bar)* is standard bar soap, and although it's fragrance-free and contains some oil, it can still be too drying and irritating for all skin types.

☹ **Obsessively Organic Start Up Exfoliating Facial Wash** *($13 for 4 ounces)* seems to be obsessive only about causing irritation! The numerous volatile oils (mostly citrus-based) and infusions of plants with little to no benefit for skin make this a cleanser to ignore.

☹ **Obsessively Organic So Refined Jojoba and Mint Facial** *($13 for 2 ounces)* proves there's nothing refining about it, because the peppermint, eucalyptus, camphor, and bergamot oils put skin on the fast track for irritation.

☹ **Obsessively Organic Balancing Act Facial Toner** *($13 for 5.3 ounces)* contains grapefruit, orange, and bergamot oils, making this one seriously irritating toner for all skin types.

☹ **Obsessively Organic Almost Butter Ultra Creme, for Dry, Chapped Skin** *($10 for 6 ounces)* contains a high amount of numerous problematic plants, including juniper, melissa, lavender, angelica, and various citrus fruits. Dry, chapped skin would fare much better with plain Vaseline or olive oil than with this product.

☹ **Obsessively Organic Cellmate 15 Facial Creme and Sunscreen** *($19 for 1 ounce)* insults skin by leaving it vulnerable to UVA damage because it doesn't contain the UVA-protecting ingredients of titanium dioxide, zinc oxide, avobenzone, Tinosorb, or Mexoryl SX. Further, why would a so-called natural product line use synthetic sunscreen agents instead of "natural" zinc oxide or titanium dioxide? It is also a problem that this product contains the irritating plant extracts lavender oil and geranium oil.

☹ **Obsessively Organic C the Change Ester C Serum** *($19 for 1 ounce)* contains lemon and grapefruit oils along with horsetail, a plant whose astringent quality can be irritating for skin.

☹ **Obsessively Organic Eyewitness Eye Repair Creme** *($17 for 0.5 ounce)* won't reduce puffiness, but may in fact cause eye-area skin to become inflamed and puffier due to the several problematic plant extracts it contains, as well as the lavender oil.

☹ **Obsessively Organic Underage Ultra Hydrating Moisturizer** *($19 for 1 ounce)* doesn't require an ID to purchase, but may entice you with its claim of slowing the skin's aging process. It cannot do that, but it may irritate your skin with plant extracts, not to mention that rose oil won't do a thing to stimulate cell rejuvenation.

☺ **Organic Hotspots SPF 30** *($9 for 0.5 ounce)* is an emollient sunscreen stick that includes avobenzone for UVA protection. Surprisingly, it is irritant-free and an excellent option for dry to very dry skin. This is not recommended for application to blemish-prone areas.

☹ **Obsessively Organic Break Out Botanical Acne Gel** *($17 for 1 ounce)* may be botanically based, but way too many ingredients in this gel will only make acne-prone skin worse. Among the biggest offenders are camphor, peppermint, and eucalyptus oils.

☹ **Obsessively Organic Pore Shrink Deep Pore Cleansing Mask** *($13 for 2 ounces)* absolutely has no effect on making pores smaller, but it will irritate skin due to the lemongrass, clove, and peppermint oils it contains.

☹ **Organic Lip Repair** *($8 for 0.25 ounce)* contains so many wonderful ingredients for dry lips, it's a shame it cannot be recommended due to inclusion of essential oils of spearmint and bitter orange, the latter capable of causing a photosensitizing reaction (Source: www.naturaldatabase.com).

OTHER KISS MY FACE PRODUCTS

☹ **Citrus Cleanser** *($10 for 3.75 ounces)* contains lime oil (and not just a dusting, either) along with a lesser, but worrisome, amount of lemon oil. Actually, the oils and emollients in this cleanser plus the citrus would make an intriguing furniture polish!

😐 **Olive & Aloe Soap** *($2 for a 4-ounce bar)* is an olive oil–based soap where the oil has been saponified (that is, it's been turned into soap). It is an OK option for normal to slightly dry skin but does not rinse easily, and the residue can lead to dull skin. It is also more drying than most water-soluble cleansers that come in a lotion form.

😐 **Olive & Chamomile Soap** *($3 for an 8-ounce bar)* is nearly identical to the Olive & Aloe Soap above, and the same review applies.

😐 **Olive & Green Tea Soap** *($2 for a 4-ounce bar)* is nearly identical to the Olive & Aloe Soap above, and the same review applies.

😐 **Olive & Honey Bar Soap** *($3 for an 8-ounce bar)* is nearly identical to the Olive & Aloe Soap above, and the same review applies.

☹ **Olive & Lavender Soap** *($2 for a 4-ounce bar)* contains lavender, and is not recommended for any skin type.

☹ **Olive & Verbena Soap** *($2 for a 4-ounce bar)* contains verbena leaf extract, and is not recommended.

😐 **Pure Olive Oil Soap** *($2 for a 4-ounce bar)* is just saponified olive oil, water, and salt. It is similar to the Olive & Aloe Soap above, and the same review applies.

😐 **Scrub/Masque** *($7 for 4.5 ounces)* is an OK scrub that contains natural ingredients as the abrasive agents. Oatmeal, almond meal, and cornmeal will help remove dead skin cells, but just aren't as elegant or easy to rinse as many other scrub-type ingredients. This is an OK option for normal to dry skin.

☹ **Citrus Essence Astringent, for Oily and Combination Skin Types** *($5 for 6 ounces)* irritates skin with witch hazel, boric acid, and pure lemon juice. This is a problem for any skin type, and lemon has no effect on unclogging pores.

☹ **Flower Essence Toner, for Dry to Normal Skin Types** *($5 for 6 ounces)* contains flowers that can be a problem for skin, but the deal-breaker is the inclusion of clove oil, making this toner too irritating for all skin types.

😐 **All Day Creme De Jour** *($10 for 3.75 ounces)* contains a tiny amount of some potentially irritating plant extracts and the jar packaging will render the antioxidants ineffective shortly after you begin using it. Without them, this is a very boring moisturizer.

😐 **All Night Creme De Nuit** *($10 for 3.75 ounces)* is a more emollient version of the All Day Creme De Jour above, and other than being preferred for very dry skin, the same comments apply.

☹ **Alpha & Aloe Oil-Free Fragrance-Free Moisturizer with 5% Alpha Hydroxy Acids** *($10 for 16 ounces)* lists fruit extracts, trying to make them sound like natural AHAs, but none of them have proof of efficacy compared to tried-and-true glycolic or lactic acids. The orange and lemon extracts in this product can be irritating, and, despite the fragrance-free claim, this contains a litany of fragrant plant extracts.

☹ **Alpha & Aloe Oil-Free Vanilla Scent Moisturizer** *($10 for 16 ounces)* is similar to the Alpha & Aloe Oil-Free Fragrance-Free Moisturizer above, but contains lactic acid alongside the fruit extracts. The amount isn't enough to exfoliate skin, nor is the pH of this lotion low enough for that to occur. Several of the plant extracts are potentially irritating, too, making this a questionable choice compared to body moisturizer options from Dove, Olay, or Neutrogena.

☹ **Chinese Botanical Moisturizer** *($4 for 4 ounces)* begs you to discover for yourself what the ancient Chinese knew about skin care—but relying on this folklore is akin to thinking a computer from 1982 is just as advanced as what you can buy today. Ancient civilizations of any kind didn't know about sun damage, the damage caused by irritation, how blemishes were formed, or the benefit of cell-communicating ingredients and skin-identical ingredients. This moisturizer has a lot of fragrance and several Chinese herbs whose effectiveness for skin is unproven. We do know that ginger can be irritating to skin, and that's a good reason to eat Chinese food rather than use this China-themed product.

😐 **Honey & Calendula Moisturizer, for Extra Dry, Chapped Skin** *($4 for 4 ounces)* would be better without the potentially irritating plant extracts, but remains an OK option for dry skin. It contains antioxidant olive oil and a tiny amount of water-binding agents.

☹ **Lavender & Shea Butter Ultra Moisturizer** *($4 for 4 ounces)* contains lavender oil, which makes it a distinct problem for all skin types. As I've stated elsewhere in this book, topical application of lavender oil can cause skin-cell death (Source: *Cell Proliferation*, June 2004, pages 221–229).

😐 **Oil Free with NaPCa Moisturizer** *($4 for 4 ounces)* contains a tiny amount of the water-binding agent sodium PCA, and is otherwise a boring, modestly effective moisturizer for normal to dry skin.

😐 **Olive & Aloe Moisturizer, for Sensitive Skin** *($4 for 4 ounces)* contains many ingredients that are helpful for dry skin, including olive oil, almond oil, vitamin E, lecithin, and even wax. However, the number of fragrant plant extracts makes it unsuitable for sensitive skin, and additional fragrance is thrown in, too.

☹ **Olive & Aloe Moisturizer Fragrance-Free, for Extra Sensitive Skin** *($10 for 16 ounces)* is not fragrance-free because it contains several fragrant plant extracts, including orange blossom and lavender (which are not great for any skin type, especially extra sensitive).

☹ **Peaceful Patchouli Moisturizer** *($10 for 16 ounces)* contains a significant amount of patchouli oil, whose volatile components (including eugenol) can be irritating to skin.

😐 **Peaches & Creme Moisturizer 8% Alpha Hydroxy** *($9 for 4 ounces)* contains glycolic and lactic acids at about an 8% concentration, but the pH is too high for them to function effectively as exfoliants. The water-and-wax base also contains some good plant oils and a tiny amount of fragrant plant extracts, making this an OK moisturizer for dry skin.

😐 **Peaches & Creme with Alpha Hydroxy Acids** *($4 for 4 ounces)* is similar to the Peaches & Creme Moisturizer 8% Alpha Hydroxy above, except without the glycolic or lactic acids. The fruit extracts do not function in the same manner as the AHAs. Otherwise, the same comments apply.

😐 **Vitamin A & E Moisturizer** *($4 for 4 ounces)* is an OK moisturizer for normal to dry skin that contains a blend of antioxidants and potentially irritating plant extracts, so they essentially cancel each other out.

KISS MY FACE SUN PRODUCTS

☹ **Every Day SPF 15 Moisturizer** *($12 for 11 ounces)* does not contain the UVA-protecting ingredients of titanium dioxide, zinc oxide, avobenzone, Tinosorb, or Mexoryl SX, and is not recommended. The fact that this sunscreen uses PABA, a sunscreen ingredient known to cause significant irritation, indicates what an antiquated formula this is. Further, why would a so-called natural product line use synthetic sunscreen agents instead of "natural" zinc oxide or titanium dioxide?

☹ **After Sun Aloe Soother** *($6 for 4 ounces)* has lots of aloe, but it also contains wild mint oil and that isn't soothing, it's irritating.

✓☺ **Face Factor Face + Neck SPF 30** *($10 for 2 ounces)* is a truly outstanding product in the Kiss My Face line! This in-part avobenzone sunscreen for normal to dry skin contains a very good array of water-binding agents, soothing agents, antioxidants, and the cell-communicating ingredient lecithin. Well done, and it's fragrance-free, too! That is a great change of pace!

☹ **Instant Sunless Tanner** *($10 for 4 ounces)* lists walnut extract as an active ingredient, but walnut extract isn't a regulated substance so the active designation is bogus. What's true is that walnut (either black or English, the source is not revealed) contains a component known as juglone, which can cause contact dermatitis when applied topically (Source: *Contact Dermatitis*, February 2001, pages 101–102).

☺ **Sun Screen SPF 30** *($9 for 4 ounces)* keeps skin well protected from UVA and UVB rays thanks to its 10% concentration of titanium dioxide. The water-resistant base formula doesn't score high on the impressive scale, but this is a good option for normal to dry or sensitive skin, and it is fragrance-free.

☺ **Sun Screen SPF 18** *($9 for 4 ounces)* has a lot in common with the Sun Screen SPF 30 above, and is preferred for those with rosacea (or easily irritated skin) because its only active ingredient is titanium dioxide. This version is also fragrance-free and water-resistant, and the anti-irritants are certainly helpful additions.

☹ **Sun Spray SPF 30** *($10 for 4 ounces)* takes a step backward from the two sunscreens above, leaving skin vulnerable to UVA damage because it doesn't contain any UVA-protecting ingredients. It is not recommended.

☹ **Sunswat Sunscreen & Natural Insect Repellent SPF 15** *($10 for 4 ounces)* lacks sufficient UVA protection, but it contains volatile essential oils to repel insects, so you might find that topical application of this product can cause reactions worse than what you'd get from a bug bite. In fact, one of the natural insect repellants (pennyroyal) has a distressing safety profile and is not recommended for topical application (Source: www.naturaldatabase.com).

✓ ☺ **Cranberry Orange Organic Lip Balm SPF 15** *($3.50 for 0.15 ounce)* is a very good lip sunscreen that features an in-part titanium dioxide sunscreen in an emollient base. You'll get sun and dryness protection while enjoying a glossy finish. The only drawback is the fruit flavor, though some may find that a plus.

☹ **Ginger Mango Organic Lip Balm SPF 15** *($3.50 for 0.15 ounce)* does not contain the UVA-protecting ingredients of titanium dioxide, zinc oxide, avobenzone, Tinosorb, or Mexoryl SX, and is not recommended.

✓ ☺ **Sliced Peach Organic Lip Balm SPF 15** *($3.50 for 0.15 ounce)* is, save for a change in fruit flavor, nearly identical to the Cranberry Orange Organic Lip Balm SPF 15 above. By the way, despite the name, the synthetic sunscreen agents in this lip balm are not organic.

✓ ☺ **Strawberry Organic Lip Balm SPF 15** *($3.50 for 0.15 ounce)* is, save for a change in fruit flavor, nearly identical to the Cranberry Orange Organic Lip Balm SPF 15 above.

☹ **Treat Mint Organic Lip Balm SPF 15** *($3.50 for 0.15 ounce)* keeps lips protected from sun damage, but causes irritation with menthol, camphor, and peppermint oil.

✓ ☺ **Vanilla Honey Organic Lip Balm SPF 15** *($3.50 for 0.15 ounce)* is, save for a change in flavor, nearly identical to the Cranberry Orange Organic Lip Balm SPF 15 above.

☹ **SwyFlotter Natural Tick & Insect Repellent** *($8 for 4 ounces)* contains several essential oils whose smell repels insects, but topical application can be irritating to skin. Synthetic insect repellants such as DEET aren't much better for skin, which is why wearing protective clothing is the best defense.

LA MER

LA MER AT-A-GLANCE

Strengths: Sunscreen provides sufficient UVA protection; effective cleansers; one very good serum, though less-expensive options are available from other Lauder-owned lines; mostly good foundations; supremely good powders; the makeup brushes.

Weaknesses: Outlandish claims; ultra-pricey; several products contain irritants, including eucalyptus oil and lime; no AHA or BHA products; the Blanc De La Mer products don't contain ingredients capable of diminishing skin discolorations; an incomplete makeup selection; one of the foundations with sunscreen does not provide sufficient UVA protection.

For more information about La Mer, owned by Estee Lauder, call (866) 850-9400 or visit www.cremedelamer.com or www.Beautypedia.com.

Note: Supposedly, the La Mer products are worth the money because most of them contain declustered water. Declustered water is water manufactured to have smaller ions, which supposedly makes the water penetrate the skin better. There is no proof that this synthetic water does what the company claims, but even if the water could penetrate better, is that better for skin? There is definitely research indicating that too much water in the skin can make it plump, but that could also prevent cell turnover and renewal, and inhibit the skin's immune response. Either way, skin likes taking on water—it plumps to a thousand times its normal size just from taking a bath—and it doesn't need special water to help the process along, nor would that be good for skin in the long run. Moreover, if the declustered water were indeed capable of carrying La

Mer's miracle broth further into skin, that would only make matters worse because some of the components in this broth are documented irritants.

LA MER SKIN CARE

LA MER BLANC DE LA MER PRODUCTS

☺ **$$$ Blanc De La Mer the Cleansing Foam** *($60 for 4.2 ounces)* is a foaming, water-soluble cleanser for normal to oily or normal to slightly dry skin, and it does remove makeup swiftly. But ... the gemstones do not have a brightening effect on skin, although that's the claim you're paying dearly for; all you're getting is an ordinary cleanser.

☺ **$$$ Blanc De La Mer the Whitening Essence** *($210 for 1 ounce)* is a water- and silicone-based serum that contains some yeast extract and a tiny amount of vitamin C, neither of which is "the ultimate in deep whitening." They're not even good at superficial whitening! Although this serum contains some impressive antioxidants and a few notable skin-identical ingredients, it doesn't best products from Estee Lauder's Perfectionist or Clinique's Repairwear lines. At the drugstore, Olay's Definity and Regenerist products stand a much better chance of reducing skin discolorations, because they contain niacinamide. The mica and titanium dioxide in this serum provide a soft glow to skin, but that is strictly a cosmetic effect.

☺ **$$$ Blanc De La Mer the Whitening Lotion** *($75 for 6.7 ounces)* is what you're supposed to use prior to the other Blanc De La Mer products, because it is supposed to prepare skin to "readily receive the ultimate benefits" of your regimen. By any name, this is just a standard toner that contains some good water-binding agents for all skin types, along with a few antioxidants (and packaging that does keep them stable during use). The Whitening Lotion will make skin feel soft and smooth, but any whitening is coincidental. This does contain a small amount of volatile fragrance components that may cause slight irritation.

OTHER LA MER PRODUCTS

😐 **$$$ The Cleansing Fluid** *($65 for 6.7 ounces)* removes makeup quickly due to its emollient ingredients. However, they're standard to most cleansing lotions and creams for dry skin, while the "extras" in this version (such as tourmaline and pearl powder) have no established benefit for skin. I suppose the algae extracts provide additional hydration, but that still doesn't justify the price.

☺ **$$$ The Cleansing Gel** *($65 for 6.7 ounces)* is an exceptionally standard, detergent-based, water-soluble cleanser that would be an option for normal to oily skin. But at this price, can anyone's skin really feel better?

☺ **$$$ The Cleansing Lotion** *($65 for 6.7 ounces)*. Supposedly, this milky emulsion derives its remarkable cleansing powers from magnetized tourmaline and declustered water, but there is no proof such water makes a cleanser any better. This is a standard, wipe-off cleanser for dry skin that is not all that different from Neutrogena's Extra Gentle Cleanser ($7.19 for 6.7 ounces).

☹ **The Refining Facial** *($75 for 3.4 ounces)* is a relatively standard clay mask. The "sea stuff" is in here, as are tourmaline and diamond powder. If you feel that scrubbing with microscopic amounts of gemstones (and then rinsing them down the drain) is the way to go, that's your decision—but doing so with this product will irritate your skin because of the mint and citrus ingredients. Estee Lauder and Clinique sell less expensive and less inoffensive versions of this product.

☹ **The Mist** *($50 for 4.2 ounces)* contains a euclyptus derivative called eucalyptol, which is a skin irritant. It would have been an OK toner without that irritant, but the price is a joke given the basic ingredients and the small amount of antioxidants.

☹ **The Radiant Infusion** *($90 for 4.2 ounces)* comes with fascinating claims describing its "radical, fluid architecture" that delivers "extraordinary activity on demand," all to set in motion a "continuous wave of radiance-enhancing benefits." Quite honestly, you'd get more radiance from a brisk jog around the block than from applying this toner-like product. Considering the price, it's disheartening (and not the least bit helpful for skin) that the second ingredient is alcohol. Several of the plant extracts have benefit as water-binding agents and/or antioxidants, but the lime extract can be irritating, and nothing in this product will noticeably change skin discolorations. This should be renamed The Radiant Impediment.

😐 **$$$ The Tonic** *($60 for 6.7 ounces)* is an alcohol-free toner for normal to dry skin that's worth considering only if you believe La Mer's claims about declustered water (discussed in the introduction above). It's otherwise standard fare that contains a minimal amount of ingredients that are beneficial for skin.

☹ **Creme De La Mer** *($110 for 1 ounce; $195 for 2 ounces; $1,200 for 16.5 ounces)* is the original product created by Max Huber, as described above in the introduction to La Mer. As enticing as this dramatic story sounds, the reality is that this very basic cream doesn't contain anything particularly extraordinary or unique, unless you want to believe that seaweed extract (sort of like seaweed tea) can in some way heal burns and scars. Even if it could, burns and scars don't have much to do with wrinkling, and this product is now being sold as a wrinkle cream. According to Susan Brawley, professor of plant biology at the University of Maine, "Seaweed extract isn't a rare, exotic, or expensive ingredient. Seaweed extract is readily available and [is] used in everything from cosmetics to food products and medical applications." Creme de la Mer contains mostly seaweed extract, mineral oil, Vaseline, glycerin, waxlike thickening agents, lime extract, plant oils, plant seeds, minerals, vitamins, more thickeners, and preservatives. This rather standard moisturizer also contains some good antioxidants, but the jar packaging won't keep them stable during use. This also contains a skin-stressing amount of eucalyptus oil, as well as Kathon CG, a preservative that is recommended for use only in rinse-off products. Consumers who have a "steadfast devotion" to this product are not only wasting their money but also hurting their skin.

☹ **The Moisturizing Gel Cream** *($195 for 2 ounces)* is simply a lighter version of the original Creme De La Mer above, and promotes a silkier finish due to the silicone it contains. Despite a light texture, this contains a lot of lime extract and enough eucalyptus to be more irritating than miraculously healing, as claimed.

☹ **The Concentrate** *($325 for 1.7 ounces)* is, first and foremost, not worth even a fraction of its price. All you're getting is a nonaqueous product containing mostly silicones, seaweed extract, glycerin, film-forming agents, and several plant extracts, some of which (lime, lavender, and basil extracts, and also eucalyptus oil) are irritating to skin. The formula is rounded out by trace amounts of minerals and some additional plant extracts, but none of these, and definitely not in the amounts used here, are particularly helpful for skin, be it wrinkled or not. Seaweed (also known as algae) extract has antioxidant and anti-inflammatory properties, but it is not the magical elixir of youth La Mer makes it out to be, nor is it expensive to include in skin-care products. Bulk liquid seaweed extract costs an average of $1.50 per liter, and the amount used in this product barely amounts to a teaspoon, despite being the second ingredient listed. Like all silicone-based serums, this product will leave skin feeling incredibly smooth and silky. But knowing you can achieve this same feeling with other products that cost $250 less than La Mer's version (and that still have beneficial antioxidants) is a sobering fact, to say the least! The eucalyptus oil makes this too irritating for all skin types, and overall this serum pales in comparison to those from other Lauder-owned lines, all of which cost considerably less.

☹ **The Eye Balm** *($120 for 0.5 ounce)* is a good moisturizer for normal to dry skin, but the supposed benefits of fish cartilage and malachite? Well, it's up to you to decide, because there is no research showing they're worth this kind of investment for skin. What should give you something to think about is the inclusion of eucalyptus oil (a considerable amount) and mint, which are both unnecessary and very irritating to delicate eye-area skin.

☹ **The Eye Concentrate** *($160 for 0.5 ounce)* contains some incredibly helpful, state-of-the-art ingredients for creating and maintaining healthy skin. What a shame so many of them are subject to reduced potency because of jar packaging! Moreover, how depressing that La Mer included a troubling amount of eucalyptus oil, which only serves to irritate skin. Without that and in better packaging, this really would have been an "ultraluxe eye treatment."

The Lifting Duo *($285 for the two products when purchased together)* must be filling in a gap that the other La Mer products leave, but my goodness this routine is expensive! The Duo in question consists of ✓☺ **$$$ The Lifting Face Serum** ($210 for 1 ounce if purchased separately) and ☹ **The Lifting Intensifier** ($135 for 0.3 ounce if purchased separately). Given the name of the Intensifier ("Lifting") and the claims made for the Face Serum, you have to wonder why this pair wasn't combined into one super-potent product. As it turns out, neither of these is the face-lift-in-a-bottle they're made out to be. The showcased ingredient is a rare species of blue algae. La Mer claims their special biofermentation process unleashes blue algae's lifting energy to boost its performance "far beyond anything previously imagined." Further claims of this ingredient being able to uphold the skin from within turn standard fantasy cosmetic claims into blatant quackery, though it's all carefully framed with words such as "appears" and "looks" rather than directly stating that skin is physically lifted. The Lifting Face Serum is a souped-up version of Lauder's Advanced Night Repair Protective Recovery Complex ($46.50 for 1 ounce), with the extras being more antioxidants and algae and a greater complement of skin-identical ingredients. Blue algae are present, but there is no substantiated research anywhere stating that they can lift sagging skin or increase collagen synthesis so skin becomes less wrinkled. However, in terms of providing skin with some state-of-the-art ingredients, this excels, assuming you don't mind the price. Once again, several other Lauder-owned companies offer similar versions of this product at more realistic prices.

The Lifting Intensifier is mostly water and alcohol with tiny amounts of plant extracts and a slip agent. The algae and gemstones are barely present, and do not have any miraculous benefits for aging skin. This product is not recommended.

☹ **The Moisturizing Lotion** *($165 for 1.7 ounces)* would have been a good moisturizer for normal to dry skin, but for the inclusion of lime and eucalyptus extracts, which are potentially irritating and sensitizing for all skin types. And the price is just outrageous!

☹ **The Oil Absorbing Lotion** *($165 for 1.7 ounces)* is the lotion version of the original Creme de la Mer, and it does have a much lighter texture. However, the emollients and the lack of absorbents in this product won't keep oily skin in check. That's forgivable, but the inclusion of a significant amount of eucalyptus oil and lime is not.

☺ **$$$ The SPF 18 Fluid** *($65 for 1.7 ounces)* is a good, in-part avobenzone-based sunscreen in a rather standard emollient base that would be an option for normal to dry skin. Remember, you have to use sunscreen liberally to gain the SPF benefit. How liberally are you going to apply this product given the price? The volatile fragrance components in this sunscreen keep it from earning a higher rating. It is available in various tints, and all of them are acceptable.

unrated **The Essence** *($2,100 for 3 0.5-ounce vials; 1.5 ounces total)*. I wonder sometimes if the cosmetics industry simply has a sardonic sense of humor or whether it's possible they merely don't like women very much. How else can you explain La Mer launching a product that costs $2,100 and whose primary ingredient is seaweed? At least according to the ingredient list it has a lot of seaweed—well, as much as can be present in a 1.5-ounce product—along with a huge list of other ingredients. The primary ingredient in this nonaqueous serum is seaweed extract, but what type of seaweed was used is unknown so there is no way to evaluate its benefit for skin. (There are endless kinds of seaweed extracts, some potentially quite dangerous.) Actually, I wonder how the FDA lets Lauder get around this generalized ingredient identification because it is definitely not according to the regulation.

This product also contains silicones, emollients, more seaweed (this time listed by type), ingredients that mimic the structure of skin, an assortment of antioxidants, a tiny amount of niacin (the form of vitamin B that can cause flushing, which is actually a problem for skin), and acetyl hexapeptide-3. The peptide is the ingredient that's supposed to work like Botox, but of course, it can't—even Botox can't work like Botox when applied topically to skin. And just in case you weren't sure the product was doing anything for your skin, they included a few irritating, skin-tingling plant extracts, including eucalyptus, lime, and citronella, to create the impression that it is doing something on your face. For this kind of money it should really be doing something other than irritating skin. Other than that, it's not possible to ascertain any other information because Lauder has no published studies and offers no clinical evidence (other than press releases, which fashion magazines use as if they were factual information) to support the value of the product or the efficacy of the claims.

Along with seaweed, The Essence also contains an assortment of yeast extracts: saccharomyces lysate, micrococcus lysate, artemisia extract, and bifida ferment lysate. But whether or not seaweed or yeast in any form can affect wrinkles is still not known. Indeed, that ability is something ingredient manufacturers do claim, but there are no supporting published or substantiated double-blind studies showing this to be true. Research from ingredient manufacturers is interesting, but obviously self-serving; somehow all their ingredients are always miracles. Trying to find independent research about these substances is difficult, and what does exist involves in vitro or animal studies (Sources: *Journal of Burn Care and Rehabilitation*, March–April 1999, pages 155–162; and *Wound Repair and Regeneration*, January 2002, page 38). I could carry on about how these various ingredients are theoretically supposed to affect skin without any research to even rationalize them for skin care, but at some moments in my career I just have to throw my hands up in the air and say, "I give up, the cosmetics industry is just crazy and I have no words left to explain why." I think I'll go get a Starbucks latte.... I don't understand $5 for a cup of coffee either, but at least I know exactly what I'm getting!

☹ **The Radiant Facial** *($320 for the kit)* should leave me speechless, but two words come to mind right away: Don't bother. This kit includes **Radiant Primer** and **Radiant Mask**, and both have the same ingredients because the Mask is premoistened with the Primer (which basically negates the need to apply the Primer first). The mask is just two pieces of cloth intended to fit over the upper and lower halves of the face. The whole system is as misguided as it gets, so the duplication is just silly. For over $300, you're getting mostly water (it's La Mer's "declustered" water, but simply making water less clustered doesn't translate into outstanding skin care), alcohol, and yeast. These ingredients cannot bring your skin to its utmost clarity, luminosity, and brightness in eight minutes. There are several skin-identical ingredients, plant extracts (most with antioxidant ability), and gemstones in the formula, all claiming to work in biofermented synergy to perform miracles for your skin. None of them will do much for your skin in the presence of this much alcohol, and none of them is capable of lightening skin discolorations and preventing their return. There's no reason at all to consider this occasional-use product over an alcohol-free, antioxidant-laden serum or moisturizer for daily use.

☹ **The Lip Balm** *($45 for 0.32 ounce)* ranks as one of the most expensive lip balms sold, and the first ingredient is Vaseline. Amazing! The seaweed and plant seeds may make this seem like more than it is, but the amount of eucalyptus oil is not lip-friendly, and it also contains the menthol derivative menthyl PCA.

LA MER MAKEUP

FOUNDATION: ☺ **$$$ The Fluid Foundation SPF 15** *($75)* brings consumers "the legendary La Mer cream now in a light foundation," but remember that the original La Mer moisturizer is not worthy of legendary status, and actually this foundation has more skin-beneficial ingredients, albeit in mostly small amounts. Yes, it includes the same seaweed broth as the original Creme De La Mer, but seaweed isn't the be-all and end-all for skin (it does have antioxidant and soothing properties—but lots of other ingredients do too). This water-in-silicone foundation is indeed fluid. It blends easily and leaves skin feeling silky-smooth while providing light to medium coverage and a satin-matte finish. Ten shades are available, and almost all are admirable. The only problem shade is Beige, which is slightly peach for its intended skin tone. The darkest shade (Caramel) is not that dark, but is suitable for tan skin. This product is recommended for normal to slightly dry or slightly oily skin, and I am pleased to report that the sunscreen includes titanium dioxide for sufficient UVA protection. By the way, this foundation is remarkably similar to Estee Lauder's Equalizer Makeup SPF 10 ($32.50). It would be better if Lauder's foundation had a higher SPF rating, but with the money you'll save you can splurge on a lightweight facial moisturizer rated SPF 15 or higher to wear underneath.

☺ **$$$ The Treatment Creme Foundation SPF 15** *($85)* isn't as creamy as the name suggests, but the treatment portion is fairly accurate, at least in terms of all the bells and whistles in this slightly thick but silky foundation. Like The Fluid Foundation, this is also a water-in-silicone emulsion, although a few emollients that make it better suited for normal to dry (but not very dry) skin have been added here. It offers medium coverage (and is difficult to sheer out, so be sure you are comfortable with this), and sets to a satin-matte finish that feels slightly moist but doesn't look dewy. The in-part titanium dioxide sunscreen provides broad-spectrum protection, but the nine shades have a few problematic colors. Avoid Golden (too orange), Beige (rosy), and Tan (too peach). Creme and Caramel are slightly peach, but still worth considering. Natural, Buff, Bronze, and Neutral are the best of the bunch. Although this is an elegant foundation with a higher-than-usual amount of antioxidants and other beneficial ingredients, its finish doesn't make wrinkles look less obvious as claimed.

☹ **The SPF 18 Fluid Tint** *($65)* doesn't have the same array of skin-beneficial ingredients as the two La Mer foundations reviewed above, nor does its sunscreen offer sufficient UVA protection. For the money, that's a real burn, and although there are some textural benefits to extol, they're not enough to make this worth considering over the tinted moisturizers with sunscreen available from Bobbi Brown, Aveda, Neutrogena, or my Paula's Choice line.

POWDER: ✓☺ $$$ The Powder *($65)* is one of the most expensive loose powders reviewed in this book, yet despite the luxurious feel of this talc-based powder, the money doesn't translate into a noticeable difference worth the price. Nonetheless, it does look incredibly skinlike and creates a beautifully natural yet polished finish from each of its four sheer shades. You can find similar loose powders from other Lauder-owned lines (including M.A.C.), but if you're attracted to La Mer's miracles-from-the-sea claims, this one is bound to impress you, especially if you have normal to dry skin.

BRUSHES: ☺ $$$ The Foundation Brush *($40)* is composed of synthetic fibers and differs little from almost every other foundation brush available. In fact, the only differences are in the price and La Mer's inflated pedigree. You won't be disappointed with it if you prefer applying foundation with a brush; you just don't need to spend this much to get the same result. **☺ $$$ The Powder Brush** *($70)* is a very good, retractable powder brush that the company maintains can be used to apply loose or pressed powder. That's hardly unique, and the fact that the bristles of this brush can be "extended" based on your powder preference doesn't make a noticeable difference during application. As a portable powder brush, this is a pricey but good option.

LA PRAIRIE

LA PRAIRIE AT-A-GLANCE

Strengths: All of the facial sunscreens include avobenzone for UVA protection; some very good serums; helpful products to smooth lines around the mouth and on lips; mostly good masks; one well-formulated AHA product; most of the makeup categories present good, though needlessly expensive, options that include foundations with reliable sun protection.

Weaknesses: Very expensive; overreliance on jar packaging; many products contain a potentially irritating amount of astringent horsetail extract; the sun products for the body are a mixed bag; no effective skin-lightening options; poor options for anyone dealing with blemishes (though La Prairie is concerned primarily with selling wrinkle creams anyway); the eyeshadow options are average, as are the pencils.

For more information about La Prairie, owned by Beiersdorf, call (800) 821-5718 or visit www.laprairie.com or www.Beautypedia.com.

LA PRAIRIE SKIN CARE

LA PRAIRIE THE CAVIAR COLLECTION

😐 $$$ Essence of Skin Caviar Eye Complex *($110 for 0.5 ounce)* is a lightweight moisturizer that doesn't instantly firm skin, but will hydrate to make superficial lines less apparent. The amount of horsetail extract may cause irritation in the eye area due to its astringent properties, while the caviar extract shows up as the last ingredient on the list.

😐 $$$ Extrait of Skin Caviar Firming Complex *($115 for 1 ounce)* would rate much higher and be worth the splurge if it did not contain problematic plant extracts (including horsetail and sage) along with volatile fragrance components. The amount of sunscreen agent included is odd, given that this product does not advertise an SPF rating. Taking these points into account, this rates as an average option for normal to slightly dry skin.

☹ **Skin Caviar** *($160 for 1.7 ounces)* is a silicone-based serum whose negatives are strong enough to make it not worth considering. In addition to some irritating plant extracts, this also contains the germicidal agent O-phenylphenol, which research has shown can cause acute skin inflammation and, potentially, ulceration (Sources: *National Toxicology Program Technical Support Series,* March 1986, pages 1–141; and *Critical Reviews in Toxicology*, 2002, pages 551–6250).

☹ **Skin Caviar Luxe Cream** *($350 for 1.7 ounces)* may have a luxe texture, but the ingredients used to create it are commonplace and do not justify the ridiculous price. This jar-packaged moisturizer contains many antioxidants that won't remain stable once you open it, and the pH of this cream is too high for the AHA it contains to exfoliate skin. Topping things off is the inclusion of the irritants sage, arnica, and horsetail, coupled with several volatile fragrance components. Buyer beware!

😐 **$$$ Skin Caviar Luxe Eye Lift Cream** *($275 for 0.68 ounce)* has an incredibly insulting price for what amounts to mostly water, thickeners, Vaseline, and vegetable oil. Many intriguing ingredients are included in this eye cream, but all of them are listed after the pH-adjusting agent, and many won't remain stable once this jar-packaged product is opened. This isn't luxe; It's a bona fide bad beauty investment, at least if you were hoping that the cost would translate to a superior product to vanquish every eye-area woe.

☹ **Skin Caviar Firming Mask** *($135 for the set)* might make skin appear firmer temporarily, but that effect results from the extreme irritation this two-step mask causes. The **Penetrating Serum** contains several fragrant oils, including rosemary, rosewood, and sweet marjoram. The **Skin Caviar Firming Complex** lists alcohol as the second ingredient, furthering the irritation from the Penetrating Serum.

😐 **$$$ Skin Caviar Intensive Ampoule Treatment** *($525 for 6 treatments)* consists of six ampoules each of **Solvent** and **Lyophilized Substance**, which you mix together to—what else—"guard against accelerated skin aging." Neither product has an SPF rating or contains a UVA-protecting sunscreen, and since that's the only reliable way to prevent accelerated aging with a skin-care product, right away you can tell things are bogus. The Solvent is a lightweight moisturizer that contains some slip agents, emollients, film-forming agent, plant extracts (some are irritating, while most of the others have no established benefit for skin), ceramide, and vitamin E. This also contains volatile fragrance components that may cause irritation. The Lyophilized Substance is a sugar-based powder that contains a salt form of vitamin C along with water, thickener, and the antioxidant superoxide dismutase. There's no reason those ingredients could not have been added to the Solvent, but I suppose the two-step process makes women think the set is somehow more special or customized. In the end, this isn't that exciting, and wouldn't be at even one-fourth the cost.

OTHER LA PRAIRIE PRODUCTS

😐 **$$$ Cellular Comforting Cleansing Emulsion** *($70 for 5.2 ounces)* is a very standard, very overpriced cleansing lotion for normal to dry skin. It does remove makeup but you need to use a washcloth to eliminate any residue. Some of the plant extracts can be a problem for skin if not completely removed.

☹ **Cellular Cleansing Water Face/Eyes** *($70 for 5.2 ounces)* contains gentle cleansing agents to remove makeup (but not waterproof formulas) and some interesting water-binding agents. However, almost all of the plant extracts can be irritating to skin, especially around the eyes, making this a poor choice at any price.

☺ **$$$ Foam Cleanser** *($70 for 4 ounces)* is a standard, but good, water-soluble cleanser that produces copious, soap-like foam. It's an option for normal to slightly dry or slightly oily skin, if the price doesn't make you faint. For the record, several drugstore lines offer similar cleansers for less than $10.

😐 **$$$ Purifying Cream Cleanser** *($70 for 6.8 ounces)* is a cold cream–style cleanser the company states can be rinsed or tissued off, but this requires effort to completely remove it. It's an OK option for very dry skin but is absurdly overpriced.

😐 **$$$ Suisse De-Sensitizing Cleansing Emulsion** *($70 for 5 ounces)* is very similar to the Cellular Comforting Cleansing Emulsion above, save for fewer plant extracts, none of which are a particular problem for skin, sensitive or not. Otherwise, the same comments apply.

☹ **Cellular Eye Make-Up Remover** *($55 for 4.2 ounces)* is a water- and silicone-based eye-makeup remover that is less impressive than similar options from Almay or Neutrogena. This version presents problems for eye-area skin because it contains astringent plant extracts and fragrance.

☹ **Cellular Microdermabrasion Cream** *($225 for 4.2 ounces)* is a thick-textured yet surprisingly abrasive scrub that is too rough for most skin types, and irritating for all skin types because of the grapefruit peel oil it contains. Moreover, at this price, you might as well go for professional microdermabrasion treatments, although even those aren't turning out to be all that great.

😐 **$$$ Essential Exfoliator** *($70 for 7 ounces)* is an OK scrub for normal to dry skin, and features apricot seed powder as the abrasive agent. Plant seeds or shells are not preferred to synthetic polyethylene beads because the former typically do not have perfectly smooth surfaces, and therefore can cause tears in the skin and trigger inflammation.

☹ **Age Management Balancer** *($70 for 8.4 ounces)* contains lactic acid and has a pH of 3.6, but the amount of AHA present is too low to exfoliate skin. This toner has some very good ingredients for all skin types, but the amount of horsetail can be irritating, and the lavender extract isn't good news either.

☹ **Cellular Purifying Dual-Phase Toner** *($70 for 8.4 ounces)* lists alcohol as the second ingredient—so, dual-phase or not, this is too irritating for all skin types and won't "nourish" skin as claimed.

☹ **Cellular Refining Lotion** *($70 for 8.4 ounces)* contains irritating horsetail and ivy extracts as well as several volatile fragrance components that won't firm or hydrate skin in the least.

☹ **Cellular Softening and Balancing Lotion** *($125 for 8.4 ounces)* should be brimming with ingredients that put skin in its optimum state, but La Prairie couldn't resist including the irritants horsetail, arnica, witch hazel, and eugenol, among others.

😐 **$$$ Suisse De-Sensitizing Soothing Mist** *($70 for 4.2 ounces)* could have been a very good toner for dry skin, but the balm mint, horsetail, and rose extracts are potential skin irritants, while the other plant extracts and oils are anti-irritants. I suspect that there isn't enough of any of these to make a difference, but at this price and given the claims, it's disappointing.

☹ **Cellular Retexturizing Booster** *($160 for 1 ounce)* is not the way to enjoy the benefits of glycolic and salicylic acid in one product. Although the pH is within range for exfoliation to occur, the amount of alcohol is needlessly irritating and the lavender oil damages otherwise healthy skin cells. It's insulting to the consumer that La Prairie refers to this Booster as non-irritating.

☹ **$$$ Advanced Marine Biology Cream** *($175 for 1.4 ounces)* has a name that sounds more like a college course than a moisturizer! The big to-do with this product is about the marine proteins, which are meant to protect skin from age-accelerating free radicals. But the amount of antioxidants in this product isn't as impressive as it should be for the price, and it's utterly discouraging when you consider that the jar packaging won't keep them stable once this product is in use. Far from being advanced, this moisturizer for normal to slightly dry skin stops at grade school; only its claims are at the Ph.D. level.

☹ **$$$ Anti-Aging Complex** *($195 for 1.7 ounces)* has over a dozen state-of-the-art ingredients for skin, but what precedes them isn't exciting, and the amount of irritating horsetail is larger than the amount of beneficial ingredients. Then, the jar packaging renders the retinol ineffective shortly after you open the product. Considering the price, this is very disappointing!

☹ **$$$ Anti-Aging Emulsion SPF 30** *($175 for 1.7 ounces)* contains avobenzone for reliable UVA protection and has a lotion base that those with normal to slightly oily skin will appreciate. My concern, however, is twofold. One, how liberally are you going to apply this each day considering the cost? Two, the horsetail in this product is in a larger amount than the antioxidants and cell-communicating ingredients. Of lesser concern are the volatile fragrance components, but the tiny amount in here is unlikely to cause trouble. Still, this is a tricky product to enthusiastically recommend.

☹ **Anti-Aging Eye Cream SPF 15** *($135 for 0.5 ounce)* is an emollient eye cream with an in-part avobenzone sunscreen that has a lot of potential; however, most of the really helpful ingredients are undermined by jar packaging. The horsetail and balm mint can cause irritation (along with the many volatile fragrance components in this product), making it one to skip.

☺ **$$$ Cellular Anti-Spot Brightening Serum** *($160 for 1 ounce)* doesn't contain a high enough concentration of ingredients that research has shown can inhibit melanin production, but it is an excellent serum for normal to dry skin. It contains stabilized vitamin C along with soothing agents, antioxidants, some good water-binding agents, and a couple of cell-communicating ingredients. The inclusion of horsetail extract keeps this from earning a higher rating, but it's nice that this is fragrance-free.

☺ **$$$ Cellular Anti-Wrinkle Firming Serum** *($160 for 1 ounce)* is a very good, antioxidant-rich moisturizer for normal to slightly dry skin. The truly helpful ingredients outnumber the problem-children additions, making this a contender if you prefer to spend in the upper echelon for your skin-care products.

☹ **$$$ Cellular Day Cream** *($120 for 1 ounce)* is a lot of money for a product that is mostly thickeners, vegetable oil, and Vaseline, but La Prairie was undoubtedly hoping you wouldn't notice. Plus, without a sunscreen it is a definite no-no for daytime. This would be good for dry skin, but doesn't compare with some of the other more interesting products in this line or from many other lines, because it lacks the array of antioxidants, skin-identical ingredients, and anti-irritants the others contain.

☹ **$$$ Cellular De-Sensitizing Serum** *($160 for 1 ounce)* is a poor choice for sensitive skin because of the irritating plant extracts horsetail and balm mint. These irritants are outnumbered by the anti-irritants and several antioxidants, but for this kind of money there shouldn't be any problems; and, at any price, your skin deserves the best ingredients possible.

☹ **$$$ Cellular Eye Contour Cream** *($110 for 0.5 ounce)* cannot help prevent more lines from forming, as claimed, because it does not contain sunscreen. This is a very standard, emollient moisturizer for dry skin anywhere on the face, although the amount of horsetail extract may prove problematic if used in the eye area. Antioxidants are in short supply, but the number of skin-identical ingredients is good.

☺ **$$$ Cellular Eye Moisturizer SPF 15, "The Smart Eye Cream"** *($135 for 0.5 ounce)* has an in-part avobenzone sunscreen, but it isn't inherently smarter than other eye creams, including many that cost much less. The amount of balm mint is likely too small to cause irritation, but why put it in a product meant to be used around the eyes? More disappointing is that jar packaging ensures that the many antioxidants in this product will be less potent shortly after you open it.

☺ **$$$ Cellular Hydrating Serum** *($160 for 1 ounce)* would rate a Paula's Pick if it did not include more horsetail extract than it does several other ingredients that are of value for all skin types. The amount of horsetail is unlikely to be problematic, but without it, this serum would be a slam-dunk recommendation because it is loaded with antioxidants, cell-communicating ingredients, and ingredients that mimic the structure and function of healthy skin. The texture makes this best for normal to slightly dry or slightly oily skin.

☺ **$$$ Cellular Intensive Anti-Wrinkle Age-Spot Cream** *($175 for 1 ounce)* purports to offer continuous management of "age" spots while you sleep, but that's just making a claim without really saying anything at all. I'd rather get rid of my age spots—which are really sun damage spots—than manage them (do age spots get their own 401(k) portfolio?) Regardless, this product cannot do anything for these dark spots because the potentially effective amount of vitamin C will be compromised once this jar-packaged cream is opened. The citrus and other fruit extracts in this product will not exfoliate or lighten skin, and the volatile fragrance components (present in tiny amounts) are potential troublemakers. Somehow, none of these features is exciting for a product that costs this much money.

☹ **Cellular Moisturizer SPF 15, "The Smart Cream"** *($150 for 1 ounce)* contains a frustrating mix of spectacular and suspect ingredients, complete with an in-part avobenzone sunscreen. The sunscreen is smart, but the decision to package such an antioxidant-rich formula in a jar was not, nor was the inclusion of balm mint and horsetail. Those irritants are present at more than a dusting, and when combined with the many volatile fragrance components ... well, it would be smarter to avoid it.

☺ **$$$ Cellular Night Cream** *($120 for 1 ounce)* isn't nearly as impressive as many of La Prairie's other moisturizers, so if you're going to spend this much money, at least choose one that offers skin more than a standard assortment of emollients, thickeners, and vegetable oil. Plain Vaseline or olive oil on very dry skin would be a much less expensive way to get the main benefit this moisturizer provides.

☺ **$$$ Cellular Night Repair Cream** *($185 for 1.7 ounces)* improves on the lackluster formula of the Cellular Night Cream above, but jar packaging will render most of the exciting ingredients ineffective shortly after you begin using the product. Still, the peptides, oil, and silicones will make dry skin look and feel better (though for this much money every last bit of potency should be preserved).

☹ **Cellular Normalizing Serum** *($160 for 1 ounce)* lists alcohol as the fourth ingredient, and that downgrades the overall effectiveness of this serum. Adding to that is the inclusion of a significant amount of neem leaf extract, which has questionable benefit for skin (it certainly doesn't normalize it) and can contain toxic components.

☹ **$$$ Cellular Nurturing Complex** *($225)* is sold as a set, and features a tiny amount of **Balm** and a standard size of **Serum**. The Balm is packaged in a flip-top component that sits atop the bottle that houses the Serum. Formula-wise, the Balm is a very good blend of waxes, nonvolatile plant oils, fatty acids, and a tiny amount of antioxidants. The Serum is silicone-based and contains some good water-binding agents, but the amount of horsetail extract may cause irritation. The anti-irritants in the Serum may seem impressive, but they're barely present, and as such have little to no impact on reducing surface redness. Although this duo has potential for dry to very dry skin, it really isn't worth the expense.

☹ **$$$ Cellular Nurturing Cream** *($175 for 1.7 ounces)* is a standard, slightly emollient moisturizer that contains a minimum amount of soothing agents coupled with some irritating plant extracts, so they cancel each other out. Don't expect this jar-packaged moisturizer to make quick work of facial redness, though it will relieve dryness-related discomfort.

☺ **$$$ Cellular Purifying Hydrating Fluid SPF 15** *($115 for 1.7 ounces)* is another very good, in-part avobenzone daytime moisturizer that would rate a Paula's Pick if it did not contain a potentially irritating amount of cypress and neem extracts. Neither extract has documented evidence of being able to balance and purify skin. This is otherwise recommended for normal to oily skin. It contains many water-binding agents and some unique antioxidants.

☺ **$$$ Cellular Purifying Hydro Repair** *($135 for 1 ounce)* deserves a happy face rating for being a very good AHA product that contains approximately a 10% concentration of glycolic and lactic acids at a pH of 3.5. The base formula is suitable for normal to dry skin, and features some very good water-binding agents. The antioxidants are compromised by the jar packaging, while the fragrance components pose a slight risk of causing irritation, especially given the acidic pH of this product. Without question there are equally good or better AHA products that cost far less than this one.

☹ **$$$ Cellular Radiance Concentrate Pure Gold** *($525 for 1 ounce)* sounds like it's the quick-fix solution for those who want to look younger in a hurry. This is said to plump lines and wrinkles within an hour, speed exfoliation, and immediately reduce age spots, but nothing in this formula will make these claims a reality. The formula contains mostly water, silicones, alcohol, solvents, slip agents, thickener, water-binding agents, plant extracts, vitamin C, and several more plant extracts. Yes, it does indeed contain gold (it's the third to last ingredient listed), but that has no established benefit for skin, especially when it comes to turning back the hands of time. (What a waste of good metal!) Most of the plant ingredients in this serum show up in all of the La Prairie moisturizers above, so I suppose those can make you look younger in an instant, too. Considering that this formula cannot make good on its claims (not even a little), the price is nothing less than absurd.

☹ **$$$ Cellular Radiance Cream** *($525 for 1.7 ounces)* is a water- and Vaseline-based moisturizer that takes an everything-but-the-kitchen-sink approach to moisturizers by including tiny amounts of dozens of plants along with gemstones and natural ingredients believed to be helpful for women experiencing skin changes due to menopause (though there is little research to support that line of thinking, at least in terms of using tiny amounts of such ingredients topically rather than orally). The price is ridiculous for what amounts to an emollient moisturizer for dry to very dry skin, and jar packaging renders the many antioxidants unstable shortly after you begin using it. The mineral pigments in this moisturizer are what give skin a luminous finish, which is strictly cosmetic, not skin care.

☹ **$$$ Cellular Radiance Eye Cream** *($265 for 0.5 ounce)* contains some good emollients for dry skin, but none that you won't find in hundreds of other moisturizers throughout the price spectrum. There is more mica (a mineral pigment that adds shine to skin) in this eye cream than there are state-of-the-art ingredients, and most of those will be compromised by jar packaging, which doesn't leave you with much for your money.

☹ **Cellular Revitalizing Eye Gel** *($135 for 0.5 ounce)* contains a large amount of horsetail extract as well as lesser amounts of chemical components of the plant. Horsetail has research on its ability to relax veins when taken orally, but that does not translate to mean it can reduce puffy eyes and dark circles when applied topically. The volatile components in horsetail (including trace amounts of nicotine) can be irritating to skin. It has potential antioxidant ability, but isn't preferred to other antioxidants that provide a benefit without the potential risk (Source: www.naturaldatabase.com). This product also contains a preservative that is not recommended for use in leave-on products.

☹ **$$$ Cellular Skin Conditioner** *($80 for 4.2 ounces)* is a very boring, truly ordinary emollient lotion for normal to dry skin that is comparable to products that cost only $5 at the drugstore.

☹ **$$$ Cellular Time Release Moisture Lotion SPF 15** *($135 for 1.7 ounces)* is an in-part avobenzone sunscreen in a lotion base suitable for normal to dry skin not prone to blemishes. It contains some good water-binding agents and tiny amounts of antioxidants that will likely be compromised due to the translucent glass bottle that holds them.

☹ **$$$ Cellular Time Release Moisturizer, Intensive** *($135 for 1 ounce)* claims to moisturize for up to 16 hours, and has an oil-rich formula that likely lasts that long. However, time-released or not, many emollient moisturizers can keep skin comfortable all day and prevent moisture loss. This overall unimpressive formula doesn't break new ground and the antioxidants won't last long due to jar packaging.

☹ **$$$ Cellular Wrinkle Cream** *($120 for 1 ounce)* is yet another emollient moisturizer for normal to dry skin that, just like all of the other options from La Prairie, claims to fight wrinkles. The emollients and thickeners can make wrinkles look less apparent, but all told this water-, oil-, and wax-based formula is drastically overpriced.

☹ **Cellular Balancing Mask** *($125 for the kit)* is a two-part mask: the **Solvent** consists of water, citric acid, slip agents, and plant extracts, and the **Powdered Substance** is mostly baking soda, clay, silica, and the film-forming agent PVP. The Solvent is acidic while the Powdered Substance is alkaline, so they cancel each other out and haven't a snowball's shot in you-know-where of balancing skin. If anything, these ingredients will leave your skin wondering what you could have possibly been thinking!

☹ **$$$ Cellular Cycle Ampoules for the Face** *($325 for 7 treatments)* is a less-expensive, slightly stripped-down version of the Skin Caviar Intensive Ampoule Treatment above. The ingredients in this version are truly an embarrassment, but not because they're irritating. Rather, they're so ordinary that it's almost funny, although when I think that lots of women are wasting their money on this overpriced mixture, it's actually rather depressing.

☹ **$$$ Cellular Deep Cleansing Mask** *($125 for 1.7 ounces)* is an exceptionally standard clay mask for normal to oily skin that contains token amounts of plant extracts, most of which are beneficial. The AHAs in this product cannot exfoliate skin because the pH is too high.

☹ **Cellular Energizing Mask** *($125 for 1.7 ounces)* contains a solvent that enhances penetration of the other ingredients, but that's not good news for skin because this mask contains irritating amounts of horsetail, lemon peel oil, orange oil, and juniper, and you don't want them penetrating any more than you want them on the surface of your skin.

😐 **$$$ Cellular Hydralift Firming Mask** *($125 for 1.7 ounces)* won't firm skin, but will reinforce its moisture barrier as claimed because of the Vaseline it contains, along with triglycerides and silicone. Several very good antioxidants are included, but their potency will be diminished due to jar packaging.

☹ **Cellular Purifying Blemish Control** *($70 for 0.5 ounce)* contains an unknown amount of salicylic acid as the active ingredient, but the base formula is mostly alcohol, and that's too irritating and drying for all skin types. Further, many of the plant extracts in this product can cause inflammation.

☺ **$$$ Age Management Stimulus Complex Lip Repair** *($65 for 0.5 ounce)* is a beautifully packaged, water- and silicone-based product for lips. It boasts of its retinol content, and it is present, but not in a larger amount than what you'll find in products from Lauder, Neutrogena, or RoC, among others. However, this product cannot exfoliate skin as claimed because the AHA content is minimal and the pH is too high.

✓☺ **$$$ Cellular Lip Line Plumper** *($75 for 0.075 ounce)* is, in some ways, a more interesting formula than the Age Management Stimulus Complex Lip Repair above. There's no retinol in this version, but it does contain a blend of silicones and silicone polymers that do a better job of serving as a soft spackle for lip lines. This also contains some very good water-binding agents and cell-communicating ingredients, and omits the irritants typically found in lip-plumping products. It's not as miraculous as the claims imply, but it does work temporarily to fill in lines around the mouth and makes lips look and feel noticeably smoother.

😐 **$$$ Cellular Lip Renewal Concentrate** *($85 for 0.5 ounce)* is the weakest of La Prairie's three lip products, and makes the odd claim of being able to revive natural lip color (which it cannot do; stick with lipstick for that!). It's essentially a lightweight moisturizer for lips that has more flavor than antioxidants or other helpful ingredients for lips.

LA PRAIRIE SUN PRODUCTS

😐 **$$$ Cellular Anti-Wrinkle Sun Cream SPF 30** *($135 for 1.7 ounces)* protects skin from UVA radiation with its in-part avobenzone sunscreen, and has an antioxidant-laden base formula suitable for normal to dry skin. What a shame jar packaging won't keep the numerous antioxidants stable during use. The tiny amount of lavender extract is not likely to be a problem for skin.

☺ **$$$ Cellular Protective Body Emulsion SPF 30** *($135 for 5 ounces)* includes an in-part avobenzone sunscreen and has a silky base formula built around silicone and emollients. The formula is also loaded with antioxidants, though all of them are listed after the potentially irritating horsetail extract, which is what keeps this pricey sunscreen for normal to dry skin from earning a Paula's Pick rating.

☹ **Cellular Self Tan For Face and Body SPF 15** *($110 for 3.4 ounces)* does not contain the UVA-protecting ingredients of titanium dioxide, zinc oxide, avobenzone, Tinosorb, or Mexoryl SX, and is not recommended. Self-tanner-wise, dihydroxyacetone shows up in almost every sunless tanning product being sold, and for far less money than this misguided formulation.

☹ **Cellular Luxe Lip Treatment SPF 15** *($40 for 0.12 ounce)* has deluxe packaging, but leaves lips vulnerable to UVA damage because the sunscreen is sans titanium dioxide, zinc oxide, avobenzone, Tinosorb, or Mexoryl SX. The base formula couldn't be more ordinary, and is a further insult at this price.

LA PRAIRIE MAKEUP

FOUNDATION: La Prairie does not offer shades for darker skin, but their foundations are relatively easy to test without asking a salesperson for assistance.

☺ **$$$ Cellular Treatment Foundation Powder Finish** *($75)* is a talc-based wet/dry powder foundation that has a wonderfully smooth texture and a gorgeous silky finish. It would work best for normal to slightly dry or slightly oily skin types. Companies such as Laura Mercier, Lancome, Chanel, and M.A.C. offer even more impressive powder foundations for much less money, but if you're stuck on La Prairie, this won't disappoint. Four of the six shades are great, but avoid Rose Beige (too rose), and if you have a medium to tan skin tone, consider Soleil Beige carefully.

☺ **$$$ Cellular Treatment Foundation Satin SPF 15** *($70)* costs less than half of the Skin Caviar Concealer/Foundation SPF 15 below, yet this provides an in-part titanium dioxide sunscreen. It has a fluid yet creamy texture and blends from sheer to medium coverage with a satin finish. The La Prairie salesperson was steering me away from this option, indicating that it uses "older technology" and isn't as advanced as their other foundations. However, getting the sunscreen right (as this one does), along with the comparably lower price point, makes this not only advanced but also the only La Prairie liquid foundation worth considering. Among the nine shades, the four best avoided are 1.0, 3.2, 4.0, and 4.5.

☹ **Skin Caviar Concealer/Foundation SPF 15** *($165)* deserves credit for its convenient packaging of a liquid foundation and creamy concealer (the concealer is housed in the cap), but does not deserve your attention because its sunscreen does not contain the UVA-protecting ingredients of titanium dioxide, zinc oxide, avobenzone, Tinosorb, or Mexoryl SX. Despite its silky texture and a few bells and whistles in the base formula, I can't recommend such an expensive foundation that leaves your skin vulnerable to UVA damage.

CONCEALER: ☺ **$$$ Light Fantastic Cellular Concealing Brightening Eye Treatment** *($60)* has a silky, silicone-enhanced texture and is dispensed onto a synthetic brush via a click-pen component. The product comes with a refill cartridge, which is seemingly generous for La Prairie. In terms of camouflage, this doesn't conceal more than very minor discolorations. It works best as a subtle highlighter. The "powerful" anti-aging complex is barely present, and there is no research anywhere to support the claim that glycoproteins and plant extracts, especially in the tiny amounts here, can have an antiwrinkle effect. Although this has an attractive creaseless finish and comes in three good colors, I wouldn't choose it over similar, less-expensive highlighters from Estee Lauder or Yves St. Laurent.

POWDER: ☺ **$$$ Cellular Treatment Loose Powder** *($70)* has an ultra-fine, talc-based texture and a sheer, minimalist finish that leaves skin looking polished and dusted with sparkles. If shiny, expensive powder is your thing, here's a good option, and both shades are translucent. ☺ **$$$ Cellular Treatment Pressed Powder** *($40)* is just a regular, talc-based pressed powder with a silky feel. It has a smooth finish that normal to dry skin will appreciate. The three shades are slightly peachy pink, but are sheer enough to work for most light skin tones.

😐 **$$$ Cellular Treatment Bronzing Powder** *($50)* features two attractive tan colors in one compact, but this pressed bronzing powder's texture is noticeably dry, and although the shine is soft it doesn't cling well, making this a below-average option, especially for the money.

BLUSH: ☺ **$$$ Cellular Radiance Cream Blush** *($70)* would be enthusiastically recommended were it not for the ridiculous price. It's a very good, nontraditional cream blush that applies and blends nicely, leaving a soft, transparent wash of color. Skin looks healthy and glowing

The Reviews L

from each of the four colors, and the shine level is almost on mute. If you're going to indulge in some La Prairie makeup and have dry skin, this would be something to seriously consider, but only for a splurge, because your cheeks won't look like you spent this kind of money on your face (sort of like buying Manolo Blahnik shoes that look like they came from Macy's).

😐 **$$$ Cellular Treatment Powder Blush** *($50)* doesn't impress with its drier-than-usual, slightly grainy texture, though it still applies smoothly. Every shade is shiny, but the effect is closer to a soft glow than sparkles, which is a nice change of pace. Still, countless cosmetic lines offer less-expensive powder blushes that have a superior texture and better array of shades.

EYESHADOW: 😐 **$$$ Cellular Treatment Eye Colour Ensemble** *($65)* provides four eyeshadows in one compact, with one shade in each being dark enough to use as eyeliner. These have a smoother, silkier feel and apply better than the Cellular Treatment Eye Colour below, though still a bit unevenly. Every set has quite a bit of shine, and that's not the best for wrinkled eye-area skin; the least shiny (and most workable) set is called Les Bruns.

☹ **Cellular Treatment Eye Colour** *($40)* is La Prairie's name for their powder eyeshadow singles, and is the most enticing thing about this otherwise unremarkable product. The smooth but dry texture and too-soft pressing lead to a chunky, flake-prone application, and there are far too many pastel tones that do little to shape or shade the eye.

☹ **Cellular Eye Colour Effects** *($35)* has a slick, cream-to-powder texture that leaves a silky, very shiny finish. The sheer colors impart much more shine than pigment, which won't deemphasize wrinkles or a drooping eyelid. Given the price and the "mature" positioning of this line, a product like this doesn't make much sense, nor does it last that long without creasing.

EYE AND BROW SHAPER: ☺ **$$$ Cellular Treatment Wet/Dry Eyeliner** *($35)* presents classic black and brown shades in a very good, deeply pigmented formula that works best when used wet (dry application poses a slight risk of flaking). The finish is mostly matte, but you will notice a bit of shine, which La Prairie just can't seem to do without.

☺ **$$$ Luxe Eye Liner Automatique** *($45)* is an automatic, retractable eye pencil, but the sleek metal component is what you end up paying for. Each color goes on smoothly and leaves a slightly creamy finish that won't be impervious to smearing unless set with a powder eyeshadow. Of course, you could just line with a powder eyeshadow and be done, but this is a decent option for those who prefer pencils. Avoid Lavande, which is way too purple. ☺ **$$$ Luxe Brow Liner Automatique** *($45)* comes in the same type of retractable metal component as the Luxe Eye Liner Automatique above, and also features a brow brush on the other end. This is a very good brow pencil that has a smooth but dry application and a soft powder finish that won't budge. The only issue (beyond the price) is that it takes some effort to get the colors to show up.

LIPSTICK, LIP GLOSS, AND LIPLINER: ☺ **$$$ Cellular Lip Colour Effects Luminous Transparent Glaze** *($40)* has an elegantly smooth, not-too-thick texture and a minimally sticky, sparkling finish. Featuring a brush applicator, this gloss does have movement—despite claims to the contrary—so don't expect it to not feather into lines around the mouth, just like most glosses do.

☺ **$$$ Luxe Lipliner Automatique** *($45)* has a luxurious metal component and above-average brush on the opposite end to soften and blend the line from this automatic, retractable pencil. Because it stays creamy it can't help keep lipstick from migrating into lines around the mouth, so if that's a concern, it's best to skip this one. The Nude shade is a versatile color.

😐 **$$$ Cellular Luxe Lip Colour** *($50)* leans to the greasy side of creamy, which doesn't bode well for those prone to lipstick traveling into lines around the mouth. These light- to medium-coverage shimmer-laden lipsticks leave no stain, so their wear time is relatively brief. All told, there isn't a strong argument to consider these over many other creamy lipsticks, but they're not terrible either.

☹ **Cellular Luxe Lip Enhancer** *($40)*. This slightly dry, waxy, peach-toned lipstick claims to prevent every problem you've ever had using a lipstick, but it's just a barely passable concealer that can lightly smooth the lip's surface. Don't bother with this unless you get a thrill out of wasting money.

MASCARA: ☺ **$$$ Cellular Treatment Mascara Instant Curl** *($40)* doesn't do anything instantly, but with patience this extends lashes to fluttering length and leaves them with a soft, fringed curl. Thickness is harder to come by, but the application is clump-free and wearability is uneventful.

😐 **$$$ Cellular Treatment Mascara Instant Build** *($40)* won't clump at all and leaves lashes remarkably soft, but otherwise takes a long time to produce meager lengthening. This isn't any more of a treatment for lashes than most mascaras, and the amount of La Prairie's Cellular Complex is minuscule compared to the standard waxes seen in this and most mascaras available today.

BRUSHES: La Prairie's handsome **Brushes** *($28–$65, $125–$250 for collections)* are frustrating because only four of the nine are sold separately. If you want more than that, you have to buy one of the kits. In or out of the kits, most of these brushes are nicely shaped and have comfortable handles, but you will find similarly priced and far more appealing brushes from Trish McEvoy and Stila. The best single brush is the ☺ **$$$ Professional Concealer Brush** *($30)*, which can double as an eyeshadow brush. The 😐 **$$$ Art of the Brush Collection** *($250)* gets you every brush in a sleek, roll-up case, but a few of these brushes are low quality and don't make this complete set a value.

SPECIALTY PRODUCTS: 😐 **$$$ Cellular Treatment Rose Illusion Line Filler** *($100)* supposedly works to make wrinkled skin look smooth and line-free, but don't get your hopes up and don't open your pocketbook. This thick but silky gel-cream is mostly silicone and has an opalescent pink tint to slightly brighten skin. Silicone primers have a softening effect—and that's it; they don't erase lines. If you're curious to try this type of product, I encourage you to test Prescriptives Magic Invisible Line Smoother ($35) first, which is almost identical to this and, as you can see, the price is far less mind-numbing.

LA ROCHE-POSAY (SKIN CARE ONLY)

LA ROCHE-POSAY AT-A-GLANCE

Strengths: Very good cleansers; well-formulated, stably packaged options for those seeking products with hydroquinone or retinol or stabilized vitamin C; many fragrance-free options; a unique lip moisturizer; the best assortment of well-formulated skin-care products in L'Oreal's vast stable of brands.

Weaknesses: Some problematic, overly irritating exfoliants; lack of anti-acne products that target blemishes effectively, yet gently; several ho-hum moisturizers and sunscreens that are stably packaged but don't contain light- or air-sensitive ingredients.

For more information about La Roche-Posay, owned by L'Oreal, call (888) 577-5226 or visit www.laroche-posay.com or www.Beautypedia.com.

LA ROCHE-POSAY BIOMEDIC PRODUCTS

☺ **$$$ Biomedic AntiBac Acne Wash** *($22.95 for 6 ounces)* is a very standard, water-soluble cleanser that contains 1.8% salicylic acid as the active ingredient, though its benefit in a cleanser is negligible because it is rinsed from skin before it has a chance to work. This is still a good option for normal to oily skin, provided you keep it away from the eye area.

☺ **$$$ Biomedic Purifying Cleanser** *($27 for 6 ounces)* is an excellent, water-soluble cleanser for all skin types except very dry. It doesn't purify skin better than similar options, but it's gentle, removes makeup well, and does not contain fragrance. The tiny amount of glycolic acid functions as a water-binding agent, not as an exfoliant.

☹ **Biomedic Micro Exfoliating Scrub** *($28 for 6 ounces)* is an overly abrasive scrub that contains almost every irritating volatile oil known, including lemon, lime, and grapefruit. Ouch!

☹ **Biomedic Conditioning Gel** *($30 for 2 ounces)* lists 2% hydroquinone as the active ingredient, but this effective, time-proven skin-lightening agent is joined by enough alcohol to make it too irritating and drying for all skin types. The glycolic acid and pH of 3.5 make the alcohol that much more problematic.

☹ **Biomedic Conditioning Gel Plus** *($40 for 2 ounces)* is similar to the Biomedic Conditioning Gel above, except this contains more glycolic acid. Otherwise, the same comments apply.

☹ **Biomedic Conditioning Solution** *($28 for 6 ounces)* contains a lot of alcohol and also includes irritating eucalyptus oil, neither of which will help the glycolic and salicylic acids increase skin's health or renew skin.

😐 **Biomedic AntiBac Protection** *($29 for 1 ounce)* claims to reduce breakouts while you sleep, but does not contain any effective anti-acne ingredients. An unusual ingredient in this product is lysozyme HCL. This is an enzyme typically extracted from egg whites that is used as a skin-conditioning agent. There is no research proving it has disinfectant properties against acne-causing bacteria.

☺ **Biomedic Conditioning Cream** *($34 for 2 ounces)* is a very standard 6% glycolic acid moisturizer best for normal to dry skin. The low pH makes it very effective for exfoliation, but the other ingredients are no different from what you would find in AHA products at the drugstore from Alpha Hydrox or Neutrogena Healthy Skin.

✓☺ **$$$ Biomedic C-Recovery Treatment** *($50 for 1 ounce)* is similar to but has a less absorbent finish than the Active C, for Dry Skin, reviewed below. This version adds a good amount of the cell-communicating ingredient niacinamide to the mix, making it a better-rounded product. It is fragrance-free.

😐 **Biomedic Extra Mild Protection** *($33 for 2 ounces)* consists of little more than water, several silicones, slip agent, and preservatives. It's a very basic, protective, fragrance-free moisturizer for normal to slightly dry skin. It would have been nice if it contained at least one antioxidant, but no dice.

☹ **Biomedic Extra Rich Moisturizer** *($49.95 for 2 ounces)* contains an excellent complement of ingredients for dry, sensitized skin, but the inclusion of sage oil and lavender makes it impossible to recommend. Although sage oil has antioxidant ability, two of its main volatile components (thujone and camphor) are skin irritants.

☺ **Biomedic Facial Shield SPF 20** *($29.50 for 2 ounces)* is a very basic, but effective, daytime moisturizer for normal to slightly oily skin. It contains avobenzone for UVA protection, and some absorbent ingredients to create a soft matte finish. It is fragrance-free.

😐 **Biomedic Facial Shield SPF 30** *($31.50 for 2 ounces)* includes an in-part avobenzone sunscreen in a lightweight, water-and-silicone base. The amount of alcohol poses a slight risk of irritation. Although the sunscreen is effective, this is pricey and doesn't contain any beneficial extras save for an inconsequential amount of vitamin E and some soybean oil.

😊 **$$$ Biomedic Gentle Moisturizing Lotion SPF 15** *($30 for 2.5 ounces)* is an exceptionally basic, but effective, daytime moisturizer for normal to minimally dry skin. It features an in-part titanium dioxide sunscreen and is fragrance-free, but that's about it.

😊 **$$$ Biomedic Hydrating Serum** *($52 for 1 ounce)* is a good, lightweight serum for all skin types that provides a small selection of water-binding agents and antioxidant vitamins.

😐 **Biomedic Hydro Active Emulsion** *($32 for 2 ounces)* claims to be antioxidant-rich, but contains only a small amount of vitamin E, which is hardly exciting. This is otherwise an average emollient moisturizer for normal to dry skin. It is fragrance-free.

😊 **$$$ Biomedic Potent-C 10.5 Concentrate** *($60 for 1 ounce)* contains 10.5% stabilized vitamin C, and comes in packaging that preserves the stability of this antioxidant. There's not much else to say about this product, other than that the glycol base will enhance penetration of the vitamin C, which could pose problems for those with sensitive skin.

☹ **Biomedic 21 Day Intensive Acne Treatment** *($130 for the kit)* is La Roche-Posay's needlessly pricey version of parent company L'Oreal's Special Care Acne Response Daily Adult Acne Regimen ($23.99 for the set). There are slight variations, but both sets share the problem of being incapable of helping blemish- or blackhead-inflicted skin. The **Micro-Dose Peel** and **Keratolytic Serum** in the Biomedic set contain mostly alcohol. The **Barrier Cream** is another boring La Roche-Posay moisturizer (though it is fragrance-free), while the **Effaclar K Acne Treatment Fluid** doesn't contain nearly enough salicylic acid to keep blemishes at bay and dislodge blackheads. What a waste of money!

😐 **$$$ Biomedic 21 Day Intensive Wrinkle Treatment** *($130 for the kit)* comprises four separate products, which, as a system, are designed to reduce wrinkles and discolorations. Step 1 is the **Micro-Dermabrasion Cream**, a creamy, fragrance-free scrub that contains alumina as the abrasive agent. It works well to manually exfoliate skin, but no better than using a washcloth with a gentle cleanser. Next is the **Collagenist Preparation Serum**, which contains 8% glycolic acid at an effective pH level. This is to be mixed with the **Collagenist Preparation Powder**, which is just free-flowing ascorbic acid (vitamin C) along with the stable form of this vitamin and pH-adjusting agents. You apply this mixture to your skin with the included brush, leave it on for a few minutes, then rinse. The third step is to apply the **Barrier Cream**, which is basically water, glycerin, and several silicones. It's fragrance-free and helps make skin feel smoother. After this you're done, but on alternate nights you're directed to use the Active C, for Normal to Combination Skin (reviewed below) as a supplemental nighttime treatment.

Although none of the products in this kit is a problem for skin (well, unless you get carried away with the scrub), the system is misguided. Why leave the AHA product on for only a few minutes when you'd get better results leaving it on overnight? (Though don't try that with this mixture, which begins to feel tacky within moments—you'll definitely *want* to rinse it.) And while the Barrier Cream is OK, other moisturizers outshine it by offering just-exfoliated skin a lot more. Exfoliating skin with a well-formulated AHA product and using a stabilized vitamin C product can result in smoother, more even-toned skin and help stimulate collagen production. But it doesn't take a pricey, multistep kit like this for your skin to reap these benefits.

☹ **$$$ Biomedic Collagenist Powder** *($31.50 for 0.5 ounce)* is similar to the Collagenist Preparation Powder included in the Biomedic 21 Day Intensive Wrinkle Treatment above, except this contains three instead of two forms of vitamin C. It is designed to be added to any moisturizer to customize it, but doing so will alter the pH of this powder, potentially making the vitamin C ineffective. Moreover, an excess of ascorbic acid can be irritating to skin, and you'd have no way of knowing how much you're adding in terms of potency. It is far better to stay with a serum or moisturizer whose vitamin C content has been calibrated and stabilized within that formula rather than experimenting with this do-it-yourself powder.

☹ **Biomedic Maximum C** *($19 for 0.25 ounce)* is identical to the Biomedic Collagenist Powder above, and the same review applies.

☹ **Biomedic Pure Enzyme** *($28 for 1 ounce)* relies on enzymes to exfoliate skin, but enzymes are notoriously unstable and not nearly as reliable as a standard topical scrub or, better yet, a well-formulated AHA or BHA product.

☺ **$$$ Biomedic Retinol 15**, ☺ **$$$ Biomedic Retinol 30** *($39.95 for 1 ounce)*, and ☺ **$$$ Biomedic Retinol 60** *($41.95 for 1 ounce)* all come in the same lotion base with varying amounts of retinol in what La Roche-Posay refers to as a Customizable Step-Up system. Retinol 15 contains the lowest amount of retinol (0.15%), Retinol 30 contains 0.30%, and, as expected, Retinol 60 contains 0.6%. All are fragrance-free and packaged so the air- and light-sensitive retinol remains stable. Which one you choose isn't of much importance given that there are no formulary standards for retinol concentrations. However, it is a very good antioxidant and cell-communicating ingredient for skin because it helps create better, healthier skin cells and increases the amount of skin-support substances. Keep in mind that retinol should not be the only ingredient you look for in a moisturizer. Skin needs a combination of ingredients to function optimally, including cell-communicating ingredients (of which retinol is one), an array of antioxidants (to reduce free-radical damage), and substances that mimic skin structure. Together, all these various ingredients and elements combine to create a powerful part of any skin-care routine. Biomedic Retinol is best for normal to dry skin.

LA ROCHE-POSAY TOLERIANE PRODUCTS

☺ **Toleriane Dermo-Cleanser** *($18 for 6.76 ounces)* is a very simple, fragrance-free cleansing lotion for dry skin. It poses no risk of irritating skin unless you know you're sensitive to one of the ingredients it contains, and it does a decent job of removing most types of makeup.

☹ **Toleriane Gentle Cleansing Bar** *($6 for a 4-ounce bar)* doesn't contain fragrance, which is good; however, this is standard-issue bar soap and as such is too drying and irritating for all skin types.

✓ ☺ **$$$ Toleriane Purifying Foaming Cream** *($20 for 4.22 ounces)* is a very good water-soluble foaming cleanser with a soft cream texture suitable for normal to slightly dry skin, and it removes makeup quickly. The detergent cleansing agents are not bad, but they're also not the best for "intolerant" skin, as La Roche-Posay asserts.

☺ **Toleriane Eye Make-Up Remover** *($16 for 30 0.2-ounce ampoules; 6 ounces)* is a basic, fragrance-free eye-makeup remover packaged in single-use ampoules so it does not need to contain preservatives. Although it's an effective option for sensitive skin around the eyes, the honey in this product (it's the third ingredient) lends a somewhat tacky finish that must be rinsed.

☹ **Toleriane Soothing Protective Skincare** *($20 for 1.35 ounces)* is a very basic, fragrance-free moisturizing lotion for normal to slightly dry skin. It does not contain a single anti-irritant or antioxidant, so it ends up being neither protective nor any more soothing than any other ordinary moisturizer.

☺ **Toleriane Facial Fluid** *($22 for 1.35 ounces)* is an average, fragrance-free moisturizer for normal to dry skin not prone to blemishes. Given the simplicity of the formula, this may indeed be a good option for those dealing with rosacea and the sensitivity it entails.

OTHER LA ROCHE-POSAY PRODUCTS

☺ **$$$ Effaclar Deep Cleansing Foaming Cream** *($18 for 4.2 ounces)* produces a foamy lather, but contains a high amount of the alkaline ingredient potassium hydroxide, making this an option only for very oily skin, and even those folks may find this too drying.

☺ **Effaclar Purifying Foaming Gel** *($18 for 5.1 ounces)* is similar to the Biomedic Purifying Cleanser above, and aside from producing a more copious lather and containing fragrance, the same comments apply.

☺ **Hydraphase Hydrating Cleansing Milk** *($19 for 6.76 ounces)* is a good cleansing lotion for normal to dry skin. It contains more thickening agents than detergent cleansing agents, but removes makeup well. This may require a washcloth for complete removal, and is not recommended for blemish-prone skin.

☹ **Lipikar Surgras Lipid-Enriched Cleansing Bar, for Severely Dry Skin** *($7 for a 5.2-ounce bar)* has a fancy name and affordable price, but it's still old-fashioned bar soap and can be drying and irritating for all skin types.

☺ **$$$ Rosaliac Gelee Micellar Make-Up Removal Gel** *($22 for 6.76 ounces)* is a gentle, water-based eye-area cleanser that removes most types of eye makeup (though some waterproof mascaras may prove resistant to this formula). It is great for sensitive eyes because fragrance, fragrant plant extracts, and coloring agents are excluded.

☹ **Effaclar Astringent Lotion Micro-Exfoliant** *($18 for 6.76 ounces)* lists alcohol as the second ingredient, and the amount of salicylic acid is too low for exfoliation to occur.

☺ **$$$ Hydraphase Hydrating Toner** *($26 for 6.76 ounces)* doesn't do much to impress, but its basic formula will help remove the last traces of makeup and make normal to dry skin feel softer.

☹ **Thermal Spring Water** *($6 for 1.7 ounces)* comes with claims of soothing, toning, refreshing, and providing antioxidant protection to skin, yet all it contains is water and nitrogen. Thermal Spring Water is just water and some extra nitrogen. This product is said to be "rich in selenium, a powerful antioxidant." Whether or not that is true (though obtaining pure selenium as an oral supplement is preferred) is irrelevant because the nitrogen used as a propellant to create a mist of water can generate free-radical damage and cause cell death (Sources: *Mechanisms of Ageing and Development*, April 2002, pages 1007–1019; *Toxicology and Applied Pharmacology*, July 2002, pages 84–90; and *Cellular and Molecular Biology*, April 15, 2007, pages 1–2).

☺ **$$$ Active C, for Dry Skin** *($40 for 1 ounce)* would be an outstanding way to see if a 5% stabilized vitamin C product (packaged to ensure stability and potency) improves your skin. The silky, silicone-enhanced base with its nearly matte finish is ideal for normal to oily skin. Just to be clear, vitamin C is a very good, well-established antioxidant for skin, but it isn't the only one to consider, and in that sense you are getting a one-note product by choosing this.

☺ **$$$ Active C, for Normal to Combination Skin** *($40 for 1 ounce)* is similar to the Active C, for Dry Skin above, and the same review applies.

☺ **$$$ Active C Eyes** *($31 for 0.5 ounce)* is a silky, silicone-enriched lightweight moisturizer for slightly dry skin anywhere on the face. It contains a good amount of vitamin C (as ascorbic acid) and contains fragrance in the form of bitter orange flower extract.

☺ **Anthelios SX Daily Moisturizing Cream with Sunscreen SPF 15** *($29 for 3.4 ounces)* made a big media splash with overblown stories that one of its active ingredients (ecamsule, also known as Mexoryl SX) was a new UVA filter approved by the FDA. What wasn't routinely mentioned was that the FDA approved this active ingredient for only one product, which is the subject of this review. What's noteworthy about this sunscreen is its combination of ecamsule with avobenzone, as stabilized by octocrylene. You can be assured of sufficient UVA protection if you apply this liberally and long enough before venturing outdoors. What's disappointing is that the excitement starts and stops right there. Nothing else about this silicone-enhanced sunscreen is that intriguing, and it doesn't contain even a single antioxidant. For the money and with all the hype this product has generated, you should expect more. Still, it deserves a happy face rating for its sunscreen alone, and the formula is suitable for normal to slightly dry or slightly oily skin. One more thing: Although Mexoryl SX is a good UVA sunscreen, it does not provide the highest level of UVA protection as claimed on the label. Lest we forget, titanium dioxide and zinc oxide can screen UVA rays well beyond their measurable threshold, so Mexoryl SX, while viable, is not intrinsically the best.

😐 **Hydranorme Hydrolipidic Emulsion, for Severely Dry Skin** *($20 for 1.35 ounces)* contains mostly water, mineral oil, squalane, water-binding agents, wax, preservatives, and fragrance. It's an option for dry skin, just not a particularly interesting one.

😐 **$$$ Hydraphase Eyes** *($22 for 0.5 ounce)* is a lightweight, fragrance-free moisturizer for slightly dry skin anywhere on the face. It contains antioxidant vitamin A and soy.

😐 **Hydraphase Light Facial Moisturizer** *($26 for 1.7 ounces)* is a substandard, rather lackluster moisturizer for normal to slightly dry skin. The amount of alcohol is unlikely to cause irritation, but antioxidants are conspicuously absent.

☹ **Nutritic Ultra-Fine Cream, Transforming Care for Very Dry Skin** *($26 for 1.35 ounces)* contains an unwelcome amount of coriander oil, making it too irritating for all skin types. The volatile compounds in this oil (mostly linalool) can cause photosensitivity.

☹ **Nutritic Ultra-Fine Emulsion, Transforming Care for Dry Skin** *($26 for 1.35 ounces)* is a more emollient, Vaseline-based version of the Nutritic Ultra-Fine Cream, Transforming Care for Very Dry Skin above, and the same review applies.

☺ **$$$ Redermic Daily Fill-In Anti-Wrinkle Firming Care, Face and Neck, for Dry Skin** *($42 for 1.35 ounces)* differs little from La Roche-Posay's Active C, for Dry Skin above, though this one doesn't ballyhoo its vitamin C content. Otherwise, the comments above apply.

☺ **$$$ Redermic Daily Fill-In Anti-Wrinkle Firming Care, Face and Neck, for Normal to Combination Skin** *($42 for 1.35 ounces)* is similar to, but less desirable than, the Active C, for Dry Skin above due to its alcohol content. However, it's still an option if you're curious to try a vitamin C product and you have combination skin.

☺ **$$$ Redermic Eyes, Daily Fill-In Anti-Wrinkle Firming Care** *($35 for 0.5 ounce)* is a basic, lightweight moisturizer that contains a good amount of vitamin C. The silky, nearly matte finish is suitable only if skin around the eyes is minimally dry. Think of this as a fragrance-free way to supply skin with vitamin C (though it would be better if a variety of antioxidants were included).

☹ **Rosaliac Skin Perfecting Anti-Redness Moisturizer** *($30 for 1.35 ounces)* is a product I am asked about fairly often, and the questions come from the product's target audience: women dealing with the redness and sensitivity of rosacea. Rosaliac Skin Perfecting Anti-Redness Moisturizer is said to neutralize redness while calming and soothing inflamed skin. It does have a mint green color, but that has minimal to no effect on reducing or covering facial redness of any kind. A sheer foundation or tinted moisturizer with real skin tone shades would do a better job of softening skin's reddened appearance. Overall, this is a simply formulated, fragrance-free moisturizer for normal to slightly dry skin. It's just not the solution or even a great option for someone with rosacea. Anyone dealing with rosacea is likely aware that it is wise to avoid topical irritants, especially since many cases of rosacea react to various seemingly benign ingredients with no rhyme or reason. It is therefore best to shop for skin-care products without known irritants or potentially "active" ingredients, particularly when they're intended to be left on the skin. In the case of this product, it does not make sense to include alcohol, caffeine, and niacinamide. Alcohol and caffeine have irritant properties, while niacinamide is derived from niacin, which, although it can be beneficial, has the potential to cause facial flushing—not what someone with reddened skin needs.

☹ **Effaclar K Acne Treatment Fluid** *($19 for 1 ounce)* is discussed in the review of La Roche-Posay's Biomedic 21 Day Intensive Acne Treatment above. The company claims this product contains 1.5% salicylic acid, but the ingredient list does not bear that out, leaving this a lightweight moisturizer for normal to oily skin, and that's it.

☺ **$$$ Mela-D Skin Lightening Daily Lotion** *($40 for 1 ounce)* contains 2% hydroquinone in packaging that will keep it stable during use. Interestingly, the base formula contains several sunscreen agents (including avobenzone), but does not sport an SPF rating, so you should not rely on this for daytime protection. (Note that if you opt to use this product at night, the sunscreens are useless and may cause irritation.) The amount of salicylic acid in this product is too low to exfoliate skin. Still, this is an option for daytime wear if you pair it with another product that is rated at least SPF 15 and includes UVA-protecting ingredients.

✓ ☺ **Ceralip Lip Repair Cream** *($10 for 0.5 ounce)* is a sufficiently creamy lip moisturizer that differs from the usual wax-based sticks or oil-based balms. It is definitely an option for dry lips, and is fragrance- and flavor-free.

☺ **Lipolevres Lip Protector** *($12 for 0.1 ounce)* is a standard, oil-based lip balm whose ingredients protect lips from dehydration and keep them soft. It isn't quite as elegant as the Ceralip Lip Repair Cream above.

LANCOME

LANCOME AT-A-GLANCE

Strengths: Some good cleansers; well-formulated scrubs; almost all of the sunscreens contain either avobenzone, ecamsule (Mexoryl SX), or titanium dioxide for sufficient UVA protection; an outstanding retinol product; large selection of self-tanning products; several excellent foundations with beautiful shades for almost every skin color; some great concealers; well-deserved reputation for mostly outstanding mascaras; the Absolue powder; the liquid eyeliner; all of the powder eyeshadows; one fantastic lipstick and automatic lipliner; Lancome's counter personnel is typically well-trained and approachable.

Weaknesses: Skin care is expensive for what amounts to mostly mediocre to below-average products dressed up in attractive packaging; no AHA or BHA products; no products to effectively treat blemishes or lighten skin discolorations; average toners; moisturizers that are short on including state-of-the-art ingredients; jar packaging; several foundations with sunscreen do not provide complete UVA protection; the pressed bronzing powder; average powder blush, eye pencils, and long-wearing lip color; none of the lipsticks with sunscreen include adequate UVA protection; relatively unimpressive makeup brushes.

For more information about Lancome, owned by L'Oreal, call (800) 526-2663 or visit www.lancome.com or www.Beautypedia.com. Note: Unless mentioned otherwise, all Lancome products contain fragrance.

LANCOME SKIN CARE

LANCOME ABSOLUE PRODUCTS

😐 **$$$ Absolue Absolute Replenishing Cream Cleanser** *($50 for 6.7 ounces)* is an insanely priced creamy cleanser that consists primarily of water, mineral oil, thickeners, and corn oil. Plain mineral oil or baby oil would work just as well for dry to very dry skin, though neither they nor this product are easy to rinse from skin without using a washcloth. The packaging for this cleanser is much more impressive than what's inside.

☹ **Absolue Absolute Replenishing Toner** *($40 for 5 ounces)* does little to justify its price due to what amounts to an exceedingly banal formula that's mostly water, slip agents, silicone, and coloring agents. All of the intriguing ingredients are mere window dressing, while the amount of fragrance components can be irritating.

☹ **Absolue Anti-Age Spot Serum** *($98 for 1.35 ounces)* promises immediately clearer, more even-toned skin, but with denatured alcohol listed as the second ingredient, you're getting a fairly potent dose of irritation, which will certainly add to skin's dullness. What is important to point out is that brown skin discolorations are not caused by aging, but by unprotected sun exposure. Considering the price and unimpressive formula, you have to wonder, what was Lancome thinking?

☹ **Absolue Masque Absolute Replenishing Concentrated Cloth-Mask** *($90 for 6 masks)* is concentrated with alcohol and doesn't offer anything that would be considered luxurious or indulgent for skin.

😐 **$$$ Absolue Progressive Cure Absolute Intensive Replenishing Program** *($225 for 4 0.23-ounce vials)* is a progressive treatment meant to be used over a four-week period. Included are four vials, one for each week, but all are variations on the same basic formula of water, silicone, glycerin, thickener, slip agent, titanium dioxide, and coloring agents. How any of this is supposed to make skin luminous, even-toned, resilient, and "fully renewed" (let alone be some kind of cure for wrinkles) is a mystery. It's essentially an expensive waste of time and doesn't contain anything of significance that's not found in all of the other Absolue products above (and those are a disappointment all by themselves).

LANCOME ABSOLUE PREMIUM BX PRODUCTS

This subcategory of Absolue products brags that it is "the new standard in skincare to fight the visible effects of age and hormonal changes" and that it "revolutionizes skin replenishment." Given the embarrassingly boring formulas for these pricey products, these claims are on par with Bill Gates heralding a typewriter as the next generation of portable computers.

☹ **$$$ Absolue Eye Premium Bx, Absolute Replenishing Eye Cream** *($73 for 0.5 ounce)* is said to combine two advanced discoveries: Lancome's patented Pro-Xylane and their "intensely replenishing" Bio-Network. According to a report on www.happi.com (the *Household and Personal Products Industry* magazine Web site), Pro-Xylane is derived from xylose, a type of sugar that has water-binding properties for skin. L'Oreal Senior Vice President Alan Meyers reported that in vitro skin tests and testing on human skin showed that their Pro-Xylane co plex stimulated the production of glycosaminoglycans in the skin. Glycosaminoglycans are one part of the intricate network that makes up the skin's intercellular matrix. Topical application of substances that mimic what's found in skin's intercellular matrix do help reinforce the skin's barrier function, thus allowing the intercellular matrix to function normally. L'Oreal (Lancome's parent company) may be convinced that Pro-Xylane has some wonderful effect on skin, but lots of other ingredients can do the same thing, and as it turns out, this product doesn't contain all that much Pro-Xylane. Moreover the tiny amount of Lancome's Bio-Network—consisting of soy, wild yam, sea algae, and barley—won't have the slightest rejuvenating effect on skin, nor counteract changes in skin that result from menopause. As is true for many of Lancome's skin-care products, this is yet another lackluster moisturizer. There's more titanium dioxide, mica, and iron oxides (all mineral pigments that are included in this product to create a radiant glow, which is strictly a cosmetic effect) than anything that could be considered innovative or of "premium" benefit for your skin, and the price for such a mundane formula has everything to do with market positioning, not real, revolutionary results.

☹ **$$$ Absolue Night Premium Bx, Absolute Night Recovery Cream** *($132 for 2.6 ounces)* makes additional claims for the Pro-Xylane discussed in the previous review, such as that it restores essential moisture deep in the structure of the skin's surface. Talk about something that sounds a lot better than it is! Moreover, there are lots of ingredients found in other products that do the same thing. Actually, there's not much of anything substantial in this moisturizer, given that alcohol, wax, and coloring agents are listed well before anything interesting or even remotely worth the money. This is one to leave on the shelf!

☹ **$$$ Absolue Premium Bx, Absolute Replenishing Cream SPF 15** *($108 for 1.7 ounces)* features an in-part avobenzone sunscreen and has a slightly better base formula than the Absolue Premium Bx products reviewed above, but for the money this should be brimming with state-of-the-art ingredients, and it's not. In addition, the effectiveness of the few antioxidants present in this product is diminished by the jar packaging, which is disappointing. Last, if you're considering this for sunscreen (and that's the only claim you can bank on with this product), ask yourself how liberally you'll apply a sunscreen that is this expensive. And if you're still not convinced, at least put yourself in front of the Estee Lauder counter because their moisturizers with sunscreen have formulas that are way ahead of those from Lancome and many of them cost a lot less.

☹ **$$$ Absolue Premium Bx, Absolute Replenishing Lotion SPF 15** *($108 for 2.5 ounces)* has an in-part avobenzone sunscreen, and its opaque, pump-bottle packaging will keep the vitamin E stable (that's the only antioxidant of note in this product). Those are the positives. The bad news is that alcohol is the fourth ingredient. That isn't terrible, but it isn't what you want to see in a costly product meant to combat the visible signs of aging. Despite all the ballyhoo for Pro-Xylane and the Bio-Network (consisting of algae, soy, and wild yam), these ingredients are barely present. The salicylic acid in this product does not function as an exfoliant.

LANCOME AQUA FUSION PRODUCTS

😐 **Aqua Fusion Cream, Continuous Infusing Moisturizer** *($37 for 1.7 ounces)* contains more coloring agent than anything exciting for skin, though at least the price isn't too out-of-line. The amino acids and minerals are but a dusting, leaving this as an average, jar-packaged moisturizer for normal to slightly dry skin.

😐 **Aqua Fusion Cream SPF, Continuous Infusing Moisturizer SPF 15** *($37 for 1.7 ounces)* wins points for its in-part titanium dioxide sunscreen and is overall the most impressive of the Aqua Fusion products. The letdown is jar packaging, which compromises the effectiveness of the vitamin E, the only antioxidant of note in this moisturizer for normal to slightly dry skin.

😐 **Aqua Fusion Lotion, Continuous Infusing Moisturizer, for Normal/Combination Skin** *($37 for 1.7 ounces)* touts the essential minerals it contains as being able to charge skin and keep it hydrated all day. Not only are the minerals not essential for skin (at least not topically; oral consumption as part of a healthy diet is another story), but there is also more artificial color in this moisturizer than ingredients such as calcium or zinc. At best, this is a very standard, lightweight hydrating option for normal to oily skin. You should be aware, however, that this product lacks significant levels of antioxidants or water-binding agents. Glycerin is the second listed ingredient, but alcohol is the third, so the classic ability of glycerin to moisturize skin is compromised. Aqua Fusion Lotion does contain fragrance.

😊 **Aqua Fusion Lotion SPF, Continuous Infusing Moisturizer SPF 15, for Normal/Combination Skin** *($37 for 1.7 ounces)* has a formula that's similar to the Aqua Fusion Cream SPF, Continuous Infusing Moisturizer SPF 15 except with a thinner texture and with stable packaging. Otherwise, the same comments apply.

LANCOME BRIGHT EXPERT PRODUCTS

😐 **$$$ Bright Expert Intense Brightening Cleansing Foam** *($30 for 3.4 ounces)* is a creamy, pearlescent foaming cleanser that contains enough potassium hydroxide to make it too drying an option, except possibly for someone with oily skin. None of the many plant extracts in this cleanser have a proven track record for brightening skin, intensely or otherwise, and most of them are listed after the preservatives and fragrance, meaning they can't do much other than look enticing on the label. Besides, even if they could be helpful in some way, they would just be rinsed off the skin before they had a chance to have an effect. This is an OK cleanser for someone with oily skin but the price is unwarranted for what you get, and it's easily replaced by far less expensive and less drying options.

😐 **$$$ Bright Expert Intense Brightening Toner, Hydrating & Conditioning** *($36 for 6.7 ounces)* has an appreciable amount of the vitamin C–derived ingredient ascorbyl glucoside, but there's only limited research indicating this ingredient can improve hyperpigmentation (what Lancome refers to as "dark spots"). Also, the peppermint extract can be a problem for irritation, though there's not a lot of it in this toner. This is an OK option for normal to dry skin as long as you don't expect significant lightening of sun- or hormone-induced skin discolorations.

😐 **$$$ Bright Expert Intense Brightening Moisturizing Night Cream** *($72 for 1.7 ounces)* is a jar-packaged moisturizer that contains mostly water, glycerin, silicone, alcohol, thickener, vitamins, amino acids, and fragrance. It's hardly an exciting or breakthrough formula, and the amount of alcohol keeps it from being too moisturizing, making this an OK, but overpriced, option for someone with normal to slightly dry skin. None of the ingredients in this moisturizer has a lightening effect on skin discolorations, and the jar packaging would not be helpful for the vitamins or amino acids.

☹ **$$$ Bright Expert Intense Brightening Spot Correcting Serum** *($88 for 1 ounce)* ranks as the most expensive product in the Bright Expert lineup, but unless you're convinced ascorbyl glucoside is the skin-lightening answer, there's no reason to consider this water- and silicone-based, alcohol-free serum. Even as a moisturizer this is a fairly boring formulation with minimal beneficial (meaning state-of-the-art) ingredients for skin. The amount of ascorbyl glucoside is sufficient for it to function as an antioxidant and the opaque tube packaging will help keep it stable, but if you know this won't lighten skin discolorations, why choose it over less-expensive, better-formulated serums from Olay, Clinique, or Neutrogena?

LANCOME CLARTE PRODUCTS

☺ **$$$ Gel Clarte, Clarifying Gel-to-Foam Cleanser** *($21 for 4.2 ounces)* is a very good, water-soluble cleanser for normal to oily skin. It rinses easily, removes makeup quickly, and leaves skin feeling refreshed. The fragrant plant extracts prevent this from earning a Paula's Pick rating.

✓☺ **$$$ Mousse Clarte, Self-Foaming Mousse Cleanser** *($27 for 6.8 ounces)* has a unique, foamy mousse texture some may find appealing, but at its core this is just another good water-soluble cleanser for all skin types except very dry.

☺ **$$$ Eau De Bienfait Clarte, Cleansing Water with Extracts for Face & Eyes** *($30 for 6.8 ounces)* is a simply formulated watery cleanser that is best for removing makeup rather than removing excess oil or perspiration. It's fine for normal to slightly dry skin.

☹ **Tonique Clarte, Fresh Clarifying and Revitalizing Toner, for Normal/Combination Skin** *($21 for 6.8 ounces)* lists alcohol as the second ingredient, and is not recommended.

☺ **$$$ Exfoliance Clarte, Clarifying Exfoliating Gel** *($23 for 3.4 ounces)* is a cleanser/scrub hybrid that is a good option for normal to oily skin. The exfoliating agent is polyethylene. The amount of papaya is barely worth mentioning, and has no effect on removing dulling impurities.

LANCOME HIGH RESOLUTION PRODUCTS

☹ **$$$ High Resolution Eye with Collaser-48, Deep Collagen Anti-Wrinkle Eye Serum** *($56 for 0.5 ounce)* makes much ado about the fact that it is the only Lancome eye treatment that can "accelerate the production of collagen in just 48 hours." This begs the question of why Lancome would keep selling its myriad other eye-area products if they don't work as well. After all, if this one works so expediently to push up and plump wrinkles, why bother with anything else? But Lancome doesn't have to worry, because there's nothing special or unique in this product to put their other options to shame. This ends up being a decent, though mundane, water- and silicone-based serum that contains a lot of film-forming agents. It also includes titanium dioxide and mica to make the under-eye area look brighter and shimmery. In fact, these pigments make up a much larger part of the formula than the caffeine and other ingredients Lancome claims are responsible for this product's ability to diminish dark circles and puffiness. Without question this serum-type moisturizer will smooth the appearance of wrinkles, but on dry skin it will look just like any other moisturizer. Accelerating the production of collagen is an easy claim for any moisturizer because skin that isn't dry or irritated does make collagen, so this and lots of other moisturizers would net the same result, depending on how you made the measurements or controlled the testing. And the Collaser part of this product, which is there to make you think this is replacing laser resurfacing that you'd get at a doctor's office—well, just to be clear, and I'm sure this won't surprise you, it doesn't.

☺ **$$$ High Resolution Eye with Fibrelastine, Intensive Recovery Anti-Wrinkle Eye Cream** *($52 for 0.5 ounce)*. The backbone of the formula is a standard but good mix of water, glycerin, silicone, and emollients. The excitement both starts and stops there, however. As far as the rest of the formula goes, despite all manner of wrinkle-smoothing and elastin-boosting claims, there are more cosmetic gimmicks than real state-of-the-art ingredients. For example, the talc, titanium dioxide, and mica leave a slightly reflective finish, but that's a cosmetic effect, not a skin-care benefit. And the manganese gluconate—which Lancome maintains has a relaxing effect on expression lines despite the lack of any research showing that to be the case—is a waste! Other than that, there is nothing else in this product worth mentioning or worthy of purchasing.

☺ **$$$ High Resolution with Collaser-48, Deep Collagen Anti-Wrinkle Serum** *($62 for 1 ounce)*. Despite the eye-catching words like "Collaser" and "Deep Collagen," this moisturizer is not only incapable of substituting for any type of laser or collagen injection treatment, but also a poor substitute for a well-formulated moisturizer of any kind. With the claim that this can renew collagen "in just 48 hours" and its alleged ability to make wrinkles "appear pushed up and out as though plumped from within," you'd bet there would be some fairly state-of-the-art ingredients in this product, but that is a bet you won't win. Unfortunately, there is nothing in High Resolution with Collaser-48 that can stimulate collagen production or have a prolonged effect on the appearance of wrinkles.

The backbone of this formula is water, silicone, glycerin, aluminum starch, synthetic polymer (PTFE), more silicone, buffering agent, titanium dioxide, and coloring agents. The product contains meager amounts of vitamins E and C and, of course, collagen—but the jar packaging means the antioxidants will be ineffective shortly after the product is opened. And besides, topically applied collagen won't stimulate skin to make more of its own. A roster of antioxidants, cell-communicating ingredients, and sophisticated skin-identical ingredients would have been much more impressive, but that must not be Lancome's goal. This remains an OK moisturizer for normal to slightly dry skin. It contains ingredients that make skin feel silky and let it reflect light better, but it's all surface—and for the money, your skin deserves better, deeper, and longer-lasting results.

☺ **$$$ High Resolution with Fibrelastine, Intensive Recovery Anti-Wrinkle Cream** *($74 for 1.7 ounces)* has a base formula that's similar to most of Lancome's emollient formulas for dry skin. Isn't it funny how this option claims to renew elastin and reduce deep wrinkles, while similar formulas with similar ingredients in Lancome's Renergie and Primordiale lines claim to act on different facets of aging, such as sagging and skin tone improvement? In any event, the jar packaging won't keep the vitamin E or tiny amounts of other antioxidants stable, and this cannot reduce forehead wrinkles even close to the manner in which Botox does.

☹ **High Resolution with Fibrelastine, Intensive Recovery Anti-Wrinkle Cream SPF 15** *($74 for 1.7 ounces)*. In some ways it is just shocking that Lancome is still launching sunscreens that don't include UVA-protecting ingredients, just like this one doesn't. It's also ironic that a product like this is being sold side-by-side with Lancome's UV Expert 20 (reviewed below) that makes a big deal out of the "extraordinary protection" it provides from UVA rays. For this High Resolution product, the base formula has a great texture, but it fails to impress because it has only minimal state-of-the-art ingredients, and the jar packaging just makes this an expensive mistake.

LANCOME OLIGO MINERALE PRODUCTS

☹ **$$$ Oligo Minerale Multi-Mineral Multi-Vitamin Fortifying Cleansing Mousse** *($53.50 for 4 ounces)* contains a tiny amount of vitamins and minerals, but even prodigious amounts wouldn't matter in a cleanser because it is quickly rinsed from skin. This is a fairly drying cleansing mousse that uses soap-like, potassium-based cleansing agents. It is an OK option for oily to very oily skin, and definitely removes makeup.

☹ **Oligo Minerale Multi-Mineral Multi-Vitamin Fortifying Toner** *($43.50 for 6.8 ounces)* is an embarrassing formulation that lists alcohol as the second ingredient. That makes it too drying and irritating for all skin types—and Lancome knows better! What a shame, because sans alcohol, this would have been a very good moisturizing toner for dry skin.

☹ **$$$ Oligo Minerale Multi-Mineral Multi-Vitamin Fortifying Creme** *($127 for 2.5 ounces)* is a silky, emollient moisturizer that would be a fine option for normal to dry skin, but there is nothing especially unique in this that makes it worth the investment. It does contain some good antioxidants, but the amounts are minuscule, and jar packaging won't keep them stable once this moisturizer is in use.

☹ **$$$ Oligo Minerale Multi-Mineral Multi-Vitamin Fortifying Eye Creme** *($80 for 0.5 ounce)* has some good emollients for dry skin around the eyes or elsewhere, but the amount of sunscreen agent makes this potentially sensitizing if used as directed. The antioxidants are all for naught thanks to the poor choice of jar packaging.

☺ **$$$ Oligo Minerale Multi-Mineral Multi-Vitamin Fortifying Lotion** *($100 for 1.7 ounces)* is a very good, lightweight lotion for normal to slightly dry skin, featuring an effective blend of water, silicones, slip agent, mineral oil, anti-irritant, vitamins E, C, and A (antioxidants), minerals, preservatives, and fragrance. You don't have to spend this much money for a good moisturizer, but this is certainly the most worthy among the Oligo Minerale options.

LANCOME PRIMORDIALE PRODUCTS

☹ **$$$ Primordiale Cell Defense, Double Performance Cell Defense & Skin Perfecting Serum** *($62 for 1 ounce)* was launched with much ballyhoo about how it is supposed to fight aging by blocking 99% of free radicals in an effort to attain visibly perfect skin, but then Lancome offers no explanation or proof of just how this product goes about blocking nearly all free-radical damage. And logically, given the constant onslaught of the sun, air, pollution, and free radicals generated naturally inside your body there is no way any product or substance can live up to that claim. Moreover, the claims made for this product go beyond any alleged benefit Lancome has previously attributed to the same or similar antioxidants in their products. But what's most maddening is that this isn't even a very good formula!

The primary ingredients are water, silicones (which create a silky finish), and alcohol. The amount of alcohol is potentially irritating, while the main antioxidant (ascorbyl glucoside, a form of vitamin C) doesn't play more than a moderate supporting role in a lackluster formula. In fact, coloring agents get more prominence in this serum than the other antioxidants included, so really, how serious is Lancome about this product's prodigious free radical–scavenging ability? Getting back to the testing Lancome uses to make the free-radical claim, the only details were that it was in vitro and that the free-radical reduction was in response to UVA light exposure. But what about free radicals generated by UVB light, smog, car exhaust, air, heat, and so many other things? UVA light is but one source of damage. In reality, Lancome's test results don't indicate any benefit for skin.

☹ **Primordiale Optimum Cream, Visibly Correcting Moisturizer Thermo-Control SPF 15** *($62 for 1.7 ounces)* lacks sufficient UVA-protecting ingredients, so who really cares if this can protect skin from daily temperature variations? Those might feel uncomfortable, but they have nothing to do with how skin ages.

😐 **$$$ Primordiale Optimum Eye, Visibly Correcting Eye Treatment** *($48 for 0.5 ounce)* contains mostly water, silicones, glycerin, silicone polymer, film-forming agent, honey, plant oil, coloring agents, and vitamin E. Yet the touted vitamin E (a hallmark of the Primordiale line) is given short shrift, appearing down next to ingredients that add color. This is an OK moisturizer for slightly dry skin, but the fragrance isn't the best for the eye area.

☹ **Primordiale Optimum Lotion, Visibly Correcting Moisturizer Thermo-Control SPF 15** *($62 for 1.7 ounces)* is a dud for daytime use because it lacks adequate UVA protection. Lancome products with sunscreen are the equivalent of an on-again, off-again relationship. Just when you think they have their act together with the launch of new sunscreens or foundations that include sufficient UVA protection, their next round of new products with sunscreen disappoints. Without an effective sunscreen, those who use this product daily in the hopes of it being antiwrinkle are only setting themselves up for more wrinkles and other telltale signs of aging.

😐 **$$$ Primordiale Optimum Night, Visibly Renewing Night Treatment** *($64 for 1.7 ounces)* is said to fight the first signs of visible aging with beech bud extract and vitamin A. The latter is barely present, and there is no research anywhere proving beech bud (a tree leaf) can pull even one punch against wrinkles. It's another emollient moisturizer for dry skin whose antioxidants are compromised by jar packaging.

☺ **$$$ Primordiale Optimum Lip, Lip Revitalizing Treatment** *($33 for 0.5 ounce)* can slightly fill in and smooth lines on the lips and around the mouth thanks to its strong silicone base. The amount of vitamin E is token and won't reduce lines and wrinkles, but at least the packaging helps keep it stable during use. Consider this an expensive lip moisturizer, period.

LANCOME PURE FOCUS PRODUCTS

☹ **Pure Focus Cleansing Gel with Micro-Beads** *($21 for 4.2 ounces)* contains the potent menthol derivative menthoxypropanediol as well as cinnamon bark, which makes it too irritating for all skin types.

☺ **$$$ Pure Focus Deep Pore Refining Scrub with Purifying Micro-Beads** *($23 for 3.4 ounces)* is a gel-based scrub that contains polyethylene (plastic) as the abrasive agent. The small amount of detergent cleansing agents makes this a good choice for normal to oily skin.

☹ **Pure Focus Pore Tightening Toner with Matifying Powders** *($21 for 6.8 ounces)* lists alcohol as the second ingredient and contains the potent menthol derivative menthoxypropanediol. The focus is purely on irritation here!

☹ **Pure Focus Matifying Skin Revitalizing Gel-Cream** *($46 for 1.7 ounces)* includes some good absorbent ingredients such as silica and clay, but the amount of alcohol is cause for concern, and the inclusion of irritant menthoxypropanediol is a problem, even for oily skin.

☹ **Pure Focus Matifying Moisturizing Lotion** *($34 for 1.7 ounces)* barely moisturizes thanks to its alcohol content, and irritates with the menthol derivative menthoxypropanediol. Skin does not need to tingle or be irritated to look matte!

😐 **$$$ Pure Focus T-Zone Powder Gel for Instant Shine Control** *($26 for 1 ounce)* is just silicone with fragrance and volatile fragrance components. It provides a silky matte finish, but is not preferred to Clinique's Pore Minimizer Instant Perfector ($16.50 for 0.5 ounce) or Paula's Choice Skin Balancing Super Antioxidant Mattifying Concentrate ($21.95 for 1 ounce).

☹ **Pure Focus Self-Heating Deep Clean Mask with Marine Extract** *($27 for 3.4 ounces)* contains menthol, which makes it too irritating for all skin types. The warming sensation this mask produces may feel nice, but has no effect on skin's oil output or clogged pores.

LANCOME RENERGIE PRODUCTS

☺ **$$$ Renergie Cream, Anti-Wrinkle and Firming Treatment** *($74 for 1.7 ounces)* remains a perennial favorite of Lancome customers, but it doesn't increase skin's firmness or reduce the appearance of wrinkles better than most emollient moisturizers, which is all this product is. It's a decent option for dry skin, but definitely leaves it wanting more for the money, and the various fragrance components pose a risk of inflammation.

☺ **$$$ Renergie Eye, Anti-Wrinkle and Firming Eye Creme** *($52 for 0.5 ounce)* is a good, fragrance-free, emollient moisturizer for dry skin anywhere on the face. Nothing in it will firm skin, but its rich texture will soften the appearance of wrinkles. Jar packaging doesn't make this an optimum choice if you want to provide skin with antioxidants.

☺ **$$$ Renergie Lotion, Anti-Wrinkle and Firming Treatment** *($74 for 1.7 ounces)* is a silicone-enhanced lightweight lotion for normal to slightly oily skin. Although the packaging will keep the vitamin E stable, there's barely a drop of it in here.

☹ **Renergie Microlift Flash Lifting, Instant Effect Serum** *($70 for 1.35 ounces)* has enough alcohol to cause skin to constrict and become temporarily tighter, but the resulting irritation is neither healthy nor recommended. There is far more red dye in this serum than anything uniquely beneficial.

☺ **$$$ Renergie Microlift Neck, Active Redefining Neck Treatment** *($74 for 1.7 ounces)* has a formula that is so similar to almost all of the other Lancome moisturizers for normal to dry skin that they should have to concede that those options will also lift and firm the neck, and that you don't really need this product at all. This moisturizer is an option for slightly dry to dry skin, but nothing in it is specific to skin on the neck.

☺ **$$$ Renergie Microlift Eye R.A.R.E., Superior Lifting Eye Cream** *($58 for 0.5 ounce)* has aspirations to defy gravity's pull on skin, and is said to be inspired by "the latest vertical surgery techniques" which grant this cream "exceptional lifting power." Such claims may make you think twice about booking a consultation with a cosmetic surgeon, but let me assure you such an appointment would be time well spent compared to using this inferior product. Apparently a "breakthrough" oligopeptide in this product is able to double the synthesis of protein linked to shoring up collagen. If that was true, the result would be smoother, less lined, plumped skin. The only peptide in this product is acetyl tetrapeptide-9, and it is barely present. In fact, there are far more preservatives and volatile fragrance components in this jar-packaged cream than peptide (and the amount of alcohol, while not likely irritating, is still disappointing). Acetyl tetrapeptide-9 is part of a trademarked complex known as Dermican manufactured by Laboratoires Sérobiologiques. That company's research shows that this peptide acts on a certain proteoglycan (a sugar molecule that forms the ground substance of connective tissues such as collagen) known as lumican, which is said to play an important role in the synthesis and organization of collagen fibers in skin. The kicker is twofold: the company's research is not substantiated, and the usage level they recommend (1%–3% Dermican) is not even remotely close to what Lancome chose to use. Even if Dermican could work as claimed, you're barely getting any of it in this product, which leaves you with another mundane moisturizer for normal to slightly dry skin. One last note regarding lumican: there is research showing that this proteoglycan's deterioration in skin over time likely plays a role in skin's aged appearance. In addition, animal research suggests that lumican expression is reduced as estrogen levels decrease, such as occurs after menopause (estrogen plays a role in collagen synthesis and organization).

(Sources for the above: *Journal of Dermatological Science*, September 2007, pages 217–226; Molecular *and Cellular Biochemistry*, September 2005, pages 63–72; and *Glycoconjugate Journal*, May–June 2002, pages 287–293).

☹ **Renergie Microlift R.A.R.E., Superior Lifting Cream SPF 15 Sunscreen** *($78 for 1.7 ounces)* doesn't deserve consideration because it does not contain the UVA-protecting ingredients of titanium dioxide, zinc oxide, avobenzone, Mexoryl SX (ecamsule), or Tinosorb. Lancome knows better and should be ashamed to offer such an inferior product as a means of making collagen-depleted skin look better. By the way, the base formula is as boring as watching paint dry.

😐 **$$$ Renergie Night, Night Treatment** *($88 for 2.5 ounces)* claims to accelerate surface cell renewal so that skin is "re-energized" and "looks well-rested." Sounds great, but those benign claims can be made for just about any moisturizer no matter what it contains. All in all, Renergie Night is a very expensive basic moisturizer whose jar packaging won't keep the good ingredients (which there are woefully little of) stable. It contains mostly water, squalane, silicone, glycerin, thickeners, coloring agent, and wax. The formula may be exclusive to Lancome, but no one else would want it anyway.

☹ **Renergie Intense Lift Masque, Cooling Lifting Masque with Vegetal Protein** *($41 for 3.4 ounces)* lists alcohol as the second ingredient and contains more coloring agents and mineral pigments than helpful ingredients for any skin type. What an all-around bad product that's an absurd waste of money!

LANCOME SOLEIL EXPERT & ULTRA PRODUCTS

☺ **Soleil Expert Sun Care SPF 15 Face & Body Lotion with Pure Vitamin E** *($27.50 for 5 ounces)* is a good, in-part avobenzone sunscreen in a lightweight moisturizing base. It's not "expert" sun care because the formula is short on antioxidants to help boost skin's environmental defenses, but it's still an option for normal to slightly oily, breakout-prone skin.

☺ **Soleil Expert Sun Care SPF 25 Face & Body Lotion with Pure Vitamin E** *($27.50 for 5 ounces)* is similar to the Soleil Expert Sun Care SPF 15 above, except it contains a higher amount of active ingredients to achieve its SPF rating. Otherwise, the same review applies.

☺ **$$$ Soleil Expert Sun Care SPF 30 High Sun Protection Face Creme with Pure Vitamin E** *($26.50 for 1.7 ounces)* contains a very small amount of vitamin E, so, "pure" or not, it's of little benefit to skin. The inclusion of balm mint extract isn't a plus, but the small amount is unlikely to cause irritation. This is otherwise a good option for normal to oily skin, and shields skin from UVA rays with its in-part avobenzone sunscreen.

☺ **$$$ Soleil Expert Sun Care SPF 15 Oil-Free Sun Protection Face Creme with Pure Vitamin E** *($26.50 for 1.7 ounces)* is, save for a reduced amount of active ingredients, similar to the Soleil Expert Sun Care SPF 30 High Sun Protection Face Creme with Pure Vitamin E above, and the same review applies.

☺ **$$$ Soleil Expert Sun Care SPF 15 Water-Light Body Spray with Pure Vitamin E** *($27.50 for 5 ounces)* leaves skin wanting more in terms of antioxidants, but is otherwise a very good, spray-on sunscreen that includes avobenzone for UVA protection. The water-resistant liquid lotion formula is best for normal to slightly dry skin.

😐 **$$$ Soleil Ultra Expert Sun Care SPF 50 Sunscreen Face and Body Lotion, for Sensitive Skin** *($32.50 for 5 ounces)* contains too many sunscreen actives to be considered a viable option for sensitive skin, and the propylene glycol can enhance their penetration into skin, another minus for sensitive skin. And why add fragrance? Someone at Lancome must have missed Skin Care 101 if they thought that would be good for sensitive skin! An in-part titanium dioxide sunscreen helps provide broad-spectrum protection, but the base formula is mundane and not worth the expense.

😐 **$$$ Soleil Ultra Expert Sun Care SPF 50 Sunscreen Face Cream, for Sensitive Skin** *($29.50 for 1.7 ounces)* is a lighter version of the Soleil Ultra Expert Sun Care SPF 50 product above. It also features an in-part titanium dioxide sunscreen, and contains fragrance. Another point of contention for those with sensitive skin is the amount of alcohol in this product, not to mention the amount of preservatives, listed well before any type of soothing agent.

LANCOME FLASH BRONZER PRODUCTS

☹ **Flash Bronzer Airbrush, Multi-Angle Self-Tanning Spray** *($28 for 4 ounces)* is an aerosol self-tanning mist that allows you to spray skin from any angle, but what's sprayed on is mostly alcohol. That, coupled with the many irritating fragrance components, does not make this a self-tanner to consider above most others.

☹ **Flash Bronzer Custom Color Tinted Self-Tanning Face Lotion** *($29.50 for 1.7 ounces)* is a sheer self-tanning lotion with a tiny amount of dihydroxyacetone, so unless you apply this haphazardly, it's pretty much mistake-proof. However, it isn't worth considering over similar options from Dove or Olay because this one contains volatile fragrance components, including eugenol and citronellol.

☺ **$$$ Flash Bronzer Deep Colour Self-Tanning Face Gel with Pure Vitamin E** *($26 for 1.7 ounces)* is a basic but effective self-tanning gel that's a good option for oily skin. It contains dihydroxyacetone, just as most self-tanners do. The amount of alcohol is not cause for concern.

☺ **$$$ Flash Bronzer Medium Colour Self-Tanning Face Gel with Pure Vitamin E** *($26 for 1.7 ounces)* is nearly identical to the Flash Bronzer Deep Colour Self-Tanning Face Gel above, except it contains more dihydroxyacetone, so the result is darker color.

☹ **Flash Bronzer Glow N' Wear Natural Tan** *($29 for 5 ounces)* lists alcohol as the second ingredient and contains a bevy of potentially irritating fragrance components. This is not worth considering over other fast-drying self-tanning products, though it's nice that you get to choose between Natural Tan and Shimmer Tan options.

☺ **$$$ Flash Bronzer Instant Colour Self-Tanning Leg Gel with Pure Vitamin E** *($28.50 for 4.4 ounces)* is very similar to the Flash Bronzer Deep Colour Self-Tanning Face Gel above, and there's no reason this "leg" product cannot be applied to skin anywhere on the body, including the face. The main difference, beyond price and size, is the mica this version contains. It lends a soft shimmer to skin, which you may or may not want for your face.

☺ **$$$ Flash Bronzer Medium Colour Oil-Free Tinted Self-Tanning Lotion for Face with Pure Vitamin E** *($26 for 1.7 ounces)* is a standard self-tanning lotion for normal to dry skin. It contains dihydroxyacetone as well as caramel color, which provides an instant sheer tint, while mica lends a soft shimmer finish.

☺ **$$$ Flash Bronzer Medium Colour Self-Tanning Lotion for Body with Pure Vitamin E** *($27 for 5 ounces)* may be used on the face, too, so don't let the "body" designation dissuade you. This is a standard, but good, self-tanning lotion for normal to dry skin that contains dihydroxyacetone to turn skin a darker color.

✓ ☺ **$$$ Flash Bronzer Tinted Self-Tanning Moisturizing Mousse with Pure Vitamin E** *($29.50 for 5.3 ounces)* is an excellent self-tanner for dry to very dry skin. The creamy mousse contains a beneficial amount of petrolatum and glycerin and the dihydroxyacetone turns skin tan. Mica provides a soft shimmer finish, and the iron oxides provide some instant-gratification color. In addition, this product omits the irritating fragrance components that are present in some of the other Flash Bronzer products. Well done, and truly unique!

OTHER LANCOME PRODUCTS

☺ **$$$ Ablutia Fraicheur, Purifying Foaming Cleanser** *($27 for 6.8 ounces)* is a very standard, detergent-based, water-soluble cleanser that can be drying for some skin types, though it is appropriate for someone with normal to oily skin.

☺ **$$$ Clarifiance, Oil-Free Gel Cleanser** *($27 for 6.8 ounces)* is an exceptionally basic water-soluble cleanser for normal to slightly oily skin. The price is completely out of whack for what you get, but it is an option if you want to overspend and ignore the better options from L'Oreal or Neutrogena.

😐 **$$$ Galatee Confort, Comforting Milky Creme Cleanser** *($27 for 6.8 ounces)* remains a standard, creamy cleanser for dry to very dry skin. It does not rinse without the aid of a washcloth, and is not for anyone with blemishes, however small. The amount of fragrance components demands complete removal from skin lest you risk irritation.

☺ **$$$ Mousse Confort, Comforting Creamy Mousse Cleanser, for Normal to Dry Skin** *($21 for 4.2 ounces)* is a standard, detergent-based cleanser that can be an option for normal to oily skin. It would be too drying for dry skin.

☺ **$$$ Bi-Facil, Double-Action Eye Makeup Remover** *($24 for 4.2 ounces)* is a good water- and silicone-based makeup remover that would be rated higher if it were fragrance-free and left out the questionable preservative quaternium-15. Still, this works well to quickly remove stubborn and waterproof makeup.

😐 **$$$ Effacil, Gentle Eye Makeup Remover** *($24 for 4.2 ounces)* is not gentle due to the amount of detergents and fragrance it contains. It's essentially a watered-down water-soluble cleanser, and not really worth adding to your routine unless you're a soap devotee.

☺ **$$$ Exfoliance Confort, Comforting Exfoliating Cream** *($23 for 3.4 ounces)* is a rich, creamy topical scrub for dry to very dry skin. It contains polyethylene as the abrasive agent, which is great. The only drawback is that the emollients and silicone don't rinse well from skin, so you may need to use this with a washcloth, which exfoliates too (so why use the scrub at all?).

😐 **$$$ Resurface-C Microdermabrasion, Skin Polishing and Radiance Renewing System** *($85 for the kit)* marks Lancome's contribution to the group of microdermabrasion-at-home kits. The twist they provide here is a vitamin C serum in place of the more standard soothing moisturizer or battery-operated polishing sponge. As it turns out, this serum is the best part of the kit, though it's a surprisingly one-note product, as I'll explain in a moment.

Sold as a two-step system, Step 1 is the **Polishing Cream**. It contains aluminum oxide crystals, just like most microdermabrasion-in-a-jar products. Lancome's up-sell is something the company refers to as Physio-Polish Enhancer, which is described as "a safe and gentle exfoliation process that breaks the bonds holding the dead skin cells to the surface." The skin cells then "travel to the top layer so the mechanical exfoliator, Aluminum Oxide Crystals, can sweep them away more effectively." A washcloth can provide the exact same benefit. There is nothing special about the scrub particles that enhance this process. It appears that Lancome's claim is nothing more than marketing nonsense. At its heart the Polishing Cream is merely a mechanical scrub, though the abrasiveness of the aluminum oxide crystals is softened by the emollient base of mineral oil, silicone, glycerin, and shea butter. The mineral oil slightly impedes rinsing, but the instructions do correctly indicate to "rinse thoroughly," so it's a minor issue.

After rinsing, you're directed to apply the **Radiance Renewing Vitamin C Serum**. This somewhat thick serum makes skin feel wonderfully silky thanks to its silicone content, and it contains 5% ascorbic acid (vitamin C) in very stable packaging. It would be better, however, if this serum contained an array of antioxidants as well as some cell-communicating ingredients and an anti-irritant or two. As is, it's noteworthy as a vitamin C product, but as beneficial as this ingredient is for skin, it takes more than one good antioxidant (or any other "buzz" ingredient) to take the best care of skin. Of more concern for use following the Polishing Cream is that the acid component of ascorbic acid can irritate skin. That's not the best thing to do immediately following a topical abrasive scrub, though this serum can be used separately if you're curious to see what vitamin C does for your skin. Immediately following the Polishing Cream, you would be wise to apply a soothing moisturizer loaded with antioxidants, such as those from the Clinique Repairwear line.

☺ **$$$ Tonique Confort, Comforting Rehydrating Toner, for Normal to Dry Skin** *($21 for 6.8 ounces)* is a very good toner for its intended skin type. It contains plenty of water-binding agents, plant oil, and antioxidant vitamin E, all in stable packaging.

😐 **$$$ Tonique Douceur, Alcohol-Free Freshener** *($21 for 6.8 ounces)* is mostly water, glycerin, and rose water. This product is basic and minimally effective for normal to dry skin, unless your only objective is to use a toner to remove the last traces of makeup.

😐 **$$$ Bienfait Multi-Vital SPF 30 Sunscreen Cream** *($41 for 1.7 ounces)* has avobenzone for sufficient UVA protection, but that's the only highlight of this daytime moisturizer for normal to oily skin. Alcohol is the fourth ingredient, which isn't great but is not abysmal, and the antioxidants are subject to deterioration due to jar packaging. What a shame, because this moisturizer has more antioxidants than Lancome typically offers.

☺ **$$$ Bienfait Multi-Vital SPF 30 Sunscreen Lotion** *($41 for 1.7 ounces)* would rate a Paula's Pick if not for the many volatile fragrance components. Although these aren't predominant, they're a potential cause for concern and don't add anything helpful to this in-part avobenzone sunscreen. The base formula is antioxidant-rich and stably packaged, two uncommon traits for a Lancome product. This is still appropriate for normal to oily skin.

😐 **$$$ Bienfait Multi-Vital Night, High Potency Night Moisturizing Cream** *($46 for 1.7 ounces)* makes a big deal out of the vitamins it contains, which are said to help with skin's nightly recovery process. Don't bet on it, because the jar packaging won't keep them stable once this product is in use, and the amount of vitamins is paltry—there's actually more coloring agent. (What would you rather have, a pretty tinted moisturizer or an antioxidant-rich one?) This has the requisite silky, moist texture for normal to dry skin, but that's not enough to justify the price or jibe with the state-of-the-art claims being made for this average moisturizer.

😐 **$$$ Glow Sensuelle, Daily Luminous Face Moisturizer** *($30 for 1.7 ounces)* is a basic moisturizer for normal to dry skin. It has an elegant texture and includes a tiny amount of the self-tanning ingredient dihydroxyacetone for a hint of color. The number of volatile fragrance components is cause for concern due to their irritation potential, and they make this less desirable than similar, less-expensive options from Dove or Olay.

😐 **$$$ Hydra Zen, Advanced De-Stressing Moisturizing Cream, for Normal/Combination Skin** *($46 for 1.7 ounces)* is supposed to be relaxation in a jar, or at least that's what the name and ad copy suggest. Even if you could apply something to the face to make it calmer, according to Hydra Zen that would only take a moisturizer, because that's all this product is. The only unique thing about Hydra Zen is the name. If mind over matter works, then you will feel calmer, but it probably isn't from applying this good, but rather ordinary, ho-hum, silicone-based, lightweight moisturizer that contains minimal water-binding agents and antioxidants.

😐 **$$$ Hydra Zen, Advanced De-Stressing Moisturizing Cream, for Dry Skin** *($46 for 1.7 ounces)* has a lot more going for it formula-wise than the version for Normal/Combination Skin above. Unfortunately, most of the intriguing ingredients are going to break down shortly after this jar-packaged product is opened. What a shame, because it is otherwise a great option for normal to dry skin.

😐 **$$$ Nutrix Royal, Intense Lipid Repair Cream, for Dry to Very Dry Skin** *($52 for 1.6 ounces)* contains a terrific blend of emollients to address the needs of its intended skin types. Jar packaging won't keep the tiny amount of antioxidants stable, so this ends up being a fairly expensive moisturizer whose benefits are easily obtained from other products that offer dry skin even more.

☺ **$$$ Nutrix, Soothing Treatment Cream, for Dry to Very Dry/Sensitive Skin** *($42 for 1.9 ounces)* was brought back by Lancome due to popular demand. First launched in 1936, this remains a very good, though basic, moisturizer for very dry skin. The fragrance components (and fragrance itself) are not suitable for sensitive skin. Two forms of lecithin are nice for skin, but skin needs more and, when you think about it, you wouldn't now be using just about anything that was made in 1936, from a washing machine to a typewriter (and TVs and microwaves weren't even invented).

😐 **$$$ Platineum Hydroxy(a)-Calcium, Re-Densifying and Strengthening Cream SPF 15** *($108 for 1.7 ounces)* has an in-part titanium dioxide sunscreen, which is great. What's disappointing is the mundane formula and jar packaging that won't keep the tiny amount of vitamin E stable. The ingredient hydroxyapitate is what's said to be responsible for making mature skin stronger and denser. This mineral (distantly related to pure calcium) is used in dermal fillers (Radiesse) and other plastic surgery procedures such as chin augmentation. Just because injecting something into the skin has benefit doesn't mean that rubbing it on the skin has benefit, or any effect at all for that matter. As it turns out it doesn't, and there is no research demonstrating that topical application can make aging, thinned skin stronger, which leaves you with a needlessly expensive daytime moisturizer for normal to dry skin.

☹ **Progres Eye Cream** *($52 for 0.5 ounce)* is an emollient moisturizer for dry skin anywhere on the face. It is not recommended because it contains two preservatives that are contraindicated for use in leave-on products, not to mention that the fragrance is overkill for the delicate eye area.

✓☺ **$$$ Re-Surface Eye, Retinol Concentrate Wrinkle Corrector for Eyes** *($47 for 0.5 ounce)* is a very good, fragrance-free moisturizer that is an option for use around the eyes. It contains a good amount of vitamin E and retinol, and in packaging that keeps them stable during use. Why can't more Lancome products be as well-formulated as this one?

😐 **$$$ Secret De Vie, Ultimate Cellular Reviving Creme** *($225 for 1.7 ounces)*. The major secret here is how utterly ordinary this ultra-pricey moisturizer is. I suppose Lancome didn't want to be left out of the burgeoning group of moisturizers with high-tech claims and staggering price tags. Describing itself as "Lancome's ultimate luxury," Secret De Vie asks you to believe that its key ingredient complex, Extrait de Vie (extract of life), "delivers intense restorative action to six major cell types for instant, visible, exceptional results." Notice that Lancome is trying very hard in this seductive wordplay to attempt to convince consumers that spending this much on a special formula (one that is shockingly similar to almost every other Lancome cream being sold) is somehow worth the extra expense. The company didn't even bother to use stable packaging, instead choosing a futuristic, orb-like jar.

Extrait de Vie does sound romantic and exotic, but there is nothing in this product that is in any way unique or even moderately interesting. The majority of the product consists of water, silicones, glycerin, thickener, silicone polymer, aluminum starch, wax, vitamin E, and several plant extracts, including peppermint leaf (though the amount is likely too small to cause irritation). Paying significantly more for this versus almost any of Lancome's other moisturizers, none of which are as impressive as what most other Lauder-owned companies are offering, is not good skin care.

😐 **$$$ Secret De Vie Eye, Ultimate Cellular Reviving Eye Creme** *($135 for 0.5 ounce)* is an emollient moisturizer for dry skin anywhere on the face, but the price is outrageous for what you get. Here, there's no reason to comment on the jar packaging, because there are no light- or air-sensitive ingredients in this far-from-ultimate eye cream.

☹ **Sensation Totale, Continuous-C Perfecting Complex** *($47.50 for 1 ounce)* is positioned as Lancome's premier vitamin C product, but there isn't much vitamin C in here, and the amount of alcohol (it's the third ingredient after water and silicone) makes this a potentially irritating product. This is not worth considering over countless other products whose vitamin C content bests this and that don't present the risk of needless irritation.

☺ **UV Expert 20, Face & Body Protection Daily Moisturizing Cream SPF 20** *($35 for 3.4 ounces)* got a lot of press as L'Oreal blitzed the media with claims that their ecamsule (Mexoryl SX) sunscreen is the preferred active sunscreen for UVA protection. Ecamsule is a very effective, worthwhile UVA sunscreen. However, it is not a must-have. It also doesn't offer the best protection under the sun (titanium dioxide and zinc oxide still provide more protection than ecamsule, especially when you consider that they also provide UVB protection). And it isn't preferred to avobenzone, provided the avobenzone is carefully formulated so it remains stable. This sunscreen lotion contains ecamsule, avobenzone, and titanium dioxide as actives (along with octocrylene, which primarily provides UVB protection and helps to stabilize avobenzone), so the UVA spectrum is definitely covered. What's disappointing is that the base formula is so boring. Not a single antioxidant, elegant water-binding agent, or cell-communicating ingredient shows up. Compare this to the Estee Lauder and Clinique sunscreens that provide broad-spectrum protection and have an array of skin-identical substances plus antioxidants, and honestly, what's all the fuss about?

☹ **Hydra-Intense Masque, Hydrating Gel Mask with Botanical Extract** *($27 for 3.4 ounces)* lists alcohol as the second ingredient, which doesn't make this mask the least bit hydrating. This is about as do-nothing (except irritate) as do-nothing products get!

☹ **Pure Empreinte Masque, Purifying Mineral Mask with White Clay** *($27 for 3.4 ounces)* has the makings of a very good clay mask for oily skin, but the inclusion of camphor was unwise and makes this not preferred to almost any other clay mask being sold.

LANCOME MAKEUP

FOUNDATION: ✓☺ $$$ Teint Idole Ultra Enduringly Divine and Comfortable Makeup *($36)* is a notable improvement over the original Teint Idole Makeup. As one of the genuine ultra-matte foundations, the latter provided long wear and proficient coverage, but application had to be quick and precise because mistakes were not easy to correct. I am thrilled that those negatives have been banished with this updated formula. It has a near-weightless, silky texture with a fluidity that makes blending a breeze. It sets to a strong matte finish (and still does so faster than other foundations for oily skin), but you have enough play time to get it blended on smoothly and evenly—and if you don't, mistakes can be buffed out.

The latest pigment technology allows Lancome to achieve a long-wearing, oil-absorbing matte finish without creating a flat or masklike appearance. Seventeen medium-to-full-coverage shades are available, and here's where things start to decline a bit. Most of the fair to light shades are excellent, but the deeper shades have an orange to copper cast that even the Lancome counter makeup artist commented were "bad shades" that "need more work." I love it when cosmetics salespeople openly agree with me; after all these years I still savor those moments. You should be cautious with the following shades: Suede 2, which can turn peach, and Suede 1, Suede 4, and Bisque 8, which are all blatantly peach or copper. Suede 5 is the only good option for dark skin tones, and, overall, the Buff range of shades (also known as Intensity II) is the most workable for light to medium skin tones. Does this foundation last for 14 hours? Yes, but those with very oily skin will still need to blot and powder before the end of the day.

✓☺ $$$ Dual Finish Versatile Powder Makeup *($34.50)* has been part of Lancome's foundation lineup for years and has deservedly attained classic status. This talc-based wet/dry powder foundation offers a soft matte finish and a selection of 25 beautiful colors for fair to very dark skin. The application, especially when used dry, is smooth and even with a silky, almost creamy-feeling texture that's best for normal to dry skin. The squalane and mineral oil in the formula are not the best ingredients to temper shine, but they keep this powder from looking too dry or chalky. Using Dual Finish wet is tricky because these types of foundations tend to go on streaky. It is best used dry, and applied with a brush for sheer coverage or a makeup sponge for medium coverage.

✓☺ $$$ Dual Finish Fragrance Free Versatile Powder Makeup *($34.50)* has the same formula as the original Dual Finish Versatile Powder Makeup above, minus the fragrance. An interesting point is that this version comes in only eight shades, but they're all excellent and correspond exactly with the same-named shades in the fragranced Dual Finish.

☺ $$$ Color Ideal Precise Match Skin Perfecting Makeup SPF 15 *($35)* does have impressive UVA protection (titanium dioxide is the sole active ingredient). The big claim is that the pigments in this makeup adapt to your skin tone to provide a perfect match. Although the selection of 15 shades is a mostly neutral lot that includes options for fair to dark skin, it turns out that Lancome's "precision matching" isn't that precise. I tried a couple of shades on my skin, one of which initially matched quite well. Yet the final result revealed that the color lightened noticeably as it dried, making me look unnaturally pale. The darker shade (too dark to match my skin exactly) also lightened a bit, but remained an obvious mismatch. This was very unlike my experience with Cover Girl's TruBlend Make-Up ($8.99), a foundation that makes similar shade-matching claims that in that case are legitimate.

Still, there is much to love about this Lancome foundation. It has a supremely silky, nearly weightless texture that meshes well with skin, setting to a satin-matte finish that does a great job of keeping excess shine in check. Given that, it's not surprising that those with normal to very oily skin will appreciate this foundation the most. Coverage goes from sheer to medium, and building coverage doesn't create a thick or heavy appearance. The following shades are too pink, peach, or copper for most skin tones: I-40C, III-20C, and IV-20C. Shade II-20W may be too yellow for some medium skin tones, while shades IV-30W and IV-40N are beautiful options for dark skin tones. The bottom line is that this, like all foundations, demands careful evaluation in natural light so you can be sure you're getting the best match. The good news is that most Lancome counters offer trial samples, an option I encourage!

☺ **$$$ Magique Matte Soft-Matte Perfecting Mousse Makeup** *($37)* is Lancome's version of sister company Maybelline New York's Dream Matte Mousse Foundation ($8.99). The formulas are nearly identical, and perform the same. With either foundation you get a silky, whipped texture that glides over skin and feels ultra-light. Coverage goes from sheer to medium and the finish is slightly powdery and matte, making it best for normal to oily skin (those with very oily skin will need something more absorbent, such as Lancome's Teint Idole Ultra Enduringly Divine and Comfortable Makeup). Be cautious if you have even the slightest bit of dry skin, because this type of silicone-based foundation will exaggerate it to the nth degree. Otherwise, you'll get a smooth, long-wearing foundation that comes in 12 mostly excellent shades. Although Lancome usually bests Maybelline (and L'Oreal) for neutral foundation shades, that's not the case here. Both versions provide equal numbers of viable, real skin tones. If you're considering Magique Matte (perhaps because Lancome is offering a free gift with purchase), watch out for Buff 3, Bisque 4, and Bisque 6, all of which are slightly peach. Suede 2 and Suede 4 are great shades for dark (but not very dark) skin tones.

☺ **$$$ Renergie Lift Makeup SPF 20** *($38)* is positioned as Lancome's anti-aging makeup (which it isn't), but thankfully it does have excellent sun protection and that goes a long way toward reducing the development of wrinkles and skin discolorations when worn daily! All the anti-aging claims and statistics in the world don't mean a thing without a sufficient sunscreen in your daily routine, and this in-part titanium dioxide foundation is a great way to get it. This silky liquid foundation is smooth and a pleasure to blend. The finish is natural and slightly moist, and provides medium coverage without creasing into lines. You probably guessed that this won't lift the skin anywhere, but by creating the illusion of smoother, even-toned skin it can make wrinkles (we're talking superficial lines, not pronounced wrinkles) look less apparent—silicone technology comes through again! Twelve shades are available, with the only missteps being the slightly peach Lifting Dore 10, Lifting Clair 30, and slightly orange Lifting Dore 30. If you have normal to dry skin and want to experience a state-of-the-art foundation with effective sun protection, this is highly recommended.

☺ **$$$ Bienfait Multi-Vital Teinte High Potency Tinted Moisturizer SPF 30** *($42)* is one of the few tinted moisturizers with a high SPF rating and sufficient UVA protection, thanks to its in-part titanium dioxide sunscreen. Although closer to a light-coverage foundation than a tinted moisturizer (it isn't as sheer as you might think given the name), it has a light lotion texture that blends easily and would be suitable for normal to slightly dry skin. It has a soft, dewy finish and blurs minor flaws nicely. The main issue is that all but one of the four shades lean toward the peachy side, and this isn't sheer enough to accommodate for the color shift. This is definitely one to test at the counter, though if you have a light (not fair) skin tone, Shade 1 is worthwhile. By the way, Lancome's claim that this product is vitamin-enriched makes it sound like it's bursting with antioxidants, and it isn't. They're in here, but not in amounts that will make a discernible difference.

☹ **$$$ Absolue Makeup Absolute Replenishing Cream Makeup SPF 20** *($55)* is Lancome's most expensive foundation. Is it worth it? The disappointing lack of sufficient UVA protection doesn't get this foundation off to a good start. However, its creamy application and silky, slightly moist finish are bound to please those with dry skin. Ironically, for a creamy foundation this isn't an ideal formula for someone with very dry skin. That's because it contains silicone and water-binding agents rather than the oils or emollient ingredients that would provide the extra moisturizing necessary to make very dry skin feel smooth and comfortable.

The real reason to consider this foundation is that it provides full coverage without looking heavy or too thick. It conceals without looking too conspicuous, so if you need significant coverage, have dry skin, and are willing to pair this with a broad-spectrum sunscreen, it is an option. The shade selection is smaller than Lancome's typical assortment. With ten colors, you'd hope every one would be a winner, but watch out for Absolute Almond 10 (too pink), and use caution with Absolute Caramel 10 (slightly peach, but may be OK for tan skin tones). Absolute Pearl 10 is excellent for fair skin, and the remaining shades are fittingly neutral. One last comment: Lancome's justification for this foundation's high price is its claim that the product's "exclusive bio-network" (featuring wild yam and algae) helps "revitalize and restore skin elasticity." Unfortunately, there's no proof anywhere that those ingredients can do that. Just as their Absolue skin-care products are ineffective for this purpose, so is this foundation that shares the Absolue name and overhyped ingredients. Any anyway, there's more fragrance in this makeup than yam or algae.

☹ **$$$ Adaptive All-Day Skin-Balancing Makeup SPF 10** *($33)* is one of the few Lancome foundations that offers sufficient UVA protection with a titanium dioxide sunscreen, although the SPF 10 is disappointing and ultimately what prevents this otherwise excellent foundation from earning a higher rating. Just like similar foundations from the Lauder companies, Lancome's Adaptive claims to be *the* foundation solution for combination skin because it mattifies oily areas and hydrates dry areas so that skin is unified. There is no way a foundation can sense where your skin may be dry or oily and adjust itself accordingly. If extreme combination skin is the issue, you need to adjust what you do before making up (such as applying an emollient moisturizer over the dry areas), choose a foundation that is designed to handle oily areas (which is precisely how Adaptive measures up), and use an absorbent powder over the oily areas to touch up your makeup. Texture-wise, this is one of the silkiest foundations I have experienced. Lancome has really raised the performance bar when you also consider this foundation's superb blendability, natural matte finish, and sheer to light coverage that evens skin tone without masking it. Unfortunately, Lancome has reduced the color choices for Adaptive to only a handful of shades, with no options for darker skin tones.

☹ **$$$ Photogenic Skin-Illuminating Makeup SPF 15** *($35)* may be, at least if you believe Lancome's assertions, the foundation that puts your skin in its best light. Featuring Photo-Flex Complex, this makeup supposedly self-adjusts so your skin looks radiant in any light. I didn't see that happening, but that doesn't mean this isn't a worthwhile foundation. Disappointingly, the sunscreen lacks sufficient UVA protection. However, this has a lovely smooth texture that blends superbly and sets to a satin-matte finish. Photogenic provides light to medium coverage and is best for normal to slightly dry skin. Among the nine shades, avoid Bisque 2. Ivoire 2 is a great shade for fair skin, though using this foundation demands a reliable sunscreen that provides skin with sufficient UVA protection.

☹ **$$$ Aqua Fusion Teinte Continuous Infusing Tinted Moisturizer SPF 20** *($37)* lacks the UVA-protecting ingredients of titanium dioxide, zinc oxide, avobenzone, Tinosorb, or Mexoryl SX, which is a shame—because this is otherwise an excellent sheer-to-light-coverage foundation for normal to oily skin. It begins creamy, but dries to a matte finish that remains slightly moist to the touch (it appears matte but feels moist). All four shades are terrific—if only this could be a one-step product for color, coverage, and sufficient sun protection! Since it isn't, this is best for someone with normal to slightly dry skin willing to wear an effective sunscreen underneath, which seems unnecessarily redundant.

☹ **Imanance Tinted Day Creme SPF 15** *($41)* has some positives, including an in-part titanium dioxide–based SPF 15 and natural-looking sheer coverage. Yet what outweighs these traits is that almost all of the shades are appalling and the formula contains the preservatives methylisothiazolinone and methylchloroisothiazolinone (also known as Kathon CG), which is not recommended for use in leave-on products, particularly any to be used around the eye area.

CONCEALER: ✓ ☺ $$$ Absolue Concealer Radiant Smoothing Concealer *($30)* is a creamy concealer with a deceptively light texture. It easily smooths over skin, offering moderate coverage and a soft satin finish that is slightly prone to creasing into lines under the eye. Setting this with a light dusting of powder negates the creasing, and the overall result is quite attractive. There is nothing in this formula to justify the price, but this is a natural-looking concealer. Four of the five shades are exceptional; Absolute Ecru Medium is a bit too peach for its intended skin tone, but may be worth testing.

✓ ☺ $$$ Photogenic Skin-Illuminating Concealer SPF 15 *($25.50)* remains one of the best concealers available. Its titanium dioxide–based sunscreen is a wonderful counterpart to your regular sun protection, whether from a moisturizer or your foundation. Second, it has an incredibly soft, ultra-light texture that blends beautifully—almost melting into the skin—yet covers quite well. The finish is soft matte, and it has only a slight tendency to crease into lines. The six colors are mostly superb. Camee (too peach) should be avoided, and the Correcteur shade is noticeably yellow, but may be suitable for those with light to medium skin struggling with dark circles.

☺ **$$$ Flash Retouche Perfecting Brush-On Concealer Radiance & Anti-Fatigue** *($28)* is a slightly creamy liquid concealer housed in a pen-style applicator. A push button at the bottom of the component sends the product onto the built-in synthetic brush. The application is smooth and even, and it dries to a matte finish that has a soft sheen. Coverage isn't significant, so this is best used as a complexion highlighter. Three shades are available, and although Rose Lumiere is slightly pink, the sheerness negates that. As nice as this is for highlighting, Estee Lauder's Ideal Light Brush-On Illuminator ($24.50) is better because it has a larger shade selection and provides enhanced coverage (meaning you can use it as a concealer or highlighter).

☺ **$$$ Effacernes Waterproof Protective Undereye Concealer** *($25.50)* has a creamy texture that provides significant coverage and allows for smooth blending. The squeeze tube takes some getting used to (it's easy to dispense too much product), but once you acclimate, this concealer is aces, and it doesn't crease! The four shades are mostly neutral, though Porcelaine I is slightly pink. Contrary to the name, this concealer is not waterproof.

☹ **$$$ Maquicomplet Complete Coverage Concealer** *($25.50)* is a smooth, liquidy concealer with excellent, crease-free, medium to full coverage, though each shade suffers from too much shine, and adding shiny particles to a concealer won't distract anyone from what you're trying to hide. What a shame, because most of the ten shades are impeccably neutral.

If you decide to try this, avoid the slightly ash-pink Clair II and use caution with the yellow Correcteur shade.

POWDER: ✓ ☺ $$$ Absolue Powder Radiant Smoothing Powder *($50)* carries a price that may make you look anything but radiant, but wait until you feel its ultra-silky, otherworldly texture. This is one of the most elegant loose powders available. Although the talc-based formula isn't too different from many other powders, the milling process does create a slight difference. This has a non-drying sheer finish suitable for normal to dry skin. All seven shades resemble real skin tones, but watch out for the very shiny Absolute Peche and Absolute Golden—both are suitable for nighttime glamour only, unless you want showgirl shine while at the office or out shopping.

☺ $$$ Colour ID Precise Match Weightless Portable Powder *($29; $19.50 for refills)* comes in a self-contained package that feeds powder onto a built-in brush. It's the brush that's the problem, because for a powder in this price range the brush is not nearly as soft or tapered as it should be. The talc-based loose powder itself is wonderful, with a weightless texture that practically floats over skin without ever looking dry or cakey. Applying this with the brush allows for a sheer dusting, often just the right amount to minimize breakthrough shine. All eight shades are flawless, and include options for fair to dark skin.

☺ $$$ Photogenic Sheer Loose Powder *($32)* and **☺ $$$ Photogenic Sheer Pressed Powder** *($29)* claim to contain the "Photo-Flex Complex of 2-D reflecting powders and 3-D diffusing powders." That's a great hook for these pricey powders! Admittedly, both powders have a soft, finely milled, sumptuous texture and a smooth, dry finish (the Pressed Powder version is slightly drier), but the special effects are nothing more than subtle shine, plain and simple. Although the shine is barely discernible, those hoping to reduce shine may want to look elsewhere. The Loose version comes in nine shades, while the Pressed offers seven. With either powder, almost all of the shades are beautifully soft and neutral, including options for darker (but not very dark) skin tones. Only Soft Bronze stands out as too peachy for dark skin, while Deep Bronze would make a great bronzing powder.

😐 $$$ Star Bronzer Magic Bronzing Brush-Automatic Powder Brush for Face and Body *($31)* is a soft, tapered powder brush whose handle is a reservoir for a sheer, shiny golden copper powder. A push button at the base of the handle shoots powder into the brush, and from there it can be dusted over the face or body. A clever execution to be sure, but this pricey product has little impact other than the sparkling shine it leaves.

☹ Poudre Soleil Sun-Kissed Bronzing Powder *($34.50)* is a pressed bronzing powder that comes in three shiny, overtly copper shades. The Bronze Solaire shade is the best of the colors, but the too-dry texture and flaky shine are disappointing at any price.

BLUSH: ☺ $$$ Magique Blush Soft-Radiant Mousse Blush *($28.50)* is the pricier version of Maybelline New York's Dream Mousse Blush ($6.99) (Maybelline is also owned by L'Oreal, which owns Lancome). The whipped formula has a soft, spongy texture that gives way to a superior application for what's essentially a modified cream-to-powder blush. Almost all of the shimmer- or sparkle-infused shades blend on soft and sheer out quickly, so you can experiment without imparting too much color. Building more color is easy because this layers well. Just like Maybelline's version, this really stays in place after it sets, and you'll experience only minimal fading. It is a fun yet functional departure from powder blush, and is best for normal to slightly dry or slightly oily skin (provided you don't mind having shiny cheeks).

☹ **$$$ Blush Subtil Delicate Oil-Free Powder Blush** *($28.50)* has gotten pricier, but its formula hasn't kept pace with the latest and greatest powder blushes from Estee Lauder and, more importantly for the budget-conscious, L'Oreal. The latter's True Match Super-Blendable Blush ($9.99) is superior to Blush Subtil's dry texture and slightly choppy application. If you decide to try this, it includes mostly matte options and each of the colors goes on quite sheer. Miel Glace and Bronze Glow are shiny. ☹ **$$$ Blush Subtil Shimmer Delicate Oil-Free Powder Blush** *($28.50)* has the same texture as the original Blush Subtil above, but each shade is imbued with sparkles (this isn't a low-glow shimmer). The good news is the sparkles cling well and the colors apply softly, but this isn't enough to make it worth choosing over better blushes that cost less. ☹ **$$$ Blush Subtil Sheer Delicate Oil-Free Powder Blush** *($28.50)* is identical to the original Blush Subtil Delicate Oil-Free Powder Blush above, but the colors are more translucent and the range of shades is smaller.

EYESHADOW: ☺ **Colour Design Sensational Effects Eye Shadow Smooth Hold** *($15)* adds to Lancome's impressive roster of powder eyeshadows, and for the first time in a long time the shades are divided by finish on the tester unit, a very helpful concept. The formula (sold as singles) feels quite silky and applies smoothly without flaking or skipping. Medium to deep shades are easy to soften, and overall this eyeshadow takes full advantage of advances in powder technology. The shades and finishes are divided into matte, sheen, shimmer, metallic, and intense. The matte shades are my preference (no surprise there) and the best ones are Daylight, Positive, Faux Pas, Ciel du Soir, Waif, and Page 6. The sheens have a low-luster finish, appropriate unless your eyelid skin is noticeably wrinkled. Shimmer and Metallic are the shiniest group, while the Intense group is primarily deep shades best for eye lining. Among them, avoid Pink Carpet and Garment, unless you want people to notice your for-shock-value eyeshadow rather than your eyes! As much as I liked this eyeshadow formula, it isn't *quite* on par with the latest options from Clinique and Estee Lauder.

☺ **$$$ Colour Focus Palette 4 Ombres Exceptional Wear EyeColour Quad** *($40)* are sold as preselected quads and although there are several smart groupings, every shade in each has some degree of shine. If your wrinkles are few and your eyelids are taut, this won't be an issue (keep in mind that shine always makes wrinkles more noticeable). The talc-based texture has a supremely smooth application, yet doesn't have quite the buttery smoothness of similar powder eyeshadows from Clinique and Dior. The quads to explore include 4 Style, 4 Romance, 4 Dreaming, 4 Innocence, and 4 Sunset.

☹ **$$$ Ombre Perfecteur Perfecting EyeShadow Base** *($22)* is a waterproof concealer for the eyelid area that is also supposed to extend the wear of eyeshadows. The nude, matte color is applied from a pen outfitted with an angled sponge tip. It tends to go on thick, but does blend evenly. It's OK, but not really necessary if you already use a matte-finish concealer.

☹ **Aquatique Waterproof EyeColour Base** *($23)* is still around and that means Lancome is succeeding at convincing some women to use a separate product (beyond foundation or concealer) to even out the skin tone on their eyelids and to prevent eyeshadows from creasing. The opaque, thick formula creases, and what's worse is that the single color is strongly peach, not exactly what all women need or want.

EYE AND BROW SHAPER: ✓ ☺ **$$$ Artliner Precision Point EyeLiner** *($27)* remains one of the best liquid eyeliners around thanks to its easy-to-apply, quick-drying, long-lasting formula and superior brush. For considerably less money, you can get the same results from L'Oreal's Line Intensifique ($7.99). Regardless of whether you overspend or save, both liquid liners are top picks. Among the Artliner colors, watch out for Action (green) and Blueberry.

☺ **$$$ Modele Sourcils Brow Groomer** *($21)* is a brow mascara available in clear or with a tint. The lightweight formula keeps the brow groomed without being sticky, and the densely bristled brush is best for thicker, unruly brows.

😐 **$$$ Brow Expert Design Kit Powder and Pomade Duo** *($39.50)* includes a pressed brow powder and lightweight brow wax (the pomade) plus mini tools in one compact. The idea is to use the brow powder to shape and fill in brows, then apply the pomade for additional shading and to keep unruly hairs in place. Both products have a dry texture that lays down very soft color, so you'll need several applications to build a noticeable result. The tools are well-shaped but so tiny they're awkward to hold. All told, this is a pricey way to groom and define your brows, and I imagine it's more than most women will want to deal with on a daily basis.

😐 **$$$ Le Crayon Kohl** *($22)* needs routine sharpening, which is why it is not rated higher; but for those willing to tolerate that drawback this is a very good eye pencil. It applies smoothly and is minimally prone to smudging or smearing. There are some wild colors that do little to emphasize eyes, but the classics are there as well. 😐 **$$$ Le Crayon Poudre Powder Pencil for the Brows** *($23)* is one of the best needs-sharpening brow pencils. It goes on easily, if a bit creamy, and the colors (with options for all but black brows) are matte and soft. There's even a good brush at one end for softening and blending the color. This would be rated better if not for the need to keep it sharpened, which isn't convenient.

😐 **$$$ Le Stylo Waterproof Long Lasting EyeLiner** *($22)* is a smooth-textured, automatic, nonretractable eye pencil with mostly shiny colors that all tend to smudge, though no more so than most creamy pencils. This is fine for a smoky look, but it breaks down readily when wet.

😐 **$$$ Color Design Defining and Brightening Eye Pencil Duo** *($28)* is a standard, dual-ended pencil with both ends needing routine sharpening. Each side has a texture that's creamy without being thick, and once set it stays in place surprisingly well (smudging is minimal). The color pairings are clearly more for fun or shock value than for creating a sophisticated makeup design, and one shade in each pencil duo is glittery. Although the pencil itself is good, the colors aren't for everyone, and at this price you should be able to get full use of a product.

LIPSTICK, LIP GLOSS, AND LIPLINER: ✓☺ **$$$ Color Design Sensational Effects Lipcolor Smooth Hold** *($21)* has a smooth, creamy texture that hydrates lips without feeling too thick or greasy. Lancome offers a gorgeous range of shades, divided by finish (though all have the same creamy feel). Shimmer shades impart soft shine, Sheens impart a metallic iridescence, Metallics offer a strong metallic finish, and Creams have a soft, semi-gloss finish. Each shade, particularly the reds, has a great stain so these last longer than standard cream lipsticks. Quite simply, this is Lancome's most impressive lipstick, and at this price it should impress!

✓☺ **$$$ Le Crayon Lip Contour** *($21)* is an above-average automatic, retractable lip pencil with good colors and a smooth application. This lipliner really stays put and is an ideal choice for those prone to having lipstick feather into lines around the mouth.

☺ **$$$ Rouge Sensation Multi-Sensation LipColour** *($22.50)* has a supremely creamy, emollient texture and soft glossy finish. This isn't as greasy as it used to be, but it will still travel into lines around the mouth. The opaque colors are simply stunning.

☺ **$$$ Juicy Rouge Lasting Juicy Shine LipColour** *($21.50)* is a sheer lipstick infused with lots of sparkles for glistening, soft color. Application is slick, but comfortable, though don't expect this to last more than an hour or two before needing a touch-up.

☺ **$$$ Color Fever Lipstick** *($24)* has a name that may make you think the shades are richly opaque, yet that's not the case with this lightweight, semi-creamy lipstick. Color saturation is moderate even when layered. This lipstick's appearance is helped considerably by the light-catching shimmer particles in it, which give each shade an alluring glow that doesn't look over-the-top (meaning you won't have pieces of glitter dotting your lips). Contributing to the price is the debut of Lancome's sleekest lipstick component yet, a gunmetal gray mirrored surface flanked on each side by translucent deep amber panels.

☺ **$$$ Color Fever Gloss** *($22)* is billed as a lip gloss, but is closer to a liquid lipstick thanks to its smooth, moist feel and pigment level. A glossy, non-sticky finish is part of the deal, and most of the colors are striking. Paying this much for gloss is definitely not necessary, but at least Lancome provided exquisite packaging and a cleverly angled sponge-tip applicator that lets you apply more color in less time.

☺ **$$$ Juicy Wear Ultra-Lasting Full Colour and Shine Lip Duo** *($25.50)* is Lancome's version of Max Factor's Lipfinity. You get a lipstick (**Juicy Wear Full Colour Stick**) and a moisturizing top coat (**Seal and Shine**) for use after the lipstick color has set. The concept and application are identical to that of Lipfinity: apply the lip color to clean, dry lips and let it set for 60 seconds. The lipstick initially feels smooth and slightly creamy, but becomes increasingly uncomfortable as it dries. That side effect is why the top coat is vital, because it restores a moist, smooth feel without disrupting the color underneath. Lancome's top coat is largely silicone-based, and as such feels ultra-smooth and imparts a high-gloss shine. Both the lipstick and top coat contain shimmer, and most of the lipstick shades have large particles of glitter, supposedly to offset the matte effect they leave on the lips, although that should be what the top coat delivers.

The obvious question is, Does it last? Yes, it does, and for a good length of time, too. However, just like Lipfinity and all of its imitators, the top coat needs to be applied regularly to maintain a comfortable feel on the lips. Unlike Lipfinity, however, Juicy Wear Ultra-Lasting is not transfer-resistant. A small amount of color does come off on cups, utensils, and after kissing (though light pecks don't seem to disrupt it—I tested that myself). That's a slight strike against Lancome's version, but certainly not a deal-breaker. By the way, L'Oreal's Endless Kissable Shinewear Lip Duo is nearly identical to this product, for nearly one-third the price.

☺ **$$$ Juicy Gelee Crystal Clear Lip Gloss** *($17.50)* is an adorably packaged pot gloss that has a spongy, gel-like texture and a somewhat thick, slightly syrupy application that smooths on and feels surprisingly non-sticky. The translucent, fruit-themed colors may look too bold and bright in the package, but each goes on very soft. If you're a fan of lip gloss, it's a great way to experiment with color without looking too made up or dramatic, and this is considerably less slippery than many others. Just test it first if you have noticeable lines around your mouth.

😐 **$$$ Le Rouge Absolu Reshaping & Replenishing LipColour SPF 15** *($25)* not only continues the trend of department-store lipsticks' prices hitting higher and higher price tags, but also continues Lancome's pattern of launching makeup products with insufficient UVA protection. I could begin to justify the high price of this lipstick if you were at least getting superior sun protection from it, but since that's not the case you're left with a smooth, standard creamy lipstick that, while indeed pleasant, isn't reason enough to indulge. Lipsticks from L'Oreal, Revlon, and Clinique feel just as good as this one, and for considerably less money. If you're curious about how the alleged reshaping of lips is supposed to work, it's impossible to say. If you have uneven lips, applying this lipstick won't correct that, and there's nothing in it that can make lips more plump—this isn't a mini collagen injection in the form of a lipstick. Lancome refers to their "plumping polymer," but it's all wordplay without proof.

☹ **$$$ Rouge Absolu Desir Reshaping & Replenishing LipColour SPF 15** *($25)* has a price that means everything about it should be perfect, but this disappoints from the get-go because it lacks UVA-protecting ingredients. As I checked out the colors I couldn't help but shake my head in exasperation as I overheard the Lancome salesperson discuss the importance of UVA protection with another customer. This creamy lipstick feels great and has some stunning (and stunningly packaged) colors, but with incomplete sun protection, why bother?

☹ **$$$ Le Lipstique LipColouring Stick with Brush** *($22.50)* is a standard pencil with a tapered blending brush at the other end. That's convenient, but not worth the price. This does have some staying power, leaving a slight stain on the lips, and the shade selection is plentiful.

☹ **$$$ Juicy Tubes Ultra Shiny Lip Gloss** *($17.50)* has a thick, viscous application and a moderately sticky, high-gloss finish. It comes in a squeeze tube and offers a range of sheer, trendy colors, many of which seem off-putting in the tube but go on practically colorless. Even the brightest oranges and yellows (yes, yellow) go on very softly.

☹ **Le Rouge Absolu Base Revitalizing Lip Treatment SPF 10 Sunscreen** *($25)* is a very standard clear, pearlized lip balm in lipstick packaging. Not only is the sunscreen SPF rating too low for sufficient daytime protection, but in addition it does not contain the UVA-protecting ingredients of titanium dioxide, zinc oxide, avobenzone, Tinosorb, or Mexoryl SX. This product is not recommended.

MASCARA: ✓☺ $$$ Fatale Exceptional Volume Sculpting 3D Comb Mascara *($23)* takes some getting used to, but once you've mastered the tricky application process, you'll be rewarded with unbelievably long, supremely thick lashes that seem too good to be true. Using a three-sided comb rather than a traditional brush, Fatale demands precise application to avoid clumps and a too-heavy appearance. The instructions tell you to rotate the wand so you're using different sides of the comb, which does help. There's no doubt that applying mascara with a brush is faster, but if you're looking to build dramatically long, lush lashes with minimal clumps, this product should be on your short list. In case you're curious, Fatale is very similar to L'Oreal's Volume Shocking Mascara ($12.95), except that Lancome's version eliminates the lash primer step and offers even more oomph, which is why it is rated higher.

✓☺ **$$$ L'Extreme Instant Extensions Lengthening Mascara** *($23)* is positioned as a lengthening mascara, and it does just that. With a brush similar to mascara hall-of-famer Definicils ($23), L'Extreme quickly elongates lashes with barely a clump. It allows you to create long, fringed lashes with subtle thickness and wears well throughout the day. As impressive as this mascara is, you don't have to spend this much for such results, because other L'Oreal-owned lines have excellent options. Maybelline New York Lash Discovery Mascara ($5.99) and L'Oreal Voluminous Volume Building Mascara ($6.99) are equally adept at lengthening and expertly defining lashes, but that doesn't mean this entry from Lancome is undeserving of a Paula's Pick rating!

✓☺ **$$$ Definicils High Definition Mascara** *($23)* is an extraordinary lengthening mascara that builds some thickness with minimal to no chance of clumping. The only drawback, and this is a minor complaint, is it can go on a bit too wet, which increases the chance of it smearing before your lashes dry.

✓☺ **$$$ Definicils Waterproof High Definition Mascara** *($23)* does everything Lancome's regular Definicils mascara does to lengthen, lightly thicken, and separate the lashes, but with a waterproof formula that wears and wears. It is Lancome's premiere waterproof mascara, and the formula now leaves lashes feeling soft (an uncommon trait for waterproof mascaras).

✓☺ **$$$ Cils Design Pro Custom Design Double Mascara** *($35)* is Lancome's most expensive mascara, but, to their credit, you are getting two mascaras in one package. Step 1 involves sweeping the Define and Lengthen Mascara through lashes, which creates soft separation and elongates lashes without thickening them. Step 2 is a mini comb saturated with a slightly different mascara formula. The directions indicate to begin at the lash root, which deposits a lot of mascara to create a defined, fuller look. If desired, the comb can be used on the outer corner of the lashes to create a thickened, false lash effect. The results can be stunningly dramatic, making the most of every last lash without clumping or smearing. It wears well, too, yet comes off with a water-soluble cleanser. Those who aren't willing to spend this much for mascara should check out L'Oreal's very similar Volume Shocking Mascara ($12.95). Cils Design Pro has a slight application edge, but the price difference should give you pause.

☺ **$$$ Definicils Pro High Definition Curved Brush Mascara** *($23)* has a curved brush with different lengths of bristles on either side. Although not as instantly impressive as original Definicils, this produces long, noticeably thicker lashes after several coats. It also has a slight lifting and curling effect on lashes, and wears all day without flaking or smearing. I agree with Lancome's claim that, compared to regular Definicils, this does create fuller lashes. However, the results aren't so spectacularly better that you should switch to this version, though if it's included in a free gift with purchase, why not give it a try?

☺ **$$$ Hypnose Custom Volume Mascara** *($23)* dares you to go "up to 6 times the volume" for "hypnotic eyes," but real-world testing confirmed this mascara doesn't perform as claimed. This is far from being a poor mascara because it does do a reasonably good job of separating, lengthening, and slightly thickening lashes without a single clump, leaving lashes soft rather than brittle. It also removes well with a water-soluble cleanser. But if you were expecting impossibly long, voluminous lashes, this isn't the mascara for you, especially if you're currently a fan of Lancome's classic Definicils High Definition Mascara.

☺ **$$$ Flextencils Full Extension Curving Mascara** *($23)* claims that its "ultra-curving PowerSHAPE formula with patented brush gives lashes up to 30% more visible length with an eye-opening 30° curve." They then go on to say their claim is based on an in vitro study, which is curious because it is hard to imagine how they duplicated a person's eyelashes in a petri dish, not to mention how that relates to real-life use! Flextencils isn't as out-of-the-box impressive as Lancome's top mascaras, but it is a good choice for a natural look with equal parts of modest length and thickness. This doesn't clump no matter how heavily you apply it, and it does leave lashes softly curled yet no more so than other Lancome, L'Oreal, or Maybelline mascaras.

☺ **$$$ Cils Booster XL Super-Enhancing Mascara Base** *($20)* is a lash primer that really works, and is much better than Lancome's original Cils Booster Mascara Enhancing Base (reviewed below). A pre-mascara, it adds bulk and length to lashes, allowing the actual color-enhancing mascara to cling better and apply evenly. What you'll notice is more thickness and oomph to lashes than using just mascara alone. This type of product isn't for everyone (most women won't want to bother with two steps), but those with short or sparse lashes should give this a try and see for themselves what a difference it makes.

😐 **$$$ L'Extreme Waterproof Instant Extensions Lengthening Mascara** *($23)* marks one of the few times I have been disappointed by a Lancome mascara. Although this withstands tears and swimming (actually, it's so tenacious that it takes more effort than usual to remove it), it builds minimal length and thickness. At best you'll achieve moderate length and a smidgen of thickness with lots of effort, and for this price (and Lancome's reputation as a mascara leader) that's disappointing. If you insist on using a waterproof mascara from Lancome, try their Definicils Waterproof before this unexciting option.

☺ **$$$ Hypnose Waterproof Custom Volume Mascara** *($23)* disappoints compared to its non-waterproof counterpart, but is nevertheless a respectable mascara for length and clean lash separation. Thickness (referred to in the name as "volume") is fairly scarce, but at least this holds up well under water or during a good tear-jerker film.

☺ **$$$ Cils Booster Mascara Enhancing Base** *($19)* is a mascara primer meant to pump up your lashes before you sweep on mascara. Honestly, Lancome is the last line you would expect to offer such a product. The majority of their mascaras are amazingly adept at enhancing lashes all by themselves, making this step completely unnecessary.

☹ **Courbe Virtuose Divine Lasting Curves Mascara** *($23)* comes with beguiling claims, but is a rare letdown from Lancome. I'll even go so far as to say that this is their most disappointing mascara in years. The full, slightly curved brush eventually produces long, curvy lashes, but what a mess to apply! Things are uneven from the start, trying to comb through the clumps only seems to make them worse, and this begins flaking almost as soon as it dries. As for applying this to the lower lashes? Forget about it, unless you want to look like you went to sleep without washing off your mascara!

FACE AND BODY ILLUMINATING/SHIMMER PRODUCTS: ☺ **$$$ Star Bronzer Bronzing Highlighter Radiance and Healthy Glow** *($32)* is a lightweight fluid lotion infused with golden peach shimmer. The shine is intense, but this stays put better than powder-based products and finishes silky-smooth. Although pricey, it's an excellent way to add lots of shine to emphasize a (hopefully sunless) tan.

☺ **$$$ Star Bronzer Magic Golden Spray** *($31)* is a mineral oil–based liquid with yellow-gold shimmer particles. It is an easy way to moisturize dry skin while also adding shimmer, but it remains slick and greasy, and comes off easily on clothing, car seats, and the like. There are more elegant ways to add glisten and gleam to skin than this product.

BRUSHES: Lancome offers a decent assortment of ☺ **$$$ Brushes** *($20.50–$47.50)*, but, although many of them are worthwhile, the overall collection is disappointing compared to those from Bobbi Brown, Stila, Laura Mercier, M.A.C., or Paula's Choice. A consistent issue is the overall size of the brush, with an overriding tendency to be either too small or too large for the intended area. Still, there are some winners here, including the ☺ **$$$ Foundation Brush #2** *($32)*, ☺ **$$$ Bronzer Brush #5** *($35.50)*, ☺ **$$$ Concealer Brush #8** *($23)*, ☺ **$$$ Retractable Lip Brush #9** *($22.50)*, ☺ **$$$ Angle Shadow Brush #13** *($23)*, and ☺ **$$$ Angle Brow Brush #15** *($20.50)*.

SPECIALTY PRODUCTS: ☺ **$$$ Matte Finish Shine-Control Blotting Sheets** *($15.50 for 50 sheets)* are standard, tissue paper–style, non-powdered blotting sheets. They do a great job absorbing excess oil and perspiration and the simple packaging is portable. You don't need to spend this much for oil-absorbing papers, but at least if you choose to do so, you won't be disappointed with the results.

LAURA MERCIER

LAURA MERCIER AT-A-GLANCE

Strengths: Many fragrance-free products; top-notch water-soluble cleansers; very good eye-makeup remover; the serum and serum-type moisturizers are worth a look; some extraordinary foundation and powder products; great powder blush, cream blush, and powder eyeshadows; one impressive mascara; the Liquid Crystal Lip Glace; mostly great shimmer products; the makeup brushes; the Bronzing Gel.

Weaknesses: Expensive; some of the products with sunscreen lack sufficient UVA-protecting ingredients; no product to treat acne or lighten skin discolorations; jar packaging; none of the makeup products with sunscreen contain the right UVA-protecting actives; the various Primers are merely OK; average eye pencil, brow-enhancing, and lip pencil options; tester units are cluttered and not labeled well, though the sales pressure is low key.

For more information about Laura Mercier, call (888) 637-2437 or visit www.lauramercier.com or www.Beautypedia.com.

LAURA MERCIER SKIN CARE

✓☺ **$$$ Foaming One-Step Cleaner** *($35 for 5 ounces)* is a liquid-to-foam, water-soluble cleanser that's an excellent option for normal to dry skin. It removes makeup and rinses easily, and is fragrance-free. The tiny amount of witch hazel is not a cause for concern.

✓☺ **$$$ Oil-Free Gel Cleanser** *($35 for 8 ounces)* is pricey, but is nevertheless an outstanding gentle cleanser for normal to oily skin. The fragrance-free formula contains over a dozen water-binding agents and also some very good soothing agents, though their brief contact with skin doesn't allow them to do much. However, such additives are much better than the exotic and/or potentially irritating plant extracts that most cosmetics include!

✓☺ **$$$ One-Step Cleanser** *($35 for 8 ounces)* is nearly identical to the Foaming One-Step Cleanser above, except this one doesn't have the liquid-to-foam dispensing system. Which one you use is a matter of personal preference, but you get more cleanser for your money here, and the consistency makes this one easier to stretch, which helps offset the expense.

😐 **$$$ Purifying Oil – Light** *($40 for 6.7 ounces)* is an oil-based cleanser and makeup remover for dry to very dry skin. The main ingredients are not "light," and this should not be used by anyone with oily skin. Mercier claims this "leaves less oil molecules on the surface of skin," but that's impossible. The mineral oil base doesn't rinse easily without a washcloth, and no matter how you slice it, more oil molecules will be left on your skin than when you began.

😐 **$$$ Purifying Oil – Rich** *($40 for 6.7 ounces)* is more oily than the Purifying Oil – Light above, and is appropriate only for dry to very dry skin. This removes makeup easily, just like most oil-based cleansers, but leaves a greasy film. It contains fragrant plant extracts.

☹ **Gentle Eye Makeup Remover** *($18 for 4 ounces)* is a below-standard, detergent-based eye-makeup remover that is not gentle because it contains comfrey extract and methylisothiazolinone, a preservative not recommended for use in leave-on products.

✓☺ **$$$ Waterproof Eye Makeup Remover** *($18 for 4 ounces)* is a very good, water- and silicone-based eye-makeup remover. The fragrance-free formula is ideal for all skin types, and not a single irritating ingredient was used. You'll find similar options from Almay and Neutrogena for less money, but this is still a winner.

☺ **$$$ Face Polish** *($28 for 3.5 ounces)* is a standard but good topical scrub for normal to slightly oily or slightly dry skin not prone to blemishes. The tiny amounts of irritating plant extracts are not likely to be a problem.

😐 **$$$ Perfecting Water – Light** *($38 for 6.7 ounces)* claims to temporarily "over-hydrate" skin, which isn't a benefit. Too much water isn't healthy for skin, but the reality is that this toner is a fairly basic option for normal to slightly dry skin. The amount of alcohol is not likely to cause irritation, but this fragrance-free toner would be better without it.

☺ **$$$ Perfecting Water – Rich** *($38 for 6.7 ounces)* is a better option than the Perfecting Water – Light, above. The alcohol- and fragrance-free formula contains some good skin-identical ingredients and soothing agents for normal to dry skin.

☹ **$$$ Eyedration Firming Eye Cream** *($38 for 0.5 ounce)* features an absolutely huge ingredient list—but the "meat" of this product is mostly water, emollient, thickener, glycerin, several more thickeners, silicone, and film-forming agents. Barely weighing in for a supporting role are several plant extracts (mostly nonirritating) and antioxidants, along with a few water-binding agents. Had these ingredients been included in greater amounts (and not in jar packaging), this would have been a more impressive formula. It does contain fragrant plant extracts, and nothing in it will significantly firm the skin or reduce puffiness.

☹ **$$$ Flawless Skin Creme, Anti-Aging Treatment** *($95 for 1.7 ounces)* has a great name—is there any doubt what this product promises? Yet the miracle ingredient is "deep sea water." Regardless of depth, water of any kind is not the key to flawless skin. The majority of ingredients in this product appear in hundreds of other moisturizers, which is all this "treatment" really is: a basic moisturizer. What's particularly dismaying is that the many antioxidants and cell-communicating ingredients won't stay potent for long because of jar packaging. Spending this much for what amounts to a letdown isn't advised, but it still has potential for normal to dry skin.

☺ **$$$ Illuminating Brightener** *($68 for 1 ounce)* purports to work on sun spots (brown skin discolorations) while improving skin's clarity. It contains a small amount of sodium ascorbyl phosphate, a stable form of vitamin C—but unlike other forms of vitamin C, this one doesn't have any research proving its skin-lightening ability (though it does function as an antioxidant). In fact, none of the ingredients in this product can act on skin discolorations. It's just a lightweight moisturizer with some good water-binding agents and antioxidants. This would be appropriate for normal to slightly oily or slightly dry skin.

☹ **$$$ Mega Moisturizer Cream with SPF 15** *($42 for 2 ounces)* is a silky moisturizer that features an in-part avobenzone sunscreen. The silicones are suitable for normal to oily skin, but the emu oil and wax are not for anyone prone to breakouts. Unfortunately, jar packaging undermines the effectiveness of the antioxidant vitamins this contains.

☹ **$$$ Moisturizer Cream with SPF 15** *($42 for 2 ounces)* includes avobenzone for UVA protection, and wraps it in a decently emollient base for normal to dry skin. The vitamins will be subject to deterioration shortly after this jar-packaged product is opened.

☺ **$$$ Multi-Vitamin Serum** *($65 for 2 0.6-ounce bottles)* is a two-part product consisting of water-based **Phase 1** and silicone-based **Phase 2**. Both contain ingredients that will smooth and hydrate skin, and both contain several antioxidants, although Phase 2 has slightly more. From a formulary standpoint, there was no need for this product to be split into two phases. The explanation I was given by a Mercier salesperson was that the water in Phase 1 doesn't mix with the plant oils in Phase 2, but that is an issue that any cosmetics chemist could overcome by choosing the correct ingredients to keep them blended together. I suppose Mercier simply wanted her serum to seem different and more scientific, and so consumers are directed to mix several drops from both phases before applying it to the skin. If the mixing step doesn't bother you, this is a very well-formulated, antioxidant-rich serum that is recommended for all but blemish-prone skin. Its packaging ensures the antioxidants will remain stable during use. The firming sensation you get from this product comes from the film-forming agent in Phase 1, which can temporarily make skin feel tauter and look smoother. This product does not contain fragrance, but does contain a small amount of orange oil, which imparts a scent (and may cause irritation, the only misstep in an otherwise superb product).

😐 **$$$ Night Nutrition Renewal Creme, for Normal to Dry Skin** *($55 for 1.7 ounces)* is an OK, rather standard moisturizer for someone with normal to dry skin. The tiny amounts of antioxidants and water-binding agents make the price a bit of a burn. For this amount of money, you should expect much more and it should be in packaging that keeps the antioxidants stable.

😐 **$$$ Night Nutrition Renewal Creme, for Very Dry and Dehydrated Skin** *($55 for 1.7 ounces)* is similar to the Night Nutrition Renewal Cream, for Normal to Dry Skin, above, except this contains slightly more emollients, including canola oil. As such, it is preferred for very dry skin, although the shortage of state-of-the-art ingredients, coupled with the steep price, makes it a less-than-satisfactory choice.

😐 **$$$ Night Nutrition Renewal Eye Creme** *($45 for 0.5 ounce)* is a more emollient version of the Eyedration Firming Eye Cream above, and would work well for dry to very dry skin anywhere on the face. The same comments made above for Eyedration about the antioxidants, skin-identical ingredients, and jar packaging apply here as well.

☹ **Oil Free Moisturizer SPF 15** *($42 for 4 ounces)* lacks sufficient UVA-protecting ingredients and contains enough lavender extract to make it potentially irritating, which isn't good news for any skin type.

😐 **$$$ Renewal Serum** *($75 for 1.5 ounces)* claims to stimulate skin-cell turnover, but it doesn't contain ingredients capable of doing that. It's a water-based serum for all skin types that does contain an impressive amount of green tea. Yet all by itself green tea is a one-note song and not nearly as interesting for skin as healthy amounts of other antioxidants, skin-identical ingredients, and cell-communicating ingredients. This is fragrance-free and an option, just not an exciting one.

☹ **Deep Cleansing Clay Mask** *($32 for 3.7 ounces)* contains a significant amount of irritants, including arnica, balm mint, and orange oil. The clay is joined by emollients, making this both confusing and irritating for all skin types.

☹ **Hydra Soothing Gel Mask** *($32 for 3.7 ounces)* contains lavender oil, which isn't soothing due to its negative effect on skin cells. Without it, this would be a recommended mask for normal to slightly dry skin.

✓☺ **$$$ Intensive Moisture Mask** *($32 for 3.7 ounces)* promises immediate firming, but doesn't deliver. However, what this does do brilliantly is make dry to very dry skin look and feel replenished. More than just a moisturizing mask, the formula contains some very good antioxidants, plant oils, and soothing agents.

☹ **Lip Balm SPF 15** *($20 for 0.12 ounce)* does not contain the UVA-protecting ingredients of titanium dioxide, zinc oxide, avobenzone, Tinosorb, or Mexoryl SX, and is not recommended. What a shame, because this is otherwise a stellar lip balm.

☺ **$$$ Lip Silk** *($20 for 0.4 ounce)* is a very good, Vaseline-based lip balm that contains silicone for a silky finish and lighter texture. This also contains vitamin E and a cell-communicating ingredient. The glycolic and salicylic acids do not function as exfoliants.

LAURA MERCIER MAKEUP

FOUNDATION: ✓☺ **$$$ Flawless Face Silk Creme Foundation** *($40)* has a name that not only makes you want to try it immediately (Flawless? Silk? Yes, please!), but also happens to be 100% accurate. One of the hallmarks of Mercier's foundations is how well they mesh with skin. Her formulas, even this one that provides significant coverage, somehow manage to look very skinlike, primarily because they don't settle into lines, pores, and minor crevices. Flawless Face Silk Creme Foundation's silicone base blends expertly and sets to a silky matte finish. It is one of the few almost-full-coverage foundations that doesn't look too thick and that doesn't dull down healthy skin's natural luminosity. Granted, as exceptional as these qualities are, this foundation still looks like makeup—no one will believe you're sporting a sheer look—but if that's the kind of coverage you're looking for, this deserves serious consideration by those with normal to oily skin. Each of the seven shades is impeccable, but there are no options for someone with dark skin.

✓☺ **$$$ Moisturizing Foundation** *($40)* would be suitable for normal to dry skin seeking medium to almost full coverage. The texture is elegantly light and creamy, leaving a beautiful, slightly dewy finish. Six of the seven colors are excellent, although shades for darker skin tones are absent. Avoid Shell Beige, which is too pink.

✓☺ **$$$ Foundation Powder** *($40)* is a superlative powder foundation that comes in seven gorgeous shades, including options for light and dark (but not very dark) skin tones. This talc-based powder offers a suede-smooth texture, even application, and light to medium coverage when used dry. If you use it wet it provides fuller coverage, but you also run the risk of streaking if you're not careful. If the price isn't too off-putting and you have normal to oily skin, this is a must-try and it's on the very short list of today's best pressed-powder foundations. One caution: Each shade has a hint of shine. While the shine isn't distracting, you should be aware of it if you're looking for a completely matte finish.

✓☺ **$$$ Mineral Powder SPF 15** *($35)* is the first loose-powder mineral makeup from a makeup artist–based line, and right out of the gate Mercier's option trounces the competition. The drawbacks of mineral makeup (potential discoloring over oily areas, making dry skin or dry areas look and feel even drier, messy application—after all, it is loose powder) do apply here to some extent. However, this product's overall excellent attributes balance those negatives and make this a mineral makeup worth exploring. The broad-spectrum sunscreen is provided by 20% zinc oxide, an amount that also lends this powder its opacity and ability to provide nearly full coverage and an absorbent finish. The zinc oxide is joined by pearl powder and lesser amounts of other ingredients common to mineral makeup, including mica and bismuth oxychloride. Together they create a silky, dry texture that blends better on skin than any other mineral makeup I've tested (and I've tested them all!).

Its finish is matte in feel, but the pearl powder lends an attractive, non-sparkling, dimensional glow to skin that keeps it from looking too dull or flat. Only five shades are available (with no options for tan to dark skin tones), but they demand careful testing because they apply either lighter or darker than they appear in the container. Speaking of the container, the sifter has a clever closure that keeps the powder from spilling out during travel, a thoughtful touch. Applying this with a brush nets the most natural results; applying it with a sponge provides a noticeably opaque finish.

☺ **$$$ Oil-Free Foundation** *($40)* still has a lot going for it, but as foundation technology has improved this product has stayed the same, so it is no longer the "top dog" so to speak. But it is definitely worthy of consideration by anyone with normal to oily skin. The fluid, densely pigmented texture blends out to a seamless, soft matte finish with medium coverage that can appear thick unless you blend it meticulously. Twelve shades are on hand, with options for very light but not for very dark skin tones. The only shades to consider avoiding are Shell Beige (slightly pink) and Suntan Beige (slightly peach). Porcelain Ivory is a very good shade for fair skin.

😐 **$$$ Stick Foundation SPF 15** *($40)* shares the same drawback present in most of Mercier's foundations with sunscreen: a lack of sufficient UVA-protecting ingredients. That's always disappointing, but even more so here because this is an otherwise fantastic stick foundation. Its silicone base smooths over skin easily and blends to a natural-looking finish that is skinlike, while still providing light to medium coverage. The formula is perfect for those with normal to dry skin not prone to blemishes (the high wax content that keeps this foundation in stick form is the culprit). As usual, Mercier's shade range is nearly flawless. Among the eight options (no colors for darker skin tones), the only slightly suspect shade is Tawny, but it's still worth testing. If you'd prefer a stick foundation that does provide sufficient sun protection, consider Shiseido Stick Foundation SPF 15 ($35) instead.

☹ **Tinted Moisturizer SPF 20** *($40)* isn't worth considering, despite its light, creamy texture and its easy-blending application, because the SPF lacks UVA-protecting ingredients and because many of the colors, while sheer, tend to le be an too pink or peach. Until Mercier gets the sunscreen right, look to Bobbi Brown, Aveda, or Stila for superior tinted moisturizers.

☹ **Tinted Moisturizer Oil-Free SPF 20** *($40)* is oil-free but is also unfortunately free of the UVA-protecting ingredients of titanium dioxide, zinc oxide, avobenzone, Tinosorb, or Mexoryl SX, and is not recommended.

CONCEALER: ☺ **$$$ Secret Concealer** *($22)* is meant for the eye area and is far more user-friendly than the Secret Camouflage below. It comes in a small pot and offers three decent shades, each with a very creamy-smooth, petrolatum-based texture. It covers well but does tend to crease during the day. Give this a test run before you decide to purchase, and be sure to set it with powder.

☺ **$$$ Undercover** *($22)* comes in a mirrored compact and provides one pan of Secret Concealer and one pan of the Secret Camouflage reviewed below. It's actually a workable combination because the creamy texture of the Secret Concealer mixes well with the stiff, dry Secret Camouflage. A dab of each smooths onto skin easily and provides significant coverage that doesn't call attention to itself (assuming you've blended the edges well). Setting this with powder offers prolonged, nearly creaseless wear and all of the color combinations are workable when mixed (used alone each tends to be too yellow or peach).

☺ **$$$ Secret Brightener** *($30)* is a creamy highlighting pen with a brush-tip applicator. It goes on so sheer you're left wondering if you've really applied anything, but you will see a subtle shimmer finish. When used correctly, this product can create extremely subtle highlights under the eyes, on the brow bone, down the bridge of the nose, or on the collarbone. Both shades are suitable for their intended purpose.

😐 **$$$ Secret Camouflage** *($28)* is a two-sided compact concealer with a thick, dry texture and truly opaque camouflage coverage. All of the duos have yellow to beige or peach to copper colors that can work if mixed in the right proportions, but why would you want to do that when there are so many excellent one-step concealers available? Secret Camouflage was designed as a cover-up for facial blemishes, dark circles, or birthmarks, and if all else has failed, it is an option because of the high level of coverage you'll get. SC4 and SC6 are too peach or copper to recommend; SC3 is the most neutral duo.

😐 **$$$ Flawless Fix Pencil** *($20)* needs routine sharpening (hence the neutral face rating because there are so many great pencils that don't take work to use) and isn't my favorite format for a concealer, but its texture is creamy without being slick, so it stays in place better than similar options and manages to provide medium to full coverage without looking thick. This type of concealer is a no-no for use over blemishes, but is ideal for camouflaging red spots or minor, sun-induced skin discolorations. All four shades are neutral and best for fair to medium skin tones.

POWDER: ✓☺ $$$ Loose Setting Powder *($32)* has an out-of-this-world silky texture that blends beautifully over the skin and leaves a satiny-smooth, dry finish. All of the shades are workable and have a subtle yellow undertone. The formula is talc-based and also includes a small amount of cornstarch, but likely not enough to be problematic for blemish-prone skin. All three shades are beautiful.

✓☺ Pressed Setting Powder *($30)* has many of the same qualities as the Loose Setting Powder above, minus the cornstarch. The texture is smooth and dry but the sole Translucent shade is recommended only for fair to medium skin tones.

☺ $$$ Secret Brightening Powder *($22)* is a weightless, talc-based loose powder that is meant for (and does a great job of) highlighting skin, especially under the eyes—but again, the effect is subtle. There is no reason a similar effect cannot be created by the artful use of a standard concealer and powder, but for those inclined to experiment (and especially for makeup artists) this product, though pricey, may be worth experimenting with.

☺ $$$ Pressed Powders *($32)* are either bronze, shimmery, or both. They have a silky, non-flaky texture and apply evenly, imparting a soft shimmer finish and healthy color. Matte Bronze Light has the least amount of shine, while the intense shine of Matte Bronze is best for evening glamour only.

😐 $$$ Bronzing Powder *($30)* goes on smoothly, but the amount of shine and a color that is too orange for most skin tones are too distracting to look natural, so consider this carefully.

BLUSH: ✓☺ $$$ Creme Cheek Colour *($22)* ranks as an outstanding cream blush for normal to dry skin. Its creamy without being greasy, has enough slip to blend evenly, and offers a smooth satin finish from each of its three sheer colors. Those who find this type of blush appealing may wish there were more shades available, but each one is excellent.

☺ $$$ Cheek Colour *($22)* suffers from too many very shiny shades, but it does have a smooth, tightly pressed texture that allows you to apply color sheer and build from there. The least shiny, more attractive colors are Azalea, Opera, Rose Bloom, and Wild Bouquet.

☺ $$$ Face Tint *($20)* has the same formula as Mercier's Loose Setting Powder above, with blush colors. This is not as easy to use as a pressed-powder blush, but the few colors (each of which looks more intense in the container than on skin) are attractive and leave a hint of shine and sheer, flushed finish.

EYESHADOW: ☺ $$$ Eye Colour Matte *($20)*. These have a silken, non-powdery yet slightly sheer texture that apply smoothly though softer than they look. More intense shading or crease color will require some layering, but the result is flattering from most of these almost-matte shades. Several have noticeable shine, but the best ones are American Coffee, Buttercream, Caramel, Cashmere, Fresco, Margaux, Paris by Night, Toasted Almond, and Whiskey.

☺ $$$ Eye Colour Shimmer *($20)* shares the same texture and application traits as the Eye Colour Matte above, except these shades have either soft shine or sparkle, depending on which one you choose. The nude to brown tones are easiest to work with; watch out for the greens, which tend to be too distracting.

☺ $$$ Evolution of Colour - Eye *($36)* is Mercier's collection of quad eyeshadows, and although there's not much to choose from, every grouping is expertly coordinated and includes a shade dark enough for use as powder eyeliner. The texture and application are identical to that of the Eye Colour Matte and Eye Colour Shimmer above (the quads feature a mix of matte and shimmer shades, with the shine being relatively low key), which means they start a bit sheer but layer well for more intensity and apply smoothly. Plum Velvet and Brown Velvet are particularly workable, depending on whether you want cool or neutral tones.

☺ **$$$ Eye Basics** *($22)* are liquid eyeshadows that come in a tube with a sponge-tip applicator. Each neutral yet shiny shade has a lightly creamy, sheer texture that blends easily and dries to a natural matte (in feel) finish. This works almost as well as a matte-finish concealer over the eyelids.

☺ **$$$ Basic Colour** *($22)* has a formula that's nearly identical to the Eye Basics above, along with the same texture and application points. The difference here is that half the shades are medium tones meant for shading the eyes.

☺ **$$$ Metallic Creme Eye Colour** *($22)* is the one to choose if you want strong colors with a metallic finish but don't want to get it from a powder eyeshadow. This silky cream blends seamlessly, with just the right amount of slip. Its powdery (in feel) finish doesn't hold up all day, so expect some movement and a bit of creasing, though blending it with a powder eyeshadow all but eliminates this side effect.

😐 **$$$ Creme Eye Colour to Go** *($20)* makes for one too many cream-to-powder liquid eyeshadows in the Mercier lineup, and this silicone-based version is quite slippery and more difficult to blend than the Eye Basics or Basic Colour above. If you're up for a challenge, the sheer, very shiny shades work well for highlighting the brow bone.

😐 **$$$ Eye Colour Duo** *($22)*. These have a formula different from the single eyeshadows above, being silky yet drier and depositing even less color, so they're best when you want a sheer effect with moderate shine. Bamboo and Violet are the best duos; the others are too pink, green, or blue if your goal is to shape and shade the eye.

😐 **$$$ Mineral Eye Powder** *($20)* is a loose powder packaged in a pot with a sifter to control how much is dispensed. The sifter consists of one hole in the center, which keeps this from being too messy, but it still dispenses too much powder at once, and this is concentrated, pigment-rich stuff! The shine is intense and clings reasonably well, though is way too much for aging eyelids or use near wrinkles. If that's not a problem for you, this is worth a look.

EYE AND BROW SHAPER: ☺ **$$$ Eye Brow Gel** *($18)* is a basic, efficient, clear brow gel. It's a great way to keep unruly brows in place, but there is no reason to spend this much when there are equally good options available from several drugstore lines.

😐 **$$$ Eye Pencil** *($18)* and **Eye Brow Pencil** *($18)* are both utterly standard, with traditional colors, and are not worth more than a fraction of this price. Mercier apparently developed "an exact texture" for these, but there isn't any difference between these and most other pencils. Each has a dry, stiff texture that isn't the easiest to work with, but the finish stays in place so smearing is much less likely. Avoid the Bleu Eye Pencil shade because it is too intensely blue and will compete with your eye color. 😐 **$$$ Long Wear Eye Pencil** *($18)* needs no sharpening (though a built-in sharpener is included), and it is retractable. Its texture is creamy and application is quick, though it's slightly smudge-prone and not for anyone battling oily eyelids.

😐 **$$$ Brow Powder Duo** *($23)* features two dry-textured brow powders in one compact. The color combinations are quite good, and there are suitable options for redheads and blondes, along with traditional options for brunettes—but all the colors are sparkly. Why the eyebrows need to shine is beyond me, but if this appeals to you, these brow powders do apply and blend well.

😐 **$$$ Eye Liner** *($20)* is a standard powder-cake liner that must be used wet with an eyeliner brush. The texture is the same as most cake liners, except that these all have a bit of sparkle to them and the shiny particles can flake off and get in your eye, which is annoying to say the least.

😐 **$$$ Caviar Eye Liner** *($22)* is sort of like a soft-textured kohl pencil in compact form. It begins slightly creamy and sets to a dry finish. Application is smooth but sheer, so you'll need to layer for the best definition. A matte powder eyeshadow or one of the cream-gel eyeliners produces longer-lasting results with less effort.

😐 **$$$ Kohl Eye Pencil** *($18)* has a creamy, soft texture and must be applied gently or the pencil tip will break. The creamy finish is meant to be smudged for a smoky look, but you can get similar results from many other pencils that don't require sharpening.

😐 **$$$ Brow Definer** *($20)* is sold in tiny glass pots and is accurately described as a wax/gel formula. The wax content lends a stiff texture to this product and also makes for a less-than-smooth application. However, with a good brush and some patience, this is an option to fill in, groom, and define brows with soft color and a non-sticky finish. All three shades are recommended but are best for brunettes.

LIPSTICK, LIP GLOSS, AND LIPLINER: ✓☺ **$$$ Liquid Crystal Lip Glace** *($22)* provides a striking, unique finish, all in a silky-feeling, non-sticky gloss. The shade selection is limited, but this deserves an audition because it is something fresh in the overcrowded, extremely repetitive lip gloss category.

☺ **$$$ Lip Colour Creme** *($20)* is pricey for a standard cream lipstick with a slightly glossy finish. However, the colors are beautiful and it isn't slippery or greasy, so it's unlikely to migrate into lines around the mouth (and even less likely if you use an anti-feather lipliner with it).

☺ **$$$ Lip Colour Shimmer** *($20)* has the same formula as the Lip Colour Creme above, though each shade has a soft to moderate shimmer finish and the colors aren't as rich. Otherwise, the same review applies. ☺ **$$$ Lip Colour Sheer** *($20)* is exactly that, a sheer lip color with a glossy finish and marvelous, versatile colors that all have a slight stain. ☺ **$$$ Lip Colour StickGloss** *($20)* is aptly named! This is truly a lip gloss in lipstick form, and it provides a very glossy, non-sticky finish from each of its sheer but juicy colors. ☺ **$$$ Lip Stain** *($20)* is said to provide the visual effect of a stain along with the comfort and sheen of a gloss. A pot-packaged lip gloss is what this is; the stain effect is minimal yet the sheer colors are great and bound to please those looking for a softer lip color to wear alone or over lipstick. It has a slightly sticky yet glossy finish.

😐 **$$$ Lip Glace** *($20)* costs too much to make it worth strong consideration over many other standard lip glosses, but if you decide to indulge, this is a moderately sticky, sparkling wet gloss applied with a sponge tip. 😐 **$$$ Lip Pencil** *($18)* has a standard creamy texture and a dry finish. The expansive color range includes options that coordinate well with the lipsticks. Less-expensive pencils abound, but these work well if you don't mind routine sharpening. 😐 **$$$ Long Wear Lip Pencil** *($18)* is an automatic, retractable lip pencil. This has a smooth, silicone-enhanced application and feels slightly creamy, but otherwise is no different from many other automatic lip pencils, and Mercier's shade selection is not extensive. 😐 **$$$ Lip Sheer Pencil** *($18)* is meant to be used with sheer lipsticks or lip glosses because it imparts softer (fleeting) color. The creamy texture is comfortable to apply, but don't expect much longevity from this needs-sharpening pencil.

☹ **Lip Kisses SPF 15** *($20)* lacks sufficient UVA protection, and the colors are too sheer to provide the opacity necessary to shield lips from sun damage. What a shame, because the colors are lovely.

MASCARA: ✓☺ **$$$ Thickening and Building Mascara** *($19)* is a pleasure to apply, and it builds impressively long, lifted lashes with a fair amount of thickness. Lashes look full, soft, and fringed—all without clumping or smearing.

☺ **$$$ Waterproof Mascara** *($19)* has a formula that is easy to apply, makes it through the day without flaking, and really is waterproof (though you may notice slight smearing). It takes some effort to build long, thick lashes, but the result is worth it and your lashes aren't left feeling stiff or brittle.

😐 **$$$ Mascara** *($19)* creates subdued definition and average length. Thickness is a foreign concept to this mascara, and overall the payoff isn't worth the price. Watch out for Navy, which is much brighter than the name suggests.

FACE AND BODY ILLUMINATING/SHIMMER PRODUCTS: ✓☺ **$$$ Shimmer Bloc** *($38)* deserves consideration if you're looking for a shiny pressed powder to highlight or add a glow to your skin. You get four colors in one compact, and the tightly pressed formula is not flyaway, which makes application that much easier. Even better, the prismatic shine clings well and tends to not flake. Very well done!

☺ **$$$ Illuminating Quad** *($35)* presents four squares of color in one compact, without dividers between them. The result from either of the two quads is akin to a shimmery blush, with the shine level being moderate and best for evening. This has a silkier, more refined texture than Mercier's powder blush, and applies smoothly. ☺ **$$$ Illuminating Stick** *($25)* offers a lot more than a healthy glow, because this is one intensely shiny (almost metallic) finish! Application of this cream-to-powder stick is quite good, although the colors are intense and require careful blending. Illuminating Stick is best for normal to very dry skin.

😐 **$$$ Loose Shimmer Powders** *($34)* comprise the long-standing Star Dust and Sun Dust powders, each with a sheer, silky texture and sparkling, dimensional finish. The formula doesn't cling as well as it should, so you'll get some flaking, but if you're going for all-over shine, that's not such a big deal.

BRUSHES: Mercier has done her homework when it comes to ☺ **$$$ Brushes** *($10–$52; $45–$250 for Travel, Mini, or Master Sets with portfolio)*. Most of these are masterfully shaped and are dense enough to hold and deposit color evenly on the skin. Almost every brush is available with a long or short handle, which is an attractive option. The best among this collection of either natural or synthetic hairs are the **Powder Brush** *($52)*; the synthetic hair **Camouflage Powder Brush** *($28)*, which is more appropriate for eyeshadows; **Bronzer Brush** *($45)*; and the **Cheek Colour Brush** *($45)*. Almost all of the **Eyeshadow Brushes** *($24–$29)* are worth a closer look, particularly the **Eye Crease Brush** *($29)*, **Smudge Brush** *($24)*, and **Corner Eye Colour Brush** *($25)*. The Brush Sets are pricey, and the **Micro Mini Brush Set** *($45)* is lacking for the money, so make sure you're going to use every brush in these sets regularly.

SPECIALTY PRODUCTS: ☺ **$$$ Bronzing Gel** *($30)* is a standard, sheer gel bronzer that's infused with particles of shine that call attention only to themselves in daylight. If you're a fan of shine you'll find this a tempting option, and the color is utterly believable, even on fair skin tones. It has just enough copper-red pigment to closely mimic a natural tan, but the consistency makes it best for use over bare or lightly moisturized skin rather than blended over foundation (especially matte-finish foundation, which causes the gel to grab and look dotted on the skin).

☺ **$$$ Mineral Primer** *($30)* is a silky loose powder with a natural affinity for skin. Although the color is pure white, it applies sheer and creates a slight brightening effect without looking chalky or too shiny. Despite this, it's not for everyone and is definitely something you'll want to test before purchasing. This mica-based powder is said to boost the effectiveness of the sunscreen(s) in other mineral formulas, but it cannot do that. In fact, that's a sketchy claim to make since this powder does not sport an SPF rating or active sunscreen ingredients.

😐 **$$$ Foundation Primer** *($30)* is a thin, lightweight cream-gel that contains some antioxidants whose effects are counteracted by too many fragrant extracts. It's supposed to contain light-reflecting ingredients that protect the skin, but it doesn't (unless you consider the emollient shine from the finish protecting). It is a good, simple, matte-finish moisturizer for someone with slightly oily skin, but that's about it. It does not, as claimed, "act as a buffer to outside elements," especially when you consider that the major outside element is sunlight.

😐 **$$$ Foundation Primer Oil-Free** *($30)* has a thinner, less silky texture than the original Foundation Primer above, and the formula is less exciting, too. It is oil-free, but it lacks absorbent ingredients and contains too many thickeners to make someone with oily skin happy. It is best viewed as an ordinary, lightweight moisturizer to remedy slightly dry skin.

😐 **$$$ Foundation Primer–Hydrating** *($30)* contains a minimal amount of hydrating ingredients and more witch hazel than should be applied to normal to dry skin, though overall the amount is unlikely to cause irritation. All of the antioxidants and other intriguing ingredients are listed well after the preservatives. At best, this water- and silicone-based lotion will create a silky-smooth surface for makeup application, but so will many other serums and moisturizers that, while not officially sold as primers, will perform the same function while providing greater benefit.

😐 **$$$ Secret Finish** *($25)*. The real secret is that this ordinary, overpriced, lightweight moisturizer will not make a discernible difference in how your makeup wears. It is merely water, slip agent, thickener, rice starch (for a soft matte finish), plant extracts (including witch hazel, an irritant), vitamins, preservatives, more silicone, fragrance, and coloring agents. If anything, this formula isn't nearly as modern or effective as the less pricey handful of silicone-based mattifiers sold by M.A.C., Smashbox, and Prescriptives.

😐 **$$$ Lip Plumpers** *($30)* contain a flavoring agent that works with other ingredients in the gloss to build a progressive cooling sensation. Within several minutes of applying this lip gloss–like product (which comes in a small but pleasing range of sheer to clear shades), your lips will be tingling like church bells on Sunday and may be a bit plumper as a result. Of course, that tingling and any increased fullness is the result of irritation, and that's not the best thing to do to lips on a routine basis. For occasional use (or applied over lipstick, which blocks most of the active minty flavor from causing irritation) this is an option, and it does have a rich, glossy finish that feels smooth and surprisingly light, though the subtle difference isn't really worth the money.

LAUREN HUTTON'S GOOD STUFF

LAUREN HUTTON'S GOOD STUFF AT-A-GLANCE

Strengths: The makeup fares much better than the skin care; one good moisturizer and lip balm; the oil-blotting sheets; almost all the foundations are worthwhile; top-notch powder; improved mascara; company provides complete ingredient lists on its Web site.

Weaknesses: Lack of a comprehensive skin-care routine; no sunscreens; many products tainted by irritating ingredients that have no established benefit for skin; average makeup brushes and concealer; some of the makeup products contain irritating ingredients.

For more information about Lauren Hutton's Good Stuff, call (888) 395-3469 or visit www.laurenhutton.com or www.Beautypedia.com. Note: All prices listed below are suggested retail. Lauren Hutton's Web site advertises the retail price and, for most items, a sale price that is anywhere from 15% to 50% lower. Combinations of various products reviewed below can also be found in discounted kits sold on the Home Shopping Network (www.hsn.com).

LAUREN HUTTON'S GOOD STUFF SKIN CARE

☺ **$$$ Facial Cleanser and Gentle Facial Scrub** *($40 for the set)*. The **Facial Cleanser** is a standard, water-soluble option that has an overall gentle formula, but the addition of lemon and orange extracts high on the ingredient list keep it from being a better option, especially for use around the eyes. It is a good, though pricey, option for all but very oily skin types. Aside from the aforementioned citrus extracts and a few other plant ingredients, this is not a "natural" cleanser in the least, unless you consider yellow 5 dye and sodium laureth sulfate garden-worthy plants! The **Gentle Facial Scrub** combines mildly abrasive oat flour and polyethylene (plastic) beads in a lightly moisturizing gel base. It does contain the drying detergent cleansing agent TEA-lauryl sulfate, but the amount is so low it's unlikely to be problematic. That makes this just a standard, easy-to-rinse scrub product that isn't as impressive as just using a plain washcloth. However, this is still an OK scrub product for all but dry to very dry skin types.

☹ **AquaPress HydraInfuse** *($15 for 6 ounces)* lists lavender as the second ingredient, and is an overall ordinary toner that's not worth considering over most others.

☹ **AquaPress HydraSeal** *($18 for 4 ounces)* would have been a good, soothing toner for all skin types if it weren't for the lavender and geranium oils. Although they are not a major part of the formula, their irritant potential diminishes the capabilities of the anti-irritant ingredients listed before them, which is frustrating to say the least.

☹ **AquaPress HydraCream** *($22 for 0.5 ounce)* is supposed to help improve fine lines and plump skin to reduce the appearance of wrinkles. Talk about an unoriginal claim and an even more unoriginal formula! Sadly, this product is more reminiscent of the '70s than present-day formulary standards. Rather than state-of-the-art ingredients, it contains more like "state-of-the-boring" ingredients: water, plant extracts, thickener, slip agent, film-forming agent, wax, water-binding agent, preservatives, fragrant oil (can be a skin irritant), and aloe. Considering the amount of product you get for the price, this mediocre formula makes it not worth considering at all.

☺ **Matte Moisturizer** *($15 for 2 ounces)* contains too many thickeners and too much wax to allow it to have a true matte finish, though it does contain some great antioxidants and is an acceptable moisturizer for normal to dry skin. True to claim, this would work well under makeup (as long as you're not anticipating a matte finish).

☺ **$$$ Phyto Face Firm** *($30 for 0.75 ounce)* is mostly water and the absorbent ingredient magnesium aluminum silicate. That's what causes this product to make skin feel tighter and "lifted," but in the long run, overuse of this can lead to dryness and flaking. The antioxidants and minerals are a nice touch, but cannot overcome the disadvantage this product presents.

☺/☹ **Tamanu Oil with Bonus Tamanu Massage Bar** *($40 for the set)* provides a 2-ounce bottle of body oil along with a standard bar soap. The oil is just fine for dry to very dry skin.

However, all of the claims attributed to tamanu oil are unsubstantiated. It does not heal acne or acne scars, nor can it promote thicker hair or make nails stronger. The soap is as standard as it gets, and too drying for all skin types, especially since it includes pumice.

☹/☺ **Lauren's Lip Balm Pot** *($10 for 0.08 ounce)* comes in your choice of clear or sheer tints, but the tinted ones are not recommended because they contain menthol. The Clear version is lanolin-based and a rich experience for dry, chapped lips. The plant oils are nonirritating and are helpful for lips, while the chamomile oil is soothing. The formulary differences explain the dual face rating.

☹ **24/7 SPF 18 Hydrating Face Mist** *($19.95 for 2 ounces)* promises spray-on convenience that allows you to apply a fine mist of sunscreen under or over makeup (the product's mist is so fine it does not need to be massaged into skin). However, despite innovative packaging and a lightweight formula, Hutton neglected to add the UVA-protecting ingredients of titanium dioxide, zinc oxide, avobenzone, Tinosorb, or Mexoryl SX. Therefore, this is not recommended.

LAUREN HUTTON'S GOOD STUFF MAKEUP

FOUNDATION: ☺ **$$$ No Shine Tinted Moisturizer** *($30)* comes with Lauren Hutton's Sheer Concealer built into its cap. Despite the "No Shine" name, this product's description also says it will "keep your face looking dewy," which is contradictory. Discrepancies aside, this moisturizer has a slightly creamy, easy-to-blend formula that provides sheer-to-light coverage and sets to a light matte (not the least bit dewy) finish. It is appropriate for normal to slightly dry skin—those with dry to very dry skin will want to apply a moisturizer first. The three shades are mostly great; only Dark shows signs of being slightly peach, although the sheerness of the product makes that a minor issue. The creamy concealer is built into the cap in a clever design that includes a mirror for on-the-go convenience. Although the concealer has a thicker texture, it blends smoothly and doesn't look heavy or cakey on skin. It does have a slight tendency to crease into lines around the eyes (or anywhere else where lines are prominent), but otherwise it works well and provides good coverage. The concealer shades that accompany the Light and Medium moisturizer colors are beautiful, but the Dark concealer is way too peach for deeper skin tones. Both the moisturizer and the Sheer concealer are fragrance-free.

☺ **$$$ Weightless Foundation** *($35)* is an emollient, creamy, compact-type foundation that is best for those with normal to dry skin not prone to blemishes. Despite the claim of "complete coverage" (odd from a cosmetics company that supposedly created foundations because other foundations looked or felt too heavy), this product provides light to medium coverage unless you really pile it on, which I don't recommend. Four shades are available. Among them, only Medium (Yellow) is a disappointment, and that's because while it may work for some medium skin tones, it is too peach for anyone with a light to medium skin tone.

☺ **$$$ Soft Cover Wet Foundation Dry Powder** *($40)* is a talc-based powder foundation with more silicone than usual, which makes for a very silky texture and a smooth, seamless application when used dry. Wet application is another story. Included with the foundation is a bottle of Hutton's **Soft Cover Face Mist**. This highly fragrant spray-on toner is supposed to turn the foundation into a "sheer, creamy emulsion," but all it does is cause it to go on streaky and choppy. It actually gets chunky on the sponge, and is a mess to blend evenly. Therefore, this is recommended for dry application only, with which you'll net sheer to light coverage and a soft, non-powdery matte finish. The formula contains oils and emollients that make it best for normal to slightly dry skin not prone to blemishes. All three shades are neutral, though they appear borderline yellow-to-peach in the compact.

😐 **$$$ Custom Blend Foundation** *($29)* has a formula that's identical to the Weightless Foundation above and the same texture, application, skin type, and coverage comments apply. The only difference is that with Custom Blend Foundation you get two coordinating colors in one compact. The idea is that having two shades not only allows you to come closer to creating an exact match, but also allows you to adapt your foundation as your natural skin tones change with the seasons (paler in winter, darker in summer). The problem lies with the shades themselves. In contrast to the colors for Weightless Foundation, this product's shades are mostly too pink or peach. Strangely, the two shades in the lighter (Pink) option represent only a one-shade difference (the darker shade is a natural depth progression of the lighter shade). Yet in the Brown compact, the two shades are much farther apart in terms of light and dark. If you have dry skin and are willing to experiment with blending two shades together (and can somehow manage with these non-neutral colors), this is an option. Despite the formula's similarity to the Weightless Foundation, this product is not worthy of a happy face rating because of its poor shade selection.

CONCEALER: 😐 **$$$ Concealer Kit** *($35)* has the distinction (at least according to Lauren Hutton) of being "the one product that is never in our office because we're always sold out." An interesting comment, considering that I found it readily available, even after checking back now and then when working on this book. The kit includes eight shades of Spot Concealer and two shades of Sheer Concealer, which is essentially identical to the Weightless Foundation reviewed above. The Spot Concealer is included in the Face Disc product reviewed below. In short, this kit gets you a lot of two products that don't go past average in terms of application and performance. There are many other concealers (appropriate for "mature" skin) that are preferable to this one.

POWDER: ✓☺ **$$$ Texture-Light Loose Powder** *($25)* has a wonderfully light, airy texture and a seamless application that makes skin look radiantly polished rather than too matte or dry. The talc-based formula is ideal for normal to dry skin; someone with oily skin (whether all over or just in the T-zone) will likely find this powder not absorbent enough. The four sheer shades are beautiful and well-suited to a range of skin tones. In particular, Brown is a great non-ashy shade for dark skin tones, or it could be used by medium skin tones as a bronzing powder.

EYESHADOW: 😐 **$$$ Eye Do's Trio** *($57)* gets you three liquid eyeshadows that are relatively easy to apply, but go on so sheer that if you're aiming for a true shaping-and-shadowing effect, you'll need several layers of color. The water-based formula dries quickly but allows time for blending, and these do last longer than cream or cream-to-powder eyeshadows. You may be OK with the sheer application, but the colors in each kit are strange and contrasting. My kit had pink grapefruit, russet, and eggplant colors that were difficult to blend together, although each had minimal shine.

LIPSTICK AND LIPLINER: ☺ **$$$ Lip Treatment Duo** *($20)* doesn't offer any more "treatment" benefit than other lipsticks; it's just two lipsticks: one opaque and creamy, the other sheer and glossy. Both are very nice, but, contrary to claim, neither formula is truly non-feathering (the lanolin oil and castor oil don't stay in place easily), so think twice about ordering this if you have lines around your mouth.

☺ **Clear Lip Balm Pot** *($10)* is a standard, but effective, lip balm whose lanolin and petrolatum base will protect and soothe dry lips. It would be even better without the fragrance, but at least it also contains anti-irritants.

☺ **Lip Pencil** *($14)* is a standard, needs-sharpening lip pencil that applies evenly and has a smooth, semi-creamy finish that is not prone to feathering into lines around your mouth. Only three shades are available, but they coordinate with the Face Disc color palettes reviewed below. Of course, there are many other excellent lip pencils available with better color selections and that don't require sharpening.

☹ **Tinted Lip Balm Pot** *($10)* imparts barely any color, but the menthol in it will cause your lips to tingle from irritation, which isn't good. What a shame, because this lanolin-based balm otherwise would take good care of dry, chapped lips.

MASCARA: Hutton's ☺ **Mascara** *($12)* has changed since I originally reviewed it, and for the better. The former bushy brush was replaced by a much smaller brush so it is easier to reach every lash. You'll get appreciable length and thickness without much drama. If that's what you're looking for, this mascara is recommended.

BRUSHES: ☺ **$$$ 7-Piece Professional Brush Set** *($60; also sold individually, prices vary)* is a reasonably effective brush collection. Each brush is color-coded to match its corresponding product in Lauren Hutton's Face Disc, a nice touch for those who are never quite sure which brush goes with which product. Most of the brushes are made of natural hair, but a few are made of Taklon, a synthetic fiber that is excellent for applying creamy (moist) products. The synthetic brushes (Spotter, Concealer, and Eyebrow) are preferred to the natural-hair brushes in this set because the hair is not as soft as it should be, at least not for this price. Each brush serves its purpose, but the three synthetic options feel better. If you're interested in this brush set and the Face Disc reviewed below, Hutton's Web site offers them together at a discount.

SPECIALTY PRODUCTS: ☺ **$$$ Face Disc** *($60; $5–$8 for individual shade/product refills)* is the star product of Lauren Hutton's Good Stuff, and it is the item from this line I am asked about most often. Housed in a giant compact that's roughly the size of a compact disc are seven products, each color-coded so you know, step-by-step, where to apply them. The how-to-apply part is explained in the detailed brochure that accompanies each Face Disc, and if that's not clear enough, an instructional videotape is included as well.

Step 1 is the lanolin- and Vaseline-based Lip Balm. Nice enough, but nothing special. It does not contain needless irritants like menthol, which is a plus. The logic for applying this first is to let lips soak it up while you apply the rest of your makeup, but that is a misguided notion. The occlusive ingredients in the Lip Balm are not absorbed into your lips—they can only remain on the surface. Then there's the issue of wearing the Lip Balm while applying makeup. If you happen to touch your lips while applying your foundation or powder, it can be a greasy, slippery mistake. Plus, if you have any problem with lipstick bleeding into lines, this balm will speed up the process.

Step 2 involves applying the Spot Concealer. Each Face Disc includes four shades of this product, with the goal being to mix and match according to variances in your skin tone and the imperfections you're trying to cover. For the most part, each shade on its own is not the easiest to work with because (depending on which Face Disc you have) they are too light, too peach, too yellow, or too copper. However, if you mix two or three of them together in proportion to your skin tone (definitely not an easy task), the results can be okay and the coverage full. The main issue I have with Spot Concealer is its heaviness. The mineral oil–based formula isn't as greasy as I thought it would be, but is still thick and moderately difficult to blend. Its finish is semi-matte, but the texture tends to look heavy on skin, while slipping easily into lines, wrinkles, or large pores.

Step 3 brings us to the Light Concealer, which Hutton feels is the best product in the Face Disc. It is recommended that you use this concealer to erase shadows formed in the corner of the eye (near the nose bone) and to create the illusion of a straighter nose. However, this emollient, waxy concealer applies, looks, and feels heavy on the skin. Countless other concealers are available that far outperform this product, and I promise they do not make your skin look older (which this product will do because it slips into lines and indentations so quickly).

Things improve slightly with Step 4, the Contouring Shadow. This powder-based, matte-finish product has a silky texture that applies evenly and blends easily. It is recommended that you use this shadow to sculpt the face (at the jawline, on the neck, and around the hairline), but this effect rarely looks convincing. It is a common technique professional makeup artists use for camera work, but for everyday makeup it can look obvious or contrived unless you're skilled with proper application and can blend the darker shade without destroying the illusion of shadow/contour. In all of the Face Discs, this product is best used as eyeshadow rather than for trying to make your face look slimmer or your chin less doughy.

Next up is Blush. Each matte shade has a texture and application that is identical to the Contouring Shadow, except the colors are blush-appropriate. This is a very nice powder blush that wears without fading or streaking. Step 6 is the Eyebrow step, and with each Face Disc you get one powder color to do the job. This is a limitation (for example, in the lightest kit, someone with fair skin and dark brown eyebrows would find the Eyebrow powder useless). However, as the directions explain, you can use one of the other powder colors in the Disc to match and fill in your brows. In each Disc, the palette of tan to brown shades should meet the needs of all brow colors, except those of true redheads.

Pooch & Nose follows and is a step Hutton claims is "model stuff ... because it takes some time, but it's great for a night out." This is a powder-based product meant to be used for lighter contouring jobs. For example, the powder can be used to visually minimize puffy corners of the eye or to contour the nose. Compared to the Contouring Shadow shades, each Pooch & Nose color is more muted, and as a result easier to work with. Yet the art of creating convincing contour demands patience and practice. If you're not up to the task, at least all of the Pooch & Nose colors make wonderful eyeshadows, and all are matte. The last step in the Face Disc is Wet/Dry Eyeliner, a densely pigmented powder with a dry but still smooth texture. It can indeed be used wet or dry, with wet application intensifying the effect; it's best to use it wet on the upper lash line and dry on the lower lash line.

Four Face Discs are available, for different depths of skin tone. Pink is designed for fair skin, Yellow for light to medium skin, Olive for light to medium ethnic skin, and Brown for African American or Indian skin tones. The Pink and Yellow kits have the best palettes, while the Olive selection pairs peachy concealers with charcoal-brown contour powder and mauve blush. The Brown kit contains concealer shades (remember, there are five in all) that do provide coverage, but they are also too dark, making deeper skin tones look muddy rather than flawless.

All told, the Face Discs' blend of products, with very good to below-average textures, makes them tough to recommend. That's because in kits like this, you should expect to get reasonable use from all (or at least most) of the items. As it stands, half the products are worthy of a happy face rating and half a sad face, leading me to assign a neutral face rating to the entire set. The color-coding and thorough application instructions go above and beyond what comes with most makeup kits; it's just unfortunate that not all of the products are as state-of-the-art as they could be.

☹ **$$$ Try Me! Trio** *($25)* is a condensed version of what you get in the Face Disc product reviewed above. Included are Hutton's Lip Balm, one shade of Blush, the Light Concealer, and Contouring Shadow. Please refer to the Face Disc review above for comments on these products. The same shade concerns and textural comments apply here, too.

☺ **$$$ Blush/Lip Trick Trio** *($64)* is often on sale for less than half its retail price, and that's a good thing, because $64 is ridiculous for three powder blush shades and one strip of lip balm. The "trick" of this trio is that you can use the powder blush as lip color. You're supposed to apply the lip balm, then (with a clean finger) dab on one of the powder blush shades to tint the lips. This trick is neither new nor that advantageous. Depending on how the balm was applied, you'll likely end up with unevenly colored lips because the areas with more lip balm will grab the blush's pigment first. Further, the finish this combination provides isn't all that attractive: moist underneath, dry and powdery looking on top. And just try pressing your lips together ... Yuck! If you find this trio on sale and are attracted to the blush colors, consider a purchase—the blush's texture and application are excellent, and each shade is 100% matte. It is for these reasons that this product deserves a happy face rating.

☺ **$$$ Suck Ups Oil Blotting Paper** *($12 for 50 sheets)* are standard blotting papers, thin sheets of tissue-paper material that do a really good job of absorbing excess oil or perspiration buildup without leaving a powder finish behind. There is nothing negative to report about this product except that the price is steep for what you get, especially when you consider that identical versions of this product are available for a lot less.

LORAC

LORAC AT-A-GLANCE

Strengths: Mostly great foundations in a neutral shade range; beautiful pressed powder and bronzing powder; several super blush and lipstick options; one superior lip gloss; awesome collection of shimmer products; the makeup brushes.

Weaknesses: Limited, average skin-care options; average to problematic concealers; unimpressive eyelining and brow-enhancing options; the Lotsa Lip products; the mascaras are a mixed bag with mostly disappointing results.

For more information about Lorac, call (800) 845-0705 or visit www.loraccosmetics.com or www.Beautypedia.com.

LORAC SKIN CARE

☹ **$$$ MakeupPREP Gentle Skin Resurfacer** *($32 for 3.7 ounces)* is an at-home microdermabrasion topical scrub product that contains aluminum oxide as the main abrasive agent. This gritty-feeling scrub is formulated in a creamy base to help cushion your skin as you apply it. Even so, it should be used very gently because you can easily go overboard with this type of harsh scrub. Rinsing is a bit difficult due to the oil in the formula. Aluminum oxide is not a "gentle" scrub ingredient, so the name is misleading, and it doesn't work any better than (and is definitely not as gentle as) a washcloth.

☹ **$$$ Oil-Free Moisturizer** *($37.50 for 2 ounces)* is a basic, lightweight, truly oil-free moisturizer for normal to slightly dry or slightly oily skin. It contains good water-binding agents, but lacks antioxidants. The small amount of comfrey is not likely to be a problem for skin.

LORAC MAKEUP

FOUNDATION: ✓☺ $$$ Satin Makeup *($35)* has a sheer, elegantly moist texture that is a treat for normal to dry skin, and the formula contains some skin-beneficial ingredients. This foundation offers better coverage than the Oil-Free Makeup below, but still blends well. The colors tend to go on lighter than they appear. To avoid an overly jaundiced or peachy look, avoid M6, M7, and M8.

✓☺ $$$ Oil-Free Wet/Dry Powder Makeup *($35)* is fantastic. This ultra-smooth, almost creamy, talc-based pressed-powder foundation is a joy to apply. It blends imperceptibly over the skin and creates a sheer, polished finish. All five shades are superior, with options for light to tan skin. Few pressed-powder foundations look this beautiful on skin, and wet application is a step above the rest, too (but be careful to avoid streaking).

☺ $$$ Oil-Free Makeup *($30)* has a fluid, lightweight texture that blends very well, merging into skin to create a natural matte finish with sheer coverage. The colors have improved slightly, though the best ones (you'll know which ones those are immediately because the tester bottles at the counter are almost empty) have remained the same. Among the ten options, only S6 and S8 are a bit too peachy orange to look convincing. The darkest shade, S10, isn't quite dark enough for most African-American skin tones, but is still a beautiful color.

☹ ProtecTINT SPF 30 Oil-Free Tinted Moisturizer *($30)* has a water-fresh, moist texture with lots of slip and a dewy finish suitable for normal to dry skin. The five shades are very sheer and workable for all but very dark skin tones, but this is not recommended because it lacks sufficient UVA-protecting ingredients. With so many tinted moisturizers with sunscreen that get this fundamental element right, why choose one that puts skin at risk for more sun damage?

CONCEALER: 😐 Coverup *($16)* comes in a pot and offers great emollient coverage, but it also tends to crease almost immediately and keeps on creasing. If creasing isn't a concern for you, the range of shades (which apply less yellow than they appear) is quite good.

☹ Undercover Lover *($22)* is a slightly thick liquid concealer housed in a pump bottle that tends to dispense much more product than you're going to need. In addition to problematic packaging, the concealer itself is subpar, looking too thick and heavy on skin and not being nearly as silky as it could be. For the money, this is disappointing.

POWDER: ✓☺ $$$ Translucent Touch Up Powder *($32)* is a talc-based pressed powder that has a smooth-as-silk texture and three very good colors, each with a slight amount of shine. It provides a bit more coverage than traditional pressed powder, and blends on easily.

☺ $$$ Bronzer *($28)* comes as a pressed powder and is available in two attractive, shine-infused shades. A natural tan doesn't add shine to skin, but at least this silky powder applies evenly and lasts, plus the shine stays put.

😐 $$$ Face Powder *($28)* is a talc-based loose powder that has a very dry texture, smooth finish, and five workable colors. The dry finish is only for normal to very oily skin and, for the money, isn't as elegant and seamless as many other loose powders.

BLUSH: ✓☺ $$$ Blush *($16)* offers a small, but very good, palette of colors. Plum, Rose, Soul, and Peach are particularly great. Avoid Desire and Crimson unless the goal is extreme shimmer on your cheeks. The texture and application are beautiful, and the color begins sheer but builds well. **✓☺ $$$ Sheer Wash** *($17.50)* has been downsized and is now much easier to use as a lip stain due to the smaller applicator. Comparable to but slightly better than Benefit's BeneTint, Sheer Wash comes in three beautiful colors suitable for a wide range of skin tones.

As is true for all liquid stains, this dries almost immediately and tends to work best on smooth, flawless skin. If you can master the application quirks inherent to this type of product, it lasts all day without fading.

☺ **$$$ Cheek Duo** *($28.50)* offers a pressed-powder blush and bronzer in one compact, and the pairings are well done. Both colors have noticeable shine, but can work for evening glamour or to highlight younger skin. ☺ **$$$ Multiple Rush** *($20)*. The "multiple" in the name is because Lorac created this product for use on both cheeks and lips. This is a swivel-up stick with a cream-to-powder texture that is smooth and non-greasy. It blends so well as to almost become a second skin, producing a believable flush on cheeks (hence the happy face rating). On lips, the results are mixed: the color (Crush Rush) is fine, but the finish leaves lips feeling parched. I also wouldn't recommend using the other shade (Love Rush) either as a blush or lipstick because it's too pale. It is best as a highlighter for the top of the cheeks or the underbrow area.

☺ **$$$ Portable Paints** *($24)* come in clever, interlocking packaging and are designed as palettes of sheer, shimmering colors to make you look radiant and polished but not made-up. Each product has a soft, creamy texture that slips over skin and offers more shine than color payoff (they are not for anyone who wants to use color to shape and shade their features). The moist texture is best used on bare skin or with a dewy foundation; trying to blend them over a matte or powder foundation will produce uneven, messy results. All told, this is an expensive way to look like you're not wearing makeup at all, but the compacts are discreet, easy to stash in a makeup bag, and, dare I say, cute.

☺ **$$$ It Kits-Lip & Cheek** *($28)* come in a compact and provide a cream blush that doubles as lip color and a shiny powder blush. The colors are well coordinated, and the sleek case makes it easy to transport, especially for low-key, monochromatic summer makeup.

☺ **$$$ Cheek Stamp** *($22)* is a unique way to apply powder blush. Housed in a round container is a sponge applicator. When the container is closed, it comes into contact with a powder cake built into the product's cap. Dabbing and blending this weightless, silky-textured blush on skin produces smooth, sheer color that you can easily build for more intensity. It also blends surprisingly well using just your fingers (though the sponge or a brush is preferred). The best, most flattering shades (each with some shine, but it's not distracting) are Coral, Golden Glow, and Island Spice. Avoid Pink Paradise unless vibrant, Barbie-doll pink cheeks are what you're after.

EYESHADOW: The excellent ☺ **$$$ Eye Shadows** *($16)* go on incredibly smooth and are a bit on the sheer side, but building intensity is easy enough. If only there weren't such an overwhelming assortment of intensely shiny shades, this would be a slam-dunk recommendation. Still, the shine tends to not flake, which is always helpful. The least shiny options include Beige, Black, Cappuccino, Dark Brown, Nude, and Suede. Interestingly, the green-toned shades tend to apply more gold or khaki than they appear, making them blendable with several of the line's brown- or beige-toned colors. Avoid the green apple–tinged Lush and the violet-toned Delight. **It Kits-Eye Duos** *($28)* have the same formula and application traits as Lorac's single Eye Shadows above, but these are sold in slim compacts as duos. The pairings are primarily tone-on-tone and as such are easy to work with, though the Denim & Diamonds set is skewed a bit too blue to recommend.

EYE AND BROW SHAPER: 😐 **Eye Pencils** *($12)* are standard fare and more or less available to appease pencil lovers. You can find comparable pencils that don't need routine sharpening at the drugstore.

☹ **$$$ Creamy Brow Pencil** *($18)* has a texture that's more thick than creamy, though it does leave a moist finish. This needs-sharpening pencil comes in four excellent shades that with practice can be feathered through brows to create a natural, defined appearance. Application can drag a bit if the pencil is not kept consistently sharp, while the mascara-type brush on the opposite end helps complete the brow-enhancing result.

☹ **$$$ Brow Wax** *($16)* is basically a soft brow-pencil color in a pot. In contrast to pencils, this starts moist and dries to a soft powder finish, but it can still go on heavier than a matte brow powder. The three available colors are excellent, particularly Blonde and Auburn. However, this type of product won't be to everyone's taste and really isn't worth the extra expenditure over just an appropriate shade of matte powder eyeshadow.

☹ **Eye Shadow/Liner** *($16)* needs sharpening and, although that may be tolerable, you likely won't want to put up with this chunky pencil's too-creamy application and the fact that the large particles of glitter built into each color flake.

LIPSTICK, LIP GLOSS, AND LIPLINER: ✓☺ $$$ Lip Intensity Lip Gloss *($16)* is a great choice if you want the opacity of a traditional lipstick with a non-sticky, gloss finish. I wish there were more colors, because the result is striking and a perfect all-in-one option that moisturizes without feeling slick or greasy.

✓☺ **$$$ Co-Stars** *($19)* are a late entry into the ring of long-wearing, two-part lip colors—but it was worth the wait, because Co-Stars is one of the best to come along since M.A.C.'s equally impressive Pro Longwear Lipcolour ($20). The color coat feels creamier than most when first applied, and imparts rich, nearly opaque color. It feels remarkably less creamy as it sets, which is why the glossy top coat is necessary for comfortable wear. Staying power is where this product excels. Lorac pledges eight-hour wear, and this delivers. Aside from reapplying the glossy top coat, the color stays on through eating, drinking, smooching—anything that causes traditional lipstick to transfer or come off. Removing this requires an oil-based product, because silicone makeup removers do not work well. The shade selection is smaller than that offered by other lines, but if you find one you like (and there are some very good nude pink and rose tones), this is something to check out!

☺ **$$$ Cream Lipstick** *($17.50)* is a light, decadently creamy lipstick with a slightly greasy finish that goes on smoothly and imparts rich color. The large selection of shades is stunning, although most of the celebrity-inspired shades have disappeared.

☺ **$$$ Matte Lips** *($17.50)* are not matte, but these do have a less creamy texture than the Cream Lipstick above, and offer more intense colors that last without feeling dry or cakey on the lips. Although the color selection is limited to only three shades, Explore is one of the best red hues you'll find. ☺ **$$$ Sheer Lipstick** *($17.50)* is the exact same formula as the Cream lipstick, but with less pigment, so these tend to fade quickly. The soft colors work for a variety of skin tones.

☺ **$$$ Lip Polish** *($17.50)* is, by any other name, just lip gloss. The twist to this one is its fluid texture and its a tiny nail-polish bottle. You apply it with the built-in brush and you're left with smooth, sheer color and a slightly sticky, shimmering finish. The vanilla-mint flavor is refreshing without being irritating. ☺ **Lip Gloss** *($15)* is a slick, petrolatum-based, highly fragrant pot gloss. It is lighter and less sticky than many lip glosses, though very slippery. The small selection of shades are sheer and versatile. ☺ **Gloss Stick** *($15)* is presented in a ChapStick-style container as a light-textured lip balm with just a hint of glossy color and a slick finish. Sheer Berry is a good "your lips but better" shade, while Sheer Shine is colorless. The other shades are also commendable.

😐 **Lip Pencil** *($12)* is just a standard pencil with a great color selection that coordinates nicely with the majority of Lorac's lipsticks. The application is creamy but these have a drier finish, which keeps them in place longer, though you still have to sharpen them.

😐 **$$$ Mocktail** *($18)* is a series of lip glosses named after and flavored to taste like various cocktails. I don't quite get the association of lip gloss and cocktails, never mind that flavored lip glosses tend to encourage the wearer to lick her lips, which promotes dryness and means you have to reapply the gloss more often. This is an OK gloss with a moderately thick texture and slightly sticky feel. For the money, it's not worth choosing over numerous drugstore lip glosses. If the novelty of flavored gloss speaks to you, Jane and Bonne Bell have copious options available.

😐 **$$$ Vitamin E Stick** *($16)* is available in tinted or untinted versions. The former isn't really tinted, it's just an emollient lipstick that's loaded with white iridescence. Used alone, this can make lips look ghostly. The untinted version is a standard, emollient lip balm. Both versions contain a meager amount of vitamin E.

☹ **Lotsa Lip Plumping Lipstick** *($18.50)* is disappointing. The lipsticks reviewed above are quite lovely, with elegant textures and enticing colors, but not so here. This sheer, slick lipstick is infused with large glitter particles that look silly, not seductive, and they actually claim that this provides "long-lasting color." Don't believe it for a second—this slips off before you know it, leaving behind noticeable pieces of glitter. Does this lipstick have a plumping effect to offset its inadequacies? Lorac uses Maxi-Lip, an ingredient mixture from Croda (a large supplier of raw materials to the cosmetics industry). Maxi-Lip is a blend of standard thickeners and emollients along with palmitoyl oligopeptide, which is said to reduce lines, add moisture, and increase the lip's volume. There is no substantiated research showing that Maxi-Lip has a legitimate plumping effect on lips. The only supportive information is from Croda, and that's hardly impartial. Peptides can help bind moisture to skin (and lips), but for now we have no idea whether or not they can affect collagen in any way, and for certain this product can neither duplicate nor come close to the results you get from lip injections of collagen or hyaluronic acid. ☹ **Lotsa Lip Plumping Lip Gloss** *($18.50)* has much more pigment than the Lotsa Lip Plumping Lipstick above, as well as a smooth, non-sticky texture and sexy gloss finish. The problem is it contains capsicum extract. This ingredient, typically extracted from peppers, is a counterirritant when used in topically applied arthritis treatments. It works by confusing the pain receptors (creating inflammation on the skin, which "tricks" the nerves around the joints), but in a lip gloss it's just a potent irritant (Source: www.naturaldatabase.com). While it can temporarily swell lips, the long-term results are not pretty (irritation is bad for skin).

MASCARA: ☺ **$$$ Lorac Lashes** *($17.50)* hasn't changed a bit over the years, but that's OK if all you need is a lengthening mascara that applies cleanly and wears all day without flaking or smudging, which is pretty good. The Aubergine color is an attractive deep plum shade for those who want a more experimental color, while the Auburn shade is a new twist on standard black or brown, especially for redheads.

😐 **$$$ Publicity Stunt Lashes** *($18.50)* is billed as a breakthrough formula because it lasts for days and is gym-proof, cry-proof, and waterproof. The formula eschews standard waxes in favor of the film-forming agent polyester-3, which is what ensures long wear and makes this mascara impervious to water and water-soluble cleansers. It's not much different from standard waterproof mascaras, except that when you use an oil- or silicone-based remover, it comes off in flakes and chunks. That's messy, and this mascara's performance isn't good enough to make the odd removal tolerable. You'll get longer, separated lashes (the built-in lash comb is a nice but unnecessary touch), but the real publicity stunt is in convincing consumers that this mascara really is a breakthrough and that it is OK to keep mascara on for days!

☹ **Lotsa Lash Fiber Mascara** *($19)* has one of the largest mascara brushes I've ever seen, and it doesn't make for better application. If anything, it demands extra vigilance because it's too easy to get excess mascara on the skin around your lashes, and it makes it nearly impossible to reach the lashes at the inner corners of your eyes (at least not without some risk of hurting yourself). This formula does contain fibers, which Lorac claims "cling to lashes like mini lash extensions" for "baby doll–like lashes." It turns out this mascara is *lotsa* talk and very little action because it takes longer than usual to build mediocre length and minimal thickness. The fibers don't create baby-doll lashes, nor do they have a curling effect. Instead, they make lashes feel brittle and the fibers tend to flake off, which is a problem for eyes in general, and especially for those who wear contact lenses.

☹ **Waterproof Lashes Waterproof Mascara** *($18.50)* is waterproof, but it smears with little provocation (even after lashes have dried) and tends to flake, making it an expensive mistake. Even without those surprising setbacks, the application is uneven, looking too heavy in one place and too sparse in others. In short, this is a mess of a mascara!

FACE AND BODY ILLUMINATING/SHIMMER PRODUCTS: If you're looking for long-lasting shimmer products that cast an attractive glow on skin, Lorac's small selection is par excellance! ✓☺ **$$$ Oil Free Luminizer** *($28)* is a sheer liquid shimmer product that has a silky, lightweight texture and very smooth application. This leaves a shiny finish that is noticeable without being distracting, perfect for dressing up evening makeup with hints of sparkle and a soft radiance. Perhaps best of all, this stays put without flaking and doesn't feel slick or greasy. Two shades are available: L1 (sheer white with pale pink and gold undertones) is more versatile, especially for lighter skin tones. Shade L2 is a peachy gold tone that would look appealing on medium to dark skin tones. One caveat: This product is packaged in a pump bottle that dispenses more product than you're likely to need. A little of this stuff goes a long way and too much can look too obvious—so dispense carefully.

✓☺ **$$$ TANtalizer Body Bronzing Luminizer** *($30)* basically takes the concept of the Oil-Free Luminizer above and parlays it into a bronze-toned body lotion laced with radiant shimmer. This sheer-tinted lotion feels silky and light, and its finish on skin (especially medium to tan skin) is gorgeous. This is sure to be a summertime favorite, especially for evening. One caution: The lotion comes off on clothing, so apply carefully.

✓☺ **$$$ Glam Rocks Loose Metallic Eye Shadow** *($16)* should be completely problematic, because most loose-powder eyeshadows tend to be a flaky mess with minimal ability to cling to skin. Not this one! The powdered-sugar texture smooths over the eye area and blends beautifully. The effect is definitely metallic and meant for dramatic accents. If that's your aim, this loose powder clings well (it flakes only if you apply too much at once) and won't crease if your lids are prepped with a separate powder eyeshadow.

BRUSHES: Another strong point of the Lorac line is the excellent, well-edited assortment of **Brushes** *($9–$35)*. Check out the eyeshadow options, including ✓☺ **Brush 106** *($15)* and ✓☺ **$$$ Brush 108** *($26)*, both of which are outstanding. ☺ **$$$ Brush 103** *($24)*, which has synthetic hairs, works well for more detailed concealer or blending jobs. Avoid ☹ **Brush 110** *($35)* and ☹ **Brush 109** *($25)*, both of which are floppy and hard to control for applying loose powder and crease color.

SPECIALTY PRODUCTS: Carol Shaw has launched a few of her key colors as ☺ **$$$ Greatest Hits CDs** *($48)*. These cleverly named color collections feature four eyeshadows, one blush, one lip/cheek tint, and a lip gloss. Not bad, considering that purchasing these items singly (instead of as an "album") would cost over twice as much. CD1 showcases warm colors, while CD2 (which is more attractive) spotlights cool tones. Depending on your preferences, both are worthwhile.

😐 **$$$ Oil-Free Neutralizer** *($30)* is supposed to even out any blue or red discolorations. It works to some extent because of its semi-opaque coverage and whitening effect (the green tinge has been minimized), but the same results can be achieved with a single foundation—though not with Lorac's liquid foundations, which are too sheer to conceal bothersome redness.

😐 **$$$ aquaPRIME Oil-Free Makeup Primer** *($30)* departs from the typical silicone-based, nonaqueous foundation primer with its simple formula of water, acrylate film-forming agent, water-binding agent, and preservative. It has a super-light gel texture and is oil-free, yet can make skin feel slightly tacky, and this much acrylate can cause irritation.

L'OREAL PARIS

L'OREAL PARIS AT-A-GLANCE

Strengths: Inexpensive, quality makeup (the entire range is overall the best at the drugstore); some good to outstanding water-soluble cleansers; nice assortment of self-tanning options; effective AHA option (in the form of an at-home peel kit); one of the best, most comprehensive makeup collections at the drugstore, with superb options in every category except eyeshadow, shimmer products, and specialty products; L'Oreal's mascaras (along with those from sister company Maybelline New York) are a tough act to follow.

Weaknesses: Jar packaging; almost all of the daytime moisturizers with sunscreen lack sufficient UVA protection; terrible adult acne management kits; no product to successfully combat blemishes (at least not without causing more irritation); no skin-lightening options; boring to problematic toners; several foundations with sunscreen still lack sufficient UVA protection despite L'Oreal's media push for Mexoryl SX; the Lineur Intense Liquid Eyeliner.

For more information about L'Oreal, call (800) 322-2036 or visit www.loreal.com, www.lorealparisusa.com, or www.Beautypedia.com. Note: Unless mentioned otherwise, all L'Oreal skin-care products contain fragrance.

L'OREAL PARIS SKIN CARE

L'OREAL PARIS ADVANCED REVITALIFT PRODUCTS

☹ **Advanced Revitalift Complete Day Cream SPF 15** *($16.49 for 1.7 ounces)* does not contain the UVA-protecting ingredients of titanium dioxide, zinc oxide, avobenzone, Tinosorb, or Mexoryl SX, and is not recommended.

☹ **Advanced Revitalift Complete Day Lotion SPF 15** *($16.49 for 1.7 ounces)* is the lotion version of the Advanced Revitalift Complete Day Cream SPF 15 above, and the same review applies.

☹ **Advanced Revitalift Complete Day Lotion SPF 15, Fragrance-Free** *($16.49 for 1.7 ounces)* is indeed fragrance-free, but what it's also lacking is sufficient UVA protection, making it a poor choice for daytime (and it's a really boring moisturizer, too).

😐 **Advanced Revitalift Double Eye Lift** *($16.99 for 0.5 ounce)* packages two products in one dual-chambered pump container. You're supposed to apply both products in sequence, because one is designed to reduce wrinkles while the other firms and lifts—an odd instruction given how many individually packaged L'Oreal moisturizers claim to do the same thing at once. Step 1 is the **Under Eye Anti-Wrinkle Cream**. This emollient, cushy moisturizer with a silky finish will improve the appearance of dry skin (and fine lines caused by it) under the eye. However, the only compelling antioxidant is retinyl palmitate (not retinol, as claimed), so this isn't as exciting as it could have been, though it is fragrance-free. Step 2 is the **Upper Eye Lifting Gel**, a mix of water, silicone, glycerin, thickener, film-forming agent, vitamin E, and the cell-communicating ingredient adenosine. This won't lift skin but it is a decent lightweight moisturizer. Combined, this duo is more impressive than what L'Oreal usually produces, but that isn't saying much. Of course, this won't "stop the signs of aging... for 40ish skin," or any *ish* skin.

☹ **Advanced Revitalift Double Lifting, Intense Re-Tightening Gel & Anti-Wrinkle Treatment** *($16.49 for 1 ounce)* can make skin feel tighter temporarily because of the amount of alcohol and absorbent magnesium sodium silicate it contains, but that's about drying up skin and causing irritation, which is actually wrinkle-inducing. There isn't much else to extol in this gel, and calling it advanced must be L'Oreal's idea of sarcasm.

😐 **Advanced Revitalift Eye Day/Night Cream** *($16.49 for 0.5 ounce)* is a water- and silicone-based moisturizer for normal to dry skin anywhere on the face. It is fragrance-free, as claimed. The tiny amount of vitamin A is the only antioxidant, though jar packaging won't keep it stable. Of course, nothing in this product will lift skin or reduce puffy eyes.

😐 **Advanced Revitalift Face & Neck Day Cream** *($16.49 for 1.7 ounces)* has some emollient properties and a silky texture suitable for normal to dry skin, but it's inappropriate for daytime use unless you pair it with a foundation rated SPF 15 or greater. The soy and vitamin A antioxidants won't last long once this jar-packaged product is opened, and the volatile fragrance components may cause irritation.

😐 **Advanced Revitalift Night Cream** *($16.49 for 1.7 ounces)* doesn't differ significantly from the Advanced Revitalift Face & Neck Day Cream above, but it has a thicker texture. Otherwise, the comments for skin type, jar packaging, and fragrance components apply here, too.

☹ **Revitalift Intense Lift Treatment Mask** *($16.49 for 4 masks)* contains enough alcohol to be irritating to all skin types, and is a completely uninspired, ineffective formula that doesn't stand a chance of lifting skin.

L'OREAL PARIS AGE PERFECT PRODUCTS

☺ **Age Perfect Anti-Fatigue Lotion Cleanser** *($5.49 for 6.7 ounces)* is a standard, mineral oil–based cleanser that is an option for dry skin, but it tends to leave a greasy feel. It's nearly identical to Galatee Confort, Comforting Milky Creme Cleanser ($27 for 6.8 ounces), so if you enjoy that Lancome cleanser, there is no reason you won't like this product too, and for a fraction of the cost.

☹ **Age Perfect Anti-Sagging & Ultra Hydrating Day Cream SPF 15** *($15.99 for 2.5 ounces)* is imperfect for skin of any age because it lacks active sunscreen agents that provide sufficient UVA protection. As you may have guessed, this is not the solution for sagging skin.

😐 **Age Perfect Anti-Sagging & Ultra Hydrating Night Cream** *($15.99 for 2.5 ounces)* is nearly identical to the Advanced Revitalift Face & Neck Day Cream above, except this one contains vitamin E instead of vitamin A. Otherwise, the same review applies.

☹ **Age Perfect Double Action De-Crinkling & Illuminating Treatment** *($19.99 for 1 ounce)* invites you to brighten and "de-crinkle" mature skin in one step, and features a dual-chamber container to keep the two products separate until the pump dispenser mixes them just prior to use. Is any of this necessary? L'Oreal claims that this packaging keeps the vitamin C (ascorbyl glucoside, an antioxidant with minimal research on its effectiveness) stable before each use, but an opaque airless pump component would have worked just as well, assuming the product's pH level would keep the vitamin C stable. L'Oreal also claims this product helps alleviate age spots and discolorations, but it contains nothing that can improve such pigmentation problems. This is just a light-textured moisturizer suitable for normal to dry skin of any age, with an antioxidant content that is meager, at best. That doesn't mean this product should be ignored; rather, its capabilities are limited to smoothing and softening the skin while leaving behind a subtle, moist finish. This fragranced product contains salicylic acid, but it is not formulated at the proper pH level to allow exfoliation.

☹ **Age Perfect Eye Anti-Sagging & Ultra-Hydrating Cream** *($15.99 for 0.5 ounce)* is an emollient moisturizer for normal to dry skin that loses points for its jar packaging and the mere dusting of antioxidants. This contains mineral pigments that leave a soft shine finish on skin, but that won't diminish wrinkles (though it does "brighten").

☹ **Age Perfect Pro-Calcium Day Cream SPF 15** *($24.99 for 1.7 ounces)* is yet another anti-aging moisturizer from L'Oreal that lacks sufficient UVA-protecting ingredients. This is maddening given that they clearly know about the issue. But what's really disheartening is that women who use such a product are putting their skin at risk for more wrinkles. Adding insult to injury is a pathetic formulation that is about as state-of-the-art as Wonder Bread. And by the way, the calcium in here (in the form of calcium pantethene sulfonate) cannot be absorbed through skin and has no benefit for skin (or bones) when applied topically.

☹ **Age Perfect Pro-Calcium Day Cream SPF 15, Fragrance Free** *($24.99 for 1.7 ounces)* is the fragrance-free version of the Age Perfect Pro-Calcium Day Cream SPF 15 above, and the same review applies.

☹ **Age Perfect Pro-Calcium Eye Cream** *($24.99 for 0.5 ounce)* is a very thick moisturizer for dry to very skin anywhere on the face. The combination of water, thickener, silicone, glycerin, and wax isn't exciting, but it does make dry skin smoother and soften the appearance of wrinkles. The same comments about calcium for the Pro-Calcium Day Cream above apply here. This is fragrance-free.

☹ **Age Perfect Pro-Calcium Night Cream** *($24.99 for 1.7 ounces)* promises users will wake up with crease-free skin thanks to L'Oreal's double calcium blend. Calcium isn't an antiwrinkle wonder, and this moisturizer ends up being remarkably similar to several others from L'Oreal and sister company Lancome. Its emollient formula is suitable for dry to very dry skin, but the few antioxidants won't survive long once this jar-packaged product is opened. This also contains potentially irritating fragrance components.

L'OREAL PARIS PURE ZONE PRODUCTS

☹ **Pure Zone Deep Action Cream Cleanser** *($6.49 for 6.5 ounces)* is a 2% salicylic acid cleanser in lotion form, but the pH (over 5) is too high for the BHA to be effective as an exfoliant. The menthol is a problem for all skin types.

☹ **Pure Zone Skin Clearing Foaming Cleanser** *($6.49 for 6.7 ounces)* contains menthol, which makes this water-soluble cleanser too irritating for all skin types. Menthol has no effect on skin purity, nor does it help breakouts; it just hurts skin.

☹ **Pure Zone Unclogging Scrub Cleanser** *($6.49 for 6.7 ounces)* contains a lot of alcohol and adds menthol to the mix, making for a skin-irritating experience.

☹ **Pure Zone Pore Tightening Astringent** *($6.49 for 6.7 ounces)* lists alcohol as the second ingredient, making it too drying and irritating for all skin types. Plus the castor oil in here is not what you want to stroke across blemishes.

😐 **Pure Zone Skin Relief Oil-Free Moisturizer** *($6.49 for 2.5 ounces)* is an interesting option for a "moisturizer." This lotion is mostly water, silicone, glycerin, clay, thickeners, preservatives, and fragrance. It will leave a matte feel on skin and the 0.6% salicylic acid would be suitable for someone with normal to oily skin and minimal problems with breakouts. However, the pH of 6 means the salicylic acid is ineffective for exfoliation.

☹ **Pure Zone Continuous Action Spot Check** *($6.26 for 0.5 ounces)* lists 2% salicylic acid as the active ingredient, but the pH is too high for it to function as intended, and the amount of alcohol in this "spot" treatment makes it a problem for all skin types.

L'OREAL PARIS SKIN GENESIS PRODUCTS

😐 **Skin Genesis Multi-Layer Cell Strengthening Daily Moisturizer, Oil-Free Lotion** *($24.99 for 1.7 ounces)* has a brilliant name, one that implies that this rather ordinary lotion can bring about the rebirth of healthy, glowing, beautifully smooth skin. Skin will be smoother and softer thanks to the silky silicone base and similar ingredients, but that's about it. A more flawless complexion is what's promised, but what's delivered is not as state-of-the-art as the claims. Mineral pigments titanium dioxide and mica are on hand to create a subtle glow, and are present in greater amounts than the couple of antioxidants L'Oreal included. For a moisturizer that purports to work deep within the skin's surface, this formula is pretty superficial stuff.

☹ **Skin Genesis Multi-Layer Cell Strengthening Daily Moisturizer, SPF 15 Lotion** *($24.99 for 1.7 ounces)* not only leaves skin vulnerable to UVA damage because it lacks the right active sunscreen ingredients, but also lists alcohol as the third ingredient, making this moisturizer about as moisturizing as using vodka as a toner. What a disappointing, skin-detrimental product!

☹ **Skin Genesis Multi-Layer Cell Strengthening Daily Moisturizer, SPF 15 Lotion, Fragrance Free** *($24.99 for 1.7 ounces)* is, save for the omission of fragrance, identical to the Skin Genesis Multi-Layer Cell Strengthening Daily Moisturizer, SPF 15 Lotion, above, and registers the same disappointment!

☹ **Skin Genesis Multi-Layer Cell Strengthening Daily Treatment, Serum Concentrate** *($24.99 for 1.7 ounces)* lists alcohol as the third ingredient, and this watery product contains nothing of substantial value to the health and appearance of your skin. The couple of potentially worthwhile ingredients in this serum are found in countless others whose formulas (even from those that have been around for years) are a huge improvement over this.

L'OREAL PARIS SUBLIME BRONZE PRODUCTS

☹ **Sublime Bronze Any Angle Self-Tanning Spray, Medium** *($9.99 for 3.9 ounces)* lists alcohol as the first ingredient and also contains some unfavorable fragrant plant extracts, which doesn't make this aerosol self-tanner worth considering over dozens of others.

☺ **Sublime Bronze Dual Action Instant Bronzer and Self-Tanning for Face, Medium** *($10.07 for 1 ounce)* is a lightweight self-tanning lotion for normal to oily skin. Dihydroxyacetone provides the tan, while cosmetic pigments provide instant color that washes off with a standard cleanser.

☺ **Sublime Bronze Self-Tanning Gelee, Medium-Deep, for Body** *($9.39 for 5 ounces)* has a smooth, nearly weightless texture and thus is ideal for normal to oily, blemish-prone skin. The tan comes from dihydroxyacetone, while caramel coloring leaves a sheer tint. This can be used on the face, too!

☺ **Sublime Bronze Self-Tanning Gelee, Deep, for Body** *($9.39 for 5 ounces)* is nearly identical to the Sublime Bronze Self-Tanning Gelee, Medium-Deep for Body, above, except this version contains more dihydroxyacetone for darker skin tones.

☹ **Sublime Bronze Self-Tanning Glove, Medium Natural Tan** *($9.99 for 4 single-use gloves)* is a clever way to apply self-tanner and eliminates the concern about getting tan palms or nails; you just slip on a glove and massage the self-tanner (the exterior of the glove is pretreated; the interior is dry) over your body. Despite the ingenious application method, this self-tanner is not recommended because it contains far too many irritating fragrance components. Why risk irritation when so many dihydroxyacetone-based self-tanners don't pose this problem? Plus, wearing plain old plastic gloves works just as well to prevent your palms and cuticles from getting tan, and would give you a lot more than four applications.

😐 **Sublime Bronze Self-Tanning Lotion SPF 15, Deep** *($9.39 for 5 ounces)* includes avobenzone for sufficient UVA protection, and is otherwise a fairly standard self-tanning lotion for normal to oily skin. The amount of alcohol poses a slight risk of irritation. Keep in mind you will need to apply this tanner liberally if it is going to be your only source of sun protection.

😐 **Sublime Bronze Self-Tanning Lotion SPF 15, Light-Medium, for Face/Body** *($9.39 for 5 ounces)* is remarkably similar to the Sublime Bronze Self-Tanning Lotion SPF 15, Deep, above, yet likely contains a bit less dihydroxyacetone for a tan that's not as dark as the above product would provide.

☺ **Sublime Bronze Self-Tanning Lotion, Deep** *($9.39 for 5 ounces)* is a very standard, but good, self-tanning fluid for normal to oily skin. It contains dihydroxyacetone to color your skin tan, while mica adds a soft shine.

☺ **Sublime Bronze Self-Tanning Lotion, Medium-Deep** *($9.39 for 5 ounces)* is nearly identical to the Sublime Bronze Self-Tanning Lotion, Deep, above, except with more dihydroxyacetone for a darker tan.

😐 **Sublime Bronze Self-Tanning Perfector & Corrector** *($9.99 for 8 0.06-ounce packettes; 0.48 ounce total)* is an emollient scrub that contains alumina as the abrasive agent, along with a lesser amount of pumice. Both will help remove self-tanning mistakes, but this can be irritating to skin unless applied with a gentle touch (and can you be gentle if you're panicked about removing a blotchy application of self-tanner?). A washcloth with a gentle cleanser would work as well with less risk of irritation. In the long run, there really is no reliable way to remove a self-tanner except with time.

☹ **Sublime Bronze Self-Tanning Towelettes, for Face, Light-Medium** *($9.99 for 6 towelettes)* may seem convenient, but these single-use cloths are an expensive way to self-tan! The cloths are steeped in a solution that contains the self-tanning agent dihydroxyacetone, but the number of volatile fragrance components (and the expense—six uses and you'll have to buy more) makes them not worth considering.

☺ **$$$ Sublime Bronze Self-Tanning Towelettes, for Body, Medium** *($9.99 for 6 towelettes)*. Assuming you don't mind the added expense of self-tanning with disposable towelettes, these are a better option than the Sublime Bronze Self-Tanning Towelettes, for Face, Light-Medium, above. That's because they do not contain volatile fragrance components and so are much less likely to cause irritation.

☺ **Sublime Bronze Sunless Scrub, Body** *($7.89 for 6.7 ounces)* is a standard scrub that contains polyethylene (plastic) as the abrasive agent and also a detergent cleansing agent. This dual-purpose product works well to prep skin before applying self-tanner.

☺ **Sublime Glow Daily Moisturizer, for Fair Skin Tones** *($9.99 for 8 ounces)* is a lightweight moisturizer for normal to oily skin. The glow comes from the mica, while a relatively small amount of the self-tanning agent dihydroxyacetone provides a hint of tan color.

☺ **Sublime Glow Daily Moisturizer, for Medium Skin Tones** *($9.99 for 8 ounces)* is nearly identical to the Sublime Glow Daily Moisturizer, for Fair Skin Tones, above, except this one contains more dihydroxyacetone. Otherwise, the same comments apply.

☹ **Sublime Glow for Face Daily Moisturizer SPF 15, for Fair Skin Tones** *($9.99 for 2.5 ounces)* lacks the UVA-protecting ingredients of titanium dioxide, zinc oxide, avobenzone, Tinosorb, or Mexoryl SX, and is not recommended.

☹ **Sublime Glow for Face Daily Moisturizer SPF 15, for Medium Skin Tones** *($9.99 for 2.5 ounces)* lacks the UVA-protecting ingredients of titanium dioxide, zinc oxide, avobenzone, Tinosorb, or Mexoryl SX, and is not recommended.

☹ **Sublime Glow Moisturizing MicroFine Mist, for Medium Skin Tones** *($9.99 for 4.2 ounces)* would be a slam-dunk for all skin types if it did not contain so many volatile fragrance components. The mist facilitates application, but other self-tanners offer this format without the risk of irritation. A great one to try instead is Banana Boat Summer Color Self-Tanning Mist, for All Skin Tones ($6.77 for 5 ounces).

L'OREAL PARIS WRINKLE DE-CREASE PRODUCTS

All of the Wrinkle De-Crease products with L'Oreal's Boswelox complex contain small amounts of the ingredients *Boswellia serrata* and manganese gluconate, which together are allegedly responsible for the wrinkle-smoothing ability of these products. *Boswellia serrata* is also known as Indian frankincense. The active part of this plant is the resin, which contains the anti-inflammatory agents boswellic acid and alpha-boswellic acid. The research pointing to *Boswellia serrata* extract's anti-inflammatory properties was based on its oral consumption. There is insufficient evidence to support its use topically, and it definitely has no effect on muscle contraction or wrinkles (Source: *Natural Medicines Comprehensive Database*, 8th Edition, 2006, page 705). Manganese gluconate is a mineral salt that is found in trace amounts in body tissues. However, there is no evidence that it has any effect on wrinkles, and it definitely has no effect on muscle contractions when applied topically!

☹ **Wrinkle De-Crease with Boswelox Advanced Wrinkle Corrector & Dermo Smoother SPF 15** *($19.99 for 1.7 ounces)* lacks the UVA-protecting ingredients of titanium dioxide, zinc oxide, avobenzone, Tinosorb, or Mexoryl SX, and is not recommended.

😐 **Wrinkle De-Crease with Boswelox Advanced Wrinkle Corrector & Dermo Smoother** *($18.99 for 1.7 ounces)* doesn't work to systematically reduce expression lines, but is an OK, slightly emollient moisturizer for normal to dry skin. The jar packaging won't keep the vitamin E stable.

😐 **Wrinkle De-Crease with Boswelox Daily Smoothing Serum** *($20.32 for 1 ounce)* is a thinner version of the same basic formula L'Oreal recycles for most of their moisturizers. It is primarily water, silicone, glycerin, thickener, slip agent, film-forming agent, vitamin E, plant extract, preservatives, and fragrance. It will make normal to slightly dry skin smoother, but the Boswelox duo will not reduce expression lines.

☹ **Wrinkle De-Crease with Boswelox Eye Wrinkle Corrector & Dermo Smoother** *($19.99 for 0.5 ounce)* contains what L'Oreal refers to as a "breakthrough phyto-complex, combining a powerful dose of boswellia extract and manganese," all of which are said to reduce the appearance of lines around the eye resulting from "facial micro-contractions." Please refer to the introduction to this section for an explanation of these ingredients. This is a simple, but effective, moisturizer for dry skin anywhere on the face. It contains mostly water, silicone, mineral oil, glycerin, thickeners, plant extract, manganese, more thickeners, vitamin E, film-forming agent, and preservatives. It does not contain fragrance, but because *Boswellia serrata* extract is derived from the same family of plants as frankincense, it has a trace of that scent.

☹ **Wrinkle De-Crease with Boswelox Night** *($20.01 for 1.7 ounces)* functions well as a run-of-the-mill moisturizer for normal to dry skin, but it cannot correct wrinkles or expression lines caused by furrowing one's brow, squinting, or smiling. This product will make dry skin feel smooth and soft, just like most moisturizers, but that's where the benefits start and stop.

☹ **Wrinkle De-Crease Collagen Filler, Targeted Wrinkle Reducer** *($19.99 for 1 ounce)* is meant to give the impression that it's a substitute for collagen injections. It isn't. The "technology targeted to wrinkles" sounds new, but it is nothing more than a new spin on the old notion that topically applied collagen can somehow penetrate and supplement your skin's own collagen—it can't. We know collagen damage and depletion lead to wrinkles and other signs of skin aging, but whether it comes in special "bio-spheres" or not, collagen applied in a cosmetic isn't the same substance as the collagen that physicians inject; they have different properties. Even if collagen in a cosmetic could somehow attach to and build up your own collagen, this L'Oreal product contains barely any of it (though you may wonder, if it really worked wouldn't your face change its shape from the buildup of too much collagen?). At best, this is a decent moisturizer for normal to slightly dry skin.

☹ **Wrinkle De-Crease Collagen Filler Eye Illuminator, Targeted Eye Treatment** *($19.99 for 0.5 ounce)* lists alcohol as the third ingredient, which means this "treatment" puts your skin on target for irritation. The amount of collagen and vitamin E is meager, and the collagen can absolutely not work in any way, shape, or form to fill in crow's feet or expression lines.

OTHER L'OREAL PARIS PRODUCTS

☹ **Hydra Fresh Foaming Face Wash, for Normal to Dry Skin** *($6.26 for 6.5 ounces)* is a creamy, foaming, water-soluble cleanser whose potassium hydroxide content, while not a deal-breaker, isn't the best for normal to dry skin. This can, however, be an OK cleanser for normal to very oily skin, and the amount of corn oil is unlikely to exacerbate blemishes.

☺ **Ideal Balance Foaming Cream Cleanser, for Combination Skin** *($6.49 for 6.5 ounces)* is a gentle, basic, lotion-style cleanser that professes to deep clean and reduce the appearance of pores, though it really isn't capable of making pores look any smaller than any other good water-soluble cleanser. The standard detergent cleansing agent in here is quite mild, but it's also not adept at removing makeup, so this is best used in the morning or at night if you wear minimal to no makeup. This cleanser contains several absorbents, including cornstarch, silica, and kaolin (clay), though in a cleanser they won't have much time to absorb oil; instead they'll serve merely as thickening agents.

☺ **Ideal Balance Foaming Gel Cleanser, for Combination Skin** *($6.89 for 6.7 ounces)* is a good, water-soluble cleanser that would be a better choice for makeup removal than the Ideal Balance Foaming Cream Cleanser above. This product does contain a higher than normal level of potassium hydroxide, which can be drying, so this is best reserved for combination to oily skin. The salicylic acid is present more for show than effect, because in a cleanser it's rinsed away before it has time to work on the skin.

😐 **Nutri-Pure Foaming Cream Cleanser** *($5.49 for 6.5 ounces)* features myristic and palmitic acids as the main cleansing ingredients, and although they both produce copious foam (something many consumers appreciate), they can be drying and are the wrong choice for use in a cleanser designed for dry skin. This also contains a higher than normal amount of potassium hydroxide, which will further enhance the drying effects of the cleansing agents. This would be an OK cleanser for someone with oily skin, but better options abound from L'Oreal and most other lines.

✓😊 **Nutri-Pure Self Foaming Cleanser, for Normal to Dry Skin** *($5.86 for 5 ounces)* would be a much better choice for someone with dry skin than the Nutri-Pure Foaming Cream Cleanser above. This water-soluble, fragrance-free cleanser contains gentle but effective detergent cleansing agents coupled with mild foam boosters for a soft, cushiony lather. It is indeed appropriate for someone with sensitive skin, including those with rosacea. In fact, this is L'Oreal's best water-soluble cleanser and a beauty bargain to boot!

😊 **Visibly Clean Foaming Gel Cleanser** *($6.89 for 6.7 ounces)* is a standard, detergent-based water-soluble cleanser that would work well for normal to oily skin. Although it contains salicylic acid, the pH of the cleanser is too high for exfoliation to occur. Even if the pH were low enough, the salicylic acid would be rinsed away before it had a chance to work.

😐 **Refreshing Eye Makeup Remover, Oil-Free** *($6.11 for 4 ounces)* is a standard, detergent-based eye-makeup remover that works best before cleansing and removes most types of eye makeup. It is not rated as highly as others because it contains fragrance.

😊/☹ **ReFinish Micro-Dermabrasion Kit** *($25.12 for the kit)* includes a topical scrub that contains the same aluminum oxide ingredient used in spa- or dermatologist-performed microdermabrasion treatments. Labeled **Gentle Micro-Dermabrasion Exfoliator**, the abrasive agent is in a base of emollients and oils, so its somewhat buffered effect is suitable for someone with dry skin. There are inherent problems to watch for when using this type of scrub, however, such as scrubbing too aggressively or using it too often, which can injure skin. Perhaps more important, however, is that these types of scrubs do not in any way mimic or take the place of microdermabrasion done by a trained professional. That's because just scrubbing the skin is unrelated to the way the microdermabrasion machine works and the way that service is performed. Moreover, microdermabrasion (the real deal) is turning out to be a somewhat disappointing procedure to endure, showing diminishing returns with repeated treatments. This scrub ends up being a standard, somewhat abrasive scrub, nothing more.

The second part of this set includes a **Post-Treatment SPF 15 Moisturizer**. Skin needs sun protection whether it's exfoliated or not (but even more so if it has been exfoliated), so including a sunscreen makes sense. However, and this is a big *however*, it lacks sufficient UVA-protecting ingredients in its rather mundane moisturizing base. Overall, this scientific-sounding kit is really just a very expensive topical scrub with a sunscreen that no one should be using.

😊 **Visibly Clean Foaming Cream Scrub** *($6.49 for 6.5 ounces)* is a good option for a topical scrub product. The moisturizing base will leave normal to dry skin feeling soft, and this contains the tried-and-true ground-up plastic (polyethylene) as the abrasive ingredient. Although it does contain fragrance, it does not include common irritants often found in scrubs, particularly menthol and citrus oils. This does have a mild foaming action, even though the foam has nothing to do with how well the product exfoliates.

☹ **HydraFresh Toner** *($6.17 for 8.5 ounces)* lists alcohol as the third ingredient, which isn't terrible, but it's not helpful either. What follows is barely interesting for skin and makes this a toner you should ignore.

☹ **Ideal Balance Pore Clarifying Toner** *($6.49 for 6.7 ounces)* lists alcohol as the second ingredient, which is a shame, because this would otherwise be a gentle (and basic) soothing toner for normal to dry (but not combination) skin.

☹ **Nutri-Pure Soothing Toner, for Dry Skin** *($6.29 for 6.7 ounces)* would have been a decent, though boring, toner for normal to dry skin were it not for the inclusion of alcohol (it's the third ingredient). Although the amount of alcohol is likely too small to be a big problem, your skin deserves better. This toner has no other significant redeeming qualities to make it worth auditioning.

☹ **Visibly Clean Skin Renewing Toner, for Normal Skin** *($6.49 for 6.7 ounces)* is yet another toner that lists alcohol as the third ingredient, and that makes it a problem for any skin type. This does contain some good water-binding agents (including silicones) along with vitamin C, but the alcohol, even in this small amount, makes this a problem for skin, and your skin deserves better. Doesn't L'Oreal's tag line for their hair products say "Because I'm Worth It?"

☹ **ReNoviste Anti-Aging Glycolic Peel Kit** *($24.75 for the kit)* is L'Oreal's version of their department-store relative Lancome's Resurface Peel ($145 for kit containing 8 applications). Guess what? It's a slightly better system than Lancome's and at a significantly lower price; unfortunately it still has problems to avoid. ReNoviste consists of three steps (Lancome's has four), beginning with the **Soft Glycolic Peel**. This liquid solution contains primarily water, alcohol, and 10% glycolic acid. Its pH of 3.6 allows exfoliation to occur, but there is no reason for your skin to tolerate the irritation from the alcohol when effective AHA products sans alcohol are available. You're instructed to leave this solution on your face for no more than five minutes, at which time you apply the **Post Peel Neutralizer**. This simple, toner-like formula has a pH of 6.3, enough to neutralize the acidic pH of the Soft Glycolic Peel. Yet because rinsing with plain tap water has the exact same effect (tap water has a pH of 7), the Post Peel Neutralizer is an unnecessary product. Besides, after applying the Neutralizer, the instructions indicate you should rinse the skin anyway, which essentially confirms the "why bother?" premise of this step.

After the peel, you finish with an application of **Rebalancing Moisturizer**. Unlike the boring Comforting Cream in Lancome's Resurface Peel, L'Oreal's peel kit contains a thoughtfully formulated, fragrance-free moisturizer that actually bests many of their stand-alone options. The formula contains mostly water, silicone, glycerin, emollients, mineral oil, water-binding agents, antioxidants, thickeners, petrolatum, plant oils, and preservatives, and is good to use whether or not you go through this two-step rigmarole. Its lightweight texture and silky finish are suitable for normal to slightly dry or slightly oily skin, and the opaque tube packaging will help keep the antioxidants stable.

All in all, there's not much reason to consider buying this product. Even though the kit is not much of a financial investment, there are better ways to exfoliate skin, soothe it, and moisturize it. More important, this is absolutely not similar to the type of AHA peel you can get from a dermatologist or at a medical spa. You can find the 10% concentration of glycolic acid in several creams and lotions at department stores, salons, and the drugstore that are much simpler to use. Plus for most skin types daily use of an AHA product is far better than only once a week. If you want a streamlined approach, consider the 10% glycolic acid products from Alpha Hydrox, Peter Thomas Roth, M.D. Formulations, or my product line, Paula's Choice.

☹ **Active Daily Moisture Lotion SPF 15, for All Skin Types** *($8.14 for 4 ounces)* isn't good for those who are active or even for couch potatoes to use daily because it lacks the UVA-protecting ingredients of titanium dioxide, zinc oxide, avobenzone, Tinosorb, or Mexoryl SX.

😐 **Eye Defense** *($13.74 for 0.5 ounce)* is a simply formulated, fragrance-free moisturizer for dry skin anywhere on the face. It contains mostly water, glycerin, plant oil, cholesterol, caffeine, thickener, anti-irritant, and preservative.

☹ **Hydra-Renewal Continuous Moisture Cream, for Dry/Sensitive Skin** *($7.99 for 1.7 ounces)* contains the preservatives methylisothiazolinone and methylchloroisothiazolinone, which are contraindicated for use in leave-on products due to their irritation potential. Needless to say, this product is ill-advised for use on all skin types, but especially sensitive skin.

☹ **Futur-e Moisturizer SPF 15, for Normal to Oily Skin** *($11.03 for 4 ounces)* does not contain the UVA-protecting ingredients of titanium dioxide, zinc oxide, avobenzone, Tinosorb, Mexoryl SX, and is not recommended.

☹ **Futur-e Moisturizer SPF 15, for Normal to Dry Skin** *($10.98 for 4 ounces)* isn't the future for anyone's skin unless you want to make your skin vulnerable to UVA damage. This daytime moisturizer with sunscreen does not have the right active ingredients to protect skin.

😐 **Nutrissime Reactivating Dry Skin Cream** *($10.86 for 2.5 ounces)* doesn't really break any new ground as far as moisturizers go, but it's a decent formula to address the rudimentary needs of normal to dry skin (your skin deserves a more advanced formula, but that doesn't seem to be something L'Oreal can pull off). It is fragrance-free, but the jar packaging will render the vitamin E ineffective shortly after opening. More to the point, it's about time for L'Oreal to start providing more than just vitamin E for antioxidant benefits because one antioxidant isn't ideal for skin and not in the teeny amounts found in this product; not to mention L'Oreal should be providing better packaging.

☺ **Revitalift UV, Daily Moisturizing Cream with Sunscreen SPF 15** *($21.99 for 1.7 ounces)* is identical in every respect to Lancome's UV Expert 20, Face & Body Protection Daily Moisturizing Cream SPF 20 ($35 for 3.4 ounces) and Lancome's option ends up being the less-expensive option when you compare the sizes. Both sunscreens include Mexoryl SX (ecamsule), avobenzone, and titanium dioxide for excellent UVA protection. Neither formula is that moisturizing, while both of them are devoid of antioxidants or any other interesting ingredients. This is a good sunscreen for normal to slightly dry or slightly oily skin, and despite the mundane base, it's still worthy of a happy face rating due to its combination of active ingredients.

☹ **Transformance Skin Perfecting Solution** *($15.99 for 1 ounce; also available fragrance-free)* promises to create "the skin you've always wanted. Ultra-soft. Ultra-smooth. Newly even. Virtually poreless. Flawless." So are you tempted? I have no doubt many consumers will be, but alas, flawless, poreless skin will remain out of reach for anyone who uses this product. This water- and silicone-based moisturizer lists alcohol as the third ingredient. The silicones can make skin feel silky soft, but they won't reduce the size of large pores. The tiny amount of vitamin C is neither unique nor transforming in the least. This product is nearly identical to L'Oreal-owned Lancome's Sensation Totale Continuous-C-Perfecting Complex ($47.50 for 1 ounce), and the Lancome version has the same water-in-silicone base and the same type of vitamin C, namely ascorbyl glucoside. Just like Sensation Totale, Transformance Skin Perfecting Solution is a one-note product. Vitamin C is a good antioxidant, but the amount in both of these products is too small to matter for skin, and the formula lacks any other antioxidants, cell-communicating ingredients, or skin-identical ingredients, which are what really transform skin into looking better and functioning in a healthier manner.

☹ **Visible Results Eye Skin Renewing Treatment** *($19.84 for 0.42 ounce)* cosmetically diminishes the appearance of dark circles due to the amount of brightening pigments it contains. However, beyond these minimally visible cosmetic results (meaning you won't be impressed with the difference this makes), the lavender oil makes it too irritating, especially for use around the eyes.

😐 **Visible Results Skin Renewing Moisture Treatment SPF 15** *($19.09 for 1.6 ounces)* is one of the only daytime moisturizers with sunscreen from L'Oreal available in the United States that includes a UVA-protecting ingredient (titanium dioxide). Unfortunately, it doesn't add much that's new compared to the many other well-formulated sunscreens that are available from Olay, Dove, or Neutrogena. This contains mostly water, glycerin, silicone, thickeners, shine (in the form of mica), more thickeners, film former, fragrant plant oil, preservatives, and coloring agents. The lack of any significant antioxidants, anti-irritants, skin-identical ingredients, or even a vaguely interesting formulation, makes this disappointingly boring. There are far better ways to take care of your dry skin and get sun protection at the same time.

😐 **Wrinkle Defense** *($12.49 for 1.7 ounces)* is similar to most of the L'Oreal moisturizers above, all of which make various antiwrinkle claims that, for one reason or another, cannot be fulfilled. This is a standard mix of water, silicone, thickeners, slip agent, vegetable oil, sunscreen agents, water-binding agents, a tiny amount of vitamin A, fragrance, and preservatives. It's about as exciting as sitting down to do your income tax (my apologies to all of the accountants who get a thrill out of number-crunching).

☹ **Special Care Acne Response Daily Adult Acne Regimen** *($23.99 for the set)* is a seemingly sensible anti-acne skin-care routine consisting of cleanser, toner, and topical disinfectant. However, for a complete regimen during the day, you would need a separate sunscreen and at night, if needed, a gel or serum-type moisturizer for dry areas. Going product by product, you begin by washing with ☹ **Pore-Clearing Cleanser**. It contains 1% salicylic acid, but any benefit that might bring is lost because you quickly rinse this down the drain. More problematic is the amount of alcohol, and it also contains clay, which adds to the dryness and makes it tricky to rinse. Next up is ☹ **Skin-Clarifying Toner**, which contains too much alcohol to make it worth considering, though the amount of glycolic acid and the pH are just sufficient to cause some exfoliation (never mind that glycolic acid isn't nearly as effective against acne as salicylic acid). The only worthwhile product in this kit is the ☺ **Blemish-Fighting Lotion** with 2.5% benzoyl peroxide in a nonirritating, fragrance-free lotion base. It is a simple but effective option to kill acne-causing bacteria, but you don't need to spend this much money for such a product or waste your money on the other products in the kit that you shouldn't be using. Instead, consider the benzoyl peroxide–based topical disinfectants from Neutrogena, Stridex, Zapzyt, or my Paula's Choice line of products.

☹ **Special Care Acne Response Intensive Adult Acne System** *($23.99 for the set)* continues the trend of launching multistep, at-home kits designed to replicate the types of treatments typically performed under a dermatologist's or aesthetician's care. The problem with these kits—especially those from L'Oreal and its department store–owned line Lancome—is that for all their clinical posturing, the products are either poorly formulated or completely boring. Step 1 of this version from L'Oreal involves washing your face with the **Pre-Peel Prep Treatment**. It contains only 0.55% salicylic acid, which is an inadequate amount, and in a product that is quickly rinsed from the skin. Even if the amount were adequate, it wouldn't have any chance to impact your skin. Otherwise, this is a very standard, water-soluble cleanser that is easily replaced by others at the drugstore.

Next is the main event, **Intensive Peel**. With 2% salicylic acid plus glycolic acid, this would be a formidable option to combat blemishes or blackheads—if the pH weren't above 4 and the product didn't contain so much alcohol, which makes this intensely irritating and problematic for any skin type. The last step is the **Post-Peel Neutralizing Moisturizer**, a lackluster, dry-finish formula that isn't needed because the peel itself doesn't work, which negates the need to neutralize. Not to mention the fact that just rinsing with water would neutralize this type of peel. Making this even more useless is the amount of alcohol and clay it contains, especially for a product calling itself a moisturizer. The 0.6% salicylic acid is ineffective due to the product's high pH. All told, given the availability of well-formulated cleansers and pH-correct BHA products, there is no reason to invest in this kit. And it definitely is no substitute for a dermatologist-delivered BHA peel.

L'OREAL PARIS MAKEUP

FOUNDATION: ✓☺ True Match Super Blendable Makeup SPF 17 *($9.99)* is L'Oreal's best foundation for normal to very oily skin. The fluid, silky formula feels almost weightless on skin and blends superbly, setting to a natural matte finish that is translucent enough to let your skin show through, while still providing light coverage that diffuses minor flaws and redness. The original version of this foundation did not include sunscreen, but L'Oreal wisely added one with the sole active being titanium dioxide. Now True Match Super Blendable Makeup is an even better choice for those with oily skin. The palette of 24 shades is not only one of the largest shade selections for a single drugstore foundation, but also, for the first time, L'Oreal's shades take a strong cue from Lancome's typically superior selection of neutral colors. Almost all of the shades are excellent, and they cover a wide range of skin tones from porcelain to deep tan. The only shades to avoid are Natural Ivory C2 and Classic Beige C5 (both too pink), and Tawny Beige C6 (too peach).

The only drawback to this foundation is its drier finish. Although it does a good job of reducing oily shine and keeping skin looking polished, it tends to emphasize the slightest bit of dry skin, and can also make lines around the eye look more apparent. If you have dry areas or visible lines around the eye, it is imperative that you smooth and hydrate these areas before applying this foundation. An emollient moisturizer lightly applied around the eyes and regular use of an effective topical exfoliant should minimize this problem and make working with this foundation a better experience. Note: This foundation contains subtle shimmer particles that impart a barely perceptible shine to the skin. The particles are so small you have to look very closely to see them in daylight, but it's worth mentioning for those who wish to avoid any type of shimmer in their makeup.

☺ **Cashmere Perfect Soft Powdery Liquid Foundation** *($10.99)* has an accurate name, at least in terms of this nonaqueous foundation's powder attribute. It dispenses as a thick cream but once blended melts into a silky fluid that quickly sets to a smooth, powdered finish. It has so much slip that controlled blending is a challenge, but this can be remedied by carefully applying the makeup to one area of the face at a time. L'Oreal claims the powder finish lasts for 12 hours, a marker I suspect most women who use this foundation won't reach. It is appropriate for normal to very oily skin, provides light to medium coverage, and is available in nine shades, though only five actually look like skin. Classic Ivory is a good pale shade with a slight (not objectionable) pink cast, while Nude Beige, Natural Beige, Buff Beige, and Sand Beige are also recommended. Avoid Natural Ivory, Creamy Natural, Classic Beige, and Honey Beige, which are all too peach or pink to look convincing. Note: Unlike most L'Oreal foundations, Cashmere Perfect has a strong fragrance.

☺ **Ideal Balance Balancing Foundation for Combination Skin** *($12.79)* is another foundation claiming to moisturize dry areas while keeping shine in check over oily ones. Considering the number of people who readily identify with the combination skin profile, it's not surprising that products with promises to reconcile the demands of this skin type keep appearing. Despite the name, this makeup is not capable of balancing anything, though the slightly thick, noticeably silky texture glides on and feels smooth. This has a soft matte finish that won't hold back excess oil for long—you can almost sense the moisture in the formula at war with an army of dry-finish ingredients. Overall, this formula is best for someone with normal to slightly oily skin, because it is matte enough to look unflattering over dry or flaky patches. If you decide to try this, the best almost-neutral shades from the assortment of 12 colors are Soft Beige, Beige, Buff, Tan, Caramel, Mocha, and Cappuccino (the last two are excellent for dark skin tones). The remaining colors are unabashedly pink or peach.

☺ **Ideal Balance QuickStick Balancing Foundation for Combination Skin SPF 14** *($12.79)* is a slightly revised version of L'Oreal's former stick foundation, with the most notable improvement being the colors, which are now much more neutral. There really aren't any bad options among the 12 shades, primarily because each blends out so well. As stick foundations go, this has a thicker, less silky texture and tends to drag over skin a bit. You can remedy this by applying a light layer of moisturizer first, but that's not a good choice for oily areas, so blend carefully. Coverage goes from sheer to medium, and this foundation builds well without looking too heavy. The sunscreen is all titanium dioxide, and because SPF 14 is so close to the benchmark SPF 15 I opted to rate this with a happy face. By the way, this foundation is not a "fast, smart solution" for both oily and dry areas. The silicone-enriched matte finish exaggerates the slightest amount of dry skin, so be sure to prep any dry areas with moisturizer before applying this.

😐 **Infallible Never Fail Makeup SPF 18** *($13.89)* is a mixed bag. On the pro side, this is one of the few L'Oreal foundations to feature an in-part titanium dioxide sunscreen, plus it feels nearly weightless and undeniably silky on skin. The major con is the way this foundation looks on skin—in a word, heavy. I doubt most women will like the strong, dry-matte finish and full coverage of this foundation. Its silicone technology ensures long wear without fading or streaking, but also demands careful, precise, and efficient blending before it sets. It is best for those with normal to very oily skin who are seeking a long-wearing matte finish and need substantial coverage, even at the expense of looking made-up. Among the 14 shades, 4 are disappointingly pink or peach: avoid Natural Ivory, Buff Beige, True Beige, and Cocoa. The remaining shades include options for fair to dark skin, though the choices aren't as impressive as L'Oreal's True Match Super-Blendable Makeup SPF 17 above. By the way, not only do the vitamins and minerals not fight signs of facial fatigue (as L'Oreal claims), but also the amount of them in this foundation is inconsequential for providing skin with any level of benefit.

😐 **Visible Lift Firming Line-Minimizing + Firming Makeup SPF 17** *($13.49)* is meant for those concerned with wrinkles, yet immediately falls short (at least in the prevention department) by not providing a sunscreen with UVA-protecting ingredients. The advertised Pro-Retinol is not actually retinol, but rather retinyl palmitate, the fatty-acid form of vitamin A. However, both the amount of it and the pea extract (with its over-hyped, silly claims) are so tiny that your skin won't be one fraction firmer, nor will lines retreat. So, should you consider this foundation? It does have a silky application and smooth, satin-matte finish capable of providing medium coverage, and it comes in six mostly good shades—only Sand Beige may be too peach for medium skin tones. But for a foundation positioned as an advanced solution for the visible signs of aging skin, it is a disappointment. Still, if you have normal to slightly dry skin and are willing to pair this with an effective sunscreen, its better qualities make it worth checking out, though I wouldn't consider it over Revlon's Age Defying Makeup with SPF 15.

☺ **Visible Lift Line Minimizing Makeup SPF 17** *($11.29)* now sports a higher SPF rating, yet without the UVA-protecting ingredients of titanium dioxide, zinc oxide, avobenzone, Tinosorb, or Mexoryl SX it is not recommended for sun protection. Without that critical element, forget about any line minimizing! On the plus side, it does have a silky texture that melds with the skin and dries to a soft matte finish. You'll get light to medium coverage and, despite the fact that the target market for this is women with dry skin, the non-emollient formula is best for normal to oily skin. There are ten shades, including a couple of options for very light skin tones. The following shades should be avoided due to overtones of pink and peach: Pale, Buff, Creamy Natural, Golden Beige, and Sand Beige.

😐 **Visible Lift Extra Coverage Line Minimizing Makeup SPF 12** *($11.29)* does not contain adequate UVA protection, though you may notice that titanium dioxide is listed as the third ingredient on the regular (not the active) ingredient list. However, if it is not listed as an "active ingredient," that doesn't count for UVA protection. Despite the sun-protection problems, this silky, creamy formula lives up to its extra-coverage claim. The finish is natural matte, making it suitable for someone with normal to slightly dry skin who is willing to wear a separate sunscreen underneath. There are nine shades available, but six are too peach or pink and they look incredibly artificial given the opaque nature of this foundation (which tends to darken significantly as it dries). The only contenders are Nude Beige, Natural Beige, and Golden Beige.

😐 **Feel Naturale Light Softening One-Step Makeup SPF 15** *($12.79)* is a cream-to-powder makeup with a smooth, creamy application and a soft, slightly matte finish. It's an older formula that's not as elegant as today's best cream-to-powder makeups, and the lack of sufficient UVA protection makes it a tougher sell. If you decide to try this anyway, it is best for normal to slightly dry skin. Although the label makes the ubiquitous "oil-free" claim, this does have waxes that will likely aggravate the situation for those prone to breakouts. The 12 shades feature some good neutral choices; the ones to avoid are Sand Beige, Golden Beige, Buff (can be too peach), Soft Ivory (slightly pink), Sun Beige (too peach), and Cocoa (ash).

😐 **Bare Naturale Powdered Mineral Foundation SPF 19** *($14.99)* is one of the few L'Oreal foundations with sunscreen that contains the right UVA-protecting ingredients. However, the titanium dioxide and zinc oxide in this loose powder "mineral makeup" conspire to create an opaque, heavy-looking finish, no matter how well you blend. If you're considering this foundation as your sole source of sun protection you'll need to use a generous amount, which only makes your skin look coated and powdery, not bare or the least bit natural. Curiously, although L'Oreal is the first major cosmetics company to venture into the category of mineral makeup, their version, unlike most others, contains talc, which most mineral makeup lines decry as being a problem for skin. (Of course, talc is absolutely a natural earth mineral with a magnificent texture when it is finely milled.) Nonetheless, the natural sunscreen agents zinc oxide and titanium dioxide, and bismuth oxychloride—the more typical ingredient found in "mineral" makeups—are present in high enough concentrations to be comparable to others in this category of makeup, such as the options from bare escentuals. What's odd about this type of makeup is that the opacity and the dry feel seem less bothersome than they are because it leaves your skin with a soft glow. Such radiance usually denotes moisture, but not here. If anything, skin feels increasingly dry the longer this type of powder foundation is worn. Still, if you're curious to see how mineral makeup looks on your skin, L'Oreal did produce eight soft, neutral shades for light to tan skin tones, and the brush applicator is soft and dense enough to allow controlled application of the powder.

☹ **Age Perfect Skin-Supporting & Hydrating Makeup for Mature Skin SPF 12** *($16.49)* is supposed to be makeup with built-in skin-care benefits, but the most significant benefit is the titanium dioxide sunscreen (though SPF 12 still falls short of the benchmark for daytime protection). This water- and silicone-based, whipped-cream foundation has a phenomenally silky texture that smooths on like a second skin and provides light coverage with a radiant matte finish that looks beautiful. If your mature skin is dry, you'll need to pair this with a moisturizer because it isn't too "skin-supporting" in that regard. The ingredients that are supposed to support the claim of "making skin age perfect" are present in amounts too small to function as anything but window dressing, but the feel of this makeup makes it worth considering if you have normal to slightly dry or slightly oily skin and are willing to pair it with an effective sunscreen rated SPF 15 or greater. More good news: 11 of the 12 shades are suitably neutral! The only shade to avoid due to a noticeable peach cast is True Beige. Interestingly, several of the shades that appear too pink or peach in the jar set to a neutral hue. There are no shades for dark skin tones, an odd oversight given how well L'Oreal did with darker shades for their True Match liquid makeup.

CONCEALER: ✓ ☺ **True Match Concealer** *($7.89)* comes with a brush applicator (rather than the standard sponge tip), and is truly a beautiful liquid concealer thanks to its smooth, even-blending texture that feels ultra-light, yet provides fairly good coverage. It sets to a natural matte finish and does not crease, though the coverage isn't opaque enough to hide prominent dark circles. Nine shades are available, and six of them are ideal neutral options for light to medium skin tones. Avoid N6-7-8, which tends to turn peach, C1-2-3 (too pink), and C6-7-8 (too orange).

✓ ☺ **AirWear Long-Wearing Concealer** *($10.19)* is a smooth, silicone-based liquid concealer that glides on and covers well without looking heavy or thick. It has a crease-free matte finish that is a pleasure to blend, and it layers beautifully for areas that need more intense camouflage. Of the six colors, avoid Corrector (too yellow), Brightener (too pink), and Deep (may turn ash on darker skin tones).

☺ **Visible Lift Eye Line Minimizing Concealer** *($9.99)* has an elegant, creamy application that dries to a soft matte finish and it doesn't crease into lines around the eyes. This is very similar to Lancome's popular Effacernes Concealer ($25.50). The four skin-tone shades are beautiful, though Medium-Deep won't work very well for darker skin tones. Avoid the overly yellow Neutralizer and white Lightener shades. For all this concealer's good qualities, it won't minimize lines, and you can test that for yourself by applying a dab to eye-area wrinkles and blending, and leaving the other eye without concealer. The wrinkles on the bare side will be less apparent—one of the unfortunate elements of thinking that makeup will disguise wrinkles!

☺ **Infallible 16-Hour Concealer** *($9.99)* won't really last for 16 hours without minor signs of fading or creasing (when applied to the under-eye area), but it is still a formidable stick concealer with a slightly creamy texture that doesn't have too much slip. It provides good coverage and sets to a soft powder finish that does a good job of staying in place, plus each of the four shades is worth considering. This type of concealer is not recommended for use over blemishes because of the waxlike thickening agents necessary to keep it in stick form.

😐 **Ideal Balance Stick Concealer for Combination Skin** *($8.99)* is a creamy, twist-up stick concealer that goes on opaque but can be blended to achieve medium coverage. The formula remains creamy on the skin, so this isn't the best choice for use under the eyes (some creasing is inevitable, but not intolerable), or over oil-prone areas and blemishes. The six shades walk the line between acceptable and unattractive peach, which isn't the best tone to use over dark under-eye circles or reddened areas. The best shades are Cream Light, Medium, and Deep. The Corrector shade is too yellow to work for most skin tones, but may be worth a try if you have minor red discoloration or prefer a creamy texture. For best results, set this concealer with powder.

POWDER: ✓ ☺ **True Match Super-Blendable Powder** *($9.99)* has the distinction of offering the largest palette of shades available at the drugstore. That is to the advantage of almost all skin tones, because this is an outstanding, talc-based pressed powder. Its texture isn't quite as otherworldly as Estee Lauder's AeroMatte Powder ($26), but it's close, and the price difference between the powders should give you pause. True Match Super-Blendable Powder is suitable for all but blemish-prone skin (owing to the inclusion of cornstarch, a food-based ingredient that can feed the bacteria that contribute to blemishes). Among the 24 shades, divided into groups of warm (W), cool (C), and neutral (N), the only ones to avoid are W5 (too peach), N5 and N6 (too orange), C4 (too ash), and C7 (too copper). Shade C2 is great for very fair skin because it is neither too white nor too pink.

✓ ☺ **Translucide Naturally Luminous Powder** *($10.59)* is a talc-free loose powder with a marvelous, powdered-sugar texture and a smooth, even finish. It feels like silk on the skin and leaves a subtle radiant finish. The amount of vitamin C is negligible, but the packaging isn't the type to keep it stable anyway. All four sheer shades are excellent. This fragranced powder is perfect for those with normal to dry skin who hate to look powdered but want to look polished.

☺ **Visible Lift Line Minimizing Powder** *($12.49)* is a translucent, talc-based powder with a silky, very sheer finish and a hint of shine. It won't diminish one line on your face, but it nicely sets makeup and is an option for all skin types except very oily. All the shades but one are excellent; avoid Colour Lift, a pink tone that no one should be dusting all over their face.

☺ **Glam Bronze Bronzing Powder** *($12.49)* presents three shades of talc-based pressed bronzing powder. Two have a soft, radiant shine that isn't distracting, while Enchanting Sunrise is ultra-sparkly. Regardless of which shade you choose, this applies evenly and deposits soft color, though it would be nice if the shades leaned more toward tan to bronze rather than peach to copper. You may want to use this as a blush rather than a bronzer, especially if you have fair to light skin.

😐 **Ideal Balance Pressed Powder SPF 10** *($10.99)* has a supremely silky, talc-based texture and applies evenly, if quite sheer. The titanium dioxide sunscreen is a nice touch, but the SPF rating is disappointing. Oddly, not all of the four shades include sunscreen, so choose carefully. You're likely wondering whether this powder can balance the skin, keeping dry areas from looking too powdery and oily areas from showing breakthrough shine. As smooth as this no-coverage powder is, meeting two such dissimilar expectations is a dream that won't come true for anyone with combination skin. Even so, this doesn't leave a dry or powdered finish, so although skin won't be balanced, it does fare better over dry areas than many other powders.

BLUSH: ✓ ☺ **Feel Naturale Light Softening Blush** *($11.99)* remains one of the best pressed-powder blushes at the drugstore thanks to its super-silky formula, expert application, and shades with enough pigment to last all day without fading. It is recommended for all skin types, and most of the shades are matte (or nearly so). The following shades are quite shiny, and best for evening, if at all: Charmed Peach, Mauvelous, Mocha Rose, and Plume.

✓☺ **True Match Super-Blendable Blush** *($9.99)* is a collection of silky powder blushes whose sheer colors and seamless application do indeed make them super-blendable. The palette of soft colors is beautiful and is divided into warm, cool, and neutral tones just like L'Oreal's True Match foundation, powder, and concealer. You might find their blush groupings confusing (some of the cool shades go on more golden or peach than befits that description), but if you shop by the color itself rather than by its classification you should be satisfied. Each blush also indicates a coordinating shade of L'Oreal True Match foundation and powder, but blush color and foundation or powder color are unrelated so you can ignore that matching as well. Aside from those details, this is one of the better powder blushes at the drugstore. (Note: Each shade has a subtle shine, but it gives a soft glow to the cheeks, not distracting sparkles.) Compared to L'Oreal's equally impressive Feel Naturale Light Softening Blush, True Match has a lighter feel and deposits slightly less color on skin.

✓☺ **Bare Naturale Gentle Mineral Blush** *($14.49)* is a loose powder blush that is talc-based (remember, talc is a mineral, too—so you can think of this in the mineral makeup category) and has an airy, gossamer texture that looks beautiful and blends superbly. The workable, built-in brush sweeps on a sheer layer of color and imparts a glowing (not sparkling or distracting) finish to perk up the complexion. The shade selection isn't large, but each is worth considering if you don't want a matte finish blush. Best of all, this formula doesn't feel or make skin look dry or flat, and layers well if you wish to build more color.

☺ **Blush Delice Sheer Powder Blush** *($9.99)* may be sheer when it comes to color impact, but not when it comes to shine. Wearing any one of the five shades is more about adding iridescence than color, but if that's your goal or you have a disco night planned, this smooth blush won't disappoint.

EYESHADOW: 😐 **Wear Infinite Eyeshadow** *($3.99 singles, $4.99 duos, $6.99 quads)* comprise the bulk of L'Oreal's eyeshadow offerings. The colors are divided into Perle (noticeably shiny), Matte (true matte to subtle shine), and Rich (deeper matte and soft shine colors for contour or lining) finishes, and the color selection presents plenty of classic shades. For example, there are a number of viable options among the quads, although, with the exception of Wood Rose and Subtle Berries, each has at least one shiny shade. The formula is very silky, but also very sheer and almost waxy-feeling. Don't count on anything close to infinite wear from these, but for very soft color and easy application, they'll do. The best matte Singles are Sandy Shores, Brushed Suede, Deep Mocha, Lush Raven, Smooth Latte, and Midnight Sky. From the Duos, only Classic Khaki is matte.

😐 **Wear Infinite Holographic Eye Shadow Single** *($3.89)* has a creamier, thicker texture than the original Wear Infinite Eyeshadows and has a bit more pigment, too, which makes application and building intensity easier. There are only a handful of shades, each with a strong metallic sheen that's best for unwrinkled eyes. The holographic effect is just a way to describe shine that in different lighting or from different angles goes from bronze to plum to dusky pink. That can make coordinating an eye design tricky, but it's fun for special occasions.

😐 **Illumination Loose Eye Color** *($6.99)* may sound like a mess waiting to happen, but L'Oreal packaged this loose-powder eyeshadow to minimize the mess potential. Housed in a plastic container is a built-in brush to apply this shimmering powder. It goes on easily with minimal flaking, but after an hour or so you'll see how it just doesn't cling well, which causes fading and, eventually, flaking. There are better ways to achieve shiny eyes than this, despite the smart packaging.

☺ **Touch-On Colour for Eyes and Cheeks** *($10.19)* imparts minimal color but maximum shine. This soft-textured, cream-to-powder product works best to highlight the top of the cheekbone or brow bone, but only if you want intense shine. It blends well without too much slip, and the shine tends to stay put, especially compared to shiny loose powders.

EYE AND BROW SHAPER: ✓☺ **Lineur Intense Felt Tip Liquid Eyeliner** *($8.29)* used to be known as Line Intensifique, and in the previous edition of this book it was a favorite liquid liner. It still is, and one to seriously consider if you're a fan of Lancome's equally impressive but much costlier Artliner Precision Point Eyeliner ($27). The felt-tip applicator makes applying liquid eyeliner easier than ever, and the formula dries quickly and has amazing tenacity, not to mention a resistance to smudging, smearing, or flaking.

✓☺ **Voluminous Eyeliner** *($7.49)* has an applicator the company refers to as a "mistake-proof marker," which involves an even, steady flow of liquid color. It works quite well, and allows better precision than you'll get from a standard, thin liquid eyeliner brush. The versatility of the slanted tip is supposed to let you draw a thin or thick line, but I couldn't get the line as thin as L'Oreal's illustration, regardless of how I held the tip or how much pressure I applied (or didn't apply, which I also tried). Still, unless you insist on a thin line, this eyeliner is definitely recommended. Application is easier than most, the formula dries quickly and doesn't smear or flake, and it removes with a water-soluble cleanser.

😐 **Wear Infinite Soft Powder Eye Liner** *($7.19)* is a standard pencil with a swift, smooth application and a reliable powder finish. If you prefer pencils and don't mind routine sharpening, this is one to consider because it is less likely to smudge or fade than many others. However, the color selection is mostly shiny, and there are several hues that are inappropriate for lining the eyes, unless you're going for all-out techno-glamour.

😐 **Wear Infinite Waterproof Self-Sharpening Eyeliner** *($7.49)* is an automatic, non-retractable pencil with a thick tip that makes it tricky to draw a thin line. Application is easy due to this pencil's smooth glide, but its finish is somewhat sticky. It is partially waterproof and getting it wet results in some loss of color, but you'll still have some definition.

😐 **Le Kohl Smooth Defining Eyeliner** *($7.49)* is a standard, needs-sharpening pencil reminiscent of Lancome's Le Crayon Kohl ($22). It applies smoothly without being greasy and stays in place quite well. The shade selection has been edited down to just the classics, and all of them have merit. 😐 **MicroLiner Ultra Fine Eyeliner** *($8.29)* is a needs-sharpening pencil that promises "the precision of a liquid liner." Considering how tough it is to be precise with a liquid liner, that's not much of a claim! The advantage of this pencil is its slender tip that allows for a thin, discrete line, or you can build the line for more drama. Because this stays creamy, some smudging is apparent by day's end (much sooner if you have oily eyelids), but it is an option if you prefer pencil and want a very fine line. 😐 **Pencil Perfect Automatic Eye Liner** *($7.49)* isn't what I would call perfect; if anything, it tends to go on creamier than most and that means greater risk of smearing. As a plus, it doesn't need sharpening, but it's non-retractable, so don't wind up more than you need. Avoid green Sage and the self-explanatory Paris Blue.

😐 **Brow Stylist Brow Shaping Duet** *($7.49)* is marketed to women who have a difficult time finding a brow pencil to match their brows. You get two small, standard pencils in lighter and darker variations of classic colors (including options for blondes and redheads). The color pairings are thoughtful, but with the wealth of brow-enhancing options available, it really isn't necessary to use two pencils to get your perfect shade, if anything it can make an otherwise easy application step awkward and choppy looking. In addition, L'Oreal's formula is a bit too creamy to last and can make brows feel slightly matted.

😐 **Telescopic Precision Liquid Eyeliner** *($7.99)* is outfitted with an excellent slanted-tip brush that makes it relatively easy to draw an even line following the curvature of the eye. The formula takes a bit longer to dry than usual, which can encourage smearing, but what's most disappointing is the color saturation runs out before you've made it to the end of the lash line, necessitating another application. This stays in place and wears quite well once set, but it turns out to be a liquid eyeliner that demands more patience than many others, including L'Oreal's own Lineur Intense Felt Tip Liquid Eyeliner reviewed above.

☹ **Lineur Intense Brush Tip Liquid Eyeliner** *($7.99)* is a surprisingly bad liquid liner. The main problem is the stiff brush that tends to splay and deposit color unevenly. The formula dries quickly, but remains smear-prone longer than it should, which is reason enough to leave this on the shelf.

LIPSTICK, LIP GLOSS, AND LIPLINER: ✓ ☺ **Glam Shine Dazzling Plumping Lipcolour** *($8.99)* makes lips look plump only by virtue of its coverage and shimmery finish. However, do take the "glam" part of this name seriously, because each color (mauve and plum tones dominate) is definitely about putting the spotlight on lips. This lightweight, slightly creamy gloss feels supremely smooth and completely non-sticky, and has longer-than-average staying power.

✓ ☺ **Colour Riche Lip Gloss** ($5.49) is L'Oreal's best lip gloss, period. It has a silky yet moisturizing texture that imparts sheer to medium color (depending on the shade) and leaves lips with a glossy finish free of stickiness. The shades, including the goes-with-anything Rich Pink, are bound to please—and don't be nervous about trying the deeper hues; each goes on softer than it appears.

☺ **Colour Riche Nurturing and Protective Lipcolour** *($7.49)* is rich in every way except price, which is a boon for you and your lips! This decadently creamy lipstick offers intense colors that have admirable staying power, although it is creamy enough to slip into lines around the mouth. You'll find this almost identical to Lancome's Rouge Sensation Multi-Sensation LipColour ($22.50), right down to the fragrance. In terms of being nurturing and protective, it is no more so than many other creamy lipsticks. L'Oreal's in-store displays nicely divide this large collection of lipsticks into color families, making it easy to find the type of shades you like.

☺ **Endless Comfortable 8-Hour LipColour** *($9.99)* feels remarkably light and has a minimally creamy finish, yet imparts intense, pulls-no-punches color that really lasts, although not for eight hours. You'll need to touch up after coffee breaks or eating (this isn't a transfer-resistant formula), but for the most part this leaves standard creamy lipsticks behind in the longevity department. The **Endless Platinum** colors are infused with lots of silver glitter and have a slight metallic finish, but are otherwise identical to the original formula (the Platinum version is packaged in silver while the other colors come in a gold tube).

☺ **Endless Kissable ShineWear, The Glossiest Zero-Transfer Lip Duo** *($9.99)* is a two-part system that's somewhat of a spin on long-wearing lip products such as Max Factor's Lipfinity. Lancome fans will recognize this duo as being nearly identical to the company's Juicy Wear Ultra-Lasting Full Colour and Shine Lip Duo ($25.50). The concept is the same: Apply a seemingly regular lipstick, allow one or two minutes for it to set, then (because lips will feel dry and tight) slather your lips with an ultra-shiny, wet-look gloss. The gloss ensures comfortable wear without causing the lipstick color to fade, travel into lines, or smear. If you follow the instructions, this (just like Lancome's version) really does stay put for hours and transfers minimally onto napkins, coffee cups, and significant others. The all-silicone gloss coat feels slick and unlike traditional gloss, but if you find it's texture agreeable, it allows for even wear—no balling, chipping, or peeling lipstick. I still prefer Estee Lauder's and M.A.C.'s versions to this, but L'Oreal comes close, the price is right, and the shade range is tempting.

☺ **Colour Juice Stick** *($9.49)* advertises "sheer, light, luscious" as its selling points, yet this creamy lipstick isn't nearly as lightweight as L'Oreal's Endless Comfortable 8-Hour Lipcolour above, nor are the colors that sheer. Rather, this is a moisturizing, light-coverage lipstick with a soft glossy finish and an enticing range of fruit-scented colors. Despite the glossy finish, this isn't too slippery, and lasts a bit longer than standard glossy lipsticks. ☺ **Colour Juice Sheer Juicy Lip Gloss** *($7.79)* is a tube lip gloss that comes in a dazzling array of shades, from sheer cherry to sparkling pale gold and peachy bronze tones. As glosses go this is nothing exceptional, but the deeper shades impart longer-lasting color and the formula provides a minimally sticky, wet-look finish that leaves lips feeling moist rather than slippery. I actually preferred this to Lancome's Juicy Tubes Ultra-Shiny Lip Gloss ($17.50) and encourage you to compare them and walk away with the savings when you notice how much better the L'Oreal version is.

☺ **Colour Riche Anti-Feathering Lipliner** *($7.79)* is a standard, twist-up, retractable pencil with a built-in sharpener. The sharpener part isn't really necessary given the finer point that most twist-up pencils like this one already have; plus, after one use the shavings clog the sharpener and that's that. Application is smooth and creamy, and the available colors are versatile. Oh, and it does a great job of preventing lipstick from feathering into lines around the mouth!

😐 **Volume Perfect Re-Shaping Lipcolour** *($9.99)* is a dual-ended lipstick. One side is a colorless lip balm/stick that is supposed to fill in lines and ridges on the lips. This is a "primer" step, and is said to create a uniform surface that allows the lipstick to go on more smoothly, resulting in lips that appear fuller and more youthful. The ads for this lipstick (featuring the unquestionably gorgeous Andie MacDowell) make it look as if her lips have almost no lines at all. Your real-world experience will prove otherwise—the lip primer feels like a silicone and wax mixture, and makes little visible difference when the lipstick is applied over it. Actually, I preferred the way the lipstick looked *without* the primer underneath. Even though the extra step isn't warranted, this is a decent creamy lipstick whose semi-opaque colors come in a striking palette, though most are infused with large particles of silver shimmer, which tend to stay on (and around) the lips as the color fades—not the best look for the mature woman this product is targeted toward.

😐 **Endless Kissable Lipcolour** *($8.79)* promises to be a "zero-transfer, extremely long lasting" experience for your lips. I am pleased to report that this lipstick succeeds in staying put and, aside from the occasional trace of color, does not transfer onto objects (think coffee cups) or people (think a friendly "hello" kiss, not a passionate smooch). Its matte-finish formula dries quickly, leaving pigment on your lips without a trace of moisture or gloss, so your lips have color, but no slip or moistness. The instructions state that this product is not to be used with another balm, lip gloss, or lipstick, an advisory I found wise, because adding an emollient product on top of this lipstick definitely cuts its longevity. However, because this lipstick makes lips feel dry, most women will want to pair it with something that feels creamy, as I did, which only minimally affected the staying power. It's worth a try, but it's not in the same league as two-step products such as Max Factor's Lipfinity or M.A.C.'s Pro Longwear Lipcolour.

☹ **Infallible Never Fail Lipcolour** *($11.99)* is another lip paint/top coat duo, although this one is packaged to resemble a Zippo lighter (that probably wasn't the intention, but the association is impossible to ignore). The problem right off the bat is that although the base color applies sheer, it goes on unevenly, which was a problem with the darker shade. In fact, the darker shades went on so unevenly that I could not get them applied appropriately, and trying to smooth it out with the topcoat turned the whole thing into a mess that necessitated starting over. Application of the lighter, paler colors went better. The Lipcolour is, as expected, a bit drying and the color wears off unevenly, although a sheer wash of color did adhere to my lips throughout the day while eating and drinking. Reapplication of the top coat solved any dryness issues, but it did have to be reapplied several times throughout the day. Also, while the top coat is moisturizing and has a nice sheen, if you want a glossier finish for evening, you'll be disappointed with it. Back to the packaging: although it is compact and portable, it isn't as convenient as superior long-wearing lip color products from Cover Girl, Max Factor, or Maybelline New York.

☹ **Crayon Petite Automatic Lip Liner** *($7.49)* is an automatic, nonretractable lip pencil that is definitely creamier than most and offers some good colors, including a Clear version. Unlike the Colour Riche Anti-Feathering Lipliner, this doesn't stop lipstick from bleeding into lines around the mouth.

MASCARA: ✓☺ DoubleExtend Lash Extender & Magnifier Mascara *($10.49)* is a dual-ended mascara, including a lash "Magnifier" (primer) on one end and actual mascara on the other. The Lash Magnifier is just clear mascara, adding extra layers that you can't really see. It's no different from adding extra layers of the black mascara on the other end of the tube, so it's a relatively unnecessary step because this mascara does magnificently well on its own, building incredible length and thickness without clumps or flakes.

☺ **Double Extend Lash Fortifier & Extender Mascara Waterproof** *($10.49)* is a dual-ended mascara with a lash primer/conditioner on one end and mascara on the other. You apply the white "Extender" first and then sweep on the mascara. Supposedly, this pairing should bring about "lush lashes up to 60% longer," but what ends up happening is that the results with the Extender, though assuredly impressive, are the same as applying two or three coats of the mascara alone, which is exactly what I did. When I asked friends if the lashes on one eyelid looked longer, thicker, and more dramatic than the other, no one could tell a difference. Both the Extender and the mascara contain ingredients necessary for a waterproof mascara, and true to claim, this does not budge when lashes are wet, nor does it clump during application or flake during wear. This is another stellar mascara, but one that doesn't need the gimmick of a primer step to sell itself.

✓☺ **Full Definition Voluminous Volume Building Mascara** *($6.99)* is another stellar mascara from L'Oreal. This formula closely matches, if not mimics, the performance of Lancome's Definicils Mascara ($23), meaning it excels at creating long, softly fringed, and separated lashes with some thickness. It keeps lashes soft yet wears all day without smudging or flaking, and comes off easily with a water-soluble cleanser.

✓☺ **Lash Architect 3-D Dramatic Mascara** *($8.29, straight or curved brush)* remains a prime pick if your goal is long, thick, dramatic lashes. With just a few sweeps lashes go from blah to wow, with only minor clumping (and only then if you're overzealous during application). Whether you use the straight or curved brush option you will not be disappointed; either formula also leaves lashes curled in a way the Panoramic Curl Extreme Mascara below can't touch.

☺ **Waterproof Volume Shocking Mascara** *($12.99)* is a waterproof mascara that really did produce shocking results, and I mean that in a good way! Although the lash-enhancing result isn't as prodigious as its non-waterproof partner, you'll still be shocked by how long and thick this two-part mascara makes your lashes. A translucent white primer is applied first, using a standard mascara brush. This is followed by mascara, applied with a serrated comb applicator. It's the applicator that takes lashes from blah to bountiful in seconds, and the more you comb it through your lashes, the longer and thicker they get. However, if you can't restrain yourself, you'll find this produces a too-heavy look that must be smoothed out lest you go all day with thick, spidery-looking lashes. The formula wears well (an overzealous application may produce minor flaking) and takes patience to remove, so be prepared. Otherwise, if you want a false-eyelash effect that holds up to rain and tears, you've found it!

☺ **Telescopic Mascara** *($7.99)* is L'Oreal's version of Lancome's superior Fatale Exceptional Volume Sculpting 3D Comb-Mascara ($23). Lancome's version has the edge due to a better application, but results with either mascara amount to dramatically long, thick lashes. Telescopic uses a multisided comb (rather than brush) applicator and its biggest problem is immediate clumping and a too-heavy appearance. Luckily, the flipside of the comb allows for smoothing things out, but it still takes patience (and perhaps a separate lash comb or brush) to get all the clumps combed through. Although this mascara does not apply in a wink, it wears beautifully all day and keeps lashes soft.

☺ **Panoramic Curl Extreme Curl & Separating Mascara** *($8.49)* disappoints when it comes to curling lashes. It can go on a bit unevenly, but the brush allows for easy comb-through—and once dry, the formula wears and removes well. While not as perfect as L'Oreal's long-gone Le Grand Curl Mascara, this is still a worthwhile option for equal parts moderate length and thickness. ☺ **Panoramic Curl Extreme Curl & Separating Waterproof Mascara** *($8.49)* leaves lashes soft while being tenaciously waterproof and allowing you to build long lashes that maintain a slight curl. You'll get a bit of thickness, too, and no clumps or flakes, which make this one of L'Oreal's better waterproof mascaras.

☺ **Lash Out Lengthening and Separating Mascara, Curved Brush** *($7.49)* has a better brush than the original Lash Out mascara below, and that enables you to build a touch more length with a softer, cleaner separation. Thickness is not in this mascara's bag of tricks, but if that's not what you need or prefer, this is fine. ☺ **Lash Out Waterproof Lengthening and Separating Mascara** *($7.49)* produces better-than-average length and creates lifted, slightly curled lashes that remain soft. The formula is waterproof, too.

☺ **Voluminous Volume Building Mascara** *($6.99, straight or curved brush)* remains a superior lengthening mascara, but falters when it comes to creating noticeably thick, lush lashes. It doesn't clump or smear, however, and it does hold up beautifully throughout the day, making it a good choice if you're not expecting dramatic results as claimed. Results are the same whether you use the straight or curved brush.

☺ **FeatherLash Water Resistant Mascara** *($7.49)* is marginally adept at lengthening, but won't build even a hint of thickness. It goes on easily, with no globs or clumps, but be prepared to work for anything more than a subtle effect. What's best about this mascara is that lashes stay soft to the touch and the formula nicely resists water, yet is easily removed with a water-soluble cleanser. Those traits make it worthy of a happy face rating.

☺ **Volume Shocking Mascara** *($12.99)* is shocking, at least if you're used to average or natural-look mascaras! This two-step mascara includes a Lash Defining Base Coat and a

Volume Constructing Top Coat. The Base Coat is a white "primer" whose formula is similar to that of most mascaras, minus the pigment. It nicely separates and lengthens lashes, but things really get exciting when you apply the Top Coat. It goes on with a comb instead of a brush applicator, and the result is a heavier application of mascara that dramatically lengthens, thickens, and curls with a few strokes. As usual, I applied the primer step on one set of lashes and then used just the mascara on the other. Usually the difference isn't noticeable, but it was this time, albeit marginally. The side with the Base Coat produced fewer clumps when the Top Coat was applied, although some clumping was apparent with or without the Base Coat, as was minor flaking during wear. That's the tradeoff if you decide to try this product: magnificently enhanced lashes, but an application process that demands precision and, preferably, a clean brush to comb through lashes so clumps are smoothed out. This is surprisingly easy to remove with a water-soluble cleanser.

😐 **Lash Out Lengthening and Separating Mascara** *($7.49)* doesn't extend lashes as much as the name implies. This is one of the more lackluster mascaras from L'Oreal, but it serves its purpose if all you need is a satisfactory lengthening mascara that provides minimal thickness. 😐 **FeatherLash Softly Sweeping Mascara** *($7.49)* has a clean, slightly wet application, but does little to magnify lashes beyond their natural state. Most women will want more than that, but for those seeking a "natural look" mascara that leaves lashes slightly gelled yet soft, this is an OK option. 😐 **FeatherLash Softly Sweeping Mascara, Curved Brush** *($7.49)* has the same traits as the original FeatherLash, but this time the curved brush makes it easier to apply an even, sheer layer for barely defined lashes.

😐 **Voluminous Waterproof Mascara** *($6.99)* won't knock your socks off with prodigious length and thickness, but it does a respectable job in both departments. The main reason to choose this is for its clump-free application and strong waterproof properties. 😐 **Lash Architect Waterproof 3-D Dramatic Mascara** *($8.29)* has the same brush as the non-waterproof Lash Architect above, but the results here prove that the best mascaras are an ideal union of brush and formula. Because this waterproof formula is thinner, you get less than half the oomph of the non-waterproof version, making for a less-impressive mascara. It lengthens well, doesn't clump, and is waterproof, which may be reason enough for you to give it a try.

FACE AND BODY ILLUMINATING/SHIMMER PRODUCTS: 😐 **Glam Bronze All-Over Loose Powder Highlighter** *($12.49)* has a formula that is nearly identical to the Translucide Naturally Luminous Powder above, but this one has a low-glow golden shimmer. It feels weightless and can be an attractive way to highlight large areas of skin, but it comes off easily and you're guaranteed to lose your gleam within an hour or two. How disappointing!

BRUSHES: L'Oreal's collection of short-handled **Makeup Artiste Brushes** *($5.89–$12.89)* competes nicely with similar drugstore offerings from Revlon and Prestige, but these aren't in the same league as department-store brushes. The ✓😊 **All Purpose Shadow Brush** *($7.89)* is excellent, a soft, elegantly tapered brush great for applying all-over color or for softly defining the eye's crease. 😊 **All Purpose Powder Brush** *($12.89)* is a workable brush that is nicely shaped and dense enough for controlled application of powder. It isn't luxuriously soft, but does the job at an attractive price. 😊 **Precision Concealer Brush** *(7.89)* is also good, though I prefer something that is thinner and has a more pointed tip. This synthetic brush moves across the skin without pulling or dragging, and is worth a look if the shape appeals to you. Less impressive are the standard 😐 **Brow/Lash Brush** *($5.49)* and ☹ **Lip Brush** *($7.89)*. The Brow/Lash Brush is OK, and the price isn't off-putting—but softer bristles would have been better. The

Lip Brush has a decent shape, but the bristles are too soft and sparse for controlled application of lip color.

☺ **Makeup Artiste Travel Brush Set** *($13.89)* comes with four tiny brushes for applying powder, eyeshadow, concealer, and lipstick. They're housed in a thick plastic pouch, and while the small size isn't as elegant as brushes with longer handles, it's a convenient set to toss in your purse or desk drawer for quick touch-ups.

SPECIALTY PRODUCTS: 😐 **De-Crease Eye Shadow Base** *($7.99)* has its purpose, but doesn't replace a long-wearing, matte-finish concealer, which is essentially how this product works. It's a powdery liquid that comes in a single, pale peach–toned shade. You'll get light coverage and a solid matte finish suitable for powder eyeshadow application. The talc-based formula keeps lids matte, but again, so does a matte-finish concealer, and unlike De-Crease, your matte-finish concealer works elsewhere (such as under the eyes), too.

L'OREAL PARIS H.I.P. MAKEUP

✓☺ **Flawless Liquid Makeup SPF 15** *($13)* is nearly identical to L'Oreal's True Match Super Blendable Makeup SPF 17, reviewed above. The same comments for texture, application, finish, and UVA protection apply here, too. The difference is the more varied selection of shades for women of color, and these shades are a bit more intense (less is more, but don't skimp too much if you're relying on this as your sole source of sun protection). The 16 shades present options that favor medium to deep skin tones; there are no suitable shades for fair skin. The following shades are too peach, orange, or copper: Fawn, Terra, and Cappuccino (slightly orange; may work some tan skin tones). Mahogany is a beautiful shade for darker African-American skin tones. Last, but not least, the sunscreen is pure titanium dioxide.

☺ **Vibrant Shimmer Bronzing Powder** *($12)* is a talc-based pressed bronzing powder with a smooth, dry texture and relatively soft application. The shine is a bit obvious and sparkling, but clings decently. Radiant is the most versatile shade among the three; Blesses is more gold than bronze, and works best as a highlighting powder on medium to dark skin tones.

☺ **Blendable Blushing Creme** *($10)* is a somewhat thick-textured cream-to-powder blush. Each of the three shades is strongly pigmented and finishes with a soft metallic shine. Elated is suitable only for dark skin tones, the others are more versatile—but due to the color intensity, these are tricky to apply softly. They do have good staying power, though.

☺ **Concentrated Shadow Duo** *($7)* has contrasting, sometimes shocking, colors as its biggest drawback. Most of the duos have more to do with creating colorful rather than artfully shaded eyes. Application-wise, these are very smooth, so blending is effortless. They have a silky texture and moderate pigment saturation (which means that even the darkest shades may need to be layered for more intensity). Every duo has at least one shiny shade, but it clings well. The most workable duos are Shady, Mischief, Dynamic, Foxy, and Saucy.

😐 **Bright Shadow Duo** *($7)* is identical to the Concentrated Shadow Duo above, except these duos feature very colorful, bright combinations, all of which are difficult to work with if your goal is a natural eye design. These are options if you want bold colors that draw attention to themselves rather than to your eyes.

☺ **Pure Pigment Shadow Stick** *($10)*. This resembles tiny pieces of chalk and has a talc-based, slightly dry texture that applies better than you'd think. Drag is present but tolerable, and once you "draw" the shadow where you want it, you can blend a bit and soften any hard edges. Speaking of edges, using this stick on its edge allows it to function as a long-wearing powder eyeliner, too. It may also be used wet, which intensifies the effect of each shade. Alluring, Dazzling, and Majestic are the best shades for shadow, while Exquisite is an option for highlighting. The other shades aren't as impressive.

😐 **Shocking Shadow Pigments** *($12)* come packaged in a tiny jar (with a sifter to keep things tidy) and include a small but workable eyeshadow brush for application. The colors and intense shine are way too magnified and noticeable (and not in a good way), making this best for evening makeup when you really want strong shine; in daylight it looks way too obvious and overdone. Tenacious, Intrepid, and Restless are the easiest hues to work with. This would be rated higher if the shine had better cling; the texture is supremely smooth.

☺ **Color Truth Eyeliner** *($8)* needs routine sharpening, but that's the only drawback that keeps this from earning a Paula's Pick rating. It applies easily without skipping and the silicone-enhanced formula sets quickly to a smudgeproof powder finish. Try Black and Brown, but avoid Green and Navy because they are both a bit extreme.

✓☺ **Color Truth Cream Eyeliner** *($11)* is L'Oreal's version of the long-wearing gel eyeliners sold by some department-store lines, as well as my Paula's Choice line. Just like all the others, this has a soft, cream-gel texture that must be applied with a brush. A mini angled eyeliner brush is included, and is workable, but most consumers will want something more elegant or capable of drawing a thinner line. Performance-wise, this applies smoothly and sets quickly to an immovable finish. Oddly, color saturation isn't as strong as for other HIP products, so you may need to layer to get more dramatic results. Still, this matches its competitors for long wear without smearing, and requires an oil- or silicone-based remover. All five shades are worth considering, depending on whether you want a classic or trendy look.

✓☺ **Intensely Moisturizing Lipcolor** *($10)* has a luscious, creamy texture and fully saturated colors. This has a slight tendency to bleed into lines around the mouth, but is otherwise recommended for fans of creamy lipsticks with a plush, moist finish. The shade selection is beautiful, especially if you favor bold colors.

😐 **Brilliant Shine Lip Gloss** *($9)* is an average tube lip gloss that has a very thick, unusually sticky texture. This makes it last longer than many other glosses, but that's not too exciting given how uncomfortable it can feel. The shimmer-laced colors are quite pigmented and apply almost the way they look in the tube.

✓☺ **High Drama Volumizing Mascara** *($10)* has a brush that's similar to L'Oreal's Lash Architect 3-D Dramatic Mascara reviewed above, and performs about the same. You'll get long, thick, lush lashes with nary a clump, and all in a few strokes. Someone asked me if I was wearing false eyelashes or had lash extensions when I wore this out to dinner—that's how dramatic the results are, yet it keeps lashes soft. The Ultimate Blue Black shade isn't noticeably blue; it's just a very deep, inky black.

☺ **Illuminating Highlighter** *($10)* presents two complementary shades of a cream-to-powder shimmer in one compact. The shine stays on well and this sets to a finish that tends not to smear. The color saturation isn't anyone's definition of high intensity, but this blends well over foundation, blush, or eyeshadow.

LUMEDIA
(SEE BREMENN RESEARCH LABS)

LUMENE (SKIN CARE ONLY)

LUMENE AT-A-GLANCE

Strengths: Relatively inexpensive; some good serums and eye creams; every sunscreen contains sufficient UVA-protecting ingredients, though some have low SPF ratings; good selection of cleansers and eye-makeup removers.

Weaknesses: An overall mediocre assortment of products; lots of jar packaging; some sunscreens have disapprovingly low SPF ratings; no AHA or BHA products; Lumene's use of supposedly rare arctic or Scandinavian ingredients, including arctic cloudberry, peat, and water lily, lack substantiated research proving they have any benefit for skin; the Premium Beauty products are as premium as Wonder bread.

For more information about Lumene, visit www.lumene.com or www.Beautypedia.com.

LUMENE BLUE & BLUE SENSITIVE PRODUCTS

☹ **Blue Hydra Drops Moisturizing Day Cream SPF 4** *($10.49 for 1.7 ounces)* features a pitifully low SPF rating that is absolutely insufficient for daytime protection, even though its sole active ingredient is titanium dioxide. Even if the SPF were what it should be (the minimum is SPF 15 according to the American Academy of Dermatology, www.aad.org), this is a very boring moisturizer with lackluster, ordinary ingredients. This is not recommended over superior daytime moisturizers from Olay, Dove, or Neutrogena, among many others.

😐 **Blue Hydra Drops Moisturizing Eye Gel** *($10.49 for 0.5 ounce)* boasts the "freshness of pure spring water," but fresh or not, water alone isn't enough to make eye-area skin look and feel better. The only ingredient of merit in this lightweight gel is glycerin, but it's accompanied by a dry-finish ingredient that likely disrupts (at least partially) any hydrating benefits. A couple of intriguing ingredients are present, but in tiny amounts (they're listed well after the preservative), along with some potential irritants. All in all, this adds up to a below-average eye gel.

😐 **Blue Hydra Drops Moisturizing Night Cream** *($10.49 for 1.7 ounces)* is a basic emollient moisturizer for dry to very dry skin. It contains mostly water, thickeners, vegetable oil, glycerin, plant oils (including olive oil), preservative, silicone, anti-irritant, and fragrance. For basics this will do, but your skin deserves more.

☹ **Blue Hydra Luminous Matt Tinted Day Cream SPF 6** *($10.49 for 1.7 ounces)* includes avobenzone for UVA protection, but SPF 6 is embarrassingly low for anyone who takes daily sun protection seriously (and that is the only way to take it!). The base formula is almost as boring as that of the Blue Hydra Drops Moisturizing Day Cream SPF 4 above, except for its sheer, almost imperceptible tint. It also includes tiny quantities of vitamins, but your skin deserves better than a token amount.

😐 **Blue Hydra Drops Intensive Moisturizing Mask** *($10.49 for 2.5 ounces)* has claims that make it sound like a dream product for sensitive skin in need of soothing. However, this is a rather basic, fragrance-free mask that lists denatured alcohol as the fifth ingredient, meaning that it's neither that intensive nor particularly beneficial for dry skin. It's a decent though unimpressive moisturizer for normal to slightly dry skin and contains a tiny amount of oat extract to support its anti-irritant claim, but in name only.

😐 **Blue Sensitive Tender Drops Soothing Moisture Cream** *($15.99 for 1.7 ounces)* has some promising ingredients for skin, including ceramides, anti-irritants, and antioxidant vitamins. However, their presence is a mere dusting, and even if there were more significant quantities, this moisturizer's jar packaging wouldn't keep the antioxidants stable for long. This is a good, though unexciting, fragrance-free emollient moisturizer that's an OK option for dry to very dry skin.

😐 **Blue Dream Lips Age-Defying Lip Care** *($4.99 for 0.5 ounce)* doesn't list an SPF rating on the package, but the active ingredient list reads: "Titanium Dioxide SPF 4." That type of sunscreen labeling is not what the FDA mandates for sunscreens, but given that Lumene products are made in Europe (where sunscreens are not sold as over-the-counter drugs), that's forgivable. What's not as easy to overlook is the SPF rating itself, which is way too low for protection. Independent of the sunscreen issue, this is a very well-formulated lip balm that contains a blend of petrolatum (Vaseline) with other emollients and olive oil. It will nicely protect and nourish dry, chapped lips; it just isn't the best option for daytime unless you apply another lip sunscreen or opaque lipstick afterward.

LUMENE LIFTING PRODUCTS

☹ **Lifting Time Freeze Targeted Wrinkle Treatment** *($18.99 for 0.47 ounce)* is one of those products where the claims, not the quality, define the elevated price tag. Bringing "a little magic to your skin care routine … with surgical precision" is definitely a lofty assertion, but this product doesn't deliver any of that or have any line-smoothing benefits. This fragranced product also contains the menthol derivative menthyl lactate and, as such, is too irritating to use around the eyes, and is a waste anywhere else.

😐 **Lifting Magic Drops Instant Beautifyer** *($19.99 for 1 ounce)* is another water-based serum claiming to smooth fine lines, this time with a "Lumene bio-communicator compound" of natural ingredients. The minuscule amounts of seaweed, soy, and water lily extract won't reduce wrinkles. All in all, this is more of a plasticizer for skin than a state-of-the-art antiwrinkle treatment that can provide skin with beneficial ingredients.

😐 **Lifting Skin Supporter Day Firming Day Cream** *($19.99 for 1.7 ounces)* doesn't show an SPF rating other than mentioning SPF 4 on the active ingredient list (as in the Blue Dream Lips Age-Defying Lip Care above), which is not permitted for U.S.-manufactured sunscreen products. Regardless of regulatory issues, an SPF 4 (even if the product contains the UVA-protecting ingredient avobenzone) is too low for reliable daytime protection. Were this rated SPF 15 and packaged in an airtight container, it would be a good choice for those with dry to very dry skin. As is, it has more shortcomings than positives.

😐 **Lifting Skin Supporter Eye Firming Eye Cream** *($18.99 for 0.7 ounce)* is a good, though somewhat basic, moisturizer that is suitable for use around the eye area, although it would be better without the fragrance. It contains mostly water, thickeners, plant oil, algae, wax, anti-irritants, plant extracts, glycerin, and preservatives. Although light in texture, its oil content makes it best suited for dry skin around the eyes or elsewhere.

😐 **Lifting Skin Supporter Night Firming Night Cream** *($19.99 for 1.7 ounces)* is a passable choice if you have dry to very dry skin and want an emollient moisturizer that's not overly greasy. However, the rather short supply of antioxidants and the jar packaging don't add up to great skin care. Although this has merit for making dry skin look and feel better, it almost goes without saying that skin deserves more than this moisturizer provides (and it won't lift your skin in any way, shape, or form).

☹ **Lifting Time Freeze Instant Lift Mask** *($18.99 for 2.5 ounces)* contains enough alcohol and menthyl lactate (a menthol derivative) to be considered too irritating for all skin types. Its "lifting" and "freezing" ability is fictional.

LUMENE PREMIUM BEAUTY PRODUCTS

☺ **$$$ Premium Beauty Rejuvenating Day Cream SPF 15** *($29.99 for 1.7 ounces)* deserves credit for including an in-part avobenzone sunscreen, but that's about it. The overall formula is tailored to those with dry skin, although antioxidants are barely present, which doesn't jibe with this product's name or its price point. The price for this product is preposterously high given its similarity to all of the other Lumene moisturizers that cost a lot less. Lumene attributes the product's firming ability to peptides, yet they're clearly an afterthought and there isn't substantiated research proving they firm skin anyway, though they can be useful skin-care ingredients. This is an effective moisturizing sunscreen for normal to dry skin, but it isn't a premium choice by any stretch of the imagination.

☺ **$$$ Premium Beauty Rejuvenating Eye Cream** *($22.99 for 0.5 ounce)* will pique the interest of those who are endlessly trying to get rid of dark circles in the under-eye area because Lumene claims that's what this moisturizer is for. But it is merely another ordinary eye cream for normal to dry skin, containing a standard blend of water, plant oil, absorbent, and thickeners. The claimed dark circle–eliminating ingredient is the bioflavonoid hesperidin methyl chalcone. Although there is research pertaining to this ingredient's effect on edema (swelling) and capillary function when administered internally, there is no research proving it has any effect on dark circles. Darkness under the eye isn't usually due to a problem with weak capillaries or edema. Rather, under-eye skin is so thin that in some people, the blood passing through veins under the eye produces a bluish to purple discoloration. There are other causes of dark circles, too, such as lack of sleep and allergies, but the fact remains that hesperedin methyl chalcone is not the answer for treating the problem.

☺ **$$$ Premium Beauty Rejuvenating Instant Serum** *($29.99 for 1 ounce)* is premium in name only, and its rejuvenating ability is minimal due to a lackluster formula in which the only helpful ingredients are listed well after the preservative. This is an OK, serum-type moisturizer for normal to slightly dry skin, but it absolutely will not delay the formation of new lines or even-out age spots (pigment discolorations). It does contain small amounts of several fragrant components that can be problematic for sensitive skin, or for all skin types when used around the eye.

☺ **$$$ Premium Beauty Rejuvenating Night Cream** *($29.99 for 1.7 ounces)* is the cream version of the Premium Beauty Rejuvenating Instant Serum above, and the same basic review applies. The main difference is that the Night Cream adds the emollients and thickeners necessary to create the product's texture. Lumene claims the tiny amount of sea buckthorn oil in this will promote the regeneration of skin cells, but don't count on it. This is an average moisturizer that is best for normal to dry skin—but your skin deserves a lot more than this product can provide.

☺ **$$$ Premium Beauty Age Spot Treatment** *($27.99 for 0.5 ounce)* boasts of its ability to lighten and even-out age spots while keeping them from becoming darker. This is merely a moisturizer masquerading as a skin-lightening product, because none of the ingredients have a proven track record for reducing hyperpigmentation. The two types of vitamin C in this "treatment" have shown promise for helping hyperpigmentation, but in amounts substantially larger than what Lumene uses. This is barely recommended as a basic moisturizer for normal to slightly dry skin.

☹ **Premium Beauty Rejuvenating Lip Care** *($27.99 for 0.5 ounce)* is a thick-textured cream recommended to enhance the fullness of your lips as it smooths the lines around them.

The fullness effect comes from the irritation caused by peppermint and menthyl lactate. There are countless other lip balms that do not contain irritants to choose over this expensive mistake.

LUMENE VITAMIN+ PRODUCTS

😐 **Vitamin+ Energy Cocktail Fortifying Cream** *($17.99 for 1.7 ounces)* claims to pamper dry skin from the first application, and, like most moisturizers with a basic blend of vegetable oil, thickeners, and emollients, it will do just that—albeit not with the most elegant texture or interesting formula. The vitamin E that is present won't remain stable in the jar packaging once the product is opened.

😐 **Vitamin+ Energy Cocktail Pampering Drops** *($17.99 for 1 ounce)* is a decent serum consisting primarily of water, jojoba oil, thickeners, plant oils, glycerin, and vitamin E. Other antioxidants are also included, but they don't account for much of the formula. However, this is still worth it if you have dry skin, and it can be used alone or paired with another moisturizer.

😐 **Vitamin+ Radiant C-Energy with SPF 15 Age-Defying Day Cream** *($17.99 for 1.7 ounces)* contains an in-part avobenzone sunscreen in a lightweight base suitable for normal to slightly dry skin. Unfortunately, that's the most enticing part of this jar-packaged moisturizer. It contains several antioxidants, but they are listed after the preservatives. Given that, and the packaging, which exposes them to light and air, your skin won't come out ahead. The big-deal ingredient in this product is arctic cloudberry (*Rubus chamaemorus*), which Lumene maintains gives your skin energy. I couldn't find any published research supporting that claim, but did discover a German publication that examined the fatty acid content of several berry species from Finland, including those in the *Rubus* genus, and they stated that this ingredient (as it is used by Lumene in its oil form) is considered a good source of triglycerides (fatty acids) for skin (Source: www.springerlink.com/content/j4mxw0yt4cwlhyfp/). That makes it good for dry skin, but it won't change the energy or age of your skin.

😐 **Vitamin+ Radiant C-Energy Age-Defying Intensive Care** *($15.99 for 1.7 ounces)* is supposed to prevent premature aging of skin due to its reservoir of antioxidants, but the only antioxidant of note in here is vitamin E, and even that is in limited supply, not to mention that the jar packaging won't keep it stable anyway. In addition, almost all of the unique or interesting ingredients are listed after the preservatives, as seems to be the pattern for Lumene moisturizers in general.

☺ **Vitamin+ Radiant C-Energy Eye Intensive Renewing Eye Serum** *($15.99 for 0.34 ounce)* has a unique roll-on applicator and a relatively interesting formula that packs more of a skin-friendly punch than most of the other Lumene moisturizers. That makes it a standout in this line—although when compared to other well-formulated products, this would be at the end of the list. It contains a decent blend of glycerin, plant oil, soothing agents, water-binding agents, and stabilized vitamin C; is fragrance-free; and is suitable for use around the eye area.

😐 **Vitamin+ Radiant Dual Serum Energising Morning Serum & Age-Defying Night Serum** *($17.99 for 1.7 ounces)* is a two-part product that, just like all the others in the Vitamin+ line, purports to give your skin energy and renewed radiance. Energising Morning Serum (no confusion here as to when this product is to be used) is mostly water, emollient, glycerin, several film-forming agents, and preservative. The peptides and other intriguing ingredients are barely noticeable. Without sunscreen, there is no advantage to using this during the day rather than the evening. All you can expect from this serum is slight hydration. Age-Defying Night Serum is essentially a more moisturizing version of the Morning Serum. Otherwise, the same basic comments apply, and there is nothing about this serum that makes it more useful for your skin when used in the evening. The two-part system is far more gimmicky than helpful and there's no reason to believe Lumene's "instant energy" claims.

☺ **Vitamin+ Retinol Night Revitalizer Age-Defying Night Cream** *($15.99 for 1 ounce)*. In comparison to other Lumene moisturizers, this is a fairly impressive formulation and the packaging is appropriate to keep the product stable. For normal to very dry skin, this is a consideration.

😐 **Vitamin+ Vita-Nectar Vitalizing Day Cream SPF 15** *($14.99 for 1.7 ounces)* is worth considering for its in-part avobenzone sunscreen, but the rest of the formula, while not terrible, is just ordinary with no notable difference from any standard sunscreen. It is best for normal to dry skin.

😐 **Vitamin+ Vita-Nectar Eye Vitalizing Eye Cream SPF 6** *($14.99 for 0.7 ounce)* lists titanium dioxide as the only active ingredient, but on its own an SPF 6 is too low to use for daytime protection. Once again, Lumene's idea of antioxidants in skin-care products has seemingly more to do with window dressing than efficacy, although this is a well-packaged, slightly emollient moisturizer for normal to dry skin. It would earn a happy face rating if its sunscreen were at least SPF 15.

😐 **Vitamin+ Vita-Nectar Vitalizing Night Cream** *($14.99 for 1.7 ounces)* has slightly more antioxidants than the typical Lumene moisturizer, but given Lumene's overreliance on jar packaging that's not saying much. This is an average water-and-wax moisturizer that cannot forestall premature aging, though the amount of avocado oil it contains is helpful for dry skin.

😐 **$$$ Vitamin+ Radiant C-Energy Drops Beauty Capsules** *($21.99 for 28 capsules)* include an appreciable amount of vitamin C (ascorbic acid) packaged in single-use capsules to protect its potency. The silicone base will make skin feel silky, but the fragrance components are a disappointing addition. These capsules aren't as exciting as Elizabeth Arden's Ceramide Advanced Time Complex Capsules Intensive Treatment for Face and Throat ($65 for 60 capsules; 0.95 ounce), and end up costing nearly the same because Arden provides twice as many capsules.

😐 **Vitamin+ Radiant C-Energy 5-Min. Mask Invigorating Facial Mask** *($15.99 for 2.5 ounces)*. You might as well rinse this off after five minutes because your skin won't receive much benefit from this mask, no matter how long you leave it on. This very basic concoction of water, thickener, silicone, glycerin, and more thickeners is acceptable for normal to dry skin, but don't expect an application of this to rid your skin of the lingering signs from even a week's worth of fatigue!

OTHER LUMENE PRODUCTS

☺ **Express Touch Cleansing Wipes** *($2.49 for 10 wipes)* provide a quick, convenient way to remove makeup or refresh skin. Despite the low price, these aren't much of a value. The cost works out to be about 25 cents per cloth, while similar options from Pond's, Olay, Aveeno, and Dove cost less. If you opt to try Lumene's version, their formula is best for normal to dry skin not prone to blemishes.

☺ **Matt Touch Balancing Gel Cleanser** *($8.99 for 5.1 ounces)* is a very basic, water-soluble cleanser that is only capable of controlling shiny skin by removing surface oil, just like many similar cleansers. If you have naturally oily skin, you'll see shine in the same amount of time, so this option, while effective as a cleanser for normal to oily skin, isn't distinctive.

☺ **Milky Touch Gentle Cleansing Emulsion** *($8.99 for 6.8 ounces)* is a standard cleansing lotion that does not contain detergent cleansing agents. That makes it a gentler option for dry, sensitive skin, and it rinses surprisingly well (though you may need a washcloth to remove stubborn makeup). This can remove eye makeup, as Lumene recommends, but it would be better suited for the eye area if it didn't contain fragrance.

☺ **Moisture Dream Revitalizing Cream Cleanser** *($8.99 for 5.1 ounces)* is a good, water-soluble, foaming cleanser for normal to slightly dry skin. It can remove makeup and it rinses well, so don't misconstrue the cream portion of the name as meaning this is akin to a typical cold cream.

☺ **Absolute Away Eye Makeup Remover for Waterproof Makeup** *($5.99 for 4.2 ounces)* is a dual-phase, water-in-silicone eye-makeup remover that works well to break down long-wearing makeup, including waterproof mascara. The small amount of witch hazel isn't likely to be problematic even for use around the eyes.

☺ **Gentle Eye Makeup Remover** *($5.99 for 4.2 ounces)* is indeed a gentle, water- and glycerin-based liquid that removes most types of eye makeup, but it isn't as adept at removing mascara (waterproof or not) as is the Absolute Away Eye Makeup Remover above. This is worth trying, although the cleansing agents are best rinsed from the skin instead of left on it.

☺ **Arctic Touch Dual Action Exfoliating Cream** *($8.99 for 3.4 ounces)* combines a cleanser and scrub in one product whose oil content makes it preferred for normal to dry skin not prone to blemishes. Polyethylene (ground-up plastic) is the abrasive agent, and the moisturizing ingredients in this cleanser keep it on the gentle side, even if you happen to get a bit overzealous while massaging it on skin. The oils impede rinsing slightly, but their overall effect on dry skin makes this side issue easy to live with.

😐 **Dream Mist Hydrating Water Spray** *($7.99 for 5.1 ounces)* could not be a more basic toner if it were just water, which is mostly what this contains. More dreary than dreamy, this is almost not worth using at all given its limited benefit for skin, but it's an option if your skin is normal all around and you just need a little help removing excess makeup that your cleanser may have missed.

☹ **Matt Touch Balancing Facial Tonic** *($8.99 for 6.8 ounces)* lists alcohol as the second ingredient, which makes this toner too irritating for all skin types. Alcohol doesn't tighten pores, it just irritates your skin and causes it to swell, which momentarily makes pores appear smaller. That isn't helpful for skin in the least and can be problematic in the long run.

😐 **Milky Touch Alcohol-Free Facial Tonic** *($8.99 for 7 ounces)* is another ho-hum product from this poorly conceived skin-care line. It will help complete the cleansing process, but this bland blend of mostly water, castor oil, and preservative cannot balance skin functions, and castor oil can feel sticky on the skin. Think of this as Twinkies for the skin, just not as much fun.

😐 **Moisture Dream Revitalizing Facial Tonic** *($8.99 for 6.8 ounces)* has a couple of bells and whistles present in trivial amounts, but is otherwise nearly identical to the Milky Touch Alcohol-Free Facial Tonic above, and the same comments apply.

😐 **Matt Touch Balancing Moisturizer** *($8.99 for 1.7 ounces)* makes the too-good-to-be-true claim of being able to provide moisture to dry areas while keeping oily areas shine-free. This very basic moisturizer has a soft matte finish on skin, but its emollient content (the second ingredient) isn't helpful for those with oily areas. The fact that this moisturizer is marketed to teens doesn't excuse Lumene from ignoring many fundamentals about what it takes to create a state-of-the-art moisturizer, but that's pretty much what they've done. There are lots of beauty bargains that can be beautiful for skin, but this isn't one of them.

😐 **Arctic Touch Purifying Peat Facial Mask** *($8.99 for 3.4 ounces)* lists peat as the second ingredient. Peat is partially decayed vegetable matter, and although it may seem intriguing due to its organic nature, peat isn't a skin-essential ingredient in the least. This mask also contains kaolin (clay), along with several thickening agents, none of them capable of purifying skin. It's an OK absorbent mask, but that's about it.

☹ **No Spots Targeted Blemish Care** *($4.99 for 0.14 ounce)* is an anti-acne treatment containing 1.5% salicylic acid (BHA) as its active ingredient. Unfortunately, there is too much alcohol present, which makes this too irritating for all skin types. That's a shame, because without the alcohol this would have been an effective, pH-correct BHA product.

LUMENE SUN PRODUCTS

😐 **After Sun Soothing Emulsion** *($13.99 for 6.8 ounces)* comes with claims that make it sound like you can bask in the sun all day, develop a beautiful tan, and then with one application of this lotion repair any damage while enhancing your bronzed result. I despise this kind of product advertising because it crosses the line between claims that are just not true and claims that are actually dangerous for your skin. Adding insult to injury is the fact that this is a really basic, unimpressive moisturizer. It will remedy minor dry skin problems, but so will almost every other moisturizer being sold. The very small amount of cloudberry oil won't soothe or repair sun-damaged skin.

☺ **Sun Defence for Face Age-Defying Sun Cream SPF 30** *($13.99 for 1.7 ounces)* is a good moisturizing sunscreen primarily because it contains avobenzone for sufficient UVA protection. Nothing about the formula is specific to facial skin and, as is the case for most Lumene products, antioxidants are in short supply. The formula is preferred for normal to slightly oily skin.

☺ **Sun Defence Protective Sun Care SPF 15** *($17.99 for 6.8 ounces)* contains an in-part avobenzone sunscreen in an ordinary, lightweight lotion base best for normal to oily skin. Lumene's touted Sun Essence compound (consisting of antioxidant plant extracts and vitamin E) sounds promising, but there is too little of it in this product to add anything to the sun protection that the active ingredients provide.

☺ **Sun Defence Protective Sun Care SPF 45** *($17.99 for 6.8 ounces)* is nearly identical to the Sun Defence Protective Sun Care SPF 15 above in terms of its base formula, but both the percentage and number of active ingredients is greater, which gives it a higher SPF rating. Otherwise, the same review applies.

LUSH (SKIN CARE ONLY)

LUSH AT-A-GLANCE

Strengths: None… OK, they do offer complete ingredient lists in their newspaper-like catalog.

Weaknesses: Almost every product contains at least one potent skin irritant; no sunscreens to be found, nor are they recommended by the company; no products to address common skin conditions such as acne, hyperpigmentation, or eczema; jar packaging; visiting a Lush store is a disaster for anyone battling fragrance allergies.

For more information about Lush, call (888) 733-5874 or visit www.lush.com or www.Beautypedia.com.

☹ **Angels on Bare Skin** *($7.95 for a 3.5-ounce bar)* contains lavender and patchouli oils, and is not recommended. This recipe claims to be from the Middle Ages, which to my way of thinking is not a positive selling point! Back in those days, life expectancy was drastically short and bloodletting was the pinnacle of medicine!

☹ **Aquamarina** *($7.95 for a 3.5-ounce bar)* contains irritating calamine powder as well as orange and patchouli oils. This is not something you should use if your face has caught too much sun.

☹ **Baby Face** *($7.95 for a 1.2-ounce bar)* is a very fragranced bar cleanser that irritates skin with tangerine oil and concentrated narcissus fragrance.

☹ **Coalface** *($9.35 for a 3.5-ounce bar)* assaults skin with sandalwood and rosewood oils plus sodium lauryl sulfate and genuine coal powder. Washing your face in the fireplace would be preferred to this product.

☹ **Fresh Farmacy** *($7.15 for a 3.5-ounce bar)* is based around calamine powder and irritates skin with lavender oil and sodium lauryl sulfate (and how often do you see that growing on the farm?)

☹ **Sweet Japanese Girl** *($8.95 for a 1.2-ounce bar)* is a rich, buttery soap that irritates skin with lemon and juniper oils.

☹ **Ultra Bland** *($11.75 for a 1.5-ounce bar)* is indeed bland, yet it's also irritating to skin due to the iris, rose absolute, and benzoin it contains.

☹ **Ocean Salt** *($15.30 for 4.2 ounces)* rubs salt in the wound (figuratively speaking), thanks to lemon and lime additives. This would be a great way to break down skin's protective barrier and create dull skin.

☹ **Breath of Fresh Air Facial** *($14.40 for 8.4 ounces)* is better dabbed on as perfume given the amount of volatile (and irritating) fragrant oils it contains. You've been warned…!

☹ **Eau-Roma Water, for Dry to Normal Skin** *($14.40 for 8.4 ounces)* is an unexceptional toner that's mostly perfumed lavender and rose water. It is not beneficial for any skin type.

☹ **Tea Tree Water** *($14.40 for 8.4 ounces)* has tea tree oil in it, which is fine. But the grapefruit and juniper turn what was fine into irritation, and that's not helpful for "troublesome teenage problems."

☹ **Afterlife** *($38.70 for 1.5 ounces)* is a rich, honey-based moisturizer, which contains "fresh" ingredients that are subject to quick deterioration if this is not properly stored and used within a small window of time. However, it is not recommended because of the volatile fragrant oils it contains.

☹ **Almond Kisses** *($38.70 for 1.5 ounces)* is a basic emollient moisturizer for dry skin that is not recommended due to the floral perfume oils and citrus oil it contains. They smell great, but that's not going to help your skin.

😐 **Celestial, for Sensitive Skin** *($17.95 for 1.5 ounces)*. Finally a product in the Lush lineup with minimal fragrance! Though it still contains vanilla water and orchid extract, I imagine that it contains the least amount of fragrance of all the Lush products. But while this may contain the least amount for Lush, it isn't little enough to make this a good moisturizer because it doesn't contain one water-binding agent, antioxidant (vanilla water doesn't count), or anti-irritant.

☹ **Cosmetic Lad** *($17.10 for 1.5 ounces)* isn't a good choice for lads or lasses because it's based around lavender and also contains irritating sandalwood and tangerine oils.

☹ **Enchanted Eye Cream** *($18.90 for 1.5 ounces)* would be an OK emollient eye cream for dry skin if it weren't based on lavender, but that makes it is too potentially irritating for all skin types.

☹ **Enzymion** *($29.70 for 1.5 ounces)* contains enzymes naturally present in papaya juice to exfoliate skin, but those aren't reliable (not when compared to a well-formulated AHA or BHA product) and the jar packaging makes these unstable ingredients even less active. That's not good news, and things only get worse because Lush added lemon juice and lime oil.

☹ **Gorgeous** *($72 for 1.5 ounces)* claims to leave a matte feeling, but the olive and evening primrose oil base doesn't allow that. The lemon juice, orange flower, neroli, and myrrh resin are all fragrant and problems for skin, at least if you want yours to be described as "gorgeous."

☹ **Imperialis** *($17.95 for 1.5 ounces)* contains too many problematic plants and fragrant extracts to make it the "imperial majesty of moisturizers." Of particular concern is St. John's wort, which can cause a phototoxic reaction when skin is exposed to sunlight.

☹ **Mirror Mirror** *($17.95 for 1.7 ounces)* won't make you the fairest of them all, but will cause irritation thanks to sandalwood oil and other volatile fragrant extracts. Lush actually sells this for use either as a moisturizer or a fragrance!

☹ **Skin Drink** *($15.30 for 1.5 ounces)* contains neroli and rose absolute oils, which makes it too irritating for all skin types. Plain aloe vera gel and sesame oil (the main ingredients in this product) would be much better, though still far from what skin needs to function optimally.

😐 **Skins Shangri La** *($38.70 for 1.5 ounces)* is an extremely emollient moisturizer for dry skin that contains some good plant oils and a tiny amount of antioxidants. The fragrance is a bit much, but not terrible.

☹ **Ultralight** *($17.10 for 1.5 ounces)* contains the sunscreen agent octyl methoxycinnmate, but does not have an SPF rating (nor is the sunscreen listed as "active"), so it cannot be relied on for daytime protection. The sandalwood and lavender oils plus myrrh resin in this emollient moisturizer make it unsuitable for all skin types.

☹ **Mask of Magnaminty** *($17.10 for 11.1 ounces)* contains peppermint oil and African marigold oil, which can cause contact dermatitis (Source: *Encyclopedia of Common Natural Ingredients Used in Food, Drugs and Cosmetics*, 2nd Edition, John Wiley & Sons, 1996).

☹ **Chocolate Whipstick Lip Balm** *($7.20 for 0.3 ounce)*, ☹ **Dream Time Temple Balm** *($7.20 for 0.3 ounce)*, ☹ **Flying Fox Temple Balm** *($7.20 for 0.3 ounce)*, ☹ **Honey Trap Lip Balm** *($7.20 for 0.3 ounce)*, ☹ **Lip Lime Lip Balm** *($7.20 for 0.3 ounce)*, ☹ **Lip Service Lip Balm** *($7.20 for 0.3 ounce)*, ☹ **Lite Lip Balm** *($7.20 for 0.3 ounce)*, ☹ **Party On Temple Balm** *($7.20 for 0.3 ounce)*, ☹ **T Tree Simplex Lip Balm** *($7.20 for 0.3 ounce)*, and ☹ **Whoosh Balm Temple Balm** *($7.20 for 0.3 ounce)* are emollient balms meant for the lips or, as the name states, temple area (for pressure-point massage). All of them contain one or more irritating essential oils, including peppermint, lavender, rosemary, lime, lemon, ginger, palmarosa, and jasmine. Expect them to cause redness and make dry, chapped lips look and feel worse.

M.A.C.

M.A.C. AT-A-GLANCE

Strengths: Skin-care selection includes some impressive moisturizers; all the daytime moisturizers with sunscreen include sufficient UVA protection; excellent lip balm and toner; excellent foundations (some whose sunscreen includes the right UVA-protecting ingredients) in a mostly gorgeous range of shades; great concealers; the Select Sheer and Mineralized powders; the Sheertone Blush and traditional cream blush; wide selection of powder eyeshadows in various finishes; Fluidline and Technakohl Liner; dizzying array of lipstick shades in mostly sumptuous formulas; Lipgelee; all of the Pro Longwear Lipcolour options; several very good mascaras (regular and waterproof); the makeup brushes; most of the Prep + Prime products work as claimed.

Weaknesses: A few products with uncomfortably high levels of known or potential skin irritants; no AHA or BHA products; no anti-blemish products; the Lightful products can't affect sun-induced skin discolorations; some of the foundations were downgraded because their sunscreen did not offer sufficient UVA protection; several average pressed and loose powders; the pencil concealer; Cream Colour Base; the Lustre and Velvet eyeshadows; the traditional eye pencils (that need sharpening); Brow Set and Brow Finisher; Lipglass and Plushglass; the Brush Cleanser.

For more information about M.A.C, owned by Estee Lauder, call (800) 588-0070 or visit www.maccosmetics.com or www.Beautypedia.com.

M.A.C SKIN CARE

M.A.C. LIGHTFUL PRODUCTS

😐 **$$$ Lightful Cleanser** *($22 for 3.4 ounces)* claims to just about do it all: remove makeup and calm, refresh, and balance skin by managing oily areas while soothing dry spots (and reducing redness). Wow! This isn't a cleanser extraordinaire, though, it's just a standard, foaming, water-soluble cleanser that's best for normal to oily skin. The potassium-derived cleansing agents can make dry skin feel worse. This is similar to L'Oreal's considerably less expensive Hydra Fresh Foaming Face Wash, for Normal to Dry Skin ($6.26 for 6.5 ounces), and that company's Nutri-Pure Self Foaming Cleanser, for Normal to Dry Skin ($5.86 for 5 ounces) is even better.

✓😊 **$$$ Lightful Softening Lotion** *($28 for 5 ounces)* is a very good toner for normal to dry skin, which it should be for the money! M.A.C combines slip agents with vitamin C and several other antioxidants and soothing agents, along with smaller amounts of skin-identical ingredients. It won't do much to lighten skin discolorations, but certainly gives normal to dry skin what it needs to look better and feel refreshed.

😊 **Lightful Daily Moisturizer** *($32 for 1.7 ounces)* has a fluid, smooth texture that feels light, but the emollients and the amount of jojoba oil make it best for normal to slightly dry skin not prone to breakouts. It contains a smattering of antioxidants and some good water-binding agents, but some of the floral plant extracts are potentially sensitizing.

😐 **$$$ Lightful Essence** *($40 for 1 ounce)* is a decent vitamin C serum, but the form of vitamin C (ascorbyl glucoside) doesn't have nearly as much substantiated research on its side as other forms, including magnesium ascorbyl phosphate or L-ascorbic acid. Another issue is the blend of irritating and anti-irritant plant extracts, whose opposite effects cancel each other out. Although an OK option for normal to slightly dry or slightly oily skin, this pales in comparison to similar products from the other Lauder-owned lines.

OTHER M.A.C PRODUCTS

☹ **Cleanse Off Oil** *($20 for 5 ounces)* isn't any better than removing makeup with a gentle cleansing lotion or even plain olive oil because it contains irritating bitter orange and lavender oils. This is not recommended for any skin type, and would be a problem for eye-area use.

😐 **$$$ Cremewash** *($19 for 3.4 ounces)* is a water-soluble cleanser that produces copious foam. The main cleansing agent is the soap constituent potassium myristate, which means this cleanser can be drying for some skin types, rather than "super-hydrating" as claimed. It is an OK option for normal to oily skin, and removes makeup easily. Cremewash is similar to but better-formulated than Clinique's Rinse-Off Foaming Cleanser ($17.50 for 5 ounces).

☹ **$$$ Green Gel Cleanser** *($19 for 5 ounces)* is an OK, water-soluble cleanser for normal to very oily skin. The drying TEA-lauryl sulfate cleanser is third on the ingredient list, which doesn't make this preferred to several other (less expensive) gel cleansers.

✓☺ **$$$ Wipes** *($16 for 45 sheets)* are a favorite at the M.A.C counter and it's not hard to see why: these sturdy yet soft cloths easily and quickly remove all types of makeup, including long-wearing lip stains and waterproof mascara. The formula combines gentle cleansing agents with a solvent and silicones to accomplish this, and most will find it a soothing experience. Wipes are convenient, but keep in mind that a water-soluble cleanser with a washcloth is just as effective (and costs less per use).

☺ **$$$ Cleansing Tips** *($12.50 for 30 swabs)* are cotton swabs whose hollowed-out center is filled with a gentle cleansing fluid, similar to most non-silicone eye-makeup removers. One end is pointed for quick cleanup around the lash line, while the other end is rounded for cleaning up larger areas such as the eyelid. These work well and can be convenient, but they're not a cost-effective way to remove makeup, especially when you can just purchase a bottle of eye-makeup remover and a large box of pointed cotton swabs for roughly half the price. If you love the concept of pre-filled cotton swabs for makeup removal, check out the equally effective Swabplus Liquid Filled Cotton Swabs ($3.79 for 72 swabs) available online at www.drugstore.com.

☹ **$$$ Gently Off Eye and Lip Makeup Remover** *($17.50 for 3.4 ounces)* is a standard, but effective, dual-phase makeup remover with silicone. The plant extracts are a mix of fragrant rose and soothing cucumber, with rose extract not being the best for use around the eyes. Although this works very well, it doesn't best less-expensive options from Almay or Neutrogena that are available at the drugstore.

☺ **$$$ Pro Eye Makeup Remover** *($17 for 3.4 ounces)* is a standard, detergent-based eye-makeup remover that works as well as any, and is fragrance-free. The formula claims to be pro-quality, but isn't different from what most other lines offer for less money.

☹ **$$$ Microfine Refinisher** *($26.50 for 3.4 ounces)* contains "microfine crystals" of alumina to polish skin, so it's a good thing this scrub is blended with oil to cushion your skin because it can be fairly abrasive. And keep in mind, a washcloth works far better than almost any scrub.

☹ **$$$ Fix +** *($15 for 3.4 ounces)* is a standard, but good, alcohol-free toner for normal to dry or slightly oily skin. The mist application is convenient, but don't mist this over your makeup—nothing in the formula will "finish" it or prolong wear. Quite the opposite is true!

☹ **$$$ Fast Response Eye Cream** *($28.50 for 0.5 ounce)* is a silicone-based moisturizer that contains several antioxidants, but also enough caffeine to make it problematic for use around the eyes due to its irritant potential. This contains fragrance in the form of methyldihydrojasmonate.

☺ **$$$ Oil Control Lotion** *($28 for 1.7 ounces)* doesn't control oil as much as it just leaves a smooth matte finish. This is a good moisturizer for oily skin types with dry patches. It contains a few antioxidants and cell-communicating ingredients in stable packaging.

☺ **$$$ Prep + Prime Face Protect SPF 50** *($26.50 for 1 ounce)*, given the price tag, is disappointing due to the shortage of antioxidants. It is otherwise a very good in-part zinc oxide sunscreen in a silicone-enriched base that is ideal for use under makeup. The amount of zinc oxide leaves a slight white cast, but this is a non-issue if you're going to follow with foundation.

Unless you are prone to breakouts from zinc oxide, this is an excellent, fragrance-free daytime moisturizer (or primer, if you prefer) for normal to very oily skin.

✓☺ **$$$ Strobe Cream** *($29.50 for 1.7 ounces)* contains mineral pigments to optically "brighten" skin, which basically means particles of shine to make skin look radiant rather than dull. Looking beyond the light show reveals a well-formulated moisturizer brimming with the essential elements normal to dry skin needs to look and feel its best. Almost all of the antioxidants included have considerable research documenting their topical benefit for skin.

☹ **Studio Moisture Cream** *($29.50 for 1.7 ounces)* contains a large amount of *Aleurites moluccana* oil. Also known as tung seed oil, it is known to cause sweating on contact and can cause acute contact dermatitis. It is also a good source of linolenic and linoleic acids, but so is evening primrose oil, without the negatives (Source: www.naturaldatabase.com).

😐 **$$$ Studio Moisture Fix** *($28 for 1.7 ounces)* is a slightly more emollient version of the Strobe Cream above, but doesn't contain the same impressive array of antioxidants. This is still a good moisturizer for normal to dry skin, and works well under makeup (assuming your foundation is rated SPF 15 or greater).

✓☺ **$$$ Studio Moisture Fix SPF 15** *($28 for 1.7 ounces)* has an in-part zinc oxide sunscreen with a beautiful silky texture, provides a soft matte finish, and is loaded with antioxidants, skin-identical substances, and anti-irritants. It is a brilliant option for normal to oily skin, although the amount of zinc oxide (and its slight whitening effect) may prove tricky to work with on darker skin tones. This product does contain fragrance.

☺ **$$$ Blot Film** *($12.50 for 30 sheets)* is a set of 30 uncoated sheets of thin plastic material with absorbent properties. They work well to soak up excess shine and perspiration. Whether you choose them over tissue paper–style blotting papers comes down to personal preference.

✓☺ **$$$ Lip Conditioner** *($12 for 0.5 ounce)* is an exemplary, stably packaged lip balm that's based around Vaseline, but contains appreciable amounts of several antioxidants and skin-identical substances. It is highly recommended for dry, chapped lips, and the tube applicator is convenient when you're on the go.

☹ **Lip Conditioner SPF 15** *($13 for 0.5 ounce pot or 0.16 ounce stick)* leaves lips vulnerable to UVA damage because it does not contain titanium dioxide, zinc oxide, avobenzone, Tinosorb, or Mexoryl SX. Its formula is also not nearly as elegant as that of the regular Lip Conditioner above.

M.A.C. MAKEUP

FOUNDATION: ✓☺ **Studio Fix** *($25)* remains one of the top pressed-powder foundations available, despite several impressive entries from other companies. It has an exceptionally silky, talc-based texture that applies and blends like a dream. As usual, wet or dry application is possible, but using this wet poses the risk of streaking. Dry application provides light to medium-full coverage. If you prefer this type of foundation and have normal to slightly dry or slightly oily skin, it is highly recommended. Almost all of the 37 colors are impressive (albeit repetitive) for a broad range of skin tones, but the following shades are best avoided due to pink, orange, or peach overtones: C6, NC42, NW25, NW30, NW40, and NC40.

✓☺ **$$$ Studio Stick Foundation SPF 15** *($28.50)* is a stick foundation that includes an in-part titanium dioxide sunscreen for UVA protection. It has a silky, initially creamy texture that allows ample playtime before it sets, providing light to medium coverage. This layers well for additional coverage over more obvious imperfections; it also can be sheered out, but keep in mind that doing so will reduce the amount of sun protection. As usual, M.A.C.'s shade selection is mostly top-notch; among the 27 options to consider only a few shades should be avoided—NC40, NC42, NC45, and NW40 can be too peach for most skin tones, while NW23 is slightly peach. As with all foundations of this type, the ingredients that keep the product in stick form can be potentially problematic for blemish-prone or very oily skin. Studio Stick Foundation is ideal for normal to slightly dry or slightly oily skin. Just make sure any dry areas are smoothed before applying, because this foundation's somewhat powdery finish will not be kind to them.

✓☺ **$$$ Select SPF 15 Moistureblend** *($28.50)* gets everything right, from its elegantly creamy texture (those of you with dry to very dry skin, take note!) and soft glow finish to its brilliant, in-part zinc oxide sunscreen. Not a cream-to-powder makeup, but instead a plant oil–based creamy compact makeup, this blends superbly and is neither too greasy nor too slick. Coverage stays in the medium range (this isn't an easy foundation to make sheer), but the finish keeps skin looking fresh and dimensional. The range of 23 shades is remarkably good, and includes options for all skin tones. The only shades to consider carefully are the slightly pink-to-peach NC44, NW30, and NW40. Avoid the obviously peach NW25.

☺ **$$$ Studio Tech Foundation** *($28.50)* is a next-generation cream-to-powder foundation that offers a lighter, almost weightless texture, smooth application, and a soft satin finish that tends not to grab onto dry areas. It combines the super-light feel of a water-to-powder makeup with the slip and smoothness of silicone-based cream-to-powder makeups. Studio Tech applies easily and provides light to medium coverage. A staggering range of 27 shades is available, with suitable options for very light (NC15, NW15) and darker (NW50, NW55) skin tones. Although the majority of the shades lean toward neutral, six of them are too orange or peach for their intended skin tones: NC40, NC45, NC55, NW25, NW30, and NW40. This formula is best for normal to slightly dry and dry skin—the non-matte, non-powdery finish won't do much to temper shine, and even though this is not traditional cream-to-powder makeup, enough waxes and thickeners are present to make it problematic for those battling blemishes. If your skin fills the bill for this makeup, it's certainly worth checking out.

☺ **$$$ Studio Mist Foundation** *($28.50)* mists onto skin, because this super-light foundation is packaged in a pressurized metal container. That allows for a very fine application of foundation that has a see-through sheer finish yet still manages to make skin look refined and, well, better than it does without any makeup. The directions tell you to spray this foundation onto your hands or a brush before applying, and that's wise because this dispenses forcefully enough so that spraying it directly onto your face would easily get product in your eyes, nose, and all over your hair. (Of course you have to wonder why they would put it in a spray container at all.) This applies well with fingers though it is initially greasy before it sets to a semi-matte finish. Blending must be thorough to avoid splotches of color, and this is ideally for normal to slightly dry skin types. The six shades (a small assortment for M.A.C., but they're all so sheer that each shade works for more than one skin color) lean a bit toward the peachy side, but not enough to warrant avoiding any of them. If you have fair or very dark skin, you'll want to consider one of M.A.C.'s other foundations.

☹ **$$$ Hyper Real SPF 15 Foundation** *($27)* lacks the UVA-protecting ingredients of titanium dioxide, zinc oxide, avobenzone, Tinosorb, or Mexoryl SX, and so is not to be relied on for daytime protection. This is otherwise a very good foundation whose slightly thick, lotion-like texture blends to a smooth matte (in feel) finish that has enough soft shine to make skin look radiant rather than glittery. Coverage runs from light to medium and the formula is best for normal to oily skin. The range of 15 shades offers many beautiful options for fair to dark skin tones. The only shades to view cautiously are NC500 and NW500 (both are slightly peach). NW700 is a beautiful non-ashy shade for dark skin tones, while Bronze Reflections has a soft, peachy gold shimmer that's attractive on medium to tan skin.

☺ **$$$ Face and Body Foundation** *($31)* comes in a 4-ounce bottle and is very liquidy and sheer. It takes some patience to blend on because it tends to slide around a lot before drying. This can be layered for more coverage (as can most foundations) and is reasonably waterproof. For body makeup it can be a problem, however, because it can come off on clothes, and it's not a great choice for major flaws you want to fully conceal. There are 16 shades, and most are neutral and workable. The deeper shades can be sketchy because most of them have a slight peach to red cast that won't work for many skin tones; avoid N6. This also contains grapefruit oil, though likely not enough to cause irritation.

☺ **$$$ Full Coverage Foundation** *($27)* is a creamy, thick compact makeup whose level of coverage is indeed full and more akin to a concealer than a traditional foundation. The concentrated formula blends out well, leaving a cream finish. It no longer includes sunscreen, and is best for normal to dry skin that needs serious camouflage. M.A.C. offers 18 shades for fair to dark skin tones, and most are quite good. The only troublesome colors are the peachy NW25 and pink NW30. Shade C35 is excellent for concealing dark circles on light skin tones.

☺ **$$$ Studio Fix Fluid SPF 15** *($25)* has so much going for it, but it doesn't come out a winner because it lacks UVA-protecting ingredients. If you're willing to wear an effective sunscreen underneath, this has a beautifully silky texture and ultra-smooth application that sets to a natural matte finish. Best for normal to oily skin, Studio Fix Fluid provides medium coverage and comes in 23 shades, of which only 4 are poor contenders: NC55 is too ash, NW30 and NW35 too peach, and NW45 has a copper overtone that makes it a tough match for darker skin tones. NW50 and NW55 are ideal shades for dark skin, and there are options for very light skin, too.

☺ **$$$ Select SPF 15** *($25)* has a formula very similar to the Studio Fix Fluid SPF 15 above, and is another M.A.C. foundation whose sunscreen lacks sufficient UVA-protecting ingredients. If you're already using a separate sunscreen rated SPF 15 or higher and want to give this a try, it has a fluid, lightweight texture that blends easily and sets to a silky matte finish. This offers slightly less coverage than the Studio Fix Fluid and is preferred for normal to slightly dry or slightly oily skin. Among the 25 mostly excellent shades are a few duds: NC45 is slightly orange, NW25 slightly peach, NW35 very peach, NW45 a bit too coppery, and NW50 slightly ash.

☺ **$$$ Select Tint SPF 15** *($25)* is one of the oldest M.A.C. foundations and one you won't find prominently displayed at their department-store counters (it's available mostly in freestanding M.A.C. stores). Although the sunscreen lacks sufficient UVA protection, this has a very light fluid texture and blends well, setting to a soft matte finish. Being a tint, coverage is sheer, but it builds well if you need more. What a shame the sunscreen is incomplete, because this is a good formula for normal to oily skin. Among the 12 shades, avoid the peach-tinged NW35 and slightly copper NW45.

☺ **$$$ Mineralized Satinfinish SPF 15** *($26.50)* has so much going for it, yet the sunscreen lacks sufficient UVA protection. Surprisingly for this mineral-themed foundation, M.A.C. did not opt to use titanium dioxide or zinc oxide for the sunscreen, a typical standard in this category of makeup. This fluid foundation dispenses from a pump and has a beautifully smooth texture and soft matte finish that gives a good dimensional (rather than flat) quality to skin. Achieving medium coverage is easy; in fact, this is difficult to make sheer. It has a hint of shine and is available in 18 shades, of which the following should be considered carefully due to their peachy casts: NW30, NW35 (way too peach for most), NW43 (also quite peach), and NW45. This is a product to consider if you have normal to slightly dry or slightly oily skin and are willing to pair it with a separate product during the day that contains the UVA-protecting ingredients of zinc oxide, titanium dioxide, avobenzone, Tinosorb, or Mexoryl SX.

CONCEALER: ✓☺ Select Cover-Up *($14.50)* is a great concealer. Lightly creamy with a natural matte finish, this liquid concealer provides good camouflage with minimal risk of creasing. Fifteen mostly neutral shades are available, plus four color correctors, of which Colour Corrector Peach is an OK option. Colour Corrector Pink may work for some porcelain skin tones, though it has an opalescent finish. Of the regular shades, the ones to be cautious with are NC45, NW35, and NW45.

☺ **Select Moisturecover** *($15.50)* is another great liquid concealer, though this definitely has a creamy feel. Easy to control during application and providing medium to full coverage, this sets to a smooth finish that's minimally prone to creasing. The palette of 15 shades is practically a case study in neutral to yellow tones for fair to dark skin, and the only color to consider carefully is the slightly peach NW30.

☺ **Studio Finish Concealer SPF 35** *($14.50)* replaces M.A.C.'s former Concealer SPF 15, which was workable but not as refined as this version. The formidable sunscreen is in-part titanium dioxide, and the creamy texture is smoother and thus easier to blend. This is still a full-coverage concealer, and it takes practice to achieve the level of coverage you want without using too much product. It is excellent for concealing redness, dark circles, and other discolorations, but too emollient to use over blemishes. There are 16 shades, and almost all are exceptional. NC42 is too yellow for most skin tones, while NC45, NW35, and NW40 suffer from peach overtones. NW45 is too coppery for most dark skin tones, but the deeper NW50 is ideal. Fair to light skin tones will find more than one suitable shade, so be sure to test this at the counter before making a purchase.

☺ **Studio Stick Concealer** *($15.50)* is the partner product to M.A.C.'s Studio Stick Foundation above, and this creamy, full-coverage concealer nicely complements it. Smooth, even coverage is obtainable with one stroke, and this concealer blends exceptionally well considering its opacity. It's a superb option for concealing dark circles and other discolorations, but has a slight tendency to crease before the end of the day when used under the eyes. There are 15 shades amd. given the number of shades, there are some to avoid, including NC45 (too orange), NW15 (too white but may be an option for porcelain skin), and NW25, NW30, and NW40 (all three of which are too peach).

😐 **Studio Touch-Up Stick** *($14.50)* is a slightly chubby, needs-sharpening pencil concealer with a creamy, soft texture and smooth application, though it's best for on-the-spot coverage. The formula is too emollient to use over blemishes, but it nicely conceals red marks left from blemishes that have healed. It's fairly crease-prone, and not as long-wearing under the eyes as all the other M.A.C. concealers. There are 15 mostly good shades, but the following are too peach to consider: NC42, NW30, and NW35.

POWDER: ✓☺ $$$ Select Sheer Loose Powder *($20)* sets a new powder precedent by offering an ultralight texture that seems to disappear into the skin, yet provides a smooth, dimensional, polished finish. The talc-based formula has an understated shine that is visible, but that doesn't detract from this powder's incredibly light texture and fine finish. The 14 shades are typically M.A.C., meaning there are many noteworthy neutral tones. Each shade goes on very sheer and imparts just a hint of color, so getting an exact match isn't essential, and the choices are plentiful. Both NW43 and NW35 are beautiful options for bronzing powder, and shade NC5 is for the most porcelain skin tone.

✓☺ **$$$ Select Sheer Pressed Powder** *($20)* is basically a pressed version of the Select Sheer Loose Powder above, except that this powder does not have any shine and, as is true for most pressed powders when compared to loose powders, it offers more coverage. Most of the 17 shades are exceptional, although NW43 may be a touch too copper for some dark skin tones and NW50 is slightly ash. Shade NC55 makes an excellent bronzing powder color, while NW5 is nearly white. Overall, this is a wonderful pressed powder, especially if you want a finished look but aren't a fan of traditional powders. Those with oily skin may find this not absorbent enough, but it's still worth auditioning.

✓☺ **$$$ Mineralized Skinfinish** *($24.50)* is a sheer, talc-based pressed powder that looks wonderfully natural on skin. It's almost impossible to make this powder look heavy, thick, or dry. Those with normal to dry skin will appreciate the slight sheen this leaves behind (and remember, talc is a mineral, too, so M.A.C.'s name for this product is accurate). All five shades are neutral and highly recommended, but there are no options for very dark skin tones.

✓☺ **$$$ Bronzing Powder** *($20)* is a talc-based, pressed-powder bronzer with an extremely smooth texture and dry finish. It comes in five believable tan shades, three of which have a very shiny finish. Matte Bronze is truly matte and Bronze is almost matte. Looking to spend less money for similar results? Try Wet n' Wild's Bronzer ($2.99).

☺ **$$$ Hyper Real Pressed Powder** *($23)* is talc-based powder with a soft shimmer finish. Available exclusively in M.A.C. Pro stores, the six shades are best for highlighting areas of skin rather than for dusting all over. Half the shades fall into the category of color correctors, but the sheer application has minimal corrective impact (which in this case is good). The flesh-toned shades to consider include Extra Light, Light, and Medium.

😐 **$$$ Set Powder** *($22)* is a talc-based loose powder that contains silica and film-forming agent to create a waterproof finish. Sold exclusively at M.A.C. Pro stores (which, confusingly, are not the same as "regular" M.A.C. stores), it comes in several shades, many of which are color correctors. However, because this goes on so sheer and isn't much for pigment, any correction is very subtle. It does help waterproof your complexion, but so will many other powders that contain similar ingredients.

😐 **$$$ Blot Powder Loose** *($20)* is identical to M.A.C.'s Set Powder but is more widely available and comes in four classic shades for medium to dark skin tones. It leaves a soft, sheer matte finish and is absorbent enough to help manage oily areas. Still, neither this nor the Set Powder are in the same league as the Select Sheer powders above. 😐 **$$$ Blot Powder Pressed** *($20)* has been reformulated and is now a talc-free, silicone-based powder that feels silky yet looks a bit chalky and dry on skin. It is best for taming oily skin, and all five shades are worth considering—but check the finish in natural light to make sure you like it.

😐 **$$$ Iridescent Powder Loose** *($20)* comes in a tub, and this talc-free powder is appropriately named. The two sheer colors do well in terms of providing high shine, but the shine doesn't cling as well as the Iridescent Powder Pressed below, so the effect doesn't last as long. 😐 **$$$ Iridescent Powder Pressed** *($20)* has a dry, slightly grainy, talc-based texture and is available in two pale, iridescent shades that impart noticeable shine and cling moderately well.

BLUSH: Powder Blush *($17.50)* presents almost 50 shades, from the palest pinks and peaches to the deepest browns and plums. The vast palette is divided into five finishes and two formulas. The 😐 **$$$ Mattes** are a standard, pressed-powder blush with a reasonably smooth application and dry texture that causes the colors (especially the deeper shades) to grab a bit. 😐 **$$$ Frosts** have the same dry texture and application as the Mattes, but each shade has a soft to medium shimmer finish. The ☺ **$$$ Satins** feel silkier than the Mattes or Frosts and have good pigmentation with less tendency to grab. Best among the powder blushes are the ✓☺ **$$$ Sheertone** and ✓☺ **$$$ Sheertone Shimmer** shades. Although both lack the pigmentation of the other M.A.C. blushes, they apply extremely well, have a super-silky texture, and the regular Sheertone comes in a beautiful range of true matte colors. The Sheertone Shimmer version is just that: sheer colors with a soft shimmer finish. They work well for evening makeup, but most have too much shine for daytime, at least if you work in a professional environment. Both Sheertone formulas have limited options for darker skin tones, but fair to medium skin tones are well served.

✓☺ **$$$ Blushcreme** *($17.50)* brings back the old-fashioned (in a good way) true cream blush. Those with dry to very dry skin, take note: The emollient, oil-based feel and dewy finish of this blush make skin look radiant and healthy. The colors are all classics, with an equal representation of warm (peach) and cool (pink/rose) tones. The moist texture takes some getting used to during blending, so be sure to use less than you think you need and blend purposefully for best results. This does not work for those with normal to oily skin or if you have enlarged pores over the cheek area.

😐 **$$$ Cream Colour Base** *($16.50)* has been around for years, and the color collection keeps expanding, so there must be a lot of people buying these somewhat slick, crease-prone (when used as eyeshadow) colors. The shade range offers options for eyes, lips, and cheeks, and their intensity varies, so this is definitely a product to test at the counter before purchasing. The creamy base is ill-advised for blemish-prone skin, but normal to dry skin looking to add a soft, radiant (or iridescent, depending on the shade) glow may want to give this a try. The best shades to use for blush are Virgin Isle, Fabulush, Flighty, Bronze, and Premeditated.

EYESHADOW: The ☺ **Eye Shadows** *($14)* maintain the same almost-smooth, dry texture they've had for the past several years. The only real difference this time around is that many of the colors go on softer and more sheer. You'll notice less of this with the medium to dark shades, which tend to go on grainier and deeper than they look and don't blend as evenly as the best eyeshadows, but there is minimal flaking. These are not the smoothst shadows in town, but they do the job. Although the shades are labeled Satin, Frost, Lustre, Matte, Velvet, Veluxe, and Veluxe Pearl, they are arranged by color, not formula or finish, on the tester unit. Among the various finishes and formulas, the most problematic are ☹ **Lustre** and **Velvet** due to their grainy, difficult-to-blend texture and flaky shine. The large number of ☺ **Matte** (most of the shades are indeed matte) and ☺ **Satin** shades apply much better, though the darker Matte shades drag a bit, so blending must be precise. The ✓☺ **Veluxe** shades (don't ask me what Veluxe means; I assume it's a combination of velvet and luxurious) have the most beautifully silky texture and even application. I wish there were more shades, but the following shades are excellent: Dovefeather, Llama, Samoa Silk, Mink Pink, and Brown Down. The 😐 **Veluxe Pearl** shades have a drier texture and slightly flaky application, and the colors have a strong metallic finish. Not bad, but a couple steps down from the regular Veluxe.

M.A.C. stores carry an extended selection of shocking shades such as opaque orange, taxicab yellow, and vivid green, but these strong tones are really best for fantasy or theatrical makeup.

☺ **$$$ Paint** *($16)* is essentially a cleverly named and packaged cream-to-powder eyeshadow. Dispensed from a tube (don't apply too much pressure because you'll end up wasting product), the concentrated formula blends very well and has a natural opacity that can almost take the place of your foundation or concealer as a means for evening-out skin on the eyelid and underbrow area. Most of the 20 colors are neutral and workable yet supply intense shine. There are a few softer shades that can work for a mildly shiny look. Paints can be used alone or mixed with other products, and they sheer out well if you prefer a subtle wash of color. Regardless of color or shine intensity, these tend not to crease and last all day without fading or smearing.

😐 **$$$ Shadestick** *($16)* is a twist-up, retractable eyeshadow stick whose texture is neither creamy nor too dry. Unfortunately, it is still dry enough to make using it as eyeshadow a problem because it tends to drag and pull over eyelid skin, though it creases surprisingly little. This works best to emphasize the lower lash line, or to dot across the upper lash line and blend with a brush or your fingertip for a smoky, deliberately smudged look. Each shade is shine-laden, a finish that is not kind if you have moderate wrinkles. For the most versatility, I still prefer M.A.C's powder eyeshadows, used wet or dry with all manner of eyeshadow and eye-lining brushes.

EYE AND BROW SHAPER: ✓☺ **Fluidline** *($14.50)* is nearly identical to Bobbi Brown's Long-Wear Gel Eyeliner ($19), a once-unique product of which I am a fan because of its remarkably easy application and tenacious wear. Long Wear Gel Eyeliner, M.A.C. Fluidline, and Stila's Smudge Pots are the only eyeliners that can stand up to oily eyelids without fading, smearing, or running. All of these have a slightly moist application that sets to a long-wearing matte finish. Fluidline is every bit as tenacious as Brown's Long-Wear Gel Eyeliner, but the colors are mostly … well, they're odd. Yes, classic browns and black are available, but the majority of the shades are not meant to define the eye so much as to add a shock of color. Peacock blue and bright purple are indeed eye-catching, but neither fulfills the main purpose of eyeliner, which is to define and accent the eye and enhance the depth of eyelashes. Not surprisingly, the M.A.C. counters and stores I visited while researching this book were consistently sold out of the black and brown shades, but had plenty of the Halloween-appropriate tones! Rich Ground, Dipdown, and Blacktrack are the most versatile choices.

✓☺ **Eye Brow Pencils** *($13.50)* are automatic, nonretractable, ultra-sleek pencils that apply easily and impart soft color without being greasy or smudging. The colors are brow-perfect, but don't ask me to explain the sexually charged names such as Stud, Lingering, and Fling! ✓☺ **Technakohl Liner** *($14.50)* is the eyeliner pencil to choose if you want a smooth application that doesn't drag or skip while imparting rich color. Initially creamy, this automatic, retractable pencil's formula sets to a soft powder finish that remains smudge-resistant. All but one of the shades is laced with shine, so if that's not on your must list, stick with Brownborder. And unless your eye-lining goal is to draw attention to the liner rather than to your eyes, skip Jade Way, Auto-de-blu, and Smoothblue.

☺ **$$$ Liquidlast Liner** *($16.50)* has a thin, flexible brush to ensure even application (assuming you have a steady hand). Dry time is average, so this isn't a liquid liner for anyone who flinches easily. Once set, it wears quite well, fading only slightly, and without smearing or flaking. Coco Bar and Point Black are the classic colors for a variety of eye-makeup designs. The remaining shades have a strong shimmer or metallic finish that is best for evening makeup and not appropriate for wrinkled eyelids. ☺ **$$$ Liquid Eye Liner** *($15)* is fairly straightforward, applying nicely with a thicker, firmer brush than the Liquidlast Liner above, yet with a faster dry time. You're unlikely to experience flaking or smearing, and all three colors are good.

☺ **Brow Shader** *($15)* pairs a pressed brow powder with a powder eyeshadow in shades best for highlighting with a satin (slightly shiny) finish. All five brow powders are workable (mostly for various brunette tones), but all have sparkles. Do brows need to sparkle, too? Really? All right, M.A.C.—but only because these apply so smoothly and the pigmentation allows gradual building of color for an elegantly defined rather than overdrawn brow.

The 😐 **Eye Pencils** *($12.50)* are utterly standard (right down to the commonplace colors) and comparable to most of the other pencils out there. For lining the eyes, M.A.C.'s matte eyeshadows or Fluidline shades are a better alternative. 😐 **Eye Kohl** *($13.50)* is another group of pencils that are an unnecessary addition, but here's one more twist on the creamy, standard pencil formula. The chance of smearing is slightly less than for the Eye Pencils above, but don't bet on them not smearing, despite their powdery finish.

😐 **Powerpoint Eye Pencil** *($13.50)* glides on with no tugging or skipping, but smears easily before it sets. Allow a minute or two for this to set, and you will be treated to several hours of fail-safe wear. As usual, M.A.C.'s shade selection is a mix of classic (brown and black) shades with trendy and unusual shades (jade green) meant to satisfy a wide variety of tastes. The soft, creamy texture of this pencil means it is difficult to create a fine, thin line, but it works great for thicker or smokier lines. The only other drawback? It needs to be sharpened, which keeps it from earning a happy face rating.

😐 **Brow Set** *($13)* is a basic brow gel formula that comes with a very good brush and has a minimally sticky finish. The Clear option is best; the others imbue brows or lashes with noticeable shimmer and have a tacky finish that can feel strange. ☹ **Brow Finisher** *($14.50)* is a twist-up, waxy, tinted stick that's packaged like a brow pencil. The texture is so waxy that application is difficult and it tends to stick brow hairs together, not to mention the waxy smell (all of the testers I played with had an "off" odor). This also feels tacky on brows and isn't something most women would want to tolerate given the variety of other options (including clear and tinted brow gels) that groom and define while being almost imperceptible.

LIPSTICK, LIP GLOSS, AND LIPLINER: M.A.C.'s ☺ **Lipsticks** *($14)* remain one of the major attractions of this line. The majority of the formulas provide lush textures and feel comfortable, and the color range is nearly unparalleled. Here is how they break down: ✓☺ **Satins** are softly creamy with a rich, opaque texture and moist finish, and offer the best compromise of long wear and desirable creaminess. The ✓☺ **Amplified Cremes** have an overall texture and application very close to the Satin Lipsticks, but these offer enhanced opaqueness and a touch more gloss. ☺ **Frosts** are creamy lipsticks with medium coverage and a soft shimmer to true frost finish, available in over 40 colors. ✓☺ **Mattes** are not true mattes, but come pretty close with their deeply pigmented, full-coverage colors and non-glossy finish. ☺ **Lustre Lipsticks** are M.A.C.'s largest collection of sheer lipsticks, each with a glossy finish and enough slip to easily make its way into any lines around the mouth. If that's not an issue for you, these are worth checking out. The ☺ **Glazes** were the predecessors to Lustre Lipsticks and present a much smaller shade selection. The colors are more sheer and less glossy than the Lustres. Last, ☺ **Lip Treatment** is a standard, colorless lipstick designed to work as a lip balm. It does just that, but no better than any of the lipsticks above.

✓☺ **$$$ Pro Longwear Lipcolour** *($20)* is M.A.C.'s version of Max Factor's Lipfinity. It is a dual-sided product, one end holding the lip color and the other a brush-on, glossy top coat. Although the concept is the same as Lipfinity, Outlast from Cover Girl, and all the other imitators, M.A.C.'s version excels because the colors go on so easily and evenly with a single application and, more important, because the top coat feels better than those of competing products. It actually goes a long way, not only keeping lips glossy, but also in preventing the color beneath from chipping or peeling as the top coat wears off. As a result, you get amazingly long-lasting lip color combined with a superior top coat that keeps up appearances, and that makes this option from M.A.C. a must-try. You could argue that M.A.C. has attempted to mimic the technology Procter & Gamble developed for their Max Factor and Cover Girl long-wearing lipsticks, but the way I see it, M.A.C. took a good thing and made it even better—improvement is the new sincerest form of flattery!

✓☺ **$$$ Pro Longwear Lustre Lipcolour** *($20)* is a departure from the original Pro Longwear in two ways: the colors (they're less opaque, though not sheer) and the accompanying top coat, called Mirror (which is infused with mutlicolored glitter rather than being clear and glossy). The application process and impressive wear time are the same, but I am not a fan of the glittery top coat because it limits the use of the striking but soft colors of the Pro Longwear Lustre Lipcolour. The good news is you can purchase one of M.A.C.'s other top coats to accompany the Lustre shade you like—the bad news is it must be purchased separately for $12.50 (it screws onto the color-base component so you can alternate top coats as needed). See if you like the glittery top coat before committing to this. Otherwise, this product is highly recommended.

✓☺ **Lipgelee** *($14)* is a far cry from the thick, sticky feel of M.A.C.'s Lipglass or Tinted Lipglass reviewed below. Packaged in a tube with an angled plastic applicator, Lipgelee is wonderfully smooth, completely non-sticky, and provides a high shine finish. The shades appear much bolder than they look on the lips, so if you're looking for a sheer gloss, this should be on your short list.

☺ **Pro Longwear Gloss Coat** *($13)*, described in the reviews above for Pro Longwear Lipcolour, is available in five finishes to be purchased separately. Whichever one you choose, each fits the component for either of M.A.C.'s Pro Longwear formulas. The **Crystalizer** is clear with large flecks of glitter; **Pink Iridescence** is just as the name says; **Mirror** adds a sparkling shine with multicolored glitter; **Pearlizer** adds soft gold shimmer; and **Clear** is the original top coat, which adds a wet-look shine without shimmer or glitter.

☺ **Slimshine Lipstick** *($14.50)* is for women who prefer sheer, glossy colors. That's exactly what this smooth, lightweight lipstick provides, and the color range is a smart blend of the trendy along with the tried-and-true. These slim lipsticks have a very glossy finish but aren't the least bit sticky. They're not much for longevity (and not for anyone prone to lipstick bleeding into lines around the mouth), but if those concerns don't apply to you, this is another sheer lipstick to consider.

☺ **$$$ Lacquer** *($16.50)* is a thick-textured liquid lipstick with a sticky, high-gloss finish and a tantalizing range of medium- to full-coverage colors. The wand applicator has a brush instead of an angled sponge tip, and the brush holds up well without splaying.

☺ **Lustreglass** *($14)* has the same wet-look shine as M.A.C.'s original Lipglass, but the Lustre version kicks up the color, so this is more of a lipstick/gloss hybrid than standard gloss. The brush applicator helps the gloss glide on, and considering this gloss's thicker texture, it is comparably non-sticky. The shimmer-infused shades feature mostly conservative (meaning softer and less intense) choices that should please most gloss fans, especially if they plan to apply this over a regular lipstick.

☹ **Clear Lipglass** *($13)* and **Tinted Lipglass** *($14)* are very thick, tenacious glosses whose heavy, syrupy texture is not for everyone. The tinted version has a slightly thinner texture and comes in a tube with a wand applicator; original Lipglass is packaged in a squeeze tube. The extensive shade range for Tinted Lipglass goes from sheer to dramatic.

☹ **Lip Pencils** *($12.50)* have a superior color selection, but that's the only thing that separates these standard, needs-sharpening pencils from nearly identical pencils found in almost every other line. ☺ **Cremestick Liner** *($14)* is an automatic, retractable lip pencil that has a creamy, glide-on application and soft cream finish that is slightly prone to smearing. The shade range is beautiful and complements dozens of M.A.C. lipstick colors.

☹ **Tinted Lip Conditioner SPF 15** *($14.50)* is an emollient tinted lip balm whose petrolatum and castor oil base will make dry, chapped lips feel better. If only the sunscreen included sufficient UVA-protecting ingredients, this would be recommended. As is, the colors are too sheer to provide any natural protection. ☹ **Plushglass** *($17.50)* is similar to Clinique's Full Potential Lips Plump and Shine, but omits the peppermint oil. Still around to irritate lips into a plump state are ginger root and capsicum (pepper) oils, neither of which are great to use consistently. This is otherwise a standard sheer lip gloss with a smooth feel and minimally sticky finish (it does feel nicer than Clinique's version). Compared to Clinique's plumping option, the omission of peppermint oil makes this the lesser of two evils, though it's still difficult to recommend for anything but occasional use.

MASCARA: ✓☺ **Pro Lash Mascara** *($11)* is in a league all its own! This home-run mascara builds dramatic thickness and length, while being only slightly difficult to control. It's almost too easy to over-apply this mascara, so be sure to exercise restraint to avoid a heavy, clumped appearance. Otherwise, you will be impressed at how quickly this revs up your lashes! M.A.C. also offers **Pro Lash Colour**, and although it performs identically to the regular Pro Lash, the green and blue colors are for extreme or costume-party makeup only.

✓☺ **Zoom Lash Mascara** *($11)* can go on a bit too heavily (especially if you're too zealous while applying it), but it builds impressive thickness with minimal effort and does so without bothersome clumps or smudges. This is also supposed to curl lashes, but the effect is subtle—you'll still need your eyelash curler (assuming you ordinarily use one). This mascara is best for those who want lash drama, not demureness.

☺ **Pro Longlash Mascara** *($11)* is touted as extreme lengthening mascara, and it does lengthen—just not that well or that fast. It adds no thickness and finishes lashes with a soft curl. But for all the promises, it just doesn't have the "wow" factor of the Pro Lash Mascara above.

☺ **Splashproof Lash Waterproof Mascara** *($11)* allows you to create lasting thickness and length with minimal effort, though it can clump slightly as it builds. This is also tenaciously waterproof, and a bit difficult to remove (have a silicone- or oil-based makeup remover handy). This mascara competes nicely with the top choices from drugstore lines Maybelline New York, L'Oreal, and Jane, and is only a bit more expensive.

☺ **Loud Lash Mascara** *($11)*, despite the name, isn't loud in the least, at least not in terms of the colors, which are only classic black or brown. This is primarily a lengthening mascara and with some effort it does a beautiful job of making lashes fringed, separated, and long with no clumps or smears. The "extra-strength" claim is accurate because this mascara wears and wears and wears. It is waterproof (it didn't budge on me after two showers) and as a result requires an oil- or silicone-based makeup remover (water-soluble cleansers are no match for this formula). It's definitely recommended if you need worry-free wear and don't care for much thickness.

😐 **Mascara X** *($12.50)* is said to deliver dramatically longer, thicker lashes, but it isn't nearly as impressive as M.A.C.'s newer mascaras, not to mention that several L'Oreal and Maybelline New York mascaras outperform this one at half the cost. 😐 **Fiber Rich Lash Mascara** *($11)* does contain tiny, hairlike fibers, but unlike similar mascaras from a decade or more ago, these fibers tend to stay on the lashes rather than flake off (and into your eyes) throughout the day. Why M.A.C. needed this mascara is a question worth asking because, aside from the fibers, it doesn't distinguish itself from their Pro Lash or Pro Longlash Mascaras. It does just an OK job and doesn't impress with its lengthening ability.

😐 **Prep + Prime Lash** *($13.50)* is meant to smooth and condition lashes, but doesn't do much better in this regard than most mascaras—there is nothing in this product that is all that conditioning for lashes, though it does make them feel soft. It is also supposed to intensify "the build and lengthening quality of all [mascara] formulas," but that didn't happen. Side-by-side testing confirmed what is true of almost all lash primers: they tend to make mascara trickier to apply and don't help lengthen or thicken lashes anymore than simply applying two or three coats of regular mascara. I suppose this is an OK option if you're using a lackluster mascara, but the bigger question is why you're not using a superior mascara, given how many there are! This does make a noticeable difference with average mascaras.

FACE AND BODY ILLUMINATING/SHIMMER PRODUCTS: ☺ **$$$ Pigment** *($19.50)* comes in small jars of shiny loose powder, available in almost every color imaginable and with a shininess scale that goes from sheer to POW! Most of the colors cling surprisingly well and allow you to create an array of effects. The shades labeled **Glitter** cling terribly and flake everywhere. Although Pigments can be messy to use, they add some kick to evening or special-occasion makeup. The best colors include Gold, Rose Gold, Deep Brown, Copper, Naked, Dark Soul, Black Black, Melon, Tan, Vanilla, Chocolate Brown, Lily White, and Apricot Pink.

BRUSHES: As stated in previous editions of this book, M.A.C. has one of the best selections of brushes you'll find anywhere *(over 40 different brushes, ranging from $10–$71)*. The big brushes are a little pricey, but they last forever if you take care of them. Though there are indeed good, inexpensive brushes to be found, if you're going to splurge, this is one area where the extra expense won't be wasted. Be sure to check out M.A.C.'s variety of eyeshadow brushes, particularly the ✓☺ **#275 Medium Angled Shading Brush** *($24)*, an excellent, versatile eyeshadow brush. Also, test the ✓☺ **#217 Blending Brush** *($21.50)*. Other top choices include the ✓☺ **#168 Large Angled Contour Brush** *($32)*, ✓☺ **#192 Cheek/Face Brush** *($32)*, ✓☺ **#194 Concealer Brush** *($18.50)*, ✓☺ **#208 Small Angled Brow Brush** *($18.50)*, ✓☺ **#219 Pencil Brush** *($22.50)*, ✓☺ **#239 Eye Shading Brush** *($24)*, ✓☺ **#242 Shader Brush** *($22.50)*, ✓☺ **#249 Large Shader Brush** *($26.50)*, and all of the various ✓☺ **Angled Shader Brushes** *($16.50–$24)*.

The only brushes to really avoid are the ☹ **#202 Replaceable Sponge Tip Applicator** *($18.50)*, which comes free in most eyeshadow kits, and the 😐 **#204 Lash Brush** *($10)*, which is easily duplicated by washing off an old mascara wand.

The freestanding M.A.C. stores sell pricier brushes known as M.A.C. Pro brushes, and these are definitely worth a look, especially if you're a working makeup artist with a generous budget. In particular, ✓☺ **$$$ Brush #174** *($71)* and ✓☺ **$$$ Brush #136** *($62)* are softer, more refined versions of M.A.C.'s regular loose-powder brushes.

SPECIALTY PRODUCTS: ✓☺ **Prep + Prime Lip** *($14.50)* is a base that is applied before lipstick to facilitate application and prevent it from feathering into lines around the mouth.

Guess what? It works! The silicone- and wax-based stick forms a great barrier to keep color in place, in a way similar to long-discontinued products such as The Body Shop's No Wander and Coty's Stop It! As good as this product is, keep in mind that it won't prevent greasy, slippery lip glosses from migrating into lines around the mouth. It works best with moderately creamy or satin matte lipstick formulas, of which M.A.C. has plenty!

☺ **$$$ Prep + Prime Skin** *($22)* is an ultralight, fragrance-free lotion meant to be applied to skin before foundation. This product doesn't necessarily prime skin better than similar products labeled as moisturizers, gels, or serums, but it does indeed create a silky-smooth, non-greasy surface that facilitates makeup application. Whether it's for you depends strictly on whether your skin needs help in this regard. Compared with other products sold as primers, this formula goes a bit further by being more than a mixture of silicones and water. Prep + Prime Skin contains appreciable amounts of plant extracts that serve as antioxidants and anti-inflammatory agents. It is a suitable formulation for normal to slightly dry or slightly oily skin, but has one potential drawback: shine. Rather than the subtle radiance you get from such products as Revlon SkinLights or a foundation such as L'Oreal True Match Super Blendable Makeup, this M.A.C. product's shine is more obvious and more glittery than shimmery. If you don't mind added shine under your makeup (or on bare skin), this won't be an obstacle. All others are encouraged to sample this product with foundation to make sure the amount of shine is not objectionable.

☺ **Prep + Prime Eye** *($16)* works well as a cream-to-powder concealer for the eye area as well as for other discolorations. Its creamy texture quickly morphs into a silky, weightless matte finish that is minimally prone to creasing. The finish can look slightly powdery, but the effect is canceled once eyeshadow is blended over it. The five shades present options for light to dark skin tones, but nothing for someone with porcelain to fair skin. But that's OK, because although this product has its purpose, it is easily replaced by a matte-finish concealer, such as M.A.C. Select Cover-Up ($13.50).

☺ **$$$ Matte** *($17.50)* is a thick, but silky, silicone-based gel that creates a smooth skin texture and has a long-wearing matte finish. It isn't as absorbent as other products in this category (Smashbox's Anti-Shine trumps this one), but is nevertheless worth a try.

😐 **Brush Cleanser** *($9)* is an alcohol-based solution that does remove makeup and excess oil from brushes, but will eventually make natural hair dry and stiff. Although it's OK for occasional quick clean-ups, washing your brushes with a gentle shampoo and water is preferred.

☹ **Clear Gloss** *($17.50)* is a thick, clear gloss meant to add "polish, shine and highlights to bare or made-up skin." It certainly adds shine, but why anyone would want to tolerate this product's sticky finish is a good question, especially when there are so many smooth, non-sticky shine alternatives. Applying this over makeup will ruin any careful blending, and if you have long hair, expect it to get stuck in this gloss.

MAKE UP FOR EVER

MAKE UP FOR EVER AT-A-GLANCE

Strengths: A couple of good cleansers and makeup removers; one good lip balm; the newer foundations have many wonderful qualities; impressive options (and shade ranges) for powders, powder blush, and powder eyeshadow; some extraordinary lip glosses and lipstick/lip color options (and again, the shade ranges are remarkable); a few formidable mascaras; good shimmer options; the huge selection of makeup brushes.

Weaknesses: Expensive; a few products suffer from needlessly irritating ingredients; average toner; the foundations and concealers that have been in this line longest are behind the times; mostly average eye and lip pencils; the Transparent Mascara; the Diamond Powder and Lipstick Sealer; mostly lackluster specialty products.

For more information on Make Up For Ever, call (877) 757-5175 or visit www.makeupforever.com or www.Beautypedia.com. Note: The product assortment below is typical of what you will find at Sephora boutiques across the country. If you wish to view the complete collection of Make Up For Ever, the only place to do that is at their freestanding store in New York City (or their European stores).

MAKE UP FOR EVER SKIN CARE

☹ **Extreme Cleanser, Balancing Cleansing Dry Oil** *($30 for 6.76 ounces)* is a lotion-textured creamy cleanser that contains a dry skin–compatible amount of oil, which also helps dissolve makeup. Despite this, it is not recommended for any skin type because it contains rosemary oil, pepper extract, and volatile fragrance components that can cause irritation.

😐 **$$$ Gentle Milk, Moisturizing Cleansing Milk** *($23 for 6.76 ounces)* omits most of the irritants found in the Extreme Cleanser above, and is an OK option for normal to slightly dry skin not prone to blemishes. The milky cleanser removes makeup easily and leaves minimal residue. It would be better without the volatile fragrance components, but their presence is minor.

☺ **$$$ Pure Water, Moisturizing Cleansing Water** *($23 for 6.76 ounces)* is a basic liquid cleanser that combines slip agents with gentle detergent cleansing agents. It's an option for normal to slightly dry or slightly oily skin when minimal makeup is used, or as a morning cleanser.

😐 **$$$ So Divine, Moisturizing Cleansing Cream** *($27 for 4.4 ounces)* is a cold cream–style cleanser for very dry skin, and requires a washcloth for complete removal. The tiny amount of plant extracts either have a soothing quality or impart subtle fragrance.

☺ **$$$ Sens'Eyes, Waterproof Sensitive Eye Cleanser** *($23 for 3.38 ounces)* works well to remove waterproof eye makeup, but isn't preferred for sensitive eyes over similar but less-expensive options from Almay, Neutrogena, or Clinique. This product is fragrance-free.

😐 **$$$ Cool Lotion, Moisturizing Soothing Lotion** *($23 for 6.76 ounces)* costs a lot for what amounts to an average toner that's primarily water, grape water, solvent, and slip agent. It's a mediocre option for normal to dry skin.

😐 **$$$ Mist & Fix, Make-Up Fixer Mist** *($27 for 4.22 ounces)* coats skin with an acrylate-based film-forming agent, similar to those in firm-hold hairsprays. It can, to some extent, prolong makeup wear (especially if you're going to be exposed to rainfall), but not without a slightly stiff, sticky feel and potential irritation. This contains a minimal amount of hydrating ingredients and absolutely cannot protect skin from pollution.

😐 **$$$ All Mat, Face Matifying Primer** *($45 for 1.01 ounces)* creates a smooth matte finish thanks to its formula of silicone, slip agent, silicone polymers, and mineral-based absorbents. It is an option for normal to very oily skin looking to prolong a matte finish, but what a shame this pricey product lacks truly helpful ingredients for skin.

☹ **Stop Shining+ Matifying Gel** *($16 for 0.5 ounce)* is similar to the All Mat, Face Matifying Primer, above, and even though the price makes it more attractive, the inclusion of several volatile fragrance components makes this not worth considering.

☺ **$$$ Moisturizing Lip Balm** *($18 for 0.12 ounce)* is a lipstick-style clear lip balm that has a strong wax base along with lesser amounts of dryness-quelling emollients. It's a good but needlessly pricey option to take care of dry, chapped lips.

MAKE UP FOR EVER MAKEUP

FOUNDATION: ✓☺ $$$ Powder Foundation *($40)* is talc-based and has an outstanding, finely milled texture that sweeps over skin, providing a flawless, soft powder finish with sheer coverage. All four shades are exemplary. Note: Some shades list SPF 8, but the ingredient list does not indicate any sunscreens, so don't rely on this powder foundation for any amount of sun protection. This is recommended for all skin types except very dry.

✓☺ $$$ Duo Mat Powder Foundation *($32)* provides everything a pressed-powder foundation should, and excels in each area. The talc- and silicone-based formula feels buttery smooth and blends on like a second skin. The slightly dry, non-chalky matte finish is ideal for normal to very oily skin, and this provides light to medium coverage that doesn't mask skin, but does make it look refined and polished. The selection of 11 shades is first-rate; the only questionable colors are the slightly orange 209 Warm Beige and the slightly peach 214 Dark Beige. Shades 216 Caramel and 218 Chocolate are beautiful for darker skin tones or used as matte bronzing powders. Shade 200 Beige Opalescent has a soft shine that will magnify oily areas. This powder foundation does contain fragrance.

✓☺ $$$ Mat Velvet + Mattifying Foundation *($34)* has a thin, fluid texture with enough slip to allow smooth blending before setting to a strong matte finish. Coverage goes from medium to almost full, and this foundation camouflages diffuse redness on skin quite well. The absorbent formula is ideal for oily to very oily skin, with the only caveat being the prominence of cornstarch and its potential for feeding the bacteria responsible for blemishes. Sixteen mostly impressive shades are available. The ones to avoid due to obvious peach or orange tones are Sand, Neutral Beige, and Golden Beige. Soft Beige and Honey Beige may be too peach for some skin tones, but are worth a look. Alabaster is a superb shade for very fair skin, while the Brown and Chocolate shades are gorgeous, non-ashy shades for ebony skin tones.

☺ $$$ Face and Body Liquid Makeup *($38)* is a liquidy, water-based foundation that also contains a blend of silicone and mineral oil, so this has a good amount of slip on the skin, yet blends readily to a natural matte finish. Coverage can go from sheer to medium, and allows you to build coverage without it looking thick. The collection of ten shades is deceiving, because many of them look too peach or pink in the bottle, yet almost all of them end up being soft and neutral on the skin—plus there are equally good options for light and dark skin tones. Test Natural 3 and Bronzed Beige 26 carefully, as both finish slightly peach. This can be used on the body if desired, but it isn't as tenacious or clingy as products like DermaBlend, so the results can be mixed. This lightweight formula works best for normal to slightly dry or slightly oily skin.

😐 $$$ Mat Velvet Oil-Free Foundation SPF 20 *($37)* contains effective sunscreen agents, but they're not listed as active so they cannot be relied on for daily protection. That's a shame, because this offers a slightly thick but smooth texture, a powdery matte finish, and light to medium coverage that would appeal to those with oily skin. The nine colors are very good, but advertising a sunscreen without listing active ingredients shows flagrant disregard of FDA and European regulations, making this not worthy of a better rating.

😐 $$$ Liquid Lift Foundation *($41)* is overpriced for what amounts to a very basic formula that absolutely cannot lift skin or impart a tightening effect. It has a fluid, silky texture and nice slip, which makes blending easy. Coverage is medium and it leaves a slightly dewy finish suitable for someone with normal to dry skin. Among the six shades (best for fair to medium skin) only Golden Beige 5 stands out as too peach.

😐 **$$$ Corrective Makeup Base SPF 18** *($24)* is essentially a lightweight, slightly moist liquid foundation that comes in the color-correcting shades of mauve, white, yellow (labeled as "blue"), and orange. The sunscreen is in-part titanium dioxide, which is great, but I am not a fan of color correctors because they don't work, so this is hard to recommend. However, because these colors are very sheer, mesh quite well with the skin, and leave a soft matte finish, the corrective effect is all but gone once foundation, concealer, and powder are applied on top. If you're curious to see how a product like this would work for you, definitely test it before purchasing. The Blue 5 shade is actually a pale yellow tone (don't ask me why) that may work as a foundation for some fair skin tones.

😐 **$$$ Pan Stick** *($30)* has a thick, petrolatum- and wax-based creamy texture that's not too far removed from traditional theatrical makeup. Unless you need full coverage and are willing to trade that for a makeup that doesn't look natural no matter how well it's blended, this has limited appeal. Considering the ingredients, it doesn't feel or look as oily as you'd think. Five shades are offered, and only Caramel 5W is slightly peach. The others, while heavy, are surprisingly neutral.

CONCEALER: ☺ **$$$ Lift Concealer** *($21)* begins liquidy, but dries quickly to a long-lasting, powdery matte finish. It provides good coverage that you can build to move up from light to medium coverage. This water-, talc-, and silicone-based formula comes in a tube and is best for oily skin or for use over oily areas. Five shades are available, with the best ones being Medium Beige 2, Neutral Beige 3, and Matte Beige 4. By the way, this won't lift skin in the least, so don't bank on that benefit.

😐 **$$$ 5-Camouflage Cream Palette** *($36)* comes in a palette with four flesh-toned colors that veer slightly to the peachy side, along with a green color corrector. You can blend the shades together to create a custom match, but unless you need significant coverage and are willing to put up with this difficult texture, this is easy to pass up. The waxes in this concealer are a poor choice for use over blemishes, but do lend an opacity that helps conceal red marks, dark circles, or flat scars.

☹ **Concealer Pencil** *($18)* is a dual-sided pencil that comes in two different skin tones, one for lighter skin and one for medium skin. It's greasy, looks heavy, and is unsuitable for use over blemishes.

POWDER: ✓ ☺ **$$$ Super Mat Loose Powder** *($24)* has a super-fine, ultralight texture and a soft, dry finish that's ideal for oily skin. This talc- and silica-based loose powder looks beautiful on skin, and each of the three translucent shades are great.

☺ **$$$ Compact Powder** *($30)* is talc-based and has a silky, dry texture and sheer finish that doesn't look chalky or too powdery on skin. The three shades are all decent, but this isn't quite as good as the Super Mat Loose Powder above. ☺ **$$$ Velvet Finish Compact Powder** *($29)* has a talc- and kaolin (clay)–based texture that feels slightly thick and dry, but it applies smoothly, leaving a velvety matte finish. Failing to blend carefully or brushing on too much of this powder results in a chalky appearance, so use restraint. Each of the eight shades applies lighter than they appear in the compact, but all of them are very good. Caramel and Chocolate are great for dark skin tones or for use as bronzing powder on medium to tan skin tones.

☺ **$$$ Sun Tan Bronzing Powder SPF 8** *($32)* is a very good, talc-based pressed bronzing powder available in two believable tan shades, with only a hint of shine, and a third matte option (labeled Natural Gold 1). No active ingredients are listed to back up the SPF claim, but it takes more than a dusting of bronzing powder for substantial sun protection anyway, so for this product the sun protection claim is disregarded in the rating.

BLUSH: ✓☺ $$$ Sculpting Blush Powder Blush *($24)* ranks as Make Up For Ever's best lineup of powder blush in the last ten years. The talc- and clay-based formula feels gossamer smooth and applies evenly. Almost all of the colors are matte but still beautifully enliven skin, and the pigmentation is strong (so begin with a sheer application and build color as needed). Shade #2 Matte Blue Pink has the faintest hint of pink and won't show up as "blush," even on someone with very fair skin (but it's OK as a highlighting powder). Shades #24 Matte Fawn, #26 Matte Sienna, and #28 Brown Brick are workable, warm-toned hues for women of color.

☺ $$$ Powder Blush *($18)* comes in a bountiful array of shades, from the pinkest pinks to the most understated neutrals. These are strongly pigmented shades, and without careful, sheer application they tend to grab on the skin, which is a side effect of this blush's drier texture. Use restraint and you will likely be pleased with the results and the long wear. Several shiny shades are also available, and the good news is the shine clings well and applies evenly.

EYESHADOW: ☺ $$$ Eyeshadow *($18)* has a texture, application, and intensity that is nearly identical to that of the Powder Blush above. The range of shades is staggering (125 in all, though most Sephora boutiques only stock a fraction of them), with some of the most imaginative (and largely unnecessary) shades right next to the earth and neutral tones that are universally flattering. These apply evenly, and most of the shades provide opaque coverage, which lets them last without creasing or fading.

😐 $$$ Pearly Waterproof Eyeshadow Pencil *($18)* is a standard chubby pencil with a creamy texture that glides over the skin and imparts sheer, shimmering color. This pencil is not preferred to the Eyeshadow above, but some will undoubtedly find it intriguing, and the formula is waterproof.

EYE AND BROW SHAPER: ☺ $$$ Color Liner *($19)* is a good liquid eyeliner that features a soft but firm-textured brush and a formula that applies easily and dries quickly. All of the colors have a strong iridescent finish, making them best for evening makeup on unwrinkled eyelids. Best of all, once dry, the formula holds up remarkably well.

😐 $$$ Eye Pencil *($16)* needs routine sharpening and has a slightly stiff, fine-tipped application that finishes slightly creamy. It's OK, but rather basic for the money. Avoid Dark Blue 11 and Bright Blue 31. **😐 $$$ Waterproof Eyeliner Pencil** *($16)* needs sharpening and has an unusual base of cottonseed and jojoba oils, neither of which are as waterproof as silicone-based pencils, though it does hold up to minimal water exposure (think crying versus swimming). Although the application is creamy, this sets to a tacky finish that stays put. All of the shades are laced with shine, so choose carefully. Turquoise 7L is recommended only if you're a performer in Cirque de Soleil.

😐 $$$ Waterproof Eyeliner *($21)* has an ultra-thin brush that applies the slow-drying liquid liner well. It is reasonably waterproof once set, but has a tendency to fade, making it an average choice and not really worth its price. **😐 $$$ Eyebrow Pencil** *($18)* has to be sharpened, which is a pain, but it applies very smooth and has a lightweight, non-waxy texture and a soft powder finish that won't smear or smudge. All of the colors are workable (and matte), making this an easy recommendation if you don't mind sharpening.

☹ Kohl Eye Pencil *($17)* is a substandard pencil that applies too thick, flakes a bit, and is very prone to smearing. Avoid it unless you like eye makeup that demands constant upkeep!

LIPSTICK, LIP GLOSS, AND LIPLINER: ✓☺ $$$ Liquid Lip Color *($18)* remains a favorite, but the shade selection has been streamlined since the previous edition of this book. The ultra-smooth texture imparts intense, opaque color and a completely non-sticky, high-gloss finish. This lipstick/gloss hybrid comes in a tube with a brush applicator, and the opening of the tube is large enough to prevent the brush from splaying—a major plus. Consider this a must-try if you like the opacity of lipstick with the finish of a lip gloss.

✓☺ **$$$ Super Lip Gloss** *($16)* is a favorite of Make Up For Ever fans, and it's not hard to see why. This is one of the smoothst, least sticky glosses you're likely to find. It comes in a tube and is silicone-based, so it can feel slippery (and can encourage lipstick feathering if you're prone to that), but women who have a problem with bleeding lipstick should stay away from glosses in the first place. The available shades are beautiful and include some unconventional (but sheer) options.

✓☺ **$$$ Fascinating Lip Gloss** *($18)* is applied with a sponge tip and is just as smooth and refreshingly non-sticky as the Super Lip Gloss above. It has a slightly lighter texture and all of the sheer colors are infused with glitter, but it doesn't feel grainy on the lips.

☺ **$$$ Lipstick** *($18)* is the general name for Make Up For Ever's newest lipstick option, available in four finishes, each with the same basic formula (what differs is the level of pigment). The **Creams** (shades numbered in the 200s) are lightweight yet sufficiently creamy, with medium coverage and a slight gloss finish. **Pearly** (shades numbered in the 300s) are identical to the Creams, but with a soft, pearlescent finish. The **Transparents** (shades numbered in the 400s) offer sheer to light coverage and a gorgeous selection of colors, each with a soft glossy finish and minimally greasy texture. Last, the **Mattes** (shades numbered in the 500s) provide opaque coverage and opulent colors, but do not have a true matte finish—it's definitely creamy—but these last the longest due to the high level of pigment. The red shades in this range are stunning!

☺ **$$$ Moisturizing Lip Balm** *($18)* is a colorless, emollient, glossy lip balm that works well to remedy and prevent dry, chapped lips. It does not contain any irritants and it does not feel too thick or waxy.

☺ **$$$ Lip Palettes** *($39)* feature the new lipstick formula in its various versions packaged in a slim palette with a workable brush. The mix of shades is complementary, allowing you to blend two or three together for an attractive custom color.

😐 **$$$ Lip Pencil** *($16)* is a standard pencil with a good creamy application and some unique but wearable shades among a few stand-bys. It's longer than most, so keep in mind that that makes it a tough fit for small makeup bags.

☹ **Lip Care Pencil SPF 16** *($16 for 0.12 ounce)* is a colorless, needs-sharpening lip pencil meant to moisturize and protect lips from sun damage. The in-part titanium dioxide sunscreen helps ensure broad-spectrum protection, but the emollient formula suffers from the inclusion of menthol, which is present in a much greater amount than typically found in lip products.

MASCARA: ✓☺ **$$$ Lengthening Mascara** *($19)* has a small brush that provides big results, and quickly. This is a fantastic lengthening mascara that just doesn't know when to stop, making lashes impossibly long, all without clumps. Thickness is incidental, but for lash-fluttering length that wears all day, this excels!

✓☺ **$$$ Waterproof Lengthening Mascara** *($20)* has been improved and is an excellent lengthening mascara that is indeed waterproof. The tiny, tailored brush allows easy access to every lash, extending them beautifully, but building little in the way of thickness. Clumps are absent though, so if length and waterproofing are what you're after, this works beautifully.

😐 **$$$ Mascara Volume** *($19)* comes off easily with a water-soluble cleanser, but is otherwise very boring, and doesn't live up to its enticing name, at least if your expectation is thick, voluminous lashes.

☹ **Transparent Mascara** *($18)* is basically a styling gel formula in mascara form. The small brush works for lashes and brows, but the clear gel is too sticky for either. Considering the number of inexpensive non-sticky and minimally sticky brow gels, this isn't worth the bother.

FACE AND BODY ILLUMINATING/SHIMMER PRODUCTS: ☺ **$$$ Shine-On Powder** *($26)* has an honest name, as most powders with shine also claim to keep skin matte while concurrently adding sparkles to the skin. This talc-based loose powder has a pleasant texture and its finely milled shiny shades work well for a low-key evening look.

☺ **$$$ Compact Shine On** *($29)* is a smooth-textured, talc-based pressed powder with a shine that has elements of subtle glow (finely milled shimmer pigments) and visible sparkles (which, while visible, aren't gaudy). The shine clings better than you'd expect, and all three shades are soft, sheer options for highlighting areas of the face or body.

☺ **$$$ Star Powder** *($18)* is simply a very shiny loose powder that comes in a wide variety of shades, from gold and silver to lots of pastel hues, as well as finishes ranging from soft shimmer to metallic. They're versatile and include several deeper colors for dramatic effects, and they cling reasonably well. Be forewarned, however, a little goes a long way and even tiny amounts can be messy to use, so build slowly.

☺ **$$$ Diamond Cream** *($36)* presents shimmer in lotion form and it's another concentrated product, so apply sparingly until you get the desired effect. It does have a slightly tacky finish, but the shine doesn't flake. It actually works best mixed with a standard body lotion for a soft glow.

☹ **Diamond Powder** *($24)* offers truly diamond-like shine in the form of another messy loose powder. Unfortunately, although the effect is very cool, the powder flakes endlessly and feels slightly grainy.

BRUSHES: You will find that Make Up For Ever's ✓☺ **Brushes** *($13–$54)* have something to offer everyone, whether you're a makeup brush neophyte or connoisseur. The brushes include both natural and synthetic hair options, and the majority are expertly shaped and sized appropriately for their intended purpose. There are some superfluous ones to consider carefully, but that chiefly depends on what your needs are. All in all, the choices are plentiful and the prices are comparatively reasonable. The only unfortunate element is that most Sephora stores sell only a small portion of this company's brushes. To view the entire collection, you need to find a Make Up For Ever counter in a department store or visit their flagship store in New York.

The ☺ **Professional Brush Case** *($32)* holds several brushes and its tri-fold design has pockets and zippered pouches for other small makeup odds and ends. Considering the variety of items you can carry, this case ends up being quite a value. In contrast, the 😐 **$$$ Brush Set** *($55)* is incomplete and far from any makeup artist's definition of a complete brush "set." Included are only three brushes (for powder and eyeshadow, plus a sponge-tip eyeshadow applicator) in a flimsy case. You'll be left wanting (and, in fact, needing) more for even the most basic makeup application.

SPECIALTY PRODUCTS: ☹ **Lip Plus Lipstick Sealer** *($19)* is a clear solution of alcohol, silicone, film-forming agent, more alcohol, thickener, and fragrance. It's meant to be applied over a lipstick or lip gloss to net all-day wear. Not only does this brush-on liquid burn upon application (even over a thick layer of lipstick), but it barely works. Lipstick still comes off on cups or even with a light peck on the cheek. This is one to leave on the shelf!

☺ **Eyelashes Individual** *($14)* are sold in a kit that includes several smaller bunches of eyelashes rather than a single strip. If you're adept at applying false eyelashes (or are willing to learn), these are a good way to dramatize your natural lashes without going overboard. The individual pieces can be cut to size, but before you attempt that, make sure you have the hang of the application and removal process.

☺ **$$$ Matte Lip** *($20)* is designed to be used over lipstick to minimize a glossy or creamy finish. It's somewhat odd given that you can achieve this finish by simply choosing a demi-matte or regular matte lipstick. Dabbing this colorless, cornstarch-based cream over lipstick can be a messy task, but it does mattify and is an option if applied very carefully.

☺ **$$$ Stop Shining** *($16)* is a thick, nonaqueous, silicone gel with absorbent properties meant for use over oily areas. It doesn't hold up all day, nor is it as effective as similar products from Clinique and Smashbox that combine silicones with absorbent magnesium, but it may be worth a try if your oily areas aren't too out of control.

☺ **$$$ Mist & Fix** *($27)* is supposed to be used not only to touch up makeup but also to protect skin against external damage. This spray-on product consists primarily of water, slip agent (methylpropanediol, which absolutely won't refresh makeup), and film-forming agent, similar to what's used in hairsprays. This has a slightly sticky finish that can feel odd, but I suppose it does provide some protection from makeup fading and slipping. Overall, this is a gimmicky product that's a poor solution for those looking to reinforce or touch-up makeup on-the-go. A good oil-blotting paper and quick dusting of pressed powder (and lipstick touch-up, of course) are much better.

☹ **Glossy Full** *($20)* adds a striking vinyl sheen to lips when applied over any lipstick. Essentially a colorless lip gloss, this product loses points for its undeniable mint flavor and for containing fragrance components that can be irritating to lips. The amount of pentapeptide won't plump lips even a little.

MARY KAY

MARY KAY AT-A-GLANCE

Strengths: Most of the products are fragrance-free; some noteworthy cleansers, serums, and sunscreens; every sunscreen offers sufficient UVA protection; packaging that keeps light- and air-sensitive ingredients stable during use; very good eye-makeup remover and topical disinfectant with benzoyl peroxide; two good foundations; the MK Signature Concealer; the eyeliner pencils; the MK Signature Lip Gloss; the Brush Set (individual brushes are sold separately but these are a mixed bag); well-packaged samples are available for selected products.

Weaknesses: The overall collection is a mixed bag of exciting and disappointing products; several outdated moisturizers and greasy cleansers; no AHA or BHA products; no products that can successfully address skin discolorations; unexceptional topical scrub; irritating lip balms; average powder blush; the Medium Coverage Foundation; the Waterproof Mascara; the Eye Primer isn't necessary.

For more information about Mary Kay, call (800) 627-9529 or visit www.marykay.com or www.Beautypedia.com. Note: Unless mentioned otherwise, all Mary Kay products are fragrance-free.

MARY KAY SKIN CARE

MARY KAY TIMEWISE PRODUCTS

☹ **TimeWise 3-In-1 Cleanser, for Combination to Oily Skin** *($18 for 4.5 ounces)* lists the drying detergent cleansing agent TEA-lauryl sulfate as the second ingredient and also contains a couple of irritating plant extracts, making this expensive cleanser a poor choice for anyone.

😐 **$$$ TimeWise 3-in-1 Cleanser, for Normal to Dry Skin** *($18 for 4.5 ounces)* is a very standard and somewhat greasy cleansing lotion for dry to very dry skin. The mineral oil, Vaseline, and clay make this difficult to remove with a washcloth, and this should be avoided if you have dry skin with blemishes.

☹ **TimeWise 3-in-1 Cleansing Bar** *($18 for a 5-ounce bar)* is a standard, drying bar soap that does not contain a single ingredient capable of exfoliating skin as claimed. On that same note, this soap cannot "reduce the visible signs of aging." What a ridiculous claim for a product that's basically a bar of Dove Soap!

😐 **$$$ TimeWise Age-Fighting Eye Cream** *($26 for 0.65 ounce)* is a decent, lightweight-moisturizer for slightly dry skin anywhere on the face. The lack of antioxidants and skin-identical ingredients is disappointing, but this contains peptides, which theoretically function as cell-communicating ingredients.

😐 **TimeWise Age-Fighting Moisturizer, for Combination/Oily Skin** *($22 for 3.3 ounces)* has a fluid texture and silky feel. It's a suitably light moisturizer for its intended skin types, and leaves a soft matte finish. Regrettably, it lacks a good selection of antioxidants and ingredients that mimic the structure of healthy skin. And, of course, without a sunscreen, this product cannot fight aging any more than an ant can drive a car.

😐 **TimeWise Age-Fighting Moisturizer, for Normal/Dry Skin** *($22 for 3.3 ounces)* has a creamy but light texture and contains some helpful ingredients for normal to dry skin, but most of the impressive ingredients are listed after the preservatives, so they're barely functional. Moreover, antioxidants are in very short supply.

😐 **TimeWise Age-Fighting Moisturizer Sunscreen SPF 15** *($22 for 3 ounces)* deserves kudos for its in-part zinc oxide sunscreen, but the base formula for normal to slightly dry skin is rather boring, with insignificant amounts of antioxidants and water-binding agents.

✓☺ **TimeWise Day Solution Sunscreen SPF 25** *($30 for 1 ounce)* is the most impressive daytime moisturizer in the TimeWise collection. The in-part zinc oxide sunscreen provides sufficient UVA protection, while the fluid but creamy formula contains a great selection of antioxidants, skin-identical ingredients, and lightweight emollients for normal to dry skin. This also has a silky finish that wears beautifully under makeup.

☺ **$$$ TimeWise Firming Eye Cream** *($30 for 0.5 ounce)* is a very emollient, Vaseline-based moisturizer for dry to very dry skin anywhere on the face. Lots of thickening agents combine with smaller amounts of peptides and a few antioxidants to round out the skin-beneficial traits of this product (but, regrettably, it won't firm skin).

☹ **TimeWise Night Solution** *($30 for 1 ounce)* is a clear, slightly tacky serum that's loaded with antioxidants and peptides. The unhappy face rating is because these ingredients are joined by several fragrant plant extracts that cause irritation, including geranium, wild mint, rose, orange, and jasmine. The tingling sensation this causes is not good news for aging skin.

✓☺ **$$$ TimeWise Even Complexion Essence** *($35 for 1 ounce)* promises to restore a natural, even tone to skin while helping to reverse skin discolorations. Eschewing the established skin-lightening agent hydroquinone, this water-based serum contains niacinamide and ascorbyl glucoside instead. There is some research showing that niacinamide can interrupt the transfer of melanocytes (pigmented skin cells) to keratinocytes (regular skin cells that make the protein keratin), which would essentially cut the discoloration process off at the pass. However, these studies were done in vitro (test tube) rather than on human skin. Moreover, while the researchers pointed out that a positive outcome was dose-dependent, the dosage was not revealed (Source: *Experimental Dermatology*, July 2005, pages 498–508). A smaller study, which was done on human skin, revealed that a 5% concentration of niacinamide produced a noticeable effect on discolorations after four weeks of use (Source: *British Journal of Dermatology*, July 2002, pages 20–31). It should be noted this previous study was done on only 18 women, and was from Procter & Gamble, whose Olay and SK-II lines are big on the use of niacinamide.

There is no substantiated research concerning the ability of the vitamin C derivative ascorbyl glucoside to lighten skin, although vitamin C in other forms has shown potential. So what we have here is a potentially good alternative skin-lightening product, though Mary Kay is definitely not using 5% niacinamide. Nonetheless, this product is worth considering by all skin types as a lightweight serum that contains several vitamin- and plant-based antioxidants as well as water-binding agents, including peptides.

😐 **$$$ TimeWise Microdermabrasion Set** *($55 for the set)* is Mary Kay's contribution to the growing number of at-home microdermabrasion kits. Just like its numerous competitors, this two-part product features a topical scrub and post-treatment moisturizer. **Step #1–Refine** *($30 for 2 ounces; may be purchased separately)* contains alumina crystals as the abrasive agent, and yes, this is the same ingredient used in professionally administered microdermabrasion treatments. But there's a difference between massaging a scrub on your skin and how the microdermabrasion machine works (and the way it's operated). Further, recent research has shown that microdermabrasion doesn't appear to have a cumulative benefit.

Either way, products like this (when used gently) are indeed viable topical scrubs. What I like is that Mary Kay's version is free of added irritants and that it rinses easily (many microdermabrasion scrubs are difficult to remove with water).

Step #2–Replenish *($25 for 1 ounce; may be purchased separately)* is to be applied after Step #1–Refine, though I can think of many other serum-type moisturizers that have formulas superior to this, including those from Aveda, Clinique, Estee Lauder, Olay, and Paula's Choice. Rather than create a product brimming with antioxidants, anti-irritants, and cell-communicating ingredients, Mary Kay created a functional, but ordinary, product that is just an OK option for normal to slightly oily skin. It's being marketed for dry or oily skin, but if you have dry skin, Replenish will leave your skin wanting more, and for oily skin it may prove too emollient. It has some good antioxidants and the packaging will keep them stable, but the amounts are likely too small to bring much benefit to your skin. Overall, there is nothing about the scrub in this kit that can't be replaced by a washcloth, and there are better moisturizers than this. But if you're still interested in trying a microdermabrasion-at-home product, consider Neutrogena's At-Home Microdermabrasion Kit ($25), which comes with a rotating brush applicator and cleanser.

☹ **TimeWise Targeted-Action Eye Revitalizer** *($35 for 0.34 ounce)* asks you to "imagine a product so powerful, it can reduce the appearance of both dark circles and under-eye puffiness in just two weeks." That's something many people would love to achieve given how common these eye-area skin conditions are. But can this product and its roller-ball applicator produce such results? Sadly, it cannot. The water- and film-forming agent–based fluid contains some state-of-the-art ingredients, but neither they nor the numerous plant extracts (some of which are irritating) have been proven to lighten dark circles and make puffiness recede. This is actually more of a problem for skin around the eyes because it contains the irritating menthol derivative menthyl lactate (for the cooling sensation mentioned in the claims).

✓ ☺ **$$$ TimeWise Targeted-Action Line Reducer** *($40 for 0.13 ounce)* deserves a Paula's Pick rating for its elegant formula laced with several antioxidants, soothing agent, and a cell-communicating ingredient. The antiwrinkle claims for this product are far-fetched because this click pen–dispensed product works poorly and doesn't really act like spackle, especially if you smile. This will not fill in deep, etched lines like those that occur along the naso-labial folds. Wrinkles aside, the formula as a whole is very good for normal to dry skin, whether around the eyes or on other areas that need temporary smoothing. And thank you, Mary Kay, for not implying in the least that this product is better than Botox or dermal injections!

✓ ☺ **TimeWise Age-Fighting Lip Primer** *($22 for 0.5 ounce)* is a silicone- and wax-based spackle for filling in lines on the lips and around the mouth. It works to a minor extent, but the effect is temporary and diminishes faster if you wear greasy or overly glossy lipsticks. What's particularly impressive is the amount of antioxidants and cell-communicating ingredients this contains. Those help skin repair itself while reducing inflammation, and earn this product a Paula's Pick. By the way, this is worth considering over Lauder's more expensive Perfectionist Correcting Concentrate for Lip Lines ($35 for 0.08 ounce).

OTHER MARY KAY PRODUCTS

😐 **Creamy Cleanser Formula 2** *($10 for 6.5 ounces)* is an exceedingly standard water- and mineral oil–based cleanser for normal to dry skin not prone to blemishes. It requires a washcloth for complete removal.

✓ ☺ **Deep Cleanser Formula 3** *($10 for 6.5 ounces)* is a very good water-soluble cleansing lotion for normal to slightly oily skin. It rinses cleanly, removes makeup, and does not contain fragrance.

😐 **Gentle Cleansing Cream Formula 1** *($10 for 4 ounces)* is a cold cream–style cleanser for dry to very dry skin. It removes makeup easily but you need a washcloth to make sure you don't leave a greasy residue.

☹ **Velocity Facial Cleanser** *($10 for 5 ounces)* uses TEA-lauryl sulfate as the main detergent cleansing agent, which makes this too drying and irritating for all skin types. In addition, several of the plant extracts are irritants, and the fragrance is not needed.

✓ ☺ **Oil-Free Eye Makeup Remover** *($14 for 3.75 ounces)* works quickly and beautifully to remove all types of makeup. The silicone-enhanced formula may be used before or after cleansing and, unlike many makeup removers, this one omits the fragrance.

☹ **Blemish Control Toner Formula 3** *($11 for 6.5 ounces)* won't control blemishes, but will instead cause irritation and redness due to the alcohol, eucalyptus oil, and menthol it contains.

☹ **Hydrating Freshener Formula 1** *($11 for 6.5 ounces)* consists primarily of water, slip agent, and preservatives, but the menthol makes it not worth considering over dozens of other toners.

☹ **Purifying Freshener Formula 2** *($11 for 6.5 ounces)* lists alcohol as the second ingredient, making this too drying and irritating for all skin types.

😐 **Advanced Moisture Renewal Treatment Cream** *($19 for 2.5 ounces)* covers the basics for replenishing dry to very dry skin, but is an overall lackluster (not advanced) moisturizer whose token amounts of antioxidants and the cell-communicating ingredient lecithin are a too little, too late approach.

😐 **Balancing Moisturizer Formula 2** *($16 for 4 ounces)* is similar to Clinique's original Dramatically Different Moisturizing Lotion, and just as boring. It is an outdated, inadequate option for normal to dry skin.

😐 **Enriched Moisturizer Formula 1** *($16 for 4 ounces)* is a thicker, more emollient version of the Balancing Moisturizer Formula 2 above, and the same comments apply, except that this is suitable for dry to very dry skin.

☹ **Extra Emollient Night Cream** *($11 for 2.1 ounces)* is basically Vaseline and mineral oil along with several waxes. Yes, it will make dry skin feel smooth and lubricated, but the inclusion of menthol is a burn.

☹ **Indulge Soothing Eye Gel** *($15 for 0.4 ounce)* contains a frustrating mix of helpful and skin-hindering ingredients, with the negatives (comfrey, witch hazel, and eyebright) outweighing the positives and making this more a problem than an indulgence for skin.

😐 **Intense Moisturizing Cream** *($30 for 1.8 ounces)* is a very standard, humdrum moisturizer that is primarily water, mineral oil, Vaseline, and waxes with little to no antioxidants or water-binding agents. In the end, this is an OK moisturizer for dry to very dry skin. However, in this price range, far better options are readily available.

😐 **Oil Control Lotion Formula 3** *($16 for 4 ounces)* doesn't carry a high price, which it shouldn't, because this is a very ordinary mix of water, silicone, slip agent, thickener, and film-forming agent. It is a substandard option for normal to oily skin, and does not do a remarkable job at keeping skin shine-free.

😐 **Oil-Free Hydrating Gel** *($30 for 1.8 ounces)* is considerably more modern than the Intense Moisturizing Cream above, and has a wonderfully silky, lightweight texture for normal to oily or combination skin. The drawback is jar packaging, which won't keep the antioxidants in this product stable once it's opened.

😐 **Oil Mattifier** *($15 for 0.6 ounce)* is much better at curtailing surface shine (oiliness) than the Oil Control Lotion Formula 3 above. The tiny amount of alcohol isn't cause for concern. The solvent isododecane and the silicones help promote and maintain a lightweight matte finish. It would have earned a higher rating had it included antioxidants, cell-communicating ingredients, or skin-identical ingredients, something all skin types can benefit from immensely.

☹ **Velocity Lightweight Moisturizer** *($12 for 4 ounces)* offers minimal benefit for skin and contains enough alcohol to be potentially irritating. It also contains several irritating plant extracts, including cinnamon and sandalwood.

✓ ☺ **Acne Treatment Gel** *($7 for 1 ounce)* lists 5% benzoyl peroxide as the active ingredient, and is a very good, gel-based topical disinfectant for those battling blemishes.

😐 **Clarifying Mask Formula 3** *($12 for 4 ounces)* is a standard clay mask that is an OK option for oily to very oily skin, but contains potentially problematic lavender along with a tiny amount of TEA-lauryl sulfate. It's not terrible, but better clay masks abound.

☹ **Moisture Rich Mask Formula 1** *($12 for 4 ounces)* ranks below standard because it lacks state-of-the-art ingredients for dry skin and contains menthol, which serves no purpose other than to cause irritation and convince you the product is "working."

😐 **Revitalizing Mask Formula 2** *($12 for 4 ounces)* may cause your skin to be confused due to its contrasting mix of absorbent clay with moisturizing agents, waxes, and exfoliating walnut shell powder. I don't know who to recommend this mask for—it's too drying for normal to dry skin and too emollient for oily skin.

😊 **Beauty Blotters Oil-Absorbing Tissues** *($5 for 75 sheets)* are non-powdered thin sheets of linen-type material that do their job to absorb excess oil and perspiration. The price is good, too.

☹ **Satin Lips Lip Balm** *($18 for 0.3 ounce)*. Your lips will thank you if you skip this menthol-laced balm in favor of plain Vaseline, which is the main ingredient in this pricey product.

☹ **Satin Lips Lip Mask** *($9.50 for 0.3 ounce)* isn't satiny in the least and lips don't need a clay mask with the kind of aggressive exfoliation this causes when massaged over the mouth. Furthermore, the menthol in here isn't the least bit helpful, and may make chapped lips worse.

MARY KAY SUN PRODUCTS

😊 **After-Sun Replenishing Gel** *($12 for 6.5 ounces)* is a lightweight, soothing gel that contains mostly water, slip agent, glycerin, silicone, green tea and other antioxidants, thickener, preservatives, fragrance, and coloring agents. It is recommended for normal to slightly dry skin, and the green tea may help skin repair itself to some extent from sun exposure—though it's far better to not let sun-exposed skin get to a point where a "repair" product is needed.

✓😊 **Lip Protector Sunscreen SPF 15** *($7.50 for 0.16 ounce)* combines an in-part zinc oxide sunscreen with petrolatum and other lip-smoothing emollients and antioxidant soybean oil along with vitamin E. This smart lip balm is a beautiful option for keeping lips smooth and protected year-round. The addition of yellow coloring agents helps offset the slight white cast from the zinc oxide, a thoughtful touch.

✓😊 **SPF 30 Sunscreen** *($14 for 4 ounces)* is a water-resistant sunscreen for normal to oily skin. It includes avobenzone for UVA protection and contains a nice selection of vitamin-based antioxidants (plus green tea) known to help skin defend itself better from sun exposure. This is an outstanding sunscreen formulation that's priced right; it does contain fragrance.

😊 **Sun Essentials Sunless Tanning Lotion** *($10 for 4.5 ounces)* is a standard self-tanning lotion for normal to dry skin. Dihydroxyacetone is what causes the color change, and this fragranced lotion leaves a moist finish.

MARY KAY MK SIGNATURE MAKEUP

FOUNDATION: 😊 **$$$ Creme-to-Powder Foundation** *($14 for foundation, $9 for refillable compact)* is smooth without feeling greasy or too thick, and provides medium coverage with an effect that's not too powdery or too creamy. This is more akin to traditional cream-to-powder foundation, which means it is best for normal to slightly oily skin without dry patches—which this foundation's finish exaggerates. Nine shades are available; among them, Ivory 2, Beige 2, Bronze 1, and Bronze 2 are best avoided due to overtones of rose or orange.

😊 **$$$ Dual Coverage Powder Foundation** *($14 for foundation, $9 for refillable compact, $4 for powder brush)* has the requisite smooth, dry texture that characterizes most pressed-powder foundations, but this talc-based formula goes on sheer and blends exceptionally well, leaving a satin finish. The nine shades aren't the most neutral around, but they're really too sheer to be problematic. Mary Kay has removed the noticeable shiny particles that used to mar this foundation.

☺ **Tinted Moisturizer with Suncreen SPF 20** *($18)* has a fluid, beautifully smooth texture that blends easily, providing sheer to light coverage and a satin matte finish. The in-part zinc oxide sunscreen makes this a smart choice for daytime use by those with normal to slightly dry or slightly oily skin. The six shades could have been more neutral (for a newer product the overtones of pink and peach are odd), but the good news is that this is sheer enough so that the lesser shades (which would be Beige 1 and Bronze 1) are still options should one of the other colors not work for you.

😐 **Full Coverage Foundation** *($14)* has a smooth, emollient formula that is suitable for those with normal to dry skin. It provides medium to full coverage and is relatively easy to blend, but it can look masklike on the skin, though the overall effect is more attractive than that of the Medium Coverage Foundation below. This is an option if you need significant coverage, but the tradeoff is a finish that makes skin look covered rather than enhanced. Twenty shades are offered, with options for very light to dark skin. The following shades are too pink, peach, or rose for most skin tones: Beige 304, Beige 404, Bronze 500, Bronze 507, and Bronze 607. Due to this makeup's high talc content, the darkest shade, Bronze 808, can look slightly ash, but this effect can be minimized by mixing the foundation with a dab of moisturizer.

☹ **Medium Coverage Foundation** *($14)* feels (and looks) like a giant step backward compared to the marvelous foundations from the Lauder companies, L'Oreal, Cover Girl, and many others. It is a fairly smooth liquid foundation, but it doesn't blend all that well and ends up having a dry, slightly chalky, flat finish that can look artificial and masklike on skin. Rather than floating over or merging with the skin, the pigments in this foundation tend to creep into every crevice, which magnifies dry areas and can make skin look tired and older than it is. Twenty shades are available; although most of them are just fine, the overall look of this foundation isn't one I'd encourage you to explore.

CONCEALER: ✓☺ **MK Signature Concealer** *($9.50)* comes in a squeeze tube and is very concentrated. This has an excellent, silicone-enhanced texture that blends without slip-sliding all over your face. It provides almost full coverage without looking thick or creasing, so it's a top choice if you have very dark circles. The six colors are fairly good, with the best ones being Light Ivory, Ivory, and Beige. The Yellow shade is too yellow for just about everyone.

😐 **$$$ MK Signature Facial Highlighting Pen** *($18)* is housed in a pen-style component with a built-in synthetic brush applicator. Although labeled a highlighter, its finish and coverage on skin are closer to that of a true concealer, as are the four shades. Among those, shades 1 and 3 have a peach cast that's tricky to soften. Estee Lauder's Ideal Light Brush-On Illuminator ($24.50) costs slightly more, but is an overall much better product if your goal is to highlight skin and reflect light to make shadowy areas brighter.

POWDER: ☺ **MK Signature Loose Powder** *($14)* is a talc-based powder with a soft, dry consistency and sheer finish. Five of the six colors are quite good—only Bronze 1 can be too peach for most skin tones.

😐 **$$$ MK Signature Bronze Highlighting Powder** *($16; $9 for refillable compact)* has a smooth, non-powdery texture and even application, but the result is shine to the extreme, which won't convince anyone you have a real tan. This is workable for evening makeup if shiny cheeks and temples are what you're after, but many other pressed bronzing powders have a better balance of pigment and shimmer (or you could go for a matte finish, but that's personal preference).

BLUSH: 😐 **$$$ MK Signature Cheek Color** *($10 for blush tablet, $8 for refillable compact)* has a smooth, dry texture and an application that begins sheer, but builds nicely for color that is more vibrant. However, many of the shades are quite sparkly, and that's too distracting for daytime wear. The only matte option is Desert Bloom. Several shades are dual-toned, meaning that half of the powder tablet is a lighter color and the other half is a darker color or tonally different. It's an interesting concept, but you're most likely to apply it as one color anyway, because a standard-size blush brush sweeps over both shades.

EYESHADOW: ☺ **MK Signature Eye Color** *($6.50 for each eyeshadow, $8–$16 for the various compacts)* is utterly silky, and these apply beautifully without flaking or streaking. They are pigment-rich, too, so it only takes a tiny amount to shape and shade the eye. Just keep in mind that the shine level is intense and, although that can be suitable for evening makeup, it's none too flattering if you have wrinkled or drooping eye-area skin. The ☺ **MK Signature Eye Color Duets** *($6.50; $8 for refillable compact)* share the same positive traits as the single MK Signature Eye Color above, with the caveat that almost all of the duos are dated, contrasting color combinations that do nothing to shape and shade the eye. If you're looking for this type of product and don't mind its shiny finish, the best couplings are Double Espresso and Onyx.

EYE AND BROW SHAPER: ☺ **MK Signature Eyeliner** *($9.50)* is an automatic, retractable pencil that has a smooth application, smear-proof finish, and a reasonable price. There are some attractive soft colors available along with classic brown and black. This requires an oil- or silicone-based makeup remover.

☺ **MK Signature Liquid Eyeliner** *($11)* has been improved and now sports a brush that's easier to control and a formula that dries faster and lasts. This liner is water-resistant as claimed, but note that if you swim with this and then rub your eye, it comes off immediately.

😐 **MK Signature Classic Blonde Brow Definer Pencil (wood)** *($8.50)* is a standard pencil that is a bit stiff yet has a long-lasting powder finish. The blonde shade is suitable for blonde eyebrows, and the color goes on sheer but builds if you need more intensity. 😐 **MK Signature Brow Definer Pencil** *($10)* is a standard brow pencil that needs routine sharpening, but if you're OK with that, the results are great, as is the soft powder finish. Application and color deposit are good, and in fact the shades themselves are impressive with options for blondes and redheads. This would get a happy face rating if sharpening wasn't a requirement.

LIPSTICK AND LIPLINER: ☺ **MK Signature Nourishine Lip Gloss** *($13)* isn't as impressive as the original MK Signature Lip Gloss, but this replacement formula offers colors that are much more sheer, while keeping the formula smooth (though it has become thicker and now finishes with a slight stickiness) and the shimmer intact. A few of the colors work well over any shade of lipstick.

☺ **MK Signature Creme Lipstick** *($13)* leans heavily toward the greasy side of creamy, and has a semi-opaque, soft gloss finish. The range of over 35 shades is nicely divided into Berries, Reds, Neutrals (which are not neutral at all—they are popular cool tones), Metals (which are largely unattractive), Pinks, Reds, and Chocolates. Note: This has a potent fragrance that some may find disagreeable. ☺ **MK Signature Lip Liner** *($10)* is recommended as a good, automatic, retractable lip pencil whose shade selection has been attractively expanded. The packaging is nicely color-coded, too, and this would be a Paula's Pick if it were more adept at keeping lipstick from feathering into lines around the mouth.

MASCARA: ☺ **MK Signature Ultimate Mascara** *($15)* doesn't reach the status of being worthy of its "ultimate" name, but it's nevertheless a good mascara that builds length and thickness quickly and in equal measure. Subsequent applications yield diminishing returns, which is why this isn't the one to choose if your objective is "ultimate" lashes. ☺ **MK Signature Lash**

Lengthening Mascara *($10)* does just what the name says, and accomplishes its task without clumping, flaking, or smearing. You won't notice any thickness, but if longer lashes are all you're after, this is one to try.

☺ **MK Signature Waterproof Mascara** *($10)* works just as most waterproof mascaras do, meaning it lengthens lashes, doesn't do much to thicken, yet holds up when lashes get wet. The average aspect of this mascara is that it takes longer than it should to provide any noticeable difference in your lashes.

BRUSHES: ☺ **MK Signature Brush Set** *($45)* includes five brushes in a well-constructed synthetic leather case that includes extra pouches so you can add more brushes in the future. The **Powder Brush** and **Blush Brush** are quite soft and appropriately dense, though the Blush Brush would work better if its head were larger. The **Eye Definer Brush** and **Eye Crease Brush** don't fare as well, but aren't terrible, while the dual-sided **Eyeliner/Eyebrow Brush** is practical and functional (though the Eyebrow Brush is a bit too stiff). It's an overall worthwhile brush set that is priced fairly for what you get.

☺ **Retractable Powder Brush** *($10)* is an OK powder brush option if you need a secondary choice to stash in your purse or overnight bag. It isn't elegant or as well-shaped as it could be for everyday use. ☺ **Round Powder Brush** *($4)* is a short, flat powder brush that fans out to apply powder over one section of the face at a time. This is one of those rare cosmetic instances where you really do get what you pay for, so keep your expectations low.

☹ **Cheek Color Brush** *($2.50)* is a compact-size blush brush similar to many pre-packaged powder-blush brushes. It's not recommended over a regular, full blush brush.

SPECIALTY PRODUCTS: ☺ **MK Signature Eye Primer** *($12)* is a slightly thick, water- and talc-based white cream meant to prevent eyeshadows from creasing or smudging. Despite the prominence of talc, this remains slightly moist and doesn't work as well for its intended purpose as a flesh-toned matte finish concealer. It's OK, but not suitable for anyone who has trouble getting eyeshadows to stay put.

MAX FACTOR (MAKEUP ONLY)

MAX FACTOR AT-A-GLANCE

Strengths: Colour Adapt Foundation; the Lipfinity products; some great mascaras; good powder eyeshadows; two fabulous lip glosses.

Weaknesses: Most of the foundations have dated formulas and terrible colors; bad concealer; OK pressed powder; average brushes; the sleek packaging update can't disguise the plethora of still-unimpressive products.

For more information about Max Factor, owned by Procter & Gamble, call (800) 526-8787 or visit www.maxfactor.com or www.Beautypedia.com.

MAKEUP REMOVER ☺ **Remover for Long Lasting Makeup** *($4.29 for 2 ounces)* is a very standard, mineral oil–based lotion that will definitely remove just about any makeup, but then so will plain, fragrance-free mineral oil, and for mere pennies.

FOUNDATION: ☺ **Colour Adapt Foundation** *($11.99)* is a unique, silicone-in-water foundation that contains what Max Factor refers to as Microscopic Color Adapt technology, which is basically a fancy way to say that the pigment particles have been micronized. The major claim made for this foundation is that it adjusts to 95% of a person's skin tone. Procter & Gamble

(Max Factor's owner) states that a "regular" foundation adapts only to 23% of a person's facial skin tones. (How they came to this conclusion is not revealed, but I'd love to know—no one in the company I talked to seemed to know either.) Regardless of how well this foundation adapts to your skin versus what those other brands can do, the point is that Colour Adapt proves itself to be a foundation that's worthy of its hype.

It's dispensed through a pump, and comes out somewhat thick and opaque. Yet once you apply it to skin it softens immediately and blends effortlessly. Few foundations feel so incredibly light and silky on the skin, and there is no question you will be amazed at how Colour Adapt conceals minor flaws without camouflaging your underlying skin tone. This makes for a matte finish that truly can be called natural.

Still, there are a couple of drawbacks. The tradeoff for such a remarkably natural-looking foundation is that more pronounced flaws are never really concealed enough, even when this foundation is layered. Of course, you can use a separate concealer to remedy this, but if you're used to a foundation providing adequate coverage for flaws such as red spots, dark under-eye circles, or sun-induced brown discolorations, this is not the foundation for you.

Those who aren't concerned about concealing, but instead want a smooth foundation to even their skin tone will be most pleased with Colour Adapt. It is also worth mentioning that it can crease on the eyelids if not set with powder, though if it's left alone on the face (meaning no powder), it does a better-than-average job of keeping skin shine-free, and it does not break up on the skin, as some silicone-based foundations can. It's an option for all but very dry skin.

Nine shades are available and, due to the pigment technology in this foundation, you may find you can wear more than one! For example, I purposely applied a shade that, in the bottle, was unquestionably too dark for me. Yet on my skin, it looked just a touch darker, having lightened as I blended, but that's due to the sheer coverage. Overall, the shades are suitable for light to medium-deep skin tones, though the middle shades can pull a bit toward the peachy gold side, a fact that is of little consequence due to Colour Adapt's finish and sheer-to-light coverage. Last, Cover Girl's less expensive TruBlend Foundation is identical to Colour Adapt in every respect, except that Cover Girl offers more shades.

😐 **Powdered Foundation** *($7.89)* feels light and silky, but its talc-based formula is too sheer to function as more than a standard pressed powder. It is fragrance-free, and although most of the colors appear too peach or pink, they apply softer and blend out well. I wouldn't choose this over pressed powders from L'Oreal, but it's not deserving of an unhappy face rating either.

☹ **Pan-Cake Water-Activated Foundation** *($6.99)* and **Pan-Stik Ultra-Creamy Makeup** *($6.99)* are both old-fashioned foundations dating to the 1920s, with textures that are too heavy, thick, or greasy. Even if you have very dry skin and want something really emollient, almost all of the colors for both products are unabashedly peach and pink.

☹ **Whipped Creme Fluid Makeup** *($6.59)* has also been around for years, and isn't as creamy as the name implies. The most offensive things about this liquid makeup are the embarrassingly bad colors (though the three Shimmering shades are OK) and its pervasive fragrance.

☹ **Lasting Performance Liquid Makeup** *($7.89)* claims it will wear for eight hours, but although its matte finish holds up well (especially if you have normal to oily skin) it tends to look too heavy and chalky on skin, not to mention settling readily into lines and large pores. Although Cream Beige and Rich Beige are too pink to consider, the other shades (including the misnamed Cool Bronze, which is very light) all suffer from the chalky appearance. Revlon's

ColorStay foundations are much better, and most have an SPF 15 rating, too, which means someone with oily skin doesn't have to layer products for sun protection.

☹ **Silk Perfection Liquid to Powder Foundation** *($6.69)* is another poor Max Factor foundation that has remained in the line for years. This old-fashioned cream-to-powder makeup is waxy, looks artificial on the skin, and comes in only one salvageable color, Light Champagne. Cream-to-powder foundation has made some great strides (check out the stellar options from Prescriptives, Clarins, and M.A.C.), making this effectively obsolete.

CONCEALER: ☹ **Erace Secret Cover Up** *($5)* hasn't been updated in years, and desperately needs to be. Its titanium dioxide–based formula goes on heavy and offers significant coverage at the expense of a heavy appearance and somewhat chalky finish.

POWDER: 😐 **Lasting Performance Loose Powder** *($7.99)* is hard to find, and although it's a decent, talc-based loose powder, it's not worth seeking out given the prevalence of other outstanding powders that are available.

BLUSH: ☺ **Natural Brush-On Satin Blush** *($5.79)* is a soft, exceedingly smooth blush that allows you to brush on sheer color that you can build to a deeper tone. The shade selection favors warm tones, and all of them have shine, though it's subtle except for Cinnamon. If you find a color you like, it's worth a try.

EYESHADOW: ☺ **MAXEye Shadows** *($4.69)* now come as trios in one compact, with no dividers between the colors. You get a light shade for lid color and highlighting along with two mid-tone shades for contouring. A deeper shade to line the eyes is not included, which is a shortcoming. The good news is the texture has improved and this applies smoothly, without flaking or skipping. The less exciting news is that the sheerness of each shade makes shading and shaping the eye difficult, but it's an option if you want a really subtle, and I mean really, really subtle, look. The best sets, all with some amount of shine, are Compass Rose, Toast to That, Cocoa Crazy, Connoisseur, Beach Brown, and Vintage Vixen. The other trios are too bright, bold, or contrasting, unless you want to use eyeshadow for shock value.

EYE AND BROW SHAPER: 😐 **MAXeye Liner** *($5.89)* is an automatic, retractable eye pencil whose many glitter-infused shades are tailor-made for the nightclub scene. There are a couple of traditional, non-shiny shades to consider, and it's an OK option for a creamy eyeliner that is mildly prone to smudging unless set with powder.

☹ **Linemaker Waterproof MAXeye Liner** *($5.49)* is a liquid liner with a thin, long, flexible brush that makes it tricky, but not impossible, to draw an even line. Things get messy because this takes too long to dry—and it is prone to chipping.

LIPSTICK, LIP GLOSS, AND LIPLINER: ✓☺ **Lipfinity** *($10.89)* started the long-lasting, two-step lip paint craze that has inspired dozens of imitators, some of whom have improved on Lipfinity. Both this product and Cover Girl's Outlast use PermaTone technology, a "revolutionary new color bond complex which provides semi-permanent color by gently attaching color pigments to lips in a 'flexible mesh' effect." The formula, researched and developed by Procter & Gamble, resists normal wear and will not come off while you are eating, drinking, or even kissing. Sign me up! This really is a breakthrough lipstick in terms of long and comfortable wear, though you need to remember a few important tips. Lipfinity consists of a lip gloss–like product that puts a layer of opaque color over the lips. and is accompanied by a top coat. The colored portion of the product is applied separately to the lips with a sponge-tip applicator and then the color needs about a minute or two to dry completely. Once dry, you can slick on the glossy top coat, and voilà—you get the long wear and coverage of an ultra-matte lipstick and the familiar feel of a traditional creamy lipstick.

Along with the pros, there are some considerable cons to keep in mind before trying Lipfinity or any of its imitators. First, application of the "paint" layer can be tricky. The color goes on thick and opaque and must be smoothed out immediately or you will be left with an uneven layer. Application needs to be almost perfect, because any irregularity can quickly turn into a permanent mistake, though mistakes and the entire lip color can be removed with pure mineral oil or plain Vaseline. Finally, your lips must be absolutely clean, smooth (any flaking, no matter how minor, will be greatly exaggerated), and dry before you use this.

The moisturizing top coat does indeed make this feel great, and for the most part the color stays on and stays true, even through meals (as long as they aren't greasy or oily meals). You may notice some color fading toward the inner part of the lips, but you weren't expecting perfection were you? Note that the color swatch on the box (and the product itself) does not provide an accurate indication of what the color will actually look like once applied. Although you should not need to touch up the color for most of the day (really!), the top coat does need to be reapplied at regular intervals to avoid dry lips.

The **Lipfinity Moisturizing Top Coat** *($5.99)* is also sold separately, which is convenient, as you will likely go through this long before the partnered lip color is gone. For a touch of pizzazz, you may want to consider the glistening **Lipfinity Top Coat Shimmer Finish** *($6.39)*. ✓☺ **Lipfinity EverLites** *($10.29)* share the same long-wearing, semi-permanent color technology as the original Lipfinity formula, but EverLites offer a collection of softer, more sheer shades. As wonderful as the original Lipfinity is, many women felt that the shades were too intense or opaque. Lipfinity Everlites solve that complaint with colors that last as long as the original Lipfinity, but without the intensity. The only compromise is that the EverLites shades do not last quite as long due to the decreased amount and finer texture of the pigments. It still goes the distance when it comes to long wear without chipping or peeling, but the original Lipfinity remains the one to use when you want to get as close to all-day wear as possible. Given that most women prefer softer lip colors, I don't imagine slightly decreased wear time will be a deal-breaker here, especially since the palette of EverLites shades is beautiful.

✓☺ **Colour Perfection Luxe Gloss** *($5.89)* is a renamed version of Max Factor's former Colour Perfection Gloss. With the exception of a few deeper colors, it remains the same. The cake frosting–smooth texture doesn't feel the least bit goopy or sticky, while the shimmer-to-metallic finish puts the spotlight on lips. The Ibizia Ice shade is clear and without shimmer. This is a surprisingly well-done product! ✓☺ **Maxalicious Glaze** *($5.99)* is a very good tube lip gloss available in two sets of shade. The Nice range of shades includes softer pinks and sheer nude tones, all with innocent-sounding names such as Falling in Love and First Kiss. The Naughty range pumps up the color (though most are still on the sheer side) and includes suggestive shade names such as Too Much Wine. Each has a beautifully smooth texture and shimmer-infused gloss finish that isn't the least bit sticky.

☺ **Lipfinity Lustre** *($10.89)* is identical to Max Factor's original Lipfinity, and the same comments apply—it's an amazing product (once you master the application) for truly long-wearing lipstick. This new version adds shades with considerably more iridescence than the other Lipfinity colors, but they suffer from feeling a bit grainy if you're not diligent about applying the shimmer-infused top coat.

☺ **Colour Perfection Lipstick** *($7.19)* is promoted as a unique creamy lipstick because the network of "micro-layers" within its gel-based formula are said to contain micronized pigments in multiple layers. The idea is that as each layer of lipstick wears off, a new layer of color takes its place. So you get hour after hour of color that looks as if it's just been applied. As interesting as it sounds, you won't find this happening when you wear this lipstick. This is merely a good, lightweight creamy lipstick that comes in many enticing colors (including some gorgeous reds), but the described technology doesn't play out in reality. This lipstick wore about the same as most creamy lipsticks, meaning I needed a touch-up after a couple of hours. It came off on coffee cups, and missing a touch-up meant uneven wear. Despite the claims, it isn't any different from most cream lipsticks.

☺ **Max Wear Lipcolor** *($8.79)* is meant to be a Lipfinity-like long-wearing lip gloss. The dual-sided wand features a sheer lip color (the shades look bright and bold but go on softer than they appear) and a coordinating gloss top coat. Once the liquid lipcolor has had a couple of minutes to set, you slick on the gloss. Different in feel from the stick-type top coat that accompanies Lipfinity (and Cover Girl's Outlast), the gloss top coat has a thicker texture and sparkling finish. It lingers longer than the stick-type top coat, but the color beneath doesn't have the surprising longevity of Lipfinity. Still, it lasts longer than traditional lipstick and even makes it through a light meal (meaning nothing too oily) without fading. Once again, Cover Girl's competing, almost identical product (Outlast Double LipShine) costs less and offers more approachable shades, though the accompanying top coat is colorless.

😐 **High Definition Lip Liner** *($5.29)* is a very standard, creamy lip pencil that needs routine sharpening and comes in a limited range of colors, most of which are surprisingly dark. Not bad, but not great.

MASCARA: ✓☺ **Lash Perfection Mascara Waterproof** *($6.99)* wins high marks for being an overall excellent mascara if your goal is equal parts length and thickness without results that are too excessive. If your mascara mantra is "longer, thicker, drama ..." well, this doesn't impress to that extent. But it is waterproof, shows its stuff quickly without clumps, and wears all day without a hitch.

✓☺ **Volume Couture Mascara** *($6.99)* requires a bit more patience than usual during application, but the rewards are great. You will be impressed with how well the spiky, rubber-bristled brush separates lashes while building very good length, moderate thickness, and curl. Clumping is barely an issue, and when it occurs the brush allows nimble comb-through for a clean result. Although there are more dramatic mascaras available (such as L'Oreal Volume Shocking), this is definitely a top choice and it too wears without a hitch.

☺ **Volume Couture Waterproof Mascara** *($6.99)* has the same brush as the original Volume Couture Mascara above, and although that's great, the formula itself isn't as outstanding, though it is definitlely waterproof. Application is surprisingly uneven in terms of how much mascara is deposited. Clumps aren't an issue, but you will need a lash brush or comb to ensure a smooth, defined outcome. This is still recommended if you need a good lengthening waterproof mascara that doesn't smear of flake.

☺ **Lash Perfection Mascara** *($7.80)* is excellent unless your main goal is to create dramatically thick lashes. The rubber-bristled brush coats your lashes evenly without clumps while allowing you to make them long, slightly thick, and softly fringed.

☺ **2000 Calorie Straight Brush Mascara** *($5.95)* doesn't provide as much thickness as it used to, at least not compared to the best thickening mascaras from L'Oreal and Maybelline. It's still worth considering but performs best as a lengthening mascara. The Deep Auburn color is excellent for redheads! ☺ **2000 Calorie Curved Brush Mascara** *($5.95)* adds more oomph to lashes than the Straight Brush version above because the curvature of the brush deposits slightly more mascara at the base of the lashes. You'll get more length than thickness, but this shows its stuff quickly, wears well, and leaves lashes with a soft, fringed curl.

☺ **Lash Lift Waterproof Mascara** *($6.19)* produces beautifully elongated lashes with effort, and is very waterproof yet not any more difficult to remove than most waterproof mascaras. This would rate a Paula's Pick if it didn't take so long to apply. ☺ **2000 Calorie Aqua Lash Mascara** *($5.96)* performs similarly to the non-waterproof versions of 2000 Calorie Mascara above, except this stays on through swims and rainy days. You'll get longer lashes with Max Factor's Lash Lift Waterproof Mascara, but more thickness with this one. ☺ **Lash Enhancer Mascara** *($5.69)* is meant to enhance lashes for a natural look, and it does just that. This quickly darkens and separates lashes while building modest length and no thickness. Clumping, flaking, and smearing are not an issue, and this comes off easily with a water-soluble cleanser.

😐 **Lash Lift Mascara** *($6.19)* is billed as a lightweight mascara, which it is, but that's about its only trick. The slightly dry, uneven application must be combed through to look presentable, and lengthening is marginal, albeit noticeable. 😐 **Stretch & Separate Waterproof Mascara** *($6.19)* separates lashes but with little fanfare. It's an OK option for a minimalist lash look that is indeed waterproof yet not inordinately difficult to remove. 😐 **No Color Mascara** *($5.51)* is a very standard clear mascara that offers minimal lash enhancement and actually works better as a brow gel. This formula is identical to Cover Girl's Professional Natural Lash Mascara, which sells for slightly less money.

☹ **Stretch & Separate Mascara** *($6.19)* will separate lashes, but it stunts more than stretches and tends to apply unevenly. This doesn't do much to impress, and isn't worth considering.

BRUSHES: The stubby-handled 😐 **Blush Brush** *($4.09)* splays a bit and isn't all that soft, but it's an inexpensive option if you need a blush brush for travel or want something portable to apply loose or pressed powder. The 😐 **MAXeye Shadow Brush** *($4.69)* features a synthetic, slightly tapered shadow brush on one end and a sponge-tip applicator on the other, making this only 50% useful.

MAYBELLINE NEW YORK (MAKEUP ONLY)

MAYBELLINE NEW YORK AT-A-GLANCE

Strengths: The line earned Paula's Pick ratings for products in almost every category; many excellent foundations; superior mascaras; inexpensive makeup brushes; some terrific concealers, powders, blush, eyeshadow, eyeliner, lipstick, and bronzer options.

Weaknesses: The makeup removers; the foundations with sunscreen lack the right UVA-protecting ingredients; disappointing lipliners; average lip gloss; the loose powder eyeshadow; Great Lash mascaras.

For more information about Maybelline, owned by L'Oreal, call (800) 944-0730 or visit their www.maybelline.com or www.Beautypedia.com.

MAKEUP REMOVER ☺ **Expert Eyes Eye Makeup Remover Towelettes** *($6.49 for 50 wipes)* are small cloths packaged in a resealable pouch. The simple, gentle formula works well to remove makeup unless the formula is long-wearing or waterproof, in which case too much "elbow grease" is needed, and that's not great for skin around the eyes. The tiny amount of lavender extract is not cause for concern. ☺ **Superaway Lipcolor Remover** *($4.99)* is a tube of makeup remover with an angled tip that's meant to take off long-wearing lip color, either from Maybelline or any other company. The silicone-enriched formula feels silky and, as long as you let it sit on lips for a moment after application, it works great to remove tenacious color while leaving a smooth finish.

😐 **Expert Touch Moisturizing Mascara Remover** *($4.49 for 2.3 ounces)* is an incredibly simple concoction of mineral oil, emollient thickener, lanolin oil, and preservative. This greasy liquid will indeed remove mascara and most other makeup as well—but the greasy film it leaves behind is not something most women would want to put up with.

☹ **Expert Eyes 100% Oil-Free Eye Makeup Remover** *($4.49 for 2.3 ounces)* is an antiquated eye-makeup remover with too much boric acid and isopropyl alcohol to use it around the eyes. It is not recommended.

FOUNDATION: Maybelline's shade palette for foundations tends to have the most neutral, workable options at the lightest and darkest end of the spectrum. For some reason, their medium shades are more often than not noticeably peach or peachy pink, which definitely leaves a large group of consumers under-served. Sister company L'Oreal's foundation range (as well as competitor Revlon) are much more reliable for someone with a medium skin tone.

☺ **Pure Makeup** *($5.99)* is a simply formulated, lightweight liquid foundation that smooths beautifully over skin and sets to a soft matte finish. The level of coverage is light but can be built up to medium if needed. The formula and finish are ideal for someone with normal to oily skin. Twelve shades are available; the lightest and darkest hues are the best options. Among the mid-tones, Light 3 and Medium 2 are slightly peach; Light 5, Medium 3, and Medium 4 are strongly peach; and Dark 1 is too rosy. By the way, despite the "won't clog pores" claim, this foundation contains enough titanium dioxide so that this is not a worry-free choice for the blemish-prone.

☺ **Dream Matte Mousse Foundation** *($8.79)* has a smooth, whipped texture that feels wonderfully light on the skin and blends impeccably, setting to a slightly powdery matte finish. Coverage can go from sheer to medium, and this foundation layers well for additional coverage without a heavy or caked appearance. The nonaqueous silicone formula's main drawback is that it exaggerates any degree of dry skin. Therefore, either exfoliate your skin before using it or make sure your skin is prepped by applying a moisturizing sunscreen. Of course, applying a moisturizer negates this matte makeup's benefit for oily skin, but someone with very oily skin (who is unlikely to have any dry patches) can skip this step. Twelve shades are available, with options for light and dark (but not very dark) skin tones. The only shades to steer clear of due to strong overtones of pink or peach are Creamy Natural, Pure Beige, Medium Beige, and Tan. Porcelain Ivory is a good shade for fair skin tones, while Cocoa is a deep brown shade that doesn't turn ashy on skin, always a plus! Classic Ivory may be too peach for some light skin tones. This foundation is remarkably similar to Lancome's Magique Matte Soft-Matte Perfecting Mousse Makeup ($37).

😐 **Superstay Silky Foundation SPF 12** *($10.99)* is a two-part foundation that combines a primer and foundation with a pure titanium dioxide sunscreen and a too-low (but not terrible) SPF rating (SPF 15 would have been best). The first time you use this, the primer is dispensed before the foundation, which is wasteful. But when the foundation joins the primer (each is packaged in its own chamber, visible through the plastic component) they mesh together well—until you notice the colors. Almost all of them are noticeably pink, peach, orange, rose, or copper. What you see in the bottle is very close to what you get on your skin once this foundation sets to its silky matte finish. It has a very good lightweight texture that allows plenty of time to blend, and the finish holds up quite well, providing medium coverage and a slightly too-opaque look. But among the 12 colors, the only recommended shades are Light 2, Light 4, and Medium 1—and even these aren't as stellar as what you'll find at L'Oreal.

☹ **Instant Age Rewind Foundation SPF 18** *($7.39)* has a great name! Maybelline even included the classic VCR "rewind" symbol as part of this product's logo. But clever names and logos don't relate to fact: no one's skin will be any firmer or "look younger instantly" with this water- and silicone-based foundation. And any age-rewinding credibility this foundation hoped to have is lost in advance because its sunscreen does not provide sufficient UVA protection. That lack of protection is disappointing, because this foundation's texture and application are beautiful. It provides medium coverage and sets to a smooth matte finish that is laced with shiny particles. The shine isn't as subtle as that of similar products from Revlon or M.A.C., so consider this factor carefully. The selection of 12 shades includes some excellent options for fair to light and tan to dark skin tones, including Porcelain Ivory, Classic Ivory, Tan, Caramel, and Cocoa. Those with medium skin tones will be disappointed, however, because those shades (Creamy Natural, Honey Beige, Sandy Beige, and Pure Beige) all lean toward or are blatantly peach. In summary, this foundation has more pros than cons, but is an option for normal to slightly dry or slightly oily skin if you're willing to pair it with a sunscreen that provides better UVA protection.

☹ **Instant Age Rewind Cream Foundation SPF 18** *($8.99)* is remarkably similar to the original Instant Age Rewind Foundation above, right down to its insufficient amount of UVA protection. This has a slightly thicker texture and slightly moist finish, but isn't what most people (especially those with dry skin) would consider creamy. This version also has the same noticeable sparkles as its predecessor, and they're very obvious in daylight. Among the 12 mostly good shades, the problematic colors include Medium Beige, Creamy Natural, and Honey Beige. This foundation is best for normal to slightly dry skin and must be paired with a sunscreen that provides sufficient UVA protection.

☹ **PureStay Powder Plus Foundation SPF 15** *($8.69)* is a talc-based pressed powder with slightly heavier coverage so it can double as a foundation. It has a superior, smooth texture, an even application, and a soft matte finish that can go from sheer to medium coverage. What a shame the sunscreen lacks significant UVA-protecting ingredients! Still, if you're already using a well-formulated sunscreen rated SPF 15 or higher, this is worth considering by those with normal to very oily skin. Most of the eight shades are excellent neutrals; the ones to avoid due to pink or peach overtones are Soft Cameo, Golden, and Sand.

CONCEALER: ✓☺ Instant Age Rewind Under Eye Concealer *($5.39)* is a superb matte-finish concealer that provides substantial coverage without creasing, caking, or making skin look dry and pasty. It blends well and has enough slip so that mistakes (including over-applying) are easy to soften or buff away. There are five shades; the best options are Fair, Light, and Medium. Dark is strongly peach and not recommended, while Yellow is suitable only if you have prominent dark circles.

✓☺ Instant Age Rewind Double Face Perfector *($8.99)* provides a liquid concealer and coordinated highlighter in one sleek, dual-sided package. The concealer has a supremely lightweight texture that is easy to apply, but blending must be quick because it sets to a crease-less matte finish in short order. Coverage-wise, this really excels. It's meant to camouflage "adult imperfections" such as discolorations from the sun or broken capillaries, and does so without calling attention to itself. The highlighter has a thinner texture, more slip (so you have more time to blend), and offers a sheer finish with a hint of shine. It is ideal for highlighting small areas and may be used around the eyes. Among the four shade duos, only Medium falls short because it's borderline peach. This remarkable duo is otherwise highly recommended.

😐 **True Illusion Undetectable Concealer SPF 10** *($5.39)* has no UVA-protecting ingredients and the SPF 10 is too low for all-day protection, so it is unreliable for sunscreen; but it is a very good concealer with a smooth texture and a semi-opaque, natural matte finish. It blends easily and does not crease. True Ivory and True Beige are both great options for light skin tones.

😐 **Pure.Concealer** *($4.99)* is an automatic, nonretractable pencil concealer, the type that makes pinpoint application to red spots and blemishes a cinch. The silicone-based formula applies smoothly and provides sufficient, non-cakey coverage, but it does contain waxes and waxlike ingredients that aren't the best for routine use on blemishes. This contains 2% salicylic acid (BHA), but a pH cannot be established in a waterless medium, so there's no way the BHA will exfoliate. Pure.Concealer comes in three very good shades (for light to medium skin) and is an option to spot-conceal redness or minor discolorations. Benefit's Galactic Shield! ($18), however, remains the preferred pencil-type concealer for use over blemishes because it contains fewer waxlike ingredients.

☹ **Coverstick Corrector Concealer** *($5.49)* is a dated, oil- and wax-based formula that is too greasy to stay put for long, and it creases easily. It also tends to look too thick and heavy on skin, even when blended thoroughly. Maybelline claims this is their #1-selling concealer, and while that may be true in volume, it is not so in performance, especially when compared to their other concealers.

POWDER: ✓ ☺ **Finish Matte Pressed Powder** *($5.59)* is an exceptional talc-based powder with two beautiful colors and a silky, even texture. It does contain a tiny bit of mineral oil, but not enough for your skin to notice one way or another. This is best for normal to slightly dry skin that is fair to light. Avoid Medium Beige, which is too peach.

✓ ☺ **Dream Matte Face Powder** *($7.99)* has a silky-smooth yet dry texture, allowing it to make good on its claim of providing an air-soft matte finish. It is a very good pressed powder for normal to very oily skin. Application is sheer, and applying more doesn't lend a thick, powdery look (though it can make skin look dull, so do use some restraint). Eight shades are available, all of which are beautiful, including options for very fair to tan skin tones. Well done!

☺ **Shine Free Oil-Control Loose Powder** *($5.49)* is a talc- and clay (kaolin)–based powder that comes in two translucent colors and has a soft texture and sheer matte finish. It isn't quite as elegant as L'Oreal's Translucide Naturally Luminous Powder ($10.59), but for half the price you may not mind! This powder is suitable for normal to very oily skin. ☺ **Shine Free Translucent Pressed Powder** *($5.49)* can't control shine any more than most powders, but it is a suitably soft, dry-finish powder that applies smooth and sheer and is indeed oil-free. The talc-based formula is available in four colors. Natural Beige 04 is too pink, especially for those battling excess oil, but the other three shades are fine.

☹ **Pure.Powder** *($6.25)* feels silky, but tends to roll and ball up in the compact, which negatively impacts application, although once you get it on, it has a very sheer finish, imparting minimal color. Nothing about it will make skin look blemish-free. In fact, if you're using this to conceal blemishes, you'll be disappointed. I'm not quite sure who this powder would work best for because its limitations mean it isn't worthy of any sort of recommendation, and certainly not when so many exceptional pressed powders are available, including those from L'Oreal and Cover Girl.

BLUSH: ✓☺ **Dream Mousse Blush** *($6.99)* is accurately described as "air-whipped." It has a soft, spongy texture that gives way to a superior application for what's essentially a modified cream-to-powder blush. Each shimmer-infused shade blends on soft and sheers out quickly, so you can experiment without imparting too much color. Those who want to add more color will find this product layers well. Even better, this really stays in place after it sets, and you'll experience only minimal fading. It is a fun yet functional departure from powder blush, and is best for normal to slightly dry or slightly oily skin (provided you don't mind having shiny cheeks). You will find this identical to Lancome's pricier Magique Blush Soft-Radiant Mousse Blush ($28.50).

✓☺ **Dream Mousse Bronzer** *($6.99)* has the same formula and thus deserves the same accolades as the Dream Mousse Blush above, only here you get two shiny bronze tones. Glistening Sun is preferred for fair to light skin, while Sun Glow is ideal for medium skin tones. This is one to try if you don't mind a tan with noticeable shine.

😐 **Expertwear Blush** *($5.29)* doesn't deserve its silky-smooth description because this pressed-powder blush is a bit too dry and thus tends to apply a bit unevenly. The less-than-ideal application isn't a deal-breaker because each shine-infused shade goes on sheer, but I wouldn't choose this over L'Oreal's True Match Super-Blendable Blush ($8.99). Maybelline's shade selection does not offer deeper hues for women of color.

😐 **Expertwear Blush Duo** *($5.29)* has the same formula and application issues as the Expertwear Blush above, but here you get a slightly shiny powder blush paired with a shinier highlighting powder. The Two to Glow duo is an option as a bronzing powder for someone with fair skin. 😐 **Expertwear Blush Bronzer** *($5.29)* also has the same formula as the Expertwear Blush above, except that the two shades are meant to be used as bronzing powder. The Salsa Sun shade is matte and can work as a bronzer or for contouring.

EYESHADOW: ☺ **Expertwear Eye Shadow** *($3.49 singles; $4.39 duos; $4.99 trios; $5.79 quads)* is a notable improvement over previous versions of Maybelline powder eyeshadows, though it doesn't surpass the top picks in this category. What's missing from these shadows is that lush, almost suede-like smoothness and impeccable blending found in superior options. Expertwear Eye Shadow does have a nice silkiness, but also has a waxy feel that prevents smooth, even blending. Pigmentation has improved, as have these eyeshadows' ability to cling to skin. You won't get as much color payoff as you will with eyeshadows from M.A.C. or Stila, but the sheerness is bound to please those looking for softer eyeshadow shades.

There appear to be some matte options among the singles, but closer inspection reveals that even these have some shine, so avoid them if matte is your goal. The almost-matte single shades include Vanilla, Earthly Taupe, Champagne Fizz, and Creme de Cocoa. All of the duos have a soft shine, but if that doesn't bother you, the best pairings are Indian Summer, Browntones, and Grey Matters. Two of the three shades in each trio set are shiny, but again, there are some attractive combinations, including Almond Truffles, Chocolate Mousse, and Impeccable Greys.

Among the quads, most sets have at least one matte shade, and at least one shade is suitable for use as powder eyeliner. The most workable quads include Mocha Motion, Designer Chocolates, Sunlit Bronze, and Time for Wine. ☺ **Expert Eyes Designer Selections Shadow** *($7.39)* provides eight powder eyeshadows in one compact, though you get just a small amount of each. Four of the shades are matte and four are shiny. These apply and feel just like Maybelline's Expertwear Eye Shadow above, which means they're good but not great. If you decide to try this, the best set is Sunbaked Neutrals.

☺ **Dream Mousse Shadow** *($6.50)* continues Maybelline's mousse makeup theme with eyeshadows. Each shade of this soft-touch mousse is infused with shine, though if it's applied sheerly it can appear rather subtle. The formula applies well, with enough slip to blend where you want it, but not so much that it travels where you don't want it. It also wears well, without flaking or creasing. Although you can achieve the same effect from a standard, powder-based eyeshadow, this is a novel approach that, with practice, is almost as easy to use. Unless you're going for a retro-look, avoid Mint Dream and Blue Heaven, and use caution with the pinks and lavenders. The limited shade selection keeps this product from earning a Paula's Pick rating.

☺ **Cool Effect Cooling Shadow/Liner** *($5.69)* feels cool due to the water and glycol base, and although this glides on easily, it sets quickly. That means using any of the shine-infused shades as eyeshadow or highlighter (there are lots of pale colors) requires quick, precise blending. You'll find that as eyeliner these last all day without smearing, though the amount of shine is too strong for someone with wrinkled or drooping eyelids. The following shades are either too contrasting or odd for an attractive eye makeup design: Cool as a Cucumber, Frosty Pink, Sugar Plum Ice, and Midnight Chill.

☹ **Shadow Stylist Loose Powder** *($6.49)* is packaged like the inkwell-style liquid eyeliners, but this is loose powder eyeshadow that's applied with a synthetic, pointed sponge tip. Although the powder's texture is smooth and blendable, the application method causes way too much flaking, even if you dab off excess product. Given that the results are comparable to what you can achieve with a powder eyeshadow that doesn't flake, there is no reason to consider this.

EYE AND BROW SHAPER: ✓☺ **Expertwear Defining Liner** *($5.79)* used to go by the name Expert Eyes Defining Liner, and it remains a great automatic, retractable eye pencil whose dry finish isn't as smudge-prone as most eye pencils, though it's not quite as worry-free as lining with a matte powder eyeshadow. It's definitely worth a look for pencil lovers, and the smudge-tip concealer has a built-in sharpener for those desiring a finer point.

✓☺ **Unstoppable Smudge-Proof Waterproof Eyeliner** *($6.59)* is an automatic, retractable pencil that applies swiftly without skipping and really doesn't smudge, even with provocation. It's waterproof, too, yet removes easily. The only drawback is its slightly tacky finish. That's a minor issue for such an outstanding pencil, and with the exception of Jade, the color selection is reliable.

✓☺ **Line Stylist Eyeliner** *($6.95)* is another excellent automatic pencil, though this one isn't retractable. However, the wind-up is calibrated, so there's little chance you'll break the pencil tip. The tip allows you to draw a thin or thicker line, and application is smooth and even. Once set, this feels powdery and stays in place all day. Most of the shades have shimmer or sparkle, but those looking for classic colors will appreciate Onyx and Espresso. Note: This tenacious product is difficult to take off without an oil- or silicone-based remover.

☺ **Define-A-Line Eye Liner** *($5.55)* is supposed to glide on smoothly, and it does. This automatic, retractable pencil needs no sharpening, but includes a built-in sharpener (housed under the sponge-tip smudger) if you desire a finer point. Because this pencil's finish is quite smudge-prone on its own, it is best for creating a smoky eye effect. The shade range offers several variations on brown along with gray and black. Khaki Green is an intriguing departure: a shiny golden olive that can look alluring blended with (or over) a black or deep brown eyeliner (or powder eyeshadow).

☺ **Brow Styling Gel** *($5.69)* is a standard brow gel that is very easy to apply and feels light and non-sticky. There are two sheer colors, which would work for dark blondes and brunettes, as well as a clear shade for just holding unruly brows in place. It's a good, inexpensive option if you're looking to tame your brows or add a soft sheen.

☺ **Expertwear Brow and Eyeliner** *($5.79)* is an automatic, retractable pencil that can be sharpened to a finer tip than most (the sharpener is built into the pencil). This pencil has a dry texture, which means less smudging. The sheer application and drier finish is well-suited to brows.

☺ **Ultra Liner Waterproof Eyeliner** *($5.89)* is a liquid liner with a brush that only allows you to draw an intense, thick line. It takes a bit longer to dry than it should, but once it does it won't move, even under water. If you're going swimming and want thickly lined, dramatic eyes, here's your solution! ☺ **Waterproof Liquid Eyeliner** *($6.59)* has a finer tip and thus allows for a more versatile application (you can easily go from thin to thick) than the Ultra Liner Waterproof Eyeliner above. Another plus is that this formula dries almost instantly, which reduces the chance of smearing. It stays on well, too, and is waterproof. The only issue is that it tends to apply unevenly, so you have to smooth out the line before it sets. It would otherwise be rated a Paula's Pick.

☺ **Ultra Brow Brush-On Brow Color** *($5.69)* is a standard, matte brow powder that comes packaged with the standard hard brush that you should toss away and replace with a good soft professional brush. There are two shades, which is limited to say the least, but what's available works if it matches your brow color.

😐 **Expert Eye Twin Brow and Eye Pencil** *($3.99)* has been part of the Maybelline line for decades, and it's still a standard small pencil whose dry, stiff texture is somewhat workable for brows. However, it would still net you a dated look, and you don't want to use this for eye-lining because it is so dry, it would actually hurt as you tried to move it along the skin. There are ample colors for all brow colors, from blonde to black, and the dry finish really stays put. If you don't mind sharpening and you prefer pencil to powder, this is one to consider. 😐 **Expertwear Softlining Pencil** *($4.29)* is a standard "sharpen me again" pencil that goes on creamy but doesn't smudge or smear as readily as it once did. It isn't exceptional, but is worth considering if you don't mind routine sharpening.

LIPSTICK, LIP GLOSS, AND LIPLINER: ✓☺ **Superstay Lipcolor** *($9.99)* brings us another Lipfinity imitator, though I must admit that a few of these "me-too" products have wound up performing better (at least in one aspect or other) than the originator. Superstay Lipcolor is one such example: It bests Lipfinity by the way it wears more evenly. The now-familiar two-step application process involves applying the color coat, then waiting two minutes for it to set (it feels very sticky as it dries, unlike most of the other long-wearing lip paints out there). Next you apply a glossy top coat to ensure a shiny finish and, more important, comfortable wear. Whereas Lipfinity, like Cover Girl's identical Outlast Lipcolor, tends to wear off at the inner portion of the lips, Superstay Lipcolor stays and stays. There's just one caveat: This is not a liquid lipstick that makes it through a meal, although it's fine with just drinks. This is partially because Maybelline's shade range is so soft. Most of the colors, even those that appear intense, apply sheer, and layering doesn't build significantly more color. Removing this product requires mineral oil, Vaseline, or an oil-based cleanser. The top coat is in stick form, and feels similar to the top coats that accompany Lipfinity and Outlast. Although I disagree with Maybelline's claim that Superstay Lipcolor lasts 16 hours (only if you hold perfectly still, don't talk, and don't eat anything), it is another terrific alternative to traditional lipstick. Maybelline also deserves kudos for packaging the two steps in one component, similar to what M.A.C. and Estee Lauder have done with their competing products.

☺ **Superstay Gloss** *($9.99)* claims to deliver "double-duty beauty" because one end is a sheer liquid lip color and the other is a clear, patent leather–shiny gloss. This Max Factor Lipfinity–like product is applied in two steps. You paint on the lip color, let it dry for two minutes, then brush on the thick, clear gloss. This is an option if you're looking for long-wearing sheer colors and want a super glossy finish; however, it is not preferred to Maybelline's original Superstay Lipcolor above because the Gloss version's top coat is sticky and doesn't do a great job of making the liquid lip color increasingly comfortable. Great colors, though, including "your lips, but better" shades. Wear time is definitely longer than a traditional gloss, which is the main reason to consider this product.

☺ **Shine Seduction Glossy Lipcolor** *($6.99)* takes a standard sheer lip gloss and packages it in a sleek tube with a click-dial that feeds product onto an angled applicator. The high-shine gloss has a moderately thick texture and a wet, slightly sticky finish with fair tenacity. Seduction-wise, this is easily kissed off, but it will look alluring, and that may be all it takes!

😐 **Moisture Extreme Lipcolor SPF 15** *($6.49)* provides lips with lots of emollient moisture, but disappoints with a sunscreen that fails to deliver sufficient UVA protection. This creamy-bordering-on-greasy lipstick feels almost like a slick balm when applied to lips, and leaves a glossy finish. The shade selection is plentiful (almost 40 colors), but none has much staying power, especially if you're prone to lipstick feathering into lines around the mouth. 😐 **Lip Polish Hi-Shine Color** *($5.59)* provides a somewhat creamy, but also powdery, texture that spreads sheer, colored glitter over the lips. It isn't as greasy or messy as some glosses, but it also isn't as smooth—it just has lots of sparkle.

😐 **Moisture Extreme Lipliner** *($5.59)* needs sharpening and is creamy enough to be worthy of its name. The application is ultra-smooth, but the downside is this pencil is too creamy to last as long as many others, and it puts up little resistance when your lipstick starts migrating into lines around the mouth. 😐 **Line Stylist Lip Liner** *($6.49)* is an automatic, very thin–tipped, nonretractable lip pencil with a smooth but dry application that goes on a bit unevenly. It finishes dry rather than creamy, and although that helps it last longer, the shades are pigment-shy and tend to fade sooner than they should. There are better lip pencils at the drugstore from L'Oreal, Cover Girl, and others.

☹ **Shiny-Licious** *($5.69)* has a smooth application and a glossy finish that isn't too slick or slippery, but the formula has mint in it, as evidenced by the tingling feel after it's applied. There is little question that this gloss irritates lips, making it not worth choosing over dozens and dozens of others that don't have this problem.

MASCARA: ✓☺ **Full 'n Soft Mascara** *($6.79)* ranks as Maybelline's best mascara for those desiring equal parts impressive length and thickness. The balanced application sweeps on without clumps, separates lashes evenly, and wears all day. Marvelous!

✓☺ **Lash Discovery Mascara** *($6.79)* has a very small brush that initially made me skeptical. Yet this tiny, short-bristled brush let me be adept not only at getting to each and every lash, but also at expertly lengthening, separating, and providing appreciable thickness without clumping or smearing. ✓☺ **Lash Discovery Waterproof Mascara** *($6.79)* lacks the noticeable thickness of its non-waterproof counterpart, but this is otherwise an extraordinary mascara that lifts, lengthens, and leaves lashes with a soft, fringed curl. It's also waterproof and the tiny brush makes application to the lower lashes a cinch.

✓☺ **Sky High Curves Extreme Length and Curl Mascara** *($6.79)* almost lives up to its lofty name. This is a thoroughly impressive mascara! The easy-to-wield brush allows for ample (not extreme) lengthening and almost instant, high-impact thickness that just keeps getting better the longer you apply it. Perhaps the best news is that for all this lash-building, clumping is barely a problem.

✓☺ **Sky High Curves Extreme Length and Curl Mascara Waterproof** *($6.79)* isn't much for creating curled lashes, but wow, does this make lashes incredibly long, and quickly, too! The smearproof formula holds up beautifully to water exposure, yet isn't overly difficult to remove. It is one of the better lengthening waterproof mascaras at the drugstore.

✓☺ **Volum' Express Mascara 3X** *($6.79; regular or curved brush)* isn't the best thickening mascara in Maybelline's lineup anymore, but it still excels at creating long, thick lashes without clumps. Results are noticeable immediately, and layering makes lashes slightly more dramatic. The curved brush version is similar, except that it produces even faster results and makes lashes look slightly more lifted. ✓☺ **Volum' Express Turbo Boost Mascara 7X** *($6.99)* advertises that users will achieve seven times the volume in one stroke, and guess what? It works! This is far and away Maybelline's most impressive thickening mascara, with an application that's quick and clump-free and a lash look that's only for those who covet long, impossibly thick lashes.

✓☺ **XXL Volume + Length Microfiber Mascara** *($7.59)* is similar to L'Oreal's excellent DoubleExtend Lash Extender & Magnifier Mascara ($9.99). Both are dual-ended mascaras: one end contains a lash primer and the other a mascara. Just as I did with L'Oreal's version, I applied the "microfiber basecoat" to my left eyelashes and followed with the mascara. Results were impressive. On my right lashes I applied two coats of the mascara only. As expected, both sides looked nearly the same, with the slight length and thickness edge going to the mascara-only lashes. The bottom line is that Maybelline's XXL Microfiber Mascara (which, by the way, doesn't contain any fibers) is an outstanding lengthening/thickening mascara all by itself. The basecoat is no more effective than applying two coats of regular mascara, and, if anything, including the basecoat wastes space that could be filled with mascara instead! Whether you use this product's two steps or just apply the mascara, you're not likely to be disappointed.

✓☺ **Intense XXL Volume + Length Microfiber Mascara** *($7.59)* is similar to L'Oreal's Volume Shocking Mascara ($12.95), but (despite the name) this is less intense. It involves a two-step process of base plus top coat, although—just like Maybelline's other XXL mascaras—the basecoat makes little difference, assuming you're willing to apply two or three coats of the mascara itself. The best news is that whether or not you use the basecoat, you'll get beautifully long, nicely separated, and moderately thickened lashes with absolutely no clumps. The formula wears well and removes easily, making for hassle-free work all around.

☺ **Define-A-Lash Mascara** *($6.99)* uses a spiky-looking, rubber-bristled brush first seen from Cover Girl (Lash Exact, Volume Exact). Promising zero clumps with stunning definition and length, this mascara really delivers! It isn't much for creating thicker lashes, but each stroke makes them longer without any mishaps. The brush doesn't take as much getting used to as does the fact that the wand is too flexible. Sweeping this through lashes causes the wand to bend more than it should, which can affect application, but for the most part it wears without a hitch, keeping lashes exceptionally soft.

☺ **XXL Volume + Length Microfiber Mascara Waterproof** *($7.59)* is indeed a tenaciously waterproof version of the XXL Microfiber Mascara above. One end of this dual-sided product is a lash primer and the other a lengthening mascara. I applied the primer and mascara combination to one set of my eyelashes and used just the mascara on the other. The mascara alone produced copious length and beautifully defined, clump-free lashes. However, if you apply mascara immediately after using the primer, you'll notice slightly more length than with the mascara alone. It's not enough of a difference to justify two steps, but at least it's something.

☺ **Lash Expansion Waterproof Mascara** *($6.79)* builds instant length and clean separation, but it's impossible to continue building because it dries too fast, so you're out of luck if you want any additional thickness or longer lashes than the first coat provides. This leaves lashes softly curled and is waterproof, but is best for those whose lashes are naturally long and don't need much enhancement.

☺ **Unstoppable Full Length Mascara** *($6.79)* claims to lengthen up to 50%, a refreshingly modest statistic considering the disproportionate numbers often touted for cosmetics ("makes skin 450% smoother!" and "lashes are 800% fuller!"). This does indeed make lashes remarkably longer, without clumps, and it builds easily. You won't notice any thickness, but its lengthening ability surpasses Maybelline's former (discontinued) champ, Illegal Lengths Mascara.

☺ **Volum' Express Waterproof Mascara 3X** *($6.79)* builds quickly and makes lashes moderately longer and noticeably thicker without clumps. It is waterproof. ☺ **Full 'n Soft Waterproof Mascara** *($6.39)* is said to build "full, soft thick lashes." It does a decent job of fulfilling that claim, albeit with less thickness than you may be expecting. Still, it bests several other waterproof mascaras that make thicker-lashes claims, and this one won't come off in the pool or inclement weather.

☺ **Great Lash Clear Mascara** *($3.59)* is a multipurpose clear mascara that adds a touch of length and a glossy finish to lashes while also grooming unruly brows. The standard formula is similar to that of most other clear mascaras and brow gels, but it does its job without flaking or feeling sticky. It does take a bit longer than usual to dry, but that's a minor quibble for this versatile, affordable product.

😐 **Lash Expansion Mascara** *($6.79)* promises dimensional lash volume and length but at best this works as a lengthening mascara that doesn't distinguish itself as a must-have. If you're curious, it's good that this formula doesn't flake or clump. 😐 **Volum' Express** 😐 **Turbo Boost Mascara Waterproof 5X** *($6.79)* is said to make lashes five times thicker in one stroke. Its turbo effect is more akin to a standard 4-cylinder engine because it takes its time to get going, and you will be dealing with clumps and uneven application along the way. It builds reasonable length, but is really more for thickening lashes, an area where it does not perform as well as Maybelline's other Volum' Express mascaras (reviewed above). The best reason to consider this is because it's tenaciously waterproof. It requires a silicone- or oil-based makeup remover—a water-soluble cleanser (even those with some oil) won't do the job.

☹ **Lash Stylist Mascara** *($6.79)* is another brushless mascara that, instead of a brush, uses tiny, comblike teeth arranged in a V-pattern, which is said to lift and lengthen lashes. It definitely does that, and dramatically so. You'll quickly achieve long, lightly curled lashes that have impact—this isn't a mascara for a natural look. So why the unhappy face rating? Because, despite the impressive application, it consistently flakes and smears easily. What a shame, because it is otherwise a premier option. For a similarly dramatic effect without the problems, try L'Oreal's Volume Shocking Mascara ($12.95). ☹ **Lash Stylist Waterproof Mascara** *($6.79)* has the same comb applicator as the regular Lash Stylist Mascara, but it deposits too much product on lashes, leaving them looking too heavy and wet. This takes longer than it should to dry, and also tends to smear, making it not recommended despite the fact that once it sets, it holds up well under water.

☹ **Great Lash Mascara** *($4.99; regular or curved brush)* builds some length, though it takes a good deal of effort to get anywhere, and pales in comparison to most of Maybelline's other mascaras. Great Lash does not build any thickness and it has a tendency to smear. The curved brush version does little to make an unimpressive mascara any better. It may (shockingly) be the #1–selling mascara, but that doesn't mean it's the best. ☹ **Great Lash Waterproof Mascara** *($4.99)* is an utterly boring mascara that takes lots of effort for an "Is that all there is?" result. It stays on in the rain or pool, but so do Maybelline's other waterproof mascaras—all of which are preferred to this.

BRUSHES: Maybelline's name may not be synonymous with brushes, but if you're on a budget and are ready to toss out your miniature sponge applicators and other inferior tools, you'll find the ☺ **Eyeshadow Brush** *($4.99)* and ☺ **Blush Brush** *($4.99)* are extremely soft, but firm, and that they work decently well. The synthetic ☺ **Eye Contour Brush** *($4.99)* is an option for brows or eyelining, but not for eyeshadow. The ☺ **Retractable Lip Brush** *($6.39)* is a standard lip brush that travels well, though it could be firmer. The ☺ **Expert Eyes Brush 'n Comb** *($3.99)* is a standard, feasible brow and lash comb that's affordably priced. Less impressive is the 😐 **Face Brush** *($7.99)*, which feels soft but is too floppy for controlled application of powder, though some women may prefer a "looser" powder brush.

M.D. FORMULATIONS (SKIN CARE ONLY)

M.D. FORMULATIONS AT-A-GLANCE

Strengths: The entire line is fragrance-free; some well-formulated AHA products featuring glycolic acid and ammonium glycolate; a selection of very good cleansers; some extraordinary moisturizers and serums; very good toner; an oil-rich lip balm with broad-spectrum sunscreen; a skin-lightening product with retinol and arbutin.

Weaknesses: Some AHA products that include alcohol and other irritants; jar packaging; sunscreens without sufficient UVA protection; the at-home peel kit is an irritation waiting to happen; adhering to a routine of several M.D. Formulations products may expose skin to an excessive amount of exfoliation; incomplete routine(s) for blemish-prone skin.

For more information about M.D. Formulations, call (800) 451-3940 or visit www.md-formulations.com or www.Beautypedia.com.

M.D. FORMULATIONS CONTINUOUS RENEWAL PRODUCTS

☺ **$$$ Continuous Renewal Complex** *($35 for 1 ounce)* is a basic, fragrance-free, pH-correct AHA moisturizer for normal to dry skin. Bells and whistles are absent, but it does the job to exfoliate skin and renew its texture. Between the glycolic acid and ammonium glycolate, the AHA content is at least 10%.

😐 **$$$ Continuous Renewal Complex, Sensitive Skin Formula** *($35 for 1 ounce)* contains enough AHAs to exfoliate, but the pH of 4.4 doesn't allow that to occur; AHAs do best at a pH of 3 to 4. So this product really isn't worth considering for any skin type (Source: *Cosmetic Dermatology*, October 2001, pages 15–18).

☺ **$$$ Continuous Renewal Serum** *($53 for 2 ounces)* claims to deliver the same benefits of glycolic acid without the irritating side effects. However, this doesn't contain anything too different from the other products in this line that contain glycolic acid. Despite the contradictory claim, this is an effective (meaning pH-correct), no-frills AHA product for all skin types. It contains approximately 12% AHA.

😐 **$$$ Continuous Renewal Serum, Sensitive Skin Formula** *($53 for 2 ounces)* has a more elegant formula than the Continuous Renewal Serum above, but the pH of 4.4 reduces the potential for the AHAs it contains to exfoliate skin.

M.D. FORMULATIONS MOISTURE DEFENSE PRODUCTS

✓☺ **Moisture Defense Antioxidant Spray** *($28 for 8.3 ounces)* is pricey, but in this case you're getting a well-done spray-on toner. It supplies skin with very good skin-identical ingredients, antioxidants, and a couple of notable soothing agents, all without any irritants or fragrance.

😐 **$$$ Moisture Defense Antioxidant Comfort Creme** *($44 for 1 ounce)* is a basic moisturizer for normal to dry skin. The meager amount of antioxidants will become less effective once this jar-packaged product is opened.

😐 **$$$ Moisture Defense Antioxidant Creme** *($55 for 1.7 ounces)* contains a selection of ingredients capable of reinforcing skin and rebuilding its protective barrier as claimed, and that's excellent. What's not so great is that jar packaging will render the many antioxidants ineffective shortly after you begin using this cream. In better packaging, this would be a slam-dunk recommendation for normal to slightly dry skin.

😐 **$$$ Moisture Defense Antioxidant Eye Creme** *($35 for 0.5 ounce)* contains too few impressive ingredients and earns its stripes primarily via cosmetics trickery. The amount of titanium dioxide and iron oxides create a whitening, slightly pearlescent finish that helps mask the appearance of dark circles. It's not as effective as a concealer, and overall not worth considering over many other eye creams.

✓☺ **$$$ Moisture Defense Antioxidant Hydrating Gel** *($45 for 1 ounce)* contains effective, state-of-the-art water-binding agents, antioxidants, and cell-communicating ingredients in an ultralight base suitable for all skin types (or for very oily skin seeking an antioxidant-laden gel). This would also be worthwhile for someone with rosacea. This is a lighter-weight product than Prescriptives' similar Redness Relief Gel ($50 for 1 ounce).

✓☺ **$$$ Moisture Defense Antioxidant Lotion** *($50 for 1 ounce)* lists urea as the fourth ingredient, and thus has some exfoliating properties; it is also a very good moisturizing agent for dry skin. A lesser amount of lactic acid (likely 2%) boosts the exfoliation potential, and the pH of 3.8 is within range. Even better, this lotion for normal to dry skin is loaded with antioxidants and ingredients that reinforce skin's healthy functioning. A beautiful formulation that's packaged right, too!

☺ **$$$ Moisture Defense Antioxidant Treatment Masque** *($26 for 2.5 ounces)* contains approximately 8% AHAs, but the pH of 4.4 reduces the potential for effective exfoliation. This is otherwise a thick, creamy mask for dry skin that contains some good antioxidants and soothing agents. These ingredients are best left on skin rather than rinsed off.

😐 **Moisture Defense Soothing Eye Gels** *($8 for 1 pair)* are fluid-filled patches cut to fit under the eyes. The formula is mostly water, glycerin, and sugars. There's not much reason for those ingredients to be placed on the skin in patches, but there really isn't any reason for those ingredients to be on the skin in general (at least not without some other really interesting beneficial ingredients).

M.D. FORMULATIONS THE TEMPS PRODUCTS

☹ **The Temps Brighten & Tighten Eye Serum** *($36 for 0.16 ounce)* comes packaged with a roller-ball applicator that allows this water-based solution to glide onto the under-eye area. Contrary to claims, this product doesn't contain any ingredients that can vanquish dark circles or puffiness. Actually, it's a problem for use around the eye area because it contains arnica extract, which can cause contact dermatitis and be very irritating to mucous membranes (Source: www.naturaldatabase.com). By the way, this also contains PVP/polycarbamyl polyglycol ester (a hairspray-type ingredient) that can also be a skin irritant.

😐 **$$$ The Temps Wrinkle Filler & Deep Crease Relaxer** *($36 for 0.06 ounce)* is basically positioned as a "Botox-on-the-go" product that is packaged in a pen-style applicator. This nonaqueous blend of silicones feels great on skin, but the peptides in this product won't relax expression lines, although it is reasonable to expect them to attract moisture to skin and, therefore, make lines look less apparent by virtue of hydration. Unlike the ill-advised The Temps Brighten & Tighten Eye Serum above, this product is gentle enough to use on wrinkles around the eye area.

☹ **The Temps Lip Plumping Treatment** *($28 for 0.27 ounce)* is an emollient lip balm that contains some excellent moisturizing ingredients for dry, chapped lips. Unfortunately, the plumping comes from the irritating, potent menthol derivative menthoxypropanediol. The inflammation this causes will make lips swell a little, but causing such inflammation daily isn't a good idea for the health of your lips.

M.D. FORMULATIONS VIT-A-PLUS PRODUCTS

😐 **$$$ Vit-A-Plus Anti-Aging Eye Complex** *($53 for 0.5 ounce)* contains 10% AHAs, but the pH of 4.4 limits their exfoliating properties, though they will serve as water-binding agents. This lightweight moisturizer is an option for slightly dry skin. Vitamins A and E are the only antioxidants on board, but the packaging will keep them stable during use.

😐 **$$$ Vit-A-Plus Anti-Aging Serum** *($50 for 1 ounce)* is a heavier (but not occlusive) version of the Vit-A-Plus Anti-Aging Eye Complex above, with an improved selection of helpful ingredients for normal to dry skin. The pH is too high for the 10% concentration of AHAs to exfoliate, but the vitamin A (as retinyl palmitate) content is good.

✓☺ **$$$ Vit-A-Plus Illuminating Serum** *($65 for 1 ounce)* combines the benefits of AHAs (15%) at a pH of 4 with retinol and other cell-communicating ingredients, plus a good complement of antioxidants, all in packaging that keeps them stable during use. This is highly recommended for normal to dry skin not prone to breakouts (the plant oil and wax may prove problematic for blemishes). The AHA content is likely to be problematic for those with sensitive skin.

😐 **$$$ Vit-A-Plus Intensive Anti-Aging Serum** *($55 for 1 ounce)* is similar to the Vit-A-Plus Anti-Aging Serum above, except it has a higher concentration (20%) of AHAs. Once again, the pH does not permit optimal exfoliation; however, the amount of retinyl palmitate is good.

✓☺ **$$$ Vit-A-Plus Night Recovery** *($50 for 1 ounce)* is a combination AHA/BHA product with 8% glycolic compound (consisting of ammonium glycolate and glycolic acid) and 2% salicylic acid. The pH of 4 is borderline for exfoliation, but you should net some results. The lightweight texture and reduced amount of thickening agents is preferred for normal to slightly oily skin, but this can be used by all skin types. The amount of antioxidants and water-binding agents isn't expansive, but the concentration of each are above average.

☹ **Vit-A-Plus Clearing Complex** *($39 for 1 ounce)* lists alcohol as the second ingredient. Without it, the blend of AHAs and salicylic acid plus retinol in this product would have been great for battling blemishes.

😐 **$$$ Vit-A-Plus Clearing Complex Masque** *($30 for 2.5 ounces)* contains lactic acid and sodium lactate at a pH of 3.6, so some exfoliation will occur. This is first and foremost a clay mask for oily skin, and the amount of exfoliation won't be great because you'll want to rinse this off after several minutes. The small amount of rosemary oil may cause irritation.

😐 **$$$ Vit-A-Plus Firming Treatment Masque** *($36 for 2.5 ounces)* contains a small amount of vitamin A and not enough AHA or BHA to function as an exfoliant. This is otherwise an OK clay mask for normal to oily skin not prone to blemishes (the amount of ceresin, a waxlike thickening agent, isn't the best for blemish-prone skin).

✓☺ **$$$ Vit-A-Plus Illumination Spot Treatment, for All Skin Types** *($38 for 0.11 ounce)* is an outstanding option (though an exceptionally pricey one) if you're looking for a pH-correct AHA product that combines about 5% glycolic acid with the skin-lightening agent arbutin. This deserves further praise for packaging that keeps the retinol stable and for the inclusion of other antioxidants. The only downside is the claim that this works to fade red marks left from blemishes. I admit, those marks can be very stubborn. However, because they are not related to melanin production, they do not respond to skin-lightening agents. Using a well-formulated exfoliant can help speed the healing process, so in that regard this product can be helpful for post-inflammatory hyperpigmentation.

☹ **Vit-A-Plus Illuminating Masque** *($42 for 2.5 ounces)* contains 5% AHAs at a pH of 4, so some exfoliation will occur. However, this moisturizing mask for normal to dry skin is not recommended because it contains irritating lavender oil.

OTHER M.D. FORMULATIONS PRODUCTS

☺ **$$$ Facial Cleanser** *($32 for 8.3 ounces)* is a basic, slightly creamy but water-soluble cleanser that contains 12% glycolic acid at a pH of 3.8. That's nice, but it's all for naught because the benefit is rinsed from your skin, when in fact it should be left on (though you wouldn't want to do that with a cleanser). It's an option for normal to oily skin, provided you avoid the eye area.

✓☺ **Facial Cleanser Basic, Non-Glycolic** *($18 for 8.3 ounces)* is a very good, extremely gentle cleansing lotion for normal to dry skin. The fragrance-free formula contains a reduced amount of detergent cleansing agent, but still does an overall good job of removing most types of makeup.

✓☺ **Facial Cleanser Foaming, Non-Glycolic** *($18 for 8.3 ounces)* is an excellent water-soluble cleanser for normal to very oily skin. It is fragrance-free and doesn't leave a trace of residue.

✓☺ **$$$ Facial Cleanser, Sensitive Skin Formula** *($32 for 8.3 ounces)* is a cross between the Facial Cleanser Basic, Non-Glycolic, and the Facial Cleanser Foaming, Non-Glycolic, above, except that this one includes a tiny amount of glycolic acid and some soothing agents. The glycolic acid isn't helpful in a cleanser and is an odd choice in a product meant for sensitive skin. Still, this is a gentle, effective cleanser for normal to dry skin, and it's fragrance-free.

☺ **$$$ Facial Cleansing Gel** *($32 for 8.3 ounces)* is similar to the Facial Cleanser Foaming, Non-Glycolic, above save for a much higher price and the inclusion of glycolic acid (not helpful in a cleanser). This works well but isn't worth considering over the less-expensive version.

☹ **$$$ Face and Body Scrub** *($35 for 8.3 ounces)* is a standard, detergent-based scrub that contains plastic beads as the abrasive agent. The inclusion of 15% glycolic acid (in a base with a pH of 3.8) guarantees exfoliation only if this is left on skin for a prolonged period—much longer than a product like this should be. There's nothing about this product that isn't easily replaced by a washcloth.

☹ **Daily Peel Pads** *($30 for 40 pads)* would be recommended as pH-correct glycolic and salicylic acid pads if the formula did not include several irritants, including alcohol, juniper oil, lavender oil, and witch hazel.

☹ **Glycare Acne Gel** *($30 for 2.5 ounces)* lists alcohol as the second ingredient, which makes it too drying and irritating for all skin types.

☹ **Glycare Lotion** *($40 for 2 ounces)* contains too much alcohol and causes further irritation due to eucalyptus oil. This is not the way to control excess oil or reduce the appearance of large pores.

✓☺ **$$$ Critical Care Calming Gel** *($39 for 1 ounce)* is designed to minimize redness and irritation, and contains impressive levels of ingredients research has shown do just that because of their anti-inflammatory properties. This is an outstanding, fragrance-free gel moisturizer for all skin types that contains lots of antioxidants and a cell-communicating ingredient.

☹ **$$$ Critical Care Shielding Creme** *($85 for 1 ounce)* has a beautifully silky texture built around silicones, and also includes some well-researched antioxidants and ingredients that reinforce skin's structure. Yet for the money, it ends up being a disappointment because of the jar packaging, which won't allow the antioxidants to stimulate skin's healing process.

☹ **$$$ Critical Care Skin Repair Complex** *($100 for 1 ounce)* promises to restore the smooth, beautiful skin you were born with, but it cannot replace what time and years of sun damage take away. It's just a lightweight, silky-textured moisturizer in which the effectiveness of the antioxidants is diminished due to jar packaging. M.D. Formulations should have taken "care" to get this "critical" aspect right!

☹ **Sun Protector 20** *($24 for 6 ounces)* lacks the UVA-protecting ingredients of titanium dioxide, zinc oxide, avobenzone, Tinosorb, or Mexoryl SX, and is not recommended.

☹ **Sun Protector 30 Spray, SPF 30** *($24 for 4 ounces)* lacks the UVA-protecting ingredients of titanium dioxide, zinc oxide, avobenzone, Tinosorb, or Mexoryl SX, and is not recommended. Even if it had the right UVA protection, this would be a problem for all skin types because it contains cedarwood bark and lavender oils.

☺ **Total Daily Protector 15** *($20 for 2.5 ounces)* is one of two M.D. Formulations sunscreens that provide sufficient UVA protection. This in-part zinc oxide sunscreen with SPF 15 is formulated in a generic base suitable for normal to dry skin. It is disappointingly short on antioxidants.

☺ **Total Protector 30** *($22 for 2.5 ounces)* is similar to the Total Daily Protector 15 above, except it contains a greater concentration of zinc oxide to achieve its higher SPF rating. Otherwise, the same review applies.

☺ **Benzoyl Peroxide 10** *($20 for 2 ounces)* works swiftly to kill acne-causing bacteria with its 10% concentration of benzoyl peroxide. You shouldn't start with such a high concentration, but it may be worth stepping up to if your blemishes don't respond to 2.5% or 5% concentrations.

☹ **My Personal Peel System** *($85 for the kit)* consists of five separate products meant to be customized according to your skin's needs; however, all of them contain at least one irritating ingredient. The **Power Peel Pads** contain 20% AHAs, but irritate the skin with alcohol, witch hazel, lavender oil, and juniper oil. The **Firming Anti-Wrinkle Booster** only boosts skin inflammation because it contains the menthol derivative menthoxypropanediol. The **Extra Clear Booster** contains irritating grapefruit oil (which won't promote clear skin, but can cause a phototoxic reaction). The **Brightening Booster** contains menthoxypropanediol and lavender oil. And the **Post-Peel Restorer** contains strawberry oil, which can cause contact dermatitis and has no established soothing benefit for skin, particularly if it's as irritated as it will be after proceeding through the steps of this at-home peel.

☺ **$$$ Lip Balm SPF 20** *($12 for 0.33 ounce)* contains an in-part titanium dioxide sunscreen, but the amount (0.8%) is on the low side in terms of providing superior UVA protection. This is still worth considering as a unique lip balm that contains some very good emollients and oils to stop chapped lips.

MD SKINCARE BY DR. DENNIS GROSS (SKIN CARE ONLY)

MD SKINCARE AT-A-GLANCE

Strengths: Almost all of the products are fragrance-free; several serums and moisturizers contain a brilliant assortment of beneficial skin-care ingredients; all of the sunscreens contain sufficient UVA protection; almost all of the antioxidant-rich products are packaged to ensure stability and potency.

Weaknesses: Expensive; no effective AHA or BHA products (including the at-home peel the line is "known" for); problematic toner; incomplete selection of products to treat acne, and what's available is more irritating than helpful; a few "why bother?" products; although there are some remarkable products, none of them can provide results equivalent to Botox, dermal fillers, chemical peels, or laser treatments (and definitely not a face-lift).

For more information call (888) 830-7546 or visit the Web site at www.mdskincare.com or www.Beautypedia.com. Note: Unless mentioned otherwise, all MD Skincare products are fragrance-free.

☺ **$$$ All-in-One Cleansing Foam** *($36 for 5 ounces)* is a good water-soluble cleanser for normal to oily skin, but would be rated higher if it did not contain witch hazel bark, leaf, and twig extract. The amount is not likely cause for concern, but why include it at all?

😐 **$$$ All-in-One Facial Cleanser with Toner** *($36 for 8 ounces)* is an exceptionally standard, detergent-based cleanser that is an option for someone with normal to oily skin. The teeny amount of emu oil provides no emollient benefit for skin, but the witch hazel base is potentially irritating.

☹ **Hydra-Pure Mist** *($32 for 5 ounces)* has a lot going for it, including some very effective water-binding agents and a few antioxidants. But the inclusion of comfrey extract makes this problematic for all skin types. Please refer to Chapter Seven, *Cosmetic Ingredient Dictionary* in this book for an explanation of comfrey's negative impact on skin.

☺ **$$$ All-in-One Tinted Moisturizer Sunscreen SPF 15** *($42 for 1.7 ounces)* contains an in-part avobenzone sunscreen in a silicone-enhanced moisturizing base for normal to dry skin. The six sheer shades are all worth trying, each providing a hint of color but no meaningful coverage. A higher amount of antioxidants would have netted this tinted moisturizer a Paula's Pick rating.

☹ **$$$ Auto-Balancing Moisture Sunscreen SPF 10** *($42 for 1.7 ounces).* A dermatologist selling a sunscreen with an SPF 10 is very disappointing. This sunscreen does contain avobenzone, but the gold standard for sunscreens today is SPF 15 (Source: American Academy of Dermatology, www.aad.org). The base formula is appropriate for normal to dry skin, though it doesn't automatically balance skin.

✓☺ **$$$ Continuous Eye Hydration** *($42 for 0.5 ounce)* has what it takes to address the needs of slightly dry to dry skin anywhere on the face. The formula includes effective emollients along with several antioxidants, water-binding agents, and a cell-communicating ingredient. The claims that this can reduce puffy eyes with caffeine and cucumber are unfounded, and this also cannot lighten dark circles (though the mica cosmetically "brightens" shadowed areas). Still, there's no denying that this is a well-formulated, stably packaged product.

✓☺ **$$$ Hydra-Pure Antioxidant Firming Serum** *($95 for 1 ounce)* has a texture that's more lotion than serum, and it contains a brilliant assortment of ingredients to help normal to dry skin look and feel its best. The amount of lactic acid is impressive, but the pH of 4.7 significantly reduces any potential for exfoliation. The lactic acid still has merit as a water-binding agent, however, and the formula contains appreciable amounts of several well-researched antioxidants, plus retinol and other cell-communicating ingredients. One more thing: Dimethyl sulfone is the fourth listed ingredient. Also known as methylsulfonylmethane (MSM), there is limited research supporting its benefit for skin. The only published study was a single case report of a man with a rare skin disorder (ichthyosis) who responded well to topical treatment with a moisturizer that contained, among several other ingredients, MSM. The case report did not elucidate if it was the MSM or another ingredient (or a synergistic combination) that provided relief (Source: *Ostomy/Wound Management*, April 2006, pages 82–86).

☹ **Hydra-Pure Firming Eye Cream** *($90 for 0.5 ounce)* contains some incredibly helpful, state-of-the-art ingredients for all skin types, but jar packaging won't keep them stable, and lavender oil (of which there is a significant amount) only wreaks havoc on skin cells, not to mention being problematic for use around the eyes. What was Dr. Gross thinking?

☹ **Hydra-Pure Intense Moisture Cream** *($120 for 1.7 ounces)* shares the attractive points and drawbacks of the Hydra-Pure Firming Eye Cream above, and the same comments apply.

✓☺ **$$$ Hydra-Pure Oil-Free Moisture** *($75 for 1 ounce)* is said to be a best-seller for the brand, but it also makes the claim that it removes unwanted heavy metals left on skin from tap water. How it goes about doing that isn't explained, other than that it works via the company's Chelating Complex. Chelating agents prevent metals from binding to other substances, but the amount of metals in tap water (and their potential subsequent effect on skin) isn't cause for concern. In the end, this is a very good moisturizer for normal to slightly dry skin. It contains a nice array of antioxidants, cell-communicating ingredients, and a tiny amount of water-binding agents.

✓☺ **$$$ Hydra-Pure Radiance Renewal Serum** *($95 for 1 ounce)* is designed to address skin discolorations from sun damage, and handles this task beautifully. This water-based serum has a silky texture and contains arbutin and uva ursi leaf extract in amounts that are likely to have an effect on hyperpigmentation (assuming your routine includes daily application of sunscreen rated SPF 15 or greater). The formula also contains numerous antioxidants and the cell-communicating ingredients creatinine and retinol, and it's fragrance-free. This is suitable for all skin types.

✓☺ **$$$ Hydra-Pure Redness Soothing Serum** *($85 for 1 ounce)* contains efficacious amounts of several well-researched soothing agents, including bisabolol, green tea, and licorice root extract. This fragrance-free, water-based serum's only misstep is the inclusion of witch hazel, though the amount is most likely too small to be of concern for irritation. This is recommended for any skin type dealing with redness or irritation, and would indeed be suitable for post-laser treatment or after other cosmetic procedures, such as peels or waxing.

✓☺ **$$$ Hydra-Pure Vitamin C Serum** *($90 for 1 ounce)* has a beautifully smooth silicone base and contains an impressive amount of vitamin C (as ascorbic acid, whose acid component can be a skin irritant). Two other stabilized forms of vitamin C are also in the formula, along with the antioxidants quercetin, vitamin E, willow bark, and kudzu. Gross also added cell-communicating ingredients and salicylic acid, but the amount of the latter is too low (and the pH of this product too high) for exfoliation to occur. All in all, this is a well-formulated antioxidant serum that is packaged to ensure potency.

☹ **Lift & Lighten Eye Cream** *($58 for 0.5 ounce)* is one of the least impressive MD Skincare products because it contains far more fragrance than it does the bells and whistles that he wisely added to most of the other moisturizers and serums in this line. This also contains arnica, which is a problem for all skin types, and even more so in a product meant for application to the eye area.

😐 **$$$ Maximum Moisture Treatment** *($45 for 1 ounce)* is an effective but comparably basic moisturizer for normal to dry skin not prone to blemishes. It does not contain the same amount or selection of antioxidants or other goodies present in other MD Skincare moisturizers.

✓☺ **$$$ Powerful Sun Protection SPF 30 Sunscreen Lotion** *($42 for 5 ounces)* claims it is the only sunscreen that addresses the increased risk of sun damage caused by iron that's left on your skin from tap water. Of course, this statement isn't backed up by any research on Dr. Gross's Web site, so we're left to take his word for it.

This product does contain chelating agents, which can possibly prevent iron from damaging skin in the presence of sunlight. Chelating agents are compounds that bind with a metal (such as iron) and change its function by affecting its molecular makeup. Chelating agents are often used in laundry detergents to prevent trace metals in the water from binding to clothing. Left on clothing, these trace metals can react with perspiration and cause clothing to discolor, so in that context preventing this is a good thing and chelating agents are helpful.

The chelating agents in Gross's product are tetrasodium EDTA and disodium EDTA, common chelating agents found in hundreds of products, from shampoos to moisturizers. They are not unique to his product and there is no reason to choose this over another well-formulated sunscreen because of its allegedly special protective ability. Gross focuses on chelating agents to keep iron from damaging your skin, although it's likely the amount of iron left on your skin (if any) from tap water is completely insignificant. What he doesn't mention is that there is research showing that the antioxidants present in skin-care products do a great job of keeping the iron in our skin from converting to reactive oxygen species (ROS) and causing free-radical damage in the presence of sunlight (Source: *Free Radical Biology and Medicine*, October 2006, pages 1197–1204). In addition, although there is research showing that specific iron chelators added to a sunscreen increase its ability to protect skin from sun damage, Gross didn't use either of the above compounds in this product (Source: *The Journal of Investigative Dermatology*, October 2006, pages 2287–2295). That said, if you ignore the "one-of-a-kind" claims, this is a very good, fragrance-free, in-part avobenzone sunscreen that comes in a lightweight lotion base and contains several potent antioxidants. It's expensive, but is nevertheless an excellent option for normal to slightly dry skin.

✓☺ **$$$ Powerful Sun Protection SPF 30 Sunscreen Packettes** *($42 for 60 packettes)* makes the same iron-squashing claims as the Powerful Sun Protection SPF 30 Sunscreen Lotion above, and is also the same product, just packaged in single-use, take-along packets. Although pricey, it's a good way to pack extra sunscreen for unanticipated long days outdoors or for use after washing your hands when you're away from home.

☹ **All-Over Blemish Solution** *($84 for 1.7 ounces)* has a jaw-droppingly ridiculous price that's even more insulting when you find out that the pH is above 5, so the 2% salicylic acid won't function as an exfoliant. Want more bad news? The menthol will cause irritation and possibly worsen the appearance of reddened, blemished skin.

☹ **Alpha Beta Daily Face Peel Two-Step System** *($75 for the kit)* is the system that made Dr. Gross famous, or so the company says. Step 1 involves the salicylic, glycolic, and lactic acid–infused **Alpha Beta Peel Refining**. The amount of AHAs pales next to the BHA content, but none of these exfoliants function as expected because the pH of the pads is 4.4. Step 2, the **Neutralizing System**, has been improved, but it's still superfluous (plain tap water can neutralize a peel). This is basically a good toner formula in pad form, and includes several antioxidants and retinol, but the jar packaging won't keep them stable during the lifespan of this product. In the end, this is a great big "why bother"?

☹ **Correct & Perfect Spot Treatment** *($28 for 0.5 ounce)* will irritate and aggravate thanks to the 3.25% concentration of the potent disinfectant sulfur and the inclusion of menthol. Sulfur can be helpful for blemish-prone skin, but its side effects and irritation potential are more problematic than beneficial. I have no idea why Dr. Gross chose sulfur over an effective topical disinfectant with benzoyl peroxide, but in any case, this product is not recommended.

☺ **$$$ Intense Hydra Mask** *($60 for the kit)* is not intense in the least. And what is it with dermatologist lines and their two-step kits? And why, almost without exception, do these kits feature products that are either inferior to or the equivalent of other products in the line (yet the products in the kit claim to do something completely different or better)? Gripes aside, Step 1 of this duo is the **Hyaluronic Gel**, which purports to plump skin and fill in wrinkles. Its name (and the claims) implies hyaluronic acid, which is the ingredient used in dermal fillers such as Restylane, so you'll think it will work the same. However, it actually contains sodium hyaluronate, the less-expensive salt form of this ingredient, which doesn't work even vaguely in any way, shape, or form like Restylane. It does contain a good selection of antioxidants with this skin-identical ingredient, but it's still nothing that isn't found in most of the other MD Skincare moisturizers and serums reviewed above.

Once you've brushed the Gel on (a brush is included in the kit), you apply the **Self-Heating Mask**. This is simply a mixture of slip agent, mineral, thickener, and antioxidants. The sodium silicoaluminate reacts with water and causes a warming sensation, though it has little effect on skin other than feeling pleasant. I suppose that is intended to reinforce the treatment angle for which this kit is striving. Both steps contain helpful ingredients for all skin types, but if you're using one or more of MD Skincare's best products, this kit isn't a must-have.

😐 **$$$ Serious Lip Treatment** *($58 for 2-0.27 ounce tubes)* claims to be a two-step process for plumping lips, but it ends up being two steps too many and a waste of money. Step 1 consists mostly of water, glycerin, honey, and preservative; Step 2 is mostly water, a plant oil copolymer, thickener, silicones, honey, film-forming agent, and several nonvolatile plant oils.

The ingredients in both tubes can smooth and soften lips, but that's about it. Honey appears to be the link between the two, but it has no plumping or anti-aging effect on lips; it's merely a good water-binding agent and likely contributes the flavor to both products. The only serious thing about this product is its name, although its benign, ho-hum formula doesn't deserve an unhappy face rating. But the price did make me bite my lip!

MEDERMA (SKIN CARE ONLY)

MEDERMA AT-A-GLANCE

Strengths: None, unless you want to hang your hopes on anecdotal evidence.

Weaknesses: There is no research proving that the "active" ingredient in Mederma works as claimed.

For more information about Mederma, call (888) 925-8989 or visit www.mederma.com or www.Beautypedia.com.

☹ **Mederma Skin Care for Scars** *($16 for 0.70 ounce)* is said to work by using onion bulb extract as the scar-changing ingredient. It contains water, thickeners, onion bulb extract, anti-irritant, fragrance, and preservative, and it seems that only Mederma believes their claim. An article in the *Archives of Dermatology* (December 1998, pages 1512–1514, "Snake Oil for the 21st Century") from the Department of Dermatology, Harvard Medical School, stated that "With the current promulgation of skin 'products' and their promotion and even sale by dermatologists, and the use of treatments of no proven efficacy, this association between dermatology and quackery is set to continue well into the 21st century. The list of offending treatments includes silicone gel sheets and onion extract cream (Mederma) for keloids...."

Other studies compared the results of Mederma to those of a placebo and treating scars with Vaseline. The results were as follows: "Treated [Mederma] and placebo [untreated] subjects were compared on all covariants: age, gender, ethnicity, scar age, and use. No significant difference exists between treated and placebo groups for any of these variables.... More placebo patients than treated patients reported improvement with a less noticeable scar [after] 1 week and a less red scar after 1 month." Interestingly, "More treated patients reported improvement with a softer scar after 2 months. There were no differences in improvement for either of the physician-related measures between the two groups." Additionally, "In this side-by-side, randomized, double-blind, split-scar study, the onion extract gel did not improve scar cosmesis or symptomatology when compared with a petrolatum-based ointment."

Regarding Mederma's alleged ability to reduce the unsightly redness some scars present, a detailed study revealed that "Computer analysis of the scar photographs demonstrated no significant reduction in scar erythema [redness] with Mederma treatment."

Mederma must have seen these studies and taken their disappointing results seriously, because they are now using cosmetic claims, such as "can help them appear softer, smoother, and less noticeable," rather than stating directly that their product eliminates or flattens scars to the point where they're not a visible distraction. In summary, there is no reason to use Mederma to try to improve the appearance of scars. Those who have used it and seen results would likely have gotten the same results using a placebo or nothing at all. Remember, even after a scar is formed, it can and often does improve in appearance over a period of several months (the exception to this is, unfortunately, stretch marks and indented, ice-pick scars from acne) (Sources: *Cosmetic*

Dermatology, March 1999, pages 19–26; *Plastic and Reconstructive Surgery*, July 2002, pages 177–183; and *Dermatologic Surgery*, February 2006, pages 193–197).

METROGEL, METROCREAM, AND METROLOTION (SKIN CARE ONLY)

METROGEL, METROCREAM, AND METROLOTION AT-A-GLANCE

Strengths: Fragrance-free; the active ingredient (metronidazole) has substantiated research proving its effectiveness for managing the symptoms of rosacea.

Weaknesses: Some rosacea patients won't be able to tolerate this prescription topical drug; the most common side effects include a burning sensation, dryness, transient redness, a metallic taste in the mouth, and nausea; metronidazole is not recommended for use by pregnant or lactating women.

For more information, call (866) 735-4137 or visit www.metrogel.com or www.Beautypedia.com. Note: If metronidazole does not work for you, talk to your dermatologist about other prescription options for rosacea, including azelaic acid (Finacea), oral antibiotics such as tetracycline and its derivatives, and topical products containing sulfur (though these tend to be the most irritating and drying and should be considered a last resort, assuming your skin can tolerate this ingredient at all).

☺ **$$$ MetroGel 0.75%** *($54.99 for 60 grams)* contains the active ingredient metronidazole in a simple, water-based gel formula that is excellent for someone with oily skin. It is indicated for twice daily usage.

☺ **$$$ MetroGel 1%** *($94.99 for 45 grams)* is similar to the MetroGel 0.75% above, except the base formula contains a tiny amount of the cell-communicating ingredient niacinamide. This higher concentration of metronidazole is recommended for use once per day. Promotional materials for this drug mention the term *betadex*. This ingredient is based around b-cyclodextrin, which is derived from starch and enhances penetration of the active ingredient into the skin.

☺ **$$$ MetroCream 0.75%** *($113.26 for 45 grams)* contains the active ingredient (metronidazole) in a simple emollient base that is best for someone with dry skin.

☺ **$$$ MetroLotion 0.75%** *($101.53 for 59 ml)* is great for someone with normal to dry skin and contains the same active ingredient as the MetroCream and MetroGel above. This version has the silkiest finish thanks to its silicone content.

MINERAL MAKEUP

Mineral makeup has become a sizzling hot topic. Infomercials glorify its attributes demonstrating magic results with a swift brushed-on application, and there are online chat rooms dedicated to the topic. With all this buzz, it's no wonder that cosmetics companies of all sizes are being created, or simply jumping on the mineral makeup bandwagon, all launching their own versions to try and catch the consumer's eye.

When all is said and done, mineral makeup is truly nothing all that revolutionary or failsafe. By any name, technically speaking, mineral makeup is simply a type of powder foundation. If you wear a light layer as a finishing powder or if you put a little more on, it basically works like a layer of foundation providing light to medium coverage. In essence, mineral makeup is merely loose or pressed powder created from a blend of "powdery" substances.

While the minerals in many mineral makeup products are not run of the mill, it is important to know that most pressed powders, whether they are called mineral makeup or not, are made of minerals. Talc is the primary ingredient in most standard powders, and talc, most assuredly, is as natural a mineral as you can get. However, the clamor over "mineral makeup" argues that the minerals being in those special products are unique, natural, and far better for skin, and that is absolutely not the case!

More than any other makeup product, mineral makeup's claims revolve around what it does not contain, rather than around what it does contain. The companies that sell mineral makeup often warn consumers about how other companies' loose or pressed powders are tainted by the presence of talc (even though it's a natural earth mineral), fragrance, fillers, and "harsh chemical dyes," and that is also not true. According to most of the catalogs and Web sites selling mineral makeup I've seen, they all want you to believe that their's is the ideal product, and that it contains only the good and none of the "bad," while simultaneously being the perfect choice for every skin type and skin-care problem or concern.

Here is what you need to know: Of the more popular mineral makeup lines—such as Youngblood, bare escentuals, Jane Iredale, Monave, Larenim, Baresense, Sheer Cover by Leeza Gibbons, Glominerals, Pur Minerals, Emani, Colorflo, Skin Alison Raffaele, Aromaleigh, Colorscience, Neutrogena, L'Oreal, and Everyday Minerals—whether their powder is pressed or loose powder, they tend to contain the same basic ingredients: bismuth oxychloride, mica, titanium dioxide, and zinc oxide.

The standard primary ingredient in most mineral makeups is bismuth oxychloride, which is not found in nature and is not any better for skin than talc. In fact, talc is natural, and in many ways a far more unadulterated and pure ingredient than bismuth oxychloride. Bismuth oxychloride is manufactured by combining bismuth (which rarely occurs in its elemental form in nature), obtained as a by-product of lead and copper metal refining (dregs of the smelting process if you will), with chloride (a compound of chlorine) and water. The *International Cosmetic Ingredient Dictionary and Handbook* (11th Edition, 2006) lists bismuth oxychloride as a synthetic. It's used in cosmetics because it has a distinct shimmery, pearlescent appearance and a fine white powder texture that adheres well to skin. On the downside, bismuth oxychloride is heavier than talc and can look cakey on skin. And for some people, the bismuth and chloride combination can be irritating.

Bismuth itself is a metallic element chemically similar to poisonous arsenic. However, that is more shocking than it is significant, but that is the kind of fact that mineral makeup companies use to scare you about the ingredients in other powders not deemed "mineral makeup." Just like cosmetic-grade mineral oil is not related to the crude petroleum from which it originates, neither is bismuth oxychloride identical to bismuth; therefore, its association to arsenic is irrelevant. So the bismuth oxychloride used in cosmetics is indeed non-toxic. This is just a good example of how skewed a company's definition of "natural" can be, and how companies twist factual information to make other cosmetic company ingredients sound harmful.

It is interesting to note that bismuth oxychloride can cause skin irritation (Source: www.sciencelab.com/xMSDS-Bismuth_oxychloride-9923103). Although talc has the same potential for slight irritation, bismuth oxychloride is more likely to cause an allergic contact dermatitis because of its pearlescent nature (Source: www.emedicine.com/derm/topic502.htm). This is more of a concern when bismuth oxychloride is the main ingredient in a cosmetic, as it is for many mineral makeups.

Companies that sell mineral makeup (i.e., mineral makeup that does not contain talc) often claim that the talc other companies use in their pressed and loose powders is harmful and carcinogenic, but let me assure you that there is absolutely no research to support that hysteria, not in the least. There is epidemiological evidence that frequent use of pure talc over the female genital area may increase the risk of ovarian cancer (Sources: *International Journal of Cancer*, November 2004, pages 458–464; and *Anticancer Research*, March–April 2003, pages 1955–1960), but this evidence does not prove a direct link, and further research has shown that this epidemiological evidence is questionable. A comprehensive review of several studies in *Regulatory Toxicology and Pharmacology* (August 2002, pages 40–50) notes that "Talc is not genotoxic, is not carcinogenic when injected into ovaries of rats. There is no credible evidence of a cancer risk from inhalation of cosmetic talc by humans."

Dismissing talc as a cheap, inelegant, less desirable, filler material is inaccurate because talc is the essential backbone for a number of the most luxurious-feeling powders from dozens of lines ranging from L'Oreal to Chanel. The best among those powders have a softness and virtually seamless finish on the skin that most mineral makeup lines should envy. The higher grades of talc are not "filler" materials; they are essential to creating a powder's gossamer texture and skinlike finish.

Some mineral makeup powders contain a 25% concentration of titanium dioxide and/or zinc oxide for sunscreen protection, and that's great because these are excellent non-irritating sunscreen ingredients (Sources: *Cosmetics & Toiletries*, October 2003, pages 73–78; and *Cutis*, September 2004, pages 13–16 and 32–34).

Most mineral makeups provide opaque coverage (which can be blended to achieve light to medium coverage), yet the claim is that they do so while looking extremely natural, like a second skin or better than your own skin. This does appear to be the case in pictures and on TV infomercials (just like every other makeup application created for advertising), but in real life, that is not what you will actually see. These powders (most of which are tricky to blend because they tend to "grab" onto skin and don't glide very well once they are in place) can be applied sheer, but the very nature of their ingredients results in a textured application that can look powdery and "made-up" on the skin. This is especially true if you have patches of dry skin because these mineral powders exacerbate dryness and flaking despite the fact that many claim to be moisturizing, which is just ludicrous given the properties of all powder materials, which are absorbent not moisturizing.

For those with oily skin, mineral makeup can pool in pores and look thick and layered, just like any powder. Generally speaking, mineral makeup is best for normal to slightly oily skin (meaning no signs of dryness and little to no problem oily areas).

Most of the skin-care attributes ascribed to mineral makeup are due to some tangential research about zinc oxide. There is no question that zinc oxide has healing properties for skin (it is FDA-approved as a skin protectant, and is a common active ingredient in ointments to treat diaper rash), but those healing properties have to do with skin whose barrier has been compromised, such as with wounds, ulcers, or rashes. In those cases, zinc oxide facilitates healing (Source: *Wound Repair and Regeneration*, January/February 2007, pages 2–16). But those studies don't use other minerals, such as mica or bismuth oxychloride, or have anything to do with healthy, intact skin. Zinc oxide is definitely a great sunscreen ingredient and protects skin from both UVA and UVB sun damage, with minimal to no risk of irritation, and that has immense value. But that can be said of any product that contains enough zinc oxide to deserve a decent SPF rating.

Mineral makeup is often recommended for those with rosacea, but the irritation potential from bismuth oxychloride is something to pay attention to. Many women may have success using powder as a foundation, and mineral makeup is included in this category. Mineral makeup, especially those rated SPF 15 or greater, can be a three-in-one product (foundation/powder/sunscreen) that can be somewhat easy to apply once you get the knack of it, but it is not a slam-dunk or panacea for all skin types.

One word of warning: As is true for any product with an SPF rating, to get the right amount of thorough protection, liberal application is essential, which means a sheer, light layer of mineral makeup, no matter its SPF rating, won't provide your skin with enough protection from the sun.

MURAD (SKIN CARE ONLY)

MURAD AT-A-GLANCE

Strengths: A few good water-soluble cleansers; a selection of well-formulated AHA products centered on glycolic acid; most of Murad's top-rated products are fragrance-free; the sunscreens go beyond the basics and include several antioxidants for enhanced protection.

Weaknesses: Expensive; no other dermatologist-designed line has more problem products than Murad and no conscientious doctor would or should be selling products using the ludicrous claims Murad makes; irritating ingredients are peppered throughout the selection of products, keeping several of them from earning a recommendation.

For more information about Murad, call (888) 996-8723 or visit www.murad.com or www.Beautypedia.com.

☹ **Clarifying Cleanser** *($26 for 6.75 ounces)* contains essential oils that have antibacterial properties, but they're also very irritating. In addition to the lemon, bitter orange, and lime oils, this irritation-waiting-to-happen cleanser contains menthol.

☹ **Energizing Pomegranate Cleanser** *($25 for 5.1 ounces)* irritates rather than energizes because this liquid-to-foam cleanser lists alcohol as the second ingredient. Further, it doesn't even do a good job at cleansing!

☹ **Essential-C Cleanser** *($35 for 6.75 ounces)* states it is designed to soothe environmentally stressed skin, but the orange, basil, and grapefruit peel oils do just the opposite, making this a nonessential cleanser.

☺ **$$$ Moisture Rich Cleanser** *($27 for 6.75 ounces)* is one of the only Murad cleansers that does not contain one or more problematic ingredients. This is a slightly creamy but water-soluble cleanser for normal to dry skin not prone to blemishes. The rosemary and grapefruit extracts aren't the best additives, but they're not going to bother skin like they would if they were used in their essential oil form.

☺ **$$$ Refreshing Cleanser** *($29 for 6.75 ounces)* is a very standard, but good, water-soluble cleanser for normal to oily skin. It does not contain fragrance, but does include fragrant plant extracts. The amount of glycolic acid will not function as an exfoliant.

☹ **Renewing Cleansing Cream** *($35 for 6.75 ounces)* isn't that creamy and will cause irritation because it contains lime, orange, tangerine, rosewood, and buchu oils (the buchu oil includes camphor).

☹ **Soothing Gel Cleanser** *($25 for 6.75 ounces)* irritates rather than soothes due to the number of volatile fragrant oils, along with the potent menthol derivative menthoxypropanediol. Murad sells this as their redness-relieving cleanser, which is unbelievable.

☺ **$$$ AHA/BHA Exfoliating Cleanser** *($35 for 6.75 ounces)* can be a good cleanser for normal to dry skin, but the amount of jojoba oil makes it slightly difficult to rinse without the aid of a washcloth. This contains dissolving beads which exfoliate skin; the AHAs and BHA will not exfoliate because this cleanser is rinsed from the skin before they can be of much benefit.

☹ **Clarifying Toner** *($21 for 6 ounces)* lists witch hazel as the second ingredient and also contains menthol and its derivative, menthoxypropanediol. The citronella oil doesn't help matters, and certainly isn't clarifying.

☹ **Essential-C Toner** *($30 for 6 ounces)* contains a lot of witch hazel and lesser, but still problematic, amounts of citrus and basil oils. This will not balance stressed skin!

😐 **$$$ Hydrating Toner** *($23 for 6 ounces)* offers skin some helpful water-binding agents, but the amount of witch hazel is potentially problematic and keeps this otherwise well-done toner for normal to dry skin from earning a higher rating.

☺ **$$$ Intensive Wrinkle Reducer** *($150 for 1 ounce)* may be one of the most expensive AHA products around, though it's definitely an effective one, containing at least 10% glycolic acid in a gel base with a pH of 3.2. The formula also contains several outstanding water-binding agents and plenty of antioxidants along with some good anti-irritants. It's a suitable option for all skin types, but you don't need to spend this much money to enjoy the benefits of AHAs. This product did not rate a Paula's Pick because it contains cinnamon bark extract and fragrance components that can be irritating to skin. Cinnamon has antioxidant ability, but its irritation potential when applied topically doesn't help move this product to the top of the must-have list.

☹ **Age-Balancing Night Cream** *($80 for 1.7 ounces)*. Age Balancing? At what age does age become imbalanced? And, more to the point, can a moisturizer do anything to balance one's age? Of course not. This is another moisturizer with wild yam extract, directed toward those with peri-menopausal and menopausal skin. You might as well use the wild yams for your Thanksgiving feast because they have not been demonstrated to have any effectiveness when used on skin.

Murad also puts the spotlight on chaparral extract, stating that it is clinically proven to slow down the growth of facial hair. Chaparral is extracted from a desert plant whose leaves (like those of most plants) contain antioxidant compounds. Topical application of chaparral is known to cause contact dermatitis (Source: www.naturaldatabase.com), and it's the fourth ingredient listed in this product. There's not a shred of published research on chaparral's alleged ability to slow facial hair growth, though according to Murad it can reduce hair growth by 22%. Even if that were true, is a 22% reduction what you would consider significant? This moisturizer is also a perplexing mix of good-for-skin and bad-for-skin ingredients, including several antioxidants and retinol as well as several irritating essential oils. There is no logical reason to consider this product.

☹ **Age-Diffusing Serum** *($70 for 1 ounce)* does have a lot going for it when you consider this water-based AHA serum's level of silicones, range of antioxidants, and several water-binding agents. Yet, like so many Murad products, too many irritating ingredients that have no benefit for skin corrupt its good start. Clove flower and iris extracts are the prime offenders, and further down on the ingredient list orange, lime, tangerine, and rosewood oils are joined by buchu leaf oil, which contains camphor as a major constituent. How disappointing!

☹ **Cellular Replenishing Serum** *($49 for 1 ounce)* is a water-based serum that contains a bountiful selection of water-binding agents and some good antioxidants. Why Murad added irritants such as ivy, arnica, and the allergenic plant pellitory-of-the-wall is a good question, because they keep this product from being recommended.

☹ **Combination Skin Treatment** *($55 for 3.4 ounces)* lists alcohol as the second ingredient, which isn't the way to treat oily and dry areas of skin. The amount of glycolic acid is enough to prompt exfoliation, but the alcohol makes this an irritating way to get smoother skin.

☹ **Correcting Moisturizer SPF 15** *($35 for 1.7 ounces)* provides broad-spectrum sun protection via its in-part zinc oxide sunscreen. The base formula isn't too exciting, and this is a poor option for all skin types because of the peppermint extract and lemon peel oil.

☹ **Day Reform Treatment** *($65 for 1 ounce)* is a silky, silicone-based serum with retinol and tiny amounts of a few other antioxidants. It is not recommended over other retinol serums because it contains too much tannic acid. According to www.naturaldatabase.com, "Tannic acid has astringent effects. It dehydrates tissue, internally reducing secretions, and externally forming a protective layer of harder, constricted cells." That's not what you want from a product that pledges to reverse the damage caused by environmental elements.

☺ **Energizing Pomegranate Moisturizer SPF 15** *($30 for 2 ounces)* contains an in-part avobenzone sunscreen in a lightweight lotion formula suitable for normal to slightly oily skin. Pomegranate is a very good antioxidant; it's a shame there isn't more of it in here. Still, this is one of the few Murad products not waylaid by needless irritants, and it contains some effective soothing agents. It does contain fragrance.

☹ **Essential-C Daily Renewal Complex** *($90 for 1 ounce)* is another formula that should make you question Dr. Murad's formulary expertise. This silicone-based moisturizer contains several light- and air-sensitive ingredients (including retinol), yet it's packaged in a jar. The orange, grapefruit peel, basil, and galbanum oils included here may smell nice, but they also may cause skin irritation.

☹ **Essential-C Day Moisture SPF 15** *($55 for 1.7 ounces)* contains the same irritating essential oils as the Essential-C Daily Renewal Complex above, and the same review applies.

☹ **Essential-C Eye Cream SPF 15** *($65 for 0.5 ounce)* lacks the UVA-protecting ingredients of titanium dioxide, zinc oxide, avobenzone, Tinosorb, or Mexoryl SX, and is not recommended.

☹ **Essential-C Night Moisture** *($58 for 1.7 ounces)* isn't the least bit essential despite containing some proven antioxidants for skin. The pros are just overwhelmed by the cons, which include irritation from the inclusion of several fragrant oils, including lavender, thyme, and grapefruit.

☺ **$$$ Eye Treatment Complex SPF 8** *($58 for 0.5 ounce)* includes an in-part titanium dioxide sunscreen, but an SPF rating that's embarrassingly low, especially from a dermatologist-developed line. The pH of 4 is borderline but still allows the approximately 8% concentration of glycolic acid to exfoliate. The SPF rating is the only weak spot in an otherwise well-formulated, antioxidant-rich, fragrance-free product for normal to dry skin.

☹ **Moisture Silk Eye Gel** *($49 for 0.5 ounce)* has many excellent, skin-friendly ingredients such as silicones, water-binding agents, and an anti-irritant, all in a silky gel-based formula. Yet all of this is for naught because Murad couldn't resist adding cassia, grapefruit peel, orange, and bitter orange oils—all potent skin irritants that should not be used near the eye area. This also contains a greater amount of caffeine than many products, which won't wake up the eye, but will increase the potential for irritation.

☹ **Moisturizing Acne Treatment Gel** *($42 for 2.65 ounces)* contains a less-than-desirable amount of salicylic acid, as well as a pH that's too high for exfoliation to occur. But the biggest offense is the inclusion of skin cell–damaging lavender oil.

✓☺ **$$$ Night Reform Treatment** *($65 for 1 ounce)* is an outstanding fragrance-free AHA product for all skin types, but the texture is best for normal to very oily skin. Approximately 10% glycolic acid and a pH of 3.5 help create smoother, softer, even-toned skin, while the numerous antioxidants and anti-irritants provide further benefit. The cost is the only drawback, but at least you're getting more for your money than just another functional AHA product.

☹ **Perfecting Day Cream SPF 30** *($44 for 1.7 ounces)* contains hydrogen peroxide and lavender oil, two ingredients capable of causing skin-cell death and free-radical damage. There are plenty of well-formulated sunscreens with avobenzone that omit problematic ingredients, so choosing this option would just be an expensive mistake.

☺ **$$$ Perfecting Night Cream** *($46 for 1.7 ounces)* is a very good, fragrance-free moisturizer for normal to dry skin. It would be rated a Paula's Pick if it contained more antioxidants. However, this contains some outstanding plant oils, and a few good water-binding agents.

😐 **$$$ Perfecting Serum** *($60 for 1 ounce)* provides normal to very dry skin types with many of the ingredients needed to ensure a healthy barrier and allow skin to repair itself. It's a shame the clear glass bottle will compromise the effectiveness of the vitamin A and antioxidant-rich plant oils. However, the ceramides and lipids will make dry skin look and feel better.

☹ **Recovery Treatment Gel** *($50 for 1.7 ounces)* is supposed to fortify delicate, sensitive skin and make it feel comfortable, but that's not going to happen when you add peppermint, lemon peel oil, and hydrogen peroxide to the mix.

😐 **$$$ Renewing Eye Cream** *($70 for 0.5 ounce)* includes some good moisturizing agents for normal to dry skin, though none of them are capable of firming skin or diminishing puffiness. The amount of iris and clover extracts is potentially irritating, while the amount of the most intriguing ingredients isn't as impressive as it could have been.

☹ **Sheer Lustre Day Moisture SPF 15** *($67 for 1.7 ounces)* is an in-part avobenzone sunscreen that contains far too many problematic, and often photosensitizing, ingredients to make it a smart choice for daytime wear. Putting lemon and tangerine oils in a sunscreen is just asking for trouble. Price notwithstanding, this would have been highly recommended if it did not contain so many irritants.

☹ **Skin Perfecting Lotion** *($33 for 1.7 ounces)* would be a much better moisturizer with retinol if it did not contain so much arnica extract. Arnica does not reduce redness or clogged pores, as claimed. It can cause irritation due to its volatile components and the amount of data compiled for this ingredient isn't sufficient to support its use or efficacy (Source: *2007 CIR Compendium*).

☺ **$$$ Firming Bronzer SPF 15, for Face and Body** *($48 for 3.4 ounces)* is a good, though pricey, sunscreen for normal to dry skin, and it's cost means you probably won't apply it liberally, which in turn means that you won't be getting sufficient sun protection. Avobenzone is on hand for sufficient UVA protection, and cosmetic and mineral pigments are included for a sheer bronze tint and shimmery finish. (The color is fairly natural, but it can be too peachy for very fair skin.) This sunscreen does not contain a self-tanning ingredient, just cosmetic pigments for color. Murad claims this increases skin's firmness by 32% in just 15 minutes, but because none of the ingredients in this product make skin firmer, you'll be waiting a lot longer than that for no improvement. However, keeping skin protected from sunlight will discourage the breakdown of collagen and elastin, and that helps prevent skin from sagging.

☹ **Oil-Free Sunblock SPF 15 Sheer Tint** *($25 for 1.7 ounces)* has so much going for it, including a pure titanium dioxide sunscreen, soft tint, and copious antioxidants to keep skin protected from inflammation, so it doesn't make a shred of sense that several irritating ingredients were included, too. Grapefruit, lavender, thyme, and orange oils all have their share of problems for skin, and make this sunscreen impossible to recommend.

☹ **Oil-Free Sunblock SPF 30** *($30 for 1.7 ounces)* is built around synthetic sunscreen ingredients, including avobenzone for UVA protection. However, the roster of irritants is the same as for the Oil-Free Sunblock SPF 15 Sheer Tint above; therefore, this is not recommended.

☹ **Waterproof Sunblock SPF 30 for Face and Body** *($30 for 4.3 ounces)* is similar to the Oil-Free Sunblock SPF 30 above, except it is water-resistant. The irritants still make this an ill-advised product for all skin types.

☹ **Acne Spot Treatment** *($17 for 0.5 ounce)* lists 3% sulfur as the active ingredient, which makes this spot treatment an irritating, drying experience for skin (though sulfur can kill acne-causing bacteria). This has merit as a pH-correct AHA product, but it isn't worth considering over other AHA products that don't contain additional irritants.

☹ **Age Spot and Pigment Lightening Gel** *($58 for 1 ounce)* is a very expensive skin-lightening product that contains 2% hydroquinone. The problem is the alcohol base, which makes this gel too irritating for all skin types. Paula's Choice Clearly Remarkable Skin Lightening Gel ($14.95 for 2 ounces) contains the same amount of active ingredient along with salicylic acid to help exfoliate, and no needlessly irritating ingredients.

☹ **Anti-Aging Acne Treatment** *($53 for 1.7 ounces)* contains approximately 1% hydrogen peroxide, an ingredient that is problematic as a topical disinfectant because it can greatly reduce the production of healthy new skin cells (Source: *Plastic and Reconstructive Surgery, September* 2001, pages 675–687). Moreover, as an unstable oxidizing agent, it is a significant generator of free-radical damage. A dermatologist selling an antiwrinkle product that can generate free-radical damage is like an oncologist selling cigarettes. In addition, this product also contains several plant oils (including grapefruit, clove, and sage) that are irritating to skin and can delay the healing process for those with acne. All of this amounts to an expensive risk for skin from a product that won't keep blemishes at bay and can cause undue irritation.

☹ **Clarifying Mask** *($35 for 2.65 ounces)* lists 4% sulfur as the active ingredient, which makes this an incredibly drying, irritating mask for acne-prone skin, or for any skin. Sulfur is joined by camphor and lavender oil, which are as appropriate for blemishes as using bacon grease to absorb excess facial oil.

☹ **Exfoliating Acne Treatment Gel** *($53 for 3.4 ounces)* features 1% salicylic acid as the active ingredient, but it's in a base that's mostly water and alcohol, and the arnica extract isn't helpful for any skin type. The anti-irritants in this gel can't compete with the problematic ingredients.

☹ **Exfoliating Fruit Enzyme Mask** *($30 for 1.7 ounces)* contains the enzymes papain and bromelain, both of which are unstable, and both of which have no substantiated research indicating they could be as adept at exfoliating as well-formulated AHA or BHA products, or even a topical scrub. That's not a deal-breaker, but the inclusion of geranium and pine oils is.

☹ **Lighten and Brighten Eye Treatment** *($75 for 0.5 ounce)* contains 1.5% hydroquinone as the active ingredient. Hydroquinone is adept at lightening melanin-based skin discolorations, whether they result from sun exposure or hormonal influence. However, this product is positioned as being able to lighten dark circles under the eyes, and hydroquinone cannot do that. Some people may have darkness under the eyes that results from excess pigmentation, but most cases of dark circles result from microscopic blood vessels showing through the very thin skin under the eyes. There's also the fact that this area is naturally shadowed just because of the way our skulls are shaped, as well as the fact that the infraorbital fat pads thin over time, which creates a sunken, hollow appearance. None of this is affected by topical application of hydroquinone. Not only is that disappointing in regard to this product, but also the inclusion of several irritating oils is completely wrong for use anywhere on skin, especially near the eyes.

☹ **Post-Acne Spot Lightening Gel** *($58 for 1 ounce)* could have been an effective option for treating hyperpigmentation because it contains 2% hydroquinone along with a good amount of glycolic acid. However, the amount of alcohol makes this too irritating for all skin types. If you're keen on spa or salon lines, the skin-lightening products from Peter Thomas Roth (reviewed in this book) are much better formulations.

☹ **Energizing Pomegranate Lip Therapy SPF 15** *($16 for 0.5 ounce)* lacks the UVA-protecting ingredients of titanium dioxide, zinc oxide, avobenzone, Tinosorb, or Mexoryl SX, and is not recommended.

☹ **Soothing Skin and Lip Therapy** *($13 for 0.5 ounce)* lists benzyl cinnamate as the second ingredient. This is the chief fragrant component of balsam peru, and can be very irritating to skin and lips.

☹ **Firm and Tone Serum** *($65 for 6.75 ounces).* The ingredient list for this product is a "who's who" of skin-beneficial and skin-detrimental additives. Firm and Tone Serum claims to minimize body imperfections ranging from cellulite to stretch marks and sagging skin, leaving you "proud to show off." I wouldn't bank on this water- and alcohol-based concoction for any amount of body perfection, especially when you consider the amount of irritation your skin will experience from the peppermint, menthol, and several fragrant, volatile oils that have no established benefit for skin. Last, but not least, this product also contains esculin, a component of horse chestnut, which is considered toxic and is not recommended for topical application (Source: *Ellenhorn's Medical Toxicology: Diagnoses and Treatment of Human Poisoning*, 2nd Edition, Baltimore, MD: Williams & Wilkins, 1997).

NARS

NARS At-a-Glance

Strengths: One good cleanser and lip balm; great range of foundation shades; the powder blush; the lipsticks, including a sheer option with broad-spectrum sunscreen; some of the makeup brushes are excellent.

Weaknesses: Expensive; jar packaging; drying cleansers and irritating toners and mask; no exfoliants; no sunscreens; ineffective skin-lightening products; average to poor pencils; the liquid liner; single eyeshadows; mascaras that are not impressive given their cost.

For more information about NARS, owned by Shiseido, call (888) 903-6277 or visit www.narscosmetics.com or www.Beautypedia.com.

NARS Skin Care

😐 **$$$ Balancing Foam Cleanser** *($33 for 4.2 ounces)* is a standard, detergent-based cleanser that can be more drying than most due to the amount of potassium hydroxide. The orange oil prevents this cleanser from being a safe bet for use around the eyes. It's an OK option for normal to oily skin.

😐 **$$$ Gentle Cream Cleanser** *($35 for 4.2 ounces)* is gentle in name only. This water-soluble cleanser is quite similar to the Balancing Foam Cleanser above, except it contains some additional thickening agents. Otherwise, the same comments apply.

☹ **Purifying Soap** *($22 for a 6.7-ounce bar)* is a standard, detergent- and tallow-based, highly alkaline soap that can be drying and irritating for most skin types.

😐 **$$$ Softening Milk Cleanser** *($35 for 6.7 ounces)* is the best among NARS's cleansers, but that isn't saying much. This basic, cold cream–style milky cleanser removes makeup with mineral oil and other emollients, and contains a small amount of detergent cleansing agents. A washcloth may be needed for complete removal, but this is an option for normal to dry skin.

☺ **$$$ Eye Makeup Remover** *($24.50 for 3 ounces)* is a very standard, but effective, water- and silicone-based fluid that removes most types of makeup. The inclusion of fragrant plant extracts isn't the best, and the price is extraordinary for what amounts to ordinary. This is easily replaced with better formulas for far less money.

☹ **Balancing Toning Lotion** *($32.50 for 6.7 ounces)* lists alcohol as the second ingredient and contains isopropyl alcohol, too, for a double whammy, plus camphor and eucalyptus oil. Ouch!

☹ **Hydrating Freshening Lotion** *($35 for 6.7 ounces)* omits the camphor and eucalyptus oil in the Balancing Toning Lotion above, but contains too much alcohol to be even a little hydrating. This is just irritating.

☹ **Balancing Moisture Lotion** *($55 for 2.5 ounces)* contains more alcohol and potassium hydroxide than it does any beneficial ingredients. The antioxidants are present in such teeny amounts that they are meaningless for skin.

😐 **$$$ Brightening Serum** *($59 for 2.5 ounces)* contains enough talc to leave a slight white cast on skin, which is what "visibly brightens skin after one application." This is otherwise a standard, overpriced, silicone-based moisturizer that lacks truly beneficial ingredients for skin.

☹ **Essential Vitamin Serum** *($75 for 2.5 ounces)* irritates skin with alcohol and contains more film-forming agents (the same kind used in hairstyling products) than vitamins or anything else beneficial for skin. This is just an overpriced waste of time.

😐 **$$$ Hydrating Moisture Cream** *($72 for 3.4 ounces)* is an OK emollient moisturizer for normal to dry skin. The jar packaging won't keep the tiny amount of antioxidant vitamins stable.

😐 **$$$ Lightening Cream** *($98 for 3.5 ounces)* does not contain any ingredients capable of lightening skin discolorations. Even the form of vitamin C used (ascorbyl glucoside) has minimal research proving its worth for pigmentation issues, and the jar packaging won't keep it stable during use. That leaves you with a very expensive silicone-based moisturizer for normal to slightly dry skin.

😐 **$$$ Nourishing Eye Cream** *($75 for 0.5 ounce)* is an average, jar-packaged moisturizer for normal to slightly dry skin anywhere on the face. The iron oxides (a cosmetic pigment) are what create the "radiant luminosity" the company brags about.

😐 **$$$ Aqua Gel Hydrator** *($76 for 3.4 ounces)* is a water- and silicone-based moisturizer with many of the same problems as the other moisturizers in this line, including jar packaging (a true disappointment with this product, as it contains more antioxidants than other NARS moisturizers). The claim that it contains 87% water is basically letting you know that there isn't much of anything else in here. Plus your skin doesn't need water (healthy skin is only 10% water, and too much water destroys the skin's structure). Rather, the skin needs ingredients that support and enhance its structure, antioxidants to reduce free-radical damage, and sunscreen to prevent sun damage—something this line almost completely ignores.

☹ **Mud Mask** *($45 for 3.4 ounces)* is an exceptionally standard clay mask whose alcohol content makes it even more drying, while the eucalyptus oil causes irritation. The Masada Mud from the Dead Sea may sound impressive, but your skin wouldn't know the difference between mud from that part of the world and mud from Lake Michigan.

☺ **$$$ Rain Lip Treatment** *($23 for 0.14 ounce)* is essentially a colorless emollient lipstick NARS sells as a lip moisturizer. It contains oils and waxes to ensure smooth, flake-free lips, has a nice selection of antioxidants, and is fragrance-free.

😐 **$$$ Sabrina Lip Balm** *($23 for 0.14 ounce)* claims an SPF 20 but because it doesn't list active ingredients you can't rely on it for sun protection. It is otherwise very similar to the Rain Lip Treatment above, and the same basic comments apply. The neutral face rating is for this balm's misleading claim of sun protection.

NARS MAKEUP

FOUNDATION: ☺ **$$$ Powder Foundation SPF 12** *($45; $35 for refills)* has a silky texture and seamless application that is far more advanced than either of NARS other liquid foundations reviewed below. Even better, the talc-free formula's sunscreen is in-part zinc oxide, though SPF 15 is preferred for minimum daytime protection. Still, this deserves a happy face rating for those seeking a pressed-powder foundation to wear over a regular sunscreen or over a foundation with sunscreen. It provides sheer to light coverage and leaves a soft matte finish with a hint of shine. The range of ten shades is mostly gorgeous and suitable for a wide range of skin tones; only Jamaica pulls a bit too copper for its intended dark skin.

☺ **$$$ Balanced Foundation** *($40)* is a very standard water- and oil-based foundation who has a rich but fluid creamy feel and finish. This is appropriate only for those with normal to very dry skin that prefer medium coverage. There are 12 shades, most of which are wonderfully neutral. Avoid Sahara (slightly peach) and Sedona (a bit too red). There are some good options for darker skin tones.

😐 **$$$ Oil Free Foundation** *($40)* really should be updated to make it feel smoother and look more natural on skin. It is oil-free and is best for normal to oily skin, but the liquid texture takes longer than it should to set to a matte finish that still ends up feeling tacky. You'll get light to medium coverage and this is an overall safe foundation to consider if blemishes are an issue. Otherwise, the best attribute of this makeup is the impressive selection of colors—just avoid Sahara, which is too pink and peach for most skin tones. Just as with the Balanced Foundation above, there are some good shades for darker skin tones.

CONCEALER: Those looking to combine concealer and highlighter may enjoy the dual-ended ☺ **$$$ Eye Brightener** *($22)*. Although positioned as a specialty product, it's really just a good liquid concealer with a light, sheer texture and a soft matte finish. Paired with it is a soft, off-white highlighter that can be used on its own or blended with the flesh-toned concealer shade. This duo covers minor imperfections reasonably well, but isn't what you want if hiding blemishes or dark circles is the goal. Six shades are available (the highlighter shade is the same for each) and four are great. Praline is too peach and Toffee is slightly gold, but still worth testing.

The lipstick-style 😐 **$$$ Concealer** *($20)* provides creamy, opaque coverage that can look heavy, as though it's just sitting on skin rather than melding with it. NARS claims this is crease-resistant, but it can indeed slip into the lines around the eyes. If you prefer creamy, lipstick-style concealers, there are some decent colors, but avoid Honey and Praline (both too peachy pink). Toffee is an OK option for darker skin, but may turn slightly copper.

POWDER: ☺ **$$$ Loose Powder** *($33)* remains one of the messier loose powders to use due to its awkward, over-sized packaging and lack of a sifter. This is otherwise a gorgeous talc- and cornstarch-based powder that looks beautifully natural on the skin, with only a trace of shine. The six shades are exemplary—Snow is ideal for very fair skin, but watch out for Mountain, which can be too ash on dark skin (though applied sheer this becomes a non-issue).

☺ **$$$ Pressed Powder** *($28)* has been improved and as a result has been given a higher rating. The talc-based formula shares most of the attributes of the Loose Powder version, including a sheer finish that looks natural rather than powdered. The texture is drier than the Loose Powder, too, but that doesn't affect how nice this looks on skin. All eight shades are superb, though Mountain is tricky due to its stronger yellow tone.

☺ **$$$ Bronzing Powder** *($28)* shares the same positive traits as the pressed powder, and is also talc-based. Two shades are available, each with moderate shine. Laguna is best for fair to light skin, while Casino meshes well with medium to tan skin colors. Although a real tan doesn't sparkle, at least the shine in this bronzer adheres well to skin.

BLUSH: ✓☺ **$$$ Blush** *($25)* is definitely the star attraction of this line and it's easy to see why. These have a splendid texture and apply beautifully with a sheer initial application that builds to any depth of color you want because most of the 25 colors have strong pigment (a plus for women with dark skin). The following shades are almost matte and highly recommended: Amour, Desire, Exhibit A, Gina, Gilda, and Mata Hari. The very shiny shades, which you should consider carefully include Angelika, Crazed, Lovejoy, Mounia, Outlaw, and Torrid. The remaining palette feature shiny shades that aren't the best for daytime makeup, but are great for a sultry evening look.

✓☺ **Color Wash** *($25)* is the NARS version of Benefit's BeneTint liquid blush, but NARS bests Benefit by offering more color choices, and each is suitable for a natural, flushed appearance or subtle lip stain.

☺ **$$$ Creme Blush** *($23)* is definitely creamy but not too thick or greasy. It smooths over skin, delivering sheer color and a radiant finish. Although the colors look way too intense in their compacts, each goes on translucent and layers well if you want a bit more color. You will find that this works best on dry to very dry skin.

EYESHADOW: ☺ **$$$ Duo Eye Shadow** *($31)* has an improved texture and formula that is different (and preferred) to the Single Eye Shadow below. What those lack in silkiness, these more than compensate for, and each duo applies color-true. The number of duos, all of which have some shine, is a bit overwhelming, though the majority of them feature pairings that are too contrasting or just too colorful for day-to-day makeup. The most attractive, versatile duos include All About Eve (great name, even better film), Bellissima, Charade, Key Largo, Madrague, Pacifica, and Tokyo.

😐 **$$$ Single Eye Shadow** *($21)* has a dry but smooth texture, but a somewhat choppy application. Part of the application issue has to do with how deeply pigmented and chalky these shadows are. Stronger colors aren't inherently a problem and can be easily blended if the silkiness and slip is there. Regrettably, that is exactly what is absent here. The good news is there are some nearly matte options and that the shine- and glitter-infused shades cling better than they used to. If you want to experiment with these, the almost-matte shades include Bali, Bengali, Blondie, Lulu, New York, and Sophia.

☺ **$$$ Cream Eye Shadow** *($21)* and ☺ **$$$ Duo Cream Eyeshadow** *($31)* are quite shiny but have a smooth texture and just enough slip to make application and blending easy. However, because the finish stays moist, it won't stay in place and it will fade and crease slightly. If creamy eyeshadows are what you're after but you want longevity, look to Revlon or M.A.C. first.

EYE AND BROW SHAPER: ☺ **$$$ Eyebrow Pencil** *($18)* needs sharpening, but if you're OK with that, all of these have a suitably dry texture and smooth powder finish that stays in place. The three shades present options for blondes and brunettes, but nothing for redheads or those with raven brows.

☹ **Eye Liner Pencils** *($19)* have a too creamy application that is very prone to fading and smearing, and the colors are too unnatural or too clownish to take seriously, at least for most women. ☹ **Glitter Pencil** *($24)* is a fairly creamy, thick pencil infused with flecks of glitter. The glitter tends to separate from the pencil's base formula and chip off onto your face. ☹ **Liquid Liner** *($27.50)* is absurdly priced given the number of superior liquid liners available for less than $10. The NARS version comes in a nail-polish bottle and features an OK brush (that must be assembled prior to use) and mostly wild colors that go on too sheer. Repeated applications are necessary to build intensity, and that increases the odds against precise, even application. Why anyone would bother with this is beyond me—if you want to spend this kind of money on liquid liner, I suggest Lancome's fantastic Artliner ($26.50), but there are less expensive options at the drugstore from L'Oreal and Maybelline.

LIPSTICK, LIP GLOSS, AND LIPLINER: The NARS lipstick collection is supremely good, and if you're willing to tolerate the prices you won't be disappointed by the opulent colors and reasonable wear time. Although there are three kinds of lipsticks, the NARS counter display doesn't separate them, which is frustrating. However, for some reason, if you shop this line at Sephora, you'll find that the various formulas are grouped together and a pleasure to navigate.

✓☺ **$$$ Semi-Mattes** *($23)* are the real standouts here; they have an opaque, slightly creamy finish and a good stain. Creamy lipsticks don't get much better than this, and this formula is available in over 20 colors, including some of the best reds available. ☺ **$$$ Satins** *($23)* are creamy, bordering on greasy, and are fairly opaque yet have a soft gloss finish. ☺ **$$$ Sheers** *($23)* finish glossy, aren't too slick, and offer coverage that is light rather than genuinely sheer. The colors are great.

☺ **$$$ Lip Stain Gloss** *($23)* is for those who love the opacity of traditional lipstick but also want the shiny finish of a lip gloss. This two-in-one product has a slick, silicone-based texture without a trace of stickiness and provides a high gloss shine. The intense colors leave a good stain, but are not for the timid. Think glam to the max and you'll love this!

☺ **$$$ Lip Lacquer** *($23)* isn't the easiest to use due to its glass jar packaging, but its thick, lanolin oil–based texture leaves lips heavily moisturized and beaming, although with a slightly sticky finish that won't be to everyone's liking. The large color palette includes both sheer and strongly pigmented colors, making this one to test before purchasing (the shade names are no help in determining this—what does "Chica Boom" tell you about opacity or color shade?).

☺ **$$$ Lip Therapy SPF 20** *($22.50)* now lists SPF 20 along with active ingredients (something that was a problem for this product in the past) and the sunscreen is in-part titanium dioxide, so this is now recommended as a good, sheer, glossy lipstick that provides broad-spectrum sun protection.

😐 **$$$ Lip Gloss** *($23)* features several bold colors in a sticky, thick formula whose price is unwarranted for what you get, which is just a gloss, and a rather tacky-feeling one at that. If you're going to indulge in a NARS gloss, go for the Lip Lacquer.

😐 **$$$ Velvet Matte Lip Pencil** *($23)* has a beautifully smooth texture that goes on silky and feels light, and has enough creaminess to look soft and still wear comfortably. It isn't a true matte, but velvet matte is a fairly accurate description of this pencil's finish. The shade selection is nicely varied. This pencil's creaminess is enough to pose a slight problem for those prone to lipstick bleeding into lines around the mouth, and the sharpening and resharpening is just not fun, hence the neutral face rating.

😐 **$$$ Lipliner Pencil** *($19)* claims it won't bleed or feather, and although that won't hold true for everyone, this does have a drier finish that should keep those problems in check at least for a few hours. The color selection has been expanded and coordinates well with the many lipsticks (and glosses) this line offers. This would rate a Paula's Pick if it didn't require routine sharpening.

MASCARA: 😐 **$$$ Mascara** *($22)* just doesn't impress enough, at least not for what it costs. You'll be able to build decent length, but this mascara takes time to show its stuff and can be slightly clumpy. There are at least a dozen or more mascaras at the drugstore that significantly out-perform this one.

☹ **Waterproof Mascara** *($22.50)* has characteristics similar to the Mascara above, only this one tends to stick the lashes together and creates a spiky look. This is hardly waterproof either, which is a real letdown given the price.

FACE AND BODY ILLUMINATING/SHIMMER PRODUCTS: 😐 **$$$ The Multiple** *($36.50)* is a chunky, wind-up stick with a creamy yet lightweight texture and soft, sheer colors that would work for cheeks, eyes, and, in some cases, lips. Although all of the colors have varying degrees of shine (and go on softer than they appear in the stick), these are an option for a fun evening look, though the price is extraordinary for what amounts to a soft wash of glow-y color. Sonia Kashuk's namesake line at Target uses the same concept for her Illuminating Color Stick, which is just as worthwhile and sells for one-fourth the price. 😐 **$$$ Body Glow** *($59)* comes in a heavy glass bottle and is just coconut oil with golden bronze shimmer and potent fragrance. It adds a sexy, though oily-feeling, sheen to bare skin and will definitely complement a tan (which hopefully came from a bottle and not from the sun). Be careful, this will rub off on clothing. 😐 **$$$ Monoi Body Glow II** *($59)* was launched because presumably the original Body Glow needed a sequel. Unlike the original, this version has a different scent (it's still very perfume-y) and is colorless. It retains the original's coconut oil base and is a workable, though pricey, body oil option for dry skin. 😐 **$$$ Sparkling Loose Powder** *($35)* is identical to the NARS Loose Powder above, only the single shade is infused with a subtle but sparkling shine. It clings OK, but isn't really worth the money given the number of shiny powders available at the drugstore that work far better. 😐 **$$$ Sparkling Pressed Powder** *($30)* doesn't do much to impress other than adding sparkling shine to skin. It has a smooth but dry texture and a shine that tends to apply unevenly and not stay in place for long. It's an option, but only if you're willing to pay more for fewer positives. As a plus, the three shades are versatile and sheer.

BRUSHES: The **Brushes** *($21--$55)* almost all have a lovely, soft feel and are appropriately shaped for a variety of application techniques. The only ones to steer clear of are the stiff, scratchy ☹ **Brow Brush 05** *($21)* and the ☹ **Retractable Lip Brush 11** *($25)*, which is really too small for most women's lips. ☺ **$$$ Push Eyeliner Brush 02** *($25)* is identical to those found in many other lines, except that NARS charges more, and the 😐 **$$$ Loose Powder Brush 01** *($50)* should have better-quality hair for the money. The best brushes are the synthetic ✓☺ **$$$ Flat Concealer Brush 07** *($25)*, the pricey but luxurious ✓☺ **$$$ Eye Shader Brush 03** *($55)*, and the ✓☺ **$$$Liquid Eyeliner Brush 09** *($21)*.

The ☺ **$$$ Smudge Brush 15** *($24)* has a unique cut and shape that works for smudging or other eyeshadow detail work. It's worth testing if you're in the mood for something different.

SPECIALTY PRODUCTS: ☺ **$$$ Makeup Primer with SPF 20** *($33)* contains an in-part titanium dioxide sunscreen and as such can protect your skin from UVA rays whether worn alone or under a foundation. Because this is a primer, most women will use it under foundation, so the question of whether or not this product "primes" the skin needs to be addressed. The water-in-silicone base formula will leave skin feeling silky-smooth, which will facilitate foundation application and, depending on your skin type and condition, potentially improve wear time. However, many other lightweight moisturizers (with or without sunscreen) do this, too, as such combinations of silicone and lightweight hydrating ingredients are becoming increasingly common. For example, a less expensive option that provides the same feel and finish (minus sunscreen) is Olay's Regenerist Perfecting Cream ($18.99 for 1.7 ounces). This NARS product might have been worth the splurge if it contained an array of antioxidants and other bells and whistles to help skin, but they're in short supply. The orange oil has a slight potential to cause irritation, but is included mostly for fragrance. If you want to audition this, the formula is best for normal to slightly dry or slightly oily skin.

😐 **$$$ Makeup Primer** *($33)* is just an ultra-light moisturizer that supposedly "primes" the skin for foundation. As a moisturizer, it lacks any state-of-the-art water-binding agents or antioxidants and isn't worth considering over the state-of-the art gel-creams and serums offered by many other lines, from Olay to Estee Lauder.

NATURA BISSE (SKIN CARE ONLY)

NATURA BISSE AT-A-GLANCE

Strengths: A few cleansers and eye-makeup remover with intelligent formulations, but prices are outrageous; handful of sun-care products are recommended.

Weaknesses: Very expensive; none of the daytime moisturizers with sunscreen provide sufficient UVA protection; none of the AHA products have pH that allows exfoliation; Brilliance line will not lighten skin; several of the toners are irritating; the masks are redundant and average at best; no products to successfully combat blemishes; jar packaging; ignore the Oxygen and Cytokines products.

For more information about Natura Bisse, call (800) 7-NATURA or visit www.naturabisse.com or www.Beautypedia.com.

NATURA BISSE BRILLIANCE LINE

😐 **$$$ Brilliance Lightening Milk** *($40 for 6.5 ounces)* is shockingly overpriced (a theme that runs through this entire line) for what amounts to a very standard water- and mineral oil–based cleanser. It's an OK option for normal to dry skin not prone to breakouts (the castor oil and thickeners can be a problem), but it will not lighten skin one bit.

☹ **Brilliance Lightening Toner** *($40 for 6.5 ounces)* contains enough alcohol to cause irritation, and that won't firm or balance skin in the least. The lemon extract is also a problem.

☹ **Brilliance Intensive Lightening Complex** *($125 for 1 ounce)* could have been an excellent skin-lightening product because it contains glycolic acid and 2% hydroquinone. However, alcohol as the second ingredient makes this too irritating for all skin types, and the price is a burn, too.

😐 **$$$ Brilliance Nourishing Lightening Cream** *($83 for 1.7 ounces)* is an embarrassingly standard moisturizer that's mostly water, slip agent, and thickeners. The only ingredient with the potential to lighten skin discolorations is the kojic acid (of which there is only a dusting), but the jar packaging will not keep it stable after opening.

☹ **Brilliance SPF 15 Protective Lightening Cream** *($83 for 2.5 ounces)* lacks the UVA-protecting ingredients of titanium dioxide, zinc oxide, avobenzone, Mexoryl SX, or Tinosorb and is not recommended.

😐 **$$$ Brilliance Lightening Finishing Mask** *($49 for 2.5 ounces)* is a very standard moisturizer for dry skin sold as a special mask. The amount of antioxidants is OK, but none of the ingredients offer help for hyperpigmented skin.

NATURA BISSE C+C VITAMIN LINE

😐 **$$$ C+C Vitamin Complex, Concentrate Serum with Double Vitamin C** *($145 for 4 0.2-ounce vials)* is a ridiculously overpriced product that contains ascorbic acid in powder form as the source of vitamin C. You are supposed to mix it into a solution of slip agents, fragrant orange extract, silicone, soy, glycoproteins, more vitamin C, film-forming agent, and preservatives. If you're looking for vitamin C this is fine, but lots and lots of products contain it with a lot less cumbersome application process. The soy has antioxidant ability and the glycoproteins are good water-binding agents, but no better than lots of other water-binding agents.

☹ **C+C Vitamin Cream SPF 10** *($92 for 2.5 ounces)* lacks the UVA-protecting ingredients of titanium dioxide, zinc oxide, avobenzone, Mexoryl SX, or Tinosorb and is not recommended.

☹ **C+C Vitamin Fluid SPF 10** *($86 for 1.7 ounces)* lacks the UVA-protecting ingredients of titanium dioxide, zinc oxide, avobenzone, Mexoryl SX (ecamsule), or Tinosorb and is not recommended.

NATURA BISSE CYTOKINES LINE

The Cytokines Line products are supposed to contain "Skin Growth Factor," but there isn't one ingredient in them that functions as, is similar to, or has any relation to any type of growth factor. While these do contain some good water-binding agents and tiny amounts of antioxidants, they are not capable of affecting cellular growth or cellular activity in the way cytokines do. In fact, because two of the products contain mostly alcohol and because the sunscreen has an inadequate SPF and is ineffective for UVA protection, your skin cells will be decreasing, not increasing.

In regard to cytokines, these are not a type of specific ingredient, rather they are diverse, potent, and extremely complex, multifaceted chemical messengers (there are thousands) secreted by the cells of the immune system that stimulate the production of other substances to help protect the body. Cytokines encourage cell growth, promote cell activation, direct cellular traffic, and destroy target cells—including cancer cells. Interleukins, transforming growth factor, and interferon are types of cytokines. It is also important to point out that cytokines can also cause unwanted, potentially serious side effects (Sources: www.medlineplus.com; and National Cancer Institute, www.nci.nih.gov or www.cancer.gov). Even the notion that skin-care products can directly affect cytokine production in a way to change the appearance of skin is a scary thought, given that cosmetic ingredients are not tested for safety in any way like pharmaceuticals or drugs are. There is nothing in these products that can positively affect the skin's immune system or growth structure, but what they do contain are ingredients that are detrimental to skin all on their own.

☹ **Cytokines Top Ten Complex** *($135 for 1 ounce)* lists alcohol as the third ingredient and contains the Kathon CG preservative duo that is not recommended for use in leave-on products due to its sensitizing potential.

☹ **Cytokines Top Ten Cream SPF 10** *($75 for 2.5 ounces)* lacks the UVA-protecting ingredients of titanium dioxide, zinc oxide, avobenzone, Mexoryl SX, or Tinosorb and as such doesn't belong in anyone's top ten! This also contains problematic preservatives.

☹ **Cytokines Top Ten Eye** ($75 *for 0.8 ounce)* lists alcohol as the third ingredient, which kills, not renews, skin cells. This is too irritating to use anywhere near the eye, and does not contain 5% growth factor as claimed, an omission that is actually a good thing for your skin.

NATURA BISSE DIAMOND LINE

☺ **$$$ Diamond Bio-Lift Eye Contour Cream** *($137 for 0.8 ounce)* claims to inhibit the progressive loss of firmness, reduce the appearance of wrinkles (that's what almost every moisturizer claims to do), and protect against new wrinkles. For daytime, the latter cannot be accomplished without a sunscreen, something this emollient moisturizer for dry skin lacks. Although this contains some good antioxidants, they can't stop skin from losing firmness and the jar packaging won't keep them stable during use.

☺ **$$$ Diamond Cream** *($250 for 1.7 ounces)* is similar to the Diamond Bio-Lift Eye Contour Cream above, except this has even more antioxidants and some good cell-communicating ingredients. It's actually an impressive formula, but the jar packaging means that the high-tech ingredients won't remain stable during use, making this a very expensive disappointment.

☹ **Diamond Drops** *($300 for 1.7 ounces)* contains DNA, but thankfully this cannot alter your skin's DNA (doing so could lead to all kinds of problems, including cancer or tumors). The main drawback (besides the ridiculous price) is the inclusion of cell-damaging lavender oil. Between that and the lack of elegant ingredients in this serum, it's a great big "Why bother?"

☺ **$$$ Diamond Extreme** *($300 for 1.7 ounces)* is said to apply a global approach to anti-aging, but what does that mean and how does it help skin? As far as this product is concerned, it ends up being gibberish because this is merely a standard, banal moisturizer for dry to very dry skin. It is recommended only if you relish wasting money on skin-care products that can't deliver results. The few antioxidants in here are compromised by jar packaging, thus leaving your skin begging for more. All in all, this is about as extreme as a macaroni and cheese dinner.

☺ **$$$ Diamond Gel-Cream** *($250 for 1.7 ounces)* has a silky, lightweight texture those with normal to oily skin will appreciate, but the numerous antioxidants will soon deteriorate because of the jar packaging. The amount of alcohol in here carries a small risk of causing irritation.

☹ **Diamond Ice-Lift DNA Cryo-Mask** *($140 for 3.5 ounces)* has a fancy name that may make you think you're getting a futuristic product to vanquish wrinkles, but that's not the case. Instead, skin is inflamed and irritated because this standard, peel-off mask contains polyvinyl alcohol (a hair-spray type ingredient), lavender oil, and the menthol derivative menthyl lactate.

NATURA BISSE ESSENTIAL SHOCK PRODUCTS

☺ **$$$ Essential Shock Complex + Isoflavones, Intensive Anti-Aging Firming Treatment** *($170 for 1 ounce)* is based around fermented bacteria derived from lactic acid, but there is no research anywhere proving this is an essential ingredient for skin or that it is capable of restoring firmness or elasticity. The company brags that this product contains collagen and elastin in their free form, but free or not, these molecules cannot penetrate skin and restore supplies of age-depleted collagen and elastin. At best, this is a lightweight serum for all skin types that contains a frustrating mix of antioxidants (good) and volatile fragrance components (not good).

😐 **$$$ Essential Shock Cream + Isoflavones, Firming Cream for Excessively Dry Skin** *($100 for 2.5 ounces)* contains a tiny amount of soy, which is where the isoflavone part comes in. However, the soy's antioxidant ability is compromised by jar packaging and this ends up being an overpriced, ordinary moisturizer for dry skin, nothing more.

☹ **Essential Shock Eye and Lip Treatment SPF 15** *($55 for 0.5 ounce)* lacks the UVA-protecting ingredients of titanium dioxide, zinc oxide, avobenzone, Mexoryl SX, or Tinosorb and is not recommended.

☹ **Essential Shock Gel Cream + Isoflavones, Intensive Firming for All Skin Types** *($95 for 2.5 ounces)* contains mostly water, slip agents, pH adjuster, aloe, and thickener. The amount of iris extract can be irritating. The only real shock about this product is how preposterously overpriced this substandard moisturizer is.

NATURA BISSE GLYCO LINE

According to Natura Bisse's brochure for this line of AHA products (each contains glycolic acid), safe exfoliation is guaranteed because each product has a pH of 4.5. However, that's above the effective range for exfoliation to occur, which means that none of these products will work as well as considerably less expensive AHA products from Alpha Hydrox, Neutrogena, Paula's Choice, or Neostrata (Exuviance). Considering the steep prices and the fact that a well-formulated AHA product provides numerous benefits for skin, we're talking serious disappointment.

☹ **Glyco Balance Exfoliating Fluid, for Oily Skin** *($68 for 1.7 ounces)* contains glycolic acid and lactic acid, but the pH is too high for them to exfoliate well. The alcohol and volatile fragrance components are unnecessarily irritating.

😐 **$$$ Glyco Eye Hydro-Exfoliating Eye Cream** *($52 for 0.8 ounce)* doesn't offer much for skin beyond a good amount of glycolic acid, but the pH of 4.5 prevents it from functioning as an exfoliant. It's an OK option for normal to slightly dry skin.

😐 **$$$ Glyco Face Hydro-Exfoliating Cream, for Dry Skin** *($80 for 2.5 ounces)* is a slightly more moisturizing version of the Glyco Eye Hydro-Exfoliating Eye Cream above, and the same review applies. Both products contain volatile fragrance components that may cause irritation.

☹ **Glyco Peeling 25%** *($130 for 1 ounce)* states that it contains 25% glycolic acid, an amount usually reserved for professionally administered peels. Although the amount of AHA sounds impressive, the pH renders it incapable of exfoliating. In addition, the amount of alcohol is irritating to skin, and without the benefit of exfoliation, this product isn't worth a second glance.

☹ **Glyco Peeling Plus 50%** *($170 for 1 ounce)* is similar to the Glyco Peeling 25% above, but with double the amount of glycolic acid. It's a good thing the pH is too high for the glycolic acid to function as an exfoliant because at this concentration, you'd be setting your skin up for serious irritation and potentially permanent damage.

NATURA BISSE OXYGEN LINE

All of the products below "oxygenate" skin via hydrogen peroxide. Although hydrogen peroxide does have an unstable oxygen molecule that can impact skin, that action generates free-radical damage, greatly reducing the production of healthy new skin cells. The cumulative problems that can result from impacting the skin with a substance that is known to generate free-radical damage and impair the skin's healing process, cause cellular destruction, and reduce optimal cell functioning means that this is an ingredient to avoid (Sources: *Carcinogenesis*, March 2002, pages 469–475; *Anticancer Research*, July–August 2001, pages 2719–2724; and *Plastic and Reconstructive Surgery*, September 2001, pages 675–687).

☹ **Oxygen Complex, for All Skin Types** *($125 for 1 ounce)* lists alcohol as the second ingredient, which only serves to break down skin. The hydrogen peroxide in here causes free-radical damage; in fact, this product's entire contents are a complete waste of time and money for anyone.

☹ **Oxygen Cream, for All Skin Types** *($73 for 2.5 ounces)* is a poorly conceived, boring moisturizer whose hydrogen peroxide content can damage skin by generating reactive oxygen species.

☹ **Oxygen Finishing Mask, for All Skin Types** *($30 for 2.5 ounces)* only finishes skin with irritation and free-radical damage due to its alcohol and hydrogen peroxide content.

NATURA BISSE SENSITIVE LINE

☺ **$$$ Sensitive Cleansing Cream, for All Sensitive Skin Types** *($36 for 7 ounces)* is a gentle, fragrance-free cleansing lotion that contains enough detergent cleansing agent to make it a more effective option than standard, water-and-oil cleansers. Soothing plant extracts are present, but will be rinsed from skin before they can really work. This is still a good, albeit expensive, option for normal to dry skin.

😐 **$$$ Sensitive Toner, for All Sensitive Skin Types** *($32 for 7 ounces)* is an OK moisturizing toner, but it would be better for sensitive skin if it did not contain fragrance and the irritating fragrance component d-limonene, which for a sensitive-skin product is just rude.

☹ **Sensitive Complex, for Sensitive Skin** *($120 for 1 ounce)* is an exceedingly tedious serum that contains mostly water, slip agent, aloe, castor oil, and water-binding agents. The inclusion of the preservative Kathon CG is a red flag because it is contraindicated for use in leave-on products due to their sensitizing potential.

😐 **$$$ Sensitive Cream, for Normal to Dry Skin** *($73 for 2.5 ounces)* is a basic moisturizer for normal to dry skin, but it is not a prime choice for sensitive skin because it contains fragrance. The water-binding agents are helpful, but the antioxidants won't remain stable once this jar-packaged product is opened.

😐 **$$$ Sensitive Eye Gel** *($68 for 0.8 ounce)* features what can only be called a mind-numbing formula that provides skin primarily with wax and water-binding agents. The tiny amount of antioxidants won't have much, if any, effect due to jar packaging. This also contains fragrance, which isn't ideal for sensitive skin.

☹ **Sensitive Gel Cream** *($68 for 2.5 ounces)* contains the preservatives methylisothiazolinone and methylchloroisothiazolinone (Kathon CG) and is not recommended for any skin type, especially sensitive. In fact, the amount and variety of preservatives in this moisturizer are not good news.

😐 **$$$ Sensitive Mask, Soothing Mask with Papaya Enzymes** *($31 for 2.5 ounces)* is a very standard moisturizing mask for normal to dry skin. The papaya enzymes are unstable and not likely to have any positive impact on skin.

NATURA BISSE SPECIAL FX LINE

☹ **Blemish Focus Acne Spot Treatment** *($44 for 0.5 ounce)* ranks as one of the most expensive anti-acne products around, but its alcohol content makes it too drying and irritating for any skin type.

☹ **Eye Illuminate Eye Brightening Gel** *($52 for 0.5 ounce)* includes a mix of helpful and potentially irritating plant extracts in a gel base, but the inclusion of the irritating menthol derivative menthyl lactate makes this a poor choice, especially for use around the eyes.

😐 **$$$ Line Refine Line Eraser** *($50 for 0.5 ounce)* is primarily silicones and film-forming agent (typically found in hairsprays to hold hair in place). While this does include some very helpful ingredients for skin, the hairspray and volatile fragrance components it contains make it anything but special.

😐 **$$$ Lip Booster Lip Treatment** *($44 for 0.5 ounce)* contains pepper oil, which swells lips by virtue of irritation. There isn't much of it, but it doesn't take much for this type of ingredient to irritate skin. The only boost is to the company for getting women to think this can make a positive difference in the appearance of their lips.

☹ **Red Diffuse** *($48 for 0.5 ounce)* is sold as an emergency formula to diffuse redness and broken capillaries, but the arnica and menthyl lactate in this lightweight "treatment" product only serve to cause irritation, which makes reddened skin worse.

NATURA BISSE SUN PRODUCTS

☹ **Sun Defense SPF 10 Self-Tanning Cream** *($50 for 3.5 ounces)* is a self-tanning lotion available in Medium or Deep Tan versions, each with dihydroxyacetone to turn skin color. Neither is recommended because the sunscreen lacks sufficient UVA-protecting ingredients and the SPF rating is too low.

☹ **Sun Defense Sun Radiance Lotion** *($48 for 7 ounces)* contains the melanin-enhancing ingredient copper acetyl tyrosinate methylsilanol, which promotes a faster tan. This product is not recommended because, as claimed, it "enhances the effects of the sun," which isn't what you want to do, at least not if your goal is healthy skin with minimal wrinkles and discolorations.

☹ **Sun Defense SPF 10 Sun Bronze Spray** *($52 for 7 ounces)* provides UVA protection via an in-part avobenzone sunscreen, but the SPF rating is too low. Although this may be acceptable to some as a sunscreen, the ingredient copper acetyl tyrosinate methylsilanol is designed to act on melanocytes (skin's pigment-producing cells), thus promoting a faster tan. This is a confused, unethical product.

☹ **Sun Defense SPF 15 Special Bronze Cream** *($55 for 3.5 ounces)* has the same positives and deal-breaking negatives as the Sun Defense SPF 10 Sun Bronze Spray above, and the same review applies.

😐 **$$$ Sun Defense SPF 30 Sun Defense Fluid, Oil-Free** *($90 for 3.5 ounces)* is an OK, in-part titanium dioxide sunscreen in a silky but lackluster moisturizing base for normal to slightly oily skin. The amount of antioxidants is basically non-existent—and, how liberally are you going to apply a sunscreen that costs this much?

☺ **$$$ Sun Defense SPF 30 Sun Defense Stick** *($36 for 0.16 ounce)* is expensive for what you get, but at least what you get is a good, in-part titanium dioxide sunscreen in an oil-based stick. This is best for very dry skin or for spot-application of sunscreen to often-missed areas. It can be used on the lips, too.

☺ **$$$ Sun Defense SPF 30+ Sun Defense Cream** *($115 for 2.5 ounces)* doesn't bestow on skin anything special for the money, but does provide very good sun protection via its in-part titanium dioxide sunscreen. This is supposedly formulated with "heat shock proteins," but in essence, any sunscreen could make this clam. Heat shock proteins are cellular substances that help protect the body during times of environmental stress, including sun exposure.

☺ **$$$ Sun Defense SPF 30+ Sun Defense Sport** *($120 for 7 ounces)* is similar to the Sun Defense SPF 30+ Sun Defense Cream above, and the same basic comments apply. Both formulas are best for normal to slightly dry skin not prone to breakouts.

OTHER NATURA BISSE PRODUCTS

😐 **$$$ Dry Skin Milk, Cleansing Milk** *($29 for 7 ounces)* is an extremely basic, mineral oil and Vaseline-based wipe-off cleanser that is an overpriced option for dry skin.

☺ **$$$ Facial Cleansing Cream + AHA, for Dry Skin** *($39 for 7 ounces)* contains only a tiny amount of glycolic and lactic acids, so they only function as water-binding agents (and they're rinsed from skin before they can be of much help in that regard anyway). This is otherwise a good lotion-textured, water-soluble cleanser for normal to dry skin.

☺ **$$$ Facial Cleansing Gel + AHA, for Normal to Oily Skin** *($39 for 7 ounces)* is a good water-soluble cleanser for normal to oily skin. The same comments about AHAs made above for the Facial Cleansing Cream apply here, too.

☺ **$$$ Eye Make-up Remover** *($34 for 3.5 ounces)* is a very standard, silicone-free eye-makeup remover that contains fragrance in the form of rose extract. Needless to say, it is vastly overpriced for what you get and easily replaced by far less expensive versions at the drugstore.

☹ **Dry Skin Toner, Toning Lotion for Dry Skin** *($28 for 7 ounces)* doesn't impress with its very basic formula that shortchanges skin of antioxidants (there's more preservative and fragrance in this toner), while the preservative blend of Kathon CG is sensitizing.

☹ **Stabilizing Toner, Astringent Mattifying Lotion for Combination to Oily Skin** *($35 for 7 ounces)* lists alcohol as the second ingredient and also contains irritating witch hazel, menthyl lactate, and problematic preservatives not meant for use in leave-on products. What were they thinking?

☹ **Double Action Hydro Protective Day Cream SPF 10, for Dry Skin** *($66 for 2.5 ounces)* lacks the UVA-protecting ingredients of titanium dioxide, zinc oxide, avobenzone, ecamsule, or Tinosorb and is not recommended.

😐 **$$$ Elastin Refirming Cream, for Dry Skin** *($72 for 2.5 ounces)* is a very boring moisturizer for normal to dry skin. It's mostly emollient with thickeners, and the elastin cannot restore skin's natural supply once it has diminished.

☹ **Eye Contour Cream SPF 10** *($68 for 0.8 ounce)* lacks the UVA-protecting ingredients of titanium dioxide, zinc oxide, avobenzone, Mexoryl SX (ecamsule), or Tinosorb and is not recommended.

😐 **$$$ Green Tea Extract Facial Phyto-Firming Serum** *($48 for 1 ounce)* is an OK, one-note antioxidant serum, with green tea being the only ingredient of note. The amount of alcohol is unlikely to cause irritation, and this product for normal to slightly oily skin is fragrance-free.

☹ **Hydra A Complex SPF 10** *($120 for 1.7 ounces)* is yet another Natura Bisse sunscreen whose SPF rating is too low for daytime protection and leaves skin vulnerable to UVA damage because it does not contain UVA-protecting actives. The price is just insulting for this inadequately made product.

☹ **Rose Mosqueta Oil, Intensive Regenerating Oil** *($47 for 1 ounce)* contains several volatile fragrance components that can cause irritation, including isoeugenol, linalool, and geraniol. You'd be better off massaging pure rose hip oil over dry skin: it costs much less and poses no risk of irritating skin.

😐 **$$$ Stabilizing Complex, Oil-Free Balancing Complex with Salicylic Acid, 2%** *($105 for 1 ounce)* claims to regulate oil production while protecting skin from dehydration, but this soy protein– and water-based product cannot do anything of the sort. Oil production is controlled by hormones, and the only thing skin-care products can do is help absorb what's naturally being secreted. The salicylic acid will work as an exfoliant due to this product's pH of 3.8. It's an effective BHA option for normal to slightly oily skin, but not rated as highly because of the alcohol content (it's the fourth ingredient). By the way, the inclusion of castor oil wasn't wise given the product's oil control claims.

☹ **Stabilizing Gel Cream** *($68 for 2.5 ounces)* contains a lot of alcohol plus volatile fragrance components to irritate skin, and the jar packaging won't keep the tiny amount of retinol and numerous antioxidants stable (so much for the "Stabilizing" name!).

☹ **Stimul-Eye Active Gel** *($60 for 1 ounce)* serves only to stimulate irritation because it contains the menthol derivative menthyl PCA. This is otherwise mostly water, seaweed, slip agent, and castor oil—what's the big deal? Nothing!

☹ **Titen, Neck and Chest Firming Serum** *($65 for 1 ounce)* contains too much alcohol for any skin-care consideration, whether it is on the neck or chest.

😐 **$$$ Ananas Finishing Mask** *($31 for 2.5 ounces)* is very similar to all of the other moisturizing masks Natura Bisse makes, which means it's a mediocre option for normal to dry skin. Ananas extract comes from pineapple and holds no special benefit for skin, though it can be sensitizing.

😐 **$$$ Inhibit-Dermafill** *($385 for 1 ounce)* comes with the tag line "fore-stall that face lift" and claims to fill wrinkles "from the inside out (like micro-injections) while keeping expression lines from forming." It does nothing of the sort, and I wouldn't be surprised if the FDA begins to crack down on Natura Bisse and other companies making blatant, like-a-drug claims for their cosmetic products. Since Natura Bisse does not have to prove their claims, it is up to consumers to either ignore or fall for the puffery, and in this case I'm suggesting that you avoid tripping on this puffery by choosing not to be taken in by this expensive marketing sham and deficiently formulated product.

Inhibit-Dermafill contains mostly water, silicone, yeast (incorrectly described by the company as "black tea"), glycerin, thickener, a derivative of acetyl hexapeptide (for more information about this "works-like-Botox" ingredient, refer to Chapter Seven, *Cosmetics Ingredient Dictionary* at the end of this book), anti-irritant, water-binding agents, slip agents, fragrance, film-forming agent, and preservatives. None of these ingredients is capable of preventing expression lines from forming, nor can they penetrate to fill wrinkles from the inside out. Comparing this treatment to the type of wrinkle-filling injections a dermatologist or cosmetic surgeon offers is laughable. The only face-lift this will forestall is your ability to smile once you've realized how much money you've wasted.

☹ **Inhibit Expression Line Complex** *($135 for 0.5 ounce)* lists alcohol as the third ingredient and also contains the irritating menthol derivative menthyl PCA, making this nothing more than a pricey way to make skin unhappy.

☹ **Stabilizing Cleansing Mask** *($45 for 7 ounces)* contains menthol, and is otherwise an exceptionally standard clay mask that would still be too expensive at half the price.

☹ **Stimul-Eye Mask** *($40 for 1 ounce)* is a basic, emollient moisturizer labeled as a mask. Regardless of the name, it is just too ordinary for words, plus it's over-fragranced, which adds up to a problem for skin at any price.

NEOSTRATA (INCLUDING EXUVIANCE)

NEOSTRATA AT-A-GLANCE

Strengths: Huge assortment of AHA and PHA products, all with correct pH to exfoliate; sunscreens that include AHA and/or PHA at right pH and provide reliable broad-spectrum sun protection; good cleansers; some excellent serums and lightweight moisturizers; the Exuviance makeup products are worth a try if you need full coverage with sufficient sun protection.

Weaknesses: No BHA products (better for blemish-prone skin or for those who can't tolerate AHAs or PHA); no topical disinfectants (a basic for those with acne); all hydroquinone products have at least one major negative; irritating toners; jar packaging; potentially problematic self-tanning products; lip balms contain irritating spearmint oil; most NeoCeuticals products are terrible.

For more information about Neostrata, call (800) 225-9411 or visit www.neostrata.com or www.Beautypedia.com. Note: Neostrata's range of products is advertised as being available only through physicians. However, the entire selection is available for purchase online. The Exuviance brand is sold in select department stores and specialty beauty boutiques such as Ulta.

Caution: Keep in mind that skin needs only one reliable exfoliant at a time. Neostrata sells so many good ones, you may be tempted to double (or triple) up, but doing so can backfire and be more irritating than helpful.

NEOSTRATA EXUVIANCE PRODUCTS

The polyhydroxy acid (PHA) gluconolactone is used in many Neostrata products. It is supposed to be gentler and longer acting than glycolic acid, and its delayed penetration is attributed to its larger molecular size. However, according to an article in *Cosmetic Dermatology* (July 1998), the skin can't tell the difference between the various effective AHAs, and the possibility of gluconolactone staying on the surface of skin longer than other AHAs did not prove out. So in terms of exfoliation and potential side effects, PHA ends up being as good as AHA.

☺ **$$$ Gentle Cleansing Creme** *($20 for 6.8 ounces)* is a standard, lightweight cleansing lotion that does not contain detergent cleansing agents. It removes makeup and is best for normal to slightly dry skin. It would be even gentler without the fragrance.

☺ **$$$ Purifying Cleansing Gel** *($20 for 6.8 ounces)* is a good water-soluble cleanser for normal to very oily skin. The amount of gluconolactone and glycolic acid will be rinsed away, so their inclusion isn't helpful for skin, plus it's a potential problem for the eyes.

☹ **Moisture Balance Toner** *($19 for 6.8 ounces)* lists alcohol as the second ingredient, which makes this neither moisturizing nor balancing for skin. The pH of 4.1 keeps the AHA and PHA from performing optimal exfoliation.

☹ **SkinRise Morning Bionic Tonic** *($33 for a 30-pad jar; $15 for 12 individually wrapped packettes)* are pads (also sold in packette form) that serve only to irritate skin because of the amount of peppermint oil. Other irritants include eucalyptus, grapefruit, and menthyl lactate.

Barbara Green, Neostrata Vice President of Technical and Consumer Affairs, wrote to me that this product is "a very soothing, non-irritating formulation" and supported this point by referring to the Repeat Insult Patch Testing (RIPT) results. This test is performed by many cosmetics companies (including mine) to purportedly gauge the potential for irritation and skin reactions. However, the protocols for this test involve putting a dab of product on the arm or back of volunteers, and keeping it semi-occluded. The site is then routinely checked for signs of irritation. If minimal to no reactions are noted, the product is considered non-irritating. The problems? This test doesn't correlate with how consumers use the product on their faces, and a substance applied on the arm for a few days doesn't have anything to do with using it on the face day after day. Even more to the point, there's the issue that irritation can occur without visible proof, such as redness or flaking (think of the silent damage UVA rays from the sun cause). RIPT testing may make regulatory boards happy, but it has limited relevance for the consumer.

☹ **$$$ Soothing Toning Lotion, Sensitive Formula** *($19 for 6.8 ounces)* contains a good amount of the PHA gluconolactone, but the pH of 4.7 reduces its effectiveness as an exfoliant. This is otherwise a fairly standard toner for normal to dry skin. It would be better for sensitive skin if it did not contain fragrance or coloring agents.

☺ **$$$ Essential Multi-Defense Day Creme SPF 15** *($26 for 1.75 ounces)* works beautifully to provide sun protection (it contains an in-part titanium dioxide sunscreen) and exfoliates skin with 8% glycolic acid in a pH of 3.8. The moisturizing base is suitable for normal to dry skin. Unfortunately, jar packaging renders the plant-based antioxidants ineffective shortly after you begin using it. However, this still has merit as a dual-purpose daytime moisturizer, so a happy face rating applies.

☺ **$$$ Essential Multi-Defense Day Fluid SPF 15** *($24 for 1.75 ounces)* is similar to but has a slightly lighter texture than the Essential Multi-Defense Day Creme SPF 15 above, and the same basic comments apply, except that this one is preferred for normal to slightly dry skin. Although not packaged in a jar, the translucent glass bottle means that the antioxidants will be exposed to light, and that's not the way to keep them stable and potent.

☹ **$$$ Evening Restorative Complex** *($30.50 for 1.75 ounces)*. It's a shame jar packaging compromises the effectiveness of the numerous antioxidants in this PHA moisturizer for normal to dry skin. The amount of gluconolactone and the pH of 3.8 promises exfoliation, and this does contain some good cell-communicating ingredients, so it's worth considering as an exfoliant/night moisturizer.

☺ **$$$ Fundamental Multi-Protective Day Creme SPF 15, Sensitive Formula** *($26 for 1.75 ounces)* is preferred for sensitive skin because its PHA content is 5%, and the pH of 3.4 is effective for exfoliation. For those with sensitive skin, any AHA or PHA may prove too irritating, and the synthetic sunscreen agent in here can do the same. This does contain titanium dioxide for sufficient UVA protection.

☺ **$$$ Fundamental Multi-Protective Day Fluid SPF 15, Sensitive Formula** *($24 for 1.75 ounces)* is the lotion version of the Fundamental Multi-Protective Day Creme SPF 15 above. The same basic comments apply, except this option has a pH of 4, which still allows the PHAs to be effective exfoliants while being potentially less irritating for sensitive skin.

☹ **$$$ Hydrating Lift Eye Complex** *($25.50 for 0.5 ounce)* contains 3% gluconolactone and 1% lactobionic acid at a pH of 3.6. The amount of PHA won't prompt much exfoliation, but that's not such a bad thing for a product to be used around the eye. The fragrance-free base is silky and slightly emollient, but what a shame the numerous antioxidants will be compromised due to jar packaging.

☺ **$$$ Vespera Bionic Serum** *($55 for 1 ounce)* is a good lightweight gel moisturizer for normal to slightly dry or slightly oily skin that contains small amounts of some good antioxidants along with water-binding agents and effective PHAs for exfoliation. The packaging will keep the antioxidants stable during use. This product also contains mandelic acid, but this AHA is not as effective as others.

☹ **Blemish Treatment Gel** *($14.50 for 0.5 ounce)* has a pH above 5, which prevents the 2% salicylic acid from functioning as an exfoliant. The amount of alcohol makes this gel too drying and irritating for all skin types.

☹ **Essential Skin Lightener Gel** *($21.50 for 1.4 ounces)* would be a good 2% hydroquinone and glycolic acid skin-lightening product if it weren't for the alcohol it contains, which is unnecessarily irritating and drying for skin.

☹ **Rejuvenating Treatment Masque** *($17.50 for 2.5 ounces)* only treats skin to irritation due to its blend of alcohol and polyvinyl alcohol (a common ingredient in hair spray and peel-off masks). The alcohol is joined by some problematic plant extracts and the pH of 4.4 prevents the AHA and PHA from exfoliating.

☺ **$$$ Skin Healthy Home Resurfacing Peel System** *($65 for the kit)* proves Neostrata isn't immune to jumping on the at-home-peel kit bandwagon. This is a four-step system that consists of smaller sizes of two products sold separately from the kit (the Purifying Cleansing Gel and Evening Restorative Complex). The first step is the **Activator Pads**, which combine AHAs and the PHA gluconolactone at a combined concentration of 25% and pH of 3.6. You're directed to leave this solution on skin for no more than ten minutes (and at this concentration that seems like a long time to me), at which point you apply the **Neutralizing Solution** to stop the peel's exfoliating action. This step isn't essential considering you can net the same result by simply rinsing the solution with tap water, but I suppose it makes the kit seem more "clinical."

The amount of AHAs and PHA is indeed on par with the type of peels performed in a doctor's office or by an aesthetician. In that sense, this kit bests similar options available from drugstore lines. However, I'd caution you to use this only occasionally if you routinely use another AHA or BHA product. The skin can only handle so much exfoliation before it starts reacting negatively, so pay attention to its response and remember that the amount of exfoliants in this kit can cause noticeable irritation (and don't forget to protect your skin with an effective, broad-spectrum sunscreen).

☹ **Essential Multi-Protective Lip Balm SPF 15** *($8.50 for 0.14 ounce)* would be a brilliant lip balm with sunscreen if it did not contain irritating spearmint oil. The titanium dioxide and zinc oxide (along with other actives) ensure UVA protection, but such protection shouldn't come with the tradeoff of irritated lips.

😐 **$$$ Skin Healthy Sunless Tanning Facial Pads** *($15 for 12 individual packettes)* are difficult to recommend because the amount of gluconolactone and the pH of 3.2, which allows for effective exfoliation, are not what you want while you're waiting for your self-tan to develop (the pads contain dihydroxyacetone to turn skin color). Exfoliating before self-tanning is an important step, but combining the two at the same time can result in an uneven, blotchy color.

😐 **$$$ Skin Healthy Sunless Tanning Mousse** *($24 for 3.4 ounces)* has the same drawbacks as the Skin Healthy Sunless Tanning Facial Pads above, and the lower pH of 2.9 makes the PHA that much more effective (though also potentially too irritating).

NEOSTRATA EXUVIANCE PROFESSIONAL PRODUCTS

None of the products below are professional; all are available to the general public online and most of them have formulas that are similar to those of other Exuviance products. The "Professional" moniker appears to be mere marketing, not verification of superior formulations.

☺ **$$$ Moisturizing Antibacterial Facial Cleanser** *($22 for 6.8 ounces)* contains the antibacterial agent triclosan as the active ingredient, but it is useless in a cleanser because triclosan needs to be left on skin for several minutes in order to work (Source: *Journal of Hospital Infection*, August 2001, Supplement A, pages S4–S8), and you don't want to leave detergent cleansing agents on your skin for longer than a few seconds. This is otherwise a standard, water-soluble gel cleanser for normal to oily skin; the triclosan and other additives don't make this a "professional" option any more than renaming a Big Mac "Filet Mignon Sandwich" would change the fact that it is still just a Big Mac.

☹ **Clarifying Solution** *($19.50 for 3.4 ounces)* is an alcohol-based toner that contains 8% glycolic acid at a pH that allows it to exfoliate. Many other products have the same AHA positive without the negative that this much alcohol presents.

✓☺ **$$$ Rejuvenating Complex** *($42 for 1 ounce)* exfoliates skin with 12% gluconolactone and a pH of 3.2, all in an emollient base suitable for dry to very dry skin. The "Pro-Retinol" in this stably packaged product isn't actually retinol. It's retinyl acetate, which is the ester of retinol and acetic acid (an ester is an organic compound formed from the reaction of an acid and an alcohol). Despite the different name, it's still a retinoid, but it doesn't work as well as pure retinol. Overall, this is an excellent exfoliant that provides the additional benefit of antioxidants.

😐 **$$$ Ultra-Rich Restorative Creme** *($40 for 1.75 ounces)* is similar to the Exuviance Evening Restorative Complex above, except this contains more PHAs (12% versus 8%). Otherwise, the same review applies. The amount of sodium hyaluronate in this product isn't worthy of the company's "moisture sponge" claim.

☹ **Intense Lightening Complex** *($42 for 1 ounce)* is a souped-up version of the Essential Skin Lightener Gel above, but despite the helpful additives, this still contains too much alcohol to make it a worthwhile hydroquinone product. Additionally, this contains oxalic acid, which is corrosive to skin and nails. Maybe that's what they mean by "intense"?

NEOSTRATA NEOCEUTICALS PRODUCTS

☺ **$$$ NeoCeuticals Antibacterial Facial Cleanser, PHA 4** *($22 for 6 ounces)* is nearly identical to the Exuviance Professional Moisturizing Antibacterial Facial Cleanser above, and the same review applies.

☹ **NeoCeuticals PDS Treatment Extra Strength Cream** *($26 for 3.4 ounces)* is an emollient AHA moisturizer for dry to very dry skin, but it's not recommended because it contains irritating spearmint oil.

☹ **NeoCeuticals PDS Treatment Regular Strength Cream** *($26 for 3.4 ounces)* is similar to the NeoCeuticals PDS Treatment Extra Strength Cream above, and the same review applies.

☹ **NeoCeuticals Problem Dry Skin Gel** *($24 for 4 ounces)* contains 20% urea as the active ingredient, an amount known to cause skin inflammation and promote moisture loss from skin. Urea can be an outstanding moisturizing agent for all types of dry skin, but concentrations of 10% or less are preferred, and there is extensive research to support the therapeutic benefits of this amount (Sources: *Dry Skin and Moisturizers: Chemistry and Function*, Maibach and Loden, CRC Press, 2000, pages 243–250; and *CIR Compendium*, 2007, pages 314–315). This product will likely cause, not mitigate, problem dry skin.

☹ **NeoCeuticals Acne Spot Treatment Gel** *($15.50 for 0.5 ounce)* is identical to the Blemish Treatment Gel above, and the same comments apply.

☹ **NeoCeuticals Acne Treatment Solution Pads** *($16.50 for 40 pads)* are alcohol-based pads that include 2% salicylic acid at a pH that's too high for exfoliation. Two words: Don't bother.

☹ **NeoCeuticals HQ Skin Lightening Gel, PHA 10** *($38 for 1 ounce)* is similar to the Exuviance Professional Intense Lightening Complex above, and the same comments apply.

Other Neostrata Products

😐 **$$$ Facial Cleanser, PHA 4** *($24 for 6 ounces)* is a standard, detergent-based, water-soluble cleanser with 4% PHA (polyhydroxy acid). Even though this doesn't contain much AHA, it is still of concern in a cleanser that may get into the eye area.

☹ **Foaming Glycolic Wash, AHA 20** *($25 for 3.4 ounces)* contains a lot of glycolic acid, but that's not helpful in a cleanser because it is rinsed down the drain before it can go to work. Additional problems include the amount of alcohol and the drying detergent cleansing agent sodium C14-16 olefin sulfonate.

😐 **Face Cream Plus, AHA 15** *($29 for 1.75 ounces)* contains 15% glycolic acid at an effective pH range. The simple moisturizing base is suitable for normal to very dry skin, and is fragrance-free. One caution: Daily use of products containing more than 10% glycolic acid is of concern to the FDA, but the research isn't there to support the long-term effects of such usage, for better or worse.

☹ **Gel Plus, AHA 15** *($33 for 3.4 ounces)* lists alcohol as the second ingredient, which makes this 15% glycolic acid gel too irritating for all skin types.

😐 **$$$ High Potency Cream, AHA 20** *($40 for 1 ounce)* contains 20% glycolic acid at a pH of 3.5. This will exfoliate skin, but the kickback from irritation due to such a high concentration of AHA may not be worth the risk, at least not for daily use. There isn't any research on this issue to help point you in a safe direction. This product is only recommended if your physician advises you that such potency is necessary.

😐 **Lotion Plus, AHA 15** *($28 for 6.8 ounces)* is similar to but less emollient than the Face Cream Plus, AHA 15 above, and the same concerns apply.

☹ **Oil Control Gel, PHA/AHA 8** *($23 for 1 ounce)* won't control oil as much as it will irritate skin given the amount of alcohol it contains. Neostrata recommends this as an ideal after-shave product for men—talk about a painful ending!

☹ **Oily Skin Solution, AHA 8** *($23 for 3.4 ounces)* lists alcohol as the second ingredient, and is not recommended over other products with 8% glycolic acid that exfoliate without unnecessary irritants.

☺ **Ultra Smoothing Cream, AHA 10** *($23 for 1.75 ounces)* combines 8% glycolic acid and 2% citric acid, for a total 10% AHA product, although citric acid is not nearly as effective as glycolic acid. Still, the pH of 3.5 means this will exfoliate, and it is a good, basic, fragrance-free AHA moisturizer for normal to dry skin.

☺ **Ultra Smoothing Lotion, AHA 10** *($27 for 6.8 ounces)* is the lotion version of the Ultra Smoothing Cream, AHA 10 above and, other than being preferred for normal to slightly dry or slightly oily skin, the same review applies.

😐 **Bio-Hydrating Cream, PHA 15** *($32 for 1.75 ounces)* contains 15% PHA (using gluconolactone). Since this exfoliant works in a manner similar to glycolic acid, the same concerns about using concentrations above 10% apply. This is an OK option for intermittent use by those with normal to dry skin.

✓☺ **$$$ Bionic Eye Cream, PHA 4** *($50 for 0.5 ounce)* provides exfoliation with 4% gluconolactone in a pH of 3.5, which may be too irritating for some when used around the eye. Considering that gluconolactone has some antioxidant capacity and that this product also contains other antioxidants, it is worth considering if you have normal to dry skin. The vitamin K in here does not impact dark circles; nothing in this product will, but it has other benefits.

😐 **$$$ Bionic Face Cream, PHA 12** *($42 for 1.75 ounces)* contains 12% PHA (polyhydroxy acid) in a silicone-based moisturizer that also contains some good plant oils and small amounts of water-binding agents, which make it good for normal to dry skin. However, there is concern about using such a high concentration of AHA (over 10%) given its unknown long-term effects on skin (and jar packaging won't keep the antioxidants stable once opened).

☺ **$$$ Bionic Face Serum, PHA 10** *($47 for 1 ounce)* contains only the PHA lactobionic acid, and there is no substantiated research proving this exfoliates skin, so it's not necessarily a slam-dunk if you're hoping for that benefit. This ends up being a well-packaged, water-based, fragrance-free antioxidant serum for all skin types. For that reason, it certainly deserves consideration.

😐 **$$$ Bionic Lotion, PHA 15** *($25.50 for 3.4 ounces)* exfoliates skin with the PHA gluconolactone at a concentration of 12% and a pH of 3.8. The bland moisturizing base is suitable for normal to dry skin. Given the high concentration of PHA, this product may provide the best results when alternated with another AHA product with a lower acid concentration.

✓☺ **Daytime Protection Cream SPF 15, PHA 10** *($33 for 1.75 ounces)* is a very good fragrance-free daytime moisturizer with sunscreen (titanium dioxide is one of the active ingredients). It also contains 8% PHA at a pH that allows exfoliation to occur in a standard emollient base, and is an option for normal to dry skin.

☺ **$$$ Eye Cream, PHA 4** *($26 for 0.5 ounce)* includes 4% gluconolactone with a pH of 3.2 to prompt exfoliation. The eye area may not be able to tolerate this product, but it's fine for use elsewhere on the face where skin is dry. The antioxidants and antioxidant plant oils are a nice touch, but they're not a prominent part of the formula.

✓☺ **Oil Free Lotion SPF 15, PHA 4** *($30 for 1.75 ounces)* is very similar to the Daytime Protection Cream SPF 15, PHA 10 above, except with a 4% concentration of gluconolactone. Otherwise, the same comments apply.

✓☺ **$$$ Renewal Cream, PHA 12** *($43 for 1.05 ounces)* is very similar to the Exuviance Professional Rejuvenating Complex above, right down to its 12% concentration of gluconolactone and inclusion of retinyl acetate. The same review applies.

☺ **Ultra Daytime Smoothing Cream SPF 15, AHA 10** *($30 for 1.75 ounces)* exfoliates skin with 10% glycolic acid in a pH of 3.2, while an in-part titanium dioxide sunscreen shields skin from UVA rays. The base formula for normal to dry skin isn't terribly exciting, but this is highly recommended if you're looking for a combination AHA/sunscreen product.

😐 **$$$ Ultra Moisturizing Face Cream, PHA 10** *($28 for 1.75 ounces)* is an effective, though basic, PHA moisturizer that includes 10% gluconolactone formulated at a pH of 3.5, so exfoliation will occur. The fragrance-free formula is best for normal to dry skin; what a shame the jar packaging won't keep the selection of antioxidants stable during use.

☹ **Bionic Skin Lightening Cream SPF 15, PHA 10** *($28 for 1 ounce)* contains 2% hydroquinone, but the sunscreen actives do not provide sufficient UVA protection, making this an almost-there product that doesn't deserve a purchase.

☹ **Skin Lightening Gel, AHA 10** *($27 for 1.4 ounces)* has the same problem as all of the Neostrata/Exuviance skin lightening gels above, which is too much alcohol. That keeps this otherwise effective 2% hydroquinone product from earning a recommendation.

☹ **Lip Conditioner SPF 15** *($4 for 0.14 ounce)* is identical to the Exuviance Essential Multi-Protective Lip Balm SPF 15 above, and the same (unfortunate) comments apply. Spearmint oil can cause contact dermatitis on the lips (Source: *Contact Dermatitis*, October 2000, pages 216–222).

NEOSTRATA EXUVIANCE MAKEUP

FOUNDATION: ☺ **$$$ CoverBlend Concealing Treatment Makeup SPF 20** *($22.50)* is a remarkable full-coverage foundation that effectively conceals minor and major discolorations without feeling thick and greasy on the skin. Since this is a rather opaque makeup, I don't agree with Exuviance's claim that it provides "natural" coverage. But the effect, while perceptible, is certainly more attractive on the skin and easier to work with than DermaBlend or most other heavy-duty foundations you may have tried. The silicone-based formula features an excellent titanium dioxide– and zinc oxide–based sunscreen, and although it appears thick in the jar, it has a soft, light texture that is surprisingly easy to blend.

Concealing Treatment Makeup dries to a solid matte finish, which may not be to everyone's liking, but you will certainly get more longevity out of it than you will with traditional creamy or greasepaint-type foundations. Those with normal to dry skin will definitely need to apply moisturizer before using this makeup, and you're not likely to need any setting powder, unless you want to further enhance the matte effect (which can be a mistake). Almost complete coverage is achieved with one application, and it layers well for areas that need more camouflage. There are 14 shades, but not all of them are praiseworthy. The following colors are too pink, peach, or rose for most skin tones: Neutral Beige, True Beige, Blush Beige, Honey Sand, and Palest Mahogany. Bisque and Ivory are slightly peachy pink, but may work for some fair skin tones because the dry-down result is lighter than the color you see in the container. True Mahogany, Blush Mahogany, and Deep Mahogany are beautiful for dark skin tones, although the titanium dioxide and zinc oxide sunscreen can result in a slightly ashen finish.

☺ **$$$ Skin Caring Foundation SPF 15** *($27)* has a titanium dioxide sunscreen and a strong silicone base that starts out feeling light and silky but blends down to an ultra-matte, dry finish that only those with very oily skin will appreciate. Coverage is sheer to light and it does maintain its solid matte finish for most of the day. As with most ultra-matte foundations, it will exaggerate dry spots, however minor. There are 14 shades available, and though some of them appear too pink, peach, or rose in the bottle, most dry down to a soft, semi-sheer color. The following colors are noticeably peach, pink, or rose on the skin: True Beige, Neutral Beige, Palest Mahogany, Honey Sand, and Blush Mahogany.

☹ **CoverBlend Corrective Leg & Body Makeup SPF 18** *($18)* is more akin to traditional full-coverage makeup when compared to the Concealing Treatment Makeup above. Although this silicone- and talc-based makeup with a titanium dioxide– and zinc oxide–based sunscreen does indeed provide substantial, water-resistant coverage, three of the four shades are simply too peach or pink to look convincing on most skin tones. If you're going to wear opaque makeup on the body (presumably concealing a large area of skin), you don't want to use colors that stand out against the skin and draw attention to what you're trying to hide. If you have dark skin and need this type of camouflage makeup, Mahogany is a worthwhile deep tan shade to consider.

CONCEALER: ☺ $$$ CoverBlend Multi-Function Concealer SPF 15 *($16.50)* is a slightly creamy, full-coverage concealer that includes a titanium dioxide– and zinc oxide–based sunscreen. This applies quite well, and has only a slight tendency to crease—though the complete coverage may be of interest only to those with severe dark circles or other skin flaws that are not effectively covered by traditional concealers. If you need serious coverage and don't mind the tradeoff of a less-than-natural finish, this is worth a try. There are four shades available; the following two are problematic: Mahogany has strong peachy gold overtones that don't mesh well with most dark skin tones, while Sand dries to an ashy rose color that doesn't do anything to enhance the complexion.

POWDER: ☺ $$$ CoverBlend Anti-Aging Finishing Powder *($18)* is a fine-textured, satin-finish loose powder that contains only talc, gluconolactone, pigments, and preservatives. The gluconolactone is supposed to provide a moisturizing benefit, but don't count on significant hydration from an absorbent powder containing this ingredient. This simple formula works well with the CoverBlend foundations, and the two shades are equally good options, each imparting a sheer wash of color.

NEUTROGENA

NEUTROGENA AT-A-GLANCE

Strengths: Inexpensive; some superior water-soluble cleansers; good topical scrubs; effective AHA and BHA products; several retinol options, all in stable packaging; vast selection of sunscreens, most of which offer excellent UVA protection; good variety of self-tanning products; several fragrance-free options; most Healthy Skin products are state-of-the-art; almost all of the foundations with sunscreen provide sufficient UVA protection; pressed powder with SPF 30; the Moistureshine Gloss; a tinted lip balm with broad-spectrum sunscreen; the Shimmer Sheers.

Weaknesses: Bar soap; most toners are irritating or boring; a handful of bland moisturizers and eye creams; some sunscreens lack sufficient UVA protection or contain too much alcohol; Advanced Solutions products are advanced in name only; Blackhead Clearing and most Deep Clean products are terrible; no effective skin-lightening products; jar packaging; mostly disappointing concealers and eyeshadows; most of the lip balms with sunscreen provide inadequate UVA protection; poor mascaras; several makeup items packaged so you cannot see the color, and the shade swatch on the box is typically inaccurate.

For more information about Neutrogena, owned by Johnson & Johnson, call (800) 582-4048 or visit www.neutrogena.com or www.Beautypedia.com.

NEUTROGENA SKIN CARE

NEUTROGENA ADVANCED SOLUTIONS PRODUCTS

😐 **Advanced Solutions Daily SPF 15 Moisturizer, Skin Transforming Complex** *($25.29 for 1.4 ounces)* is a good in-part avobenzone sunscreen for someone with normal to slightly dry skin, but there isn't much about it that's advanced or worth the extra expense. Beyond the active sunscreen ingredients, this moisturizer contains mostly water, glycerin, slip agent, DMAE, thickeners, glycolic acid (as a water-binding agent, not as an exfoliant), more thickeners, absorbent, vitamin E, retinol, preservatives, and fragrance. Neutrogena touts the retinol and DMAE as state-of-the-art ingredients in this sunscreen, but the amount of retinol in this product differs little from that in Neutrogena's other, less expensive retinol-containing items, so why would you spend the extra funds? It certainly wouldn't be for the DMAE (listed as dimethyl MEA, but more commonly seen as dimethylaminoethanol). Despite many claims to the contrary, there is no substantiated evidence pointing to DMAE's effectiveness for skin care. Research on DMAE is primarily for its use as an oral supplement, where it is believed to improve mental alertness because of its similarity to choline, meaning it has the potential to help stimulate production of the brain neurotransmitter acetylcholine. As a topical agent, it may help protect the skin-cell membrane, but this has yet to be proven. Topical antioxidants are far more intriguing (and have been studied far more) than DMAE, and Neutrogena would have really created something special if they had packed this product with topical antioxidants instead of relying solely on retinol (an antioxidant) and DMAE. This product does contain fragrance.

☺ **Advanced Solutions Nightly Renewal Cream, Skin Transforming Complex** *($26.49 for 1.4 ounces)* isn't a bad moisturizer, but its formula doesn't really jibe with the "advanced solutions" name. To merit that moniker, this moisturizer should contain higher levels of several antioxidants, along with anti-irritants and unique water-binding or anti-inflammatory agents. As is, this is a good-but-should-have-been-better moisturizer for normal to slightly dry skin. Composed primarily of water, silicone, glycerin, and several thickeners, it does make the skin feel smooth, soft, and comfortable, yet it can't deliver on its promise to provide "dramatically younger-looking skin." Neutrogena boasts about the retinol content, but based on where it appears on the list, there isn't any more of it in this product than there is in other retinol-containing products from Neutrogena or RoC (both Johnson & Johnson–owned companies). As a retinol product this doesn't rise to the top of the must-have list, but the opaque tube packaging will help keep it stable. As with the Advanced Solutions Daily SPF 15 Moisturizer above, this product also contains DMAE, whose limited and unproven usefulness in skin-care products is chronicled in the review above. As a basic retinol product this works, but it's a one-note product, and that is always a limitation for skin.

☹ **Advanced Solutions Acne Mark Fading Peel** *($15.19 for 1.4 ounces)* is designed to fade post-inflammatory hyperpigmentation from acne—those telltale marks left on skin long after a blemish has healed. On lighter skin tones, the marks are traditionally pink or red, while darker skin tones typically have brown to almost black marks. These marks are the remnants of your skin's healing response to blemishes, and usually fade within 12 to 18 months—an eternity when they are staring you in the face each morning. Will this Neutrogena product be the "Advanced Solution" you've been looking for? Probably not, but the 2% salicylic acid in a base with a pH of 3.8 means you can get beneficial exfoliation, and that can help the discolorations. However, the product's directions indicate that you can use it as many as three times per week and you should leave it on for periods of 5 to 10 minutes, which means you rinse it off before it really has a chance to work. The inclusion of irritating menthol makes it inherently problematic for healing. To gain maximum benefit from salicylic acid, it is best to leave it on the skin. The anti-inflammatory effect of the salicylic acid in this product is negated when paired with menthol, which has absolutely no fading or peeling abilities. Exfoliation with glycolic or salicylic acids can indeed speed the fading of post-inflammatory hyperpigmentation, as can receiving doctor-supervised facial peels or laser treatments, but using this product in the hopes that its "Celluzyme" technology will diminish these discolorations is nothing more than wishful thinking.

☹ **$$$ Advanced Solutions at Home MicroDermabrasion System** *($39.99 for the kit)* is an all-in-one kit for those who want to try a microdermabrasion treatment at home before making a far more expensive, one-time appointment for the real-deal procedure with an aesthetician or dermatologist. Included are a battery-powered, hand-held device (batteries included) with two speeds, two sponge heads, a unit for storing the device between uses, and the Micro-Oxide Crystallized Cream. The cream product contains the same ingredient (aluminum oxide) used in professionally administered microdermabrasion treatments and, thankfully, does not contain unnecessary irritants such as menthol. You're instructed to use the sponge tip (with the device turned off) to dot the exfoliant cream on key areas of your face, then switch the device on, which causes the attached sponge head to vibrate. After moving the device over your entire face to enhance the mechanical skin-scrubbing action, you're instructed to rinse the product. That's where things got tricky for me. Massaging the Micro-Oxide Crystallized Cream into my skin wasn't difficult, though it did feel a bit gritty, almost as if I were stroking my skin with soft sandpaper. However, rinsing the cream off proved a lengthy process, and hours later I was still feeling traces of the crystals on my face. Not the best.

Because this is an effective topical scrub, there is no question your skin will feel softer and smoother after a treatment (mine had a noticeable glow). However, I am concerned that the aluminum oxide crystals may cause problems in the long run if people overdo this, because irritation is a concern. When microdermabrasion is performed with a professionally guided machine, the crystals are suctioned off the skin during treatment, which drastically minimizes their potential for causing post-treatment problems. With at-home systems like Neutrogena's, the likelihood of problems increases. Of course, it all depends on how zealous consumers are about it, but it's easy to get carried away while running the device over your face.

Neutrogena does have research, which they paid for, showing that their At Home Micro-Dermabrasion System works as well as microdermabrasion performed in an office setting (Source: *The Rose Sheet*, March 7, 2005, page 3). Their comparison is impressive; 60 women received in-office microdermabrasion treatments or used the At Home MicroDermabrasion System. The two groups felt equally happy with their results! Keep in mind the study did not examine whether either treatment was as effective as a topical scrub (including just using a washcloth) paired with regular use of an effective AHA or BHA product, which has the potential to net better results for your skin (and recent research suggests that repeated microdermabrasion treatments may yield diminishing returns). Plus, published research indicates that salon/doctor-performed microdermabrasion treatments may have either marginal benefit or diminishing results. That means that if Neutrogena's works as well as the professional version, that might not be good news (Sources: *Dermatologic Surgery*, June 2006, pages 809–814, and March 2006, pages 376–379; and *Journal Watch Dermatology*, May 2004).

☹ **$$$ Advanced Solutions Complete Acne Therapy System** *($22.99 for the kit)* features a cleansing scrub, daytime moisturizer with sunscreen, and topical disinfectant (labeled as a nighttime product, but it can certainly be used as part of your daytime routine, too). The **Skin Polishing Acne Cleanser** contains 0.5% salicylic acid, an amount really too small to provide much exfoliation, not to mention that the pH is really too high for that to occur anyway. However, this cleanser also includes polyethylene (plastic) beads, which provide manual exfoliation. The cleansing base is fairly gentle. Skin Polishing Acne Cleanser works best as a topical scrub rather than as a daily cleanser. Use caution and avoid scrubbing over raised blemishes or reddened areas.

Sun Shield Day Lotion with SPF 15 is a standard sunscreen lotion with an in-part zinc oxide sunscreen. Although zinc oxide is a great broad-spectrum sunscreen, it is not the best for use over blemished skin because its occlusive nature can contribute further to clogged pores. This means you have to experiment to see if that's true for your skin. Its base formula isn't anything special or interesting, and a couple of fragrant extracts may cause irritation, but broad-spectrum sun protection is assured.

Last up is the **Overnight Acne Control Lotion**, a 2.5% benzoyl peroxide product that is as straightforward as it gets. This works well to disinfect the skin, but would have been better if Neutrogena had added some soothing agents or anti-irritants. Still, it is an option as a topical disinfectant and does not contain needless irritants. Given that the three-piece kit above lacks a leave-on, pH-correct salicylic acid exfoliant and features a sunscreen with an active ingredient that can be problematic for someone with acne, you might ask how is this an advanced solution? In short, this collection of products, though attractively packaged, is not necessarily one-stop shopping for blemished or blemish-prone skin. A one-size-fits-all approach to treating blemishes may seem convenient, but it takes systematic experimentation to find the best combination of products for you. If Neutrogena's offerings in this kit were a bit more sensible, it would have received a higher recommendation.

😐 **$$$ Advanced Solutions Facial Peel** *($26.49 for 1.7 ounces)* is an interesting product, mainly because its "peeling" comes from the directions on the package to manually rub the skin, which in essence exfoliates the skin. Advanced Solutions Facial Peel does not contain an AHA or BHA. What it does contain is *Mucor miehei* extract, which Neutrogena refers to as "mushroom protein." From what I could find out about this ingredient, it is an acid protease (protease is an enzyme that breaks down protein—which would break down the substances that hold the cells on the surface of skin together) derived from a type of fungus. As you might suspect, the next question is whether this ingredient can exfoliate (peel) skin or have any benefit whatsoever. In this scenario you've got to take Neutrogena's word for it, because there is no research pointing the way on this one (at least not in the concentration used in this product). I suspect this product's skin-smoothing ability comes from the exfoliating beads it contains, not from a "breakthrough" ingredient capable of providing "dramatic, skin-revitalizing benefits." If you decide to try this product as a topical scrub, be forewarned that it has a lot of fragrance.

☹ **Advanced Solutions Lip Rejuvenating Treatment SPF 20** *($16.09 for 0.33 ounce)* does not contain the UVA-protecting ingredients of titanium dioxide, zinc oxide, Mexoryl SX (ecamsule), avobenzone, or Tinosorb and is not recommended for daytime protection. The lip balm itself leaves much to be desired, and isn't as good as the other lip options from Neutrogena.

NEUTROGENA BLACKHEAD ELIMINATING PRODUCTS

☹ **Blackhead Eliminating 2-in-1 Foaming Pads** *($7.89 for 28 pads)* won't eliminate a single blackhead, but will cause irritation due to the menthol in these pads, and will cause dryness because of the detergent cleansing agent chosen. Textured pads have nothing to do with remedying blackheads.

☹ **Blackhead Eliminating Daily Scrub** *($5.99 for 4.2 ounces)* is nearly identical to Clean & Clear's Blackhead Clearing Scrub (both companies are owned by Johnson & Johnson), and the same comments apply. Neutrogena's version contains menthol rather than menthyl lactate, but both are unnecessary irritants. As a reminder, using a topical scrub over blackheads removes only the top portion of them. That means that the "root" of the blackhead is still inside the pore, so the effect from the scrub is minimal at best, and for that benefit a washcloth would prove just as effective (without the irritation from the menthol).

☹ **Blackhead Eliminating Warming Cleanser** *($5.99 for 4 ounces)* produces a warming sensation when you splash your face with it because of the interaction between water and a zeolite mineral in this product. The sensation of warmth won't eliminate blackheads any more than planting roses instead of carnations will keep bees at bay. A larger problem this cleanser has is the inclusion of irritating cardamom oil, and the amount of potassium hydroxide, may cause dryness.

☹ **Blackhead Eliminating Astringent** *($6.79 for 8.5 ounces)* contains 0.5% salicylic acid, which isn't enough to have much of an effect on blackheads, but even if it were, this astringent contains a good deal of alcohol and witch hazel, as well as smaller, but still irritating, amounts of peppermint and eucalyptus. At any price, this product is a mistake for any skin type, but especially for someone struggling with blackheads.

☹ **Blackhead Eliminating Treatment Mask** *($6.79 for 2 ounces)* also contains 0.5% salicylic acid, which is minimally helpful for blackheads and blemishes (at least 1% is preferred). Here is yet another acne treatment product that is worthless for skin because it is loaded with irritating ingredients—the exact same offenders mentioned above for the Blackhead Eliminating Astringent, plus menthol.

NEUTROGENA DEEP CLEAN PRODUCTS

☹ **Deep Clean Cream Cleanser Oil-Free** *($5.99 for 7 ounces)* contains menthol and is not recommended. The minty sensation has nothing do with skin being deeply cleansed.

☹ **Deep Clean Invigorating Shine-Free Cleanser** *($6.99 for 5.1 ounces)* would be a great water-soluble cleanser for normal to dry skin if it did not contain the irritating menthol derivative menthyl lactate. By the way, the thickening agents in this cleanser don't leave skin with a shine-free finish.

☹ **Deep Clean Invigorating Ultra-Foam Cleanser** *($6.99 for 6 ounces)* has every element of a brilliantly-formulated liquid-to-foam cleanser until you get to the menthol, which is just irritating, literally and figuratively.

☹ **Deep Clean Facial Cleanser, for Normal to Oily Skin** *($5.99 for 6 ounces)* leaves out the menthol in the Deep Clean Cream Cleanser above, but is based around the drying detergent cleansing agent sodium C14-16 olefin sulfonate.

☹ **Deep Clean Invigorating Self-Foaming Cleansing Pads** *($8.09 for 28 pads)* would be a much gentler option if they did not contain menthol. A standard water-soluble cleanser used with a washcloth would be a much better choice.

☺ **Deep Clean Gentle Scrub** *($6.09 for 4.2 ounces)* is indeed gentle, and makes a very good cleanser/scrub hybrid product for normal to oily skin. The salicylic acid isn't doing the exfoliating; the polyethylene (plastic) beads do that when massaged over the skin.

☹ **Deep Clean Invigorating Dual Action Toner** *($6.59 for 6.7 ounces)* promises to give pores a tighter feel to "seal in the tingly sensation", which is a roundabout way of stating that this alcohol-laden toner with menthol causes lingering irritation.

☹ **Deep Clean Invigorating Foaming Scrub** *($7.59 for 4.2 ounces)* is not preferred to the Deep Clean Gentle Scrub above because it contains menthol.

☹ **Deep Clean Astringent, Oil-Free** *($7.19 for 6.7 ounces)* contains alcohol, witch hazel, and menthol, all of which conspire to cause skin irritation.

☹ **Deep Clean Invigorating Cleanser/Mask** *($7.39 for 4.2 ounces)* is a drying foaming cleanser that becomes an irritation to skin because it contains the menthol derivative menthone glycerol acetal.

NEUTROGENA HEALTHY SKIN PRODUCTS

☺ **Healthy Skin Anti-Wrinkle Anti-Blemish Cleanser** *($7.69 for 5.1 ounces)* contains 0.5% salicylic acid, which is too low a percentage to have much of an effect on blemishes, especially when included in a cleanser that is rinsed off shortly after it's applied. This also contains glycolic acid, but the pH of 4.5 is too high for effective exfoliation, and again, it will be rinsed off before it has a chance to work. What's best about this softly fragranced cleanser is the gentle cleansing agents it contains, which are effective for makeup removal and excellent for all but the driest skin types. The product name is a tongue-twister (and has no effect on either wrinkles or blemishes), but this is a good cleanser and that's great all by itself.

☺ **Healthy Skin Anti-Wrinkle Anti-Blemish Scrub** *($7.99 for 4 ounces)* contains 0.5% salicylic acid as an active ingredient and also includes 2% glycolic acid. Neither will exfoliate, however, given their brief contact with the skin before being rinsed down the drain. However, this is worth considering as a cleansing scrub for all skin types except very dry. It is more abrasive than several other scrubs that also contain polyethylene beads, but if used gently can be a helpful addition to your routine.

☺ **Healthy Skin Visibly Even Foaming Cleanser** *($7.19 for 5.1 ounces)* has a slightly richer texture than the Healthy Skin Anti-Wrinkle Anti-Blemish Scrub above and omits the salicylic and glycolic acids, but is otherwise a comparable product and good choice for normal to dry skin.

✓☺ **Healthy Skin Anti-Wrinkle Cream, Original Formula** *($11.99 for 1.4 ounces)* is a good, fragrance-free moisturizer with retinol for normal to dry skin. The retinol is packaged to keep it stable, the amount of green tea is impressive, and the formula includes tiny amounts of two forms of vitamin E. It is definitely one of the better retinol products at the drugstore.

☹ **Healthy Skin Anti-Wrinkle Cream, Original Formula SPF 15** *($11.99 for 1.4 ounces)* disappoints because it lacks the UVA-protecting ingredients of titanium dioxide, zinc oxide, avobenzone, Mexoryl SX (ecamsule), or Tinosorb and is not recommended.

✓☺ **Healthy Skin Anti-Wrinkle Intensive Eye Cream** *($17.69 for 0.5 ounce)* is a very good, lightweight moisturizing cream for use around the eyes or anywhere your skin is experiencing mild dryness. It contains a standard array of thickeners and emollients along with silicones, glycerin, several antioxidants (which is good, because none of them are present in any significant amount), an anti-irritant, retinol, film-forming agent, and preservatives. It is fragrance-free and packaged so the retinol will remain stable during use. This eye cream will (like any well-formulated moisturizer) reduce the appearance of fine, dry lines and wrinkles. However, contrary to Neutrogena's claim, it won't reduce the appearance of dark circles or fill in deep wrinkles. As elegant as this product is, it's not a viable alternative to cosmetic procedures such as Botox or dermal fillers.

✓☺ **Healthy Skin Anti-Wrinkle Intensive Night Cream** *($17.39 for 1.4 ounces)* is very similar to the Healthy Skin Anti-Wrinkle Intensive Eye Cream above, except for its slightly thinner, more lotion-like texture. It, too, is fragrance-free, features stable packaging, and the amount of antioxidants, anti-irritant, and retinol appears equal, making this another beneficial product to be used around the eyes or anywhere skin is normal to slightly dry. The Eye Cream and Night Cream versions each leave skin feeling silky-smooth.

😐 **Healthy Skin Anti-Wrinkle Intensive Serum** *($17.39 for 1 ounce)* has a silky, gel-cream texture rather than that of a true serum, and includes a blend of silicones, film-forming agents, anti-irritants, and retinol. The variety of antioxidants found in the two Healthy Skin Anti-Wrinkle products above is absent here, making this more of a one-note product, with retinol as the star ingredient. However, the amount of retinol appears to be the same in the three different products (several calls to Neutrogena asking about whether the Intensive Serum indeed contained more retinol didn't help answer that question). The decision about which one to use comes down to formula, and because the amount of film-forming agents in here is potentially problematic the other two are better options. Nonetheless, it is fragrance-free and comes in packaging that will definitely keep the retinol stable.

☺ **Healthy Skin Anti-Wrinkle Intensive SPF 20, Deep Wrinkle Moisturizing Treatment** *($19.99 for 1.4 ounces)* provides a convenient, elegant way for you to experience an in-part avobenzone sunscreen in a lightly moisturizing base with retinol and a tiny amount of water-binding agents. This isn't at the same level of formulary excellence as Neutrogena's tinted Healthy Skin Enhancer SPF 20 ($12.99) reviewed below, but it's worth a try if you have normal to slightly oily skin. This product will not fill in the look of deep wrinkles within two weeks. That's wishful thinking! Neutrogena should have settled for what works and left the other claim to less reputable cosmetics companies.

😐 **Healthy Skin Eye Cream** *($11.99 for 0.5 ounce)* does not contain glycolic acid, at least according to the ingredient list on the package. Calls to Neutrogena received the nonsensical answer that just because the company states that the product contains an AHA on the packaging doesn't mean they have to list it on the ingredient statement (What nonsense!). With or without an AHA (and make no mistake, it absolutely must be listed if the product contains it), this generic eye cream has a pH of 5.5, so no exfoliation will take place. It's an OK option for normal to dry skin and contains a few vitamin-based antioxidants.

☺ **Healthy Skin Face Lotion, for Sensitive Skin** *($12.59 for 2.5 ounces)* is a very good AHA moisturizer for normal to dry, sensitive skin, assuming your skin isn't sensitive to glycolic acid at a pH that permits exfoliation. AHA content is approximately 5%, which is tolerable for most skin types, though not as effective as 8% to 10% concentrations. This product is fragrance-free.

☹ **Healthy Skin Face Lotion SPF 15** *($12.59 for 2.5 ounces)* leaves skin vulnerable to UVA damage because it lacks sunscreen agents capable of shielding skin from the entire spectrum of UVA light. What a shame, because the 8% glycolic acid and pH of 3.3 allow exfoliation to occur, which would have made this a convenient, dual-purpose product.

✓☺ **Healthy Skin Face Lotion, Night** *($12.59 for 2.5 ounces)* is a well-formulated 8% AHA moisturizer for normal to dry skin. The pH of 3.3 permits exfoliation, and Neutrogena included some very good vitamin-based antioxidants. This does contain fragrance.

✓☺ **Healthy Skin Visibly Even Daily SPF 15 Moisturizer** *($13.09 for 1.7 ounces)* includes an in-part avobenzone sunscreen in a lightweight lotion formula enriched with the antioxidant soy. Although the pH of 4 is within range for the salicylic acid to function as an exfoliant, there isn't enough of it in here. Still, this is highly recommended as an antioxidant-rich daytime moisturizer for normal to slightly dry or slightly oily skin.

😐 **Healthy Skin Visibly Even Night Concentrate** *($15 for 1 ounce)* isn't concentrated with anything other than standard thickeners, slip agents, and silicones, all of which make this a good, basic moisturizer for normal to dry skin. The amount of salicylic acid is too low for exfoliation and the pH is too high, creating a second-rate combination. This contains retinol, but is overall not as impressive as the Healthy Skin Anti-Wrinkle Cream, Original Formula above.

☺ **Healthy Skin Anti-Wrinkle Anti-Blemish Clear Skin Cream** *($11.99 for 1 ounce)* sounds like a treat for consumers battling wrinkles and breakouts, an all-too-common frustration. However, the 2% salicylic acid cannot exfoliate very effectively because the pH is too high. This is worth considering as an antioxidant-rich moisturizer that also contains additional antioxidants (and not just a dusting, either). It is suitable for normal to dry skin but is not rated a Paula's Pick because it contains kawa extract, which can cause dermatitis and be sensitizing (Sources: *Alternative Medicine Review*, December 1998, pages 458–460; and *Clinical Experimental Pharmacology and Physiology*, July 1990, pages 495–507). The amount of kawa extract is likely too low for it to be problematic, but it's a needless inclusion.

☺ **Healthy Skin Visibly Even Skin Polishing Enzyme Treatment** *($11.75 for 1.4 ounces)* contains the ingredient *Mucor miehei* extract, which is a protease (a type of enzyme). There is no research proving it is a viable exfoliant, which is likely why Neutrogena includes polyethylene beads as a major ingredient in this scrub for normal to oily skin. This does not contain cleansing agents, and as such is one of the company's only "just a scrub" products.

NEUTROGENA OIL-FREE ACNE PRODUCTS

☺ **Oil-Free Acne Stress Control Power-Foam Wash** *($7.99 for 6 ounces)* contains 0.5% salicylic acid, but it's a useless ingredient in a cleanser because it is rinsed down the drain before it has a chance to work. This is otherwise a standard, water-soluble cleanser that's suitable for normal to oily skin. It removes makeup easily and does contain fragrance.

☹ **Oil-Free Acne Wash** *($5.99 for 6 ounces)* purports to be the #1 cleanser recommended by dermatologists for their patients with acne. If that's true, then lots of dermatologists are swayed by advertising and not up to speed on skin-care formulas. A dermatologist should know better than to endorse a cleanser that contains the drying, irritating detergent cleansing agent sodium C14-16 olefin sulfonate as a major ingredient, not to mention the fact that salicylic acid is wasted in a cleanser because it is just rinsed down the drain before it can be effective.

😐 **Oil-Free Acne Wash Cleansing Cloths** *($6.99 for 30 cloths)* are a better option than the Oil-Free Acne Wash above because the problematic detergent cleansing agent is a much smaller proportion of the formula. These cloths are a good option for normal to oily skin, but don't forget to rinse the solution from your skin.

☹ **Oil-Free Acne Wash Cream Cleanser** *($5.99 for 6.7 ounces)* has a slightly creamy texture, but that's not enough to keep the main detergent cleansing agent (sodium C14-16 olefin sulfonate) from drying skin. In no way is this a "gentle treatment" for acne; the 2% salicylic acid is rinsed away before it has a chance to work.

☺ **Oil-Free Acne Wash Foam Cleanser** *($6.99 for 5.1 ounces)* contains 2% salicylic acid, but that won't help acne in a cleanser because it is rinsed down the drain before it can go to work. This is still a good water-soluble cleanser for normal to oily skin.

☹ **Oil-Free Acne Stress Control Power-Clear Scrub** *($7.99 for 4.2 ounces)* contains menthol, which makes it too irritating for all skin types. The 2% salicylic acid isn't going to benefit blemish-prone skin when used in a topical scrub because it is basically rinsed down the drain right after it's applied and doesn't have time to absorb into the skin.

☹ **Oil-Free Acne Wash Daily Scrub** *($8.19 for 4.2 ounces)* is nearly identical to the Oil-Free Acne Stress Control Power-Clear Scrub above, and the same review applies.

☹ **Oil-Free Acne Wash 60 Second Mask Scrub** *($6.99 for 6 ounces)* is a 1% BHA (salicylic acid) scrub that is across-the-board standard in terms of its abrasive agent (ground-up polyethylene). True to form for almost all Neutrogena Oil-Free Acne products, this contains menthol, which makes it a problem for all skin types.

✓☺ **Oil-Free Acne Stress Control 3-In-1 Hydrating Acne Treatment** *($7.99 for 2 ounces)* gets Neutrogena back into the BHA game, and it's about time! Most of their previous BHA products either contained irritating ingredients (particularly alcohol and menthol) or had a pH that was too high for effective exfoliation to take place. This version contains 2% salicylic acid at a pH of 3.4, and comes in a nearly weightless silicone base that includes antioxidants and anti-irritants. Although the inclusion of fragrance and coloring agents is a slight disappointment, it's a relief that Neutrogena omitted menthol or its derivatives, making this an all-around ideal BHA lotion for skin of any type battling blemishes.

☹ **Oil-Free Anti-Acne Moisturizer** *($5.99 for 1.7 ounces)* contains the irritating menthol derivative menthyl lactate, and is not recommended. The amount of salicylic acid is too low to provide much exfoliation or to alleviate acne/blackheads.

NEUTROGENA RAPID CLEAR PRODUCTS

☹ **Rapid Clear Oil-Control Foaming Cleanser** *($7.39 for 6 ounces)* is a simply formulated cleanser that contains the strongly alkaline ingredient potassium stearate as the main cleansing agent. That means this cleanser is about as drying to skin as most bar soaps, and as a result is not recommended.

☺ **Rapid Clear Acne Defense Face Lotion** *($7.39 for 1.7 ounces)* is an effective BHA product option in the battle against blemishes. With 2% salicylic acid and a pH of 3.6, this can indeed exfoliate skin and help dislodge blackheads. The product features a lightweight moisturizing base that is best for normal to slightly dry skin dealing with blemishes. The only issue I have with Rapid Clear Acne Defense Face Lotion is the irritating fragrant extracts it contains (cinnamon and cedar), though they are present in amounts that are likely too low to cause irritation. Still, they are unnecessary additives and prevent this BHA product from earning a Paula's Pick rating.

☹ **Rapid Clear Acne Eliminating Gel** *($7.39 for 0.5 ounce)* is another product that means well by the inclusion of the proven blemish-fighter salicylic acid (in a 2% concentration), but it falters with the pointless inclusion of almost 40% alcohol along with witch hazel extract, cedarwood, and cinnamon. Even without the irritants, the pH of this product is too high for optimal exfoliation to occur.

☹ **Rapid Clear Treatment Pads** *($7.99 for 60 pads)* will rapidly irritate due to the amount of alcohol. The 2% salicylic acid is nice and potentially effective, but this is not a BHA shining star for Neutrogena.

NEUTROGENA VISIBLY FIRM PRODUCTS

😐 **Visibly Firm Eye Cream, Active Copper** *($18.49 for 0.5 ounce)* won't firm skin, but it's still an OK moisturizer for normal to dry skin anywhere on the face. The amount of antioxidants is paltry, and the jar packaging won't keep them (and likely the copper peptide) stable during use.

☺ **Visibly Firm Face Lotion, Active Copper SPF 20** *($18.49 for 1.7 ounces)* deserves praise for its in-part zinc oxide sunscreen, but the base formula for normal to slightly oily skin is bland, with the antioxidants and copper listed after the preservative. For the money, this doesn't measure up against any of Olay's Regenerist or Total Effects products with sunscreen, but is still an option.

😐 **Visibly Firm Lift Serum, Active Copper** *($18.49 for 1 ounce)* won't firm or lift skin anywhere, but don't let that overshadow the fact that this is a good water-based moisturizer for normal to slightly dry skin. It contains mostly water, slip agent, several silicones, emollient, glycerin, copper peptide (which functions as a water-binding agent, not as an antiwrinkle agent), vitamin E, soothing agent, film-forming agent, and fragrance. It will make skin feel silky without looking greasy and works well under foundation, but this is strictly about copper and it is a stretch of physiology to assume that copper is all skin needs to be healthy.

😐 **Visibly Firm Night Cream, Active Copper** *($18.49 for 1.7 ounces)* contains some good antioxidants, but once again jar packaging will be their undoing once you begin using this. Reformulated in mid-2007, this remains an OK moisturizer for normal to dry skin, but copper isn't the antiwrinkle, skin-firming answer. If it were, why is Neutrogena selling so many other products without copper, and also making antiwrinkle claims about them?

OTHER NEUTROGENA PRODUCTS

✓😊 **Extra Gentle Cleanser** *($7.19 for 6.7 ounces)* remains one of Neutrogena's standout cleansers. It is an excellent option for normal to dry or sensitive skin, including those with eczema or rosacea. The fragrance-free, lotion-textured formula contains mild cleansing agents and some good anti-irritants, but these aren't as effective in a cleanser as they are when they are left on the skin.

✓😊 **Fresh Foaming Cleanser** *($6.59 for 6.7 ounces)* is a superb water-soluble cleanser for normal to oily or combination skin. It removes makeup easily and rinses without a trace. This does contain fragrance.

😊 **Illuminating Foamy Cream Cleanser** *($6.99 for 5.1 ounces)* is a great choice for those with normal to oily skin seeking a foaming water-soluble cleanser that also has a mild exfoliating effect because of the microbeads (scrub particles) it contains. This would be rated a Paula's Pick if it did not contain a selection of potentially irritating citrus extracts.

😐 **Liquid Neutrogena Facial Cleansing Formula, Original** *($9.09 for 8 ounces)* is an option as a water-soluble cleanser for oily skin, but its combination of detergent cleansing agents is potentially drying. As a result this is not preferred to the Fresh Foaming Cleanser above.

😐 **Liquid Neutrogena Facial Cleansing Formula, Fragrance-Free** *($9.09 for 8 ounces)* is identical to the Liquid Neutrogena Facial Cleansing Formula, Original above, minus fragrance. Fragrance-free is nice, but the drying cleansing agents are a problem for all skin types.

✓😊 **Make-Up Remover Cleansing Towelettes** *($7.99 for 25 towelettes)* are cleansing cloths whose specialty is makeup removal, and they do an excellent job of breaking up and dissolving foundation, lipstick, and mascara (including waterproof types). These soft-textured cloths do not contain any needlessly irritating ingredients (such as menthol or arnica), making them safe for use around the eyes.

✓😊 **One Step Gentle Cleanser** *($6.20 for 5.2 ounces)* removes makeup and leaves skin feeling clean and smooth, all in one gentle step. This water-soluble cleanser feels great on skin, lathers slightly, and rinses easily. It also contains milder cleansing agents than many other cleansers. It is highly recommended for all but very dry skin types. It does contain fragrance. Note: For some reason, most mass-market stores that stock this cleanser are stocking it with Neutrogena's makeup rather than with their other cleansers, so it can be a bit tricky to find.

☹ **PureGlow Daily Cleansing Cushions, for Combination/Oily Skin** *($7.99 for 24 cushions)* are marketed as being able to give your skin facial-like results, but unless your aesthetician is swabbing your skin with a derivative of menthol, you're out of luck. The only thing obtained from this product will be due to irritation, and that's not the way to keep skin healthy and vibrant.

☹ **PureGlow Daily Cleansing Cushions, for Normal to Dry Skin** *($7.99 for 24 cushions)* are similar to the PureGlow Daily Cleansing Cushions, for Combination/Oily Skin above, and the same comments apply.

☺ **Sensitive Skin Solutions Cleansing Wash, for Combination and Sensitive Skin** *($8.59 for 5.1 ounces)* is a fairly gentle, lotion-style cleanser that contains mild detergent cleansing agents and anti-irritants. This also contains glycolic acid, although the product's pH is too high to allow exfoliation to occur—just as well, however, since it is rinsed off before it has a chance to work anyway. This is best for normal to slightly dry skin not prone to blemishes. It does have fragrance, which makes it less appropriate for someone with skin sensitivities.

☺ **Sensitive Skin Solutions Cream Cleanser, for Dry and Sensitive Skin** *($8.59 for 5.1 ounces)* is a very good creamy cleanser for dry to very dry skin. The surplus of emollients and thickening agents in this product offers a moist finish, but this cleanser does not rinse well without the aid of a washcloth. It is still a worthwhile option, but a cleanser designed for sensitive skin should ideally be fragrance-free, which this product is not. The fragrance makes this an iffy product for those dealing with rosacea.

☹ **Sensitive Skin Solutions Oil-Free Foaming Cleanser, for Oily and Sensitive Skin** *($8.59 for 5.1 ounces)* would have been a great gentle, water-soluble cleanser suitable for all but the most sensitive skin types, except that it contains *Arnica montana* extract, which can be a skin irritant as well as a problematic ingredient to use around the eyes and mucous membranes.

☹ **The Transparent Facial Bar, Acne-Prone Skin Formula**, ☹ **The Transparent Facial Bar, Dry Skin Formula**, ☹ **The Transparent Facial Bar, Dry Skin Formula, Fragrance-Free**, ☹ **The Transparent Facial Bar, Oily Skin Formula**, ☹ **The Transparent Facial Bar, Original Formula**, and ☹ **The Transparent Facial Bar, Original Formula, Fragrance-Free** *(all priced at $2.99 for a 3.5-ounce bar)* are all variations on the same standard bar soap based on the drying, irritating cleansing agent TEA-stearate and traditional soap ingredients (such as tallow that can clog pores). None of these bar cleansers are recommended for any skin type.

☺ **Extra Gentle Eye Makeup Remover Pads** *($6.20 for 30 pads)* is akin to a silicone-based makeup remover steeped in plush, slightly textured pads. Although pricier than using a liquid makeup remover on a separate cotton pad, there's no denying that the formula works quickly to dissolve makeup, including waterproof formulas. These pads do contain fragrance.

☺ **Ultra-Soft Eye Makeup Remover Pads** *($6.59 for 30 pads)* are indeed very soft pads that work to gently remove eye makeup. The formula is very similar to the Extra Gentle Eye Makeup Remover Pads above, and the same review applies.

✓☺ **Fresh Foaming Scrub** *($5.69 for 4.2 ounces)* is a very good cleansing scrub for normal to oily skin, though the amount of salicylic acid isn't enough to exfoliate. The polyethylene beads do that job, and do it well while rinsing cleanly.

☹ **Illuminating Microderm Cleansing Pads** *($7.99 for 24 pads)* are dry pads impregnated with a glycerin-based cleansing system that is activated when the pad is dampened with water. One side has mildly abrasive beads, while the other has "conditioning stripes" to complete the cleansing process. The exfoliating action of this product is not even close to what's possible from the other microdermabrasion-in-a-jar products that are available, and it ends up irritating skin because of the amount of menthyl lactate. You will feel a lingering tingle after each use, but that's definitely not an illuminating sign!

✓ ☺ **Pore Refining Cleanser** *($7.49 for 6.7 ounces)* is positioned as a cleanser, but is really a cleanser/scrub hybrid. It's less abrasive than the scrubs above, and it's the polyethylene beads doing the exfoliating, not the glycolic or salicylic acids. The gentle cleansing base is appropriate for normal to slightly dry or dry skin.

😐 **Alcohol-Free Toner** *($6.99 for 8.5 ounces)* is an average toner at best because it lacks significant water-binding agents or ingredients that support skin's structure. The formula is OK for normal to slightly dry or slightly oily skin.

☹ **Clear Pore Oil-Controlling Astringent** *($4.99 for 8 ounces)* contains 45% alcohol followed by witch hazel (which just adds more alcohol), and together these make this astringent too irritating to consider. The pH of this product prevents the 2% salicylic acid from functioning effectively as an exfoliant.

☹ **Pore Refining Toner** *($7.49 for 8.5 ounces)* lists alcohol as the second ingredient, and also contains witch hazel. It is even more irritating than the Clear Pore Oil-Controlling Astringent above because it also contains peppermint and eucalyptus.

☹ **Sensitive Skin Solutions Alcohol-Free Toner, for All Skin Types** *($7.95 for 6.7 ounces)* contains angelica root extract as a main ingredient, which makes this toner a problem for all skin types. Although some of the components of angelica have antioxidant ability, it is a risky ingredient to use on skin if it is exposed to sunlight (Sources: www.naturaldatabase.com; and *Journal of Agricultural and Food Chemistry*, March 2007, pages 1737–1742).

☹ **Anti-Oxidant Age Reverse Day Lotion SPF 20** *($17.99 for 1.7 ounces)* claims to neutralize 90% of free radicals, but there's no supporting evidence to validate this. Besides, under what conditions was this tested? And what free radicals? Free radicals generated from sun exposure? From breathing? Exposure to secondhand smoke? The only antioxidant of note in this in-part avobenzone sunscreen is soy, and that's hardly the most powerful option (we still don't know which antioxidant, if any, will emerge with this title). Although the sunscreen element can forestall further signs of environmental aging, this product contains methylisothiazolinone, which is not recommended for use in leave-on products due to its sensitizing potential. The inclusion of feverfew extract is also a problem because it can also be sensitizing.

☹ **Anti-Oxidant Age Reverse Eye Cream** *($17.99 for 0.5 ounce)* contains the same problematic ingredients as the Anti-Oxidant Age Reverse Day Lotion SPF 20 above, and is not recommended for any skin type. What a shame, because several aspects of this formula are quite impressive.

☹ **Anti-Oxidant Age Reverse Night Cream** *($17.99 for 1.7 ounces)* contains the same problematic ingredients as the Anti-Oxidant Age Reverse Day Lotion SPF 20 above, and the same concerns apply. This formula differs little from the Age Reverse Eye Cream above, except that the more state-of-the-art ingredients are given less prominence. All the Age Reverse products contain soy as the star antioxidant; if that's of interest to you then consider the Positively Ageless products from Aveeno; they omit the irritants Neutrogena includes.

✓☺ **Healthy Defense SPF 30 Daily Eye Cream, Light Tint** *($11.99 for 0.5 ounce)* has a light tint because of the amount of zinc oxide (the sole sunscreen active) it contains. Silica keeps this from being too creamy, and makes this lightweight, fragrance-free moisturizer best for normal to slightly dry or slightly oily skin. It is recommended for use around the eyes and contains a good array of water-binding agents and lesser amounts of several antioxidants.

😐 **Healthy Defense SPF 30 Daily Moisturizer, Light Tint** ($13.29 for 1.7 ounces) is an average daytime moisturizer with sunscreen for normal to slightly dry skin. The in-part zinc oxide sunscreen is great, but the sheer tinted base formula doesn't go the distance.

😐 **Healthy Defense SPF 30 Daily Moisturizer, Untinted** ($13.29 for 1.7 ounces) is identical to the Healthy Defense SPF 30 Daily Moisturizer, Light Tint above, except without the tint. The same review applies.

☹ **Healthy Defense SPF 45 Daily Moisturizer, Untinted** *($12.49 for 1.7 ounces)* shortchanges skin on antioxidants, but does provide an in-part avobenzone sunscreen. What's problematic is the choice of the sensitizing preservative methylisothiazolinone, which is not recommended for use in leave-on products. I'd choose Neutrogena's Ultra Sheer Dry Touch Sunblock products (SPF 30 or SPF 45) reviewed below before this.

😐 **Illuminating Eye Reviver** *($12.99 for 0.5 ounce)* has a great silicone-enhanced texture and silky finish, but tactile positives aren't enough to make this jar-packaged moisturizer worth considering over many others. Mica adds a soft shine to skin, but it cannot illuminate the eye area in the same way a deftly applied highlighter or concealer can.

☹ **Illuminating Whip Moisturizer SPF 20** *($14.99 for 1.7 ounces)* achieves sufficient UVA protection thanks to its avobenzone content, but it is not recommended because it contains the preservative methylisothiazolinone, which is known to cause contact dermatitis and is contraindicated for use in leave-on products (Sources: Contact Dermatitis, November 2001, pages 257–264; and *European Journal of Dermatology*, March 1999, pages 144–160).

☹ **Intensified Day Moisture SPF 15** *($11.99 for 2.25 ounces)* lacks the UVA-protecting ingredients of titanium dioxide, zinc oxide, avobenzone, Mexoryl SX, or Tinosorb and is not recommended. The base formula is also really boring.

😐 **Light Night Cream** *($11.99 for 2.25 ounces)* remains in the Neutrogena lineup, and is still a basic, emollient moisturizer for normal to dry skin. It contains a tiny amount of soy fatty acid, but is otherwise devoid of state-of-the-art ingredients.

☹ **Oil-Free Moisture SPF 15** *($10.59 for 4 ounces)* doesn't contain oil, but also doesn't provide sufficient UVA-protecting ingredients. Given Neutrogena's sun-savvy marketing campaigns and its roster of impressive broad-spectrum sunscreens, this product should be discontinued—it's not doing anyone's skin any favors, that's for sure.

😐 **Oil-Free Moisture, for Combination Skin** *($10.59 for 4 ounces)* provides lightweight, skin-silkening moisture for its intended skin type, and doesn't contain fragrance. However, your skin deserves more than this basic formula provides.

😐 **Oil-Free Moisture, for Sensitive Skin** *($10.59 for 4 ounces)* is suitable for dry, sensitive skin (and for those with rosacea) because it contains some good emollients and a small amount of water-binding agents. This is also fragrance-free, but that's where the excitement starts and stops.

✓☺ **Pore Refining Cream SPF 15** *($14.99 for 1 ounce)* combines an in-part avobenzone sunscreen with a pH-correct AHA product and retinol. All told, this is one of Neutrogena's most impressive formulas due to its triple benefit and the fact that it contains some skin-identical substances, such as cholesterol, and additional antioxidants. The formula is best for normal to slightly dry or slightly oily skin.

😐 **Radiance Boost Eye Cream** *($14.29 for 0.5 ounce)*. Although this is a decent, albeit ordinary moisturizer (for the eye area or the face), there is nothing in it that has proven to lighten dark circles or ameliorate puffy eyes. This contains mostly water, silicones, thickeners, pH adjusters, petrolatum, wax, more silicones, water-binding agent, and preservatives. Some antioxidants or anti-irritants would have been nice, but they're absent. As is, this eye cream can handle the basic needs of dry skin, but all the other impressive elements that create a truly great product are missing, and that certainly isn't a boost, it's a let down.

☺ **Summer Glow Daily Moisturizer SPF 15** *($11.99 for 1.7 ounces)* features an in-part avobenzone sunscreen in a glycerin-based moisturizer that also contains a tiny amount of dihydroxyacetone, the ingredient most commonly used in self-tanning products for turning skin a realistic shade of brown. This product has three effects: (1) it lightly moisturizes skin, (2) it provides broad-spectrum sun protection, and (3) it adds a slight tan color to skin, which develops in a few hours. It's a good way to maintain daily sun protection while also getting a touch of color. Just be sure to wash your hands and nails after using it to avoid staining, and follow other general guidelines for self-tanner application—especially making sure your skin is exfoliated prior to application to avoid streaks and a blotchy appearance.

☹ **Clear Pore Cleanser/Mask** *($7.49 for 4.2 ounces)* can disinfect skin because it contains 3.5% benzoyl peroxide, but the clay base makes this too potentially drying, and the menthol only causes irritation. A well-formulated leave-on benzoyl peroxide product would be far better for treating blemishes.

😐 **On-the-Spot Acne Treatment** *($6.59 for 0.75 ounce)* contains 2.5% benzoyl peroxide as the active ingredient, which is helpful for blemish-prone skin. The formula's clay and wax base is a confusing mix for skin; the clay can exacerbate the drying effect of benzoyl peroxide, while the wax may make blemishes worse. Still, I suppose this is an OK option for spot-treating a blemish (which you should do only if you rarely break out—regular breakouts require treating the entire face).

😐 **Shine-Control Blotting Sheets** *($6.79 for 60 sheets)* are thin plastic polypropylene sheets. They work decently to absorb excess oil and perspiration, but the mineral-oil additive won't keep skin as shine-free as other options. If you're curious to try these, Clean & Clear's less expensive Morning Burst Oil-Absorbing Sheets ($5.19 for 50 sheets) are identical except for the fragrance they have.

☹ **Lip Boost Intense Moisture Therapy** *($6.79 for 0.3 ounce)* contains many extraordinary ingredients for dry, chapped lips—above and beyond what most lip balms offer. That's why it's so frustrating that Neutrogena also added menthol along with melissa and peppermint extracts to the mix.

NEUTROGENA SUNSCREEN PRODUCTS

✓☺ **Active Breathable Sunblock SPF 30** *($9.99 for 4 ounces)* is remarkably similar to Neutrogena's Ultra Sheer Dry-Touch Sunblock SPF 30, reviewed below. Both are formidable sunscreens containing avobenzone for sufficient UVA protection, and both have an initially creamy lotion texture that dries to a matte (in feel) finish that's far removed from the often heavy, greasy feel of high-SPF products. Active Breathable Sunblock SPF 30 has a larger proportion of film-forming agents to back up its water-resistant claim. I think you'll be surprised by this sunscreen's exceptionally dry finish. And because it has such a lightweight feel and absorbs so quickly, those who usually dislike the feel of sunscreen may find they become better about applying it daily. If you're curious about trying this sunscreen or Neutrogena's Ultra Sheer option, the Ultra Sheer has a slightly lighter texture and is a bit more elegant for facial application, not to mention it contains more antioxidants. However, if you plan to exercise outdoors during the daytime, Active Breathable Sunblock SPF 30 would be better because of its stronger water- and sweat-resisting properties.

✓☺ **Active Breathable Sunblock SPF 45** *($9.99 for 4 ounces)* is identical to the Active Breathable Sunblock SPF 30 above, only with increased levels of active ingredients to make it an SPF 45. This still maintains a smooth, dry finish that someone with oily skin would certainly appreciate, and it won't make skin feel heavy or coated.

✓☺ **Age Shield Sunblock SPF 30** *($9.99 for 4 ounces)* has a great name, and honestly describes what a well-formulated sunscreen does for your skin. This fragrance-free, in-part avobenzone sunscreen definitely has the UVA range covered, and includes several antioxidants in stable packaging. The initially creamy application dries to a soft matte finish without a hint of greasiness. It's a texture that someone with normal to very oily skin will love, and is suitable for use under makeup.

Now to address the claims. Neutrogena maintains that this product is a breakthrough in UVA protection for the United States because of their patented Helioplex technology. Helioplex is composed of avobenzone, oxybenzone, and the solvent 2-6-diethylhexyl naphthalate, a solvent that is believed to make the avobenzone more stable, and avobenzone stability has indeed been a concern. According to Neutrogena, Helioplex "blocks more UVA rays than the leading sunscreen available in the U.S. today, to give you the best anti-aging protection around." Yet, without knowing which "leading sunscreen" they are referring to (best-selling products change daily), there is no way to know what they are comparing it to. What if that sunscreen didn't even contain UVA-protecting ingredients? If it is an issue of avobenzone remaining stable, there is substantial research showing that it can be stable without the addition of the naphthalate (Sources: *Journal of Photochemistry and Photobiology*, March 2006, pages 204–213; and *British Journal of Dermatology*, December 2004, pages 1234–1244).

Neutrogena is touting this and their other sunscreens with Helioplex as a breakthrough when, in fact, it really isn't anything new under the sun. What is perplexing is that all the ballyhoo about Helioplex and avobenzone completely ignores the UVA screening ability of titanium dioxide and zinc oxide. Both of these mineral sunscreens block light beyond the UVA light range of 320–400 nanometers, screening all the way up to 700 nanometers (Source: *Skin Therapy Letter*, Table 1, 1997), and Neutrogena also sells sunscreens with these two active ingredients. Marketing claims aside, in the end what really counts is that this remains a well-formulated, broad-spectrum sunscreen that deserves consideration when shopping for water-resistant SPF 30 products.

✓☺ **Age Shield Sunblock SPF 45** *($9.99 for 4 ounces)* is nearly identical to the Age Shield Sunblock SPF 30 above, and the same review applies.

☹ **Fresh Cooling Body Mist Sunblock SPF 30** *($10.49 for 5 ounces)* comes in a pressurized can and propels a fine-mist formula that includes an in-part avobenzone sunscreen. Unfortunately, the spray is loaded with alcohol (it makes up 67% of the formula) and also includes a menthol derivative; combining the menthol derivative and the alcohol will indeed make your skin feel cool, but not in a good way. The broad-spectrum sun protection and ultra-light feel are great, but the irritants are a significant problem for skin, even more so when it is going to be subjected to long-term sun exposure—such as during a day at the beach or on a tropical vacation.

☹ **Fresh Cooling Body Mist Sunblock SPF 45** *($10.49 for 5 ounces)* has a higher SPF than the Fresh Cooling Body Mist Sunblock SPF 30 above, but that's about the only difference. The same positives (in-part avobenzone sunscreen and near-weightless feel) and negatives (too much alcohol and needless inclusion of a menthol derivative) combine to create a product that's effective, but too problematic to recommend.

☹ **Fresh Cooling Sunblock Gel SPF 30** *($11.29 for 4 ounces)* feels cooling because it contains over 70% alcohol plus menthol, but that's exactly what makes this in-part avobenzone sunscreen too drying and irritating for all skin types.

☹ **Fresh Cooling Sunblock Gel SPF 45** *($9.99 for 4 ounces)* is similar to but contains less alcohol than the Fresh Cooling Sunblock Gel SPF 30 above, but it's still irritating, as is the menthol.

😐 **Healthy Defense Oil-Free Sunblock Lotion SPF 45** *($8.99 for 4 ounces)* is a good basic sunscreen for normal to oily skin, and includes avobenzone for UVA protection. However, I am concerned that the amount of methylpropanediol (a penetration enhancer) may make this more irritating to skin than other sunscreens. After all, 26.5% active ingredients is a lot for anyone's skin to handle. This is worth trying, but is recommended with caution.

☺ **Healthy Defense Oil-Free Sunblock Stick SPF 30** *($7.49 for 0.47 ounce)* brings portable protection for oft-forgotten areas of skin, though the wax base is not the best for blemish-prone areas. UVA protection is assured with avobenzone, and this contains small amounts of vitamin-based antioxidants.

☹ **Lip Moisturizer SPF 15** *($3.29 for 0.15 ounce)* is advertised as being PABA-free, which is nice (PABA is a sunscreen active that's rarely used because it tends to be irritating), but Neutrogena forgot to include sufficient UVA protection, so this isn't a lip balm with sunscreen that anyone should rely on.

☺ **Sensitive Skin Sunblock Lotion SPF 30** *($8.99 for 4 ounces)* contains titanium dioxide as its only active ingredient, and does not contain fragrance, two points that make it suitable for sensitive skin. The amount of antioxidants is minor (there's more preservative), but this is still a good choice for those whose skin cannot tolerate most sunscreens.

☺ **Summer Glow Daily Moisturizer SPF 20** *($8.09 for 6.7 ounces)* provides sun protection with its in-part avobenzone sunscreen and comes in a lightweight lotion base that includes a bit of dihydroxyacetone, the ingredient in most sunless tanning products. It is suitable for all skin types, but best for normal to oily skin.

☹ **Ultra Sheer Body Mist Sunblock SPF 30** *($9.99 for 5 ounces)* features 3% avobenzone for sufficient UVA protection, but the base formula is mostly alcohol, and that makes it too drying and irritating for all skin types. Oddly, this product still leaves a fairly greasy, slick finish.

☹ **Ultra Sheer Body Mist Sunblock SPF 45** *($9.99 for 5 ounces)* is nearly identical to the Ultra Sheer Body Mist Sunblock SPF 30 above, except it contains a higher percentage of active ingredients to achieve its higher SPF rating. Otherwise, the same comments apply.

✓☺ **Ultra Sheer Dry-Touch Sunblock SPF 30** *($9.99 for 3 ounces)* really does have a dry finish, and is an outstanding in-part avobenzone sunscreen that begins creamy but quickly dries down to a weightless matte (in feel) finish. The high levels of active ingredients required to net an SPF 30 do leave a very slight sheen on the skin, but it's hardly worth complaining about, especially if you are dealing with oily to very oily skin and have been unable to find a stand-alone sunscreen that doesn't feel heavy or greasy. Those with normal to dry skin will likely find this sunscreen too drying, but it's a winning option for oily skin, and it does contain antioxidants.

✓☺ **Ultra Sheer Dry-Touch Sunblock SPF 45** *($9.99 for 3 ounces)* is identical to the Ultra Sheer Dry-Touch Sunblock SPF 30 above, but with increased levels of active ingredients to reach SPF 45. This still maintains a smooth, dry finish that someone with oily skin will certainly appreciate. Remember, higher SPF numbers do not supply better protection, just longer protection. And they still need to be reapplied at regular intervals.

☺ **Ultra Sheer Dry-Touch Sunblock SPF 55** *($10.49 for 3 ounces)* contains the same Helioplex ingredient mixture as the Age Shield Sunblock SPF 30 above, so UVA bases are well-covered. Although this sunscreen is fairly lightweight, it isn't as sheer and it definitely is more apparent on the skin than either of the Age Shield Sunblocks above. The formulas are similar, but this Ultra Sheer version lacks a single antioxidant and contains fragrance, which keep it from earning a Paula's Pick rating and also make it not worth considering over Neutrogena's Age Shield Sunblocks.

☹ **Ultra Sheer Dry-Touch Sunblock SPF 70** *($11.29 for 3 ounces)* achieves its ultra-high SPF number because it contains over 25% active ingredients, including avobenzone for UVA protection. The lotion texture has a smooth feel and a dry, almost weightless finish. However, this product has some problems. First, it lacks antioxidants; second, it contains the preservative methylisothiazolinone, which is not recommended for use in leave-on products due to its sensitizing potential (Source: *Archives of Dermatological Research*, February 2007, pages 227–237); and third, its SPF 70 means there are an awful lot of sunscreen ingredients for skin to handle. Also, considering that an SPF 70 product provides about 24 hours of daylight protection (assuming you don't perspire or wash your hands), there just isn't enough daylight to warrant this kind of formulation, except in Alaska or Antarctica during their long summer days. The FDA's recent sunscreen proposal to allow SPF ratings up to 50 may mean products like this will be disallowed, which wouldn't necessarily be a bad thing, for reasons stated above.

☺ **Ultra Soft Hydrating Sunblock SPF 30** *($14.49 for 6 ounces)* carries on the dry-finish pattern first seen in Neutrogena's Ultra Sheer Sunblock formulas, also with SPF 30 and SPF 45 variations. The Ultra Soft Sunblock is another excellent, in-part avobenzone sunscreen that provides light moisture while setting to a matte finish that doesn't leave skin feeling heavy or coated. It is water-resistant, but I wouldn't bank on it for dry skin. The only thing preventing this product from earning a Paula's Pick rating is that antioxidants are barely present. That would be all it would take to make it a superior option. Well, that and omitting the fragrance.

☺ **Ultra Soft Hydrating Sunblock SPF 45** *($14.49 for 6 ounces)* contains higher levels of the active ingredient to achieve its SPF rating, but is otherwise identical to the Ultra Soft Hydrating Sunblock SPF 30 above, and the same basic comments apply, with one exception: the more abundant sunscreen agents mean that this sunscreen, while matte in feel, will appear slightly greasy on skin. If you have normal to oily skin and want to keep shine to a minimum, use the SPF 30 version above instead of this one. As with all sunscreens, liberal application is necessary to achieve the level of protection stated on the label.

✓☺ **UVA/UVB Sunblock Lotion SPF 45** *($8.99 for 4 ounces)* is a very good, water-resistant sunscreen for normal to oily skin. It includes avobenzone for UVA protection, as well as some good antioxidants and soothing agents. It is also fragrance-free, which is icing on the cake!

NEUTROGENA SUNLESS TANNING & AFTER-SUN PRODUCTS

☺ **Build-A-Tan Gradual Sunless Tanning** *($9.99 for 6.7 ounces)* is a very standard, but good, self-tanning lotion for normal to oily skin. It tans skin with dihydroxyacetone, the same ingredient found in most self-tanners.

☺ **Build-A-Tan Gradual Sunless Tanning for Face SPF 15** *($10.09 for 2.5 ounces)* is a dihydroxyacetone-based self-tanning lotion that includes an in-part avobenzone sunscreen. It's an option for daytime use, assuming you apply it liberally (not always the best idea for self-tanners because the color can come out too dark or blotchy).

☺ **Instant Bronze Sunless Tanner and Bronzer in One, for the Face** *($9.99 for 2 ounces)* is a basic self-tanner with dihydroxyacetone and caramel coloring for an instant sheer tan effect. The formula is best for normal to dry skin.

☺ **Instant Bronze Sunless Tanner and Bronzer in One, Streak-Free Foam, Medium** *($9.99 for 4 ounces)* is a good, foam-textured self-tanner for all skin types. The formula dries quickly, which helps minimize streaking. Dihydroxyacetone provides the main tan color, with erythrulose (a secondary self-tanning agent) providing additional color after a couple of days.

☺ **Instant Bronze Sunless Tanner and Bronzer in One, Streak-Free Foam, Deep** *($9.99 for 4 ounces)* is similar to the Instant Bronze Sunless Tanner and Bronzer in One, Streak-Free Foam, Medium above, except this option contains more dihydroxyacetone and is better for medium to dark skin.

☺ **Instant Bronze Sunless Tanner and Bronzer in One, Streak-Free Lotion, Medium** *($9.99 for 4 ounces)* contains caramel for instant color and the universally used self-tanning ingredient dihydroxyacetone to create a lingering "tan." The base formula is best for normal to dry skin not prone to blemishes.

☺ **Instant Bronze Sunless Tanner and Bronzer in One, Streak-Free Lotion, Deep** *($9.99 for 4 ounces)* is similar to the Instant Bronze Sunless Tanner and Bronzer in One, Streak-Free Lotion, Medium above, except this contains more dihydroxyacetone and is preferred for medium to dark skin tones.

☹ **MicroMist Tanning Sunless Spray, Medium** *($11.99 for 5.3 ounces)* contains too much witch hazel to make it a good choice, especially given the huge number of self-tanning products that work without irritating skin.

☹ **MicroMist Tanning Sunless Spray, Deep** *($11.99 for 5.3 ounces)* has the same irritancy potential as the MicroMist Tanning Sunless Spray Medium above, and the same review applies.

☺ **Moisture Rich Sunless Tanning SPF 20, Medium** *($9.99 for 4 ounces)* protects skin with an in-part avobenzone sunscreen and is otherwise a standard self-tanning lotion that turns skin color with dihydroxyacetone. Keep in mind that liberal application of this product (necessary to achieve the amount of sun protection stated on the label) may result in unsatisfactory self-tan results.

☺ **Moisture Rich Sunless Tanning SPF 20, Deep** *($9.99 for 4 ounces)* is similar to the Moisture Rich Sunless Tanning SPF 20, Medium above, except this creates a darker tan because it has more dihydroxyacetone. Otherwise, the same review applies.

☺ **Sheer Body Tint** *($9.99 for 4 ounces)* is not a self-tanner but rather a cosmetic bronzer in mousse form. The lightweight formula smooths on easily and dries quickly while imparting sheer, buildable color that washes off with any cleanser. It is available in versions for fair to light and medium to dark skin tones. Both versions contain film-forming agents that help keep this on skin, not all over your clothes. However, I wouldn't recommend wearing this under your tennis whites!

☺ **Sunless Tanning Foam** *($10.09 for 4 ounces)* is a basic, ultra-light self-tanner for all skin types. Dihydroxyacetone turns skin color while erythrulose builds additional color over a couple of days.

☺ **Sunless Tanning Lotion** *($9.99 for 4 ounces)* is similar to the Build-A-Tan Gradual Sunless Tanning product above, and the same comments apply.

☹ **After-Sun Treatment with Natural Soy** *($9.69 for 5.1 ounces)* claims to soothe and revitalize sun-exposed skin, and contains several state-of-the-art ingredients to do that. Unfortunately, this also contains the menthol derivative menthyl lactate, which ruins an otherwise incredibly impressive product. Sigh!

☹ **Pre-Sunless Scrub** *($5.29 for 6.7 ounces)* contains the drying detergent cleansing agent sodium C14-16 olefin sulfonate as the main ingredient, and is not recommended.

NEUTROGENA MAKEUP

FOUNDATION: Note: Neutrogena's foundations offer limited options for women of color, although some lighter-skinned African-American women may find the darker shades will work for their skin tone.

✓☺ **Healthy Skin Enhancer SPF 20** *($10.99)* combines an in-part titanium dioxide sunscreen with retinol and a hint of color, all of which enhance skin due to their respective qualities. Moreover, there is more than just a dusting of retinol in this product, which makes it unique! It has a light, creamy texture and a satin finish appropriate for those with normal to dry skin. If an oily T-zone is an issue, this product should be set with powder to reduce the sheen it leaves on skin. The six sheer shades are great and include options for fair (but not very fair) to tan skin tones. In addition—and this is again unusual for a foundation—plenty of antioxidants are included. This product proves that Neutrogena is capable of setting new makeup benchmarks for their drugstore contemporaries to strive for, rather than just keeping up with their competitors.

✓☺ **Healthy Skin GlowSheers SPF 30** *($12.25)* is a very sheer, tinted moisturizer that's ideal for normal to slightly oily skin. It has a feather-light texture that glides over skin and sets to a soft matte (in feel) finish. Left behind is almost translucent color and a soft, natural-looking glow. Of course, the glow makes oily areas appear oilier, but if that's not a cause for concern (or if you have slightly dry skin) this will be perfect. The base has several antioxidants to help the in-part titanium dioxide sunscreen keep skin protected. One caution: The Bronze Glow shade does not offer contain any UVA-protecting ingredients (meaning titanium dioxide, zinc oxide, or avobenzone) and should be avoided. The other five shades are all recommended, but consider Light carefully because it is slightly peach, though it's likely too sheer to matter.

☺ **Visibly Even Natural-Look Makeup SPF 20** *($9.99)* is positioned as the first makeup to correct uneven skin tones not only by virtue of its coverage, but also by virtue of its skin-caring formula, which purports to treat uneven skin tone and discolorations while you wear it. First things first: This liquidy foundation features a titanium dioxide sunscreen and has a silky, slightly moist texture that dries to a soft matte finish. However, for a makeup whose selling point is to even out the user's skin tone, this only provides sheer to light coverage. It will soften minor pink or red-toned discolorations, but it does little to conceal sun-induced brown discolorations, including freckles. This is a non-issue if obtaining significant coverage is not a concern, but those hoping to hide redness associated with rosacea or post-inflammatory hyperpigmentation will be disappointed. Layering this foundation increases coverage only slightly.

The "breakthrough" ingredient in this foundation is something Neutrogena refers to as Essential Soy, which is what the company maintains is responsible for the foundation's redness- and blotchiness-reducing qualities. Visibly Even does contain a significant amount of soybean seed extract, but there are limited studies pertaining to soy's benefit as a skin-lightening agent (Source: *Dermatology*, issue 204, 2002, pages 281–286, and issue 201, 2000, pages 118–122), and those studies combined it with other known depigmenting agents. Soy can have anti-inflammatory properties (Source: *Skin Pharmacology and Applied Physiology*, May–June 2002, pages 175–183), but the effect it may have on your facial redness depends on the strength of the source of inflammation. For example, soy may be able to help soothe redness from overexposure to sun (I'm not referring to sunburn here, just a slight pinkness), but not from stubborn skin conditions such as rosacea. It's worth trying just to see if it can minimize mild facial redness, but it won't work with such conditions as melasma or broken capillaries. Still, the sunscreen in this product can help prevent further sun-induced discolorations.

Ten shades are available, and almost all are soft enough to work for fair to medium-tan skin tones. The only colors to avoid are Rose Cream, Copper Sand, and Toasted Honey. Blushing Ivory is an excellent shade for very fair skin, and its slight pink cast should not present a problem.

☺ **Healthy Skin Liquid Makeup SPF 20** *($9.99)* is Neutrogena's original foundation, and it hasn't changed at all since it hit the market several years ago. This standard, lightweight liquid foundation offers sheer to light coverage and a soft matte finish. The sunscreen's sole active is titanium dioxide, which is great. The current lineup of 12 shades eliminates a lot of the poor colors, but the following shades are too peach or pink for most skin tones: Natural Buff, Buff Blush, Spiced Almond, Rose Cream. This works best for normal to slightly oily skin.

☺ **Skin Clearing Oil-Free Makeup** *($9.99)* asks you to believe that getting clear skin from a makeup is possible. Yet the tiny amount of BHA (0.5%), combined with a high pH, won't clear blemishes or anything else for that matter. This silicone- and talc-based liquid does have a soft feel and blends on evenly, setting to a powdery matte finish that provides medium coverage. It's an option for oily to very oily skin, but be cautious if you have any dry patches because this foundation's finish will exaggerate them. The 13 shades are mostly soft and neutral, and apply lighter than they appear in the bottle. Buff Blush, Rose Cream, Spiced Almond, and Warm Beige are too pink or peach for most skin tones (particularly if your skin is oily, which tends to oxidize and darken pigments, further exaggerating an off color).

😐 **Mineral Sheers Mineral Powder Foundation** *($11.99)* marks Neutrogena's foray into the world of mineral makeup, and it's partially successful. Housed in a self-contained unit is a loose powder with a built-in applicator brush. You shake the powder into a concealed sifter piece, which then disperses it onto the brush, ready for you to dust it on. This powder foundation's main weak spot is the brush itself; it just isn't as soft as it should be given the way you are supposed to use it. If you want meaningful coverage, you need to buff this product over your skin using the head of the brush, which feels scratchy. Sweeping the powder over your skin is an option that feels better, but you'll get sheer to no coverage, since the powder is dispensed onto the head (not the sides) of the brush.

Application issues aside, this isn't too different from most mineral makeups, with the main ingredients being mica and bismuth oxychloride. The mica adds a subtle glow to the skin while the bismuth oxychloride adds bulk, opacity, and an extremely drying matte finish that tends to get drier as the day goes by. The finish is admittedly attractive at first, but I was less enamored by late afternoon, when I noticed my oily areas looking dull and somewhat flaky. By nighttime, with only one touch-up I was unusually shine-free, but my skin had a flat, drawn appearance that wasn't nearly as nice as the finish you get from some of today's best liquid foundations. I understand the appeal of mineral makeup, yet my comments about this type of makeup remain the same: It may look good at the onset, but the drying, absorbent bismuth oxychloride exaggerates even minor areas of dry skin, and on oily areas it can thicken and look very much like makeup. To Neutrogena's credit, their powder formula is lighter than many others, and its drawbacks take longer to appear. If you're curious to try this, the five available shades are all worthwhile, though the Sheer Bronzer shade leaves noticeable gold sparkles on your skin.

☹ **Skin Clearing Oil Free Compact Foundation** *($9.99)* is a thick-textured cream-to-powder makeup that contains absorbent aluminum starch as its main ingredient, which increases the odds that it will irritate skin. The thickening agents that follow aren't the best for oily skin—and that's precisely the skin type this is being marketed to. Although it does have a rather dry matte finish that would please someone with oiliness, almost all of the 12 shades are too peach, pink, or orange to recommend, especially without any testers at the store to see if they can blend unseen into your skin tone. The color swatch on the box barely resembles the actual shade, and with no testers in sight, choosing the wrong color is all but inevitable. The minimal amount of salicylic acid (BHA) comes without a pH (you cannot establish a pH in a waterless product) and, therefore, has no effect on breakouts.

☹ **Healthy Skin Cream Powder Makeup SPF 20** *($9.99)* is an outdated cream-to-powder compact makeup with an unpleasant texture that (surprisingly for Neutrogena) lacks sufficient UVA-protecting ingredients. Each of the four shades is glaringly peach or pink, making this one of the most unappealing foundations at the drugstore.

CONCEALER: ☺ **Skin Clearing Oil-Free Concealer** *($7.99)* is packaged in a click-pen that feeds this lightweight concealer onto an angled sponge tip. It blends very well (and fast) to a matte finish, and provides excellent coverage. The light, silicone- and clay-based formula is fine for use over blemishes—just don't expect the tiny amount (0.5%) of salicylic acid at this high pH to clear things up. There are four shades, three of which are beautifully neutral. Avoid Correcting Green because green does not hide red on the skin, it only adds a Kermit the Frog shade to your face.

😐 **3-in-1 Concealer for Eyes SPF 20** *($9.99)* is positioned as another multipurpose product, this time combining concealer, eye cream, and sunscreen in one convenient package. As a concealer, this provides smooth, even coverage that looks natural and has a satin finish slightly prone to creasing. Both shades are worthwhile. The sunscreen is almost 10% titanium dioxide, which also helps enhance coverage. Where it falls short is the eye-cream claim. This product isn't too creamy (not with talc as the third ingredient) and the amount of fragrance is disappointing. There are better concealers with sunscreen from Revlon, but this is still an option.

😐 **Healthy Skin Smoothing Stick Treatment Concealer** *($5.99)* wins points for providing nearly opaque coverage with one swipe, but this lipstick-style concealer also looks heavy and creases into lines around the eye. It's an OK option for camouflaging small areas of redness, and three of the four shades are decent (Medium is too peach), but the concealers from L'Oreal and Revlon have much more to offer.

☹ **Skin Soothing Undereye Corrector** *($8.49)* is a sheer highlighter available in two peachy pink shades that are dispensed onto a brush from the click-pen component. Each has a strong matte finish that does little to cast a radiant glow, but the bigger problem is the menthyl lactate, a menthol derivative and an irritant that should not be used on skin, especially around the eyes.

POWDER: ✓☺ **Healthy Defense Protective Powder SPF 30** *($10.99)* is a pressed powder with a reliable SPF 30 that contains almost 9% titanium dioxide as the active ingredient. Although this is an excellent product, you need to know that unless you apply a liberal layer of powder (which can look too thick), you will not be getting the stated (or even significant) sun protection. However, a pressed powder with sunscreen is an excellent option as a touch-up for makeup to enhance the sun protection you are already wearing (from foundation or moisturizer). The three available shades are fine, but there are no options for darker skin tones.

☺ **Healthy Skin Loose Powder** *($9.99)* and ☺ **Healthy Skin Pressed Powder** *($9.99)* have three shades each, suitable for fair to light/medium skin. Both formulas are talc-based, with a soft, silky finish. The colors are actually quite attractive, but you have to pry open the boxes to get a glimpse of them (don't tell anyone I said this). The Pressed Powder offers a bit more coverage and has a slightly silkier feel courtesy of the silicone it contains.

☺ **Healthy Skin Blends Translucent Oil-Control Powder** *($11.99)* features various color "squares" of powder in one compact, the idea being that swirling the brush over these multiple colors nets you one translucent color on skin. It does apply that way, but I completely disagree with Neutrogena's claim that this product can be used by multiple skin tones. The powder is best for fair to medium skin tones, although some medium skin tones will find it too light. The talc-based formula has a smooth texture and an even, non-powdery application, but those dealing with blemishes should avoid these products because they contain cornstarch.

☺ **Healthy Skin Blends Natural Radiance Bronzer** *($11.99)* is identical in concept, texture, and application to the Healthy Skin Blends Translucent Oil-Control Powder above, except this comes in bronze tones with a hint of shine. The effect on skin is a soft tan that's best for fair to light skin.

😐 **Skin Clearing Oil-Free Pressed Powder** *($9.99)* has a dry, smooth texture and an almost too powdery finish that is an option only for someone with oily to very oily skin. The inclusion of salicylic acid in a powder is never effective, as the very ingredients that compose a powder have too high a pH to allow the BHA to work as an exfoliant. Three shades are available, and although they appear too peach in the compact, each goes on softly.

BLUSH: ☺ **Healthy Skin Blends Sheer Highlighting Blush** *($11.99)* is identical to the Healthy Skin Blends Translucent Oil-Control Powder above, except with this product you get pale to medium pink squares in one pressed-powder compact. The result is akin to a soft pink blush with a hint of shine, and it's best for fair to light skin.

😐 **Soft Color Blush** *($9.69)* has a smooth but unusually dry texture that makes application spotty. Most of the shades are soft, matte, and muted, but the swatch on the box is not an accurate representation. Although this is an OK blush, it isn't worth considering over powder blushes from L'Oreal, Almay, or Jane.

😐 **Mineral Sheers Blush** *($12.99)* is a talc-free sheer loose blush that's packaged with a built-in brush applicator, just like Neutrogena's Mineral Sheers Mineral Powder Foundation above. The brush could be softer and tapered better, but it does the job. The problem is the way the powder is dispensed (it tends to be too dusty), and the application is so sheer you really need to pile this on to get color to show. Color takes a backseat to shine, as each shade has rather large crystalline particles that don't cling to skin as well as they should. L'Oreal did much better with their Bare Naturale Gentle Mineral Blush ($14.49).

EYESHADOW: 😐 **Mineral Sheers for Eyes** *($7.99)* capitalize on the mineral makeup trend, yet the formula is talc-based just like most powder eyeshadows. Of course, talc is a mineral but most mineral makeup lines eschew it in favor of alternatives. In any case, these eyeshadow duos have a smooth but dry texture that applies and blends fairly well. The dryness causes some flaking unless you dust these on sheer. However, sheerness is the theme here, and you'll notice most of the shades offer more in the way of shine than color. If you're curious to try this and want a duo to shade and highlight, the only ones to really consider are Shell and Clay. The others go on too lightly to shade or shape the eye.

☹ **Skin Soothing Eye Tints** *($8.99)* is sold as a jack-of-all-trades product for use on the eyelids. According to Neutrogena, this product can function as an eyeshadow base, an eye brightener, puffiness reducer, and an aid to prevent your eyeshadows from creasing. Both shades have a hint of shimmer, and a somewhat dry texture that is a bit tricky to blend. They dry to a matte finish that can help prevent eyeshadows from creasing, but the cooling sensation you feel is from the menthyl lactate, a form of menthol that can be very irritating to the eyelids.

LIPSTICK, LIP GLOSS, AND LIPLINER: ✓☺ **MoistureShine Gloss** *($6.79)* has all the best attributes of a lip gloss: it comes with a hygienic wand applicator, has a smooth, non-sticky texture that feels moisturizing but not goopy, and leaves lips looking evenly glossed rather than overly wet. The selection of shades (most are shimmer-enriched) is beautiful and each goes on sheerer than it appears. Sweet Nothing is a colorless shade without shimmer.

☺ **MoistureShine Tinted Lip Balm SPF 20** *($6.79)* is ideal for anyone seeking good broad-spectrum sun protection (though the 1% titanium dioxide content is a bit low) with soft, glossy (not greasy) color. The shade selections are well-edited, and most have a touch of sparkle for added flair. Its slick finish means that MoistureShine Tinted Lip Balm SPF 20 is not a good choice for anyone prone to lipstick feathering into lines around the mouth. But otherwise, this is recommended and one of a handful of lip color products with decent UVA protection.

☺ **Lip Nutrition Berry Smooth Balm**, **Lip Nutrition Honey Rescue Balm**, **Lip Nutrition Mango Moisture Balm**, **Lip Nutrition Passion Fruit Balm**, and **Lip Nutrition Vanilla Replenishing Balm** *($7.99 each)* come in pots, and although each balm is slightly different, all of them have an emollient base composed of the same ingredients as most lip balms. What distinguishes these balms is the inclusion of tiny amounts of honey, vanilla, or fruit flavors. All of them will address the needs of dry, chapped lips. Which one to choose is mostly personal preference because none of the distinctive extras are present in great enough quantities to impact lips beyond a taste sensation.

☹ **Lip Nutrition Soothing Mint Balm** *($7.99)* contains menthol, which is neither nutritional nor soothing for lips. This balm is not recommended. ☹ **Lip Boost Intense Moisture Therapy** *($6.79)* is a water- and Vaseline-based lip balm that contains several good-for-lips ingredients. However, that's all for naught because they are coupled with menthol and peppermint, two irritants that make this intensely irritating, not therapeutic.

☹ **MoistureShine Lip Soother Cooling Hydragel SPF 20** *($6.79)* has a unique balm/lip gloss texture and each of the sheer, juicy colors leaves lips very shiny, but the sunscreen element lacks sufficient UVA-protecting ingredients and the menthol in this product won't do your lips any favors. ☹ **MoistureShine Soothing Lip Sheers SPF 20** *($5.99)* are sheer, minimally slick glossy lipsticks with an in-part titanium dioxide sunscreen. These would be a slam-dunk (and the shades are attractive) except that the formula includes the irritating menthol derivative menthyl lactate. The tingle may seem refreshing, but it's persistent (there's not just a dusting of this ingredient in here) and not good news.

MASCARA: 😐 **Weightless Volume Mascara** *($6.79)* is a wax-free mascara that promises full, weightless lashes with no clumps or smudges. It fulfills the latter part of that promise, but is otherwise one of the most do-nothing mascaras available. The fact that this is wax-free is fine if you're bothered by waxes. If not, waxes are an essential problem-free component of most mascaras, as they add fullness and pliability, and help keep mascara on the lashes.

☹ **Full Volume Fortifying Mascara** *($6.49)* makes lashes noticeably longer but tends to stay wet too long, so some smearing is inevitable unless you're really good at not blinking every few seconds. ☹ **Clean Lash Tint** *($7.99)* is sold as a gentle tint for eyelashes, and its advertising recommends using it with Acuvue contact lens solution. (Acuvue and Neutrogena are owned by Johnson & Johnson, so this endorsement is hardly impartial.) However, it does absolutely nothing to lengthen or thicken lashes; all you'll get is slightly darker lashes. That would be fine for those blessed with naturally long lashes, but for some inexplicable reason Neutrogena added grapefruit oil to this product.

FACE AND BODY ILLUMINATING/SHIMMER PRODUCTS: ☺ **Shimmer Sheers for Cheeks, Eyes, Lips** *($8.99)* come in squeeze tubes, and dispense as a slightly thick, but lightweight, cream that, upon blending, morphs into a dry powder finish that wears well with minimal to no creasing—when used as eyeshadow. The shine level (which tends to fade slightly throughout the day) is noticeable without being overpowering, but these are still too shiny for most tastes for daytime use on cheeks. For evening cheek glimmer, they're fine. I don't recommend using these on lips, because they tend to feel very dry in a short period of time, and end up flaking and peeling off unless you add a creamy lipstick or gloss for emolliency. Shimmer Sheers are fragrance-free, but the amount of "conditioning vitamins" they contain is barely worth mentioning.

NIVEA (SKIN CARE ONLY)

NIVEA AT-A-GLANCE

Strengths: Inexpensive; excellent makeup remover; one good toner.

Weaknesses: Boring formulas; most sunscreens have SPF ratings below SPF 15 benchmark; no products to treat breakouts or lighten skin discolorations; limited options for normal to oily skin; anti-cellulite products are a joke; jar packaging.

For more information about Nivea Visage, owned by Beiersdorf, call (800) 227-4703 or visit www.nivea.com or www.Beautypedia.com.

NIVEA VISAGE PRODUCTS

Nivea uses coenzyme Q10 (ubiquinone) in many of its products. Despite their antiwrinkle and skin-rejuvenating claims for this ingredient, the research indicates that topical application of this ingredient provides antioxidant and anti-inflammatory benefit, which is helpful for skin, but not wrinkle-erasing. Interestingly, these benefits are enhanced when coenzyme Q10 is combined with carotenoid pigments, something Nivea doesn't use (Sources: *Journal of Cosmetic Dermatology*, March 2006, pages 30–38; and *Biofactors*, 2003, pages 289–297).

✓☺ **Visage Eye Make-Up Remover** *($6.13 for 2.5 ounces)* has a unique gel-cream texture and a fragrance-free formula that works to swiftly remove all types of makeup. This is one of the better products Nivea offers, and one of the top eye-makeup removers available.

😐 **Visage Gentle Cleansing Cream, for Dry Skin** *($6.50 for 6.8 ounces)* is a thick, somewhat greasy detergent-free cleansing cream for dry to very dry skin. It will require a washcloth for complete removal, and is not recommended if breakouts are an issue.

☺ **Visage Moisturizing Toner** *($5.99 for 6.8 ounces)* impresses with its normal to dry skin–friendly blend of glycerin, plant oil, soothing agent, and the cell-communicating ingredient niacinamide. It would be rated higher if a better range of antioxidants were included, but this is definitely above the norm for toners.

☹ **Visage Anti-Wrinkle & Firming Creme SPF 4** *($9.99 for 1.7 ounces)* lacks the UVA-protecting ingredients of titanium dioxide, zinc oxide, avobenzone, Mexoryl SX (ecamsule), or Tinosorb and is not recommended. And SPF 4? Come on!

☹ **Visage Q10 Advanced Wrinkle Reducer Day Creme SPF 8** *($11.61 for 1.7 ounces)* provides UVA protection with its in-part avobenzone and titanium dioxide sunscreens, and is wrapped in an emollient base for normal to dry skin. The tiny amount of antioxidants won't remain viable once this jar-packaged product is opened, and SPF 8 is below standard recommendations for sun protection, making this a daytime moisturizer to ignore.

☹ **Visage Q10 Advanced Wrinkle Reducer Eye Creme SPF 4** *($11.72 for 0.5 ounce)* lists an embarrassingly low SPF rating, though the sole active is titanium dioxide. And this is supposed to combat new and existing wrinkles?! Don't bet on it—not with this boring formula.

☺ **Visage Q10 Advanced Wrinkle Reducer Lotion SPF 15** *($11.44 for 3.3 ounces)* finally is a Visage product that has an SPF rating your skin needs, and an in-part avobenzone sunscreen to boot. Unfortunately, the base formula is yawn-inducing, and includes teeny-tiny amounts of antioxidants (coenzyme Q10 included). This is an average option for normal to oily skin, but for sunscreen without any bells or whistles, sure.

☺ **Visage Q10 Advanced Wrinkle Reducer Night Creme** *($11.67 for 1.7 ounces)* is mostly water, glycerin, lots of thickeners, and shea butter, which adds up to not a single ingredient that can reduce wrinkles. It's an OK option for dry to very dry skin, but the jar packaging won't keep the dusting of antioxidants stable during use.

☺ **Visage Q10 Gentle Spa Micro-Dermabrasion Kit** *($19.99 for the kit)* features three steps. Step 1 is the **Pre-Treatment Cleanser**, a water- and glycerin-based cleansing agent that contains additional emollients and oils that can leave a slight film. That film is essentially removed after you scrub your skin with Step 2, the **Micro-Dermabrasion Gel**, which contains polyethylene (plastic beads) as the abrasive agent. This is a pricey way to exfoliate skin and does not compare to simply using a washcloth. Plus, given that new research shows that microdermabrasion may have diminishing results, it is not a good risk for your skin. After cleansing and scrubbing, you're directed to apply Step 3, the **Post-Treatment Balm SPF 15**, which is just a basic in-part avobenzone sunscreen that doesn't contain much that's exciting for skin, but it's an OK option if you have normal to oily skin.

☹ **Visage Sun-Kissed Facial Moisturizer SPF 4** *($6.99 for 1.7 ounces)* has a pitifully low SPF rating that should embarrass Nivea, despite the inclusion of avobenzone for UVA protection (but with an SPF of 4 it hardly matters). This is not recommended for daily use because it does not provide sun protection for as long as is recommended by the American Academy of Dermatology, which is minimum SPF 15. There are better products if you're looking for a self-tanner with sunscreen (though regular sunscreen is preferred because most people will not apply a self-tanner liberally enough to get the stated level of protection).

OTHER NIVEA PRODUCTS

☹ **Nivea Creme** *($7.42 for 6.8 ounces)* remains one of the star products for this line, and Nivea describes it as "the mother of all modern creams." First made available in 1911, the jar-packaged formula with its familiar scent is an exceptionally basic blend of mineral oil, Vaseline, glycerin, and wax. All of these standbys can make dry skin look and feel better, but there are many more ingredients that have significant benefit for skin—ingredients that weren't even close to being options when Nivea Cream launched. Far from "unmatched," there are dozens upon dozens of moisturizers that offer skin more than this cream does, and without the inclusion of sensitizing preservatives methylisothiazolinone and methylchloroisothiazolinone.

☹ **Sun-Kissed Firming Moisturizer** *($6.99 for 8.4 ounces)* is another round of moisturizers with a small amount of the self-tanning ingredient dihydroxyacetone built in for a bit of color over several days. Nivea's version (available in Light to Medium or Medium to Dark versions) is not preferred to those from Dove or Olay because alcohol is the third ingredient, which makes Nivea's too potentially irritating (but none of these are firming in the least).

☹ **Good-Bye Cellulite, Smoothing Cellulite Gel-Cream** *($12.99 for 6.7 ounces)* purports to reduce cellulite because it contains L-cartinine. Also known as carboxylic acid, this ingredient is naturally present in our bodies and may be obtained from dietary sources such as red meat. It has unsubstantiated claims of being able to affect fat metabolism when consumed orally. There is no research pertaining to its anti-cellulite benefit when applied topically, although it likely functions as an antioxidant (Source: www.naturaldatabase.com). This product won't do a thing to improve cellulite, but its alcohol content will irritate your skin and cause inflammation.

☹ **Good-Bye Cellulite Patches** *($12.99 for 6 individually wrapped patches)* are gimmicky adhesive patches meant to fit over the thighs, buttocks, or stomach. The adhesive agents can be irritating to skin, there is no research anywhere proving cartinine has a cellulite-diminishing effect, and this patch system isn't preferred over just rubbing the above Gel-Cream into your skin. So don't bother to even say hello to this product, unless you're willing to say goodbye to your money and get nothing of value in return.

NO7 (SEE BOOTS)

NOXZEMA (SKIN CARE ONLY)

NOXZEMA AT-A-GLANCE

Strengths: Good clay mask.

Weaknesses: Almost all products reviewed contain a blend of irritants camphor, menthol, and eucalyptus oil; none of anti-acne or anti-blackhead products work as claimed; no topical disinfectant for acne-prone skin; no sunscreens; no moisturizers.

For more information about Noxzema, call (800) 436-4361 or visit www.noxzema.com or www.Beautypedia.com.

NOXZEMA CONTINUOUS CLEAN PRODUCTS

☹ **Continuous Clean Foaming Cleanser** *($4.49 for 6 ounces)* contains menthol and is not recommended. The 2% salicylic acid is rinsed down the drain before it can affect skin.

☹ **Continuous Clean Citrus Scrub** *($4.84 for 5 ounces)* contains menthol and is not recommended. Much better topical scrubs are available from Neutrogena, Olay, and L'Oreal.

☹ **Continuous Clean Microbead Cleanser** *($4.84 for 6 ounces)* contains menthol and is not recommended for any skin type.

☹ **Continuous Clean Citrus Toner** *($4.49 for 8 ounces)* lists alcohol as the second ingredient and contains menthol and the potent menthol derivative menthoxypropanediol. There's no citrus to be found despite the name, but your skin will be plenty irritated from the aforementioned ingredients.

✓☺ **Continuous Clean Clay Mask** *($5 for 4 ounces)* is a very good, absorbent clay mask for normal to oily skin. I am almost shocked that this product contains soothing agents rather than the irritants that plague Noxzema. This mask does contain fragrance.

NOXZEMA TRIPLE CLEAN PRODUCTS

😐 **Triple Clean Anti-Bacterial Cleanser** *($4.83 for 6.5 ounces)* contains 0.3% triclosan, which is a good antibacterial agent, but it needs to be left on skin for several minutes for best results, and that's not a great idea with a cleanser. The amount of potassium hydroxide in this cleanser makes it more drying than most, but it's an OK option for those with very oily skin who prefer a foaming cleanser.

😐 **Triple Clean Blackhead Cleanser** *($3.97 for 5 ounces)* contains 2% salicylic acid, but it won't dislodge blackheads because it is rinsed from the skin before it can exert that benefit. This is otherwise a decent water-soluble cleanser for normal to slightly oily skin, and includes scrubbing beads of polyethylene. The small amount of sodium lauryl sulfate is not cause for concern.

☹ **Triple Clean Anti-Blemish Astringent** *($4.39 for 8 ounces)* serves only to hurt skin with alcohol, peppermint oil, and menthol, which is triple irritation that won't ban one blemish. None of these ingredients offers a positive outcome for blemish-prone skin.

☹ **Triple Clean Pads Anti-Blemish Pads** *($3.49 for 65 pads)* may seem to be a bargain, but severely irritate skin thanks to the potent combination of alcohol, camphor, eucalyptus, and menthol.

NOXZEMA ORIGINAL PRODUCTS

☹ **60 Second Cleansing Whip** *($3.94 for 10.75 ounces)* puts skin on the fast track for irritation from camphor, menthol, and eucalyptus oil. Danger, Will Robinson, danger!

☹ **Deep Cleansing Cloths** *($5.96 for 30 cloths)* are similar to the cleansing cloths offered by Olay (Olay and Noxzema are both owned by Procter & Gamble), but are not recommended because they contain menthol.

☹ **Daily Cream Cleanser, for Normal/Dry Skin** *($5.49 for 7 ounces)* contains camphor, menthol, and eucalyptus oil and is not recommended for any skin type.

☹ **Deep Cleansing Cream, for Normal/Dry Skin Plus Moisturizers, Jar** *($3.79 for 10.75 ounces)* contains camphor, menthol, and eucalyptus oil and is not recommended for any skin type.

☹ **Deep Cleansing Cream, for Normal/Dry Skin Plus Moisturizers, Pump** *($4.78 for 10.5 ounces)* contains camphor, menthol, and eucalyptus oil and is not recommended for any skin type.

☹ **Deep Cleansing Cream, Original, Jar** *($4.52 for 10.75 ounces)* is a slightly modified version of the formula that started it all, when this product was launched in 1914 with its "signature scent" of menthol, camphor, and eucalyptus oil. Those irritants are still present, but at least the phenol and lye aren't included anymore. However, that doesn't bring me any closer to recommending this product.

☹ **Deep Cleansing Cream, Original, Pump** *($4.66 for 10.5 ounces)* has a slightly different base formula than the Deep Cleansing Cream, Original, Jar above, but contains the same irritants and is not recommended.

☹ **Deep Lathering Cleanser, for Combination/Oily Skin** *($4.49 for 7 ounces)* is an alkaline cleanser that, in addition to drying skin, irritates it with menthol, camphor, and eucalyptus oil.

☹ **Wet Cleansing Cloths** *($4.49 for 25 cloths)* get skin wet and irritated because the cloths are steeped in menthol, camphor, and eucalyptus oil. Noxzema advises using these to remove mascara, but that's just begging for severe eye (and eyelid) irritation.

☹ **Daily Exfoliating Cleanser** *($4.49 for 6 ounces)* is primarily a scrub, but one that irritates skin because it contains camphor, menthol, and eucalyptus oil.

NU SKIN

NU SKIN AT-A-GLANCE

Strengths: Workable AHA and BHA products; some state-of-the-art moisturizers and serums; several products are fragrance-free; almost all sunscreens include sufficient UVA protection, and most have impressive levels of antioxidants; good lip gloss, sheer powder blush, and makeup brushes.

Weaknesses: Expensive; drying cleansers; irritating toners; Tri-Phasic White products do not noticeably improve skin discolorations; unimpressive masks and "spa-at-home" products; claims are too far from reality; several categories of Nu Skin's makeup are resounding disappointments, including foundation, concealer, and eyeshadows; the brow pencil; the Eyelash Treatment product; average lipsticks; claims surrounding ingredients the company does and does not use are not supported by substantiated research.

For more information about Nu Skin, call (800) 487-1000 or visit www.nuskin.com or www.Beautypedia.com.

NU SKIN SKIN CARE

NU SKIN 180° PRODUCTS

😐 **$$$ 180° Face Wash** *($34.91 for 4.2 ounces)* is an overpriced, standard, detergent-based cleanser that contains sodium C14-16 olefin sulfate as the cleansing agent, making it potentially too drying and irritating for skin. There are plant oils in it that can cushion some of the dryness, but why use any irritants whatsoever? The vitamin C it contains will be washed away before it has a chance to have any benefit for skin.

☺ **$$$ 180° Skin Mist** *($29.45 for 3.4 ounces)* is a good but fairly basic toner in mist form for normal to dry skin. It is fragrance-free.

☺ **$$$ 180° AHA Facial Peel** *($54.39 for set)* is an expensive but effective way to exfoliate skin. The first part of this two-step kit is the **AHA Facial Peel**. This provides 18 pads, each steeped in a water-based solution of 10% lactic acid. The pH of 3.5 ensures exfoliation, and no needless irritants are included. You swipe the pad over your skin and let it sit for at least 10 minutes, at which point you use the **AHA Facial Peel Neutralizer**, which consists of pads soaked with a water-based toner that contains some very good soothing agents. The pH of the Neutralizer stops the peel action, but so would rinsing your skin with plain tap water. At least Nu Skin made these pads better than most companies that sell at-home peel kits. Although this kit will exfoliate skin, you're better off spending less money and using leave-on AHA products that contain between 8% and 10% glycolic or lactic acids, which you leave on your skin, and there are plenty of these products available. Both products in this set are fragrance-free.

☺ **$$$ 180° Cell Renewal Fluid** *($74.81 for 1 ounce)* exfoliates skin with the polyhydroxy acid (PHA) gluconolactone at a 15% concentration and at a pH of 3.2. This is a good alternative to AHA or BHA products, but research has not shown gluconolactone to be a preferred or a gentler option (at least not in a significant way), and a 15% concentration is high and can be irritating for some skin types. This fluid also contains salicylic acid, but the amount is likely too low to boost exfoliation from the gluconolactone. By the way, if you're curious to try a product with gluconolactone, those from Neostrata are just as effective for a lot less money.

✓☺ **$$$ 180° Night Complex** *($64.60 for 1 ounce)* is a brilliant serum for normal to dry skin because it combines ingredients that restore a healthy look and feel to skin while supporting its structural integrity and supplying it with plenty of antioxidants and cell-communicating ingredients. Well done, though why couldn't this be fragrance-free like the other 180° products?

☺ **$$$ 180° UV Block Hydrator SPF 18** *($53.20 for 1 ounce)* is a great in-part zinc oxide sunscreen for normal to dry skin not prone to blemishes. For the money, this should be brimming with state-of-the-art ingredients, which it's not, but at least broad-spectrum sun protection is assured and fragrance is excluded.

NU SKIN CLEAR ACTION ACNE MEDICATION SYSTEM

Note: All Clear Action Acne medication products can be purchased separately or as a set, for $97.14.

☺ **$$$ Clear Action Acne Medication Foaming Cleanser** *($21.76 for 3.4 ounces)* is a medicated liquid-to-foam cleanser that contains 0.5% salicylic acid, which in a cleanser isn't on your skin long enough to exert a benefit. Although this is a good cleanser for normal to dry skin, its oil content is not the best for anyone battling blemishes, and makes it somewhat difficult to rinse completely.

☺ **$$$ Clear Action Acne Medication Toner** *($19.81 for 5 ounces)* is a fragrance-free, pH-correct BHA toner; however, the 0.5% concentration of salicylic acid is too low to significantly impact blemishes and blackheads. This toner is fragrance-free and contains soothing agents.

☺ **$$$ Clear Action Acne Medication Day Treatment** *($36.58 for 1 ounce)* contains 0.5% salicylic acid at a pH of 3.5, and although that allows for exfoliation to occur, it would be better if there were more salicylic acid. Still, the amount of AHA lactic acid is likely around 5%, which provides additional exfoliation, and the base formula contains some good anti-irritants.

✓☺ **$$$ Clear Action Acne Medication Night Treatment** *($36.58 for 1 ounce)* is worth considering as an antioxidant serum but not as an anti-acne treatment. That's because the amount of salicylic acid is too low (0.5%) and the pH too high for exfoliation to occur. Antioxidants include green tea, alpha lipoic acid, and vitamin E. This also contains cell-communicating ingredients (including retinol) and anti-irritants.

NU SKIN EPOCH PRODUCTS

☹ **Epoch Cleansing Bar** *($10.74 for a 3.4-ounce bar)* is a detergent-based bar cleanser that is similar to Dove's original Beauty Bar. Although more gentle than true soap, it is still drying for all skin types and the ingredients that keep it in bar form can clog pores.

☺ **$$$ Epoch Calming Touch Skin Cream** *($38 for 1.7 ounces)* is a good lightweight moisturizer for normal to slightly dry skin. Nu Skin positions this as a product meant to reduce redness and scaly skin from eczema or rosacea, but the ingredients they chose show up in hundreds of moisturizers for the face and body. That doesn't mean they're not effective at reducing dry, scaly skin; rather, it's just that they're not unique to this moisturizer. Oddly, this contains the flavoring agent homoanisealdehyde, likely used to impart fragrance.

☹ **Epoch Blemish Treatment** *($12.11 for 0.5 ounce)* contains 2% salicylic acid as an active ingredient, but the pH of 4.1 prevents it from functioning optimally as an exfoliant. This is an ineffective option for blemishes, and is irritating for all skin types due to the fragrant oils.

✓☺ **$$$ Epoch Glacial Marine Mud** *($23.51 for 7 ounces)* is a mud mask whose mud is said to be mineral-rich, but minerals aren't a cure for skin problems in the least, nor are they nurturing (especially when delivered in dirt—imagine adding that to your diet). Still, this can be a good absorbent mask for normal to oily skin, and it's fragrance-free.

Nu Skin Nutricentials Products

😐 **Pure Cleansing Gel, for Combination to Oily Skin** *($14.92 for 5 ounces)* is a standard, detergent-based, water-soluble cleanser for its intended skin type, but one that's not highly recommended because of the amount of fragrant plant extracts it contains.

✓☺ **Creamy Cleansing Lotion, for Normal to Dry Skin** *($14.92 for 5 ounces)* is an outstanding cleanser for its intended skin type. Emollients and plant oils combine with a gentle detergent cleansing agent to remove impurities and makeup without leaving a greasy film. Fans of cleansing lotions, take note!

☹ **pH Balance Mattefying Toner, for Combination to Oily Skin** *($11.02 for 5 ounces)* lists witch hazel as the second ingredient and also contains some problematic plant extracts, making this toner (which doesn't set to a matte finish) too irritating for all skin types.

☹ **pH Balance Toner, for Normal to Dry Skin** *($10.69 for 5 ounces)* contains witch hazel and camphor, making this a problem toner for any skin type, and it won't restore skin's optimal pH level (our skin is quite adept at doing so on its own anyway), but the irritation this can cause will make dry skin worse.

☹ **Celltrex Ultra Recovery Fluid** *($34.20 for 0.5 ounce)* has a lot going for it, but ends up being a problem for all skin types because it contains orange and lavender oils. Lavender oil doesn't help skin cells recover, it causes cell death.

😐 **Moisture Restore Day Protective Lotion SPF 15, for Combination to Oily Skin** *($30.40 for 1.7 ounces)* is similar to the Nu Skin 180° UV Block Hydrator SPF 18 above, except this contains a greater amount of the antioxidant vitamin E. It loses points for including a tiny amount of St. John's wort, which can make skin more sun-sensitive.

☺ **Moisture Restore Day Protective Lotion SPF 15, for Normal to Dry Skin** *($30.40 for 1.7 ounces)* would rate a Paula's Pick if not for the needless inclusion of St. John's wort, which can cause a skin reaction in the presence of sunlight. The fact that this product contains sunscreen (in-part zinc oxide) helps offset this, but not enough to make it a slam-dunk recommendation for normal to dry skin.

😐 **Night Supply Nourishing Cream, for Normal to Dry Skin** *($34.44 for 1.7 ounces)* features some very good ingredients for dry skin, but the jar packaging won't keep the antioxidants and plant oils stable during use; plus the inclusion of St. John's wort wasn't wise. This is an OK option that could've been a lot better.

😐 **Night Supply Nourishing Lotion, for Combination to Oily Skin** *($34.44 for 1.7 ounces)* is a basic, lightweight moisturizer for its intended skin type. It contains mostly water, silicone, glycerin, soothing agent, emollient thickeners, a cell-communicating ingredient, vitamin E, more thickeners, fragrance, and preservatives.

NU SKIN TRI-PHASIC WHITE SYSTEM

Note: The products reviewed below can be purchased separately or as a set, for $188.10.

☺ $$$ **Tri-Phasic White Cleanser** *($28.50 for 1 ounce)* costs a lot for what amounts to a standard water-soluble foaming cleanser for normal to oily skin. Not a single ingredient in this pricey cleanser can "inhibit the expression of discoloration on the surface of skin." Even if it contained effective skin-lightening agents, they'd be of no use because they'd be rinsed down the drain before they had a chance to work.

☹ **Tri-Phasic White Toner** *($33.25 for 4.2 ounces)* lists witch hazel as the second ingredient, making this too irritating for all skin types. This cannot exfoliate away dark spots, as claimed.

☹ **Tri-Phasic White Essence** *($57 for 1 ounce)* contains a good deal of lemon peel extract, whose volatile components can cause irritation. This isn't helped by the lesser amount of peppermint extract, and to top it off, not a single ingredient in this misguided product can have even a slight impact on skin discolorations. Animal testing has shown that lemon peel can cause a phototoxic reaction on skin in as little as three minutes, even when sunscreen is worn (Source: *Photodermatology, Photoimmunology, and Photomedicine*, December 2005, pages 318–321), and it is known to cause contact dermatitis in people, making it something to avoid.

☺ **Tri-Phasic White Day Milk Lotion SPF 15** *($47.50 for 2.5 ounces)* includes avobenzone for UVA protection and wraps it in a silky lotion base for normal to slightly oily or slightly dry skin. A greater array of antioxidants and a cell-communicating ingredient would have netted this daytime moisturizer a higher rating.

😐 $$$ **Tri-Phasic White Night Cream** *($47.50 for 1 ounce)* is a lightweight, jar-packaged moisturizer formulated with the ingredient diacetyl boldine, which Nu Skin claims works to disrupt the activation phase of skin pigmentation, when melanin (skin pigment cells) is created. Diacetyl boldine appears to have antioxidant ability, but there is no independent, peer-reviewed research supporting its claim of being able to suppress melanin production. Therefore, I wouldn't count on this otherwise OK moisturizer for slightly dry skin to do anything other than make skin feel softer and smoother.

☺ $$$ **Tri-Phasic White Radiance Mask** *($67.93 for 8 masks)* provides a collection of individually packaged, fragrance-free, pre-moistened masks that contain a good blend of water-binding agents and antioxidants. None of the ingredients in these masks has substantiated research supporting Nu Skin's claims of inhibiting any phase of hyperpigmentation, but they can make skin look and feel better.

NU SKIN TRU FACE PRODUCTS

☹ **Tru Face Priming Solution** *($33.96 for 4.2 ounces)* contains some helpful, amino acid–based water-binding agents for skin, but the amount of witch hazel makes this toner too irritating for all skin types. A product like this isn't essential to "prepare" skin for the benefits of other Tru Face products.

☺ $$$ **Tru Face Essence** *($135.90 for 60 capsules)* includes mostly silicone, thickeners, plant oils, and antioxidants packaged in tiny capsules meant for single use. The packaging is a good way to keep the antioxidants stable, though it would be better if they were more prominent in this product. For the money, these aren't as elegant as the Ceramide capsules from Elizabeth Arden, which cost half as much for the same amount of product.

✓☺ **$$$ Tru Face IdealEyes Eye Refining Cream** *($42.75 for 0.5 ounce)* was designed to send under-eye bags packing, but this fragrance-free eye cream cannot accomplish what genetics, time, sun damage, and an aging face create. What it can do is moisturize and smooth, while supplying skin with a good amount of stabilized vitamin C and lesser, but still potentially effective, amounts of other antioxidants and cell-communicating ingredients.

☹ **$$$ Tru Face Instant Line Corrector** *($67.93 for 0.5 ounce)* is Nu Skin's "works like Botox" product, claiming to relax forehead wrinkles and expression lines. The company's literature for this product mentions the "heavy risks" associated with Botox injections, but the only convincing "risk" they could come up with was the ongoing expense (I admit, Botox isn't a value-driven procedure). Formula-wise, this silicone-enriched moisturizer contains aminobutyric acid, also known as GABA. However, GABA does not inhibit muscle contractions that lead to expression lines. For a detailed explanation of this ingredient, please refer to Chapter Seven, *Cosmetic Ingredient Dictionary* in this book. This product can make skin feel silky-smooth and, to a small, temporary extent, fill in superficial lines on the face. It actually could have been a lot more impressive than it is if a broader range of state-of-the-art ingredients had been included.

☹ **$$$ Tru Face Line Corrector** *($42.28 for 1 ounce)* is a basic, lightweight, silicone-based moisturizer that contains palmitoyl-pentapeptide-3. In theory, this and other peptides are cell-communicating ingredients that also function as water-binding agents. The antiwrinkle claims come from studies that were funded by the companies that sell these peptides to the cosmetics industry, so they're hardly impartial. This is still a good, basic moisturizer for normal to slightly oily or slightly dry skin.

☹ **$$$ Tru Face Revealing Gel** *($43.70 for 1 ounce)* is similar to the Nu Skin 180° Cell Renewal Fluid above, except this version contains less gluconolactone (the company did not reveal the percentage difference, but this product appears to have less than a 5% concentration). It is an OK lightweight gel moisturizer for oily skin, but isn't likely to have a noticeable impact on pores—at least not to the extent that dry-finish silicone serums can.

☺ **$$$ Tru Face Skin Perfecting Gel** *($50.35 for 1 ounce)* is a water-based serum that contains a blend of skin-identical ingredients and a small amount of antioxidants. Don't believe the claims that this can stave off the first signs of aging and restructure your skin's collagen, because it absolutely can't do that; do believe, however, that it's a good serum for normal to oily skin, and will work well under makeup.

OTHER NU SKIN PRODUCTS

☺ **Nu Colour Eye Makeup Remover** *($8.80 for 1.76 ounces)* is a silicone-in-water fluid that includes a wax-based ingredient and plant oils to thoroughly remove all types of makeup. The oils contribute a slightly greasy film, making this a product that you should use before your regular cleanser. It is fragrance-free.

☺ **Exfoliant Scrub Extra Gentle** *($13.30 for 3.4 ounces)* contains mostly water, aloe, thickener, seashells (as an abrasive), and vitamins. The seashells can be rough on the skin, so calling this product gentle is a stretch, but it is a good exfoliant for most skin types, even though a washcloth would work as well if not better.

☺ **Facial Scrub** *($13.30 for 3.4 ounces)* is gentler than the Exfoliant Scrub Extra Gentle above, despite the name difference. This one contains finely-milled walnut-shell powder and husk, which work as a scrub, and it can be good for someone with normal to dry skin.

☹ **$$$ Polishing Peel Skin Refinisher** *($26.84 for 1.7 ounces)* is a clay- and cornstarch-based scrub that isn't as elegant or as rinseable as the two Nu Skin scrubs above. The pumpkin enzymes are too unstable to provide extra exfoliation. This is not similar to a microdermabrasion procedure any more than a mansion is similar to an efficiency apartment.

✓☺ **$$$ Celltrex CoQ10 Complete** *($47.50 for 0.5 ounce)* supplies skin with a healthy dose of several antioxidants, including ubiquinone (coenzyme Q10). It also contains a cell-communicating ingredient, water-binding agents, and anti-irritants. In short, this fragrance-free, water-based serum is highly recommended for all skin types.

☹ **Enhancer Skin Conditioning Gel** *($10.93 for 4 ounces)* is an OK basic ultra-light, gel-based moisturizer for oily skin. It lacks antioxidants but contains several water-binding agents. As claimed, this can be a soothing after-shave product for men.

☹ **Face Lift, Original Formula** *($34.96 for set)* includes the **Face Lift Powder** and the **Face Lift Activator**. These two formulas are meant to be mixed together and then applied to your skin. The Lift Powder contains egg white, cornstarch, and some water-binding agents. The Activator contains water, aloe, some water-binding agents, and preservatives. This won't lift skin anywhere, and the egg white and cornstarch can be skin irritants. In addition, the cornstarch can promote bacterial growth, which isn't good news for blemish-prone skin.

☹ **Face Lift, Sensitive Formula** *($34.96 for set)* is similar to the Face Lift, Original Formula above, except the egg white is replaced by a gum-based thickener and the Activator portion is just a water- and aloe-based toner. This isn't preferred for sensitive skin because the cornstarch can be a problem, and none of this will lift skin one bit.

☺ **$$$ HPX Hydrating Gel** *($50.35 for 1.7 ounces)* contains some intriguing ingredients, but I can't imagine most consumers being impressed by the fact that this contains human placental protein, at least I hope not. Plus, there is nothing about human placental protein that has any unique benefit for skin. Beyond that gimmick, this fragrance-free blend of oil, vitamin E, fatty acids, and preservatives is a good moisturizer for dry skin.

☹ **$$$ Intensive Eye Complex** *($36.58 for 0.5 ounce)* is a decent lightweight moisturizer for slightly dry skin anywhere on the face. It's disappointing that the really intriguing ingredients barely make a showing, though this product is fragrance-free.

☹ **Moisture Restore Intense Moisturizer** *($28.74 for 2.5 ounces)* offers those with dry to very dry skin some helpful ingredients to restore moisture and radiance, but the jar packaging means the antioxidants (of which there's very little) won't remain stable during use.

✓☺ **NaPCA Moisture Mist** *($10.74 for 8.4 ounces)* is an above-average fragrance-free, spray-on toner for all skin types. The alcohol-free formula contains several skin-identical ingredients and the cell-communicating ingredient niacinamide.

☹ **NaPCA Moisturizer** *($22.33 for 2.5 ounces)* is an option for normal to dry skin, but what a shame the many antioxidants are subject to breaking down once this jar-packaged product is opened.

☹ **Rejuvenating Cream** *($29.21 for 2.5 ounces)* is very similar to the Moisture Restore Intense Moisturizer above, and the same review applies.

☺ **Clay Pack** *($13.54 for 3.4 ounces)* is a standard clay mask with small amounts of water-binding agents and antioxidants. This is an option for normal to oily skin.

☹ **Cream Hydrating Masque** *($18.53 for 3.4 ounces)* ends up being more irritating than indulgent for skin because it contains lavender and sage oils along with pinecone extract. None of these help protect dry skin from harsh environmental conditions.

☹ **Galvanic Spa** *($34.20 for 4 treatments)* is a gimmicky "treatment" system consisting of **Galvanic Spa Pre-Treatment Gel**, which is mostly water, slip agent, film-forming agent, and several plant extracts, and **Galvanic Spa Treatment Gel**, which has a similar formula but also contains an ingredient that has a warming effect on skin, along with fragrant plant extracts that can be irritating. The warming effect can stimulate circulation and cause reddened skin, but this effect is more detrimental than helpful due to the manner in which it is caused, via irritation. It would be much more beneficial to stimulate circulation by exercising rather than wasting time and money on this mostly do-nothing duo.

NU SKIN SUN PRODUCTS

☹ **Sunless Tanner** *($21.90 for 3.4 ounces)* lists witch hazel as the second ingredient, which makes this otherwise well-formulated but standard self-tanner too irritating for all skin types.

✓☺ **Sunright Body Block SPF 30** *($13.97 for 3.4 ounces)* is an excellent, in-part avobenzone water-resistant sunscreen for normal to dry skin. It not only provides broad-spectrum sun protection but also boosts the skin's defenses with antioxidants and soothing agents. Another bonus: the price isn't so high that it's going to discourage liberal application.

✓☺ **Sunright Body Block SPF 15** *($13.97 for 3.4 ounces)* is nearly identical to the Sunright Body Block SPF 30 above, except this contains a lower total concentration of active ingredients, resulting in its reduced SPF rating. Otherwise, the same comments apply.

☹ **Sunright Lip Balm SPF 15** *($5.61 for 0.15 ounce)* lacks the UVA-protecting ingredients of titanium dioxide, zinc oxide, avobenzone, Mexoryl SX (ecamsule), or Tinosorb and is not recommended.

NU SKIN MAKEUP

FOUNDATION: ☹ **Nu Colour Tinted Moisturizer SPF 15** *($26.13)* lacks significant UVA protection, which is odd given that Nu Skin's sunscreens do a good job of protecting in that range. That's unfortunate, because this has a light, elegant application that blends superbly to a dry matte finish. The five colors tend to get peachier the darker you go, but this is sheer enough that the peachiness is not an issue. What is an issue (beyond the lack of good UVA protection) is that the base formula lists the irritant witch hazel as the first ingredient, which makes this not worth considering over tinted moisturizers with sunscreen from Bobbi Brown, Aveda, or Neutrogena. ☹ **Nu Colour MoisturShade Liquid Finish SPF 15** *($21.85)*, which lacks reliable UVA protection, is a moist-finish, light-coverage foundation that comes in ten noticeably peach, pink, rose, or orange tones. Who thought any of these shades would look convincing on real skin tones? It's a shame these two major faults overwhelm an otherwise well-formulated product, but there you have it.

CONCEALER: ☹ **Nu Colour Skin Beneficial Concealer** *($18.05)* is a cream concealer with a greasy consistency and far too much slip to cover evenly and stay in place. The colors are uniformly unflattering, but even more troublesome is the inclusion of ylang ylang and sandalwood oils, which have no business being around the eyes (or anywhere on skin for that matter). The ☹ **Correctors** *($18.05)* have a similar formula but offer either strong yellow or green colors, neither of which looks convincing or the least bit natural. These also contain ylang ylang and sandalwood oils.

POWDER: 😐 **$$$ Finishing Powder** *($23.28)* is a talc-free, rice starch–based powder, so this has a drier texture that can feel a bit grainy. It comes in one shade, and while Nu Skin claims that it's translucent, this will look too white or ashen on all but fair skin, sort of like using plain baby powder to set your makeup.

☺ **$$$ Nu Colour Custom Colour MoisturShade Wet/Dry Pressed Powder** *($19 for powder cake, $7 for compact)* feels very soft, almost creamy, and blends nicely to a dry, light-coverage finish. However, this mica-based powder has shine despite Nu Skin's claim of it being matte. Four of the six shades have an unattractive peach, pink, or rose cast that's strong enough to matter, especially in daylight. The only possible contenders are Buffed Ivory and Creamy Ivory. ☺ **$$$ Nu Colour Bronzing Pearls** *($35.63)* are bronze-colored powder beads that you sweep a brush over and dust on to complete your sheer, shiny tan. The Body Shop has had this type of product for years, and if the concept appeals to you, check out their less expensive Brush-On Bronze ($17.50).

BLUSH: ☺ **$$$ Subtle Effects Blush** *($15.20 for blush tablet, $7 for compact)* is indeed subtle, as each of the six sheer colors attests. It takes some effort to build noticeable color, but the application is smooth and even with just a hint of shine. If you're looking for sheer blush, this is one to consider.

EYESHADOW: ☹ **Custom Colour Desired Effects Eye Shadow** *($10.93 per shade, $7 for refillable duo compact)* is sold as eyeshadow singles and all have a silky, silicone-based texture, but the shine (present in all of the shades, often to a sparkling degree) flakes regardless of how careful or sheer your application is. Given the number of shiny eyeshadows that don't have this problem, why would you want to consider this?

EYE AND BROW SHAPER: ☺ **Defining Effects Smooth Eye Liner** *($10.93)* is a standard, creamy eye pencil that needs sharpening. It's easy to apply, but like most creamy pencils is prone to smudging and fading before the day is done. If you're curious to try this, avoid the Sapphire and Blue Smoke shades.

☹ **Nu Colour Defining Effects Brow Liner** *($10.93)* needs to be sharpened and you'll be doing a lot of that if you choose this creamy pencil. The colors go on strong, so achieving a softly defined, natural brow is almost impossible; plus this will smudge before the end of the day, which is hardly a strong selling point.

LIPSTICK, LIP GLOSS, AND LIPLINER: ☺ **$$$ Nu Colour Contouring Lip Gloss** *($16.63)* doesn't contour the lips; it is just a shimmer-infused, semi-thick gloss dispensed from a tube that is minimally sticky and yet tenacious enough to not require a touch-up within an hour. The oligopeptide in this product is said to make lips fuller, but there is no proof of that, and even if there were, the amount of it in this product is minuscule.

☺ **$$$ Nu Colour Replenishing Lipstick** *($16.63)* contains more than enough emollient oils to replenish dry lips, but it's too much of a good thing if you were hoping for a creamy lipstick that stays in place and lasts until lunch. This does neither, as it migrates into any lines around the mouth shortly after application. Most of the medium- to full-coverage colors are very attractive, but this is one greasy lipstick!

☺ **Nu Colour Defining Effects Smooth Lipliner** *($10.93)* is nothing unique as far as pencils are concerned, but this sharpen-me tool has a smooth application and a small, but respectable, color collection.

MASCARA: ☺ **$$$ Defining Effects Mascara** *($18.05)* is an improvement over Nu Skin's former mascara, but remains an average contender, offering only modest lash enhancement even with considerable effort. It keeps lashes soft and doesn't flake or smear, but is only worth the investment if you aren't expecting much as far as length or thickness are concerned.

☹ **Nu Colour Nutriol Eyelash Treatment** *($26.13)* is a clear mascara that is supposed to be a conditioning treatment for lashes, complete with a swanky European pedigree. Ingredients like PVP (a film-forming agent typically used in hair gels), butylene glycol, and witch hazel are not conditioning in the least, and these are the backbone of this waste-of-time-and-money product.

BRUSHES: The Nu Colour ☺ **$$$ Cosmetic Brush Collection** *($59.50)* comes in a cloth case that would be better suited to housing bathroom grooming accessories (think nail clippers, disposable razors, and cuticle nippers) than the seven elegant, well-made brushes it holds. The Powder and Blush brushes are well-shaped and suitably soft while the two Eyeshadow brushes cover the basics for a classic eye design. The Eyeliner brush can double as a Brow Brush, and the rubber smudge tip at the opposite end is an option for creating soft, smoky eyes. If only the case were better, this set would have warranted a Paula's Pick rating. All of the brushes are also sold separately, ranging in price from $8 to $15.

N.V. PERRICONE, M.D. (SKIN CARE ONLY)

N. V. PERRICONE, M.D., AT-A-GLANCE

Strengths: Good cleansers; excellent lip balm; handful of very good moisturizers for eye area; outstanding tinted moisturizer with sunscreen; well-formulated moisturizing mask and topical disinfectant; some fragrance-free products.

Weaknesses: Expensive; long on claims not supported by evidence-based science (e.g., Neuropeptide range); shortage of products with sunscreen for normal to oily skin; no BHA products; no products to lighten skin discolorations; jar packaging.

For more information about N.V. Perricone, call (888) 823-7837 or visit www.nvperricone.com or www.Beautypedia.com.

Note: A detailed assessment of the Perricone phemonenon can be found on the excellent Web site www.quackwatch.org. Here is their summary of Perricone's books and products: "Dr. Perricone has mixed a pinch of science with a gallon of imagination to create an elaborate, time-consuming, expensive, prescription for a healthy life and younger skin. There is no reason to think his program is more effective than standard measures. Although some of his advice is standard, most of his recommendations are based on speculation and fanciful interpretation of selected medical literature. He makes lots of money by convincing patients and consumers, but he hasn't succeeded in convincing critical thinkers, doctors, scientists, or anyone who wants to see hard evidence. Dr. Perricone's *prescription* isn't science; it's creative salesmanship."

N.V. PERRICONE ALPHA LIPOIC ACID PRODUCTS

☺ **$$$ Alpha Lipoic Acid Nutritive Cleanser** *($35 for 6 ounces)* is a very standard but good water-soluble cleanser for normal to oily skin. It is not a cleanser and toner in one because none of the ingredients it contains is left on skin long enough to have an effect similar to a well-formulated toner.

😐 **$$$ Alpha Lipoic Acid Face Firming Activator** *($100 for 2 ounces)* does not contain anything that has been proven to firm skin, and falters as an AHA product because its pH is above 4. This product also cannot impact facial scars or large pores. The second ingredient, tyrosine, is a non-essential amino acid that has limited research proving its benefit for skin. Oral consumption is a different story, but topically it isn't a must-have by any means (Source: www.naturaldatabase.com). At best, this is a decent lightweight moisturizer for normal to slightly dry skin.

☺ **$$$ Alpha Lipoic Acid Evening Facial Emollient** *($90 for 2 ounces)* is a rather boring lightweight moisturizer for normal to slightly oily or slightly dry skin. Perricone boasts of the retinol in this product, but the amount is smaller than what's in many drugstore-line products. In fact, most of the intriguing ingredients are listed after the preservatives, and as such don't count for much (which they should at this price).

✓☺ **$$$ Alpha Lipoic Acid Eye Area Therapy** *($50 for 0.5 ounce)* ranks as the best among the Perricone's Alpha Lipoic Acid products. This emollient moisturizer for normal to dry skin anywhere on the face contains a roster of skin-identical substances and some good antioxidants. It is also fragrance-free and lacks problematic plant extracts. The claims are stretched (this won't help with puffiness or dark circles), but the overall formula is notable.

☹ **Alpha Lipoic Acid Firming Facial Mask** *($120 for the set)* claims to bring the firming benefits of alpha lipoic acid and DMAE together in a supercharged duo. Part 1, the **Firming Serum**, contains a lot of DMAE (listed as dimethyl MEA), though there is no evidence that this really has any benefit for skin. Even if it did, the lavender oil it contains is a problem for all skin types. Part 2, the **Peel-Off Mask**, doesn't fare any better because the second and third ingredients are drying, irritating alcohols. This is an embarrassing product for any cosmetics company to sell, and even more so coming from a dermatologist.

☺ **$$$ Alpha Lipoic Acid Lip Plumper** *($35 for 0.48 ounce)* is a creamy lip moisturizer that contains some good antioxidants, but those won't create fuller lips. The amount of urea may prove sensitizing to lips, which will temporarily make them look plump, but that's by virtue of irritation. Still, urea is a better choice than mint or spice irritants.

N.V. Perricone Neuropeptide Products

If you buy into Perricone's entire Neuropeptide range, your debt will be close to that of a mortgage payment, and your routine still won't include a reliable sunscreen or cleanser. When it comes to cell-communicating ingredients—substances that can tell a cell how to function better—research is still under way. It may indeed turn out that a range of peptides, and not only neuropeptides, are viable cell-communicating substances, but for now what we do know is that peptides are readily broken down by enzymes present in the skin, making it doubtful that they can have a significant anti-aging effect when applied topically.

I talked to several dermatologists to find out if any of Perricone's claims for neuropeptides make sense. Dr. Leslie Baumann, Associate Professor of Dermatology at the University of Miami, stated, "From what I see on the label, there is nothing to substantiate his claims. Peptides are the building blocks of proteins. Peptides have many effects in the body that can be seen in the laboratory [in vitro—in petri dishes]. The problem is that they are rapidly broken down by enzymes in the blood. There are lots of blood vessels in the dermis so it is really hard to get peptides to stay in the dermis long enough to function. A good example is insulin. It is a protein. Many companies have tried to deliver it topically so that diabetics would not have to inject themselves. They cannot get high enough blood levels of it when delivered topically because of all of the enzymes in the dermis that rapidly break it down."

She further explained, "The peptides used in creams claiming to work like Botox have been shown in the lab to inhibit the production of SNAP 25. SNAP 25 is the protein that Botox breaks so that acetylcholine cannot be released to cause muscle contraction. Theoretically, decreasing formation of SNAP 25 would inhibit muscle contractions. However, you have the same issue with these peptides—when placed on the skin they are degraded too fast to do anything." Moreover, there is also the issue that lots of substances in the body, from hormones to fat tissue, decrease as we age. These all affect the "youthful appearance" of skin, and neuropeptides have no impact in those areas.

I also spoke with several other dermatologists, and they all concurred with Dr. Baumann's comments. They all agreed that if Perricone had one published paper on the topic, that would help his credibility, but he doesn't have any. In fact, almost every dermatologist I spoke to said that either Perricone is really onto something that no one else knows about or he is running the biggest scam ever seen in dermatology.

unrated **Neuropeptide Eye Area Contour** *($195 for 0.5 ounce).* Perricone maintains that the peptides in this product can fight visible signs of aging, fatigue, and stress. The idea is that your wrinkles, dark circles, and sagging skin may have met their match, despite the lack of any study results, his or anyone else's. It would be nice if there were some solid science to support Perricone's prodigious anti-aging claims for neuropeptides, which go into detail about the relationship between inflammation and collagen or elastin breakdown, among other problems, but there isn't. That means you're betting a hefty sum to find out if neuropeptides are the anti-wrinkle cure. And then you have to wonder: What about all the other products Perricone sells? Do those work less effectively than his products that contain neuropeptides? After all, they're downright cheap by comparison.

Paired with the neuropeptides in this product is DMAE (dimethylaminoethanol), an ingredient said to aid in firming skin, among other assertions. Please refer to the Perricone summary above for details about DMAE.

The reason this product isn't rated is because there is no way to interpret the effect of neuropeptides when applied topically. Given that the results derived from using neuropeptides and DMAE are uncertain and likely unverifiable, the expense of Perricone's regimen is wholly illogical. On the plus side, this product is a good, soothing, lightweight moisturizer for slightly dry skin anywhere on the face. But the sobering fact is that hundreds of less expensive (in some cases, much less expensive) products also fit that description!

unrated **Neuropeptide Facial Contour** *($240 for 2.5 ounces)* is almost inappropriately named because it contains the tiniest amount of neuropeptide imaginable, especially in comparison to Perricone's Eye Area Contour version above. It does contain DMAE (discussed in the summary for this line), and is designed to optimize the results from Perricone's Neuropeptide Facial Conformer ($570 for 2 ounces), reviewed below. A review of the ingredient list reveals that this is essentially a lightweight moisturizer recommended for use "whenever there is a need to dramatically increase the appearance of the lifting, toning, contouring, and radiance of the skin." Whenever there's a need? Unless you have perennially youthful genes, have avoided the sun for years, or have already had a face-lift, what woman over 40 doesn't have these needs?

The reality-check news is that there isn't a sentence of research showing this product works as it claims. It will make skin feel softer and appear smoother and be more light-reflective (smooth skin reflects light better than rough, dry skin), and it has the potential to reduce inflammation, always a helpful benefit in a skin-care product. But nothing in this product or its actual (versus alleged) results makes it worth the price. And above all, nothing in this product is capable of resculpting or lifting skin to approximate the results attainable from cosmetic surgery.

If you want to splurge on a specialty moisturizer, consider Lauder's Perfectionist or Clinique's Repairwear lines.

unrated **Neuropeptide Facial Conformer** *($570 for 2 ounces)* is unrated because there is no way to assess the claims made about this product. On the surface, this product is a simple one that is supposed to "…stimulate the body's natural ability to retain a more youthful appearance by decreasing fine lines and wrinkles, reducing redness and discoloration, improving hydration, and plumping and firming the skin." This is something many moisturizers claim to do. Where Perricone's claim goes above and beyond is in the fine print. His product claims that it contains "41 different neuropeptides" (though only three are listed on the label) and maintains that they can be absorbed deep into skin. Perricone's theory is that the "levels of natural neuropeptides … diminish. Therefore, our body's ability to protect and repair our skin's structure declines." It is interesting that Perricone asserts that his Neuropeptide Facial Conformer, "As opposed to conventional skincare products that only temporarily nourish the epidermis … helps the skin by rejuvenating and building younger and healthier looking skin from within." Yet, Perricone continues to sell his other "nourishing" products, whose effects by his own admission fall below the efficacy of this one.

Perricone's company insists they have research to back up their claims. Their press release states: "A very reputable and well-respected independent research facility conducted a test of the effectiveness of the Neuropeptide Facial Conformer. They concluded that after a 6-week study, subjects showed significant improvement in skin roughness, dullness, laxity, hyperpigmentations, fine lines, and wrinkles. They also used a sophisticated test called skin replica analysis, which showed significant skin smoothing, and a decrease in the number and depth of wrinkles." That sounds good, but hundreds of products have a claim that their studies show the same results, and like every other cosmetics company, Perricone's won't share the actual study and it isn't published anywhere, so there is no way to evaluate how it was done or how it compares to other studies. Unpublished studies make for good press releases, but for information they are about as reliable as a chocolate cake when you're on a diet.

unrated **Neuropeptide Facial Serum Prep** *($175 for 6 ounces)* combines DMAE (discussed in the summary above) with neuropeptides and minerals in a toner-type solution meant to be used prior to Perricone's Neuropeptide Facial Conformer, reviewed above. Talk about adding financial insult to injury! After you've plunked down hundreds of dollars for the Facial Conformer, Perricone now recommends that you *prepare* your skin for the Conformer (or his other products) with his Facial Serum Prep. Together, these two products amount to a skin-care investment of $750, and it's not even a complete routine. The same comments made for neuropeptides above apply here, too. For what Perricone is charging for this product, consumers would be wise to insist on more solid science rather than just falling prey to cosmetic hyperbole.

N.V. PERRICONE OLIVE OIL PRODUCTS

☺ **$$$ Olive Oil Gentle Cleanser** *($48 for 8 ounces)* doesn't need to be nearly this expensive, but it is a very good, definitely gentle water-soluble cleanser for all skin types except very dry or very oily. It does contain fragrance and coloring agents.

😐 **$$$ Olive Oil Polyphenols Nutrient Face Fortifier** *($90 for 2 ounces)* contains mostly water, olive oil, silicone, film-forming agent, and waxlike thickener. It can be a good moisturizer for normal to dry skin, but you don't need to spend this much to get the antioxidant benefit of olive oil (open your kitchen cabinet and use that for far less money and without the film-forming ingredient). Other antioxidants are present, too, but in very small quantities.

☹ **Olive Oil Polyphenols Face Hydrator** *($70 for 2 ounces)* is nearly identical to the Olive Oil Polyphenols Nutrient Face Fortifier above, but is not recommended because of the many volatile fragrant oils it contains, including lemon, geranium, and grapefruit.

✓☺ **$$$ Olive Oil Polyphenols Hydrating Nutrient Mask** *($65 for 2 ounces)* contains several ingredients that are extremely helpful for dry to very dry skin, including olive oil and shea butter. The other state-of-the-art ingredients are less prominent, but overall this is a well-formulated moisturizing mask for dry to very dry skin.

☺ **$$$ Olive Oil Polyphenols Moist Lips** *($22 for 0.35 ounce)* is a unique lip balm that is based around olive oil and cholesterol rather than the more standard castor oil and wax. It's pricey, but if you're going to spend this much for smooth lips, at least this option is better than the norm.

N.V. PERRICONE OUTPATIENT THERAPY PRODUCTS

😐 **$$$ Outpatient Therapy Pore Refining Cleanser** *($35 for 6 ounces)* is a standard, detergent-based cleanser that contains about 5% glycolic acid. In a cleanser, any benefit from the AHA is just rinsed down the drain, but in this case the pH is too high for it to be effective as an exfoliant anyway. This is an OK option for normal to slightly oily skin.

☹ **Outpatient Therapy Pore Refining Toner Pads** *($35 for 60 pads)* lists alcohol as the second ingredient, which makes these pads a problem for all skin types, and not helpful for acne.

😐 **$$$ Outpatient Therapy Pore Refining Moisturizer Oil Free** *($55 for 2 ounces)* is a basic, fragrance-free moisturizer for normal to dry skin, but there is nothing in it that will affect pores. The amount of lactic acid is too low for it to function as an exfoliant.

✓☺ **$$$ Outpatient Therapy Acne Treatment Gel Cream** *($55 for 2 ounces)* is a very standard 2.5% benzoyl peroxide topical disinfectant. Although this would definitely be an option for treating blemishes, the price is just out of whack. There are far less expensive versions available at the drugstore, but if you're a Perricone devotee dealing with acne, this is an effective option.

😐 **$$$ Outpatient Therapy Pore Refining Concealer** *($35 for 0.5 ounce)* is Perricone's cover-up option for those battling blemishes, but he overlooked the fact that this heavy-duty concealer contains several thickeners that pose a problem when used over blemishes. For example, the second ingredient is titanium dioxide, a mineral sunscreen and opacifying agent used in many makeup products as a pigment or for increased coverage. Because titanium dioxide is occlusive, it is not the best option for use on blemishes, particularly when it's present at such a high concentration. The antioxidant glutathione is included for its anti-inflammatory effect, but there are better ways to calm blemishes than with this concealer.

N.V. PERRICONE VITAMIN C ESTER PRODUCTS

☺ **$$$ Vitamin C Ester Citrus Facial Wash** *($30 for 6 ounces)* is a very standard but good water-soluble cleanser for normal to oily skin. The tiny amount of vitamin C cannot correct a reddened or blotchy complexion, and in a cleanser it is just rinsed away before it can have any benefit as an antioxidant. Besides, sensitized skin would do better with a fragrance-free cleanser, and this one doesn't fill the bill.

☺ **$$$ Vitamin C Ester Amine Complex Face Lift** *($90 for 2 ounces)* contains a good mix of water-binding agents and antioxidants, making this a good moisturizer for normal to dry skin. Aside from that, the rating doesn't mean this will lift skin anywhere, and if you're looking for lots of vitamin C, this pales in comparison to what Jan Marini, MD Skincare by Dr. Dennis Gross, and Skinceuticals offer.

😐 **$$$ Vitamin C Ester Concentrated Restorative Cream** *($95 for 2 ounces)* is an effective, though pricey, AHA product. With approximately 4% glycolic acid and a pH of 3.3, exfoliation will occur. However, the vitamin C, while a noteworthy amount is present, won't remain stable due to the poor choice of jar packaging. For the money, I'd go with an AHA product from Alpha Hydrox or Neutrogena before this.

✓😊 **$$$ Vitamin C Ester Eye Therapy** *($50 for 0.5 ounce)* is a silicone-based moisturizer that contains an impressive amount of stabilized vitamin C and two forms of antioxidant vitamin E. It is fragrance-, colorant-, and irritant-free, and is well worth considering if you're curious to try a modern product with vitamin C.

OTHER N.V. PERRICONE PRODUCTS

☹ **Firming Facial Toner** *($35 for 6 ounces)* irritates, not firms, the skin because it lists alcohol as the second ingredient. Without it and the tiny amount of eucalyptus, this would have been a great toner for normal to dry skin.

✓😊 **$$$ Advanced Eye Area Therapy** *($95 for 0.5 ounce)* launched with the announcement that it is the evolution of eye area care, designed to address ALL concerns one might have for aging skin in this delicate place. Although you won't see that claim fulfilled, there is no denying that this is one of Perricone's best formulations. The second ingredient is stabilized vitamin C, an anti-irritant is present at a significant amount, and antioxidants are plentiful, including alpha lipoic acid, tocotrienols, and borage seed oil. Perricone also included cell-communicating ingredients and some good water-binding agents, making this an all-around fantastic (though pricey) lightweight moisturizer for all skin types. It is fragrance-free, too. Other than the overinflated claims of remedying every eye-area concern, the only other issue I have is that Perricone states this contains "unique ingredients rarely found in one product." None of the ingredients in this product are unique or exclusive to Perricone's formulas, and there is no reason several of his other products couldn't have the same blend of state-of-the-art ingredients. The real question is: Why don't they?

😊 **$$$ Advanced Face Firming Activator** *($120 for 2 ounces)* is a "ramped up" version of Perricone's original Alpha Lipoic Acid Face Firming Activator (reviewed above), and it's an improvement. Both versions contain glycolic acid, but the Advanced contains more AHA (roughly 10%) and at a pH that allows exfoliation to occur. The pH of the original Face Firming Activator prevents the glycolic acid from working as an exfoliant. Both versions contain alpha lipoic acid along with some other interesting antioxidants, though some are present in mere window-dressing amounts. Consider this a good AHA lotion for normal to slightly dry skin, though not one that's superior to many other well-formulated AHA products. The firming claim has some basis in truth because of the manner in which glycolic acid works when it's correctly formulated. Ongoing use stimulates collagen production, which will result in smoother, firmer skin. We're not talking firm as in you'll think you're in your twenties again—instead, think incremental minor improvements.

✓😊 **$$$ Active Tinted Moisturizer SPF 15** *($65 for 1.7 ounces)* ranks as one of the most expensive tinted moisturizers available, but at least all of the necessary bases (and then some) are covered. Featuring an in-part titanium dioxide sunscreen, the formula applies smoothly, and its creamy texture leaves normal to very dry skin sufficiently moist, with a fresh, dewy finish that doesn't feel greasy. The formula even includes several antioxidants, and it's packaged to ensure they remain stable after the product is opened. Two of the three shades are great; only Tint 03 is quite yellow, with an effect that is difficult to soften on medium skin. Still, it may be worth a try at the counter to see how it looks, assuming you're willing to pay the premium price. For about half as much money, equal kudos go to Bobbi Brown's SPF 15 Tinted Moisturizer ($38) and Aveda's Inner Light Tinted Moisture SPF 15 ($25). For even less money, Neutrogena's Healthy Skin Enhancer SPF 20 ($11.99) and Paula's Choice Natural Finish Oil-Absorbing Makeup SPF 15 ($12.95) are other prime options.

☺ **$$$ Anti-Spider Vein Face** *($80 for 1 ounce)* contains an impressive amount of antioxidant green tea, but not a single ingredient in this lightweight lotion will improve the appearance of spider veins beyond possibly making them less red due to green tea's anti-inflammatory property. The other antioxidants of note in this product for normal to slightly dry skin are vitamin E and alpha lipoic acid. Others are present in amounts unlikely to affect skin, including tocotreinols.

😐 **$$$ Face Finishing Moisturizer** *($55 for 2 ounces)* is an unimpressive moisturizer for dry skin. The amount of state-of-the-art ingredients is paltry, and jar packaging won't keep the antioxidants stable during use.

☹ **Face Lipid Replenishment** *($120 for 2 ounces)* contains phosphatidylcholine (PC), which is the most active ingredient in soy lecithin. Every cell membrane in the body requires PC. Nerve and brain cells in particular need large quantities of PC for repair and maintenance, and PC also aids in the metabolism of fats, regulates blood cholesterol, and nourishes the fatlike sheaths surrounding nerve fibers. It is also a major source of the neurotransmitter acetylcholine, which is used by nerves throughout the body, including in the brain in areas that are involved in long-term planning, concentration, and focus. This substance controls the rate of stimuli entering the brain, motor activity, learning and memory, and stimuli input during sleep, sex, and other functions. But all of this research has to do with the effects of ingesting PC, not putting it on the skin. So how does any of that relate to skin care? PC is considered an excellent moisturizing agent and aids in the penetration of other ingredients into the skin. It absorbs well without feeling greasy or heavy (though other ingredients perform similarly, including glycerin, which is the sixth ingredient in this formula). It also has potent antioxidant properties, which could help reduce skin damage caused by sun exposure as well as free-radical damage. Despite all this potential, this moisturizer does more harm than good because of the grapefruit, lavender, geranium, lemon, and sandalwood oils it contains. And the PC's antioxidant ability is compromised because of jar packaging.

N.V. Perricone Sun Products

☺ **$$$ Solar Protection for Body with DMAE SPF 15** *($45 for 4 ounces)* is a classic pure mineral sunscreen whose sole active is zinc oxide. The fragrance-free moisturizing base feels silky and is suitable for normal to slightly dry or dry skin. What's missing, especially for the money, are antioxidants and, at this price, the willingness to apply it liberally, which is essential to obtain the most advantageous sun protection.

☺ **$$$ Solar Protection for Face with DMAE SPF 26** *($48 for 1.7 ounces)* is nearly identical to the Solar Protection for Body with DMAE SPF 15 above, and the same review applies. If you're going to try a Perricone sunscreen, there's no reason the Body version above cannot also be used on the face.

☺ **$$$ Ceramic Skin Smoother** *($75 for 1 ounce)* has a strange name, but I assume Perricone's reference to ceramic skin is meant to evoke the idea of a porcelain complexion. However, this water-based, oil-free gel is mostly beta-glucan (a good antioxidant and soothing agent) along with absorbent ingredients that provide a smooth matte finish. How this is supposed to create skin so perfect you can toss out your foundation is anyone's guess, because the tiny amounts of some high-tech ingredients in this product (e.g., DMAE [2-dimethylaminoethanol]) cannot do that. Despite the lack of evidence that DMAE has any effect on skin, there are hundreds of Web sites claiming that it does. It is possible that DMAE can help protect the cell membrane, and keeping cells intact can have benefit, but so far that appears to be only conjecture, not fact, and recent research suggests it can actually have a negative effect on the cell. You're better off spending your money on proven ingredients than on products like this that tantalize with the promise of perfection.

OBAGI (SKIN CARE ONLY)

Obagi is "known" for his Blue Peel. This is a standard trichloroacetic acid (TCA) peel that has been performed by dermatologists and plastic surgeons for years; Obagi simply instructs the practitioner to mix the TCA with a blue-tinted base. TCA is used for peeling the face, neck, hands, and other exposed areas of the body. It causes fewer pigmentation problems than other doctor-only peels such as phenol, and is considered excellent for "spot" peeling specific areas. It also can be used for medium or light peeling, depending on the concentration and method of application. AHA and BHA peels are considered light peels, and are often done in a series of six. TCA peels are best for fine lines and can be somewhat more effective on deeper wrinkling, but they are performed only once every couple of years. Many of the dermatologists I spoke to believe that a TCA peel is a viable option for many skin types, despite consumers' fascination with AHA peels.

OBAGI AT-A-GLANCE

Strengths: Selection of good water-soluble cleansers; prescription-only products with 4% hydroquinone; well-formulated AHA products; almost all sunscreens provide sufficient UVA protection.

Weaknesses: Expensive; some products available only via prescription, which can be inconvenient; poor anti-acne products; one skin-lightening product with sunscreens does not provide adequate UVA protection; moisturizers should contain more state-of-the-art ingredients.

For more information about Obagi, call (800) 636-7546 or visit www.obagi.com or www.Beautypedia.com. Note: Obagi products are sold only through authorized physicians, plastic surgeons, and accredited medical spas.

OBAGI CLENZIDERM M.D. PRODUCTS

Note: These products may also be purchased as part of a three-step system, but because the first two are so poorly rated you would want to think twice about making this a kit.

☹ **Clenziderm M.D. Daily Care Foaming Cleanser** *($32 for 4 ounces)* would have been a good gentle water-soluble cleansing lotion if it did not contain menthol and menthyl lactate, both of which make this too irritating for all skin types.

☹ **Clenziderm M.D. Pore Therapy** *($32 for 4 ounces)* is a terrible alcohol-based toner that also contains menthol and two menthol derivatives, making for potent irritation. Note that the inactive ingredient list for this product is in alphabetical (rather than descending) order, which is permissible because this is classified as an over-the-counter drug.

☺ **$$$ Clenziderm M.D. Serum Gel** *($65 for 1.7 ounces)* is the only product in the Clenziderm routine to consider, although the cost is ludicrous for what amounts to a very standard, fragrance-free 5% benzoyl peroxide product. Obagi speaks of the delivery system for the benzoyl peroxide, but the fact is that most products that contain this active ingredient incorporate some sort of delivery system that ensures the benzoyl peroxide is effective, and there is no research showing that Obagi's system has any advantage.

OBAGI-C RX SYSTEM

☺ **$$$ C-Cleansing Gel** *($31 for 6 ounces)* is a very good, though pricey, water-soluble cleanser for normal to slightly dry or slightly oily skin. The amount of vitamin C is impressive, but its benefit is quickly rinsed down the drain. This does contain fragrance.

☺ **$$$ C-Clarifying Serum** *($94 for 1 ounce)* is a prescription-only product that lists 4% hydroquinone as the active ingredient. It is formulated in a simple gel base that contains L-ascorbic acid, a form of vitamin C that has antioxidant benefits. The pH of this serum allows the vitamin C to be efficacious, but also potentially irritating. This is a definite option for lightening skin discolorations related to sun damage or hormones, but would have been even better if Obagi had included a roster of anti-irritants.

☺ **$$$ C-Exfoliating Day Lotion** *($52 for 2 ounces)* contains 7% glycolic acid at a pH level that ensures this will exfoliate skin. The lightweight lotion base is suitable for all skin types except very oily; the only disappointing element of this AHA product is the amount and form of vitamin C. Although this is an effective option, it doesn't best less expensive versions from Neutrogena, Alpha Hydrox, or Paula's Choice.

☹ **C-Exfoliating Day Lotion SPF 12** *($52 for 2 ounces)* is supposed to contain the same amount of glycolic acid as the C-Exfoliating Day Lotion above, but if the ingredient list is accurate, that's not the case. The amount of glycolic acid is minuscule and the sunscreen actives leave skin vulnerable to UVA damage, making this a daytime product to ignore.

😐 **C-Sunguard SPF 30** *($39 for 3 ounces)* is a basic daytime moisturizer for normal to dry skin that contains an in-part zinc oxide sunscreen. Vitamin C is absent, as are any truly interesting ingredients for skin, but this will provide sun protection.

☺ **$$$ C-Therapy Night Cream** *($83 for 2 ounces)* is a prescription-only product because it contains 4% hydroquinone as the active ingredient. The water- and glycerin-based lotion includes a couple of vitamin antioxidants, and it's a good option for normal to dry skin with pigment irregularities that has not responded well to over-the-counter levels of hydroquinone.

OBAGI NU-DERM SYSTEM

☺ **$$$ Nu-Derm Foaming Gel, for Normal/Oily Skin** *($34 for 6.7 ounces)* is nearly identical to the C-Cleansing Gel above, minus the vitamin C and with the inclusion of some non-irritating plant extracts. Otherwise, the same review applies.

☺ **$$$ Nu-Derm Gentle Cleanser, for Normal/Dry Skin** *($34 for 6.7 ounces)* is similar to the Nu-Derm Foaming Gel cleanser above, except this option includes a plant oil that makes it more suitable for its intended skin type. This would be gentler without the fragrance.

☹ **Nu-Derm Toner** *($34 for 6.7 ounces)*. The potassium alum in this toner is a potent absorbent and topical disinfectant that can be a skin irritant, and the witch hazel distillate is mostly alcohol, which also can be irritating and drying for skin. Moreover, this product does not return skin to a good pH because the potassium alum has a very high pH, something that is not helpful for skin.

☺ **$$$ Elastiderm Eye Gel** *($85 for 0.5 ounce)* is said to fill in the missing pieces of the anti-aging puzzle by improving elasticity, but if that's true, then the same claim can be tagged onto almost any other gel-type moisturizer. This contains mostly water, slip agent, solvents, glycerin, thickener, film-forming agent, emollient, more thickeners, antioxidants, pH adjuster, talc, preservatives, and mineral pigments. One of the antioxidants is a synthetic ingredient, malonic acid, which is a strong skin irritant when used in pure form. Dr. Obagi claims it is part of a mineral complex clinically proven to stimulate elastic production, but there is no research (not even his own) to confirm this.

☺ **$$$ Elastiderm Night Eye Cream** *($85 for 0.5 ounce)* is mostly thickeners and film-forming agent. Although it can address the basic needs of dry skin anywhere on the face, its antioxidant content is subject to deterioration due to jar packaging. The mineral pigments can have a slight cosmetic brightening effect, but this is an expensive way to achieve such a result.

☺ **Nu-Derm Action** *($37 for 2 ounces)* lightly moisturizes normal to dry skin, but that's the only exciting action this overall bland but fragrance-free product has. If you were hoping this was somehow state-of-the-art, well … it isn't.

☺ **$$$ Nu-Derm Exfoderm, for Normal/Dry Skin** *($57 for 2 ounces)* is just a standard moisturizer that lists phytic acid as the third ingredient. Phytic acid is a good antioxidant, but not the only one or the best one. Other than that, this is mostly water and thickeners, which makes it a rather mediocre moisturizer for normal to dry skin.

☺ **$$$ Nu-Derm Exfoderm Forte, for Normal/Oily Skin** *($57 for 2 ounces)* is a good, though very basic, AHA lotion whose glycolic acid content and pH level allow it to exfoliate skin. The amount of wax makes it inappropriate for normal to oily skin; it is best for normal to dry skin not prone to blemishes. Suffice it to say that there are far better AHA products for a lot less money.

☺ **$$$ Nu-Derm Eye Cream** *($45 for 0.5 ounce)* includes some good emollients in a simple base of water and aloe gel. Water-binding agents and antioxidants are barely present, making this expensive eye-area moisturizer a less enticing consideration compared to, say, superior options from Lauder or Clinique.

☺ **Nu-Derm Healthy Skin Protection SPF 35** *($40 for 3 ounces)* is identical in every respect (except product name and SPF rating) to the C-Sunguard SPF 30 above, and the same comments apply.

✓☺ **Nu-Derm Physical UV Block SPF 32** *($40 for 2 ounces)* is an excellent sunscreen for normal to dry or sensitive skin, and for those with rosacea. The fragrance-free formula lists only zinc oxide as the active ingredient, and the silky texture provides skin with the anti-irritant benefit of willow herb extract.

☺ **$$$ Nu-Derm Blender** *($79 for 2 ounces)* is nearly identical to the C-Therapy Night Cream above, and the same review applies, including the fact that this is prescription-only.

☺ **$$$ Nu-Derm Clear** *($83 for 2 ounces)* is similar to the C-Therapy Night Cream above, except this option contains a potentially irritating amount of sodium lauryl sulfate.

☹**Nu-Derm Sunfader SPF 15** *($63 for 2 ounces)* is a 4% hydroquinone product that also contains a sunscreen with an SPF 15. That is an intriguing concept: mixing a prescription-strength skin-lightening agent with sunscreen. However, this sunscreen doesn't contain the

UVA-protecting ingredients of titanium dioxide, zinc oxide, avobenzone, Mexoryl SX (ecamsule), or Tinosorb and, therefore, provides inadequate protection. And that will do nothing but make skin discolorations worse!

😐 **$$$ Nu-Derm Tolereen** *($47 for 2 ounces)* costs a lot for what amounts to a very basic hydrocortisone product. Obagi's contains only 0.5%, while most of those at the drugstore (retailing for a fraction of this price) contain 1%. Hydrocortisone is a very good topical aid for minor redness, itching, and inflammation. Keep in mind that hydrocortisone is for sporadic, infrequent use only, because repeated, long-term application will break down the skin's collagen and elastin. This product also contains sodium lauryl sulfate, a significant skin irritant, which is an ironic ingredient to put in a product meant to reduce skin irritation.

✓😊 **$$$ Obagi Tretinoin Cream 0.05% and 0.1%** *($65–$75 for 20 grams)* are both prescription-only products that contain tretinoin, the active ingredient in Retin-A and Renova, among others. These differ little from their competitors in the pharmaceutical world, and if your skin can tolerate them, all are options for improving collagen production and minimizing signs of sun damage.

OBAGI PROFESSIONAL-C SERUMS

All of the products below claim to contain professional-strength levels of vitamin C. However, given that there are no formally established standards for what constitutes a "professional" amount of vitamin C, the claim is unfounded and merely meant to make these basic, one-note antioxidant serums appear to be more than what they really are. Vitamin C is hardly the only or the best antioxidant. If you are still looking for a vitamin C product, options from MD Skincare by Dr. Dennis Gross, Jan Marini Skin Research, and Skinceuticals all provide more well-rounded options.

😐 **$$$ Professional-C Serum 5%, for Eye Area** *($44 for 0.5 ounce)* contains 5% L-ascorbic acid in a liquid base whose main ingredient (propylene glycol) enhances the penetration of the vitamin C. However, the pH above 4 isn't likely to keep the vitamin C stable during use, so the in-usage efficacy of this serum is questionable.

😐 **$$$ Professional-C Serum 10%** *($60 for 1 ounce)* contains vitamin C (ascorbic acid) in a glycol base with water, solvent, and fragrance. Just like the 5% version for the Eye Area above, the pH of this means that the vitamin C isn't likely to remain stable during use.

☹ **Professional-C Serum 15%** *($75 for 1 ounce)* contains 15% ascorbic acid at a pH of 2.3, a combination that, while efficacious, can also be very irritating to skin. There are better ways for skin to enjoy the benefits of vitamin C than this, and the amount of sodium lauryl sulfate in this product is cause for concern.

😐 **$$$ Professional-C Serum 20%** *($95 for 1 ounce)* has a lot of vitamin C and a less irritating pH than the Professional-C Serum 15% above, though the amount of sodium lauryl sulfate is still cause for concern and doesn't make this potent option worth choosing over better formulations from Skinceuticals or Cellex-C.

OLAY (SKIN CARE ONLY)

OLAY AT-A-GLANCE

Strengths: Inexpensive (mostly); several outstanding water-soluble cleansers and scrubs; boon for any consumer in love with cleansing cloths; all sunscreens include UVA-protecting ingredients; some good BHA options (but the low pH is a concern); bountiful selection of state-of-the-art serums and some excellent moisturizers; good self-tanners that include sun protection; some of the best products offer fragrance-free version.

Weaknesses: Bar cleansers; no eye-makeup removers; no AHA products; no topical disinfectant for blemishes; random products contain menthol; toners are mostly irritating; more than a handful of dated moisturizers; jar packaging; several sunscreens don't offer skin much beyond basic sun protection; repetitive formulas make this line confusing and tricky to shop.

For more information about Olay, call (800) 285-5170 or visit www.olay.com or www.Beautypedia.com.

OLAY AGE DEFYING PRODUCTS

☺ **Age Defying Daily Renewal Cleanser** *($5.59 for 6.78 ounces)* is a good cleansing lotion/scrub for normal to dry skin, though the beta hydroxy complex will not exfoliate skin due to its brief contact and the too high pH. What will exfoliate mildly are the polyethylene beads this cleanser contains.

☺ **Age Defying Anti-Wrinkle Daily SPF 15 Lotion** *($12.99 for 3.4 ounces)* is a lightweight, water- and glycerin-based daytime moisturizer that includes an in-part avobenzone sunscreen. Olay draws attention to this product's pro-retinol and beta hydroxy acid content, but the formula contains neither retinol nor salicylic acid. What it does contain is a small amount of retinyl propionate. Similar to the more commonly used retinyl palmitate, retinyl propionate is a retinoid ester that must be converted to a more active form by enzymes in the skin. Retinyl propionate is apparently more stable and less irritating than retinol, yet offers a similar benefit to skin. However, research on this retinol alternative is scant. And with the most current information coming from dermatologist Zoe Diana Draelos, who is a consultant to Procter & Gamble (Olay's parent company), it's not exactly impartial. Assuming that retinyl propionate is more stable than retinol (and that's only an assumption because there is no substantiated proof) doesn't fully explain why Olay chose to package this moisturizer in a translucent bottle, which doesn't help keep ingredients stable. Still, it's a good option for someone with normal to slightly oily skin. And, as with most of Olay's latest moisturizers, it includes plenty of skin-beneficial niacinamide.

😐 **Age Defying Anti-Wrinkle Replenishing Night Cream** *($14.99 for 2 ounces)* is similar to the Age Defying Anti-Wrinkle Daily SPF 15 Lotion above, minus the sunscreen. It is not rated as highly because the jar packaging will not help keep the antioxidant vitamins stable during use.

😐 **Age Defying Daily Renewal Cream** *($10.19 for 2 ounces)* is an option as a BHA product due to its salicylic acid content (approximately 2%), but the pH of 2.3 is unusually low and may prove too irritating for daily use, so proceed with caution. The base formula is best for normal to slightly dry or slightly oily skin.

😐 **Age Defying Intensive Nourishing Night Cream** *($9.99 for 2 ounces)* is similar to the Age Defying Daily Renewal Cream above, and the same review applies.

☺ **Age Defying Protective Renewal Lotion SPF 15** *($9.99 for 4 ounces)* contains an in-part zinc oxide sunscreen, but that's the only exciting element in this rather bland moisturizer for normal to slightly dry skin. The moisturizers with sunscreen in Olay's Regenerist, Total Effects, and Definity lines are more exciting.

☹ **Age Defying Revitalizing Eye Gel** *($10.19 for 0.5 ounce)* lists witch hazel distillate as the second ingredient, which makes this gel too irritating for all skin types.

OLAY COMPLETE PRODUCTS

☺ **Complete All Day Moisture Cream SPF 15, for Combination/Oily Skin** *($6.99 for 2 ounces)* is a slightly more emollient version of Olay's Age Defying Protective Renewal Lotion SPF 15 reviewed above, and the same review applies.

☺ **Complete All Day Moisture Cream SPF 15, for Normal Skin** *($6.99 for 2 ounces)* is nearly identical to the Complete All Day Moisture Cream SPF 15, for Combination/Oily Skin above, and the same comments apply.

☺ **Complete All Day Moisture Cream SPF 15, for Sensitive Skin** *($6.99 for 2 ounces)* is nearly identical to the Complete All Day Moisture Cream SPF 15, for Combination/Oily Skin above, except this version omits the fragrance. Otherwise, the same comments apply.

☺ **Complete All Day Moisture Lotion SPF 15, for Combination/Oily Skin** *($10.49 for 6 ounces)* features an in-part zinc oxide sunscreen in a lightweight lotion base suitable for its intended skin type. Aside from broad-spectrum sun protection and a silky texture, skin will be left wanting more, though this works well under makeup.

☺ **Complete All Day Moisture Lotion SPF 15, for Normal Skin** *($10.49 for 6 ounces)* is nearly identical to the Complete All Day Moisture Lotion SPF 15, for Combination/Oily Skin above, and the same comments apply.

☺ **Complete All Day Moisture Lotion SPF 15, for Sensitive Skin** *($10.49 for 6 ounces)* is nearly identical to the Complete All Day Moisture Lotion SPF 15, for Combination/Oily Skin above, minus fragrance. Otherwise, the same comments apply.

☺ **Complete Defense Daily UV Moisturizer SPF 30** *($13.99 for 2.5 ounces)* is a great, in-part avobenzone sunscreen in a lightweight moisturizing base that is a fine option for normal to dry skin. The base formula isn't too exciting, but Olay did include an appreciable amount of their favorite vitamin, niacinamide, which can help skin retain moisture and may help skin cells function better. The other vitamins, antioxidants, and soothing plant extracts are barely present and don't amount to much for skin. This product does contain fragrance.

☺ **Complete Defense Daily UV Moisturizer SPF 30, for Sensitive Skin** *($13.99 for 2.5 ounces)* has a lighter moisturizing base than the Complete Defense Daily UV Moisturizer SPF 30 above, but includes 6% zinc oxide. Although zinc oxide provides excellent broad-spectrum protection, it can also leave a whitish cast on the skin when used in this amount. Because Olay included other synthetic sunscreen active ingredients, this is not a slam-dunk choice for sensitive skin (zinc oxide or titanium dioxide are the most gentle choices for this skin type). This fragrance-free daily sunscreen would be best for normal to slightly dry skin not prone to blemishes. It contains a less impressive amount of niacinamide than the Complete Defense Daily UV Moisturizer above.

☺ **Complete Multi-Radiance Daily Illuminating UV Lotion SPF 15** *($14.99 for 2.5 ounces)* is complete in the sense that it provides a good, in-part avobenzone sunscreen. But beyond that, its base formula lacks the full complement of skin-beneficial ingredients that would make this product's name more accurate. The absence of significant antioxidants and water-binding agents is disappointing, although if you're curious to see what niacinamide will do for your skin, a good amount is present. There is also a fair amount of mica, which imparts a subtle sheen to skin (what Olay refers to as "illumination"). If you have oily skin, this extra shine is not the best. Those with normal to slightly dry skin will find this product's texture most agreeable. It does contain fragrance.

☺ **Complete Multi-Radiance Daily Illuminating UV Lotion SPF 15, Fragrance-Free** *($14.99 for 2.5 ounces)* is identical to the Complete Multi-Radiance Daily Illuminating UV Lotion SPF 15 above, except this version omits the fragrance, which makes it a better choice unless you're adamant about your daytime moisturizer having a sweet scent.

😐 **Complete Night Fortifying Cream** *($12.99 for 2 ounces)* is a lightweight moisturizer for normal to dry skin, but regrettably the antioxidants it contains will deteriorate due to the jar packaging. Several other Olay products have better formulations in packaging that will keep the air- and light-sensitive ingredients well protected.

😐 **Complete Plus Ultra-Rich Day Cream SPF 15, for Extra Dry Skin** *($8.95 for 2 ounces)* is not ultra-rich in the least. In fact, this is very similar to Olay's Complete All Day Moisture Cream SPF 15, for Combination/Oily Skin reviewed above, and the same comments apply.

😐 **Complete Plus Ultra-Rich Moisture Lotion SPF 15, for Extra Dry Skin** *($10.29 for 4 ounces)* has a base formula that's way too light for someone with extra dry skin. However, this can be an OK, in-part zinc oxide sunscreen for normal to oily skin. The tiny amount of vegetable oil won't make skin more oily and certainly won't provide "intense moisture."

😐 **Complete Plus Ultra-Rich Night Firming Cream, for Extra Dry Skin** *($10.69 for 2 ounces)* contains some helpful ingredients for dry skin, but someone with extra dry skin will likely find this formula lacking. The jar packaging won't keep the vitamin E and other antioxidants stable during use.

😐 **Complete Plus Ultra-Rich Tinted Moisturizer, for Extra Dry Skin** *($10.99 for 1.7 ounces)* is a sheer tinted moisturizer that isn't all that moisturizing, especially as it lists alcohol as the fourth ingredient. There are some ingredients present that are good for dry skin, but the alcohol automatically makes this a lighter product. Olay missed an opportunity to give women an all-in-one option by not including any sunscreen—a strange oversight given how many of the Complete products have very good sunscreens. There are better tinted moisturizer options available at similar prices from Neutrogena and Revlon.

OLAY DAILY FACIALS PRODUCTS

☺ **Daily Facials Clarity Foaming Cleanser** *($7.99 for 6.7 ounces)* contains 2% salicylic acid, but its benefit is rinsed down the drain. This is otherwise a standard water-soluble cleanser that is a good option for normal to oily skin. The salicylic acid means this should not be used around the eyes to remove makeup.

☺ **Daily Facials Clarity Lathering Cloths** *($5.99 for 30 cloths)* are meant for skin that is prone to blemishes. These standard cleansing cloths are used with water. Once they're wet, the cloths produce a rich, creamy lather that cushions skin as the textured cloth exfoliates. The formula is similar to Olay's other Daily Facials Cleansing Cloths, except this option contains a high amount of petrolatum. That isn't the best ingredient for blemished skin, not because it clogs pores, but because it doesn't rinse that well. It can also leave a somewhat slick feel on your skin, something those with excess oil problems are not likely to appreciate. The cloths provide gentle exfoliation and easily remove most types of makeup, but nothing in this product is truly appropriate for blemish-prone skin. The tiny amount of salicylic acid is useless because the pH of these cloths is too high for exfoliation to occur, and, fortunately, the small amount of witch hazel is too insignificant to cause irritation. Overall, these cloths are best for someone with normal to dry skin with minor to zero blemishes. There is nothing about this product that you can't replace with a gentle cleanser and a washcloth.

☹ **Daily Facials Deep Cleansing Cloths, for Combination/Oily Skin** *($5.99 for 30 cloths)* are similar to the Daily Facials Clarity Lathering Cloths above, except this option includes menthol and, therefore, is not recommended for any skin type.

☺ **Daily Facials Express Wet Cleansing Cloths, for All Skin Types** *($5.99 for 30 cloths)* are identical to the Daily Facial Express Wet Cleansing Cloths, for Sensitive Skin, below, except that these contain fragrance. If that's important to you (it isn't important for good skin care), these are the cloths to choose. There is nothing about this product that isn't replaced by a gentle cleanser and a washcloth.

☺ **Daily Facials Express Wet Cleansing Cloths, for Sensitive Skin** *($5.99 for 30 cloths)* are an admirable cleansing option for sensitive skin, eschewing fragrance and drying cleansing agents in favor of glycerin, slip agents, and silicones. This combination does not cleanse skin or remove makeup very well, but is fine for a refresher between normal face washings with a regular cleanser. The only ingredient caution for this product is for sensitive skin because it contains DMDM hydantoin, a formaldehyde-releasing preservative. There is nothing about this product that can't be replaced by a gentle cleanser and a washcloth.

☺ **Daily Facials Hydrating Cleansing Cloths, for Normal to Dry Skin** *($5.99 for 30 cloths)* have a gentle formula that can be a very good option for their intended skin types, though the lather they produce requires thorough rinsing to avoid a slightly greasy film. The amount of salicylic acid is too little to exfoliate.

☺ **Daily Facials Night Cleansing Cloths** *($6.99 for 30 cloths)* are presumably designated for nighttime use because they contain a tiny amount of lavender extract, whose aroma is known to relax. These cloths are otherwise similar to the Daily Facials Hydrating Cleansing Cloths, for Normal to Dry Skin above, and the same comments apply. The amount of witch hazel is too low to be problematic for skin. There is nothing about this product that you can't replace with a gentle cleanser and a washcloth.

☺ **Daily Facials Self-Foaming Discs, for Combination/Oily Skin** *($7.49 for 30 discs)* are dual-sided cleansing discs whose formula is activated by pressure from your thumbs. One side has raised nubs for an exfoliating action, while the other side is smoother. The water- and glycerin-based cleansing formula is straightforward and works well to remove excess oil and makeup for its intended skin types. There is nothing about this product that isn't replaced by a gentle cleanser and a washcloth.

☺ **Daily Facials Self-Foaming Discs, for Normal to Dry Skin** *($7.49 for 30 discs)* have a gentler, more lotion-like cleansing base than the Daily Facials Self-Foaming Discs, for Combination/Oily Skin above, but the dual-sided pad is the same. These discs would work well for normal to dry skin. Again, there is nothing about this product that can't be replaced with a gentle cleanser and a washcloth.

✓☺ **Daily Facials Skin Soothing Cleansing Cloths, for Sensitive Skin** *($5.99 for 30 cloths)* are wonderfully soothing and a good, disposable cleansing option for someone with dry, sensitive skin. The fragrance-free, emollient formula is exceptionally gentle, yet thoroughly removes makeup. There is nothing about this product that you can't achieve by using a gentle cleanser and a washcloth.

☺ **Daily Facials Clarity Daily Scrub** *($7.49 for 6 ounces)* won't "deep clean" skin any better than other standard, polyethylene-particle scrubs, though this particular one can double as a cleansing scrub because it contains detergent cleansing agents. The price is more than reasonable and it is free of needless irritants, making it a good choice for all but very dry skin types. As you may expect, the benefit of the 2% salicylic acid is wasted in a product like this.

😐 **Daily Facials Intensives Smooth Skin Exfoliating Scrub** *($7.29 for 6 ounces)* is a standard scrub that contains polyethylene as the abrasive agent, though there's considerably less of it here than in many other scrub products. There's enough sodium lauryl sulfate to be potentially irritating, which doesn't make this scrub as enticing as others from Olay.

☹ **Daily Facials Clarity Purifying Toner** *($7.49 for 6.7 ounces)* contains enough alcohol to cause irritation, while the 2% salicylic acid will not exfoliate because the pH is too high.

😐 **Daily Facials Intensives Deep Cleansing Clay Mask** *($7.99 for 4 ounces)* is a very standard but good clay mask for normal to oily skin. This contains a slight amount of detergent cleansing agent that facilitates removal, but can also make this mask more drying than need be.

OLAY DEFINITY PRODUCTS

For the most part, Olay's Definity products are merely costlier versions of the company's well-formulated Regenerist lineup. Just as with Regenerist, the B-vitamin niacinamide plays a major role in all of the Definity products. Niacinamide is a very good cell-communicating ingredient that not only improves skin's hydration levels and ceramide content, but also interrupts the process that causes irregular pigmentation (Sources: *Experimental Dermatology*, July 2005, pages 498–508; and *Journal of Cosmetic Dermatology*, April 2004, page 88).

The new kids on the block that distinguish Definity from Regenerist are acetyl glucosamine (an Estee Lauder favorite discussed below) and mineral pigments (including mica, titanium dioxide, and tin oxide). Mineral pigments cast a reflective, radiant finish on skin, brightening the look of dull complexions, but that is strictly a cosmetic effect and unrelated to taking healthy care of your skin.

On the other hand, acetyl glucosamine functions primarily as a water-binding agent. The only research pertaining to its ability to lighten discolorations comes from Olay's owner Procter & Gamble, whose double-blind, split-face, placebo-controlled research revealed that 2% acetyl glucosamine improved the appearance of skin discolorations. The effect was more pronounced when 2% acetyl glucosamine was combined with 4% niacinamide, and, based on the ingredient statement, Olay very likely uses those concentrations in most of their Definity products. However, we don't know the extent of improvement (the study didn't reveal this, and what if only a 5% improvement was noted?), nor did they tell what type of placebo was used. The placebo could have been plain Vaseline, which would have no effect on discolorations (nor would it provide sun protection, which would make skin discolorations worse). I would be interested to see how the effects of this combination from Definity compare with other skin-lighteners. For example, how does it compare with the effects of hydroquinone or arbutin after eight weeks, or with the effects of other moisturizers loaded with antioxidants, or with the effects of just an effective sunscreen, especially one with just titanium dioxide or zinc oxide? It's my guess that the results from these documented skin-lightening substances would be far superior.

☺ **Definity Illuminating Cream Cleanser** *($9.99 for 5 ounces)* is said to penetrate deep into the skin's surface for an illuminating cleansing, but the skin's surface isn't that deep and the major ingredients in this cleanser (isopropyl palmitate and petrolatum) do not penetrate skin. This is recommended as a partially water-soluble rich cleanser for dry to very dry skin. You will need a washcloth for complete removal of "the smallest traces of dirt and makeup" and of the cleanser itself, as it doesn't rinse too well.

✓ ☺ **Definity Pore Redefining Scrub** *($9.99 for 5 ounces)* has more cleansing ability than exfoliating ability, because the amount of polyethylene beads that do the exfoliating is meager. Meanwhile, the salicylic acid won't work as intended because this product's pH is too high and because it is rinsed off and so has only brief contact with skin. This is still a good, easy-to-rinse cleanser with a mild scrub action for normal to oily skin.

☺ **Definity Correcting Protective Lotion with SPF 15** *($29.99 for 1.7 ounces)* is a very good daily sunscreen that provides sufficient UVA protection from avobenzone. The base formula consists of several skin-friendly ingredients, including glycerin, niacinamide, acetyl glucosamine, panthenol, and safflower seed oil. It's a worthwhile, if not quite state-of-the-art formula (a wider array of antioxidants would have been preferred, especially given the price) for normal to dry skin. The mineral pigments provide a radiant finish that's best described as a subtle glow that works fine for daytime.

😐 **$$$ Definity Deep Penetrating Foaming Moisturizer** *($29.99 for 1.7 ounces)* foams because it is pressurized with isobutene and propane gases, but that feature is more a novelty than a particularly effective delivery system because those substances have a negative impact on the stability of the beneficial ingredients. This light-textured moisturizer contains mostly water, silicone, glycerin, niacinamide, acetyl glucosamine, thickener, film-forming agent, slip agents, preservatives, aloe, plant oil, and fragrance. Mineral pigments are included for a glowy finish, but if you're using this in the evening before you go to bed, that cosmetic effect isn't really necessary. This does contain other antioxidants, but the amount is insignificant.

😐 **$$$ Definity Deep Penetrating Foaming Moisturizer SPF 15, Fragrance Free** *($26.99 for 1.7 ounces)* has a unique foam texture, but that won't enhance penetration, nor would you want it to because the active ingredients necessary for sun protection are meant to stay on the skin's surface. The sunscreen includes avobenzone for UVA protection while the base formula is the now-standard Olay blend of glycerin, niacinamide, and silicone. As with the other Definity moisturizer, mineral pigments provide a slight glow to skin, but don't mistake this cosmetic effect for a permanent change in skin's luminosity. This is best for normal to dry skin. The propellant can cause the beneficial ingredients to be unstable.

☺ **Definity Eye Illuminator, Illuminating Eye Treatment** *($23.99 for 0.5 ounce)* combines the key ingredients in the Definity moisturizers above, but at higher concentrations. This fragrance-free formula provides a silky texture and finish while also being a good source of cell-communicating ingredients and antioxidant vitamin E. More antioxidants would have catapulted this to a Paula's Pick, but it is still a good consideration for slightly dry skin, and it works well under makeup. The mineral pigments add an "illuminating" shine to skin.

☺ **Definity Intense Hydrating Cream** *($29.99 for 1.7 ounces)* is the richest of the Definity moisturizers, but its formula is most similar to the Definity Deep Penetrating Foaming Moisturizer reviewed above, minus the propellants. Since niacinamide is the chief beneficial ingredient in this product and it's not affected by exposure to light or air, the jar packaging is appropriate. Other than that, the same comments made previously for the Deep Penetrating Foaming Moisturizer apply here as well.

OLAY HYDRATE & CLEANSE PRODUCTS

☺ **Hydrate & Cleanse Antioxidant Lathering Face Wash** *($7.99 for 6 ounces)* contains a tiny amount of the antioxidant vitamin E, which is useless in a cleanser because its benefit is rinsed down the drain. Referencing any antioxidant in a cleanser is sheer marketing hype and meaningless for skin. This is a gentle, water-soluble cleanser that is a great option for all skin types except very dry or very oily. The cleansing agents it contains remove makeup well and rinse easily.

☺ **Hydrate & Cleanse Night Nourishing Cream Cleanser** *($7.99 for 6.7 ounces)* is a cold cream–like cleanser that contains several ingredients (including petrolatum and mineral oil) that don't rinse easily from skin. A higher amount of detergent cleansing agent might have allowed for better rinsing, but as is, this creamy cleanser (it definitely removes makeup) is best for dry to very dry skin and ideally should be used with a washcloth.

☺ **Hydrate & Cleanse Micro-Bead Cleansing Serum** *($7.99 for 6.7 ounces)* is similar to the Hydrate & Cleanse Night Nourishing Cream Cleanser above, except this serum is slightly less emollient and contains a greater amount of detergent cleansing agent. The cleansing agent is sodium lauryl sulfate, which can be problematic, but the small amount present coupled with the moisturizing ingredients that precede it in the ingredient list make it no cause for concern. This rinses better than the cleanser above, but you will still need a washcloth. It is best for normal to dry skin.

OLAY REGENERIST PRODUCTS

☺ **Regenerist Daily Regenerating Cleanser** *($6.99 for 5 ounces)* is a cleanser/scrub hybrid, and the lotion base allows the polyethylene beads to exfoliate without being too abrasive. It's an OK cleansing scrub for normal to dry skin, but no product can detoxify skin (exactly what toxins are we talking about anyway? and how is this measured?), especially one that is rinsed off shortly after application.

☺ **Regenerist Micro-Derm Cleansing Cloths** *($9.99 for 30 cloths)* are Vaseline-based cleansing cloths whose texture allows for manual exfoliation, similar to using a washcloth. These cloths remove makeup, though it takes more effort for eye makeup than you might like to expend. They are best for normal to very dry skin and the solution should be rinsed from skin because of the detergent cleansing agents each cloth contains.

😐 **Regenerist Micro-Exfoliating Wet Cleansing Cloths** *($7.99 for 30 cloths)* do not contain cleansing agents or anything capable of exfoliating skin, although the mechanical action of massaging these cloths over skin (similar to using a washcloth) will remove some dead skin cells. The glycol and silicone can help dislodge makeup, but I wouldn't choose these cloths to remove waterproof mascara (Olay claims they do this, but that's debatable). I suppose these are an OK option for normal to dry skin if you wear minimal to no makeup.

😐 **Regenerist Thermal Skin Polisher** *($13.99 for 4.2 ounces)* is a topical, nonaqueous scrub that lists magnesium sulfate (commonly known as Epsom salt) as the second ingredient. Massaging it over wet skin (as directed) causes an exothermic (heat) reaction. Essentially, heat is released, and you'll feel an intense warming sensation that gets stronger as you continue to massage the product over your skin. The heat doesn't really benefit skin, though I am sure some consumers would comment that their skin feels energized or invigorated as a result, but it can be a problem for capillaries, causing them to break and surface, creating red veining on the face. The polyethylene beads exfoliate skin, but the glycolic acid is useless because the magnesium sulfate keeps this product too alkaline, and AHAs need an acidic pH to exfoliate. Still, although somewhat gimmicky, this is an OK scrub for all skin types except very oily.

✓☺ **Regenerist Daily Regenerating Serum** *($18.99 for 1.7 ounces)* is a silky, silicone-based serum that contains a nice complement of water-binding agents and antioxidants. It contains approximately 2% to 3% niacinamide, and, in this amount, it can increase the skin's ceramide and fatty acid content as well as have anti-inflammatory action (Source: *Journal of Cosmetic Dermatology*, April 2004, pages 88–93). When it comes to niacinamide being able to affect aging (wrinkled) or sun-damaged (also discolored) skin, research points to a concentration of 5% as necessary to notice any improvement in skin texture and color that's consistent with what is typically seen in young skin (Source: D. L. Bissett, J. E. Oblong, A. Saud, and M. Levine, "Topical niacinamide provides improvements in aging human facial skin," presented at the 60th Annual Meeting of the American Academy of Dermatology, 2002).

Olay claims the palmitoyl pentapeptide-3 this contains can regenerate and intensely hydrate skin. However, palmitoyl pentapeptide-3 (also known as Matrixyl) is present in this product at less than 1%, and its value for skin is documented only by Sederma, the company that sells it. As it turns out, Sederma makes lots of peptides, and makes increasingly exaggerated claims about curing every skin-care woe imaginable. Of course, none of this is published research, but that doesn't stop Sederma or any of the numerous cosmetics companies from using their ingredients. In reality, it's the various types of silicones that really give this product its elegant texture and make skin feel unbelievably silky. Regenerist Daily Regenerating Serum won't give aging skin a new lease on life, but it would be a very good serum-type moisturizer for normal to slightly oily skin. This does contain fragrance.

✓☺ **Regenerist Daily Regenerating Serum, Fragrance-Free** *($18.99 for 1.7 ounces)* is identical to the Regenerist Daily Regenerating Serum above, except this option excludes fragrance, which is even better for the health of your skin, regardless of age.

☺ **Regenerist Deep Hydration Regenerating Cream** *($18.99 for 1.7 ounces)* contains ingredients capable of hydrating skin (including glycerin and niacinamide), but has a texture that those with dry to very dry skin may find too light. Overall this is a good formula whose only shortcoming is the somewhat disappointing amount of antioxidants.

✓☺ **Regenerist Enhancing Lotion with UV Protection SPF 15** *($18.99 for 2.5 ounces)* is a very good in-part avobenzone sunscreen in a moisturizing base of water, glycerin, niacinamide (about a 3% concentration), thickener, water-binding agents, antioxidants, film-forming agent, more thickeners, preservatives, and fragrance. This is definitely a state-of-the-art sunscreen formulation, and is best for normal to slightly dry or slightly oily skin. There is some in vitro research showing that topically applied niacinamide can protect skin cells from the chain reaction of UV-induced oxidative damage, and so it can also be considered a valuable (and stable) antioxidant (Sources: S. C. Shen, T. Yoshii, Y. C. Chen, T. H. Tsai, C. H. Hue, and W. R. Lee: "Niacinamide reduces DNA damage caused by reactive oxygen species," presentation at the 60th Annual Meeting of the American Academy of Dermatology, 2002; and *Journal of Dermatological Science*, May 2003, pages 193–201).

✓☺ **Regenerist Eye Lifting Serum** *($18.99 for 0.5 ounce)* is every bit as state-of-the-art as Olay's other Regenerist products. In fact, Eye Lifting Serum differs little from Olay's Regenerist Daily Regenerating Serum, Fragrance Free ($18.99 for 1.7 ounces), which provides three times as much product for the same price. Both of these products contain silicones, glycerin, niacinamide (which can increase skin's ceramide and free fatty acid content, among other benefits), several water-binding agents, antioxidants, and anti-irritants. You really can't go wrong with most of the Regenerist serums or moisturizers as long as you keep your expectations realistic. In other words, Olay's claim that these products are able to provide "dramatically younger-looking skin without surgery" is stretching the truth—plastic surgeons have not seen a decrease in new patients since the Regenerist line came on the beauty scene. But the fact remains that this fragrance-free moisturizer is an excellent option for use around the eyes or anywhere on the face. In contrast to the Daily Regenerating Serum mentioned above, this product contains mineral pigments (including mica) that impart a soft, reflective shimmer to skin. To a slight degree, this can help make dark circles under the eye look less obvious, but the effect is strictly cosmetic.

😐 **Regenerist Micro-Sculpting Cream** *($23.99 for 1.7 ounces)* purports to be the result of 50 years of Olay research, so you'd expect this to be a breathtakingly unique formula. It's not, and in fact it's very similar to all of the other Regenerist moisturizers and serums (I can't imagine what Olay was doing for 50 years, because if this is all they came up with, that would not be something to brag about). Increasing hydration can make skin cells plump, but that doesn't restore volume to a face that is sagging due to the complex process of aging. In other words, despite the name, this is not a face-lift in a jar. Actually, the jar packaging does a disservice to the range of antioxidants in this product (it does contain more antioxidants than many Olay products). That leaves you with a decent lightweight moisturizer for normal to slightly dry skin.

😐 **Regenerist Night Recovery Moisturizing Treatment** *($18.99 for 1.7 ounces)* comes in a jar, so the potency of the interesting ingredients such as niacinamide, vitamin E, and green tea is compromised. This also contains lavender and arnica extracts, which won't provide a "mini-lift" to skin, but do have the potential to cause irritation. This has a less impressive formulation than most of Olay's Regenerist products, and if you're already using one or more of those, there is no reason to add this product, especially when there are more state-of-the-art formulas in better packaging available from companies such as Clinique, Neutrogena, and Paula's Choice.

✓☺ **Regenerist Perfecting Cream** *($18.99 for 1.7 ounces)* is a lotion version of the Regenerist Daily Regenerating Serum above, and contains all the same bells and whistles, in stable packaging. This is best for normal to oily skin, but whether to use it or the Serum is a matter of personal preference (though if you're intrigued by peptides, the Serum contains more).

☺ **Regenerist Touch Of Sun UV Defense Regenerating Lotion SPF 15** *($17.49 for 2.5 ounces)* protects skin with an in-part avobenzone sunscreen and has a silky, moisturizing base that contains a small amount of the self-tanning agent dihydroxyacetone. This provides gradual color (not as much as a standard self-tanner would) and is a good option for daytime use if you have normal to slightly dry skin and are willing to apply it liberally enough to ensure sun protection. Niacinamide, present in most of the leave-on Regenerist products, is absent here.

✓☺ **Regenerist UV Defense Regenerating Lotion SPF 15** *($18.99 for 2.5 ounces)* is an even better formula than the Regenerist Enhancing Lotion with UV Protection SPF 15 above because it contains even more antioxidants and additional soothing agents. The lightweight base is suitable for normal to slightly dry or slightly oily skin, while avobenzone is on hand for UVA protection. This does contain fragrance, but is otherwise highly recommended!

☺ **Regenerist Eye Derma-Pod** *($17.99 for 24 pods)* not only capitalizes on the name of the popular iPod digital music player, but also takes a cue from its packaging. However, the Olay Derma-Pod has nothing to do with music. It is supposed to resurface, fill in lines, and decongest puffiness around the eyes. Each pod is a tiny packet filled with a silicone-based lotion. Squeezing the pod dispenses the product onto the built-in sponge pad, and you're directed to gently dab the product all around the eye, then use the sponge to massage the area in a circular motion for one minute. The sponge and massage action provides a very mild exfoliation for eye-area skin, while the silicone feels smooth and silky. Olay maintains that the massage action is what helps "remove excess under-eye fluids," but the effect is minimal at best, not to mention that puffiness from fluid buildup is usually temporary and related to diet (high in sodium), allergies, or sinus issues, and the latter two are easily remedied by over-the-counter antihistamines or decongestants. Plus you could just massage the area without the little pads and get the exact same results.

The solution dispensed onto the sponge differs little from the other serums in Olay's Regenerist line. It contains a significant amount of niacinamide and lesser amounts of peptides along with a couple of antioxidants. These pods aren't a necessary add-on to your skin-care routine, but if you're curious to try them the formula itself is definitely beneficial for skin, either around the eyes or elsewhere, and the massage action is best done carefully because massaging too vigorously can pull delicate skin.

😐 **$$$ Regenerist Microdermabrasion & Peel System** *($27.99 for the set)* is a two-part system that includes a **Microdermabrasion Treatment** and **Peel Activator Serum**. The Microdermabrasion Treatment does not contain the usual aluminum oxide crystals. Instead, this bright orange, gel-based scrub contains baking soda (sodium bicarbonate) and silica. You're instructed to apply the exfoliating gel to dry skin and massage for a minute or so. Next, you apply the Peel Activator Serum to fingertips and massage a thick layer over the exfoliating gel. Since the baking soda in the exfoliant gel is alkaline and the serum is acidic, two things happen: a mild, fizzy, foaming action occurs, and there's a slight warming sensation. This happens whenever alkaline and acidic products are mixed together. As the skin's pH acclimates to this change, the warming sensation subsides.

After another minute of massaging the mixture over skin, you rinse it off. The abrasiveness of the baking soda makes the skin quite smooth, which is where the bulk of this duo's benefit lies. Although the Peel Activator Serum contains lactic acid and has a pH of 3.6, it is not left on the skin long enough to cause a peeling effect. All of this amounts to a somewhat convoluted way to exfoliate skin with a fairly good risk of irritation given the "salt" scrub followed so closely by the lactic acid. In Olay's attempt to be innovative, they simply combined the benefits of manual exfoliation with chemical exfoliation. I wouldn't suggest using this scrub, but rather just a washcloth with a gentle cleanser that you rinse off—and then apply an AHA or BHA product that you leave on the skin.

☺ **Regenerist Targeted Tone Enhancer** *($18.99 for 1 ounce)* is meant to combine the benefits of niacinamide with what Olay refers to as pro-retinol. However, the form of vitamin A they chose, retinyl propionate, doesn't have anywhere close to the amount of research on pure retinol, so choosing it instead is somewhat of a gamble. This is otherwise a good lightweight moisturizer with niacinamide for normal to slightly dry skin.

😐 **$$$ Regenerist Thermal Contour and Lift at Home Treatment** *($24.99 for the set)* is a two-product set "inspired by popular professional Thermal Face-Lifts." So the big to-do here is this product's alleged ability to lift skin; they want you to associate this with Thermage, the medical cosmetic corrective procedure. It's good that Olay states that these products are not a replacement for the types of procedures performed by dermatologists (hey, honesty counts, especially in the cosmetics industry), but that disclaimer might get overlooked amid all the other hype and name similarity.

Step 1 involves the **Contouring Thermal Treatment**. This gel-like product is mixed with water, which causes a heat-producing reaction with the main ingredient, magnesium sulfate. This is strictly a chemical reaction, not anything beneficial for skin. How this or any of the polymers and conditioning agents in this product are supposed to contour the skin is beyond plausible, so consider this for about all it's good for, which is creating a warm sensation on skin. Hint: A warm washcloth would do the same thing. Next, you are directed to apply the **Lifting Complex**, a jar-packaged moisturizer whose formula is similar to others in Olay's Regenerist, Total Effects, and Definity lines. This water- and glycerin-based moisturizer contains a good amount of niacinamide (which isn't stable in the jar package), but there's no substantiated evidence that this vitamin can "talk" to cells and communicate with them to lead the skin to produce the same amount of collagen that is believed to be the benefit of Thermage and other heat-controlled professional treatments. You'll enjoy this if you have normal to dry skin, but don't bother with this set unless you accept the fact that it's just a pleasant warming experience with a fragranced moisturizer in bad packaging.

☺ **$$$ Regenerist Anti-Aging Lip Treatment** *($19.99 for 0.06 ounce)*, packaged in a pen-style component with a built-in brush applicator, is an emollient, shimmery balm that can't change the lines around your mouth. The niacinamide and lecithin are a nice touch, and add to the moisturizing effect of this product, but it won't change the age of your lips by even one day.

OLAY TOTAL EFFECTS PRODUCTS

☹ **Total Effects Age Defying Cleansing Cloths** *($7.99 for 30 cloths)* are pre-moistened cleansing cloths that contain menthol, which makes them too irritating for all skin types.

😐 **Total Effects Age Defying Wet Cleansing Cloths** *($7.29 for 30 cloths)* are similar to the Regenerist Micro-Exfoliating Wet Cleansing Cloths above, and the same comments apply.

😐 **Total Effects Anti-Aging Anti-Blemish Daily Cleanser** *($7.59 for 5 ounces)* contains 2% salicylic acid in a base with a pH below 4, but these positive traits are wasted in a cleanser because it is rinsed from the skin before the BHA has a chance to work, not to mention that salicylic acid should not be used near the eyes or mucous membranes. This is an OK option as a scrub cleanser (a small amount of polyethylene beads is included for manual exfoliation) for oily skin.

✓☺ **Total Effects 7-in-1 Anti-Aging Moisturizer, Mature Skin Therapy** *($17.49 for 1.7 ounces)* is Olay's answer to the needs of women whose skin is suffering from the changes it endures during and after menopause. The seven benefits in one product claim to intensely moisturize skin, reduce wrinkles, enhance skin tone and color, minimize pores, provide free-radical defense, and lift skin. Wow, all this for under $20? Sarcasm aside, this moisturizer for normal to dry skin contains several state-of-the-art ingredients that can improve the appearance and healthy functioning of skin at any age, but without a sunscreen a major necessary benefit is missing!

Antioxidant-wise, this bests all of the other Total Effects products, propelling this to the top of the list. Much of the skin appearance enhancement has to do with visual trickery—the mineral pigments add a subtle soft-focus, brightening effect to dull skin, while niacinamide encourages ceramide production for a smoother surface, which reflects light better. This isn't one-stop shopping for menopausal skin because most of the claims are at best farfetched, but it definitely has many strong points.

☺ **Total Effects 7 Signs Serum** *($18.99 for 1.7 ounces)* must have been created so that Olay's Total Effects line has a state-of-the-art product similar to their Regenerist line, but Total Effects is far removed from having anything total for skin. Just like Regenerist's Daily Regenerating Serum ($18.99 for 1.7 ounces), this Total Effects silicone-based product contains niacinamide, along with an elegant blend of water-binding agents, silicone, film-forming agents, and antioxidants. The only glaring omission is the palmitoyl pentapeptide-3 (trade name: Matrixyl) that's present in the Regenerist product. Peptides are potentially beneficial ingredients for skin (although the hype over their anti-aging prowess is overblown) and so, considering that the two Olay serums (Regenerist and Total Effects) are nearly identical formulations at the same price and size, why not buy the Regenerist Serum for the "icing on the cake" addition of peptides?

☺ **Total Effects 7X Visible Anti-Aging Vitamin Complex** *($18.99 for 1.7 ounces)* is a lightweight moisturizer that contains a good amount of niacinamide and silicones for a silky finish. While overall not as state-of-the-art as similar options from Olay's Regenerist collection, this is still a good option for normal to oily skin.

☺ **Total Effects 7X Visible Anti-Aging Vitamin Complex, Fragrance Free** *($18.99 for 1.7 ounces)* is identical to the Total Effects 7X Visible Anti-Aging Vitamin Complex above, minus the fragrance, which is always a plus for your skin. Otherwise, the same review applies.

☺ **Total Effects 7X Visible Anti-Aging Vitamin Complex, SPF 15** *($18.99 for 1.7 ounces)* keeps skin shielded from the sun with its in-part avobenzone sunscreen, but other than that the only exciting element in this lightweight daytime moisturizer for normal to slightly oily skin is niacinamide. The other bells and whistles aren't present in impressive amounts.

☺ **Total Effects Anti-Aging Anti-Blemish Daily Moisturizer** *($18.99 for 1.7 ounces)* is a wonderfully effective beta hydroxy acid option at the drugstore. The pH of 3 allows the 1.5% salicylic acid to penetrate the pore's follicle lining, exfoliating and helping to dislodge blackheads while smoothing skin and treating inflammatory acne. The fragranced base formula is nothing to write home about, but it has a silky, light texture that won't be bothersome for normal to slightly dry or slightly oily skin. The only drawback to this product is its lack of additional anti-irritants and antioxidants (the amount of vitamin E in this product is too small to matter). However, if you're looking for a well-formulated BHA product, Olay delivers with this one.

😐 **Total Effects Eye Transforming Cream** *($18.99 for 0.5 ounce)* has a formula similar to Olay's other Total Effects products, meaning you get a blend of such ingredients as glycerin, niacinamide, silicone, emollients, and antioxidants. It features a dry-finish ingredient known as isohexadecane, which prevents it from being too creamy. If you prefer a luxurious-feeling eye cream, this is not the one to choose. Another reason to reconsider before buying this: The formulation is similar to Olay's other Total Effects products, but in this case you're getting less product for your money and it's in translucent jar packaging, which compromises the effectiveness of the antioxidants even before you open it.

☺ **Total Effects Intensive Restoration Treatment** *($18.99 for 1.01 ounces)* claims to fight past damage in your most "aging-prone zones," yet its formula is remarkably similar to that of all the other Total Effects moisturizers, save for the addition of a few thickeners (none of which can turn back the hands of time). This does contain a tiny amount of retinyl propionate, Olay's version of retinol, but the research isn't there to support its use over pure retinol. However, this is still a good moisturizer for normal to dry skin, and the amount of niacinamide is beneficial.

😐 **Total Effects Night Firming Cream, Face & Neck** *($18.99 for 1.7 ounces)* is a lightweight moisturizer for normal to slightly dry skin, but one whose jar packaging won't keep the antioxidant ingredients stable during use. Niacinamide is on board as usual, but despite the positive research available for this ingredient, it cannot firm skin.

☹ **Total Effects Touch Of Sun, Daily Anti-Aging Moisturizer** *($17.49 for 1.7 ounces)* tries to combine two steps—self-tanning and exfoliation—in one product. While the concept is nice and it sounds like a time saver, it is probably far better for your skin to apply them separately. The self-tanning process is enhanced when you exfoliate before you apply the self-tanner, not during. Applying them at the same time can be counterproductive. Perhaps more problematic for skin is this product's fairly low pH of 2.3, which, while ensuring exfoliation, is potentially irritating to skin. Overall, the result (or lack thereof) isn't worth it.

OTHER OLAY PRODUCTS

☺ **Anti-Wrinkle Nutrients Daily Lathering Cleanser** *($6.49 for 5 ounces)* is a cleanser/scrub hybrid that contains very small polyethylene beads to provide a gentle polish each time you wash your face. The orange fruit extract is there for show; it doesn't provide nutrients for skin in the same manner eating an orange does for your body. The other vitamins may sound impressive, but are of little use in a cleanser because they're rinsed from your skin before they can go to work. This is a good option for normal to oily or slightly dry skin.

☺ **Deep Cleansing Face Wash, for Combination/Oily Skin** *($5.89 for 7 ounces)* is a very standard but good water-soluble foaming cleanser for its intended skin type, and one that removes makeup easily.

☹ **Dual Action Cleanser + Toner** *($6.99 for 6.7 ounces)* contains menthol, which makes it too irritating for all skin types, especially when used to remove makeup around the eyes.

☺ **Foaming Face Wash, for All Skin Types** *($4.49 for 6.78 ounces)* is a great water-soluble cleanser for all skin types except very dry. It removes makeup easily and leaves no residue. This would be rated a Paula's Pick if it did not contain fragrance.

✓☺ **Foaming Face Wash, for Sensitive Skin** *($4.49 for 6.78 ounces)* is preferred to the Foaming Face Wash for All Skin Types above because it has the same formula but without the fragrance. Considering the aesthetics and performance of this cleanser, it is one of the best values at the drugstore.

✓☺ **Gentle Foaming Face Wash, for Sensitive Skin** *($5.99 for 7 ounces)* is very similar to the Foaming Face Wash, for Sensitive Skin above, and the same review applies.

☺ **Moisture Balancing Foaming Face Wash, for All Skin Types** *($5.99 for 7 ounces)* is nearly identical to the Foaming Face Wash, for All Skin Types above, and the same review applies.

☺ **Moisture Rich Cream Cleanser, for Normal to Dry Skin** *($5.99 for 7 ounces)* is ideal for those with normal to dry skin who prefer a cleansing lotion (this isn't too rich, and rinses quite well). You'll find this removes most types of makeup easily and won't leave skin feeling dry or tight.

☹ **Olay Moisturizing Bar, for Sensitive Skin** *($2.99 for 2 4.75-ounce bars)* is a detergent-based bar cleanser that can be drying for all skin types, and the strong paraffin base doesn't rinse well, leading to residue that may clog pores or other problems inherent in bar cleansers.

☹ **Olay Moisturizing Bar with Oatmeal, for Dry Skin** *($2.99 for 2 4.75-ounce bars)* is similar to the Olay Moisturizing Bar, for Sensitive Skin above, and the same review applies.

☹ **Olay Moisturizing Bar with Shea Butter, for Extra Dry Skin** *($2.99 for 2 4.75-ounce bars)* is similar to the Olay Moisturizing Bar, for Sensitive Skin above, and the same review applies.

☹ **Olay Moisturizing Bar with Silkening Moisturizers, for Normal Skin** *($2.99 for 2 4.75-ounce bars)* is similar to the Olay Moisturizing Bar, for Sensitive Skin above, and the same review applies.

☺ **Pore Refining Mousse Cleanser** *($6.44 for 5.2 ounces)* claims to clean deep down to the pore, but if you consider that pores are right on the surface of skin, it really isn't "deep" at all. Regardless of claim, this cleanser/scrub hybrid can't go any deeper than similar products. It's an option as a water-soluble cleanser for normal to oily skin, but its only unique twist is the propellant-based formula that dispenses as a foamy mousse.

😐 **Warming Deep Purifying Cleanser** *($9.99 for 4.2 ounces)* is a cleanser and topical scrub in one. The warming portion comes from the reaction of magnesium sulfate with water, and has no benefit for skin beyond the sensation of warmth, which can possibly be a problem by causing capillaries to surface. The exfoliation comes from polyethylene beads, and overall this is an OK option for normal to dry skin, if you keep in mind that its cleansing ability isn't deeper or more purifying than any other cleanser.

😐 **Warming Hydrating Cleanser** *($9.99 for 4.2 ounces)* is nearly identical to the Warming Deep Purifying Cleanser above and the same review applies. It does not remove impurities "better than basic cleansing," unless they're referring to the exfoliating beads that provide a more thorough cleansing experience, in the same manner that using a washcloth is beyond the basics.

☹ **Refreshing Toner** *($3.99 for 7.2 ounces)* lists alcohol as the second ingredient and witch hazel distillate (which just adds more alcohol) as the third. Menthyl lactate completes the package of ingredients primed to irritate, not refresh, skin.

😐 **Active Hydrating Cream, Original** *($6.99 for 2 ounces)* is active in name only, and is one of Olay's most boring, do-nothing moisturizers. It's an average option for dry skin, nothing more.

😐 **Active Hydrating Beauty Fluid, Original** *($8.99 for 4 ounces)* contains mostly water, thickener, glycerin, oil, Vaseline, and more thickeners, plus fragrance and coloring agents to make it smell and look pretty. This is definitely a case where the original isn't the best. Instead, it's uninspiring and minimally helpful for dry skin.

☺ **Anti-Wrinkle Nutrients Daily SPF 15 Lotion** *($12.99 for 3.4 ounces)* comes in a generous size for facial application, and includes avobenzone for reliable UVA protection. The base formula is the familiar Olay blend of water, glycerin, niacinamide, and silicone, and it's suitable for normal to slightly oily or slightly dry skin. Antioxidants are in short supply, but this does provide an opalescent glow to skin thanks to the titanium dioxide and mica it contains. You may or may not like this effect (it can make oily areas look oilier), but it can be an attractive, subtle boost for dull skin. This daytime moisturizer does contain fragrance.

😐 **Anti-Wrinkle Nutrients Night Renewal Cream** *($12.99 for 2 ounces)* actually contains more antioxidants than the Anti-Wrinkle Nutrients Daily SPF 15 Lotion above, which is why the choice of jar packaging wasn't smart. Knowing these skin-defending ingredients won't last long once you begin using this moisturizer leaves you with a fairly basic formula that's an OK option for normal to slightly oily or slightly dry skin.

😐 **Night of Olay Firming Cream** *($7.79 for 2 ounces)* is sort of a stripped-down version of the moisturizers from Olay Regenerist, Total Effects, or Definity, without all of the intriguing ingredients. That leaves just an average moisturizer for dry skin.

😐 **Sensitive Moisture Therapy Cream, for Sensitive Skin** *($7.79 for 2 ounces)* is sold as an exceptionally mild cream meant to prevent irritation. This lightweight water- and glycerin-based cream is fragrance- and colorant-free. It contains a high amount of niacinamide, which can help reinforce the skin's own structure to keep skin protected from moisture loss (Source: *British Journal of Dermatology*, September 2000, pages 524–531). Niacinamide may also help skin cells function normally (Sources: *British Journal of Dermatology*, July 2002, pages 20–31; *Biomedical and Environmental Sciences*, September 1999, pages 177–187; and *Nutrition and Cancer*, 1997, volume 29, issue 2, pages 157–162). But aside from the niacinamide, all the other antioxidants (and the sole skin-soothing agent) are barely present and will likely have no impact on skin, especially since jar packaging was chosen. This can be a good moisturizer for normal to slightly dry skin, but aside from not containing fragrance, it isn't that different from most of Olay's other moisturizers.

😐 **Sensitive Moisture Therapy Lotion, for Sensitive Skin** *($7.99 for 4 ounces)* is nearly identical to the Sensitive Moisture Therapy Cream above, except with fewer thickeners, which is what gives it a lotion texture. This version is not packaged in a jar. Otherwise, the same comments apply.

☺ **Complete Touch of Sun Daily UV Facial Moisturizer SPF 15** *($13.99 for 2.5 ounces)* combines the self-tanning agent dihydroxyacetone (DHA) with an in-part avobenzone sunscreen for color with protection. Not a bad idea, assuming you'll still apply this liberally. Although labeled to imply a sheer hint of color, the amount of DHA in both the Light/Medium and Medium/Darker versions is similar to what you'd see in a standard self-tanner, so do expect more color.

☺ **Touch of Sun Body Lotion, for Dry Skin** *($8.49 for 6.7 ounces)* is a standard self-tanning lotion suitable for normal to dry skin. It turns skin color with a combination of the self-tanning ingredients dihydroxyacetone and the slower-acting erythrulose. The texture and finish of this won't leave skin feeling greasy.

☺ **Touch of Sun Body Lotion, for Normal Skin** *($8.49 for 6.7 ounces)* is nearly identical to the Touch of Sun Body Lotion, for Dry Skin above, and the same review applies.

ORIGINS

ORIGINS AT-A-GLANCE

Strengths: Almost none for the skin-care products, save for a couple of average eye-makeup removers; makeup fares better, with several great options, including liquid concealer, powder foundation, loose and pressed powders, liquid blush, bronzing options, brow enhancer, and automatic lip and eye pencils; very good makeup brushes composed of synthetic hair.

Weaknesses: Almost every skin-care product contains potent irritating ingredients that have no established benefit for skin; no products to address needs of those with acne or skin discolorations; no AHA or BHA products; although sunscreens provide the right UVA-protecting ingredients, they also contain irritating ingredients, some of which are phototoxic; the foundations contain irritating ingredients, as do most of the lip color products; average specialty products.

For more information about Origins, owned by Estee Lauder, call (800) 674-4467 or visit www.origins.com or www.Beautypedia.com.

ORIGINS SKIN CARE

ORIGINS A PERFECT WORLD PRODUCTS

☹ **A Perfect World, Liquid Moisture with White Tea** *($20 for 5 ounces)* contains several essential oils (meaning fragrant oils, because essential oils should only be those that are good for your skin) that are extremely irritating to skin, making this product impossible to recommend and far from skin's fountain of youth!

☹ **A Perfect World, Antioxidant Moisturizer with White Tea** *($35 for 1.7 ounces)* starts out strong and, at first glance, has all the elements of what other Lauder companies (of which Origins is one) know is necessary to create a great moisturizer to ease dryness and restore skin to a healthier state. What a shame Origins had to include such unnecessary and irritating ingredients as bergamot, lemon, orange, spearmint, and vetiver oils (among others). Among all of the Lauder-owned companies, there are plenty of other excellent moisturizers whose best qualities compare favorably to this one from Origins, and those thankfully omit the problematic ingredients that create anything but a perfect world for your complexion.

☹ **A Perfect World for Eyes, Firming Moisture Treatment with White Tea** *($30 for 0.5 ounce)* is the eye-area counterpart to the A Perfect World Antioxidant Moisturizer above. The formulas for both are similar, but the designated eye-area version contains a hefty amount of peppermint, which you will notice causes a tingling sensation as soon as you apply it to your skin. Peppermint is a potent irritant and is not only an unnecessary ingredient but also should never be used around the eyes. This product also contains several fragrant plant and flower oils that will make someone with allergies miserable, not to mention further the irritation from the peppermint.

☹ **A Perfect World, White Tea Skin Guardian** *($32.50 for 1 ounce)* is a silicone- and water-based serum that contains some good antioxidants (and in stable packaging), but ultimately just irritates skin due to the bergamot, lemon peel, spearmint, and rosewood oils it contains. Your face will smell great, but that has nothing to do with taking the best possible care of skin.

☹ **A Perfect World, Nighttime Antioxidant Mask with White Tea** *($30 for 2 ounces)* should not be used at any time of day, not only because it's a lackluster formula but also because it contains so many irritating essential oils. Using this at night may mean you'll awaken to a blotchy, sensitized complexion.

☹ **A Perfect World, Antioxidant Lip Guardian with White Tea** *($20 for 0.41 ounce)* contains many oils and emollients to keep dry, chapped lips feeling smooth and flake-free, but the fragrant essential oils will cause problems for lips, up to and including making them more chapped due to the irritation.

ORIGINS BY DR. ANDREW WEIL

This Origins subcategory is one I am asked about frequently. Many of my readers are concerned that integrative medicine guru Dr. Weil has "sold out" by freely endorsing skin-care products and supplements from Origins. Of course the answer to that, from my perspective, would depend solely on whether the good doctor created products that consumers can rely on to make their skin look better. Alas, that isn't the case here. Somewhere the collaboration got off course, and almost the entire product line fell prey to what sabotages most Origins products: skin-irritating essential oils that do much to contribute to each product's scent, but offer only inflammation and discomfort to skin. Given Weil's writings on inflammation and its harmful effect on the body and mind, I wonder how he ignored the research on this, or perhaps these products are in name only. Perhaps more to the point, where is the sunscreen and how did that get overlooked? There isn't a mushroom in the world as important as protecting your skin from the sun.

Showcased in many of the Origin products to which Weil has his name attached are several species of mushrooms that do have some research demonstrating their health benefits.

However, those benefits are strictly about oral consumption, although I can see that someone might assume that they could also have benefit when the isolated active components of the mushrooms are applied topically. However, it would have been far more interesting to test that out without the unwanted extras (irritating plant extracts) that end up making skin behave badly rather than better.

☹ **Plantidote Mega-Mushroom Face Cleanser** *($25 for 5 ounces)* had potential for being a good cleansing lotion for normal to dry skin, but it includes too many irritating essential oils to earn a recommendation. The various mushrooms have antioxidant ability, but even if that translated to topical application, those benefits are just rinsed down the drain.

😐 **$$$ Plantidote Mega-Mushroom Eye Makeup Remover Pads** *($20 for 60 pads)* are not as gentle and soothing as described, but they are definitely less irritating than all of the other Plantidote products from Origins. These pads are infused with a mild cleansing solution, but hit some speed bumps on the road to recommendation due to inclusion of potentially irritating ginger root and holy basil. Neither ingredient is preferred for use around the eyes, plus there are plenty of eye-makeup removers available without them, making this pricier option a tough sell.

☹ **Plantidote Mega-Mushroom Eye Serum** *($42.50 for 0.5 ounce)* lists myrtle leaf water as the second ingredient, which is not recommended for contact with skin due to volatile compounds, including 1,8-cineole, the constituent responsible for this plant's toxicity (Sources: *Journal of Natural Products*, March 2002, pages 334–338; and www.naturaldatabase.com). Even without the myrtle, this serum contains several fragrant oils that are troublesome for skin, including patchouli, orange, and lavender oils.

☹ **Plantidote Mega-Mushroom Face Lotion** *($60 for 1.7 ounces)* contains some novel and potentially effective antioxidants, but it's laced with irritants, including a tea of orange and myrtle and fragrant oils of lavender, patchouli, olibanum, and orange.

☹ **Plantidote Mega-Mushroom Face Serum** *($65 for 1.7 ounces)* is a water-based serum that contains a large number of skin-beneficial ingredients, including efficacious plant oils (the kind that aren't fragrant and protect skin), glycerin, lecithin, and many antioxidants, including olive oil, turmeric, and several species of mushrooms. Things go awry then because Origins just couldn't resist adding irritating fragrant oils to the Plantidote products. Lavender, orange, patchouli, geranium, and mandarin oils all have volatile compounds that counter the soothing, anti-inflammatory effects of the ingredients that precede them. Dr. Weil could have easily found this out from a number of sources, including the medical journal search engine at www.pubmed.com (the National Institutes of Health Web site), www.naturaldatabase.com, and other resources. The oils assuredly make this serum smell wonderful, which is great for your nose, but they aren't helpful to skin in the least, and prevent this product from being recommended. Without these questionable, problematic fragrant extras, this could have been one of the more intelligently formulated antioxidant serums available.

☹ **Plantidote Mega-Mushroom Face Cream** *($60 for 1.7 ounces)* is the cream version of the Plantidote Mega-Mushroom Face Serum above, sharing many of the same ingredients, but it omits the emollients and thickeners needed to create a cream texture. Assuming the irritating ingredients mentioned in the review of the Plantidote Mega-Mushroom Face Serum above are not present, the many antioxidants in this moisturizer for normal to dry skin are compromised by this product's jar packaging, because antioxidants are not stable in packaging that isn't airtight. As it is, this well-intentioned product has too many negatives to make it a calming, age-fighting experience for skin.

☹ **Conditioning Lip Balm with Turmeric** *($15 for 0.14 ounce)* is a substandard castor oil–based lip balm that leaves lips irritated due to lime and ginger oils. The lime oil is dangerous to put on lips that may be exposed to sunlight because a phototoxic reaction can occur that leads to discolorations.

OTHER ORIGINS PRODUCTS

☹ **Checks and Balances, Frothy Face Wash** *($17.50 for 5 ounces)* is a very drying, alkaline cleanser that's made even more troublesome because it contains spearmint, lavender, and geranium oils.

☹ **Clean Energy Gentle Cleansing Oil** *($17.50 for 6.7 ounces)* begins with several nonvolatile, gentle oils suitable for dry to very dry skin, but quickly turns from mild to irritating due to several fragrant oils, including lavender, lemon, patchouli, and cedarwood.

☹ **Cream Bar, Plant-Based Face Soap with Creamy Lather** *($10.50 for a 5.2-ounce bar)* is a standard bar soap that contains several potent skin irritants, including spruce and wintergreen oils and clove.

☹ **Get Down, Deep-Pore Clay Cleanser** *($17.50 for 5 ounces)* is based around peppermint water, and although that's not as bad as peppermint oil, Origins includes volatile oils too, in the form of eucalyptus and sage.

☹ **Liquid Crystal, the Extra Gentle Cleanser You Use with Water** *($17.50 for 6.7 ounces)* is an oil cleanser that emulsifies with water to create a cleansing fluid capable of removing any type of makeup. What a shame this otherwise fine cleanser contains peppermint oil, which you don't want to get anywhere near your eyes.

☹ **Mint Wash, Cooling Gel That Lathers Clean** *($17.50 for 6.7 ounces)* has a name that can't possibly translate to a good rating, and it doesn't because of the numerous irritating fragrant oils this cleanser contains.

☹ **Never a Dull Moment, Skin-Brightening Face Cleanser with Fruit Extracts** *($17.50 for 5 ounces)*. The only thing that isn't dull about this cleanser are irritating plant extracts—pine, eucalyptus, grapefruit, and mint oils—which will make your face glow with inflammation.

☹ **Pure Cream, Rinseable Cleanser You Can Also Tissue Off** *($17.50 for a 5-ounce tube; $18.50 for a 6.7-ounce jar)*. Regardless of how you decide to remove this cleanser, it's best not to use it in the first place because of the peppermint, tangerine, lime, and spruce oils. Ouch!

😐 **Well Off, Fast and Gentle Eye Makeup Remover** *($13.50 for 3.4 ounces)* is a simply formulated, rosewater-based eye-makeup remover (which is more eau de cologne than skin care) that is only slightly less of a problem than all the other Origin products that are loaded with unfriendly skin ingredients.

☹ **Modern Friction, Nature's Gentle Dermabrasion** *($36 for 4 ounces)* is Origins' take on the group of at-home scrub products that purport to mimic the effect of microdermabrasion treatments. Unlike other microdermabrasion scrubs, which contain aluminum oxide crystals, Modern Friction contains rice starch. Rice starch is considerably less abrasive, but before you get too excited, keep in mind that this is an Origins product. That means you can expect irritation, delivered here by a bevy of essential oils: lemon, bergamot, peppermint, and camphor. These oils are not present in meager amounts either, and you will feel a deep-down tingle (irritation) as you massage this scrub over your skin. Without these additives, this would be a great scrub for normal to dry or sensitive skin types. As is, I do not recommend it.

☹ **Never a Dull Moment, Skin-Brightening Face Polisher with Fruit Enzymes** *($23.50 for 4.4 ounces)* contains eucalyptus, pine, and mint oils, and is absolutely not recommended.

☹ **Swept Away, Gentle Slougher for All Skins** *($18.50 for 3.4 ounces)* isn't gentle in the least—not with a hefty amount of grapefruit and peppermint oils poised to irritate skin with each application.

☹ **Swept Clean, Special Sloughing for Oily-Acting Skin** *($18.50 for 3.4 ounces)* isn't any better than the Swept Away Gentle Slougher above, and adds menthol to the cocktail of irritants that keep this scrub from being recommended.

☹ **Comforting Solution, Sensitive Skin Soother** *($17.50 for 5 ounces)* includes several ingredients that are completely inappropriate for sensitive skin, such as balm mint, eucalyptus oil, and sage oil. Far from comforting, this will send sensitive skin into irritation overdrive.

☹ **Oil Refiner, Skin Purifying Tonic** *($17.50 for 5 ounces)* contains many more irritants than helpful ingredients for skin, and is not recommended.

☹ **United State, Balancing Tonic** *($17.50 for 5 ounces)* is a toner that's mostly alcohol and witch hazel, but causes further irritation due to the volatile essential oils it contains. This cannot exfoliate or balance skin.

☹ **Balanced Diet, Lightweight Moisture Lotion** *($22.50 for 1.7 ounces)* contains spearmint, lavender, and bergamot oil, all of which irritate skin while imparting zero benefits.

☹ **Constant Comforter, Calming Moisture Cream** *($22.50 for 1.7 ounces)* contains lavender oil, which causes skin-cell death, and lime oil, which can irritate and cause a phototoxic reaction when skin is exposed to sunlight. Does that sound comforting?!

☹ **Eye Doctor, Moisture Care for Skin Around Eyes** *($27.50 for 0.5 ounce)* is not what the doctor ordered! This moisturizer contains wintergreen, mint, and lemon oils, all of which are a problem for skin and increasingly so when used around the eyes.

☹ **Grin from Year to Year, Brightening Face Firmer** *($26 for 1.7 ounces)* is a water-based serum that won't induce a smile from anyone looking to avoid irritating their skin. This contains a litany of problematic essential oils and fragrance components that won't firm skin in the least. The brightening effect is from cosmetic pigments (mica and titanium dioxide) and is essentially just a way to add shine to skin.

☹ **Have a Nice Day, Super-Charged Moisture Cream SPF 15** *($32.50 for 1.7 ounces)* contains an in-part titanium dioxide sunscreen, but at only 1%, so I wouldn't bank on it for UVA protection. Beyond that issue, you won't have a nice day because this daytime moisturizer irritates skin with its peppermint base and blend of volatile citrus and mint oils.

☹ **Have a Nice Day, Super-Charged Moisture Lotion SPF 15** *($32.50 for 1.7 ounces)* is the lotion version of the Have a Nice Day, Super-Charged Moisture Cream above, and the same comments apply (though this contains slightly more titanium dioxide).

☹ **High Potency Night-A-Mins, Mineral-Enriched Eye Cream** *($28.50 for 0.5 ounce)* has an emollient, silky formula, but it has no business being used around the sensitive eye area due to the many fragrant oils it contains. Without them (and in better packaging), this would have been a Paula's Pick as an outstanding, thoughtfully formulated moisturizer for dry to very dry skin.

☹ **High Potency Night-A-Mins, Mineral-Enriched Moisture Cream** *($32.50 for 1.7 ounces)* replaces Origins' former Night-A-Mins Cream, but the formulary differences are token. What significantly hurts this product (and, in the long run, your skin) is the prevalence of several fragrant oils, including orange and neroli. All of these are on hand in greater amounts than the vitamins or the many other skin-beneficial ingredients such as linoleic acid and cholesterol. This product is not recommended.

☹ **High Potency Night-A-Mins, Mineral-Enriched Moisture Lotion** *($32.50 for 1.7 ounces)* has a lighter texture than the High Potency Night-A-Mins, Mineral-Enriched Moisture Cream above, but the same negative comments apply here, making this product one to avoid.

☹ **Look Alive, Vitality Moisture Cream** *($22.50 for 1.7 ounces)* contains basil, sweet orange, rosemary, and other essential oils, all in troublesome amounts that can be irritating to skin. Fragrance components such as eugenol are also high on the list, while the truly helpful ingredients are minimized.

☹ **Make a Difference, Skin Rejuvenating Treatment** *($32.50 for 1.7 ounces)* has a silky texture that can translate to smoother skin, but the main difference this product makes is by causing skin irritation with essential oils of citrus, spearmint, and vetiver. The redeeming ingredients can't compete with these irritants, and won't last long due to jar packaging.

☹ **Matte Scientist, Oil Controlling Lotion** *($22.50 for 1.7 ounces)* doesn't contain enough salicylic acid to help skin, and the amount of irritants is considerable, making this a product all skin types should ignore. Those with very oily skin will do much better keeping shine at bay with one of the Pore Minimizing products from Clinique or with Smashbox's Anti-Shine options.

☹ **Never Say Dry, Extra-Rich Moisture Cream** *($32.50 for 1.7 ounces)* gets a prize for its wonderfully clever name, but the formula is rife with problematic, irritating essential oils. Sweet orange, grapefruit, mint, and petitgrain all make appearances, as does camphor, which is not at all helpful for skin, be it dry or otherwise. What's so disappointing about these inclusions is that without them Never Say Dry would have been an exceptionally rich, soothing moisturizer for very dry skin. As it is, your skin will be moisturized and irritated, and it doesn't deserve the latter.

☹ **Urgent Moisture, Nature's Humidifier for Super-Dry Conditions** *($25 for 1.7 ounces)* is a rather lightweight moisturizer that's not deserving of its name. Although this has merit for slightly dry skin, the rose water and myrtle leaf–water base and essential oils of lavandin and clary sage make this too potentially irritating to consider.

☹ **Youthtopia, Skin Firming Cream with Rhodiola** *($47.50 for 1.7 ounces).* I have to hand it to Origins for coming up with some of the most clever product names around, because they convey a sense of cuteness. I wish what was inside the jars was just as clever, because—despite some very good ingredients—Origins' penchant for potent, skin-sensitizing essential oils makes almost all of their products too irritating for skin, as is the case with this moisturizer. It contains sandalwood, geranium, orange, patchouli, cinnamon, nutmeg, and thyme oils, all of which present problems for skin and won't do a thing to help it regain its youthful appearance.

☹ **Youthtopia, Skin Firming Lotion with Rhodiola** *($47.50 for 1.7 ounces)* is the lotion version of the Youthtopia, Skin Firming Cream, above, and the same basic review applies. By the way, if you're wondering what rhodiola is, it's a flowering plant that's known as an adaptogen, a term referring to an ingredient that, when consumed orally, helps the body deal with stressors such as intense exercise or a compromised immune system. Although there is a small amount of research pertaining to rhodiola's benefit when consumed orally, information about its effect as a topical application is scant, though components of this plant do have antioxidant properties (Source: www.naturaldatabase.com). Origins uses the active (root) portion of this plant, but its benefit on skin, if any, is diminished by the inclusion of so many irritating essential oils.

☹ **Clear Improvement, Active Charcoal Mask to Clear Pores** *($20 for 3.4 ounces)* is a clay and charcoal mask that would have been a good option for oily to very oily skin if it did not contain so much horsetail extract, which can constrict skin and cause irritation.

☹ **Drink Up, 10 Minute Mask to Quench Skin's Thirst** *($20 for 3.4 ounces)* offers dry skin some relief, but at the expense of causing irritation because this mask contains bitter orange and camphor oils.

☹ **Make a Difference, Skin Rejuvenating Sheet Mask** *($35 for 6 masks)* are cotton masks said to restore a youthful look to skin, whether the damage was done decades or mere days ago. Don't count on it, primarily because each mask contains a lot of problematic ingredients, including lavender, bergamot, and lemon oils.

☹ **Modern Fusion, Skin Transforming Catalyst** *($36 for 1 ounce)* wants to transform your skin with its rice refinishing complex, but this product will only transform skin from healthy to irritated due to the number of sensitizing ingredients it contains. Bergamot, orange, galbanum, field mint, lemon, and tangerine oils are indeed natural, but they are far from what is needed to enhance skin's glow and clarity, or to make pores vanish as claimed. Bergamot and the citrus oils can cause serious problems for skin if it is exposed to sunlight without adequate protection.

😐 **No Puffery, 30-Day Solution for Puffy Eyes** *($20 for 0.64 ounce)* cannot reduce puffiness by releasing "trapped fluids and toxins." What toxins are lurking under your eyes anyway? No one at Origins could explain this to me logically. Regardless, this water-based gel has a good plant extract for every bad one, essentially canceling out the effect of either and making this product a genuine "Why bother?"

☹ **No Puffery, Cooling Mask for Puffy Eyes** *($20 for 1 ounce)* contains several fragrant oils that shouldn't get anywhere near the eyes (puffy or not), and as such this rose water-based product (rose water is mostly fragrance anyway) is not recommended.

☹ **Out of Trouble, 10 Minute Mask to Rescue Problem Skin** *($20 for 3.4 ounces)* gets skin into trouble because it contains camphor. That won't rescue anyone's skin, and those with blemish-prone skin are potentially setting themselves up for more breakouts because of the high amount of zinc oxide in this mask.

☹ **Spot Remover, Acne Blemish Treatment Gel** *($10 for 0.3 ounce)* is basically a laundry list of irritants, none of which are helpful at making blemishes go away. Alcohol heads the list, but skin is also assaulted with oregano oil and witch hazel.

☹ **You're Getting Warmer, Purifying Clay Mask** *($20 for 3.4 ounces)* is a glycerin-based clay mask that contains sodium potassium aluminum silicate, also known as the mineral nepheline. Traditionally used in the manufacture of ceramics, glass, and enamels, it is occasionally used in cosmetics, but its alkaline nature makes it quite drying. This might have been a tolerable mask for oily skin had Origins not also included a battery of problematic essential oils. Cinnamon, ginger, grapefruit, lemon, and lime don't mean you're getting warmer, just seriously irritated.

☹ **Zero Oil, Instant Matte Finish for Shiny Places** *($10 for 0.64 ounce)* lists witch hazel as the second ingredient and also contains camphor oil, making this instantly irritating for all skin types.

☹ **Cover Your Mouth, Lip Protector with SPF 8** *($7.50 for 0.15 ounce)* not only features an embarrassingly low SPF rating, but also irritates lips with peppermint oil, which is present in a significant amount that definitely makes this a lip balm to keep away from.

☹ **Lip Remedy** *($11 for 0.17 ounce)* contains a lot of peppermint oil, which is the opposite of being any sort of lip remedy.

ORIGINS SUN PRODUCTS

☹ **Faux Glow, Radiant Self-Tanner for Face** *($17.50 for 1.7 ounces)* lists peppermint (ouch!) as the second ingredient, and that makes this otherwise standard self-tanner extremely irritating. And that's before you even get to the orange, spearmint, and rosemary oils—all of them irritants—that are present, too. Instead of this problematic mix, try an irritant-free self-tanner (most of them are, from Coppertone to Neutrogena), and purchase peppermint oil to inhale while waiting for the self-tanner to dry!

☹ **Let It Show, Bare Body Skin Enhancer** *($20 for 5 ounces)* only irritates body skin because of the high amount of fragrant essential oils. Grapefruit and bergamot oils are especially problematic, especially if you apply this after shaving.

☹ **Out Smart, Daily SPF 25 Naturally Protective Sunscreen** *($20 for 1.7 ounces)* includes pure titanium dioxide for sun protection, but is not recommended due to the irritation the many essential oils included can cause. Using this product is not smart, not when there are so many sunscreens that shield skin without causing needless irritation.

☹ **Sunshine State, SPF 20 Sunscreen with Natural Minerals for Face and Body** *($22.50 for 5 ounces)* will leave your skin in an irritated state due to the atypically large amount of peppermint present in this titanium dioxide–based sunscreen. The rather standard base formula contains more irritants than skin-friendly antioxidants or soothing agents, and, given the price, that's insulting.

☹ **The Great Pretender, Shimmery Self-Tanner for Body** *($17.50 for 5 ounces)* is almost identical to the Faux Glow facial self-tanner above, and the same comments apply. Without the unnecessary irritants, both of these self-tanners would have been excellent nongreasy options.

ORIGINS MAKEUP

FOUNDATION: ☺ **Silk Screen Refining Powder Makeup** *($23.50)* is the best and only foundation I recommend from Origins. This talc-free pressed-powder foundation does not contain any of the irritating essential oils that plague the options below. It has an awesome silky texture and smooth, dry finish that provides light coverage. There are 15 shades available, including options for fair to dark skin, and there's not a poor one in the lot. This is recommended for normal to oily skin, though it's not quite on par with similar pressed-powder foundations from Estee Lauder, M.A.C., and Prescriptives.

☹ **Next of Skin Modern Moisture Makeup SPF 15** *($22.50)* combines neutral colors and an elegant texture with a titanium dioxide and zinc oxide sunscreen. So why the unhappy face? Because of Origins' misguided belief that essential oils are today's anti-aging heroes; they unwisely included pine, peppermint, spearmint, and several citrus oils in this otherwise commendable foundation. And these oils aren't present just as a mere dusting, they're an integral part of the formula, as your nose will attest if you take a moment to smell this foundation. Think about it this way: If these kinds of ingredients were so good for skin, why don't any of the other 20+ Lauder companies use them?

☹ **Nude and Improved Bare-Face Makeup SPF 15** *($17.50)* has a lot going for it, from its titanium dioxide sunscreen to its mostly neutral colors and natural finish. How unfortunate that Origins chose to add problematic lemon, spearmint, and grapefruit essential oils. Among those, lemon and grapefruit oils are known to be phototoxic, which means it should not be applied to skin about to be exposed to sunlight (Sources: *Archives of Dermatological Research*, 1985, issue 278, pages 31–36; and www.naturaldatabase.com).

☹ **Reflection Perfection Mattifying Face Makeup** *($17.50)* is a liquid foundation with a strong matte finish someone with oily to very oily skin will appreciate, but the amount of alcohol, coupled with irritating clove and eucalyptus, makes this too irritating to recommend.

☹ **Stay Tuned Balancing Face Makeup** *($17.50)* has a lot in common with sister company Estee Lauder's Equalizer Makeup SPF 10 ($32.50), except the Origins version contains irritating spearmint, geranium, and lavender oils. All of these present their share of problems for skin and yet have no balancing effect whatsoever. What a shame, because the shade range is beautiful and this foundation costs significantly less than Lauder's version (but with theirs you're getting an irritant-free product).

☹ **Original Skin More Coverage** *($17.50)* is Origins' oldest foundation and although it has some positive traits, half of the six shades still offered are too peach or pink, and the lavender, cardamom, and lemon essential oils make it unacceptably irritating for all skin types.

CONCEALER: ✓☺ **Quick, Hide! Easy Blend Concealer** *($13.50)* is Origins' only concealer, but it's an outstanding version whose only plant ingredients are the soothing variety, a welcome change of pace. This lightweight, water- and silicone-based concealer provides substantial coverage without looking thick or heavy. It sets quickly to a natural matte finish, so blending must be swift—but it stays in place really well and won't crease into lines under the eye. There are seven mostly excellent shades—Dark is too peach for most skin tones and Neutralizer will be too yellow for lighter skin tones, but is still worth considering. Lightest is suitable for very fair skin, while Very Dark is good but misnamed (it's too light for very dark skin).

POWDER: ☺ **$$$ All and Nothing Sheer Finishing Powder** *($23.50)* is a talc-free loose powder whose light, airy texture feels and looks amazing on skin. Origins decided to make only one shade, which works for most light to medium skin tones; on darker skin, it can look too ashy. This powder does contain mica, which adds a subtle shine, but not enough to avoid wearing during daylight hours. If the one-shade-fits-all prospect doesn't work for you, consider M.A.C's Select Sheer Loose Powder ($20), available in several shades. The synthetic-hair brush Origins includes with this powder, though tiny, is remarkably soft and easy to use. Even better, it rests neatly inside the powder's cap, a convenient addition to a great powder. ☺ **$$$ All and Nothing Sheer Pressed Powder** *($23.50)* is, like the loose version above, also talc-free and available in only one shade. It applies sheer, but will still look too light on tan or darker skin tones. It has a smooth texture and sheer, dry finish that works best for normal to oily skin.

☺ **$$$ Sunny Disposition Powder Bronzer** *($19.50)* has been improved and now ranks as a very good pressed-powder bronzer that comes in two believable shades. They'd be more convincing without the shine, but it is comparatively subtle. A little of this goes a long way, so apply sparingly and build from there if a darker result is desired.

BLUSH: ☺ **Pinch Your Cheeks** *($10)* is a liquid cheek stain that blends nicely once you get the hang of it (expect to have to practice), and offers a transparent matte finish. This works best on normal, small-pored, even-textured skin. The original shade is now labeled Raspberry, and two additional shades (a sheer bronze and peach) are also available.

😐 **$$$ Brush-On Color** *($16.50)* is a powder blush with an unusually dry texture yet smooth, even application. Almost all of the shades are laden with shine, which makes them a questionable choice for daytime makeup. The least shiny shades include Crimson and Clover, Pink Petal, and Rose Dust. The other Lauder-owned companies have powder blushes that outperform this one, but if you're devoted to Origins, it's not a total disappointment.

EYESHADOW: Origins powder ☺ **Eyeshadow** *($12.50)* includes over 20 shiny selections ranging from subtle to striking. These have a buttery-smooth texture and very nice application that is neither too sheer nor too intense. There are no suitable options for lining the eyes or filling in brows, but at least the shine tends to remain flake-free. Be warned that applying shine over the eyelid can make any amount of wrinkles in that area more noticeable.

EYE AND BROW SHAPER: ✓☺ **Fill in the Blanks Eyebrow Enhancer** *($13.50)* is a prime pick if you prefer filling in and defining brows with pencil rather than powder. This skinny, automatic, non-retractable pencil applies with ease, isn't the least bit greasy or smear-prone, and has a soft powder finish. The two shades (one for blondes, one for brunettes) are limiting, but everything else about this brow pencil is terrific.

☺ **Automagically Eye Lining Pencil** *($14.50)* is an automatic, non-retractable pencil with one of the smoothst applications you're likely to come across. No tugging or dragging here! The pencil's soft texture makes it tricky to draw a thin line, but thicker lines are a cinch and although you'll notice some fading as the day passes, it stays in place very well. Avoid the Jade and Navy shades.

☺ **Brow Fix** *($12)* doesn't try to be anything more than what it is: a standard, clear brow gel that tames unruly hairs and provides a groomed finish. It is minimally sticky and the brush doesn't deposit too much product at once, making it a breeze to use.

😐 **Just Browsing** *($12)* is a lightweight, softly tinted brow gel with an OK brush that adds natural color and definition to the eyebrow. The number of shades now stands at two (one for blondes, one for brunettes), and overall, I'd recommend Bobbi Brown's Natural Brow Shaper ($17) over this because it has a better brush and a wider selection of shades.

😐 **Eye Brightening Color Stick** *($13)* is a chubby, stout pencil that comes in one shade—a pale, shimmery silver-blue that is intended to line the inner rims of the eye, a technique that is more theatrical than practical. Also, repeated daily applications put your eyes at risk, as cosmetic coloring agents just don't belong next to the cornea. Yes, it can look striking in photographs, but it's not worth doing on a regular (or even infrequent) basis.

LIPSTICK, LIP GLOSS, AND LIPLINER: ✓☺ **Automagically Lip Lining Pencil** *($13.50)* deserves consideration if you're looking for an automatic, non-retractable lip pencil whose soft and sheer colors have a drier application but enough stain and silicone-enhanced tenacity to stay on for hours. This is an excellent option for those prone to lipstick bleeding into lines around the mouth. However, just like any anti-feathering lipliner, it won't keep slick glosses or greasy lipsticks from straying past the mouth's border.

☺ **Creamy Lip Color** *($13.50)* is one of the few irritant-free lip products from Origins. It's a nice, traditional cream lipstick that offers semi-opaque coverage and comes in a small but well-edited selection of shades. You'll get much greater variety from Clinique or M.A.C. lipsticks, but if you find an Origins color that strikes your fancy, this is worth considering.

😐 **Matte**, **Sheer**, and **Shimmer Sticks** *($12; $2 for jumbo sharpener)* are the original "chubby sticks" that Origins has offered for years, and they're about the only cosmetic company that still does. Why these ever caught on is anyone's guess, because they need constant sharpening, and most are too soft to get a controlled lip line. They're all akin to standard, creamy lipsticks in pencil form. The Matte Stick is not matte in the least, and is actually rather greasy. The Sheer Stick is even greasier than the Matte version, but has less pigment. The Shimmer Stick is creamy without being greasy and has a soft metallic finish. This one stands the best chance of lasting beyond your mid-morning break.

☹ **Flower Fusion Hydrating Lip Color** *($15)* does contain several plant and flower waxes, and while those are harmless and contribute to this lipstick's creamy but thick texture, the jasmine, tangerine, lavender, and other citrus oils make this way too irritating to use on lips.

☹ **Rain and Shine Liptint with SPF 15 Sunscreen** *($13.50)* lacks adequate UVA-protecting ingredients and loses even more points due to the strong presence of peppermint oil. Plenty of sheer, glossy lipsticks are available that don't run the risk of irritating your lips. ☹ **Lasting Lip Color** *($13.50)* is flavored with peppermint, a trait you'll smell and feel (as in tingling, which isn't a good sign) as soon as you apply this otherwise creamy, opaque lipstick with a soft-gloss finish. Although not as potently irritating as the Origins lipsticks that contain pure essential oils, this is still too potentially troublesome to recommend. ☹ **Liquid Lip Color** *($13.50)* presents lip gloss with a bit more pigment than usual, which means you'll get a semi-opaque, glossy finish. What a shame the mint flavoring is so powerful and irritating, because the selection of colors is enticing.

☹ **Liquid Lip Shimmer** *($13.50)* contains enough mint to make lips tingle and, depending on how much or how often you apply this, burn. The irritation is not worth it when many other glitter-infused glosses are so widely available. ☹ **Once Upon a Shine Sheer Lip Gloss** *($13.50)* could just as easily be called "once upon an irritation" because that's what your lips are up against once they come into contact with this peppermint oil–infused gloss.

☹ **Smileage Plus Liptint** *($10)* is a sheer, glossy tinted lip balm that comes in some enticing, wearable colors and contains several lip-smoothing emollients. What a shame this ends up being irritating for lips due to its essential oils of lime and tangerine. The lime oil is especially problematic for lips exposed to sunlight, as it can cause a phototoxic reaction (Source: *Archives of Dermatological Research*, 1985, volume 278, pages 31–36).

MASCARA: ☺ **Fringe Benefits Lash-Loving Mascara** *($13)* hasn't changed since it was last reviewed, and remains a commendable but not extraordinary lengthening mascara that applies without clumps and leaves lashes soft and separated. It's best for those looking for natural rather than dramatic lashes.

😐 **Underwear for Lashes** *($13)* is described as a "little lash builder" and is nothing more than a colorless mascara that adds length and bulk to lashes prior to applying a regular mascara. Its formula is nearly identical to that of the Fringe Benefits Lash-Loving Mascara above, and two or three coats of that (or an even better mascara) produces the same results as using this before applying the real mascara.

😐 **Full Story Lush-Lash Mascara** *($13)* is more like a novella than a full story, at least when it comes to making the most of your lashes. You're in for a letdown if you expect this to perform as claimed because it's one of the most unexciting mascaras around. Repeated coats will provide some length, but no thickness whatsoever. In fact, trying to build anything impressive with this mascara is akin to reading the same chapter in a book over and over while expecting the story to progress.

FACE AND BODY ILLUMINATING/SHIMMER PRODUCTS: ☺ **$$$ Sunny Disposition Bronzing Stick for Eyes, Cheeks, and Lips** *($19.50)* has a smoother-than-silk texture that is easy to apply and imparts a soft, golden bronze color. The single shade is loaded with iridescence so it looks distracting, rather than beguiling, in daylight. However, it is appropriate for evening glamour, and looks particularly attractive when used over self-tanned legs, collarbone, and brow bone. The finish of this product does not feel great on lips, unless you're mixing it with a gloss or balm. For evening use, this is an excellent shimmer product that blends nicely and (best of all) tends to stay put. It is irritant-free.

☹ **Halo Effect Instant Illuminator for Face** *($16)* works as a versatile shine-enhancing lotion that has a gorgeous shimmer effect on skin, whether used alone or mixed with foundation. The problem? A plethora of irritating essential oils, including peppermint, orange, and lemon. These make Halo Effect impossible to recommend for any skin type.

BRUSHES: Origins' ✓☺ **$$$ Brushes** *($17.50–$32.50)* have always been made of synthetic hair, a boon for animal rights activists (or just for animal lovers). The latest incarnations are better than ever—you have to feel these to believe how amazingly soft and luxurious synthetic hair can be. Every brush has a renewed softness and the hairs are cut more precisely to facilitate a professional makeup application. Even the handles have been improved, making the entire collection worth looking at. The **Eye Lining Brush** *($15)* could stand to be a bit firmer, but some may appreciate its greater flexibility. The **Lip Brush** *($15)* is standard fare but the price isn't out of line, and it comes with a cap.

SPECIALTY PRODUCTS: ☺ **$$$ Sunny Disposition Liquid Bronzer** *($19.50)* has a sheer, non-sparkling, pink-bronze tint that would work well on warm or sallow skin tones that want a tanned appearance. Its matte finish makes it preferred for normal to oily or combination skin.

☺ **Brush Cleaner** *($10 for 3.4 ounces)* is a spray-on, solvent-based brush cleaner that is scented with plant extracts so it won't leave brushes smelling medicinal. It works well and dries quickly; however, this type of product is best for makeup artists who may be using the same brushes on multiple faces. If you're the only one using your brushes, an occasional cleaning with a basic shampoo or liquid soap will suffice, and in the long run will be less drying on the brush bristles.

The ☺ **Cosmetic Cases** *($10–$22)* are priced fairly for what amounts to cute, basic, but functional, makeup bags. These aren't the ones to choose if you cart around lots of cosmetics, but they're fine for keeping a few items stashed in your desk drawer or purse.

😐 **Underwear for Lips** *($13.50)* is not really necessary if you have a traditional matte-finish concealer handy. This comes in a tube with a wand applicator, and is designed to smooth the surface of the lips and make it easier to apply lipstick. Although this does have a soft matte finish, the peachy hue is not for everyone, and this works only marginally well. Depending on how matte or greasy your lipstick is, this will barely enhance application and will leave you wondering why you bothered. However, unlike most Origins lip products, this one is irritant-free.

☹ **Underwear for Lids** *($13.50)* is a creamy eyeshadow base that comes in twist-up-stick packaging. Why Origins thought this slightly greasy, crease-prone concealer hybrid would make a good eyeshadow base is a mystery. This does not come close to the long-lasting effect you can achieve using a good matte-finish concealer, including Origins' own Quick, Hide! Easy Blend Concealer above.

OSMOTICS (SKIN CARE ONLY)

OSMOTICS AT-A-GLANCE

Strengths: Provides complete product ingredient lists on their Web site; several fragrance-free products; Triceram is an outstanding moisturizer.

Weaknesses: Expensive; disappointing cleansers and toners; daytime moisturizers don't go much beyond basic sun protection; jar packaging for some antioxidant-rich products; needless irritants included in a few otherwise good options.

For more information about Osmotics, call (800) 440-1411 or visit www.osmotics.com or www.Beautypedia.com.

☹ **Balancing Cleanser, for Normal to Oily Skin Types** *($27 for 6 ounces)* has all the makings of a good (albeit pricey) water-soluble cleanser for its intended skin types, but the inclusion of lavender oil is a letdown and doesn't make this worth considering over countless others at the drugstore.

😐 **$$$ Calming Cleansing Milk, for Sensitive Skin Types** *($27 for 6 ounces)* is an OK cleansing lotion for normal to dry skin, but is not recommended for sensitive skin because it lists "aromatic oils" on the ingredient list, which, in their unknown context, may or may not be irritating. (The term *aromatic oils* does not meet FDA regulatory standards for ingredient labeling.)

☺ **$$$ Hydrating Cleanser, for Normal to Dry Skin Types** *($27 for 6 ounces)* can be a good water-soluble cleanser for its intended skin types, but the amount of orange oil means this should not be used near the eyes.

☹ **Balancing Tonic Facial Mist, for Normal to Oily Skin Types** *($35 for 6.8 ounces)* won't balance skin, but it will irritate it because of the essential oils of lavender and sandalwood. The amount of comfrey extract is also cause for concern.

☹ **Firming Tonic Facial Mist, for Normal to Dry Skin Types including Sensitive** *($35 for 6.8 ounces)* has almost the same problems as the Balancing Tonic Facial Mist above, and the same comments apply. The base formula of both of these Osmotics tonics is barely average.

😐 **$$$ Age Prevention Balancing Complex SPF 15, for Normal to Oily Skin Types** *($48 for 2 ounces)* cannot balance skin, but it does have merit as a lightweight, in-part avobenzone sunscreen. Where it fails to impress is its lackluster base formula, though the exclusion of fragrance is a plus. Considering the price, this sunscreen should be overflowing with antioxidants, anti-irritants, and other state-of-the-art ingredients, but except for some water-binding agents and a tiny helping of vitamins E and C, there isn't much to extol. If you decide to try this, it is best for normal to slightly oily skin.

☺ **$$$ Age Prevention Illuminating Complex SPF 15, for Normal to Dry Skin Types Including Sensitive Skin** *($48 for 2 ounces)* matches the broad-spectrum active sunscreen ingredients of the Age Prevention Balancing Complex SPF 15 above and has a better base formula, including multiple antioxidants in amounts that increase the chance of providing benefit to the skin. This water-based, slightly creamy moisturizer is fine for normal to dry skin, and works well under makeup (a good idea if your foundation lacks sunscreen or you don't apply it over your entire face). The amount of comfrey extract is likely too small to be cause for concern, but the product would be better without it.

😐 **$$$ Age Prevention Protection Extreme SPF 40, for All Skin Types Especially Sensitive** *($45 for 2.5 ounces)* provides sufficient UVA protection with its in-part zinc oxide sunscreen, but the fragrance-free cream base isn't that exciting for the money, merely supplying dry skin with basic emollients and some water-binding agents, but no state-of-the-art antioxidants, cell-communicating ingredients, or skin-identical ingredients. Lauder's DayWear sunscreens provide a lot more bang for your buck.

😐 **$$$ Anti-Radical Age Defense Barrier Longevity Complex** *($125 for 1.7 ounces)* has a hefty price, and quite radical story to go along with the exorbitant cost. The company claims this moisturizer is "the only product on today's market with Anti-oxidants, Anti-carbonyls and Anti-Nitrogens—to protect against all forms of free radical aging." First, there are many types of free radicals in the environment, many present in our own bodies, that all contribute to the aging process, but that is only a part of what is taking place. There are certain antioxidants that work at destroying specific types of free radicals (such as peroxidases or nitroxides), while others are better at vanquishing other types of free radicals (such as a triphenylmethyl radicals). "Anti-carbonyls" inhibit free radicals formed by reactions in the Earth's ozone layer, while "Anti-nitrogens" somehow block free radicals formed from nitrogen gas, which comprises just over 78% of our atmosphere. There is no way a single product, regardless of its content, can protect skin from every source of free-radical damage. And none of this explains why Osmotics opted to package this emollient moisturizer for dry skin in a jar, which quickly depletes the activity level of all of the antioxidants it contains.

☹ **Antioxidant Eye Therapy, for All Skin Types** *($55 for 0.5 ounce)* not only leaves its many antioxidants subject to deterioration after opening because of jar packaging, but also contains enough balm mint and lemongrass to be irritating to skin around the eyes. This misguided product is not recommended.

😐 **$$$ Blue Copper 5 Firming Eye Repair** *($75 for 0.5 ounce)* contains some intriguing and proven ingredients for helping normal to dry skin regain and maintain a healthy appearance. What a shame jar packaging subjects so many of them to quick deterioration once this lightweight moisturizer is being used. This product contains an ingredient blend known as Trylagen, manufactured by raw material supplier Centerchem. This blend consists of several peptides, wheat and soy proteins, and gel-based thickening agents. Together, they are said to increase collagen production, protect existing collagen from breaking down (not possible because this product lacks a sunscreen), and controlling collagen (by that I assume they mean controlling its growth though how this complex goes about doing that isn't explained and is in all likelihood impossible). The only research pertaining to this complex comes from Centerchem, and as such is hardly impartial. Such research is akin to Levi's doing a study that concluded their blue jeans were the best (well of course they are, if Levi's spearheaded the study)!

☺ **$$$ Blue Copper 5 Face Lifting Serum** *($75 for 1 ounce)* promises "the ultimate lifting experience," so get ready to cancel your appointment with the plastic surgeon! In all seriousness, the only lifting sensation this water-based serum provides is from the high amount of film-forming agent (the kind of holding ingredient found in hairspray) it contains. There are some good, unique antioxidants in this product, including shiitake mushroom extract. Cell-communicating ingredients are on hand, too, but what about the copper? It is present in two forms, but there is no substantiated research anywhere proving it firms or lifts skin in any manner. If you're looking for a brief tightening effect, this product can be used by all skin types except sensitive.

☹ **Blue Copper 5 Firming Elasticity Repair** *($55 for 1 ounce)* is an overpriced moisturizer that is described by Osmotics as the answer to every woman's antiwrinkle skin-care need (which begs the question, why do we need all the other Osmotics products, and why do they make the same claims about getting rid of wrinkles?). Copper has been shown to be effective in healing serious wounds, but that is unrelated to daily skin care or to preventing wrinkles. It is a good antioxidant, just not the answer for skin. Despite this, jar packaging won't keep it or the other antioxidants stable, and the lavender oil isn't a healthy additive if you're concerned with keeping skin in top shape.

😐 **$$$ Crease-Less Surgical Alternative** *($85 for 1 ounce)* is Osmotics' "works-like-Botox" product. It claims to be a surgical alternative to relax and prevent expression lines, all without needles (always good to throw that in, given that the widespread panic about needles must be why the number of Botox injections keeps *increasing* every year, right?). The company is using an "octapeptide" known as acetyl glutamyl hexapeptide-1. As expected, there isn't a shred of substantiated research proving this is the non-surgical answer to Botox. The only information about this ingredient (also known as SNAP-8) comes from the companies that sell it—hardly impartial sources—and the studies they supply to support their claims are limited, at best, and most performed in vitro. There is no reason to expect this to ease expression lines, though you may furrow your brow over the price, considering this is otherwise a basic, no-frills moisturizer.

☺ **$$$ Creme De l' Extreme, Suitable for Dry Skin Types Including Sensitive** *($48 for 1 ounce)* contains some excellent ingredients to help dry to very dry skin feel restored and comfortably smooth. It's a shame the antioxidants are subject to breaking down due to jar packaging. This fragrance-free formula, though expensive, is still worth considering for its ingredients that mimic the structure and function of healthy skin.

☺ **$$$ Cream Extreme Barrier Repair** *($75 for 1.7 ounces)* is a very emollient, balm-like moisturizer for dry to very dry or sensitive skin. It contains some outstanding ingredients to prevent moisture loss and prevent barrier destruction. It's a shame better packaging wasn't chosen because the handful of light- and air-sensitive ingredients won't survive long once the jar is opened.

☺ **$$$ Eye Surgery Under Eye Rejuvenator** *($65 for 0.5 ounce)* is "clinically proven" to work, but the clinical results are not available for public scrutiny, nor are they published, so don't bank on this product being able to "dramatically improve" your eye-area woes or anything else for that matter. Aside from misleading marketing claims, the good news is that this fragrance-free moisturizer for slightly dry skin contains some state-of-the-art peptides and several good antioxidants, though none of them are present in impressive amounts. The main peptide, acetyl tetrapeptide-5, is said by the raw material supplier to reduce under-eye puffiness. However, there is no independent, peer-reviewed research to support this claim. And it certainly cannot reduce puffiness resulting from aging as the fat pad beneath the eye begins to loosen; only cosmetic surgery can do that.

☹ **Intensive Moisture Therapy, for Dry Skin Types Including Sensitive** *($65 for 1.7 ounces)* is not recommended because the main plant extracts include irritants, and the unidentified "essential oils" will likely contribute to this irritation. Hundreds of moisturizers are available for dry skin that don't contain questionable ingredients, so why settle for this one?

☺ **$$$ Kinetin Cellular Renewal Serum, for All Skin Types** *($78 for 1 ounce)* is an OK water-based serum that contains more film-forming agent than kinetin or other antioxidants. It is suitable for all skin types. Kinetin has potential as an antioxidant, but the unknowns surrounding its long-term use should give you pause. For a detailed discussion of kinetin, please refer to the introduction for the Kinerase line, also reviewed in this book.

☺ **$$$ Kinetin Intensive Eye Repair, for All Skin Types** *($75 for 0.5 ounce)* comes packaged in a jar, which means all the spendy, trendy ingredients won't remain effective shortly after this emollient moisturizer for dry skin is opened. For the money, that's not good news.

✓☺ **TriCeram** *($30 for 3.4 ounces)* is an excellent moisturizer for dry to very dry skin. It contains some of the ingredients essential to restore a healthy skin barrier function while potent antioxidants work to minimize damage and reduce inflammation. TriCeram is fragrance-free and not only is one of the best products Osmotics offers, but also is priced sensibly.

☺ **$$$ Anti-Wrinkle Vitamin C Patches** *($48 for 12 treatments)* contain only a form of vitamin C that you can patch onto your skin. This is a strange way to apply vitamin C to skin because you can't get it all over, and there's no moisture or any other benefit. Lest we forget: vitamin C is not the most significant antiwrinkle ingredient around, and isn't worthy of this tricky, expensive mode of application.

☺ **$$$ Facial Refining Masque, for All Skin Types** *($32 for 2.5 ounces)* is an emollient mask with several plant extracts, most of which can be anti-irritants, although some can be irritants. The papaya has no exfoliating properties for skin. This standard group of ingredients can make normal to dry skin feel smooth, but they won't refine any part of your skin.

☹ **Lipoduction Body Perfecting Complex** *($95 for 6.8 ounces)* claims to reduce the appearance of cellulite by 60% to 80% in two months while at the same time firming your hips. And if you have even a trace of cellulite along the backside of your thighs, your curiosity will be piqued by their impressive pronouncement. Considering the steep price, you'd think investing in it would net the positive results described above. Alas, it's all bogus—because there is nothing in this "complex" that will even slightly alter the dimpled, orange-peel appearance of cellulite.

This contains mostly water, alcohol, and slip agents, along with caffeine, which appears in many other anti-cellulite products that cost significantly less than this one. Two studies have shown caffeine to have benefit for cellulite, but neither study can be considered unbiased. One was conducted by Johnson & Johnson, which owns RoC and Neutrogena, both of which sell anti-cellulite products that contain caffeine. The other study was conducted by the cosmetic ingredient manufacturer that sells anti-cellulite compounds (Source: *Journal of Cosmetic Science*, July–August 2002, pages 209–218). So there is no independent research showing that caffeine provides any benefit for treating cellulite. In an effort to make you think this product is working once it's applied, Osmotics included spearmint, which together with the alcohol causes irritation; that isn't helpful for cellulite or skin. Lipoduction Body Perfecting Complex does contain a couple of intriguing plant extracts, but their intrigue has nothing to do with eliminating cellulite. Instead, the research points to these plants being potentially helpful (when consumed orally) for many health issues, from asthma to heartbeat regulation (Source: www.naturaldatabase.com), but that has nothing to do with changing cellulite from the outside in.

OXY (SKIN CARE ONLY)

OXY AT-A-GLANCE

Strengths: Inexpensive; selection of fragrance-free topical disinfectants with benzoyl peroxide.

Weaknesses: Everything that's a problem for acne! Most Oxy products won't help acne, but will irritate skin with alcohol and menthol; BHA products not formulated at correct pH range to exfoliate, and also contain needless irritants.

For more information about Oxy, call (800) 688-7660 or visit www.oxynation.com or www.Beautypedia.com.

☹ **Chill Factor Daily Cleansing Pads** *($6.59 for 90 pads)* contain mostly alcohol and menthol, and are not recommended for any skin type.

☹ **Chill Factor Daily Wash** *($6.59 for 6 ounces)* is a water-soluble cleanser that contains 10% benzoyl peroxide, but any benefit is rinsed down the drain. The chill comes from the menthol added to this daily wash, making it too irritating for all skin types.

☹ **Daily Cleansing Pads, Focus: Blackheads** *($5.69 for 90 pads)* are nearly identical to the Chill Factor Daily Cleansing Pads above, minus the menthol. The low amount of salicylic acid and improper pH range means these pads won't help remove blackheads.

☹ **Daily Cleansing Pads, Maximum** *($3.89 for 55 pads)* contain a potentially helpful amount of salicylic acid, but the pH is too high for it to function as an exfoliant, and the almost 50% alcohol base is too drying and irritating.

☹ **Daily Cleansing Pads, Plus** *($6.29 for 90 pads)* contain less salicylic acid than the Daily Cleansing Pads, Maximum above, and less alcohol, too. However, the pH is still too high for exfoliation to occur and the alcohol can still be drying and irritating.

☹ **Daily Cleansing Pads, Standard** *($3.89 for 55 pads)* are nearly identical to the Daily Cleansing Pads, Plus above, and the same review applies.

😐 **Daily Wash, Maximum Strength** *($5.69 for 6 ounces)* is identical to the Chill Factor Daily Wash above, except this version omits the menthol, making it a better choice for normal to oily skin seeking a water-soluble cleanser. The 10% benzoyl peroxide will have minimal, if any, impact on acne due to its brief contact with skin.

☹ **Chill Factor Face Scrub** *($5.99 for 5 ounces)* contains menthol, sodium C14-16 olefin sulfonate, and aluminum powder, all of which make this scrub too irritating and drying for all skin types.

😐 **Face Scrub Acne Treatment, Maximum** *($5.19 for 5 ounces)* is a medicated scrub that contains 2% salicylic acid, but the pH is too high for it to exfoliate, not to mention that it is rinsed from skin before it could penetrate into the pore. The detergent cleansing base can be drying unless you have very oily skin; better scrubs are available at the drugstore.

✓ ☺ **Oxy Lotion, Vanishing Acne Medication** *($5.69 for 1 ounce)* is a very good, simply formulated topical disinfectant with benzoyl peroxide. The Standard version contains 5% benzoyl peroxide, while the Maximum and Maximum Tinted have 10% benzoyl peroxide, an amount that many will find too drying for ongoing use (but may be worth a try if your blemishes are not responding well to the 5% strength). All three strengths are fragrance-free; the tinted version looks peach in the bottle, but goes on quite sheer.

✓ ☺ **Oxy Spot Treatment** *($5.49 for 0.65 ounces)* is a slightly more silky-textured version of the Oxy Lotion, Vanishing Acne Medication above. This also comes in three versions: Clear, Light, and Dark, each fragrance-free and with 10% benzoyl peroxide as the active ingredient. The Light and Dark versions provide subtle camouflage and a matte finish, but you'll still need a liquid concealer to cover redness from blemishes.

PATRICIA WEXLER, M.D. (SKIN CARE ONLY)

PATRICIA WEXLER, M.D. AT-A-GLANCE

Strengths: Good selection of well-formulated moisturizers and serums; two highly recommended cleansers; good topical disinfectant with benzoyl peroxide.

Weaknesses: Moderately expensive; at-home AHA peel provides more irritation than help for skin; all lip products contain potent irritants; one sunscreen lacks UVA-protecting ingredients; no non-irritating salicylic acid products for acne-prone skin; skin-lightening product is alcohol-based; jar packaging.

For additional information about Patricia Wexler, M.D., call (888) 939-5376 or visit www.patriciawexlermd.com or www.Beautypedia.com. Note: Bath and Body Works is selling Patricia Wexler, M.D. Skin Care at most of their stores across the country; please refer to Chapter Seven, *Cosmetic Ingredient Dictionary*, for detailed information aboud matrix metalloproteinases (MMPs).

✓☺ **$$$ Dual Action Foaming Cleanser** *($18 for 3.4 ounces)* is an excellent, fragrance-free, liquid-to-foam cleanser for normal to oily or slightly dry skin. The water-light formula cleans and removes makeup well without leaving a residue or drying skin. The smattering of plant extracts is more for show than effect.

☺ **$$$ Universal Anti-Aging Cleanser** *($18 for 3.4 ounces)* is a standard, but very good, cleanser for normal to dry skin. It's reminiscent of Neutrogena's Extra Gentle Cleanser, except for the price, of course, which is about twice that of Neutrogena's. While nothing in this product has anything to do with fighting aging, the claim will get the attention of many. For removing makeup, you will need to use a washcloth to be sure you've gotten everything off. It does contain fragrance. By the way, if by "universal" Wexler means "all skin types" that's a mistake, because someone with oily to very oily skin won't be happy with this product. This contains fragrance in the form of methyldihydrojasmonate.

☹ **Exfoliating Cleanser with Acnostat** *($16 for 3.4 ounces)* makes claims that would be more genuine if this were a leave-on product. Because it's a cleanser, the 2% salicylic acid won't exfoliate skin and the MMPi ingredients advertised on the label are rinsed from skin before they can exert any benefit. Most bothersome is the inclusion of cypress oil. Although not much is known about this oil, its volatile compounds can be irritating and its safety and effectiveness (if any) are unknown (Source: www.naturaldatabase.com).

Resurfacing Microbrasion System *($60 for the kit)* is a two-step system. Step 1 is the 😐 **$$$ Skin Resurfacing Cream with MMPi**, which is nothing more than a scrub in an emollient base with alumina as the abrasive agent. It can be gritty, so use it carefully. As far as scrubs go, this is OK, but the claim that it can inhibit collagen breakdown is wishful thinking because the ingredients are washed away before they can be of much use to the skin. Step 2 is the ☺ **$$$ Intensive Hydrator with MMPi**, a well-formulated moisturizer with ingredients that mimic the structure of skin, cell-communicating ingredients, and some unique antioxidants. The combination of these two products doesn't hold any special benefit and more to the point, there are better, less expensive scrubs available, and there are other Wexler moisturizers more interesting than this one. Note: A reappraisal of published literature concerning multiple professional microdermabrasion treatments indicates that its overall level of improvement is marginal, at best (Source: *Dermatologic Surgery*, June 2006, pages 809–814).

😐 **$$$ Skin-Quenching Calming Mist** *($18 for 3.4 ounces)* is a decent toner, but "decent" doesn't make for great skin care. On a positive note, it does contain several plant extracts that potentially can inhibit substances in skin that cause collagen to deteriorate. But some of these extracts are also potential irritants, such as ivy, sage, pinecone, rosemary, and lemon, and that definitely causes collagen to break down. For some reason this also contains sunscreen ingredients, but the product isn't rated with an SPF, which makes them useless and just potential irritants. There is certainly a lack of great toners on the market, and this one doesn't change the situation.

☹ **Exfoliating Glyco Peel System** *($65 for the kit)*. Step 1, **10% Glycolic Peel Pads**, do, as the label states, contain 10% glycolic acid. That could have made this very effective for exfoliation, but the pH of 4.4 makes it far less effective than it would be with a lower pH, and for this kind of money it should be very effective indeed. This Peel also contains several irritating plant extracts and oils, including lemon, mandarin, and tangerine, which serve no purpose other than to add fragrance and cause irritation. There are better 10% AHA products on the market with an appropriate pH so they will actually facilitate exfoliation, and without the irritating additives. Step 2, **Skin Neutralizer**, is completely unnecessary. A neutralizer is needed only after application of an extremely potent AHA (over 20%) in a base with an effective pH, neither of which applies to the Peel part of this system. In addition, this Neutralizer has a pH of 8, and there is research showing that products with a pH over 7 can increase the bacteria content in skin. Complicating matters further are several problematic plant extracts that can potentially cause irritation. From almost every perspective this is not a good idea. Step 3, **Intensive Hydrator**, is by far the best product in this kit. It contains several state-of-the-art ingredients, but also includes cypress oil, and that is just a mistake for skin. This mistake might have been overlooked, but not when added to the other problems in this group of products.

☹ **Overnight Acne Repair Lotion with Acnostat** *($20 for 1 ounce)*. Day or night, the 1.25% concentration of salicylic acid in a pH of about 3.5 found here can be extremely helpful for combating acne, acting as both an exfoliant and a disinfectant (to kill acne-causing bacteria at the source). But this product ends up being a complete disappointment because alcohol is the second listed ingredient. To claim that this product reduces irritation, when it contains alcohol in such a prominent position, is just wrong.

😐 **$$$ Deep Wrinkle Eye Repair with MMPi** *($29.50 for 0.5 ounce)* is a fairly state-of-the-art formulation, but the jar packaging leaves much to be desired because none of the exciting ingredients fare well when routinely exposed to air.

😐 **$$$ De-Puff Eye Gel** *($19.50 for 0.5 ounce)*, with polymethylacrylamide listed as the third ingredient, raises concerns about use around the eyes. Although that ingredient can be "firming" (because it is a film former, not because it changes something in the skin), it can also be irritating, and around the eye is not the best place to apply this much of it. There are some worthwhile ingredients in here for skin, similar to those in other Wexler products, but also a few new ones. It contains something called oxidoreductases, but this is a class of ingredients rather than a specific ingredient, so there is no way to know exactly what it is or what it is meant to do (and it doesn't meet FDA regulations for ingredient lists). Generally, oxidoreductases (superoxide dismutase is an example) are meant to inhibit oxygen in some way, as in preventing free-radical damage. It also contains *Agaricus bisporous* extract from the white button mushroom you often see in supermarkets. Regrettably, it also contains an extract of peppermint, which is potentially irritating, though the amount seems so minuscule that it shouldn't be much of a problem.

☹ **Instant De-Puff Eye Gel** *($19.50 for 0.5 ounce)* won't deflate puffy eyes instantly or even after a week of diligent use. The formula is similar to that of Wexler's regular De-Puff Eye Gel above, except that this contains even more acrylate-based film-forming agent and adds caffeine to the mix (though there is no research proving caffeine wakes up tired, puffy eyes). Other than these changes, the same comments made for the De-Puff Eye Gel apply here, too. Overall, this is just too potentially irritating for the eye area.

😐 **$$$ Intensive Night Reversal and Repair Cream** *($42.50 for 1.7 ounces)* features a state-of-the-art formula, but much of what makes it an exciting option for normal to dry skin will be lost once this jar-packaged product is opened. The amount of cypress oil is potentially cause for concern; although not much is known about this plant, two of its components are camphor and d-pinene, both of which can irritate skin.

😐 **$$$ MMPi Skin Regenerating Serum** *($55 for 1 ounce)* does have a wonderful silky-smooth texture, but it lacks the impressive state-of-the-art ingredients in Wexler's other products, plus the jar packaging won't help keep the few good ingredients in here stable.

☹ **MMPi•20 Anti-Aging Acne Serum with Acnostat** *($55 for 1 ounce)* lists alcohol as the second ingredient, followed by ethoxydiglycol, a penetration-enhancing ingredient that only makes the alcohol that much more irritating and drying. What an expensive way to irritate skin.

☹ **Oil Free Hydrator SPF 30+** *($39.50 for 1.7 ounces)*. I am just stunned at this product, and it is absolutely not recommended because it lacks the UVA-protecting ingredients of titanium dioxide, zinc oxide, avobenzone, Mexoryl SX (ecamsule), or Tinosorb. Without these you leave your face vulnerable to a sizable range of damaging sunlight. Elaborate claims and scientific mumbo jumbo can't replace the need for a well-formulated sunscreen. I'm not sure how this was overlooked, as the research about sunscreen formulations shows up in more dermatological journals than you can imagine.

😐 **$$$ Skin Brightening Daily Moisturizer SPF 30+** *($39.50 for 1.7 ounces)* has what the above Oil Free Hydrator SPF 30+ sunscreen lacks, thanks to its in-part avobenzone sunscreen and some very interesting state-of-the-art ingredients. How foolish to package it in a jar, which leaves the efficacious antioxidants subject to deterioration on exposure to air and light.

☺ **$$$ Under-Eye Brightening Cream** *($29.50 for 0.5 ounce)* is an impressive blend of antioxidants, cell-communicating ingredients, anti-irritants, and ingredients that mimic the structure of skin, and it has a silky, emollient texture. This would be great for any part of the face—under eye, cheek, jaw—because there's nothing about the formulation that makes it specific for the eye area. As state-of-the-art as this formulation is, to hope that it can improve dark circles under the eye is little more than wishful thinking, though the mica (shine particles) and the whitening effect of the titanium dioxide will cosmetically give the skin a light glow. But that's makeup trickery, not a skin-care breakthrough. It does contain *Uva ursi* (bearberry) leaf extract, which in large amounts can have melanin-inhibiting properties, but at this low concentration, it will barely be noticed by your skin.

☺ **$$$ Universal Anti-Aging Moisturizer PM with MMPi** *($39.50 for 1.7 ounces)* is an emollient moisturizer for normal to dry skin. You can be assured you'll get antioxidants, cell-communicating ingredients, and ingredients that mimic the structure of skin, which is good. Unfortunately, this formula also gives you more fragrance (methyldihydrojasmonate) than any of the more fascinating components. It is still a desirable option, but there could have been more of the good stuff up front (meaning higher up on the ingredient list).

😐 **$$$ Universal Anti-Aging Moisturizer SPF 30 with MMPi** *($39.50 for 1.7 ounces)* contains avobenzone, so this nicely covers the UVA spectrum for good sun protection. While the sunscreen ingredients will remain stable in the jar packaging, the plant extracts, peptides, antioxidants, and retinol certainly won't. That's truly disappointing, because every other aspect of this formulation excels, and it would have been worth the investment for those with normal to slightly dry skin.

☺ **$$$ Acne Spot Treatment with Acnostat** *($15 for 0.5 ounce)* is a very good, absorbent cream with 10% benzoyl peroxide as the active ingredient. The addition of soothing plant extracts helps calm redness from blemishes, but that effect is counteracted somewhat by the inclusion of cinnamon bark extract, which keeps this anti-acne product from earning a Paula's Pick rating. The amount of salicylic acid is inconsequential for skin.

✓☺ **$$$ Advanced No-Injection Wrinkle Smoother** *($29.50 for 0.5 ounce)* won't replace the need for Botox or dermal filler injections, but if it really could have this effect then wouldn't it put Wexler's medical practice, which include injections of Botox and dermal fillers, out of business? Shouldn't she just be handing out this product instead of charging her patients $600 for Botox and even more for dermal injections? Despite the disingenuous claim, this is an exceptionally well-formulated serum-type moisturizer that contains several cell-communicating ingredients and proven water-binding agents. This fragrance-free product is recommended for all skin types, but not for those who are dealing with rosacea because the amount of myristyl nicotinate has a chance of triggering facial flushing if the product is not carefully formulated to avoid the release of free nicotinic acid (Source: *Journal of Pharmaceutical and Biomedical Analysis*, February 2007, pages 893–899).

☺ **$$$ No-Injection Instant Line Filler for Lips & Eyes** *($17.50 for 0.5 ounce)* contains fewer exciting ingredients than the Advanced No-Injection Wrinkle Smoother above, yet its nonaqueous silicone base is considerably silkier. Used around the eyes or on the lips, the concentrated silicone functions as a soft spackle for superficial lines. It's a bit of a letdown that most of the cell-communicating ingredients are listed after the preservative. And, of course, this doesn't have a snowball's shot in you-know-where of replacing what dermal injections do for the lips.

☹ **Spot Damage Lightening Serum** *($25 for 0.5 ounce)* lists 2% hydroquinone as the active ingredient, so you can take this product's claim of lightening skin seriously. However, you should leave it on the shelf because the second ingredient is alcohol, and farther down on the list is cypress oil, making this product too drying and irritating for all skin types. For far less money, Rodan & Fields has a 2% hydroquinone product selling at $35 for 4.2 ounces, and without the problems in this formulation.

☹ **Damage Reversal Lip Treatment** *($20 for 0.5 ounce)* has far too many potentially irritating ingredients to make this a recommendation at any price. Spearmint, lime, and peppermint oil are all too irritating for the skin (including lips). That certainly doesn't reverse damage, but it can compound the issue. The claim that the teensy amount of vitamin E in here can provide environmental protection is unfortunately an unrealistic expectation.

☹ **Advanced No Injection Lip Plumper** *($17.50 for 0.16 ounce)* joins Wexler's still-available original No Injection Lip Plumper reviewed below, but differs little from it other than being a bit more emollient and coming in a selection of sheer shades. How does it make lips plump? Not with hyaluronic acid spheres as claimed. Rather, the menthol derivative menthyl lactate slightly swells lips by irritating them. This is not in any way comparable to what dermal injections can achieve for the lips (procedures Wexler performs in her medical practice because she isn't selling this product to her patients as a way to avoid injections).

☹ **No Injection Lip Plumper** *($16 for 0.13 ounce)* is a mineral oil–based gloss that plumps the lips by irritating them with cinnamon oil (think of the candy Red Hots) and the menthol derivative menthyl lactate. Other than that there are some interesting cell-communicating ingredients and water-binding agents, but don't expect the teeny amount of collagen present to change the size of your lips in any way.

☺ **$$$ Instant Airbrush Line Smoothing Superconcealer** *($19.50)* is made to sound like an instant fix in a tube, claiming to relax wrinkles, treat dark circles, and improve skin tone, all while camouflaging flaws. The ingredients in this water- and silicone-based formula cannot relax lines (the GABA complex it includes has never been shown to be effective for this purpose, and there isn't much of it in here anyway), and the tiny amounts of plant extracts that are natural sources of arbutin won't affect skin discolorations (including dark circles) in the least. I would assume that as a dermatologist Wexler knows all this, because this kind of information has been reported on extensively in every dermatologic medical journal I've read.

Wexler's concealer has a lightweight, silky texture that covers moderately well and won't crease into lines under the eye, though its strong matte finish can accentuate these lines. It can be used over blemishes, and is a good alternative to creamy or stick-based concealers for that purpose. Both shades are very good, but are limited to those with fair to light skin tones. Last, it's a boon for skin that this brush-on, pen-style concealer contains a nice array of antioxidants and cell-communicating ingredients, all in packaging that will keep them stable.

PAULA'S CHOICE

I decided to ask for help with the introduction to my own product line, reasoning that who better than one of my own customers to describe my work and my products? So in my free email Beauty Bulletin (available at www.cosmeticscop.com) I put the word out that I was "looking for Paula's Choice customers who feel they have a strong sense of what my mission is and what my products are all about to help write an introductory paragraph for my new book." The responses were incredible and I'd like to express a special thanks to everyone who took the time to write. After going through all of the submissions, the winner was Debe Czerwiec from Raleigh, North Carolina. This is what Debe had to say about my products:

"How can you go wrong with a cosmetics line where every single item is a result of many years and hundreds of hours of detailed research into what's wrong or right about almost all cosmetics on the market today? Paula's Choice products represent the results of combining the best of the best after careful research and consultation with experts in the field of skin, hair and body care. No false promises of reduced aging, miracle cures, or repairing hair are found in Paula Begoun's line. She has exposed those false or impossible claims in other product lines, and is very clear about what her products can and cannot do for you. Her company is very consumer oriented, and does everything possible to meet the needs and requests of its customers. It also makes the very unusual offer of selling sample sizes of all products for trial use or for travel. Each product is described very carefully without exaggeration or hype, making it easy to select the one right for your needs. I cannot imagine why anyone would trust another company with their skin care and cosmetic needs when Paula's Choice is so completely transparent about its products. If you choose something you don't like, you can easily return it, and if you choose, you can be counseled in what might be a better product for you to try. They'll also be forthright with you if they do not have a product that matches your preferences. Enjoy reading about the wonderful options in Paula's Choice. You won't be disappointed!"

PAULA'S CHOICE AT-A-GLANCE

Strengths: All products fragrance-free; all products formulated based on published research on ingredients and their functions/benefits for skin; pH-correct AHA and BHA products; effective skin-lightening options; gentle cleansers; toners that go beyond the norm; all sunscreens provide UVA protection; topical disinfectants for acne; antioxidant-rich serums and moisturizers; every foundation provides sun protection and comes in a range of neutral colors; eyeshadows with a completely matte finish; sheer lipstick with sunscreen; innovative eyelining and lip paint products; superior makeup brushes.

Weaknesses: Shortage of sunscreens rated above SPF 15 (though this will be changing); limited self-tanning options (there are so many great options at the drugstore there is little reason to add more to this crowded field; if I can't come up with better options, I won't do it); limited makeup shades for darker skin tones (though this will be changing).

For more information about Paula's Choice, call (800) 831-4088 or visit www.paulaschoice.com or www.Beautypedia.com.

PAULA'S CHOICE SKIN CARE

✓ ☺ **One Step Face Cleanser, for Normal to Oily/Combination Skin** *($14.95 for 8 ounces)* is a water-soluble gel cleanser that feels silky and rinses cleanly. Skin is left smooth and refreshed, and this cleanser removes most types of makeup.

✓ ☺ **One Step Face Cleanser, for Normal to Dry Skin** *($14.95 for 8 ounces)* is a water-soluble cleanser with a milky texture and low lather. It works beautifully to remove all types of makeup.

✓ ☺ **Skin Balancing Cleanser, for Normal to Oily/Combination Skin** *($14.95 for 8 ounces)* has a pearlescent, cushiony texture that leaves skin perfectly cleansed and free of makeup. This is the cleanser to consider if you prefer lots of foam (though the foam itself has no effect on cleansing ability).

✓ ☺ **Skin Recovery Cleanser, for Normal to Very Dry Skin** *($14.95 for 8 ounces)* feels rich and soothing, and its creamy texture cleanses skin while leaving it feeling smooth and supple. It does not leave a greasy residue, nor does it require a washcloth for complete removal.

✓ ☺ **Gentle Touch Makeup Remover** *($12.95 for 4 ounces)* is a water- and silicone-based, dual-phase liquid that quickly removes all types of makeup, from long-wearing foundations to waterproof mascaras and lip stains. It contains soothing agents and is safe for use around the eyes.

✓ ☺ **Healthy Skin Refreshing Toner, for Normal to Oily/Combination Skin** *($14.95 for 6 ounces)* contains ingredients that improve skin function while reducing cellular damage, leaving skin feeling refreshed with a nearly imperceptible finish, and it also removes the last traces of makeup.

✓ ☺ **Moisture Boost Hydrating Toner, for Normal to Dry Skin** *($14.95 for 6 ounces)* helps normalize and optimize skin to function normally. It contains antioxidants, cell-communicating ingredients, and skin-softening agents that leave a satin-smooth finish while also removing the last traces of makeup.

✓ ☺ **Skin Balancing Toner, for Normal to Oily/Combination Skin** *($14.95 for 6 ounces)* is based around the cell-communicating ingredients niacinamide and adenosine triphosphate, both of which improve skin and restore balance while also improving hydration. This toner helps eliminate mild dryness and flaking skin while leaving it feeling smooth.

✓ ☺ **Skin Recovery Toner, for Normal to Very Dry Skin** *($14.95 for 6 ounces)* is truly a moisturizing toner and is ideal for restoring essential elements to environmentally compromised or sensitized skin. It contains antioxidants, anti-irritants, and essential lipids while being a perfect starting point before applying moisturizer, serum, or sunscreen.

✓ ☺ **1% Beta Hydroxy Acid Gel, for All Skin Types** *($17.95 for 4 ounces)* features 1% salicylic acid in a pH-correct formula whose gel texture feels silky-smooth. Ideal for exfoliating the skin's surface and inside the pore to improve its texture and appearance, while minimizing blemishes and blackheads.

✓ ☺ **1% Beta Hydroxy Acid Lotion, for All Skin Types** *($17.95 for 4 ounces)* contains 1% salicylic acid in a pH-correct lotion formula that contains soothing agents. It exfoliates and improves skin's texture while providing lightweight moisture.

✓ ☺ **2% Beta Hydroxy Acid Gel, for All Skin Types** *($17.95 for 4 ounces)* is similar to the 1% Beta Hydroxy Acid Gel above, but has twice the concentration of salicylic acid for those with stubborn blemishes or blackheads. This is suitable for all skin types, but best for normal to oily skin.

✓ ☺ **2% Beta Hydroxy Acid Lotion, for All Skin Types** *($17.95 for 4 ounces)* combines 2% salicylic acid in a pH-correct lotion that soothes and softens skin with its combination of water-binding agents and anti-inflammatory ingredients. This is ideal for those with normal to dry skin prone to breakouts.

✓ ☺ **2% Beta Hydroxy Acid Liquid, for All Skin Types** *($17.95 for 4 ounces)* works efficiently and quickly to remedy breakouts and dislodge blackheads, smooth the surface of skin while imparting no irritation, and improving skin tone (due to the gentle but functional exfoliation it offers). This product also can calm pre-existing irritation. You can apply this toner-like solution with fingertips or a cotton pad.

✓ ☺ **8% Alpha Hydroxy Acid Gel, for All Skin Types** *($17.95 for 4 ounces)* pairs an effective amount of glycolic acid in a pH-correct, silky gel. It exfoliates and smooths sun-damaged skin and improves signs of unevenness and minor discolorations.

✓ ☺ **HydraLight Moisture-Infusing Lotion, for Normal to Oily/Combination Skin** *($18.95 for 2 ounces)* is one of my lightest moisturizers, yet its antioxidant-rich formula provides a powerhouse of helpful ingredients skin needs to look radiant and healthy. Skin is left feeling fresh and looking matte; this works great under makeup, too.

✓ ☺ **Hydrating Treatment Cream, for Normal to Dry Skin** *($16.95 for 2 ounces)* makes skin feel luxuriously soft with its combination of skin-identical ingredients, plant oil, cell-communicating ingredients, and emollients. The texture and results make this one of my favorite products to use around the eyes when they're showing signs of dryness.

✓ ☺ **Skin Balancing Daily Mattifying Lotion SPF 15, for Normal to Oily/Combination Skin** *($18.95 for 2 ounces)* has a weightless texture someone with oily skin will love, yet it provides sun protection and supplies skin with potent antioxidants and cell-communicating ingredients, while leaving a matte finish. UVA protection is assured by avobenzone.

✓ ☺ **Skin Balancing Moisture Gel, for Normal to Oily/Combination Skin** *($16.95 for 2 ounces)* leaves skin feeling remarkably silky, while imparting necessary elements that maintain and generate healthy skin. It is ideal under makeup, assuming your foundation provides broad-spectrum sun protection.

✓ ☺ **Skin Recovery Moisturizer, for Normal to Very Dry Skin** *($16.95 for 2 ounces)* restores vital moisture to its intended skin types and has an elegantly creamy texture. Skin is fortified with emollients, peptides, antioxidants, and skin-identical ingredients, all of which combine to deliver soft, smooth, skin.

✓ ☺ **Skin Recovery Daily Moisturizing Lotion with SPF 15, Normal to Dry Skin** *($18.95 for 2 ounces)* combines titanium dioxide and zinc oxide for daytime sun protection while pampering your skin with a blend of emollients, silicones, lots of antioxidants, and cell-communicating peptides. Surprisingly moisturizing for being so lightweight, it is designed to work well under foundation.

✓ ☺ **Almost the Real Thing Self-Tanning Gel, for All Skin Types** *($12.95 for 5 ounces)* is a water-based self-tanner that contains dihydroxyacetone to turn skin color. The formula is tinted so you can instantly see where it has been applied, and it dries quickly. It is suitable for all skin colors, which is why I don't offer separate formulas for light and medium to dark skin.

✓ ☺ **Essential Non-Greasy Sunscreen SPF 15, for Normal to Oily/Combination Skin** *($12.95 for 6 ounces)* is my classic sunscreen that contains avobenzone for UVA protection and leaves skin feeling fresh, smooth, and lightly hydrated. It is ideal for use anywhere on the body, and is designed to not pose problems for blemish-prone skin.

✓ ☺ **Extra Care Moisturizing Sunscreen SPF 30+, for Normal to Dry Skin** *($12.95 for 6 ounces)* has a smooth, creamy texture that feels elegant yet provides water-resistant sun protection and includes titanium dioxide and zinc oxide, among other actives, plus antioxidants.

✓ ☺ **Pure Mineral Sunscreen SPF 15, for Normal to Very Dry Skin** *($14.95 for 6 ounces)* is my favorite sunscreen to use in sunny climates when I'm going to be outside for a long day. This gentle formula contains only titanium dioxide and zinc oxide and has a silky texture that applies easily and feels light. Green tea is the chief antioxidant, and that coupled with the non-sensitizing actives makes this a great choice for those dealing with rosacea or for use on children. Pure Mineral Sunscreen is also great for use around the eyes.

✓ ☺ **Ultra-Light Weightless Finish SPF 30 Sunscreen Spray, for All Skin Types** *($15.95 for 4 ounces)* is a non-aqueous, convenient spray that includes avobenzone for sufficient UVA protection and potent antioxidants to help boost skin's environmental defenses. This protects skin beautifully yet feels like you're wearing nothing at all.

✓ ☺ **Blemish Fighting Solution, for All Skin Types** *($15.95 for 2.25 ounces)* contains 2.5% benzoyl peroxide in a soothing lotion base. It is an ideal topical disinfectant for those battling mild to moderate blemishes and is one of the few benzoyl peroxide products that do not include irritating plant extracts or drying alcohol.

✓ ☺ **Extra Strength Blemish Fighting Solution, for All Skin Types** *($15.95 for 2.25 ounces)* is similar to the Blemish Fighting Solution above, but contains 5% benzoyl peroxide, which is recommended for more stubborn or pervasive blemishes.

✓ ☺ **Clearly Remarkable Skin Lightening Gel, for All Skin Types** *($16.95 for 2 ounces)* packs a 1, 2 punch for discolored areas with its combination of 2% hydroquinone and 2% salicylic acid (the latter speeds the results from the hydroquinone). The gel texture feels refreshingly light, and the special packaging is designed to keep the hydroquinone stable during use.

✓ ☺ **Remarkable Skin Lightening Lotion, for All Skin Types** *($16.95 for 2 ounces)* lightens sun- or hormone-induced skin discolorations with its blend of 2% hydroquinone and 7.4% glycolic acid. This smooth-textured lotion may be used alone or layered with other products as needed.

✓ ☺ **Skin Balancing Carbon Mask, for Normal to Oily/Combination Skin** *($12.95 for 4 ounces)* is a unique treatment mask that absorbs excess oil with clay and carbon. This rinses easily, and the drawing action of the mask also helps to dislodge blackheads.

✓ ☺ **Skin Recovery Hydrating Treatment Mask, for Normal to Very Dry Skin** *($12.95 for 4 ounces)* drenches skin in moisture while helping to restore a healthy barrier function and reduce inflammation. Skin is left feeling soft and looking radiant; you can leave this mask on as long as necessary.

✓ ☺ **Skin Balancing Super Antioxidant Mattifying Concentrate, for Normal to Very Oily Skin** *($22.95 for 1 ounce)* is a weightless combination of beneficial antioxidants, cell-communicating ingredients (including retinol), skin-identical ingredients, and soothing agents. It helps to normalize skin-cell function while keeping excess oil in check thanks to its long-lasting matte finish (which also allows this to work as a "primer" under foundation). It has a silky smooth finish that feels elegant and makes skin look supple and smooth.

✓ ☺ **Skin Recovery Super Antioxidant Concentrate, for Normal to Very Dry Skin** *($22.95 for 1 ounce)* revitalizes its intended skin types with copious antioxidants, cell-communicating ingredients (including retinol), and efficacious plant oils. This is a great way to improve the appearance and healthy functioning of sun-damaged skin.

✓ ☺ **Super Antioxidant Concentrate, for All Skin Types** *($22.95 for 1 ounce)* is my original Antioxidant Concentrate, and is an excellent all-purpose option that supplies skin with stabilized vitamin C and other potent antioxidants in a base formula that's neither matte nor emollient.

✓ ☺ **Exfoliating Treatment** *($9.95 for 0.5 ounce)* is a unique way to get dry skin off your lips, elbows, knees, or heels without irritation. A tiny amount gently massaged over dry skin is all that's needed. Simply keep massaging until this wax-based product starts to flake off, taking the dead, dry skin with it. Brush or rinse off what remains, and the skin is left silky-smooth.

✓ ☺ **Lip & Body Treatment Balm** *($9.95 for 0.5 ounce)* is a customer favorite. It contains protective oils, waxes, and emollients that prevent moisture loss and restore dry, chapped skin to a normal state. Applying this twice a day can guarantee you never have chapped lips again.

✓ ☺ **Moisturizing Lipscreen SPF 15** *($7.95 for 0.16 ounce)* is an in-part titanium dioxide–based lip balm in a twist-up, ChapStick–style container. Lips are protected from the sun while maintaining a glossy, balm-like finish.

✓ ☺ **Oil-Blotting Papers** *($6.95 for 100 sheets)* are thin tissue paper–style sheets that quickly soak up excess oil and perspiration without leaving a powdery residue.

✓ ☺ **Skin Relief Treatment, for All Skin Types** *($14.95 for 4 ounces)* is a unique toner-like product that contains stabilized aspirin and vitamin C to soothe skin and calm irritation. This is ideal as an after-shave product or for use before and after spa or dermatologist procedures.

✓ ☺ **All Over Hair & Body Shampoo, for All Skin & Hair Types** *($12.95 for 16 ounces)* functions as a shampoo for all hair types (including chemically treated) and works just as well as a body wash. The formula rinses cleanly and does not contain any ingredients that may be irritating to skin or scalp. It is excellent for use on babies and children, too.

✓ ☺ **Smooth Finish Conditioner, for All Hair Types** *($12.95 for 16 ounces)* moisturizes, detangles, and adds shine to hair, all without making it look or feel limp or greasy. This is one of the only fragrance-free conditioners available, and my goal was to make it every bit as elegant as any others I have reviewed. It works for all hair types, and you only need to change the amount you use to achieve the desired results of smooth, silky, combable hair.

✓ ☺ **Close Comfort Shave Gel, for All Skin Types** *($11.95 for 6 ounces)* is a cushiony, soothing shave gel that's tinted with azulene so you can quickly see any missed spots. The concentrated formula does not foam or lather, yet rinses easily from the razor blade while also protecting your skin from nicks and cuts.

✓ ☺ **Cuticle & Nail Treatment** *($10.95 for 0.06 ounce)* is an emollient blend of oils and conditioning agents dispensed from a pen-style applicator with a built-in synthetic brush tip. The applicator makes it ideal for targeted use to keep nails looking great.

✓ ☺ **Beautiful Body Butter, for Dry to Extra Dry Skin** *($14.95 for 4 ounces)* is a decadently rich moisturizer that forms a protective barrier on skin. Cocoa and shea butters dramatically improve the appearance of dry, cracked skin while preventing further moisture loss. This works perfectly on heels, elbows, and other severely dry areas of the body.

✓ ☺ **Silk Mist Moisturizing Body Spray, for All Skin Types** *($14.95 for 4 ounces)* feels ultra-light, yet this non-aqueous body moisturizer makes skin touchably smooth and soft. The formula is a blend of plant oils with silicone and antioxidants, and is ideal misted on after bath or shower.

✓ ☺ **Silky Start Sugar Scrub for the Body, for All Skin Types** *($10.95 for 4 ounces)* smooths dry, rough skin thanks to a mix of exfoliating sugarcane crystals steeped in skin-softening oils. Because the sugar granules dissolve as you scrub, there is minimal risk of being too aggressive or "overscrubbing" your skin.

✓ ☺ **Skin Revealing Body Lotion with 10% Alpha Hydroxy Acid, for All Skin Types** *($19.95 for 8 ounces)* contains 10% glycolic acid in a pH-correct base formula that supplies skin with an array of ingredients it needs to look and feel its best. This is ideal for rough, dry, sun-damaged skin.

✓ ☺ **Slip Into Silk Body Lotion, for All Skin Types** *($15.95 for 8 ounces)* contains state-of-the-art ingredients that go above and beyond what typical body moisturizers contain. This lotion leaves skin feeling unbelievably smooth while supplying it with antioxidants, cell-communicating ingredients, and proven water-binding agents.

✓ ☺ **Weightless Body Treatment with 2% Beta Hydroxy Acid, for All Skin Types** *($19.95 for 8 ounces)* is an effective BHA body lotion that contains 2% salicylic acid at a pH of 3.2. Soothing agents and antioxidants work with the salicylic acid to eliminate dry, rough skin and help improve blemishes from the neck down.

PAULA'S CHOICE MAKEUP

FOUNDATION: ✓ ☺ **Best Face Forward Foundation SPF 15** *($14.95)* is designed for normal to very oily or combination skin. It has a fluid, ultra-light texture that blends beautifully and sets to a long-wearing matte finish that doesn't look thick or feel heavy. An in-part titanium dioxide sunscreen provides broad-spectrum protection from the sun, eliminating the need for a separate sunscreen (provided you apply the foundation evenly over your entire face). Available in five neutral shades for fair to medium/tan skin, this foundation offers sheer to medium buildable coverage.

✓ ☺ **All Bases Covered Foundation SPF 15** *($14.95)* has a light, creamy-smooth texture and is ideal for normal to dry skin. It has a soft matte finish and offers light to medium coverage with excellent blendability in five neutral shades for fair to medium/tan skin tones. It protects skin from sun damage with a pure titanium dioxide SPF 15 sunscreen.

✓ ☺ **Barely There Sheer Matte Tint SPF 20** *($14.95)* has a creamy but light texture that slips flawlessly over skin and provides a smooth, satin-matte finish. Its sheer-coverage formula provides a hint of color to even out your complexion while still allowing your natural skin tone to show through. The broad-spectrum titanium dioxide and zinc oxide sunscreen included will help shield your skin from harmful UV rays, making this an ideal all-in-one option for broad-spectrum sun protection and light moisturizing, plus soft color that enhances your skin. It comes in five neutral shades for fair to medium/tan skin tones.

✓ ☺ **Natural Finish Oil-Absorbing Makeup SPF 15** *($14.95)* is a sheer foundation designed for normal to oily/combination and blemish-prone skin. The lightweight, state-of-the-art formula begins slightly creamy, but blends to a smooth matte finish that absorbs excess oil, while also providing sufficient UVA protection thanks to its in-part avobenzone sunscreen. I created four shades that are suitable for fair to medium/tan skin tones, each capable of sheer to light coverage. This is a brilliant way to combine sun protection and soft coverage to create a natural look that helps keep excess oil in check without feeling heavy or too thick.

CONCEALER: ✓ ☺ **No Slip Concealer** *($9.95)* is a creaseless concealer that you apply with a wand. The matte finish formula provides long-lasting coverage and works equally well over dark circles, red spots, or blemishes. Each of the four muted shades is meant to blend imperceptibly into your skin, and coordinates with every Paula's Choice foundation.

✓ ☺ **Soft Cream Concealer** *($9.95)* features everything I (and any self-respecting makeup artist) wants in a cream concealer: it has a smooth texture that blends easily, it covers well without looking thick or cakey, it has a natural satin finish that resembles skin rather than makeup, and it remains creaseless for hours. I created three neutral shades to complement fair to medium/deep skin tones, whether used alone or with foundation and powder.

POWDER: ✓ ☺ **Skin Perfecting Loose Powder** *($12.95)* was a product I resisted adding to my makeup line for quite some time, primarily because I think loose powders tend to be unnecessarily messy. However, once I tried this airy, silky talc-based formula and discovered a loose-powder component with a closable sifter, I was hooked. Two translucent shades are available, best for fair to medium skin. This is a loose powder that makes skin look polished and natural, not dry. ✓ ☺ **Sheer Perfection Pressed Powder** *($12.95)* has a talc-based formula that helps absorb excess oil and set makeup while making skin look refined, not powdered. You can apply it with a brush for sheer coverage or use a sponge for additional camouflage. Four neutral shades are available, best for fair to medium/tan skin.

✓ ☺ **Healthy Finish Pressed Powder SPF 15** *($14.95)* offers the option of shine control and additional sun protection, with a titanium dioxide– and zinc oxide–based sunscreen. This has a velvety feel and goes on evenly and smoothly without looking chalky or dry. You'll find this provides light to medium coverage and has a soft matte finish. It can be used as a pressed-powder foundation (best for normal to slightly dry or slightly oily skin) or simply used with a powder brush to set makeup or touch up your sun protection (over sunscreen or foundation with sunscreen) without redoing your makeup. Please keep in mind that I don't recommend relying on *any* SPF-rated pressed powder as your sole source of sun protection because it is unlikely anyone will layer it thickly enough to achieve optimal sun protection. It is best to use an SPF 15 powder in conjunction with a moisturizer or foundation that has an SPF 15 or greater and that contains UVA-protecting ingredients. Three neutral shades are available, plus ✓ ☺ **Healthy Finish Pressed Bronzing Powder SPF 15** *($14.95)*, which has the same formula but is designed to lightly bronze fair to medium skin tones.

BLUSH: ✓ ☺ **Soft Matte Blush** *($8.95)* is my original powder blush, and is available in a classic assortment of pink, peach, rose, and earth tones that complement many skin colors. It is completely matte, feels silky, applies evenly and has a long-lasting color payoff. ✓ ☺ **Barely There Sheer Matte Blush** *($9.95)* is a "goof-proof" sheer version of my Soft Matte Blush. Each shade goes on very softly, almost translucent, yet you can build more color intensity if desired. The selection of matte shades includes staples for any makeup wardrobe, and they are always in season.

EYESHADOW: ✓ ☺ **Soft Matte Eyeshadow** *($8.95)* has an ultra-silky texture that applies without flaking or skipping. Blending is easy whether you want sheer shading or all-out drama, and the finish is completely matte. Several shades work beautifully to line the eyes and define or fill in the brows. The formula may be used wet (great for eyelining) or dry. ✓ ☺ **Soft Matte Eyeshadow Trios** *($10.95)* share the same formula as the single Soft Matte Eyeshadows, but present three coordinated shades (one for highlighting, one for contouring, one for lining) in a single component. This is a foolproof way to create a basic eye design, and every Trio is matte.

EYE AND BROW SHAPER: ✓ ☺ **Ultra-Thin Eye & Brow Pencil** *($7.95)* is an automatic, retractable eye pencil with a smooth application and soft, powder finish that works equally well to line your eyes or fill in your brows. The precision tip allows you to draw a thin line that can be made thicker at the outer third of the eye.

✓ ☺ **Constant Color Gel Eyeliner** *($12.95)* is one of my personal favorites. This long-wearing, water-resistant gel-cream eyeliner has a smooth, quick-drying formula with the texture of a cream lipstick. It glides easily over the lid when applied with your favorite eyeliner brush. You get the look of liquid eyeliner and the smooth application of powder liner. Best of all, it won't smudge, fade, smear, or tear off once it has set. It's ideal for those whose regular eyeliner doesn't make it through the day or anyone with oily eyelids.

✓ ☺ **Brow/Hair Tint** *($9.95)* defines eyebrows with natural-looking color. The brush-on formula is lightweight and flakeproof, and the four shades can also be used to touch up gray hair at the roots between colorings. (This is the one product I keep in my purse, briefcase, car, and desk—if I see gray hair, I quickly cover it up and no one is the wiser.)

LIPSTICK, LIP GLOSS, AND LIPLINER: ✓ ☺ **Smooth Matte Lipstick** *($9.95)* has the long-wearing, full-coverage qualities of a true matte lipstick, but maintains a smooth, almost creamy feel on lips that makes its matte finish uniquely comfortable, never dry. It doesn't bleed or feather into lines around the mouth, a quality I insisted on so that I could wear it without worrying about a mess around my lips after an hour or two. Each Smooth Matte Lipstick shade has a coordinated color from Paula's Select Long-Lasting Anti-Feather Lipliner below. ✓ ☺ **Soft Cream Lipstick** *($9.95)* has an emollient, smooth feel with a silky texture, soft gloss finish, and opaque to semi-opaque coverage. Unlike many creamy lipsticks, this doesn't feel overly slick or slippery, and thus stays in place longer. ✓ ☺ **Sheer Cream Lipstick SPF 15** *($10.95)* offers a beautiful palette of sheer, mostly shimmering colors and includes an in-part avobenzone sunscreen to protect lips from the sun. This lipstick has a modern, lightweight texture that feels comfortably creamy while providing a soft, glossy finish. A colorless version (Invisible) is available to use alone or over your favorite lipstick when you want sun protection.

✓ ☺ **Constant Color Lip Paint** *($10.95)* is an innovative lip product I developed as an alternative to long-wearing lipsticks such as Max Factor Lipfinity and Cover Girl Outlast. Although I am a fan of both products, they have limitations. You cannot reapply the color without starting over and you can't use them with other products, such as an additional lipstick or gloss. My Constant Color Lip Paint solves those dilemmas thanks to its versatility. Applied alone, it serves as a long-wearing, full-coverage lip color with a matte finish that won't streak, chip, or make lips feel parched. Used with another lipstick, it can serve as a base color or it can be applied over any other lip color or lip gloss (without disruption) to create a unique shade or to intensify the effect. There are 11 flattering shades, some soft and some slightly more dramatic. This is a lip product I am never without! The one drawback is that it can build up and roll, so you sometimes have to remove it completely and then reapply.

✓ ☺ **Soft Shine Moisturizing Lip Gloss** *($9.95)* is a lightweight, wand-applicator gloss with an emollient, non-sticky application and moderately glossy finish. ✓ ☺ **Liquid Diamonds High Shine Lip Gloss** *($9.95)* comes in a squeeze tube and has a thick, emollient texture and very glossy, shimmer-infused finish. It's great for evening or whenever you want to add a multidimensional shine, either on bare lips or over lipstick.

✓ ☺ **Long-Lasting Anti-Feather Lipliner** *($7.95)* is a standard, automatic lipliner in colors I selected specifically to coordinate with my lipsticks. These have a smooth application but aren't greasy, and they can help prevent feathering (just like most pencils that have this kind of texture). I've also included a colorless version (Clear) that helps keep most lipsticks from bleeding (though it won't stop exceptionally greasy, glossy lipsticks from feathering).

MASCARA: ✓ ☺ **Lush Mascara** *($9.95)* quickly creates long, thick lashes without clumping, flaking, or smearing, and it will last all day. It's water-soluble for easy removal. ✓ ☺ **Epic Lengths Mascara** *($9.95)* has great lengthening ability without the intense thickening action of the Lush version above. This wears well and does not flake or smear, yet is easy to remove.

BRUSHES: My ✓ ☺ **Brushes** are very soft and dense, precisely cut for their intended purpose, and they hold their shape and place color evenly with minimal to no flaking of powder. All of them are short-handled so they fit nicely and conveniently in any makeup bag. The **Powder Brush** *($19.95)*, **Blush Brush** *($15.95)*, two **Eyeshadow Brushes, Small** and **Large** *($11.95 each)*, **Wedge/ Brow Brush** *($10.95)*, **Eyeliner Brush** *($9.95)*, **Lipstick Brush with Cap** *($9.95)*, **Shadow Softening Brush** *($11.95)*, **Crease Defining Brush** *($11.95)*, **Precision Shadow Brush** *($11.95)*, and **Concealer Brush** *($10.95)* are all professional-style brushes to help you apply makeup using the same tools on which most makeup artists rely. Additional brushes you might wish to consider based on your needs are the tapered **Contour Brush** *($14.95)*, **Soft Blending Brush** *($10.95)*, **Angled Shadow Brush** *($10.95)*, **Precision Liner Brush** *($10.95)*, **Retractable Powder Brush** *($16.95)*, and **Brow/Lash Brush** *($11.95)*.

The **Pro Basics Brush Set** *($90.65)* provides seven essential brushes tucked in a synthetic leather carrying case. The case has room for up to 12 brushes, so you can add to your collection as needed. The **Brush Carrying Case** *($12.95)* is also available separately. The **Mini Brush Set** *($32.95)* includes small yet perfectly functional versions of my Powder, Blush, Large and Small Eyeshadow, Wedge/Brow, and Eyeliner brushes inside a nylon pouch with a Velcro closure. It's great as a secondary brush set for office or travel.

SPECIALTY PRODUCTS: For those who need to keep excess shine in check, my ✓ ☺ **Oil-Blotting Papers** *($6.95 for 100 sheets with plastic case; $3.95 for refill pack of 50 sheets)* absorb oil and perspiration without leaving a layer of powder or making skin feel dry. My latex-free ✓ ☺ **Makeup Application Sponges** *($4.95 for 10 round sponges)* are for applying foundation and for blending the edges of makeup, an essential step that's all too often overlooked. Various washable makeup ✓ ☺ **Bags** and **Cases** *($4.95–$12.95)* are available as well.

PETER THOMAS ROTH (SKIN CARE ONLY)

PETER THOMAS ROTH AT-A-GLANCE

Strengths: Provides complete ingredient lists on Web site; most products are fragrance-free; very good AHA products; wide selection of water-soluble cleansers and scrubs; great makeup remover; some excellent sunscreens, skin-lightening products, and benzoyl peroxide products; many antioxidant-rich formulas; Roth avoids the use of extraneous ingredients, including plant extracts with no documented benefit for skin.

Weaknesses: Expensive; mostly lackluster toners; mostly boring to potentially irritating masks; no BHA products that do not include at least one needless irritant; jar packaging; a growing number of products claiming to work like or be similar to cosmetic corrective procedures.

For more information about Peter Thomas Roth, call (800) PTR-SKIN or visit www.peterthomasroth.com or www.Beautypedia.com.

☺ **$$$ Anti Aging Cleansing Gel** *($35 for 8 ounces)* purports to contain natural ingredients that boast antiwrinkle technology, but this is nothing more than a standard water-soluble cleanser for normal to oily skin. The amount of glycolic and salicylic acids is too low for ideal exfoliation (though they would be rinsed away before they could have an effect), and the citrus extracts aren't the best for use around the eyes. Although this is an OK cleanser, the price is way out of line for what you get.

😐 **$$$ Beta Hydroxy Acid 2% Acne Wash** *($35 for 8 ounces)* lists 2% salicylic acid as an active ingredient, but this is rinsed from the skin before it can have an effect. This is otherwise a very simple fragrance-free cleanser for all skin types except very dry.

☺ **$$$ Chamomile Cleansing Lotion with Natural Herbal Extract for All Skin Types** *($32 for 8 ounces)* would be a great water-soluble cleanser for any skin type, but because it contains fragrance those with rosacea or sensitive skin should consider it carefully. This will remove makeup well and contains soothing plant extracts.

☺ **$$$ Combination Skin Cleansing Gel, Oil-Free for Slightly Oily, Combination or Normal Skin Types** *($32 for 8 ounces)* is similar to but gentler than the Anti Aging Cleansing Gel above. It is better suited for normal to dry or slightly oily skin, and it rinses without a trace.

☺ **$$$ Extra Strength Cleansing Gel Oil-Free for Oily, Combination or Problem Skin Types** *($32 for 8 ounces)* is a very standard water-soluble cleanser for normal to oily skin, and one that removes makeup easily while also being fragrance-free.

☹ **Foaming Face Wash, for Oily Combination or Normal Skin Types** *($32 for 8 ounces)* is not preferred to any of the cleansers above because it contains lemon oil, which can be irritating, especially when used around the eyes.

✓ ☺ **$$$ Gentle Cleansing Lotion, with Azulene for Sensitive, Dry, Mature or Normal Skin Types** *($32 for 8 ounces)* has a great silky texture and is indeed a gentle cleansing lotion that rinses completely. This contains some good anti-irritants, is fragrance-free, and is an outstanding option for normal to dry skin types.

😐 **$$$ Glycolic Acid 3% Facial Wash** *($32 for 8 ounces)* may contain 3% glycolic acid, but without the right pH and given this cleanser's brief contact time with skin, it doesn't matter. It is otherwise a very standard, fragrance-free water-soluble cleanser for normal to oily skin.

😐 **$$$ Medicated BPO 5% Acne Wash** *($32 for 8 ounces)* contains 5% benzoyl peroxide in a very basic but effective water-soluble cleanser for normal to oily or slightly dry skin. The benzoyl peroxide is said to kill bacteria on contact, but for best results should be left on skin, which you don't want to do with a cleanser.

😐 **$$$ Medicated BPO 10% Acne Wash** *($32 for 8 ounces)* is nearly identical to the Medicated BPO 5% Acne Wash above, except this contains 10% benzoyl peroxide. Otherwise, the same review applies.

☺ **$$$ Sensitive Skin Cleansing Gel** *($32 for 8 ounces)* would be better for sensitive skin if it did not contain fragrance, an odd addition given the number of fragrance-free cleansers in this line. Still, this is another effective water-soluble cleanser for normal to oily or slightly dry skin, and worth considering if the price doesn't faze you.

☺ **$$$ Tissue Off Silky Rich Cleansing Cream** *($32 for 8 ounces)* does not contain detergent cleansing agents, but instead contains emollients, oil, and thickeners to dissolve makeup. This is a good option for dry to very dry skin, but you do need to use a washcloth for complete removal.

✓☺ **$$$ Gentle Eye & Face Make-Up Remover** *($22 for 4 ounces)* is an excellent water- and detergent-based makeup remover that contains some good antioxidants and soothing agents, as well as being fragrance- and coloring agent–free.

☺ **AHA/BHA Face & Body Polish** *($35 for 8 ounces)* contains only a tiny amount of AHA and BHA, so the exfoliant duties fall to synthetic polyethylene beads (the third ingredient). This is a good scrub for normal to very oily skin, and it is fragrance-free.

☺ **$$$ Botanical Buffing Beads** *($36 for 8 ounces)* is a scrub that contains jojoba beads as the abrasive agent. They're quite gentle and a good option for normal to dry skin. However, they cannot open clogged pores and emulsify sebum (oil) as claimed. In contrast, because jojoba oil's molecular structure is so similar to our skin's oil, it is much more likely to contribute to rather than remedy clogged pores.

☹ **Fresh Ripe Wild Strawberry Scrub** *($35 for 8 ounces)* isn't something you'd see at your local farmer's market. The only strawberry in this cleansing scrub is fragrance, while the addition of pumice and almond meal makes this scrub too abrasive for all skin types.

😐 **$$$ Multi-Action All-in-One Micro-Dermabrasion** *($50 for 2.3 ounces)* is a fairly gritty scrub that contains aluminum oxide as the abrasive agent. This isn't the best for daily use, and recent research has revealed that even the results of professional microdermabrasion aren't all that impressive after all. This type of scrub is best for normal to oily skin.

😐 **$$$ Pumice Medicated Acne Scrub BPO 2.5%** *($35 for 8 ounces)* is a detergent-based scrub that contains polyethylene as the abrasive agent. The inclusion of 2.5% benzoyl peroxide isn't that helpful because its contact with skin is too brief, and acne cannot be scrubbed away.

☺ **$$$ Silica Face & Body Polish** *($35 for 8 ounces)* is a water-soluble cleansing scrub with polyethylene and silica as the abrasive agents. The fragrance-free formula rinses cleanly and is a good option for normal to very oily skin.

😐 **$$$ Aloe Tonic Mist** *($32 for 8 ounces)* is a very basic, alcohol-free spray-on toner that contains mostly water, aloe (which is primarily water), soothing agents, and a dusting of antioxidants. It is fragrance-free, and suitable for all skin types.

☹ **Conditioning Multi-Tasking After Shave Tonic** *($20 for 8 ounces)* contains several irritants, including witch hazel, lauryl leaf oil, menthol, and citrus peel oils. This would be a terrible product to apply to just-shaved skin!

😐 **$$$ Conditioning Tonic** *($32 for 8 ounces)* is an exceptionally basic toner whose salicylic acid content is too low to be effective, even though the pH is within range. Countless other less expensive toners offer your skin more than this.

😐 **$$$ Glycolic Acid Clarifying Tonic** *($32 for 8 ounces)* is a substandard toner that contains a frustrating mix of helpful and irritating ingredients, plus the pH is too high for the glycolic acid to function as an exfoliant. Let me clarify by saying that there are numerous other tonics that provide your skin with more than this.

☹ **Oxygen Mist** *($37 for 8 ounces)* contains a hefty amount of hydrogen peroxide, an unstable ingredient that causes free-radical damage on contact.

☺ **$$$ Power C Firming Spritz** *($37 for 8 ounces)* is Peter Thomas Roth's best toner thanks to its blend of stabilized vitamin C and some good water-binding agents. This formula is fragrance-free and would be rated higher if it included a wider variety of ingredients for skin.

✓☺ **$$$ AHA 12% Ceramide Hydrating Repair Gel** *($48 for 2 ounces)* blends 12% glycolic acid at an effective pH of 3.2 with an impressive array of water-binding agents and lesser amounts of ingredients that mimic the structure and function of healthy skin. It is fragrance-free and suitable for all skin types.

😐 **$$$ AHA/Kojic Under Eye Brightener** *($52 for 0.75 ounce)* has an effective amount of glycolic and lactic acids at a pH of 3.5, so exfoliation will occur. The issue is that the eye area can be too sensitive to this level of exfoliation, and the jar packaging won't keep the kojic or azelaic acids stable during use.

☹ **Gentle Complexion Correction Pads** *($36 for 60 pads)* contain an unimpressive amount of salicylic acid, but would have merit as an AHA product if the base did not contain so much alcohol.

😐 **$$$ Glycolic Acid 3% Eye Complex** *($52 for 0.75 ounce)* contains 3% glycolic acid at a pH of 3.5, so this is a gentler option if you're curious to try an AHA moisturizer around the eyes. Several water-binding agents join the emollients to make this a well-rounded product, but the vitamins won't last long due to jar packaging.

😐 **$$$ Glycolic Acid 10% Clarifying Gel** *($45 for 2 ounces)* is an OK glycolic acid gel with an acceptable pH, but the amount of alcohol is potentially irritating. I wouldn't choose this over the AHA 12% Ceramide Hydrating Repair Gel above.

✓☺ **$$$ Glycolic Acid 10% Hydrating Gel** *($48 for 2 ounces)* omits the alcohol in the Glycolic Acid 10% Clarifying Gel above, and replaces it with a good water-binding agent. This is an excellent fragrance-free AHA product for all skin types, and the pH of 3.6 ensures efficacy.

✓☺ **$$$ Glycolic Acid 10% Moisturizer** *($45 for 2 ounces)* is an ideal AHA moisturizer for normal to dry skin. Glycolic acid at a pH of 3.8 ensures exfoliation, while emollients and antioxidants help dry skin look and feel better, all without added fragrance.

☹ **Max Complexion Correction Pads** *($36 for 60 pads)* share the core problems of many anti-acne pads: an alcohol-based solution and a pH too high for salicylic acid to exfoliate, which won't help blemished skin in the least. This is absolutely not recommended.

😐 **$$$ Un-Wrinkle Peel Pads** *($45 for 60 pads)* are alcohol-free pads that contain 20% glycolic acid, a level that is close to peel strength but before you get too excited, know that the pH of the solution is almost a 6, which is well beyond the level needed for the acid to exfoliate skin. There is no reason to consider these pricey pads (though they're certainly not a problem for skin); the many antioxidants and retinol will not remain stable due to jar packaging.

😐 **$$$ All Day Moisture Defense Cream with SPF 20** *($38 for 1.7 ounces)* is an overall good daytime moisturizer for normal to dry skin, but comes up short with its in-part titanium dioxide sunscreen. Although formulary standards for UVA protection don't yet exist, the 0.5% titanium dioxide (coupled with other synthetic sunscreen agents) can leave skin vulnerable to UVA damage.

😐 **$$$ Anti-Aging Cellular Eye Repair Gel** *($42 for 0.76 ounce)* is sold as a revolutionary eye treatment whose benefits for wrinkles go beyond retinol. The company's Firme-CELL-4 technology is allegedly responsible for this feat. It combines four peptides (including the works-like-Botox argireline, also known as acetyl hexapeptide-3) said to have a synergistic effect on reducing deep lines and wrinkles. Before you get too excited, there is no substantiated research to support this claim. Peptides have theoretical cell-communicating ability and likely play a role in encouraging healthy skin functioning, but whether or not they can affect wrinkles is unknown; they probably can't. In contrast, retinol has mounds of research pertaining to its ability to improve skin's appearance and stimulate collagen production. Besides, beyond the peptides, this gel is mostly slip agent, film-forming agent (a hairspray-type ingredient), and preservatives, which is hardly worth opening up your pocketbook for.

☹ **$$$ Ceramide Eye Complex** *($52 for 0.75 ounce)* includes several noteworthy ingredients for dry skin, including plant oil, shea butter, hyaluronic acid, and cholesterol. It is an impressive, fragrance-free moisturizer that is offset only by the jar packaging, which won't keep the antioxidant vitamins stable during use.

☺ **$$$ Ceramide Moisture Renewal** *($48 for 1.7 ounces)* doesn't have the same wow-factor list of ingredients as the Ceramide Eye Complex above, but it does come in much better packaging. This is a good fragrance-free moisturizer for dry to very dry skin and would be rated higher if it contained more antioxidants and a cell-communicating ingredient or two.

☺ **$$$ Ceramide Night Renewal** *($52 for 1.7 ounces)* is similar to the Ceramide Moisture Renewal above, and the same review applies.

☺ **$$$ Ceramide Ultra-Rich Night Renewal** *($54 for 1.7 ounces)* is a more emollient version of the Ceramide Moisture Renewal above, and is best suited for nighttime use (it can be too slippery to wear under makeup). By the way, if this version contains extra ceramides, that is not reflected in the ingredient statement.

✓☺ **$$$ Environmental Repair Hydrating Gel** *($40 for 2 ounces)* is an outstanding gel-textured moisturizer for normal to very oily skin. It contains a very good mix of water-binding agents, antioxidants, and a cell-communicating ingredient, all in stable packaging. This does contain fragrance.

☺ **$$$ Max All Day Moisture Defense Cream with SPF 30** *($40 for 1.7 ounces)* is a good daytime moisturizer for normal to dry skin. The in-part titanium dioxide sunscreen provides sufficient UVA protection, and the formula includes antioxidants (though they should have been given more prominence).

☹ **$$$ Max Anti-Shine Mattifying Gel** *($35 for 1 ounce)* is merely a blend of silicones and a dry-finish solvent. It produces a matte finish, although without absorbent ingredients that offer more absorbency, don't expect shine-free longevity. Also, for the money, the company could have included at least one antioxidant and a single skin-identical ingredient.

☺ **$$$ Max Sheer All Day Moisture Defense Lotion with SPF 30** *($42 for 1.7 ounces)* isn't that sheer, but it's a good daytime moisturizer with an in-part avobenzone sunscreen suitable for normal to dry skin. This product is fragrance-free.

☹ **$$$ Mega Rich Intensive Anti-Aging Cellular Creme** *($85 for 1.7 ounces)* uses the same Firma-CELL-4 technology described for the Anti-Aging Cellular Eye Repair Gel above. This time the base is creamy and only two of the four peptides are present in notable amounts. However, none of the peptides can affect deep wrinkles or expression lines. At best, this moisturizer will make normal to dry skin feel better, but the many antioxidants are subject to deterioration because of jar packaging, making this a mega waste of money.

☹ **$$$ Mega Rich Intensive Anti-Aging Cellular Eye Creme** *($65 for 0.76 ounce)* lists most of the bells and whistles after the preservatives, and the jar packaging leaves all the ingredients vulnerable to the deteriorating effects of exposure to air.

☹ **$$$ Moisturizing 24/7 Anti-Aging Cellular Repair** *($52 for 1.5 ounces)* combines argireline (acetyl hexapeptide-3) with a bevy of standard thickeners and antioxidant vitamins whose potency won't last long once this jar-packaged product is opened. Acetyl hexapeptide-3 (and the other peptides in this product) theoretically can function as cell-communicating ingredients, but whether or not they work in real life as they do in a test tube has yet to be seen.

✓☺ **$$$ Moisturizing Multi-Tasking After Shave Balm** *($24 for 3.4 ounces)* is a brilliant choice for a moisturizer to use after shaving (or anytime, anywhere skin is dry). The fragrance-free balm contains significant amounts of antioxidants, cell-communicating ingredients, and ingredients that reinforce skin's healthy barrier function. And the price is realistic, too!

😐 **$$$ Oil-Free Moisturizer** *($42 for 1.7 ounces)* remains one of Roth's more basic moisturizers, though it is indeed oil-free. This would be an OK option for normal to slightly oily or slightly dry skin. It does contain fragrance.

☹ **Oxygen Eye Relief** *($52 for 0.75 ounce)* contains hydrogen peroxide, a potent generator of free radicals and a completely inappropriate ingredient for skin care. Although the jar packaging won't keep the peroxide (or antioxidants) stable for long, the entire concept of oxygenating skin to improve wrinkles is just bonkers!

☺ **$$$ Power C20 Anti-Oxidant Serum Gel** *($85 for 1 ounce)* is an intriguing serum if you're curious to see what a high amount of vitamin C (as L-ascorbic acid) can do for your skin. Water-binding agents and tiny amounts of other antioxidants (vitamin C is the headliner) comprise the rest of this all-skin-types product. By the way, the company needs to explain what their "stabilizing complex" is. It is not an ingredient in and of itself, and shouldn't be on the ingredient list as such because that doesn't meet FDA regulations.

😐 **$$$ Power C Eye Complex** *($52 for 0.75 ounce)* is a lightweight, fragrance-free moisturizer for slightly dry skin, and although it contains some impressive water-binding agents, the jar packaging won't keep the vitamin C (or vitamin E) stable during use.

☺ **$$$ Power C Souffle** *($85 for 1 ounce)* contains a good mix of water-binding agents and antioxidants along with lesser amounts of emollients and plant oils, making this a suitable moisturizer for normal to slightly dry skin. Given the product's name, it's odd that vitamin C isn't a more prominent part of the formula.

☹ **Power K Eye Rescue** *($100 for 0.5 ounce)* includes several antioxidants front and center, but none of them will do much good for your skin because of the jar packaging. In addition, vitamin K cannot affect dark circles or brighten skin when applied topically, and although arnica has a history of being used for bruising, it is ill-suited for use around the eye, not to mention that very few cases of dark circles are actual bruises.

☹ **Power Rescue Facial Firming Lift** *($150 for 1.7 ounces)* contains a lot of film-forming agent, and also has the same formula pitfalls as the Power K Eye Rescue above—making this not worth the investment or the potential irritation to skin.

☺ **$$$ Tinted Mineral Moisturizer SPF 30** *($42 for 1.7 ounces)* contains only titanium dioxide for sun protection, and the amount of it (nearly 15%) is likely what made it necessary for this product to have a sheer, flesh-toned tint so that it doesn't look ghost white on your skin. The silicone-based formula is suitable for normal to oily skin not prone to blemishes, and it contains a couple of antioxidants as well.

☹ **Ultimate Body Sculpting Slimming Gel** *($100 for 7.5 ounces)* costs so much because of the lofty claims made for it, not because it actually works or because it contains anything worth the price. For this much money, most of what you're getting is alcohol (listed first on the ingredient statement as ethanol), water, and glycerin. The anti-cellulite cocktail that is supposed to grant firmer thighs, stomach, and buttocks consists of caffeine, escin, carnitine, and butcher's broom extract. I discuss all of these ingredients in a report entitled "Caution Cellulite: Bumpy Road Ahead" on my Web site at www.CosmeticsCop.com. Suffice it to say, there is no substantiated research that any of the above-listed ingredients will affect cellulite or firm sagging skin in any way, shape, or form. It's interesting that Peter Thomas Roth claims the cellulite-fighting ingredients in this product are used "at the max levels," when there is no formulary protocol (or independent research) documenting just what a maximum usage level for these ingredients should be. It sounds good, and I suppose it allows the company to justify their outlandish price for what's mostly alcohol and water, but your thighs won't be any less dimpled (though your pocketbook will be lighter). By the way, if you're curious to find out if the ingredients in Roth's product can make a difference, they're also present in Neutrogena's and RoC's anti-cellulite products at a fraction of this price.

😐 **$$$ Ultra-Lite 24/7 Anti-Aging Cellular Repair** *($52 for 1.5 ounces)* makes the same antiwrinkle, our-peptides-pack-a-punch claims as the Anti-Aging Cellular Eye Repair Gel above. Peptides are brimming in this product, but there is no proof they can affect collagen and elastin production or improve the appearance of wrinkles and expression lines. This is an OK option for normal to dry skin, but the smattering of antioxidants is not helped by jar packaging.

☹ **Ultra-Lite Multi-Tasking After Shave Balm** *($24 for 3.4 ounces)* lists witch hazel distillate (which is mostly alcohol) as the second ingredient, and is not recommended.

☺ **$$$ Un-Wrinkle** *($120 for 1 ounce)* is a serum loaded with peptides in a proportion that the company claims tops out at 23%, therefore enabling this product to prompt up to a 52% reduction in wrinkles after a month of use, or so goes the claim. Yet there is no research showing that higher concentrations of peptides can have such an effect. There are some intriguing (if somewhat scary) assertions made about these peptides, such as the peptide called SYNr-AKE (technically dipeptide diaminobutyroyl benzylamide diacetate), which mimics the activity of snake venom. (This is Roth's claim, not mine.) The effect of real snake venom on skin can range from swelling and redness all the way to severe infection and necrotic (dead) tissue. Why on earth would a company advertise a peptide as being akin to snake venom? Good question, and it's telling that Roth's Web site mentions the correlation to snake venom, while the same product sold on Sephora's Web site leaves this chilling comparison out. Clearly Sephora was as shocked as I was.

SYNr-AKE comes from Pentapharm, whose Web site describes it as a "peptide with an Age Killing Effect. Mimics the neuromuscular blocking properties of Waglerin 1, a polypeptide found in the venom of the snake *Tropidolaemus wagleri.*" This snake is a type of viper, and Waglerin-1 is a peptide (composed of 22 amino acids) that is derived and purified from the venom. There is information on how this peptide performs on neurons in the brain and on its relation to GABA (gamma amino butyric acid), a common ingredient in products claiming to work like Botox. However, information on how this ingredient works when blended into cosmetic products is lacking and I'm not sure anyone should be a guinea pig for a substance like SYNr-AKE. Waglerin-1 is said to be another blocker of the neurotransmitter acetylcholine, which triggers muscle contractions. But if it worked as claimed, when applied topically it would relax muscles in your fingers, too, and what would happen if you used too much at once or accidentally got it too near the area around your eyes or mouth? (Sources: *Journal of Pharmacology and Experimental Therapeutics*, July 1997, pages 74–80; and *Brain Research*, August 1999, pages 29–37).

This product also contains a peptide referred to as SNAP-8, which Roth claims targets the "wrinkle formation mechanism" in the same manner as Botox injections. Although there is no substantiated research to support that, keep in mind that not even Botox works like Botox when it's applied topically. Fear the needle or not, if you want Botox to work it must be injected into, not dabbed on, your skin. SNAP-8 (technically acetyl glutamyl heptapeptide-1) is the trade name for an ingredient manufactured by Centerchem. Yet this ingredient is not listed for Un-Wrinkle, making an already bogus antiwrinkle product even more suspect. Of course, the only efficacy studies performed for this peptide were conducted by the manufacturer, and done in vitro rather than on human skin (Source: www.centerchem.com/PDFs/SNAP-8%20Tech%20Lit%20Aug05.pdf). The best reason to consider using this water-based serum is not for its litany of peptides or antiwrinkle prowess (which it is most certainly lacking), but for its antioxidants and water-binding agents, all in stable packaging. This is a costly way to get those ingredients, but they nevertheless are the most substantiated, useful ingredients in this product.

☺ **$$$ Un-Wrinkle Eye** *($100 for 0.5 ounce)* makes the same "look years younger" claim as the Un-Wrinkle product above, but doesn't have nearly as interesting a formula, at least not if you're looking for a peptide-rich product (there's no pressing need to do that, but peptides do get a lot of buzz). This has purpose as a lightweight moisturizer for slightly dry skin anywhere on the face, and it contains some good antioxidants in packaging that will keep them stable during use. However, this will not lead to lineless eyes.

☺ **$$$ Wrinkle Preventer** *($75 for 1 ounce)* may entice you with the percentages of trade-name ingredient mixtures it bandies about, but in the end this is just another serum-type moisturizer that contains a skin-silkening blend of glycerin, soy oil, and silicones. The rose water base adds a lot of fragrance, but this product does contain lots of antioxidants. Although that's great, no amount or blend of antioxidants can "stop wrinkles before they start." That takes an effective sunscreen and routinely practicing sun avoidance, something most people would rather not do, and understandably so. In case you're wondering, Colhibin is a rice-derived peptide its manufacturers claim can inhibit matrix metalloproteinases (MMP), specifically collagenase, which left unchecked can lead to collagen destruction. Aldenine is a mixture of wheat and soy proteins with a tripeptide that is said to boost collagen synthesis, and Pepha-Protect is a "highly purified" watermelon extract said to protect DNA in skin cells from sun damage. There is no independent research available to support any of these claims; all such information comes from the companies that supply the raw materials to skin-care companies.

☹ **Acne Spot And Area Treatment** *($32 for 1 ounce)* lists 5% sulfur as its active ingredient. Although sulfur is a potent disinfectant, it is very drying and irritating for most skin types. For that reason, it is not preferred to benzoyl peroxide or even tea tree oil. The pH of 3.1 serves only to make the sulfur more irritating, but it does allow the blend of glycolic and salicylic acids to exfoliate.

☹ **AHA/BHA Acne Clearing Gel** *($45 for 2 ounces)* contains 2% salicylic acid in the correct pH range for exfoliation to occur, but the amount of alcohol makes this too potentially drying and irritating for acne-prone skin.

☺ **$$$ Aloe-Cort Cream** *($30 for 2 ounces)* is a very standard lotion that contains 1% hydrocortisone as the active ingredient. It's an option for occasional use on minor skin irritations and itching, but for the money you'll get just as much efficacy from less expensive hydrocortisone creams at the drugstore. Aloe alone doesn't justify the price.

✓☺ **$$$ BPO Gel 5%** *($24 for 3 ounces)* is an excellent topical disinfectant for blemishes, with 5% benzoyl peroxide as the active ingredient in a weightless, fragrance-free gel base.

✓☺ **$$$ BPO Gel 10%** *($26 for 3 ounces)* is nearly identical to the BPO Gel 5% above, but contains 10% benzoyl peroxide. This amount, while effective, may prove too drying and irritating for some. However, it's worth a try before progressing to prescription topicals.

☹ **BPO Gel 10% and Sulfur** *($32 for 3 ounces)* combines the potency of 10% benzoyl peroxide with 5% sulfur, and together this harms skin more than it helps. This combination of actives is very drying and irritating for all skin types.

😐 **$$$ Cucumber Gel Masque** *($45 for 5.3 ounces)* is an overpriced water-based mask that contains a mixture of irritating and non-irritating plant extracts. It should not be considered calming or capable of reducing under-eye puffiness, at least not any better than using a cold compress to relieve swelling.

😐 **$$$ Hydrating Nutrient Masque** *($45 for 5 ounces)* may end up confusing your skin due to its blend of absorbent clays with thickeners and plant oils. It is too rich for oily skin and too absorbent for dry skin, which limits its appeal. Moreover, the price is out of line for what you get.

☹ **Oxygen Detoxifying Mask** *($54 for 4.5 ounces)* lists hydrogen peroxide as the third ingredient, which is a potent generator of free-radical damage and not recommended for anyone's skin. The jar packaging won't keep it stable for long, which leaves you with a very standard moisturizing mask that cannot detoxify a single skin cell.

☺ **$$$ Post-Peeling Healing Balm** *($25 for 0.8 ounce)* is similar to but more emollient than the Aloe-Cort Cream above. Otherwise, the same review applies. For a post-peel product, this is surprisingly void of known anti-irritants (well, beyond the hydrocortisone, that is).

✓☺ **$$$ Potent Botanical Skin Brightening Gel Complex** *($50 for 2 ounces)* contains a tiny amount of alcohol, but not enough to be cause for concern. This is quite a well-formulated skin-lightening product that eschews hydroquinone in favor of azelaic acid, kojic acid, and bearberry and mulberry extracts. All of these ingredients have research proving their worth for lightening discolorations (with azelaic acid leading the pack), making this gel highly recommended for all skin types as an option to the far more effective hydroquinone (Sources: *Cutis*, February 2007, pages 4–6; *Journal of the American Academy of Dermatology*, December 2006, pages 1048–1065; and *Biological and Pharmaceutical Bulletin*, August 2002, pages 1045–1048).

☹ **Potent Skin Lightening Gel Complex** *($55 for 2 ounces)* contains the gold standard hydroquinone in a 2% concentration, but the base formula contains too much alcohol, making this more irritating than many other skin-lightening options.

☹ **Power K Skin Brightener** *($110 for 1 ounce)* is said to combat several types of discolorations, including bruises, broken capillaries, and post-inflammatory hyperpigmentation from acne. Vitamin K has never been proven to do anything of the sort when applied topically (liposome delivery system or not), and the amount of arnica oil in this product makes it a problem for all skin types due to its tendency to cause contact dermatitis (Source: www.naturaldatabase.com).

😐 **$$$ Pumpkin Enzyme Peel, for All Skin Types** *($44 for 3.3 ounces)* is a simply-formulated, non-irritating product that banks on pumpkin enzymes to provide "deep exfoliation" for skin. Most enzymes used in skin-care products are unstable, and this is no exception (and jar packaging doesn't encourage stability). It's very likely the only benefits you'll receive from this non-peeling peel is softer skin (from glycerin) and, if this appeals to you, a pumpkin scent.

☹ **Sulfur Cooling Masque** *($40 for 5 ounces)* severely irritates skin due to its 10% concentration of sulfur along with eucalyptus oil. This mask is not recommended.

☹ **Therapeutic Sulfur Masque** *($40 for 5 ounces)* omits the eucalyptus oil in the Sulfur Cooling Masque above, but maintains the irritating concentration of sulfur, and is not recommended.

✓☺ **$$$ Ultra Gentle Skin Lightening Gel Complex** *($55 for 2 ounces)* is a very good option to treat skin discolorations. It contains 2% hydroquinone to inhibit melanin production and AHAs to help speed the process (though the pH of 4.1 is borderline for exfoliation). This fragrance-free gel is suitable for all skin types.

☹ **Lips to Die For** *($25 for 0.3 ounce)* won't make strangers fall at your feet due to your inflated mouth, but it will irritate your lips because there is so much menthol-like menthone glycerin acetyl in here. The special massaging applicator only causes further agitation that temporarily swells lips, but none of this is an equitable substitute for professional lip injections.

😐 **Matte Lip Balm** *($12 for 0.25 ounce)* is a blend of silicones with antioxidant plant extracts, two of which (rosemary and ginger) can be irritating. The silicone has a protective action on your lips while feeling feather-light, and does set to a matte finish.

PETER THOMAS ROTH SUN PRODUCTS

☺ **$$$ Natural Looking Self-Tanner** *($28 for 4 ounces)* is a good self-tanning lotion for normal to dry skin. Like most self-tanners, it's dihydroxyacetone that turns skin color. This contains fragrance in the form of rose oil.

😐 **$$$ Beach & Pool Sunblock SPF 30** *($26 for 4 ounces)* contains more fragrance than beneficial extras to help boost sun protection, but provides UVA protection with avobenzone. This water-resistant sunscreen is suitable for normal to dry skin.

☺ **$$$ Instant Mineral SPF 30** *($30 for 0.32 ounce)* provides sun protection with titanium dioxide and zinc oxide, and is a mica-based loose powder packaged in a self-contained applicator with a built-in brush. Powder application is sheer, but the brush is merely OK. You'd have to apply this liberally to ensure SPF 30 protection, and doing so is difficult due to the application method. That makes Instant Mineral SPF 30 best as an adjunct to a separate sunscreen or foundation with sunscreen. The product imparts very sheer color and a subtle shine, and has an absorbent finish.

☹ **Oil-Free Hydrating Sunscreen Gel SPF 20** *($26 for 4 ounces)* not only lacks sufficient UVA-protecting ingredients, but also has an alcohol base and lavender, which conspire to cause irritation.

✓☺ **$$$ Oil-Free Sunblock SPF 30** *($26 for 4 ounces)* is a very good in-part avobenzone sunscreen whose antioxidant-rich formula is suitable for normal to slightly dry skin. This is also fragrance-free and while it does not contain any oil, some of the thickening agents may be problematic for blemish-prone skin.

✓☺ **$$$ Ultra-Lite Oil-Free Sunblock SPF 20** *($26 for 4 ounces)* is similar to but slightly heavier than the Oil-Free Sunblock SPF 30 above. That said, the same review applies.

✓☺ **$$$ Ultra-Lite Oil-Free Sunblock SPF 30** *($26 for 4 ounces)* is similar to but slightly heavier than the Oil-Free Sunblock SPF 30 above, and the same review applies.

☹ **Ultra-Lite Oil-Free Sunscreen Mist SPF 15** *($28 for 8 ounces)* does not contain the UVA-protecting ingredients of titanium dioxide, zinc oxide, avobenzone, Mexoryl SX (ecamsule), or Tinosorb and is not recommended. Even with sufficient UVA protection, this is a really no-frills formula that is completely devoid of antioxidants or other skin-beneficial ingredients. What a disappointment!

☺ **$$$ Water Resistant Sunblock SPF 30** *($26 for 4 ounces)* is nearly identical to the Beach & Pool Sunblock SPF 30 above, minus the fragrance. It is the preferred water-resistant choice in the Roth line, and provides UVA protection via avobenzone.

PHILOSOPHY

PHILOSOPHY AT-A-GLANCE

Strengths: Relatively inexpensive; some of the best products are fragrance-free; very good retinol products; selection of state-of-the-art moisturizers; skin-lightening option that includes sunscreen; great lip balms, including those with a tint; impressive specialty makeup products

Weaknesses: Irritating and/or drying cleansers; average to problematic scrubs for face and lips; at-home peel kits far more gimmicky than helpful; most sunscreens contain lavender oil; several products include irritating essential oils; insufficient options to manage breakouts; the majority of makeup items do not rise above average status.

For more information about philosophy, call (800) 568-3151 or visit www.philosophy.com or www.Beautypedia.com Note: philosophy opts to use lowercase letters for every product they sell, so the listings below are simply following suit.

PHILOSOPHY SKIN CARE

☹ **on a clear day, super wash for oily skin** *($18 for 3.3 ounces)* is super-irritating for all skin types because it contains sodium lauryl sulfate as the main cleansing agent and adds camphor and sulfur to the mix.

☹ **purity made simple** *($20 for 8 ounces)* has the beginnings of a very good water-soluble cleanser for normal to dry skin, but things quickly head south due to the inclusion of several irritating plant oils, such as rosewood, geranium, and cinnamon.

😐 **$$$ the great mystery** *($25 for 5 ounces)* is basically glycerin, water, sea salt, and thickeners, along with some token marine plant extracts and a tiny amount of lavender oil. Salt can be a problem for the skin due to its high pH and irritation potential, though it does work as a scrub, but for that purpose a simple washcloth will work even better. The only mystery is why more people don't do that instead of bothering with all these scrub particles scraping and abrading their faces.

😐 **$$$ the microdelivery exfoliating wash** *($25 for 8 ounces)* contains a gentle detergent cleansing agent, but the clay it contains can be a bit drying for all but oily skin. The apple amino acids may sound farm fresh, but they have no ability to exfoliate skin, especially not in a product that is quickly rinsed away.

☺ **the afterglow, oil-free smoothing gel** *($20 for 4 ounces)* contains an efficacious amount of the AHA lactic acid at a functional pH of 3.5, all in a supremely lightweight, fragrance-free base. This would be even better with some anti-irritants or more sophisticated water-binding agents, but it's definitely worthwhile as an AHA product for all skin types.

☹ **the microdelivery mini peel pads** *($35 for 60 pads)* contain eucalyptus, tangerine, lemon, lavender, and orange oils, which make these AHA pads (lactic acid is on hand for exfoliation) too irritating for all skin types. If you want an effective AHA product that is free of needless irritants, consider the less expensive options from Alpha Hydrox, Avon, Neutrogena, Paula's Choice, or philosophy's the afterglow product above.

☹ **the microdelivery multi-use peel pads** *($55 for 100 pads)* may have multiple uses, but skin will be irritated and sensitized wherever these pads are stroked. The same problematic ingredients mentioned in the microdelivery mini peel pads above are present here, too.

😐 **$$$ the microdelivery peel** *($65 for the kit)* is a two-step at-home peel kit that ends up being more trouble than it's worth. Step 1 involves the **Vitamin C/Peptide Resurfacing**

Crystals. This is essentially a baking soda scrub that contains silica for additional exfoliation and antioxidant vitamins, none of which will remain stable once this jar-packaged scrub is opened. You massage the Resurfacing Crystals over your skin for up to one minute, then apply Step 2, the **Lactic/Salicylic Acid Reactivating Gel**. This gel contains mostly water and lactic acid, and its pH of 2 interacts with the alkaline pH of the baking soda in the Resurfacing Crystals, which is what provides the immediate sensation of warmth. The warm feel doesn't mean the vitamin C and peptides are suddenly active, as philosophy claims; it's merely a chemical reaction. Not surprisingly, it leaves your skin very smooth after rinsing, just as it would be if you used a standard scrub with a washcloth. The lactic acid functions as an AHA product (with a pH that's definitely irritating), but its contact with skin is too brief to do much, so this is essentially a very expensive, potentially irritating baking soda scrub.

☺ **$$$ booster caps retinol capsules** *($50 for 60 capsules; 0.71 ounce total)*. Each capsule contains a blend of silicones with a plant sugar, the algae chlorella (water-binding agents), film-forming agent, retinol, and fragrance. The capsule system is a good way to keep the retinol stable until you use it, and the contents have an extremely silky texture that is suitable for all skin types. Still, this product contains no more retinol than its competitors, and the lack of other antioxidants is short-sighted. Retinol does have research showing it has antiwrinkle benefits for skin (Sources: *Skin Pharmacology and Physiology*, March/April 2005, pages 81–87; and *Radiation Research*, March 2005, pages 296–306), but research also shows that its benefit for skin is further enhanced when antioxidants and ingredients that mimic the skin's intercellular matrix are included. None of this makes this product not worth trying, but given its one-note nature, there are more interesting retinol products available.

😐 **$$$ booster serum** *($60 for 1 ounce)* was created to "give your skin the ultimate anti-aging treatment," but it seems no one at philosophy stopped to consider what that should entail because this is one of the most lackluster serums around. It contains more fragrance than antioxidants (much less the talked-up peptides), and is modestly successful at being an OK moisturizer for normal to slightly dry skin.

☺ **$$$ dark shadows, illuminating eye and upper lip cream** *($30 for 0.5 ounce)* is a good lightweight moisturizer for normal to slightly dry skin anywhere on the face. It contains a couple of unique antioxidants and peptides, which may have cell-communicating ability. What this cannot do is eliminate dark circles or discolorations above the upper lip. It contains fragrance in the form of hibiscus flower.

✓☺ **$$$ eye believe, deep wrinkle peptide gel** *($30 for 0.5 ounce)* is a thick, silicone-based gel that contains a couple of antioxidants along with retinol and peptides. It's an elegant formula that can smooth the appearance of superficial lines (those related to dryness, not permanent wrinkles), but more important, it provides all skin types with some very helpful ingredients, and does so without fragrance.

☺ **$$$ help me** *($45 for 1.05 ounces)* is a good retinol product for normal to very dry skin not prone to blemishes (the amount of wax can aggravate breakouts). Content-wise, retinol isn't given more prominence here than it is in several drugstore lines, but it is stably packaged, fragrance-free, and certainly an option.

☹ **hope in a bottle, deep pore cleansing moisturizer for congested skin** *($35 for 2 ounces)* contains an unspecified amount of salicylic acid, but regardless of the amount, the pH of this moisturizer is too high for preferred levels of exfoliation to occur. It is not recommended because it contains lavender oil and lacks any significant amounts of beneficial ingredients.

☹ **$$$ hope in a jar, original formula** *($35 for 2 ounces)* is sold as philosophy's world-famous therapeutic moisturizer, but it's a rather ordinary formula that does not contain lactic acid as claimed. Instead, this has lauryl lactate, which is the ester of lauric and lactic acids. Although the product has a pH of 3.2, lauryl lactate does not have exfoliating abilities; rather it functions as an emulsifier and enhances the spreadability of creams. Jar packaging won't keep the antioxidants in this product stable, and it's really not deserving of its alleged worldwide fame.

☹ **hope in a jar, for dry, sensitive skin** *($35 for 2 ounces)* is completely inappropriate for any skin type because it contains lavender and sage oils, both of which have components that are irritating to skin and destructive to cells.

☺ **$$$ hope in a tube, high density eye and lip firming cream** *($30 for 0.5 ounce)* is a thick, emollient-rich, fragrance-free cream that will take excellent care of dry, dehydrated skin anywhere on the body, but it won't firm skin one iota. Of course, given the small amount of product, this is best reserved for use on the face, and would work well around the eyes if that area is dry. Classic moisturizing standbys such as glycerin, petrolatum, and mineral oil comprise the bulk of the formula, and philosophy included a few antioxidants, too.

☹ **on a clear day protection cream** *($15 for 1 ounce)* is supposed to serve as a second skin for those with acne, but the lavender oil in this product can cause skin-cell death. This product won't net clear skin.

☺ **$$$ save me, p.m. retinol/vitamin C/peptide for fine lines, wrinkles, and uneven skin tone** *($60 for 1 ounce)* is first and foremost a vitamin C serum. It contains magnesium ascorbyl phosphate, a stable form of this antioxidant, and there is plenty of it present (it's the second ingredient listed). The other showcased ingredients (peptides, retinol, and additional antioxidants) make a less impressive appearance, but they are present. The opaque, airless pump bottle will help keep the vitamin C stable, but don't expect this product to lift and firm skin as claimed. This is suitable for all skin types and is worth trying if you're curious to see what a vitamin C serum does for your complexion.

☹ **shelter, UVA/UVB broad spectrum sunscreen for face and body, SPF 30** *($25 for 4 ounces)* would rate a Paula's Pick for sun protection if it did not contain lavender oil. The in-part titanium dioxide sunscreen and silky lotion base with plentiful antioxidants could have been a great option for those with normal to dry skin.

☹ **shelter, UVA/UVB broad spectrum sunscreen for the face, tinted SPF 30** *($20 for 2 ounces)* is identical to the shelter SPF 30 sunscreen above, except with a sheer tint. Unfortunately, the identical part means that lavender oil makes an appearance here, too.

☹ **the present, clear makeup** *($25 for 2 ounces)* is identical to the on a clear day protection cream above, and the same review applies.

☹ **when hope is not enough SPF, age defense UVA/UVB SPF 20 broad spectrum sunscreen** *($35 for 2 ounces)* is a pricey sunscreen that doesn't have much going for it, other than including avobenzone for UVA protection. The base formula lacks a blend of antioxidants in appreciable amounts, something that might have made the price tag more reasonable. Lavender oil is added for fragrance, but there is concern that this ingredient, even in concentrations as low as 0.25% (which may be applicable to this product) is toxic to cells (Source: *Cell Proliferation*, June 2004, pages 221–229). It is best to avoid any product, effective sunscreen or not, that features lavender oil, just as you would avoid any other expensive sunscreen—because its price might discourage liberal application.

☺ **$$$ when hope is not enough, facial firming serum with glutathione, peptides, vitamin C and E and soy** *($35 for 1 ounce)* contains mostly water, film-forming agent, slip agents, glycerin, water-binding agents, antioxidants, anti-irritant, pH adjuster, fragrance, and preservatives. It is a worthwhile, serum-type moisturizer for normal to slightly oily skin because it supplies hydrating agents, antioxidants, and cell-communicating ingredients without thickeners, oils, or oil-like ingredients. This product won't lift skin, and it won't help minimize facial hair growth as claimed, because it contains no ingredients with proven ability to do that.

😐 **$$$ when hope is not enough, replenishing cream while you sleep** *($45 for 2 ounces)* is an emollient moisturizer whose best, price-justifying ingredients will break down once this jar-packaged product is opened. This will help dry skin look and feel better, but so will many less expensive moisturizers.

✓☺ **a pigment of your imagination SPF 18** *($30 for 2 ounces)* is one of philosophy's most unique products because it combines an effective, in-part avobenzone sunscreen with ingredients that can improve hyperpigmentation. The main ingredient responsible for lightening skin discolorations is arbutin, and that's due to its hydroquinone content. Although the research describing arbutin's effectiveness is persuasive (even if almost all of the research has been done on animals or in vitro), concentration protocols have not been established. That means we just don't know how much arbutin it takes to have an effect in lightening the skin. Related information suggests that a newer compound known as deoxyarbutin also has merit as a skin-lightening agent, though this research was also done in vitro on cultured human skin cells (Sources: *Journal of Cosmetic Science*, July/August 2006, pages 291–308; and *Experimental Dermatology*, August 2005, pages 601–608). A pigment of your imagination is fragrance-free and best for normal to dry skin. It is comparable to but actually a better formulation than Shiseido's Whitess Intensive Skin Brightener ($125 for 1.4 ounces).

😐 **$$$ hope and a prayer, a.m. topical vitamin C powder** *($35 for 0.25 ounce)* consists of a bottle of vitamin C powder that contains other antioxidants, amino acids, and a couple of water-binding agents. The powder is designed to be used alone or added to a moisturizer or serum to create "a state-of-the-art vitamin C formula." There are lots of top-notch vitamin C products available that don't involve a messy powder or mixing with another product. This is a viable option if you're curious to see what a vitamin C product will do for your skin; the only issue is that the form chosen (ascorbic acid) can be irritating, while other, more stable forms of vitamin C don't have this drawback.

☹ **on a clear day, blemish serum for adult acne** *($30 for 1 ounce)* combines salicylic acid at the wrong pH with an alcohol base, so this serum ends up being more irritating to skin than helpful. Alcohol in this amount can cause free-radical damage, and that's not what acne-prone skin needs (Source: http://pubs.niaaa.nih.gov/publications/arh27-4/277-284.htm).

☹ **on a clear day, h202Cream** *($20 for 1 ounce)* purports to fight breakouts with hydrogen peroxide. Although this can indeed disinfect skin and kill acne-causing bacteria, the amount of free-radical damage it generates is more of a problem and is not preferred to the more stable benzoyl peroxide or azelaic acid (Sources: *Carcinogenesis*, March 2002, pages 469–475; *Anticancer Research*, July–August 2001, pages 2719–2724; and *Cellular and Molecular Biology*, April 2007, pages 1–2). Oddly, philosophy's choice of jar packaging won't keep the hydrogen peroxide active for long once it is opened because it breaks down quickly in the presence of light and air.

☹ **oxygen peel kit** *($45 for the kit)* is a two-step kit that contains **oxygen foam** and **catalase enzyme capsule**. The foam portion contains a good deal of hydrogen peroxide, which is not recommended for anyone, while the capsules contain the enzyme catalase, which is responsible for the elimination of peroxide. Taken together, this is a do-nothing duo that is not akin to any type of in-office professional peel.

😐 **$$$ the microdelivery peel, hydrating mask** *($25 for 1.3 ounces)* has lots of potential as a moisturizing mask for normal to dry skin, but the lavender oil it contains is a problem for all skin types. There isn't much of it in here, and this is ideally meant to be rinsed from the skin after a brief period, so the rating is more lenient.

☹ **the present, clear powder** *($14 for 1 ounce)* has absorbent properties, but contains several potent irritants, including rosewood, rosemary, and peppermint oils. Lavender oil adds to the mix, and makes this one present you don't want to receive.

😐 **$$$ unplastic surgery to go, big shots wrinkle smoothing swabs** *($25 for 36 swabs)* are liquid-filled, disposable, cotton-tipped swabs filled with a solution said to infuse deeply wrinkled areas with "cutting-edge peptide technology." This water- and slip agent–based formula contains small amounts of two peptides, but neither has substantiated research proving they can smooth etched lines or redefine the contours of an aging face. All in all, a gimmicky product that is not going to put any cosmetics surgeons out of business!

☺ **$$$ big mouth lip plump** *($22 for 0.22 ounce)* is just a very expensive lanolin oil–based, sheer tinted gloss for lips. It's great for keeping dry, chapped lips at bay, but does not contain anything to make lips look larger, though its glossy finish reflects light, which can create the illusion of slightly fuller lips.

☹ **kiss me exfoliating lip scrub and facial** *($15 for 0.5 ounce)* is an emollient sugar-based scrub for lips that works to remove dry, flaky skin and leave it smooth. The problem? Peppermint oil, which only causes irritation. You're better off mixing a bit of table sugar with a nonvolatile plant oil or mineral oil and massaging that mix over dry lips.

PHILOSOPHY MAKEUP

FOUNDATION: 😐 **$$$ the supernatural powder airbrushed canvas SPF 15** *($35)* deserves credit for its pure zinc oxide sunscreen, but this is otherwise a standard loose-powder mineral makeup that comes packaged with a built-in (and removable, if you want to clean or replace it) sponge applicator. The powder shakes onto the sponge to minimize mess, and you buff it over your skin. Like most mineral makeup, the main ingredient is bismuth oxychloride. Despite a lightweight texture, this can make skin feel increasingly dry during wear, and the strong matte finish is offset by noticeable sparkles. Coverage goes from sheer to medium, but you really have to pile this on to get to that level, which increases the dryness later on. Although the range of nine shades is mostly neutral, if mineral makeup intrigues you, consider the silkier-feeling options from bare escentuals before this.

CONCEALER: 😐 **$$$ the supernatural airbrushed color corrector** *($25)* gets you three creamy concealers in one compact, complete with a synthetic brush. The brush's square tip isn't as easy to work with as those with a rounded or tapered tip, and although the concealer applies smoothly and covers well, it creases unless carefully set with powder. Three palettes are available. Light is the best assortment, Medium is OK but two of the shades pull toward peach, and the shades in the Dark palette are too disparate to work together. This would have been better if they were sold as single colors with a slightly tweaked formula and a less creamy finish.

BLUSH: 😐 **$$$ the supernatural airbrush blush** *($25)* has the same packaging, though on a smaller scale, as the supernatural powder airbrushed canvas SPF 15 above. Whereas the foundation is talc-free, this loose powder blush is talc-based. That gives it a silky texture, but the application is so sheer it leaves skin with more sparkles than color. Considering the number of shiny blushes available for much less money (many with shine that clings to skin better than what you'll find with this product), this is one to leave on the shelf.

EYESHADOW: ☹ $$$ the supernatural all-in-one eye palette *($35)* provides three powder eyeshadows, a cream-to-powder cake eyeliner that features two shades in a split pan design, and applicators in one sleek compact. The emollient-feeling eyeshadows apply beautifully, but each has shine (lots of shine), not to mention there is only one palette (best for fair to medium skin tones). The eyeliner is OK in that application is smooth and even, but longevity isn't its strength. As for the applicators, some may find them useful, but the squared tips tend to leave hard edges of color.

EYE AND BROW SHAPER: ☹ $$$ think big big gorgeous eye pencil *($12.50)* is a standard creamy eye pencil that needs routine sharpening and comes in only one shade, a pearlescent white. The company recommends applying it to the inner rim of your lower lashline for a bright-eyed look, but it's not good to place cosmetic ingredients next to the cornea, not to mention that this look never lasts.

LIPSTICK, LIP GLOSS, AND LIPLINER: ✓☺ kiss me clear tube *($10)* is the original, colorless kiss me product and remains an excellent choice for those seeking a lip balm with a non-sticky texture and glossy finish. This lanolin-based balm is a great choice for treating dry, chapped lips and, thankfully, is irritant-free. **✓☺ kiss me red tube** *($10)* is a very good, non-sticky lip balm/gloss hybrid that has the sheerest berry-red tint that heightens, but doesn't brighten one's natural lip color.

☺ $$$ the supernatural lip gloss *($15)* is a standard lip gloss with a wand applicator that has a slightly thick, sticky feel and shimmer-infused finish from each of the sheer colors. This is flavored with mint, but it's subtle and the product does not contain direct peppermint oil so the risk of irritation is slim.**☹ lip shine** *($10)* is a philosophy lip gloss that's exclusive to Sephora stores. It comes in several tempting flavors, including cinnamon buns and mimosa. These thick, sticky glosses are loaded with shimmer and each imparts more sparkle and shine than color. Avoid the empowermint lip shine because it contains peppermint oil.

☹ kiss me – pink tube *($10)* is a very sheer pink gloss with a slick, emollient texture—too bad it is loaded with peppermint oil, so lips get a potent dose of irritation along with a glossy finish. **☹ big mouth lip sheer** *($22)* has a slightly less slick formula that contains ingredients to swell lips for "that bee stung look." It does this by including appreciable amounts of irritating menthol and camphor, neither of which is recommended for regular (or even occasional) application to the lips, though it does make them temporarily swollen.

☹ $$$ the supernatural lip pencil *($12.50)* needs sharpening and is all-around standard except for the fact that the slightly dry application doesn't smear. Otherwise, the few shades are versatile enough to coordinate with several shades of lipstick.

MASCARA: ☹ $$$ think big big gorgeous eyes mascara *($22)* has an enticing name, but the only thing "big" about this mascara is the box it comes in (which is an unreasonable waste of packaging material). If anything, applying this mascara will be a big disappointment. No matter how many times you stroke the brush through your lashes or dip it into the container hoping more product will produce "gorgeous" results, they won't appear. Minimal length and almost no thickness is all you'll achieve. If you are only interested in modest results, this will work well enough. It doesn't smear or flake during the day and washes off easily, but that is hardly worth the price.

☹ **$$$ the supernatural mascara** *($22)* has been reformulated so it's less of a do-nothing-but-darken-lashes mascara, but it still fails to wow, at least if your goal is to build length or thickness. Truly a natural-look mascara, the unconventional formula coats lashes minimally, basically creating minor improvements all around. It's an option if you're 90% satisfied with the lashes you have, but anything less will leave you disappointed, especially at this price, and you have to be careful that the wetter formula doesn't smear before it dries.

BRUSHES: ☺ **$$$ the supernatural brush** *($25)* is a dense, synthetic powder brush whose head is cut straight across. That makes it a workable choice to apply loose-powder foundation (such as the one philosophy sells) or blush. Whereas philosophy used to sell several brushes (usually in sets), they now have decided that you need only one brush for all your makeup needs. That's not possible, any more than a blouse is all you need to wear to go outside and to the office.

SPECIALTY PRODUCTS: ☺ **$$$ the supernatural face bronzer** *($25)* is a liquid bronzing lotion that really is supernatural. The fluid slips over skin and blends easily, providing a translucent wash of bronze color with a subtle glow and slightly moist finish. The sole color is best for fair to barely medium skin; if you have fair skin, this is one of the few bronzing products that looks convincing (meaning it doesn't appear too orange, copper, or deep against light complexions).

☺ **$$$ the supernatural poreless flawless tinted SPF 15** *($30)* is a nonaqueous, silicone-based primer with an in-part titanium dioxide sunscreen. It has the requisite silky texture and smooth matte finish, but is marred by a strange, though sheer, peach tint. This is best for light to medium skin tones (the peachy tinge won't make someone with fair skin happy), and as primers go, this does contain some great antioxidants.

☺ **$$$ the supernatural oil-control blotting tissues** *($10 for 100 sheets)* are standard, non-powdered oil-blotting papers with a tissue-thin texture. They do soak up excess shine or perspiration, and the dispensing method is unique.

☹ **$$$ think big big mouth lip primer** *($25)* is a semi-matte, colorless lipstick that is supposed to fill in lines on the lips and make them smoother pre-lipstick. It does this to a minor extent, but despite plumping claims, the formula doesn't contain anything that makes lips bigger, even temporarily. This is a pricey, superfluous product whose smoothing benefit you can get from many lipsticks.

☹ **$$$ the supernatural fingerpaints** *($25)* is a compact of three minimally creamy colors, each with a smooth, shiny powder finish. Although meant for use on the eyes, lips, and cheeks, the neutral or cool palettes work best as cream eyeshadows. As blush, they're too shiny and/or sheer, and the formula isn't too comfortable on your lips. Despite being named fingerpaints, philosophy included a brush applicator.

PHISODERM (SKIN CARE ONLY)

PHISODERM AT-A-GLANCE

Strengths: Inexpensive; most cleansers are excellent; some good scrubs.

Weaknesses: Bar soap; several products contain problematic ingredients, including lavender oil and alcohol; overall boring toner, moisturizers, and sunscreens; jar packaging.

For more information about pHisoDerm, call (877) 636-2677 or visit www.pHisoDerm.com or www.Beautypedia.com.

☹ **Anti-Blemish Gel Facial Wash** *($4.89 for 6 ounces)* includes sodium C14-16 olefin sulfonate as its main cleansing agent, which makes this too drying and irritating for all skin types. The salicylic acid's brief contact with skin won't allow it to exfoliate, as claimed.

☺ **Deep Cleaning Cream Cleanser, for Normal to Dry Skin** *($4.99 for 6 ounces)* is a very good detergent-based cleanser for its intended skin type. This removes makeup easily, but the mineral oil content means it is best used with a washcloth. Despite the name, this doesn't go any deeper than other cleansers. All well-formulated cleansers (of which there are hundreds) will remove dirt, excess oil, and makeup from the skin's surface.

✓☺ **Deep Cleaning Cleanser, for Normal to Oily Skin** *($4.49 for 6 ounces)* rinses much better than the Deep Cleansing Cream Cleanser above, and is a great option for normal to slightly oily skin, especially if you need to remove your makeup quickly.

✓☺ **Deep Cleaning Cleanser, for Sensitive Skin** *($4.89 for 6 ounces)* is a brilliant option for sensitive skin that is normal to dry. This gentle, fragrance-free cleanser contains enough mineral oil that rinsing may be a slight problem, but this ingredient also helps remove makeup and cushions delicate skin, even when used with a washcloth.

☹ **Foaming Facial Wash** *($6.99 for 5 ounces)* contains lavender oil, which makes this otherwise good water-soluble cleanser too irritating for all skin types, and one that should never be used around the eyes.

☺ **Gentle Skin Cleanser for Baby** *($4.79 for 8 ounces)* is similar to but with fewer ingredients than the Deep Cleansing Cream Cleanser, for Normal to Dry Skin above, and the same review applies. Considering the name and positioning of this cleanser, it should be fragrance-free, but isn't. This is a better choice for teens or adults than for babies.

✓☺ **pH2o Daily Replenishing Wash** *($6.29 for 6 ounces)* is a good, gentle, water-soluble cleanser for all but very oily skin or for those who wear heavy makeup. It won't replenish skin, but it will leave it feeling soft and smooth, not to mention clean!

☹ **Skin Cleansing Bar, Unscented** *($2.49 for a 3.3-ounce bar)* is a very standard bar soap that, unscented or not, is too drying and irritating for all skin types.

😐 **Clear Confidence Self Heating Daily Scrub** *($5.69 for 4 ounces)* is similar to Olay's Regenerist Thermal Skin Polisher, but the pHisoDerm product costs significantly less. Just like Olay's option, this scrub heats up because of an exothermic reaction when mixed with water; pHisoDerm achieves the effect with a zeolite mineral. The warming sensation does not detoxify skin or improve acne. If anything, topical scrubs should be used with extreme care or avoided completely if acne is present, and heat can cause capillaries to surface and break.

☺ **Nurturing Facial Polish** *($5.89 for 6 ounces)* won't nurture your skin (the amount of vitamins included is negligible and they will be rinsed from your skin before they have a chance to work), but it is a standard, effective topical scrub. The formula lacks irritants, which is a welcome change from the norm, and it comes in a slightly emollient base that cushions skin, but also leaves a slight film. Nurturing Facial Polish is best for normal to dry skin not prone to blemishes. This product does contain quite a bit of fragrance.

☺ **pH2o Anytime Nurturing Scrub with Gentle Microbeads** *($6.09 for 5 ounces)* is similar to the Nurturing Facial Polish above, except it adds a small amount of clay, which mostly serves to thicken the product. Otherwise, the same review applies.

😐 **Nurturing Toner** *($6.99 for 7 ounces)* has too much alcohol to make it nurturing, and the amount of intriguing water-binding agents is paltry, making this a minimally beneficial toner for normal to slightly oily skin.

☹ **Clarifying Gel Facial Moisturizer** *($8.99 for 4 ounces)* would be wholeheartedly recommended as an ultra-light gel moisturizer for oily skin with dry areas, but the amount of lavender oil it contains makes it too problematic for all skin types.

😐 **Daily Moisturizer with SPF 15** *($7.89 for 2 ounces)* has the UVA protection part right, thanks to its in-part avobenzone sunscreen, but that's the only reason to consider this otherwise ho-hum product. The lightweight lotion base will please those with normal to oily skin, but part of the lightness results from the 3% alcohol content. The fragrance and preservatives outweigh the advertised vitamins, meaning they're mere window dressing. That's a shame because if slightly more thought had gone into this sunscreen, it would have been enthusiastically recommended.

☹ **Extra Rich Nighttime Moisturizer** *($8.59 for 2 ounces)* is an uninspired moisturizer that contains lavender oil, which makes it a problem for all skin types, and the formula isn't all that exciting, which speaks to the boring nature of this product. Almost any moisturizer from Nivea bests this option.

☹ **pH2o Everyday Moisturizer** *($8.19 for 2 ounces)* is a poorly formulated moisturizer that lists sd-alcohol as its third ingredient. The jar packaging renders the vitamins (antioxidants) useless shortly after the product is opened. If you're shopping for a facial moisturizer at the drugstore, this is one to leave on the shelf.

PHYSICIANS FORMULA

PHYSICIANS FORMULA AT-A-GLANCE

Strengths: Inexpensive; almost all products fragrance-free; outstanding cleansers; one worthwhile toner; pressed powder with broad-spectrum sunscreen; several bronzing powder options (primarily for fair to light skin tones); one of the only lines at the drugstore selling matte finish eyeshadows; the loose powder; most of the blushes; good liquid liner; excellent automatic brow pencil.

Weaknesses: Dated moisturizer formulas; several sunscreens lack sufficient UVA protection; microdermabrasion kit is mixed bag; jar packaging; several of the makeup products epitomize wasteful packaging; the shade selection for almost all the foundations and concealers is awful; tons of gimmicky products that don't perform as well as you'd think but are eye-catching in their compacts; several bad eyelining options; the lip color and lip plumper; mostly average to disappointing mascaras.

For more information about Physicians Formula, call (800) 227-0333 or visit www.physiciansformula.com or www.Beautypedia.com.

PHYSICIANS FORMULA SKIN CARE

✓😊 **Gentle Cleansing Lotion, for Normal to Dry Skin** *($7.25 for 8 ounces)* is a very standard, but also very good, fragrance-free cleansing lotion for its intended skin type. It is also recommended for those with sensitive skin who cannot tolerate detergent cleansing agents. You will need a washcloth for complete removal.

✓😊 **Deep Pore Cleansing Gel, for Normal to Oily Skin** *($6.95 for 8 ounces)* doesn't go any deeper than other water-soluble cleansers, but is a standout due to its gentle, fragrance-free formula that cleanses thoroughly and rinses completely.

✓☺ **Eye Makeup Remover Lotion, for Normal to Dry Skin** *($4.75 for 2 ounces)* has a formula that's remarkably similar to the Gentle Cleansing Lotion, for Normal to Dry Skin above, except this version is marketed as a makeup remover. It works in that capacity, even removing waterproof mascara, but if you're already using or considering the Gentle Cleansing Lotion, you don't need this as well.

☺ **Eye Makeup Remover Pads, for Normal to Dry Skin** *($5.75 for 60 pads)* are an effective but greasy way to remover eye makeup, including waterproof mascara. These pads are best used before washing your face, because the residue they leave behind isn't something you want to go to bed with on your face. By the way, a cheaper version of this product that would work just as well given the ingredient list would be plain mineral oil.

☹ **Oil Free Eye Makeup Remover Pads, for Normal to Oily Skin** *($5.75 for 60 pads)* contain only a tiny amount of cleansing agents capable of removing makeup, and is mostly fragrant rose water and irritating witch hazel. That's eau de cologne, not skin care!

☺ **Vital Lash Oil Free Eye Makeup Remover, for Normal to Oily Skin** *($4.75 for 2 ounces)* isn't vital to anyone's eyelashes. It's just a standard, detergent-based makeup remover that is effective and that you'll need, particularly around the eyes, if you wear a good amount of makeup to make sure you're getting everything off.

😐 **Gentle Refreshing Toner, for Dry to Very Dry Skin** *($6.95 for 8 ounces)* is a standard, but OK, alcohol-free toner for normal to dry skin. It is fragrance-free.

☹ **Pore Refining Skin Freshener, for Normal to Dry Skin** *($6.95 for 8 ounces)* is mostly water and alcohol, and as such is an undesirable option, especially for dry skin.

😐 **Collagen Cream Concentrate, for Dry to Very Dry Skin** *($8.95 for 2 ounces)* contains a tiny amount of collagen, but no amount applied topically can impact your skin's own collagen. This is otherwise an average, jar-packaged, fragrance-free moisturizer that's mostly water, plant oil, and lots of thickeners. It's OK for its intended skin types.

😐 **Deep Moisture Cream, for Normal to Dry Skin** *($8.50 for 4 ounces)* is a very basic, fragrance-free moisturizer for dry skin. Although this is inexpensive, it's also short on anything remotely state-of-the-art.

😐 **Elastin/Collagen Moisture Lotion, for Normal to Dry Skin** *($8.50 for 4 ounces)* is similar to and earns the same review as the Deep Moisture Cream, for Normal to Dry Skin, above.

😐 **Enriched Dry Skin Concentrate, for Dry to Very Dry Skin** *($8.50 for 4 ounces)* is a blend of plant oils with Vaseline, lanolin, slip agent, preservatives, and fragrance. Nothing too exciting here, but most of these ingredients are appropriate, though exceptionally basic and passé, for dry to very dry skin (though the plant oil's potential will be lost because of jar packaging).

😐 **Extra Rich Rehydrating Moisturizer, for Normal to Dry Skin** *($8.50 for 4 ounces)* is an exceptionally basic, dated moisturizer that's an OK option for dry skin, assuming you're willing to settle for less than what skin deserves.

😐 **Luxury Eye Cream, for Normal to Dry Skin** *($5.95 for 0.5 ounce)* contains some emollient ingredients with a rich texture, but overall is a basic formula that you could easily replace just by using plain Vaseline, or even better by using a plant oil such as olive oil, around the eye area to treat very dry skin.

😐 **Nourishing Night Cream, for Dry to Very Dry Skin** *($5.95 for 1 ounce)* is an oil-based moisturizer for very dry skin, but the formula itself is quite dated and the greasy texture isn't all that appealing.

☹ **Oil Control Oil-Free Moisturizer, for Normal to Oily Skin** *($8.50 for 4 ounces)* contains a minimal amount of absorbent ingredients and the thickeners that precede them on the ingredient list won't do a thing to keep excess oil in check. This is an average moisturizer for normal to dry skin, but is not appropriate for any degree of oily skin.

☹ **Self Defense Color Corrective Moisturizing Lotion SPF 15** *($7.50 for 2 ounces)* lacks the UVA-protecting ingredients of titanium dioxide, zinc oxide, avobenzone, Tinosorb, or Mexoryl SX, and is not recommended.

☺ **Sun Shield Extra Sensitive Skin SPF 25** *($9.95 for 6 ounces)* contains titanium dioxide as the sole active ingredient, and is tinted slightly to avoid the bluish white cast common to some mineral sunscreens. The silicone-enhanced texture is suitable for normal to dry skin, while the fragrance- and irritant-free nature of this product makes it a boon for sensitive skin (including those with rosacea). What keeps this from earning a Paula's Pick rating is the paucity of antioxidants and the lack of skin-identical ingredients.

☺ **Sun Shield for Faces Extra Sensitive Skin SPF 25** *($8.95 for 4 ounces)* is very similar to the Sun Shield Extra Sensitive Skin SPF 25 sunscreen above, and the same review applies.

☹ **Sun Shield for Faces Ultra-Light Cream SPF 20** *($8.95 for 4 ounces)* lacks the UVA-protecting ingredients of titanium dioxide, zinc oxide, avobenzone, Tinosorb, or Mexoryl SX, and is not recommended.

☹ **Sun Shield Lip Care SPF 15** *($2 for 0.15 ounce)* lacks the UVA-protecting ingredients of titanium dioxide, zinc oxide, avobenzone, Tinosorb, or Mexoryl SX, and is not recommended.

☹ **Sun Shield Sunless Tanning Lotion SPF 20** *($9.95 for 6 ounces)* lacks the UVA-protecting ingredients of titanium dioxide, zinc oxide, avobenzone, Tinosorb, or Mexoryl SX, and is not recommended.

☹ **Derm@Home Mineral MicroDermabrasion System** *($29.95 for the kit)* is a two-step kit that promises professional-level microdermabrasion for skin. Before I discuss the products, it's important to note that recent research indicates that repeated professional microdermabrasion treatments have diminishing returns. First is the **Mineral MicroDermabrasion Cream**, which blends alumina crystals with buffering thickeners and some gemstones, which add no change to the outcome but sound impressive. This step is easily replaced by a washcloth. After polishing skin with this scrub, you apply the **Mineral Post-Treatment Moisturizer**, a straightforward product that's mostly thickeners and common water-binding agents. Some soothing agents are included, too, but their effects are offset by the menthol, which is never a good idea for application to skin.

PHYSICIANS FORMULA MAKEUP

Note: The shade range of this line does not cater to darker skin tones. In fact, for some products, only those with fair to light skin will find options.

FOUNDATION: ☺ **Pearls of Perfection Multi-Colored Face Tint** *($12.95)* is a sheer, gel-based face tint that has a lightly creamy texture and subtle sparkly finish. This is fine for a very soft wash of all-over or strategically placed color. The two remaining shades offer the choice of a soft gold glow or sheer bronze.

☹ **Mineral Wear Talc-Free Mineral Foundation** *($10.45)* has an odd name not only because most liquid foundations are talc-free, but also because talc is a mineral! This water- and silicone-based foundation is dispensed from its tube onto an attached sponge. The sponge is a bit small for application to the entire face, but it smooths the product well. Despite an initially attractive texture, this sets to a strong matte finish that appears chalky and tends to just sit on the skin rather than mesh with it, which is not good. Out of the six shades, the only real-skin shades are Classic Ivory and Natural Beige. Although not a total loss, this is only worth considering by those with very oily skin who desire medium coverage.

☹ **Le Velvet Film Makeup SPF 15** *($5.25 refill; $3.75 for compact)* is an old-fashioned cream-to-powder foundation that goes on surprisingly moist and creamy and can be blended out fairly sheer. The SPF is part titanium dioxide, which is great, but the finish is somewhat chalky and none of the colors resemble real skin tones, making this one to avoid.

☹ **Sun Shield Liquid Makeup SPF 15** *($5.95)* belongs in the same category as Max Factor's antiquated Whipped Creme Makeup. Insufficient UVA protection, a dated formula, and some incredibly poor colors add up to a foundation that is a must-avoid.

☹ **Beauty Spiral Brightening Compact Foundation** *($9.95)* is a cream-to-powder makeup that "spirals" two colors together. It's eye-catching, but that's all this substandard foundation has going for it. The thick texture offers sheer coverage and a dry, powdery finish that just doesn't feel or look great on the skin. The three colors are passable, but there are far more elegant cream-to-powder foundations from Cover Girl or Revlon, and their options include sun protection.

☹ **Beauty Spiral Skin Brightening Liquid Foundation** *($9.95)* is a sheer, light-textured foundation that has an uneven, slightly pasty-looking finish due to the high amount of titanium dioxide. The three shades are passable, but nothing this chalky can have any sort of brightening effect.

☹ **CoverToxTen50 Wrinkle Therapy Foundation** *($12.95)* is one of a few foundations claiming to work like Botox, without painful injections. One of the main ingredients is GABA (gamma amino butyric acid). Please refer to Chapter Seven, *Cosmetics Ingredient Dictionary*, for an in-depth discussion of this ingredient. Suffice it to say, GABA does not work to smooth wrinkles; not even Botox works for this purpose if it is applied topically rather than injected. Another anti-aging ingredient touted on the package is vitamin C (as tetrahexyldecyl ascorbate) but there is so little in this foundation, your skin won't even notice it. Although it is clever and convenient that this initially creamy liquid foundation is dispensed onto a built-in brush, it does little to enhance application. It also doesn't change the fact that no matter how much blending you do, this foundation always looks heavy and somewhat opaque, with a flat, slightly chalky finish. It is not the answer to camouflaging wrinkles; in fact, its finish tends to emphasize them and most of the colors go on too peach or pink to recommend.

CONCEALER: ☺ **Magic Cube Concealer** *($5.95)* is billed as a "high tech cream-to-powder" concealer and, although that's a bit over the top for what you get, this happens to be Physicians Formula's only worthwhile concealer. Its light, silicone-based texture glides over skin without excessive slip and provides medium coverage with minimal risk of creasing. The Yellow and Green shades are missteps and only add a strange hue to skin, but Light and Neutral Beige are good choices.

😐 **Wanderful Wand Brightening Concealer** *($6.95)* is a liquid concealer housed in a pen-style applicator with a built-in synthetic brush. It has good slip and is easy to blend, but coverage is disappointly sheer and its flat finish doesn't put skin in its best light, so to speak. The Yellow and Green shades are terrible; Light and Neutral Beige are OK, but not enough to elevate this to a happy face rating. 😐 **Gentle Cover Concealer Stick** *($5.45)* is a thick, lipstick-style concealer that provides moderate coverage with a heavy-looking, crease-prone finish. Two of the four colors are marginally acceptable, but this is only recommended for those who refuse to consider the many superior concealers at the drugstore.

☹ **CoverToxTen50 Wrinkle Therapy Concealer** *($8.95)* has the most unbelievable claims for a concealer I've ever seen, and that's saying a lot! Billed as serious care for your wrinkles, it promises to not only reduce their appearance, but also to reduce dark circles by 77%, relieve puffy eyes, and enhance collagen synthesis—all with "no prescription needed." There isn't anything remotely drug-like in this product. The wrinkle-erasing claim is tied to GABA (gamma aminobutyric acid), a neurotransmitter inhibitor whose proponents say that it works like topical Botox. Without rehashing all of the details of this ingredient (it's discussed many times elsewhere in this book and in Chapter Seven, *Cosmetic Ingredient Dictionary*), it doesn't work—not even Botox works like Botox when applied topically rather than injected. This liquid concealer comes in a tube with a built-in synthetic brush applicator. Although quite silky thanks to the high amount of silicone, coverage is sparse and the matte finish manages to creep into every crevice, line, or large pore on the skin. Couple this with mostly peachy pink colors and misleading claims and it's easy to see why this is not recommended.

☹ **Concealer Palette 4-in-1 Concealing Palette** *($7.95)* provides three shades of concealer and a pressed powder, each tiny squares in one compact whose top revolves to allow access to one shade at a time. A brush is included, but it's too small for practical use. Even if the brush were better, the creamy concealers have a dry, powdery finish that looks obvious on skin, the powder is waxy, and the whole product is more gimmicky than useful.

☹ **Instant Makeover Tool 2-in-1 Wet/Dry Concealer/Foundation** *($7.95)* is a thick, chubby pencil that needs sharpening. The concept is that you use the product dry as a concealer or mixed with a bit of water, which turns it into a sheer foundation. Neither option works very well or looks the least bit natural. Dry application produces opaque coverage and a creamy, crease-prone finish, while wet application is tricky to blend evenly and tends to streak. If the colors were more neutral this might have been workable, but they're not.

☹ **Concealer Twins Cream Concealer 2-in-1 Correct and Cover SPF 10** *($6.95)* has an admirable (though not quite high enough) titanium dioxide sunscreen, but an otherwise lackluster creamy texture. You get a flesh-toned color on one end and a yellow or green hue on the other, but both leave much to be desired.

☹ **Gentle Cover Cream Concealer SPF 10** *($5.45)* is a mineral oil– and wax-based concealer with a wand applicator and a titanium dioxide sunscreen. This formula will easily crease into any lines around the eye. The Yellow and Green shades are horrid, while Light is barely passable.

☹ **Powder Finish Concealer Stick SPF 15** *($5.45)* is a creamy stick concealer with titanium dioxide as one of the active ingredients for sun protection. This is nice, but the only flesh-toned shade (Light) is too pink to look natural (especially with this concealer's thick texture), and the powder finish is minimal—it tends to stay creamy and creases easily.

☹ **Concealer 101 Perfecting Concealer Duo** *($7.25)* doesn't make the grade as an introduction to concealers, at least not if one of your prerequisites is shades that resemble skin. The texture, coverage, and finish of this concealer are quite nice, but that doesn't mean a thing when the unnatural skin colors scream "obvious" over whatever you're trying to hide.

☹ **Beauty Spiral Perfecting Concealer** *($6.95)* is rarely seen in drugstore displays for Physicians Formula makeup, and that's fine because this creamy compact concealer comes in two awful colors (bright yellow and green) that absolutely look unnatural and unflattering on anyone's skin.

☹ **Mineral Wear Talc-Free Mineral Cream Concealer SPF 10** *($6.95)* provides sun protection via 15% titanium dioxide, but that amount also gives this liquid concealer an unusually opaque finish, which doesn't make the four awful shades look any better.

☹ **Conceal Rx Physicians Strength Concealer** *($7.95)* has a ridiculous name, because there is no such thing as a physician's strength concealer. They claim this liquid concealer is the prescription for "any and all imperfections" due to its coverage capability. This does provide full coverage that can camouflage dark circles, redness, or bruising but the result is heavy and chalky, while none of the colors resemble real skin tones in the least.

☹ **Circle Rx Circle Control Concealer** *($8.95)* is only "just what the doctor ordered" if your doctor is in favor of runny concealers that dispense too heavily and look opaque and chalky on skin. Yes, this conceals dark circles but so do many other concealers whose finish doesn't call attention to itself (and also comes in much better colors). By the way, the plastic syringe packaging is corny to the max!

POWDER: ✓☺ Loose-to-Go Multi-Colored Loose Powder *($11.95)* is a pressed powder in a loose-powder tub. The component includes a "shaver" that, with a twist, dispenses a small amount of loose powder out of the slits in the sifter. It is clever, but at times too much powder is shaved off, and the excess remains in the top, making things just as messy as most loose powders. Packaging aside, this talc-based powder has a superior smooth texture and satin finish that leaves skin with a soft glow (well, except for the Loose Bronzer, which is very shiny). As with most Physicians Formula powders, multiple colors merge into one on skin, and this follows suit. The formula and finish are best for normal to dry skin.

☺ **CoverToxTen50 Wrinkle Therapy Face Powder** *($12.95)* is a talc-based pressed powder with GABA, which is said to work like Botox to reduce wrinkles and expression lines. It doesn't work as claimed but this sheer, creamy-feeling powder is a very good option for normal to dry skin. The three shades appear slightly pink in the compact, but go on soft enough so as not to be a concern. There are no shades for medium to dark skin tones. Just to be clear: although this is recommended, it does not do a better job of reducing the appearance of wrinkles than any other recommended powder (and, generally speaking, powdering isn't the way to make wrinkles less apparent).

☺ **Retro Glow Face Lace Balancing Face Powder** *($11.95)* is an attractively packaged, noticeably decorated compact containing a talc- and kaolin-based pressed powder. Recommended for and ideally best for oily skin, it has a sheer application and dry, slightly powdery matte finish. The two shades are very good, but limited to fair/light skin tones.

☺ **Magic Mosaic Multi-Colored Custom Pressed Powder** *($12.95)* is a tightly pressed, talc-based powder that features overlapping circles of tone-on-tone colors. Applying this to skin produces a uniform color that is quite sheer and non-intrusive, though it does have a dry texture. The Light Bronzer/Bronzer and Ivory/Creamy Natural shades have noticeable shine, while the other four options have a very subtle shine that's suitable for daytime.

☺ **SolarPowder SPF 20 Face Powder** *($12.95)* is a talc-based, pressed bronzing powder that includes an impressive titanium dioxide–based sunscreen. The three shades (a Translucent shade that's best for light skin and two bronzers) go on sheer, and each has three colors, representing a picture of the sun setting over a beach (it sounds odd, but it fits the theme). Swirling a powder brush over the entire powder cake results in one uniform color with a tiny amount of shine. Although it would be nice if a greater range of skin-tone shades were available, this pressed powder with sunscreen is one to consider, especially if you want to pair it with a foundation that contains sunscreen for a touch of bronze color without the sun damage.

☺ **Mineral Wear Talc-Free Mineral Face Powder** *($12.95)* has a smoother, silkier texture and better application/appearance on skin than the Mineral Wear Talc-Free Mineral Loose Powder below. The mica-based powder contains much less zinc oxide than its loose counterpart, which contributes significantly to its natural, yet slightly powdery, look on skin. The five shades are good and include two bronzing powder choices.

☺ **Baked Pyramid Matte Bronzer** *($11.95)* is a good pressed-powder bronzer that comes in two semi-matte colors. Dry application produces sheer color and an almost matte finish that can be layered for more intensity. Wet application reveals stronger color and a shimmer finish, though you have to blend carefully to avoid streaking (this isn't a problem once the powder dries).

☺ **Powder Palette Multi-Colored Face Powder** *($12.95)* is a kaleidoscopic arrangement of different colors that all come off as the same color on the skin, as it should be. The range of shades has improved; although some look a bit odd in the compact, they blend on neutral and leave a soft, translucent finish. The Light Bronzer option is matte, while Peach-to-Glow is better as blush than an all-over powder. Avoid the Highlighter shade because of its contrasting colors, and avoid Green, for obvious reasons.

☺ **ReVined Rejuvenating Face Powder** *($12.95)*. Physicians Formula seemingly has a powder for every skin type and concern, so why not include one that claims to fight the visible signs of aging by banishing free radicals? This talc-based pressed powder contains tiny amounts of red and white wine extracts, and is embossed with a bunch of grapes as a visual tie-in to the antioxidant claim. How cute! I wouldn't count on any antioxidant benefit from this powder, but it does have a suede-smooth texture and leaves skin looking polished with a faint hint of shine. All three colors are sheer and nearly translucent, which makes getting an exact match a non-issue.

😐 **Face Aid Skin Controlling Face Powder** *($12.95)* is a dry-textured, talc-based powder that claims to prevent breakouts because it contains 1.5% salicylic acid. That active is on hand, but it's ineffective in a nonaqueous product because the pH cannot be established or maintained. As a shine-controlling powder this works very well, but the colors are limited. The most convincing shade is Beige.

😐 **Mineral Wear Talc-Free Mineral Loose Powder** *($10.45)* contains mica and zinc oxide instead of talc, which adds up to a mineral-based loose powder (but talc is a mineral, so almost all powders meet the criteria). The zinc oxide causes this light-textured powder to feel dry and look somewhat thick and pasty on skin, but that effect is offset to some extent by the mica's shine. Among the six shades, three are too peach to consider, including Creamy Natural, Natural Beige, and Sand Beige. The dry finish of this powder is best for oily skin, but you'll have to be OK with the shine it leaves behind, which kind of defeats the purpose of using powder. 😐 **Mineral Wear Talc-Free Matte Finishing Veil** *($11.95)* is a loose powder packaged in a container that is attached to a sifter which feeds the powder onto the built-in brush. The corn- and aluminum starch–based powder feels weightless and has a very dry texture and finish that is only suitable for very oily skin not prone to blemishes. Further limiting its appeal, the sole shade is only suitable for those with fair skin. The 😐 **Mineral Wear Talc-Free Bronzing Veil** *($12.95)* has the same formula and packaging as the Matte Finishing Veil above, but comes in a slightly orange/bronze shade that is an OK option for medium skin tones, but not for all-over use.

😐 **Pearls of Perfection Multi-Colored Powder Pearls** *($11.95)* are large pots of colored, talc-based powder beads, available in bronze, flesh, and shiny highlighting shades. They're fun in concept, but the execution is messy and not worth the effort. Still, if you're a fan of Guerlain's Meteorites Powder for the Face ($48), this is quite similar and only one-fourth the price.

😐 **Retro Glow Mosaic Powder** *($12.95)* brings you a "timeless arrangement of 5 translucent shades" in one compact, but whether you choose the Translucent or Bronze options, each comes off as one sheer shade on skin and leaves it laced with lots of sparkles. Although the matte finish of the powder lasts, the sparkles tend to flake off. Come to think of it, powders with shine that flake are retro, meaning that once was the norm but the best options in this category don't do that anymore.

😐 **Skinsitive Ultra-Gentle Face Powder for Sensitive Skin** *($11.95)* holds no particular advantage for sensitive skin over any other talc-based powder. In fact, including aluminum starch as the second ingredient is a disadvantage for those with sensitive skin, because aluminum starch is known to cause contact dermatitis when used in high amounts. This is best for oily skin, and the two colors are limited to fair or light skin tones.

☹ **Les Botaniques Botanical Face PowderBronzer** *($11.95)* is a talc-based pressed-powder bronzer embossed with cutesy designs of flowers and the blazing sun. It contains a few botanicals, but in very small amounts, meaning they're mere window dressing. This has a dry, almost stiff texture that applies unevenly, and both shades impart more of a yellow-orange than tan color to skin, which only makes matters worse.

BLUSH: ☺ **Powder Palette Multi-Colored Blush** *($10.95)* combines several blush shades in a mosaic pattern that is eye-catching, but the fact is the colors come off as one unified shade on skin, just like a standard powder blush. This has a smooth, impressively silky texture and dry finish laced with sparkles. The sparkly effect is subtle, which explains why each shade looks matte in the package. Blushing Mocha is suitable as a powder bronzer—as if this line needs more options in that regard!

☺ **Cheek Palette Cream-to-Powder Blush** *($7.95)* doesn't have a powder finish, so ignore the inaccurate name. This is actually a very good, sheer cream blush that blends smoothly, doesn't streak, and leaves a soft cream finish. You get three colors in one compact, but despite looking different, they all appear similar on skin. This blush is best for normal to dry skin that is not prone to blemishes.

☺ **Mineral Wear Talc-Free Mineral Blush** *($10.95)* is a mica-based pressed-powder blush that has a beautifully silky texture and smooth application. The color payoff is much better than the Magic Mosaic Multi-Colored Custom Blush below, while the radiant (rather than sparkling) finish is attractive. The Nude Glow shade is closer to overall skin color than what you'd want from a blush, but the other shades are soft and well-suited for application to cheeks.

😐 **Planet Blush Powder & Blush 2-in-1** *($10.95)* features a split compact with a shiny pressed highlighting powder on one side and a softly shiny blush tone on the other. The domed top is there to allow a tiny blush brush to stand upright in the center of the compact, but its rough texture and extremely short handle make it impractical to use. This is another gimmicky product that will take up more room in your makeup bag than it should.

😐 **Baked Blush Wet/Dry Blush** *($10.95)* is a domed pressed-powder blush whose three shades are all noticeably shiny. The fact that this powder is "baked" doesn't make it better or preferred over other options. If anything, it tends to crumble easily despite applying smoothly (though it's pigment-rich, so apply sparingly unless you want stronger color). Wet application is tricky because of streaking, but if you're careful (and want intense shine) it works.

😐 **Magic Mosaic Multi-Colored Custom Blush** *($10.95)* looks pretty and pillowy in its pressed-powder compact, but this blush is so sheer and so difficult to pick up on the brush that you'll be left wondering why you bothered unless your goal is the faintest hint of blush. Even the Soft Mocha/Mocha shade (for bronzing) goes on so soft no one will believe you've been kissed by the sun. Still, this does have a matte finish.

☹ **Pearls of Perfection Multi-Colored Blush** *($9.95)* looks cute if the idea of pressed spheres of powder blush appeals to you. Application, however, is another issue because it's difficult to pick up enough powder on your brush so that it will show on skin, and all you end up getting is noticeable shine. From concept to execution, this isn't any match for a standard pressed-powder blush.

EYESHADOW: ✓☺ **Matte Collection Quad Eye Shadow** *($6.75)* has some of the best neutral color combinations around, with a welcome silky texture and matte finish that applies and blends beautifully. There are only four quads available, but each is excellent, though each one does not have a suitable shade for eyelining.

✓☺ **Bright Collection Shimmery Quads Eye Shadow** *($6.75)* is identical to the Matte Collection Quad Eye Shadow above, except with these sets all four shades have shine (which tends to stay in place, making these highly recommended if you prefer shiny eyeshadows). Otherwise, the same basic comments apply.

☺ **Color Eyes Cream Eyeshadow Stick** *($5.95)* drags a bit during application and has a slightly tacky finish, but if you're a fan of cream eyeshadows, these stay around longer than most and don't crease. The neutral and mauve-toned shades all have shine, but if that doesn't bother you this is worth a look.

☺ **Baked Collection Wet-Dry Eye Shadow** *($7.60)* offers three well-coordinated, shiny eyeshadows (what the company refers to a "luminous matte") in one compact. Most of the trios have one darker shade to use as eyeliner, and these have smooth, dry textures that blend nicely and last, plus the shine doesn't flake. True to the name, these may be applied wet or dry (most powder eyeshadows have this feature) with wet application intensifying the color and shiny finish. Watch out for Baked Spices—the orange tones aren't the easiest to work with. Baked Sweets has the same issue with its colors.

☺ **Mineral Wear Talc-Free Mineral Fluid Powder Eye Shadow** *($6.95)* has a name that's long, confusing, and inaccurate because minerals comprise a very small portion of this loose powder eyeshadow. It comes with a pointed sponge tip applicator, and between that and the initially "wet" feel, this tends to drag over skin and not blend well. It becomes silky once it sets and does not flake or smear, which is a plus especially because the shine from each shade is intense (and slightly metallic). This is an intriguing option if you want something novel for eyeshadow and are willing to apply this with a brush.

😐 **Mineral Wear Talc-Free Eye Shadow Quad** *($8.95)* comes packaged in a compact with no dividers between the colors, though most of the sets are coordinated well and include three matte and one shiny shade. The issue is primarily texture: although these feel silky, the formula is very dry, goes on too sheer (so lots of layering is required if you want the color to show), and the dryness causes flaking and shortens wear time.

😐 **Bronze Gems Matte & Bright Bronzer, Highlighter, and Eye Shadow** *($12.95)* combines a bronzing powder with soft shine along with three smaller "sections" of complementary shades of shimmer powder. Whether blended together or used separately (such as bronzing powder on cheeks and highlighting powder as eyeshadow), the result is sheer color and shine that tends to flake. All told, this looks much better in the compact than it does on skin.

😐 **Mineral Wear Talc-Free Mineral Eyeshadow Duo** *($6.95)* is talc-free, but the mica base is a bit too dry for smooth, even application. The low-commitment colors are very sheer and the shine is almost non-existent, but there are better powder eyeshadows at the drugstore.

😐 **Mosaic Cream Eye Shadow Liquid Powder Technology** *($7.95)* provides five liquid-to-powder eyeshadows in one compact. Among the two sets, Nutmeg Mosaic is very shiny, but the Mauve/Berry Mosaic has shine, too. These apply a bit unevenly and set quickly, which makes blending trickier than necessary. But if you're looking for something different in the eyeshadow department, this fills the bill.

☹ **Eyebrightener Multi-Colored Eyelighter** *($7.95)* is definitely eye-catching. Unfortunately, this variegated display of colors ends up placing a sweep of intense shine and is powdery enough to flake excessively during application, making it more of a bother than it's worth.

EYE AND BROW SHAPER: ✓☺ **Eye Definer Felt-Tip Eye Marker** *($6.95)* looks like a fine-tipped marker and applies like a liquid eyeliner. The felt tip is firm yet comfortable, making it easy to draw a continuous thick or thin line. You'll find this dries almost immediately and wears all day without chipping, smearing, or fading. Bravo, Physicians Formula! ✓☺ **Brow Definer Automatic Brow Pencil** *($5.95)* ranks as one of the best brow pencils at any price, and the shade selection includes options for all but red or auburn brows. It applies smoothly and allows you to build color in sheer layers, which makes for natural-looking brows. The slightly thick powder finish lasts without smearing, while the brow comb (built into the cap) finishes things with precision.

☺ **MicroKohl Eye Definer Ultra-Slim Automatic Kohl Eyeliner Pencil** *($6.95)* is an automatic, non-retractable pencil that has a creamy-smooth application. The finish is creamy, too, and is meant to be smudged (a smudge tip is housed on the other end of the pencil).

😐 **Flat Liner Automatic Eyeliner Pencil** *($5.95)* is a twist-up, retractable pencil with an angled, flat, wide tip. The unique shape allows you to draw an unusually thick or traditional thin line, though the formula is creamy enough to smear and fade before the day is done.

😐 **Brow Corrector** *($5.95)* is an average clear brow gel that is an OK option for grooming the brows, but its stiff finish isn't as appealing as the brow gels from Cover Girl or Max Factor.

😐 **Fineline Brow Pencil** *($4.25)* needs sharpening and comes in three decent shades. It has a standard, dry texture. If you don't mind routine sharpening, this is one of the least expensive reliable brow pencils.

😐 **Mineral Wear Talc-Free Mineral Eye Liner Pencil** *($6.95)* contains a couple of minerals but the very same ones show up in almost every eye pencil being sold (because they help create the color or add texture to the pencil). This is not a unique option; it's just another standard, creamy eye pencil that needs routine sharpening. It is good that this is minimally prone to smearing or fading once it has set.

☹ **Eye Definer Automatic Eye Pencil** *($5.50)* is a twist-up, retractable eye pencil that is greasier than most, which means it can smear and smudge easily, and it does. ☹ **Eye Definer Metallic Automatic Eye Pencil** *($5.25)* is identical to the Eye Definer Automatic Eye Pencil above except for its metallic finish. ☹ **Retro Glow Liquid Kohl Eyeliner** *($5.95)* may have retro packaging, but that's the only interesting element of this terrible liquid eyeliner. Application is sketchy, it takes far too long to dry, and it smears readily. ☹ **Virtual Eyes Multi-Reflective Liquid Eyeliner** *($6.95)* is almost as bad as the Retro Liquid Kohl Eyeliner, the difference being that this applies choppy with intermittent sheer and intense sparkle-infused color.

☹ **Eyebrightener Brightening Liquid Eyeliner** *($6.50)* has the same issues as the Virtual Eyes Multi-Reflective Liquid Eyeliner and the same review applies. ☹ **Retro Glow Automatic Kohl Eyeliner Pencil** *($5.95)* twists up and retracts, which is nice, and the application is smooth and even. However, the texture of this pencil is thick and tacky, and not worth considering over countless other pencils. Also, for a kohl pencil this doesn't smudge easily, tending to look more sooty than smoky. ☹ **Wonder Brow Automatic Brow Wax Stick** *($5.95)* is billed as an all-in-one product for the brows, but remains a below-standard automatic, retractable pencil that doesn't apply as easily as most automatic brow pencils, and remains tacky, which can cause brow hairs to mat. What a shame, because the colors are attractive and don't apply too strongly.

LIPSTICK AND LIP GLOSS: ☹ **Plump Palette Plumping Lip Color** *($7.95)* features four sheer to moderate coverage lip colors in one mirrored compact complete with brush. The lipstick texture is subpar, feeling too waxy and looking not the least bit glossy. What's most problematic is the inclusion of cinnamon, ginger, and menthane carboxamide (a potent, synthetically derived form of menthol), which plump lips (minimally) via irritation. ☹ **Plump Potion Needle-Free Lip Plumping Cocktail** *($8.95)* is packaged to resemble a syringe (so much for allaying fear of the needle!) and only provides lips with a cocktail of irritants, including menthol and menthyl nicotinate. These ingredients cause inflammation and increase blood flow to the lips, resulting in a slight increase in fullness—but such irritation is not the key to younger-looking, smoother lips.

MASCARA: ☺ **F.L.A.T. Fabulously Long and Thick Mascara** *($6.95)* makes lashes long and thick in a wink, and the drama continues with each successive quote. This mascara would rate a Paula's Pick were it not for the intermittent flaking experienced throughout the day. If you use restraint during application, the flaking becomes a non-issue—but it's a shame those who go for the gusto must tolerate this side effect.

☺ **To Any Lengths Lash Extending Mascara** *($5.20)* is excellent for substantial but not excessive length and clean, clump-free definition. Don't expect any thickness from this, but as a lengthening formula this wins high marks, and it wears all day without smearing or flaking.

☺ **PlentiFull Thickening Mascara** *($5.20)* has improved from the last time I reviewed it because it is now a credible mascara to consider if you need primarily a lengthening mascara that, with several coats, builds moderate thickness without clumps or smearing. The tiny amount of botanicals (aloe and chamomile) have no impact on lashes.

😐 **Lash-in-a-Tube Waterproof Full Coverage Cream Mascara** *($5.95)* quickly makes eyelashes long and reasonably thick, though it suffers from some minor clumping issues you may have to work through. It wears decently throughout the day, but has a tendency to flake slightly. While the waterproof claim holds up, you can get better results from the waterproof mascaras sold by L'Oreal or Maybelline New York. 😐 **AquaWear Waterproof Mascara** *($5.20)* will build some length, but no thickness, and is fairly waterproof. Contrary to the claim here, no waterproof mascara can condition lashes, nor do lashes need conditioning. However, this does make lashes feel softer than a typical waterproof mascara. 😐 **Eyebrightener Conditioning, Brightening & Curling Waterproof Mascara** *($6.95)* would be the centerpiece on display if there were a Boring Mascara Hall of Fame. The only thing this has going for it is the fact that it's waterproof—but it does not curl lashes at all, or lengthen, or thicken.

😐 **Retro Glow Ultra-Dramatic Mascara** *($6.95)* is about as ultra-dramatic as an episode of *I Love Lucy*. This fancifully packaged mascara gradually makes lashes longer without clumps, but that's about it. 😐 **Lash-in-a-Tube Full Coverage Cream Mascara** *($5.95)* promises a false-eyelashes effect without the stiffness, yet all it delivers is appreciable length with minor clumps and some smearing along the way. If you're meticulous during application, this can be an OK lengthening mascara, and it does keep lashes soft.

😐 **Exerc'Eyes Mascara 2-in-1 Lash-Building and Magnifying** *($6.95)* definitely deserves recognition for its distinctive packaging (it looks like a mini dumbbell), but its performance isn't nearly as unique or clever. This dual-phase mascara includes a clear gel on one end and traditional mascara on the other. The gel may be worn alone or used as a primer before the mascara. I tried the mascara alone and then paired it with the gel primer to see if the results were as tremendous as Physicians Formula touted. Nope. The mascara-only side looked great: defined, separated, clump-free, and nicely elongated, slightly thickened lashes. The gel primer/mascara combination looked much worse, primarily because the gel forms a hard-to-remove coating around the lashes that hinders application of the mascara, resulting in short, spiky lashes that feel stiff. By itself, the gel primer provides minimal enhancement. Since only half of this product is recommended, it deserves only a neutral face rating.

☹ **Eyebrightener Brightening & Curling Mascara** *($6.95)* is blah all the way around, doing little of anything except making lashes feel especially brittle. This does not curl lashes or make eyes look any brighter. ☹ **Mineral Wear Talc-Free Mineral Mascara** *($7.95)* makes a strange claim, because mascaras are never made with talc (and it's not a harmful ingredient for eyelashes anyway). The mineral component comes from the mineral water, which is the main ingredient in this mascara. The product applies heavily from the get-go, and quite wet. It takes several minutes to dry, in which time you run the risk of smearing, making this a poor contender among other mascaras. Another downer is how difficult this is to remove. A water-soluble cleanser and two rounds of a silicone-based eye-makeup remover weren't enough (though the formula does wear well once it finally sets).

FACE AND BODY ILLUMINATING/SHIMMER PRODUCTS: ☺ **Summer Eclipse Bronzing and Shimmery Face Powder** *($11.95)* casts an equal amount of shimmer and sun-kissed bronze tint on the skin. The tightly pressed, talc-based powder applies sheer and evenly, and the shine clings better than you might think. It's best for evening glamour when you want shine without overdoing it.

☺ **Baked Bronzer Bronzing & Shimmery Face Powder** *($11.95)* is similar to the Baked Pyramid Matte Bronzer above, except this version is imbued with large flecks of gold shine, whether used wet or dry. The shine clings well either way, and wet application intensifies the color and won't streak, assuming you blend it carefully.

☺ **Virtual Face Powder Multi-Reflective Face Powder** *($10.95)* is a talc-based pressed powder that attempts to minimize lines and wrinkles by diffusing light. It doesn't work in that manner, however, because it is so shiny that any flaw or wrinkle it's applied over is magnified. However, this is perfect if you have smooth, unlined skin and want a shiny powder that has a dimensional effect and clings very well. All four shades are enticing if strong shine is your thing.

😐 **Jungle Fever Bronzing & Shimmery Face Powder** *($11.95)* is a shimmering pressed powder that comes in your choice of a tiger or leopard pattern. What that has to do with improving powder application is anyone's guess, but it nicely coincides with the clever jungle name. Each shade mixes light and bronze tones for a sheer tan effect on the skin, but the shine is most prominent—and doesn't stay in place well, making this a lesser option from Physicians Formula.

😐 **Retro Glow Illuminating Face Powder** *($10.95)* is supposed to be a return to the heritage of Physicians Formula. This talc-based powder contains aluminum starch as its second ingredient, so the finish is dry and absorbent though replete with shine. The shine is described as "imperceptible," but that isn't true in the least. Although the two shades are neutral and sheer, the shine doesn't cling well, but this is still an OK option for oily skin that's fair to light.

☹ **Shimmer Strips Custom Bronzer, Blush, & Eye Shadow** *($11.95)* tries to compete with Bobbi Brown's popular Shimmer Brick Compacts ($38), but fails due to its dry, thick texture that applies unevenly. The shimmer tends to sit (and look piled) on the skin no matter how little you use, whereas Brown's option (and the much less expensive version from Jane) mesh with and use shimmer to highlight skin.

POND'S (SKIN CARE ONLY)

POND'S AT-A-GLANCE

Strengths: Inexpensive; great makeup remover and topical scrubs; effective AHA product; state-of-the-art moisturizers with sunscreen in stable packaging.

Weaknesses: Some outdated cold cream cleansers and bar soap; no products to manage blemish-prone skin; no skin-lightening options; a few moisturizers contain irritants such as menthol or alcohol.

For more information about Pond's, call (800) 909-9493 or visit www.ponds.com or www.Beautypedia.com.

😐 **Cold Cream, The Cool Classic** *($8.69 for 9.5 ounces)* isn't cool, but it is classic cold cream and a very old-fashioned way to cleanse and remove makeup. It is an option only if you have very dry skin and prefer a heavy-duty, greasy texture.

☺ **Clean Sweep, Cleansing & Make-Up Removing Towelettes** *($6.39 for 30 towelettes)* offer a gentle cleansing formula on soft, disposable towels. Although not a clean sweep when it comes to removing long-wearing makeup or mascara, these work well for minor cleansing or to refresh all skin types when away from home.

☺ **Exfoliating Clean Sweep, Cucumber Cleansing Towelettes** *($7.59 for 30 towelettes)* are nearly identical to the Clean Sweep, Cleansing & Make-Up Removing Towelettes above, and the same review applies. The exfoliating part comes into play because one side of these cloths is textured, sort of like a washcloth.

☺ **Deep Cleanser & Make-Up Remover, The Cool Cucumber Classic** *($8.69 for 10.1 ounces)* is an exceptionally standard cleansing lotion that is suitable only for dry to very dry skin and requires a washcloth for complete removal. The oil and emollients can make short work of makeup.

😐 **Dramatic Results, Age-Defying Towelettes** *($6.69 for 30 towelettes)* contain a minimal amount of cleansing agent and instead exfoliate skin with approximately 8% glycolic acid at an effective pH. Retinol is included, too, but that and the AHA will benefit your skin only to a point unless you don't rinse. And that's not the best approach because you'd be leaving cleansing agents on your skin all day. There are better ways to enjoy the benefits of glycolic acid and retinol.

☹ **Multi-Talent, 3-In-1 Beauty Bar** *($5.59 for a 4-ounce bar)* is multi-talented in name only, because this is standard bar soap that contains the usual roster of ingredients (tallow being a prime offender) that make bar soaps and cleansers so problematic for all skin types.

☹ **Pristine Clean, Gentle Cleansing Foam** *($7.19 for 4 ounces)* contains sodium C14-16 olefin sulfonate as the main cleansing agent, which makes this propellant-based mousse cleanser too irritating for all skin types. What a shame, because the other ingredients of this cleanser are just fine, though it does contain fragrance.

✓☺ **Bare & Repair, Conditioning Eye Make-Up Remover** *($6.09 for 4 ounces)* is a very well-formulated, dual-phase makeup remover that works quickly and painlessly to remove all types of eye makeup and mascara. Pond's included several soothing plant extracts and anti-irritants, and left out the fragrance, which is always helpful. This product is recommended for all skin types, and may be used before or after cleansing.

☺ **Fresh Start, Daily Exfoliating Cleanser** *($7.19 for 6.7 ounces)* cleanses and exfoliates at the same time, and is best for normal to oily or combination skin. It contains polyethylene beads (ground-up plastic) as the abrasive agent, and is water-soluble so it rinses cleanly.

☺ **Purely Polished, Microdermabrasion Anti-Aging Kit** *($14.89 for 4.4 ounces)* tries to compete with other microdermabrasion-at-home products, but contains polyethylene (synthetic abrasive agent present in almost every topical scrub) instead of the aluminum oxide crystals found in other microdermabrasion-like products. Pond's included a **Skin Polishing Applicator** (synthetic sponge attached to a stubby handle) to make the procedure seem more professional, but that doesn't stop this from being a standard topical scrub. The good news is that this is an excellent, fragrance-free scrub product for dry to very dry skin. It is less abrasive than most microdermabrasion scrubs, and contains emollients to smooth and protect skin during the process. It does not need to be used with the applicator to get results, but if you're feeling experimental, go for it—just be sure to clean the applicator frequently.

☹ **Cool, Calm & Perfected, Pore-Shrinking Gel Toner** *($6.69 for 7.4 ounces)* lists alcohol as the second ingredient, closely followed by menthol and witch hazel. This gel-based toner will not shrink pores, but they may recoil from the irritation it causes.

☹ **Age defEYE, Anti-Circle, Anti-Puff Eye Therapy** *($14.79 for 0.5 ounce)* seemingly takes care of every eye-area concern, yet doesn't contain anything with a reliable track record for diminishing dark circles, deflating puffiness, or firming skin. It does have a substantial amount of coriander oil, an irritant that is even more troublesome in a product meant for use around the eyes. The irritant potential of coriander oil comes from its 70% linalool content. Linalool is the main fragrant component of lavender and is a potent skin irritant once it oxidizes, which it will do as soon as it touches your skin (Sources: *Contact Dermatitis*, May 2002, pages 267–272, and June 2005, pages 320–328; and www.naturaldatabase.com). Its inclusion here is a shame, because for the most part (claims aside), this is an elegant, antioxidant-laden formulation with stable packaging.

😐 **Dry Skin Cream, The Caring Classic** *($8.79 for 10.1 ounces)* takes the prize for the most boring facial moisturizer at the drugstore. It's a classic oil-in-water with wax formula, and although it can address the basic needs of dry to very dry skin, using it is akin to sending someone a telegram instead of an email.

✓☺ **Mend & Defend, Intensive Protection SPF 15 Moisturizer** *($9.39 for 3.3 ounces)* shows that when it comes to launching effective sunscreens and elegant moisturizers, Pond's has done its homework. This lightweight, soft-matte finish lotion features an in-part avobenzone sunscreen and its base formula contains several antioxidants and water-binding agents (ingredients that mimic the structure and function of healthy skin). In addition, the opaque, pump-bottle packaging keeps these elegant ingredients stable during use. It's a good thing there are so many of them, too, because it is likely that the amount of each one in an average application is quite small, but likely will add up to a potent boost.

✓☺ **Radiance Restore, Age-Defying Skin-Brightening SPF 15 Moisturizer** *($12.99 for 1.7 ounces)* improves on the Mend & Intensive Protection SPF 15 Moisturizer above by offering a superior formula with higher concentrations of antioxidants, still in suitably protective packaging. This in-part zinc oxide sunscreen is outstanding for normal to dry skin. Its silicone, glycerin, and triglyceride base contains almost a dozen antioxidants, ceramides, and other ingredients that mimic the structure of healthy skin. It is a far better moisturizing sunscreen formulation than any in the L'Oreal lineup, and would be giving drugstore frontrunner (in terms of state-of-the-art formulas) Dove a run for its money, except that both Dove and Pond's are owned by Unilever. So perhaps one inspired the other? This product does contain fragrance and a tiny amount of mica, which imparts a subtle shimmer to skin.

☹ **Smooth Perfection, Complexion Perfecting Moisturizer** *($13.69 for 2 ounces)* appears ideal when you read that it "takes care of all skin's little problems," from pore size to dullness and fine lines. Yet the formula pales in comparison to that of most moisturizers because it includes alcohol and menthol (What are they doing in a moisturizer, or in any product, because these two ingredients have no benefit for skin?). By the way, the emollient ingredients in this product will not make pores smaller—if anything they are problematic.

☺ **Time Rewind, Overnight Wrinkle Repair Cream** *($14.69 for 1.8 ounces)* contains about 8% glycolic acid and has a pH of 3.5, so it is an effective AHA product. The inordinately long ingredient list is fairly impressive, but the inclusion of a fair amount of absorbent aluminum starch octenylsuccinate makes this an option only for normal to slightly oily skin. The many antioxidants and retinol in this formula are wasted because of the jar packaging, but it nevertheless deserves a happy face rating because of its value as an AHA product.

☹ **Revive in Five, 5-Minute Age-Defying Moisture Treatment** *($13.89 for 4.5 ounces)* is a moisturizing mask whose hydrating properties are compromised somewhat by the inclusion of alcohol (it's the fifth ingredient) and, further down the list, menthol. Plus, the jar packaging will render the many antioxidants in this moisturizer ineffective shortly after it is opened, which is just too many strikes to make it a recommendation for anyone.

☹ **Clear Solutions, Clear Pore Strips** *($5.69 for 6 strips)* are similar to the Biore Deep Cleansing Pore Strips ($8.99 for 7 nose and 7 face strips), and consist of a sticky film-forming agent that is applied to skin and ripped off after a few moments. These can remove dead skin cells and superficial blackheads, but they don't address the root of the problem. Plus, the irritation from these strips can make their ongoing use a problem for skin, and no match for a well-formulated BHA product.

PRESCRIPTIVES

PRESCRIPTIVES AT-A-GLANCE

Strengths: As true for most Lauder-owned lines, moisturizers and serums are as state-of-the-art as it gets and designed to work well under makeup; all but one sunscreen provide sufficient UVA protection; good cleansers and makeup remover; superior moisturizing mask; unique lip moisturizer that's worth the price; several fragrance-free options; most of the foundations have remarkable qualities while the shade range is impressive; some outstanding concealers and pressed powders (including some with broad-spectrum sun protection); Custom Blend products; the gel eyeliner; the Moonbeam lip products; Magic Illuminating Potion Foundation Primer; several good makeup brushes; well-organized, accessible tester units.

Weaknesses: Expensive; Super Flight products and toners are problematic because they contain irritants; self-tanner with sunscreen leaves skin vulnerable to UVA damage; no effective products to manage acne; too many products in jar packaging; Plush Blush; Moonbeam eye product; lipstick with sunscreen lacks sufficient UVA protection; only two of the four mascaras are great, and at their prices all of them should reach that goal.

For more information about Prescriptives, owned by Estee Lauder, call (866) 290-6471 or visit www.prescriptives.com or www.Beautypedia.com.

PRESCRIPTIVES SKIN CARE

PRESCRIPTIVES ALL YOU NEED + PRODUCTS

☹ **$$$ All You Need+ Broad Spectrum Moisture Cream SPF 15** *($40 for 1.7 ounces)* provides ample sun protection and includes avobenzone in an oil-rich emollient formula for dry to very dry skin. Lots of state-of-the-art ingredients are present, but the unfortunate choice of jar packaging won't help them remain stable during use. This does contain fragrant plant extracts.

☺ **$$$ All You Need+ Broad Spectrum Moisture Lotion SPF 15** *($40 for 1.7 ounces)* isn't as chock-full of antioxidants and cell-communicating ingredients as the All You Need+ Broad Spectrum Moisture Cream above, but it's packaged better. It includes avobenzone for UVA protection and is overall a very good daytime moisturizer for normal to slightly dry skin not prone to breakouts. But, this does not contain ingredients capable of exfoliating skin as claimed.

✓☺ **$$$ All You Need+ Broad Spectrum Oil Absorbing Lotion SPF 15** *($40 for 1.7 ounces)* is an outstanding daytime moisturizer with an in-part avobenzone sunscreen. The base formula is suitable for normal to oily skin, but lacks absorbents that are strong enough to create a long-lasting matte finish. Still, it's loaded with antioxidants, cell-communicating ingredients, and skin-identical substances. It contains fragrance in the form of orange extract and methyldihydrojasmonate.

☹ **$$$ All You Need+ Fast Acting Moisture Cream, for Drier Skin** *($40 for 1.7 ounces)* contains two AHAs and the BHA salicylic acid, but not enough of either for much exfoliation, despite a pH of 3.6. This silky-textured, fragrance-free moisturizer for normal to dry skin contains some great antioxidants, but their performance will suffer due to jar packaging.

☺ **$$$ All You Need+ Fast Acting Moisturizer, for Normal Skin** *($60 for 3.4 ounces)* cannot optimally exfoliate skin because the salicylic acid concentration is too low and the pH is above 4. This moisturizer is appropriate for normal to dry skin, but it's not as antioxidant-rich as other options from Prescriptives (and other Lauder-owned lines). Still, it contains a nice blend of skin-identical substances.

☺ **$$$ All You Need+ Fast Acting Moisturizer, for Oilier Skin** *($40 for 1.7 ounces)* contains slightly less than 1% salicylic acid and has a pH of 3.6, so some exfoliation is possible. The lemon and passion fruit extracts do not perform the same way as AHAs, and lemon can be irritating, especially in a formula with a low pH. This lightweight lotion is suitable for normal to oily skin and contains ingredients that can contribute to healthy skin functioning. This would have been a Paula's Pick if it had a better assortment and larger amounts of antioxidants.

PRESCRIPTIVES ANTI-AGE ADVANCED PRODUCTS

☹ **$$$ Anti-Age Advanced Protection Eye Cream SPF 25** *($48 for 0.5 ounce)* is an incredibly well-formulated product that includes avobenzone for UVA protection, although this and the other synthetic active ingredients are not the best for use around the eyes (titanium dioxide and zinc oxide are preferred for their gentleness). What's most distressing is jar packaging, which won't help keep the copious antioxidants and other light- and air-sensitive ingredients stable during use. In opaque, non-jar packaging, this would have been a slam-dunk recommendation for normal to dry skin.

✓☺ **$$$ Anti-Age Advanced Protection Lotion SPF 25** *($60 for 1.7 ounces)* is a lighter-weight, better-packaged version of the Anti-Age Advanced Protection Eye Cream SPF 25 above, and the same formulary and sunscreen comments apply here. The packaging propels this to my highest rating, and the only issue is the claim that this product can combat the aging effects of excess sugar consumption. Sugars are a contributing factor to the formation of advanced glycation end products (AGE). AGEs directly affect the surface layers of skin as well as structures beneath the surface, such as collagen and elastin. At this point, we don't know whether or not AGEs can be stopped or even inhibited, so the claim Prescriptives makes is nothing more than a leap of the imagination, not fact.

😐 **$$$ Anti-Age Advanced Protection Moisturizer SPF 25** *($60 for 1.7 ounces)* is similar to the All You Need+ Broad Spectrum Moisture Lotion SPF 15 above, but with a higher SPF rating and an even greater array of antioxidants, which makes the choice of jar packaging even more disappointing.

PRESCRIPTIVES INTENSIVE REBUILDING PRODUCTS

😐 **$$$ Intensive Rebuilding Eye Cream** *($65 for 0.5 ounce)* is similar to—but ounce per ounce far more expensive than—the Intensive Rebuilding Moisturizer ($95 for 2 ounces) reviewed below. Interestingly, the Eye Cream version, which makes the same "progressive build and fill" claims as the Moisturizer, doesn't have the same wow-factor list of ingredients, though both suffer from jar packaging. This product will moisturize skin around the eyes or elsewhere, but there is no reason the Intensive Rebuilding Moisturizer cannot double as an eye cream, and according to its ingredient list, it's far better for skin anywhere on the face. The only real reason to use a different product around your eyes is if that area of skin is drier than the skin on the rest of your face and thus needs a more emollient rather than a lighter-weight product.

☺ **$$$ Intensive Rebuilding Instant Line Filler** *($40 for 0.04 ounce)* has wrinkle-reducing, collagen-building claims that make it seem like an at-home version of injectable line fillers. That's not surprising given the growing popularity of and impressive results from such real-life medically delivered dermal fillers as Hylaform, Restylane, and many others. Packaged in a sleek tube, this water- and silicone-based serum contains the typical Lauder assortment of state-of-the-art ingredients, including antioxidants, nonvolatile plant oils, essential fatty acids, water-binding agents, and cell-communicating ingredients. The blend of silicones forms a flexible film on skin as it temporarily fills in superficial and shallow lines (with the effect's duration depending on how expressive you are), so you will notice a smoother appearance and, of course, a silky finish, but the effect is at best temporary, and diminishes more rapidly the more you move your face. Although this Prescriptives product has advantages for improving the appearance of wrinkles and providing skin with the ingredients it needs to look and feel its best, it is not a substitute for what can be accomplished by injectable dermal fillers. This product is very similar to the Estee Lauder Perfectionist Correcting Concentrate for Lip Lines ($35 for 0.08 ounce) and Perfectionist Correcting Concentrate for Deeper Facial Lines/Wrinkles ($42 for 0.11 ounce), both of which provide give you more product for the money than Prescriptives.

😐 **$$$ Intensive Rebuilding Moisturizer** *($95 for 2 ounces)* uses words like Hydrabuild and Hylafill, claiming they can infuse skin with moisture, and features "doctor-designed complexes" to make it sound as if it can replace procedures performed in a doctor's office. This is incapable of providing that benefit; in fact, there isn't a skin-care product being sold that can do that.

This moisturizer, while exceptionally elegant, isn't too far removed from the best moisturizers in other Lauder-owned lines, including Clinique, Estee Lauder, and, yes, even other moisturizers in the Prescriptives lineup. All of these outstanding moisturizers contain a state-of-the-art blend of water-binding agents, plant oils and fatty acids, antioxidants, emollients, soothing agents (including beneficial plant extracts), and silicones. Because there are already so many excellent options, there's no need to make a beeline for the most expensive one—to do so is just giving in to marketing caprice, rather than selecting a product on the basis of what we know to be true about the ingredients, which are also present in similar products. One of those truths involves avoiding jar packaging to ensure the antioxidants and other light- and air-sensitive ingredients remain stable. Regrettably, this Prescriptives moisturizer ignored that necessity.

✓☺ **$$$ Intensive Rebuilding Lotion** *($80 for 1.7 ounces)* makes the same line-smoothing claims as the Intensive Rebuilding Moisturizer above, but comes in a lotion form and packaging that will keep the many antioxidants stable during use. This fragrance-free moisturizer is a truly elegant, of-the-moment option for normal to oily skin. Well done!

✓☺ **$$$ Intensive Rebuilding Deep Hydrating Mask** *($28 for 3.4 ounces)*. You know how most spa lines have a half dozen or so moisturizing masks, most of which are ordinary and repetitive? All of them could learn something from this product. It's an exceptional formulation for dry to very dry skin, providing it with a slew of helpful ingredients, all designed to improve moisture content and make skin radiant. There is no research proving the acetyl glucosamine (which is given strong presence in this product) can exfoliate skin, but we know it's an excellent water-binding agent. This mask does contain fragrance.

✓☺ **$$$ Intensive Rebuilding Hand Treatment SPF 15** *($38 for 3.4 ounces)* is pricey for a hand cream, but it covers the pertinent bases with its in-part avobenzone sunscreen and superior moisturizing formula loaded with antioxidants and emollients. The amount of mulberry extract (a plant whose natural arbutin content has been shown in some research to lighten skin discolorations) is likely too small to affect sun-damage spots, which often appear first and in the greatest numbers on your hands.

☹ **Intensive Rebuilding Lip Shaper Plumper/Definer** *($28 for 0.07 ounce)* sounds like a full-on lip-plumping injection in a tube, but this cannot approach what such a procedure can accomplish. It's a rather basic formula that contains more fragrance than state-of-the-art ingredients, and the menthol is irritating (not to mention that if you want to plump your lips with menthol, you don't have to pay this much for it).

PRESCRIPTIVES VIBRANT-C PRODUCTS

😐 **$$$ Vibrant-C Skin Brightening Cream Moisturizer** *($46 for 1.7 ounces)*. This jar-packaged moisturizer contains some notable antioxidants, but they won't last very long after the jar is opened. The orange and lavender pose a risk of irritation, and nothing in this moisturizer can actually fade skin discolorations, leaving you with a basic yet silky-textured moisturizer for normal to slightly dry skin.

☺ **$$$ Vibrant-C Skin Brightening Eye Cream** *($38 for 0.5 ounce)* is a good moisturizer for dry skin around the eyes or elsewhere. Compared to similar eye creams from Clinique or Estee Lauder (the latter is the parent company of Prescriptives), this one isn't as jam-packed with state-of-the-art ingredients. However, the opaque pump-bottle packaging will keep the light- and air-sensitive ingredients (including vitamin C) stable. The "micro-optic luminizers" this boasts of are a fancy way to describe the slight shimmer left on your skin from the mica in this product, which is a cosmetic effect unrelated to skin care.

☺ **$$$ Vibrant-C Skin Brightening Lotion Moisturizer** *($46 for 1.7 ounces)* would be rated a Paula's Pick if it didn't contain lavender and orange for fragrance. It is otherwise a brilliantly formulated moisturizer for normal to dry skin, featuring lots of antioxidants, cell-communicating ingredients, and ingredients that support skin structure and healthy functioning. The titanium dioxide and mica lend a soft-focus glow to skin, but that isn't about skin care, it's about shine.

OTHER PRESCRIPTIVES PRODUCTS

☺ **$$$ All Clean Fresh Foaming Cleanser, for Normal Skin** *($21 for 6.7 ounces)* produces a copious foam, yet also manages to clean skin and remove makeup thoroughly. This does contain fragrant plant extracts. It is best for normal to oily skin.

☺ **$$$ All Clean Rich Cream Cleanser, for Drier Skin** *($21 for 6.7 ounces)* is a fairly greasy, detergent-free cleansing cream for dry to very dry skin. It removes makeup easily, but must be used with a washcloth to avoid a residue.

☺ **$$$ All Clean Sparkling Gel Cleanser, for Oilier Skin** *($21 for 6.7 ounces)* is a very standard, but good, water-soluble cleanser for normal to oily or slightly dry skin. It does contain fragrant plant extracts.

☺ **$$$ Comfort Cleanser Gentle Lotion, for Sensitive Skin** *($21 for 6.7 ounces)* is similar to but has a thinner texture than the All Clean Rich Cream Cleanser above, and the same basic comments apply. This option contains some good anti-irritants, but the fragrance in the form of methyldihydrojasmonate is not ideal for sensitive skin.

☺ **$$$ Super Line Smoothing Cleanser** *($25 for 6.7 ounces)* cannot help prevent lines in any way, shape, or form. Prescriptives wants you to think so, probably because they hope in some way to justify the price of this very standard water-soluble cleanser. Although this is a fine cleanser for normal to oily skin, it is hardly unusual and will not fulfill the promise of smoothing lines. It does contain fragrance in the form of orange extract and methyldihydrojasmonate, which isn't the best, but it's not a deal breaker either.

✓☺ **$$$ Better Off, Fast-Acting Waterproof Eye Makeup Remover** *($18 for 4.2 ounces)* is a very good, dual-phase makeup remover whose solvent (isohexadecane) and silicones make quick work of dissolving all makeup, including waterproof formulas. It is fragrance- and colorant-free and does not contain a single questionable or irritating ingredient. This may be used before or after cleansing.

☺ **$$$ Better Off Instant Wipe-Off Makeup Remover** *($20 for 6.7 ounces)* contains a solvent and silicone to remove makeup quickly and easily. This should be rinsed off after use or applied before washing with a water-soluble cleanser. It does contain fragrance.

☺ **$$$ Quick Remover for Eye Makeup** *($17 for 4.2 ounces)* is a very standard, water- and detergent-based eye-makeup remover. It is fragrance-free and an option for all skin types, though similar formulas sell for less at the drugstore.

😐 **$$$ Dermapolish System** *($125 for the set)* consists of a topical scrub, a toner, and a moisturizer, and claims to deliver results that are comparable to those of a professional microdermabrasion treatment. I'm getting so tired of reviewing these kinds of kits. Do consumers ever notice the tremendous redundancy this industry offers?

This set has the endorsement of dermatologist Dr. Karyn Grossman, which may or may not mean anything to you. From my perspective, a dermatologist's endorsement is relatively meaningless if you don't know all the details. For example, was Dr. Grossman paid for her comments? And what if she's wrong, which in this case she is. Using this system once a week doesn't replace going to a salon or doctor's office for microdermabrasion treatments. Although the Dermapolish Treatment Cream contains the same type of ingredient (in this case, alumina; microdermabrasion treatments use nearly identical aluminum oxide crystals), what's missing is the device (and the technology behind it) that sprays these crystals on the skin and then vacuums them off. The device is controlled by an aesthetician or a physician, and their skill with the device is an essential component of achieving the best results from a professional microdermabrasion treatment. However, even professionally administered microdermabrasion treatments, when performed repeatedly over time, are turning out not to be as helpful as once thought.

The **Dermapolish Treatment Cream** is simply a gritty-feeling scrub that you apply by hand and then rinse off. This will exfoliate the skin, but overzealous or too frequent application can lead to chronic irritation. After all, this is abrasive, and the temptation to "scour away" wrinkles and blemishes is one many consumers won't be able to resist. Beyond the alumina, there's not much in this topical scrub that makes it different from many other scrub products, most of which are much gentler on the skin. Even using a washcloth beats what this scrub can provide.

After exfoliating, you apply the **Post Treatment Soothing Mist**, which is a toner, from a container that's way too small. This contains some very good water-binding agents and antioxidants, but also includes caffeine and fragrance, which can trigger irritation on just-scrubbed skin. If the goal was to make this product soothing, they should have excluded the fragrance.

Following the Mist, you apply the **Lipid Barrier Cream**, an emollient moisturizer similar to most of the other moisturizing options from Prescriptives (which is to say it is a well-formulated product, but jar packaging hinders the antioxidants). Again, it would be preferable if the fragrance and caffeine were left out. Although this is a very good moisturizer, it is not the specialized product it's made out to be—countless other moisturizers would work just as well to soothe the skin post-scrub. For those so inclined, the Lipid Barrier Cream is sold separately ($55 for 1 ounce).

✓☺ **$$$ Immediate Smooth Skin Conditioning Exfoliator** *($19.50 for 3.4 ounces)* cannot exfoliate skin, unless they are referring to the mechanical action of swiping a cotton pad across your face. Despite the misleading name, this is a very good toner for normal to slightly dry or slightly oily skin. It definitely goes beyond the norm to provide skin with a wide complement of helpful ingredients.

☹ **Flight Mist, Refresher for Dehydrated Skin** *($40 for 4.2 ounces)* is a fairly basic toner that's not preferred to most others (nor is it a unique option to use during airline flights) because it contains peppermint, which will only irritate already dehydrated, compromised skin.

☹ **Immediate Glow Skin Conditioning Tonic, for Normal/Drier Skin** *($18.50 for 6.7 ounces)* creates an instant glow on your skin from irritation caused by menthol, making this toner a bad choice.

☹ **Immediate Matte Skin Conditioning Tonic, for Normal/Oilier Skin** *($18.50 for 6.7 ounces)* lists alcohol as the second ingredient, followed closely by witch hazel. The alcohol can de-grease skin, but at the expense of being drying, irritating, and causing free-radical damage.

😐 **$$$ Comfort Cream 24 Hour Care, for Sensitive Skin** *($38.50 for 1.7 ounces)* is an emollient moisturizer for dry skin showing signs of sensitivity, but it's a shame the plant-based anti-irritants and antioxidants won't retain their efficacy because of jar packaging.

☺ **$$$ Comfort Lotion Oil-Free Care, for Sensitive Skin** *($38.50 for 1.7 ounces)* is a fairly impressive moisturizer for normal to slightly dry or slightly oily skin not prone to blemishes. It is not ideal for sensitive skin because it contains fragrant plant extracts, fragrance components, and coloring agents, all of which can be problematic for reactive skin.

😐 **$$$ Invisible Line Smoother** *($35 for 0.5 ounce)* is just a blend of silicones and preservatives. The spackle-like texture of this product can minimally and temporarily smooth lines, but how long the effect lasts depends on how expressive you are. For the money, it would have been nice if Prescriptives had included some antioxidants or retinol—something beneficial to help skin function in a healthier manner.

✓☺ **$$$ Skin Renewal Cream** *($60 for 1 ounce)* is an excellent fragrance-free moisturizer with retinol for normal to slightly dry skin. Prescriptives should use more packaging like this, because it does a brilliant job of keeping the light- and air-sensitive ingredients stable during use. One more thing: the amount of mulberry extract is unlikely to have an impact on skin discolorations, but the retinol should help improve things on many fronts, including minor discolorations.

☹ **Super Flight Cream** *($35 for 1.7 ounces)* contains several beneficial ingredients, but most of them are given short shrift in this overall problematic formula, which isn't unique in any way for satisfying the needs of skin battling the dryness associated with airplane travel. Several of the plant extracts can be irritating, including horsetail, balm mint, sage, and peppermint.

😐 **$$$ Super Line Corrector Firming Night Cream** *($65 for 1.7 ounces)* is a very good moisturizer for dry skin, but it's not all that different from several other moisturizers in the Prescriptives lineup. This supposedly firms the skin "dramatically" (after all, who wants "non-dramatic firming"?) and fades "age spots" while smoothing the skin's texture. There is nothing in this formula that can lighten one skin cell, let alone a patch of discoloration, and there is nothing that firms skin. If you have normal to dry skin, this is an option, but the jar packaging won't keep the many antioxidants stable during use. This does contain fragrant plant extracts.

😐 **$$$ Super Line Corrector Lifting Day Cream SPF 15** *($65 for 1.7 ounces)* won't lift the skin anywhere, and won't correct a single line. What does "correcting a line" mean, anyway? Did the line do something wrong? This cream is definitely appropriate for daytime use thanks to its in-part titanium dioxide sunscreen, but the moisturizing base isn't very exciting, especially at this price. There are some antioxidants and water-binding agents, but they're present in such small amounts (as are some plant irritants) as to be inconsequential for skin, plus the jar packaging won't keep them active. This does contain fragrant plant extracts.

😐 **$$$ Super Line Preventor+ Intensive Eye Treatment** *($45 for 0.5 ounce)* can be a good, lightweight moisturizer for the face because it contains an excellent assortment of water-binding agents and antioxidants. Still, it would be better if it came in airtight packaging to better preserve the antioxidants and cell-communicating ingredients.

✓☺ **$$$ Super Line Preventor Xtreme** *($47.50 for 1 ounce)* is the fifth version of Prescriptives' long-standing Line Preventor product. The good news is that their latest attempt is better than ever, although the water and slip agent base formula is identical to that of previous versions, which means it's not as silky-smooth as similar products from Lauder's Perfectionist line or Clinique's Repairwear line. However, if you don't mind a less silky, slightly tacky texture, this is well worth auditioning! The formula makes it suitable for all skin types and is loaded with state-of-the-art ingredients, including several antioxidants, cell-communicating ingredients, and potent anti-irritants. These ingredients contribute to making skin environmentally resilient (though not impervious to damage; you still need sunscreen), thus allowing it to repair itself. That leads to increased collagen production, because healthy, protected skin likes to make collagen. And this is what all well-formulated moisturizers do! This serum is also fragrance-free. Its only questionable ingredient is grapefruit peel extract, though that isn't nearly as inappropriate for skin as the whole fruit or oil, and likely conveys more antioxidant benefit than it does potential irritation. This product really is super, but only diligent use of a well-formulated sunscreen can actually prevent lines. Luckily, the texture of this product means it will work well under most sunscreens or foundation with sunscreen!

☹ **Acne Defense Serum** *($25 for 1 ounce)* contains only 0.5% salicylic acid as the active ingredient and the pH is too high for exfoliation to occur. Although there are some very good soothing agents in this serum, the addition of menthol counteracts them and makes this an expensive, irritating mistake for acne-prone skin.

✓☺ **$$$ Redness Relief Gel** *($50 for 1 ounce)* is an aloe- and water-based serum that is an outstanding, ultra-light moisturizer for all skin types, including someone with sensitive skin. In addition to aloe and water, this product contains mostly silicone, thickener, water-binding agents, antioxidants, cell-communicating ingredients, and anti-irritants. It is fragrance-free, making it ideal for easily irritated skin that cannot tolerate such ingredients. The tiny amount of rosemary leaf extract is unlikely to cause irritation. The opaque tube packaging of this product will help keep its antioxidants stable.

✓☺ **$$$ Lip Specialist, Triple Action Therapy** *($15 for 0.21 ounce)* is a unique lip balm that throws conventional formulas for a loop and offers an outstanding blend of vegetable oil (for a glossy finish) with other plant oils and buttery emollients. Even better is that it's loaded with antioxidants and ingredients that help reinforce skin's barrier function, which applies to lips, too. All of this is done without irritants, and the price isn't out of line either.

PRESCRIPTIVES SUN PRODUCTS

☹ **Sunsheen Custom Color Tinted Self Tanner SPF 15, for Face and Body** *($27 for 4.2 ounces)* is a self-tanner with sunscreen and pigments to provide instant sheer bronze color. Regrettably, this is not recommended because the sunscreen (undoubtedly a selling point for this product) lacks the UVA-protecting ingredients of titanium dioxide, zinc oxide, avobenzone, Tinosorb, or Mexoryl SX.

PRESCRIPTIVES MAKEUP

A major point of difference for this color line is their longstanding custom blend services. Although this is not available at every Prescriptives counter (call ahead), they offer customized foundation, concealer, powder, and lip gloss. The pros and cons of this service are described in detail below.

FOUNDATION: ✓☺ **$$$ Virtual Youth Lifting Moisture Makeup** *($32.50)* announces itself as "a revelation in makeup." Although it does have a state-of-the-art formula that surpasses the norm, it is not capable of lifting skin or restoring skin's clarity (unless by the latter claim they mean blurring imperfections, which this foundation does quite well). It has a fluid, creamy texture that those with normal to dry skin will love, and applies beautifully, managing medium to full coverage without looking masklike. This is still foundation, so don't expect natural perfection, but for this amount of coverage the satin finish is impressive and the in-part titanium dioxide sunscreen is an added bonus. There are 30 shades available, with equally good options for fair and dark skin tones. Smooth Chestnut, Smooth Pecan, and Smooth Clove are excellent shades for women of color. Avoid the following shades due to overtones of peach, gold, or rose: Smooth Champagne (may be OK for some medium skin tones), Smooth Gold, Smooth Antelope, Smooth Fawn, Smooth Cameo, Smooth Blush, Smooth Rose, and Smooth Porcelain.

✓ ☺ **$$$ Flawless Skin Total Protection Makeup SPF 15** *($39.50)* is positioned as a state-of-the-art, doctor-designed foundation courtesy of input from dermatologist Dr. Karyn Grossman. Based on its formula, I'm not quite sure how this foundation is supposed to go above and beyond by also being superior skin care because its ingredients are common to almost all newer foundations, from L'Oreal and Revlon to M.A.C. and Estee Lauder. If the skin-care element they're referring to is the sunscreen, then I get the connection. But even then, this foundation's combination of zinc oxide, titanium dioxide, and octinoxate is hardly unique, nor is it an addition that requires a dermatologist's guiding hand. Nevertheless, this foundation has some wonderfully positive traits. Its creamy-smooth, elegant texture and dewy, radiant finish are well-suited for normal to dry or even very dry skin. Flawless Skin is a fairly accurate name for this foundation because its medium to full coverage evens skin tone and conceals most flaws without making skin look pasty or thick—though the amount of titanium dioxide and zinc oxide do lend an opacity that keeps this foundation from appearing as natural as you might hope.

The roster of 30 shades means there's bound to be a few unflattering colors, and these include Bisque, Ginger, Antelope, Fawn (all too peach or will turn peach), Blush, Cameo, Porcelain (all too pink or rose), and Chestnut (an OK dark shade, but turns ashen due to the titanium dioxide and zinc oxide). Borderline shades that will likely still work for their intended skin tones include Beige, Suede, and Camellia. As usual, the most flattering shades are in Prescriptives' Yellow/Orange color family, something most sales representatives for this line will attest to, as does a quick look at the tester unit.

☺ **$$$ Virtual Matte Oil-Control Makeup SPF 15** *($32.50)* includes an in-part titanium dioxide sunscreen and treats skin to a silky, light texture that doesn't match its robust matte finish and medium to full coverage (this is not for anyone expecting light coverage or less because it is difficult to sheer down). Application is smooth and even, and there's enough playtime so that blending doesn't have to be ultra-fast. Among the 29 shades, you will find some remarkably soft, neutral colors, especially for light to medium skin. Darker skin tones should take a look at this makeup, too, because several shades (in particular Fresh Clove, Fresh Cocoa, Fresh Sienna, and Fresh Pecan) are beautifully deep and rich without turning copper or ashen on skin. The following shades have overtones of peach, rose, or pink that are likely to be too strong for most skin tones: Fresh Antelope, Fresh Blush, Fresh Hazelnut (OK but can become slightly red), Fresh Honey (may be OK for some medium skin tones), Fresh Porcelain, Fresh Fawn, Fresh Cameo, Fresh Suede, Fresh Dusk, and Fresh Chestnut (turns slightly ash). If Prescriptives had included higher levels of titanium dioxide for UVA protection (0.97% is minimal, but still effective), this would have been a slam-dunk Paula's Pick recommendation for oily to very oily skin.

☺ **$$$ Virtually Fresh Skin Refining Makeup SPF 15** *($32.50)* really does make skin look refined because it provides enhancing coverage that can approach full camouflage without calling much attention to itself. Even better, it does so while still feeling lightweight, almost like an elegant moisturizing lotion with a satin-matte finish (and Prescriptives did include some beneficial bells and whistles in this stably packaged foundation). What's somewhat of a letdown is the sunscreen. Although it does contain titanium dioxide for UVA protection, the amount is only 1% (although that's in addition to a larger percentage of another sunscreen). Better UVA protection would be assured with at least 2% or more titanium dioxide. However, because there are still no formulary percentage standards for UVA protection, it's not as though Prescriptives disregarded a guideline. A streamlined (well, at least for Prescriptives) range of 18 shades is offered, with only 4 missteps: Natural Bisque and Natural Beige are slightly peach, but may work for some skin tones; Natural Peach is accurately named and best avoided unless you want to look unnatural; and Natural Rose is slightly pink and may exaggerate a ruddy complexion. Natural Cocoa is a very good dark shade. The low amount of titanium dioxide is what keeps this foundation from earning a Paula's Pick rating.

☺ **$$$ AnyWear Multi-Finish Compact Foundation SPF 12** *($32.50)* almost makes it to the benchmark SPF 15 standard and includes an in-part titanium dioxide sunscreen. I decided to rate it with a happy face because the liberal manner in which pressed-powder foundations must be applied to net the stated level of sun protection is not how most women use them anyway. Therefore, this talc-based powder foundation was rated favorably as an adjunct to a moisturizer or foundation with sunscreen rated SPF 15 or greater with UVA-protecting ingredients, which is a great way to use this category of powder. Bottom line: It is not recommended as your sole source of sun protection. That said, this has an impressively smooth texture and even application that offers light to almost medium coverage without looking powdery or heavy. Its slightly dry, matte finish is suitable for normal to oily skin, though it does leave a slight shine. There are 24 shades available, most of which are exceptional. The following shades are best avoided because they are either too peach, rose, or ash: Cocoa, Fawn, Blush, Porcelain, Pecan, and Chestnut. This is the only Prescriptives foundation with disappointing options for dark skin tones.

😐 **$$$ Traceless Skin Responsive Tint SPF 8** *($32.50)* is merely a smooth-textured foundation that blends imperceptibly into the skin, creating an extremely sheer, ultra-natural finish. That means any imperfections you were hoping to hide will simply be glossed over, so if you have a noticeably uneven skin tone or anything more than minor discolorations, you will need a more substantial foundation. The sunscreen is meager and lacks adequate UVA-protecting ingredients. An attractive luminous finish is also left on the skin, courtesy of the mica in this product. There are only five shades, which is strange, as Prescriptives prides itself on its bountiful selection of foundation colors—but these neutral tones are so sheer, it's easy to see why they introduced so few. All of the shades will work for more than one skin tone, although this product is only for those whose skin is almost perfect.

😐 **$$$ Virtual Skin Super-Natural Finish SPF 10** *($32.50)* now ranks as Prescriptives' oldest foundation, and it's a shame that the SPF rating is too low and the active ingredients don't include UVA-protecting ingredients. That is truly disappointing because this is still one of the most natural-looking foundations available, and the elegantly light texture blends wonderfully. The range of 30 shades is wholly impressive, and this provides sheer to light coverage. The only colors to avoid are Real Cameo (very pink), Real Peach, Real Dusk, and Real Fawn (all slightly peach to orange), along with Real Porcelain, Real Rose, Real Petal, and Real Suede. Real Pecan and Real Chestnut are excellent colors for dark skin tones.

CONCEALER: ✓☺ $$$ Camouflage Cream *($17.50)* has a creamy, smooth application and only a slight chance of creasing. It has been around for years and deserves its "bestseller" status. You'll get plenty of playtime before it dries into place, and it is minimally prone to creasing. The 11 shades are divided into color families that correspond with the foundations, and every group except Red(!) has its weak shades. The following colors are too peach, pink, or rose to look convincing on most skin tones: Yellow/Orange Extra Dark, Red/Orange Medium,

Red/Orange Warm Extra Dark, Blue/Red Light (slightly pink, may be OK for some fair skin tones) and Blue/Red Medium.

✓☺ **$$$ Flawless Skin Total Protection Concealer SPF 25** *($22)* is a superb concealer option if you want a creamy texture, opaque coverage, and a gentle sunscreen composed entirely of titanium dioxide. Application is even without being too slippery, but you do need to set this with powder to prevent it from creasing into lines around the eyes. The emollient, skin-conditioning formula is not for use over blemishes, but beautifully conceals dark circles and redness. The nine shades are mostly soft and neutral; only Level 5 Dark has an orange cast that's tricky to blend with dark skin tones.

☺ **$$$ Site Unseen Brightening Concealer SPF 15** *($22)* is a liquid concealer with an in-part titanium dioxide and zinc oxide sunscreen. The sun protection is a plus, and this click pen–packaged, brush-dispensed concealer has minimal slip yet blends well (if you work fast), setting to a soft matte finish with a hint of shimmer (for "brightening," but let's call it what it is: shine). This provides good coverage with minimal to no risk of creasing. As usual, almost all of the shades are winners. Consider Level 2 Cool carefully due to its slightly pink cast, and note that the darkest shade, Level 6, suffers from being slightly ash.

POWDER: ✓☺ **$$$ Virtual Matte Oil-Control Pressed Powder** *($28)* cannot help regulate and reduce oil production as claimed because oil production is controlled by hormones, and a topically applied powder cannot change what is being generated by your body's androgens. If you can get past the implausible, inaccurate claims, this is a fantastic, talc-based powder for all skin types. It has a silky texture and a feather-light feel on skin, and finishes matte without a hint of dryness or chalkiness. Few pressed powders blend into skin as well as this, and five of the six shades are praiseworthy. Level 6, the darkest shade, is slightly ash. One caution: This powder contains cornstarch, a food-based ingredient that can be a problem if used over blemish-prone skin because it feeds the bacteria that cause acne. It is not the main ingredient, and as such is less of a potential problem, but those dealing with blemishes should be aware of it.

✓☺ **$$$ Flawless Skin Total Protection Powder SPF 15** *($30)* ranks as one of the few pressed powders with sunscreen, and this talc-based version is first-class thanks to its in-part titanium dioxide sunscreen and smooth, dry texture. It provides a sheer matte finish and offers a bit more coverage than standard pressed powders. As with any pressed powder with sunscreen, it is best used as an adjunct to another product with sun protection rather than on its own because liberal application of a powder can look dry and dull on skin. All of the shades are recommended except Level 6, which, due to the amount of titanium dioxide, is slightly ash.

☺ **$$$ Sunsheen Cooling Bronzing Powder** *($35)* has the same concept as Prescriptives longstanding Magic Liquid Powder ($35). Both powders contain a tiny amount of water, making them seem almost fluid, but still finish like a standard powder. The bronzing version is loose and comes in three sheer tan shades suitable for fair to medium skin. Each imparts a lot of sparkles, and although they cling reasonably well, a true tan doesn't shine this much. However, it's an option for a sparkling evening look. The Prescriptives salesperson remarked that this powder is best applied with a synthetic brush, which I found to be good advice. The powder's water content tends to "stick" to natural-hair powder brushes, making for uneven application.

☺ **$$$ Magic Liquid Powder** *($35)* is, as the name implies, a powder with a wet finish that dries to a sheer powder feel. It works well, and the cool feel is nice. This is an intriguing product to test, but don't count on anything even vaguely magical, unless you consider a shiny finish to be some sort of unique trickery. To its credit, the shine clings well and all three colors are workable, though they're best for evening glamour.

☺ **$$$ Pressed Powder Leaves** *($25)* is misnamed in the sense that although it is a pressed powder, the speckled arrangement of pigments produces a color on skin that's best used as blush, not a flesh-toned color applied all over. The smooth, almost creamy-feeling texture goes on easily and sheer, imparting soft color and a hint of shine.

☺ **$$$ All Skins Powder** *($26)* is a standard, sheer, talc-free loose powder available in a good selection of shades for fair to dark skin tones. It's pricey for what you get, especially when you consider some of the better loose powders sold at the drugstore.

😐 **$$$ Sunsheen Bronzing Trio** *($30)* features three colors in one pressed-powder compact: you get two believable tan shades and one complementary shade for highlighting. All of the shades are shiny, and have a dry, grainy texture that is surprisingly regressive for the usually top-notch powders from Prescriptives. Although the shades go on softly, this product pales (no pun intended) in comparison with other bronzing powders, including those from Bobbi Brown, Clinique, Laura Mercier, and Paula's Choice.

BLUSH: ☺ $$$ Colorscope Cheek Color *($17.50 + $6–$6.50 for refillable compact)* is Prescriptives collection of pressed-powder blushes, and there's some good news and some bad news (with the bad news really depending on your preferences). The good news is that the texture, application, and color deposit of this blush have been remarkably improved. It is supremely silky and applies evenly. The bad news is that every shade has some degree of shine, and several are very sparkly. The shiniest shades, ideal for evening only, include Nectar, Melon, Pompeii (erroneously labeled as "matte"), Mulberry, and Sherry. Four highlighter shades are also offered, and the shine these have is closer to a finely milled sheen rather than "Hey, look at me!" sparkles. The shade selection is plentiful, but (surprisingly) the collection is missing a few classic neutral tones, such as a good nude pink and muted tan. Still, if you don't mind the shine and want to experiment with some traditional and trendy shades, this is worth a peek.

☹ **Colorscope Plush Blush** *($20)* is a twist-up, mini stick blush that has an unappealingly moist texture that tends to drag on skin. This imparts little color, but lots of sparkling shine, which is difficult to blend evenly. I see the appeal of sheer, watercolor blush shades for summer days at the beach, but the finish this product leaves on skin will be a magnet for sand or strands of hair, and that's neither pretty nor carefree.

EYESHADOW: ☺ $$$ Colorscope Eye Color *($14 per shade + $3 for refillable compact)* has the same divine, silky texture as the Colorscope Cheek Color above, but the Eye Color at least has some almost-matte shades available. The shiny shades (and there are many) are designed for maximum sparkle. Although the multidimensional finish can be attractive on younger women, if your eyelid or underbrow area has any amount of wrinkling or sagging, these shades will enhance those problems. Those young enough to get away with as much shine as they want will enjoy that these eyeshadows tend to stay in place, so the shiny particles don't end up where you don't want them. The almost-matte shades include Adobe, Brownie, Mushroom, Peachy, Pongee, Terracotta, and Vanilla. Note that although these eyeshadows apply smoothly, the color deposit is softer, particularly so for the darkest shades (Ebony, Charcoal, Indigo). If you decide to use them as eyeliner, you may need to layer to build the best intensity.

☺ **$$$ Moonbeam Reflective Eye Color** *($16)* is a distinctive alternative to standard powder eyeshadows. Each silicone-enhanced liquid-to-powder shade is packed with sparkles, but it does set to a matte (in feel) finish and the shine tends to stay put. The colors themselves apply with more intensity than they used to, though they can be blended on sheer. If your eye area is still smooth and wrinkle-free, these are worth a look. The best shades are Solar Gold,

Zodiac Beige, Mocha Moon, and Satellite Wine. Watch out for the pastel and green shades, and be aware that this product has a lot of initial slip, so it's best applied to a larger area until you're used to its texture and application pitfalls.

☹ **Magic Eye Shadow Effects** *($25)* is a domed powder-like eyeshadow available in either gold or white. Both are loaded with shine and it's about as subtle as a racy red dress at a funeral. What's worse, the shine tends to flake and pretty much obscures any eyeshadow it's placed over (and Prescriptives offers plenty of shiny eyeshadows that don't flake, making this product completely unnecessary).

EYE AND BROW SHAPER: ✓☺ $$$ Perfect Every Line Gel Eyeliner *($17.50)* is an almost identical version of Lauder-owned Bobbi Brown's Long Wear Gel Eyeliner ($19), Clinique's Brush-On Cream Liner ($14.50), and M.A.C.'s Fluidline ($14.50). All of these are outstanding options for lining the eyes with color that won't smear, fade, or flake once set—even if you have oily eyelids. This version has the same ultra-smooth application, quick-dry finish, and comes off only when you want it to; make sure you have an oil- or silicone-based makeup remover handy. Licorice and Cocoa are classic black and brown shades without shine; Eggplant has a metallic purple sheen; and Sage has an olive-green base with khaki shimmer. One caution: The Fine Lining Brush Prescriptives recommends for use with this liner isn't as good as eyelining brush options from Bobbi Brown or M.A.C., so be sure you're comfortable with using it before purchasing. **✓☺ $$$ Groom Stick for Brows** *($18.50)* is a skinny, automatic, non-retractable brow pencil that has a great application, smooth texture, and powder-dry finish that only smears with considerable effort. The available shades are best for dark blonde to brunette brows, and this distinguishes itself as one of the better brow pencil options at any price. As a bonus, the opposite end of the pencil has a spooly brush to groom brows and soften the color.

☺ **$$$ Deluxe Eye Pencil** *($18.50)* is a standard, nonretractable, automatic eye pencil that has a soft, easy-glide texture, making application a cinch. The formula has a lot of slip before it sets, so watch out for inadvertent smudging. However, once this sets (after a minute or so), it does a good job of staying put. This won't outlast lining your eyes with a powder eyeshadow or a silicone-based gel eyeliner, but it's a good compromise for women who insist on pencils. Prescriptives has included a sponge tip to use if you want to soften or blend the line. Of the eight shades, the following are noticeably shiny: Sienna, Dusk, Midnight, and Khaki.

😐 **$$$ Softlining Pencil** *($17.50)* is a powdery eyeliner in pencil form with an effortless application, though routine sharpening is part of the deal. The pointed sponge tip is meant for smudging the line, which you should do because before long this pencil will smudge on its own, so it's best for creating smoky eyes. Iron Grey and Void are shiny.

😐 **$$$ Browshaping Pencil** *($15)* features four very good colors, but has a rather dry, hard texture and is not the best for an even application. Still, it isn't greasy and it would be difficult to apply too much because it goes on so softly.

☹ **Moonbeam Reflective Eye Pencil** *($17.50)* has an alluring name, but this needs-sharpening pencil has a finish that's too creamy, and it stays tacky. The shine-infused shades have a metallic tinge that can be attractive, but you can get the same effect from better pencils from other lines for less money.

LIPSTICK, LIP GLOSS, AND LIPLINER: ✓☺ $$$ Moonbeam Extreme Chromatic Lipcolor *($17.50)* has a completely different and better formula than the Moonbeam Reflective Gloss below, with a smoother texture and luminous, non-sticky finish. It's not really an apples-to-apples comparison, because this version is more liquid lipstick than lip gloss. The riveting colors have a gorgeous multidimensional shine and are not for the timid or sheer-preference crowd. All others should give this strong consideration, especially for alluring evening makeup.

☺ **$$$ Moonbeam Reflective Gloss** *($17.50)* has a thick, syrupy texture that contributes to a polished, multidimensional shine. Outfitted with a sleek brush applicator, this gloss is a breeze to apply and the shade selection is remarkable—a step above most other gloss offerings, especially if you prefer lots of shimmer and translucent but "still-there" colors. It is slightly sticky, but otherwise is a must-see for gloss fans with generous budgets for cosmetics.

☺ **Tint Balm for the Lips** *($14.50)* is a standard, sheer, glossy lip balm available in a range of pretty colors. The darker shades may look intimidating, but each goes on softly. The minimally sticky finish makes this gloss comfortable to wear. ☺ **$$$ Deluxe Lip Pencil** *($18.50)* gets its deluxe name because the opposite end of this automatic, retractable pencil has a well-made brush for applying lipstick or softening the line you draw. The pencil itself applies smoothly, has a soft cream finish that is minimally prone to smearing, and the colors have enough pigmentation to stick around longer than most. Cover Girl and L'Oreal have similar versions of this pencil for less money, but this pencil deserves consideration if you want to shop at the department store.

😐 **$$$ Colorscope Lipcolor** *($17.50)* replaces almost all of Prescriptives former lipsticks, including Modernista, Incredible Lip Color, and Lavish Lipstick. I'd be all for it if the replacement were measurably better, but it really isn't. The oil-laden formula is creamy bordering on greasy, and easily migrates into lines around the mouth. It is also very easy to smear and tends to come off on everything. The shade range is attractive and available in three finishes: Cream is as described above and includes ten shades; Sparkle offers the fewest number of shades and is just like the Cream, but with obvious particles of sparkle that don't feel grainy; the Shimmer shades number 19 and are identical to the Creams, save for their soft shimmer finish (a look toward which many women will gravitate). If you're a fan of one of the older Prescriptives lipstick formulas, they have a color/formula chart at the counter to suggest an alternative color (in some instances, it's identical) in the new Colorscope formula, assuming you want to give it a go.

😐 **$$$ Colourscope Custom Color Shifter** *($17.50)* is a somewhat greasy lipstick available in two shades, each of which are meant to change the color by adding a warm or cool tone. The Warm version is a pale gold shimmer, while Cool is a sheer, opalescent white with lavender shimmer. Applying either shade over lipstick changes its color, but often not to a flattering effect. Moreover, the texture of this can make an otherwise long-wearing lipstick become too slippery. Prescriptives has offered versions of this product in the past, and why they brought it back is a mystery because I suspect most women will find it fun once or twice, then forget about it.

😐 **$$$ Incredible Sheer Lipcolor SPF 15** *($17.50)* does have some incredibly pretty, pastel shades, but it is otherwise a commonplace sheer lipstick whose sunscreen lacks sufficient UVA-protecting ingredients. It has a smooth, agreeable application and a glossy finish, with the cachet that the Prescriptives name brings. But without a reliable sunscreen why spend this much on what amounts to nothing more than a basic sheer lipstick?

😐 **$$$ Rain Gloss** *($18.50)* is said to be "a wet burst of lush color with a cooling sensation," and although it does have a mild cooling effect, it is thankfully not from irritating ingredients. This is one of the lightest-feeling lip glosses you're likely to experience. It's slick on and feels smooth and, yes, it also feels wet, but is not the least bit goopy or sticky. It leaves a minimally glossy finish and the attractive colors provide light coverage. The only drawback is that the thin-textured gloss doesn't last as long as it should. The slightly moist feel dissipates quickly, making lips feel a bit parched and dry instead of moist and glossy.

☹ **$$$ Lipcoloring Pencil** *($15.50)* is a standard, creamy lip pencil whose relatively dry application takes some getting used to, but the reward is a stay-put finish. The shade selection, while small, comprises basic colors most women would want to consider.

MASCARA: ☺ **$$$ Beyond Long Maximum Length Mascara** *($19.50)* instantly makes lashes longer and creates decent thickness, too, all without clumps or smearing. This is Prescriptives best mascara (because the Eyelash Curler Shaping Mascara has unfortunately been discontinued), though its performance isn't impressive enough to make it worth considering over less expensive mascaras that received Paula's Pick ratings.

☺ **$$$ Lash Builder Mascara Basecoat** *($15.50)* is a lash primer whose ingredients are similar to what's found in a typical mascara, but this clear product does make a visible difference when paired with a mascara. You'll notice more thickness and overall oomph, making this worth considering if you normally use a natural-look mascara but occasionally want it to make more of an impact. Anyone using a mascara that dramatically enhances lashes on its own need not apply.

☹ **$$$ False Eyelashes Plush Mascara** *($19.50)* doesn't come close to mimicking false lashes. Although it certainly provides good length, it takes time to get there. Thickness is minimal, but lashes are cleanly separated. The packaging is impressive, but it's too bad the rather large, thick container doesn't translate into large, thick lashes. For a real false-lashes effect without the adhesive glue, consider L'Oreal's Lash Architect mascara.

☹ **$$$ Lash Envy Volumizing Mascara** *($19.50)* promises "Diva-esque lashes guaranteed to be the envy of all," but I can't imagine any "diva" being envied for the way her lashes would look wearing this mascara. It takes considerable effort to obtain length (at least four or five applications) and the result is decent but not exciting. This is better for elongating lashes than for thickening them, but it does last all day without flaking or smearing.

FACE AND BODY ILLUMINATING/SHIMMER PRODUCTS: ✓☺ **$$$ Magic Illuminating Potion Foundation Primer** *($30)* gets a stellar rating for being one of the best sheer, liquid-shimmer products available. A little goes a long way, which is a nice benefit when you're spending this much on soft shine. It edges out many others because of the way it melds with the skin, creating a shine that, while noticeable, is never intrusive or glittery. The claims for this are as exaggerated as it gets at the cosmetics counters, but what else would you expect from a "magic potion"? All three shades are beautiful options; Deep Translucent is a standout for medium to tan skin.

☹ **$$$ Illuminating Cream Potion** *($35)* comes in a compact and has a texture that's similar to but creamier than Prescriptives Photochrome foundation above. It retains some slip on skin so is not as long-lasting or worry-free as the Magic Illuminating Potion above, but it's an OK option if you want a really subtle highlight that's even suitable for daytime.

BRUSHES: The makeup **Brushes** *($16–$50)* continue to improve, with particularly outstanding choices among the powder and eyeshadow options. There are still a few superfluous brushes that, try as they might, the salespeople cannot convince me are worth the splurge. However, Prescriptives has plenty of traditional and innovative brushes that come highly recommended. If you don't mind the squat size, the ✓☺ **$$$ Portable Face Brush** *($28)* is wonderfully soft and dense, holding and depositing powder well. The ✓☺ **$$$ Foundation Brush** *($30)* is well-shaped to fit into the contours of the face and the ✓☺ **$$$ Powder Brush** *($35)* is soft and almost fluffy without being floppy. The ✓☺ **Soft Shadow Brush** *($24)* is also a winner.

☺ **$$$ Bronzer Brush** *($32)* is a unique powder brush because 85% of it is composed of densely packed, tapered hair that nicely holds its shape. The remaining 15% (these are rough visual estimates) is composed of longer, separated hairs that extend past the edge of the thicker hairs. This allows you to use just the tip (the longer, spaced-apart hairs) to apply a very sheer layer of powder (bronzing or otherwise) or, depending on the desired effect, the blunter side of the brush to achieve a stronger application. The longer hairs allow you to apply powder to a larger area. While strange in appearance, it ends up being quite practical. The ☺ **$$$ Cheek Brush** *($30)* has been the same for years, and it remains a suitable option for blush or, if held correctly, contouring.

😐 **$$$ Curvelinear Cheek Brush** *($30)* looks like a regular blush brush that has been flattened and had a shallow C-shape cut into it. The idea is that women who are uncomfortable with their lack of skill applying blush can simply dab the flat, wide side of this brush in their powder blush and stripe it on. However, as you might expect, what you're left with afterward is a stripe of color along the cheekbone. The Prescriptives makeup artist explained to me that she has to go back over her blush carefully to blend out the edges every time she uses this brush. I asked her if she had to do the same thing when using Prescriptives Blush Brush and she admitted she didn't, and also said she prefers it. I know you will, too. Avoid the inflexible ☹ **Eyeshadow Brush** *($22.50)*, the ☹ **Fan Brush** *($20)*, and the ☹ **Lip Brush** *($16)*, whose brush head is so tiny even women with small, thin lips will quickly tire of using it.

SPECIALTY PRODUCTS: ☺ **$$$ Invisible Line Smoother** *($35 for 0.5 ounce)* is a colorless, thick silicone cream that is virtually identical to M.A.C.'s Matte ($17.50), with the same matte-cream texture that is reminiscent of a sheer, soft spackle. It definitely can give the appearance of smoother skin, but the effect is temporary at best. Test drive this before you make the investment because I'm not convinced you will notice a difference.

PRESCRIPTIVES CUSTOM BLEND

Prescriptives has offered custom blend services for years at many of its counters. Despite offering over 300 shades of pre-made foundations, some women fall between shades and require a more precise match, at least that's Prescriptives rationale. Completely relaunched in October 2006, the Custom Blend options from Prescriptives are more extensive and involved than ever. **Custom Blend Foundation** *($62)*, **Custom Blend Powder** *($45; available in Loose or Pressed)*, **Custom Blend Concealer** *($32)*, **Custom Blend Lip Gloss** *($26)*, and **Custom Blend Lipstick** *($26)* are all worth looking into if you cannot find or are not satisfied with the vast number of makeup shades in any given department store. These products were not rated individually because the degree of customization and the expertise of the salesperson directly affect the outcome. Performance-wise, the Custom Blend options are on par with the better products Prescriptives offers in each respective category. One caution: it is critical that you find a Prescriptives salesperson who is experienced with this specialized service.

PREVAGE (SEE ELIZABETH ARDEN)

PROACTIV SOLUTION (SKIN CARE ONLY)

PROACTIV SOLUTION AT-A-GLANCE

Strengths: Effective, elegant-textured AHA, BHA, and skin-lightening options; all sunscreens provide sufficient UVA protection; good options for controlling excess oil breakthrough.

Weaknesses: Several products contain irritating ingredients that do not help acne-prone skin; some gimmicky products that no dermatologist-created line should be selling (they should know better); this is not *the* answer for acne-prone skin.

For more information about ProActiv, call (800) 876-9717 or visit www.proactiv.com or www.Beautypedia.com. Note: Unless you can find ProActiv products at a mall kiosk, I urge you to think twice before purchasing it via the infomercial or online. According to the Web site www.infomercialscams.com, ProActiv has received numerous registered complaints about its customer service and the company's auto-ship program, which is, according to some former customers, as difficult to cancel as a health club membership. Unless you know better or are explicitly clear about what you sign up for, ProActiv will continue to send you products and bill your credit card $39.95 per month as part of their Clear Skin Club program (Sources: www.proactive.com; and www.infomercialscams.com/scams/proactive_solution).

☹ **Clear Zone Body Pads** *($21.75 for 75 pads)* are dual-textured pads medicated with 2% salicylic acid. Although the pH of the solution in which the pads are soaked allows exfoliation to occur, the amount of alcohol and the inclusion of witch hazel do not make these a must-have option for blemished skin.

☹ **Makeup Removing Cloths** *($16.75 for 45 towelettes)* are not adept at removing makeup thoroughly because they lack cleansing agents or solvents, and they contain enough lavender to cause problems for skin. The cleansing cloths from Olay, Pond's, or Dove are preferred to and less expensive than this.

☹ **Deep Cleansing Wash** *($20 for 8 ounces)* cannot help unclog pores as claimed because its 2% salicylic acid is washed down the drain before it can go to work inside the pore lining. More of an issue is that this cleanser contains menthol, which won't help anyone have clearer skin.

😐 **$$$ Renewing Cleanser** *($16 for 4 ounces)* is a water-soluble cleansing lotion that uses 2.5% benzoyl peroxide as the active ingredient. A benzoyl peroxide wash may sound convenient, but it's a problem if used around the eyes, plus in a cleanser it's in contact with the skin only briefly, which makes it not nearly as potent as when it is used in a leave-on product.

☺ **$$$ Revitalizing Toner** *($16 for 4 ounces)* is a good 6% AHA liquid. However, when it comes to most kinds of breakouts, research indicates that BHA (salicylic acid) rather than AHA is the best way to exfoliate for breakout prevention. Salicylic acid can exfoliate within the pore as well as on the surface of the skin because it is lipid soluble (meaning it can penetrate oil). AHAs exfoliate primarily on the surface of the skin because they are water soluble and can't work beneath the surface. The amount of witch hazel is unlikely to be irritating, but it keeps this from earning a higher rating.

✓☺ **Clarifying Night Cream** *($28.75 for 1 ounce)* is a well-formulated BHA lotion that includes 1% salicylic acid at an effective pH of 3.6. As further enticement, the formula also includes retinol and several antioxidants, all in stable packaging. This is highly recommended for normal to dry skin battling blackheads and blemishes. Clarifying Night Cream does contain fragrance.

☹ **Daily Oil Control** *($20 for 1.7 ounces)* lists alcohol as the second ingredient and although that can de-grease skin, it is also very irritating and can cause free-radical damage.

☺ **Daily Protection Plus Sunscreen SPF 15** *($17.25 for 4 ounces)* is a good in-part avobenzone sunscreen for normal to oily skin. It provides a lightweight matte finish and contains some helpful absorbent ingredients. What's missing are antioxidants (the only one of note is a tiny amount of vitamin C). The amount of salicylic acid is too low to affect blemish-prone skin, although the pH is within the ideal range.

☹ **Green Tea Moisturizer** *($24.50 for 1 ounce)* contains a lot of green tea and vitamin A, two antioxidants with considerable value for all skin types. The problem is that the amount of iris root extract (also known as orris root) can cause allergic or sensitizing skin reactions and there is no research showing it to be beneficial for skin (Source: Botanical Dermatology Database, http://bodd.cf.ac.uk/BotDermFolder/BotDermC/CACT.html). What a shame, because this is otherwise a great moisturizer for normal to dry skin.

☺ **Nourishing Eye Cream** *($23.25 for 0.5 ounce)* is a good, lightweight, fragrance-free moisturizer for slightly dry skin around the eyes or anywhere on the face. It contains several antioxidants, which is good because none of them are present in a significant amount.

☺ **Oil Free Moisture with SPF 15** *($27 for 1.7 ounces)* is a basic, fragrance-free sunscreen for normal to oily skin. The in-part zinc oxide sunscreen may be a problem for someone struggling with blemishes, but it does contribute to this product's matte finish and UVA protection.

😐 **Replenishing Eye Serum** *($23.25 for 0.5 ounce)* lists a film-forming agent as the main ingredient, and at that concentration users may experience some irritation (and it definitely creates a firming, tightening sensation, though the effect is strictly cosmetic). The silicone-enhanced formula contains some impressive water-binding agents and antioxidants, but the potential for irritation makes this a risky consideration.

☺ **Sheer Finish Mattifying Gel** *($18 for 1 ounce)* definitely helps keep skin matte due to its combination of dry-finish silicones and clay. The inclusion of green tea and the omission of fragrance also make this a decent contender for those with oily skin who need shine control. However, it would have achieved a higher rating if it included a complement of antioxidants, skin-identical ingredients, and cell-communicating ingredients. Leaving those out shortchanges any skin type.

☹ **Advanced Blemish Treatment** *($17 for 0.33 ounce)* is a 6% benzoyl peroxide solution. However, the fourth ingredient is alcohol, which makes this unnecessarily drying and irritating. There are far more gentle 5% and 10% benzoyl peroxide products at the drugstore for a fraction of this price.

☹ **Medicated Pore Cleaning System** *($16.50 for the kit)* is further proof that the dermatologists behind this line are frustratingly endorsing both helpful and harmful products for those with acne. This two-step system includes **Pore Strips** and a **Pore Cleansing Solution**. The Pore Strips are like Scotch tape for skin, and include alcohol, peppermint oil, and menthol to further irritate and inflame skin. The Pore Cleansing Solution doesn't fare much better because it contains a lot of alcohol and irritating arnica extract. This is a mistake from any angle. There is nothing medicated about alcohol, menthol, or peppermint.

☹ **Mild Exfoliating Peel** *($18 for 1 ounce)* is mild to the point of being ineffective because the 0.5% salicylic acid won't work efficiently at this product's pH level. Further, with alcohol and witch hazel heading up the ingredient list, this peel is far from "calming"; rather it is irritating and drying.

☹ **Refining Mask** *($20 for 2.5 ounces)* is a standard clay mask that also contains 6% pure sulfur. Sulfur can be a good antibacterial agent, but its irritant properties outweigh its benefit for most people. There are better ways to disinfect skin than this.

✓☺ **Repairing Lotion** *($21.75 for 2 ounces)* is a very good topical disinfectant for acne. The active ingredient is 2.5% benzoyl peroxide and it is blended in a silky lotion base that contains an anti-irritant. It's pricey for what you get, but is definitely worth considering as part of a battle plan for blemishes. This does contain fragrance.

✓☺ **Skin Lightening Lotion** *($21.50 for 1 ounce)* combines 2% hydroquinone with approximately 4% glycolic acid at an effective pH of 3.3. This is an outstanding option to fade sun- or hormone-induced brown skin discolorations, while also improving skin's texture and reducing inflammation with antioxidants. The opaque packaging ensures the hydroquinone will remain stable during use.

☺ **$$$ Oil Blotter Sheets** *($16.50 for 130 sheets)* are standard, powder-free pieces of paper that work quickly to absorb excess oil and perspiration. They're on the pricey side, but at least you get an abundance of papers.

PURPOSE (SKIN CARE ONLY)

PURPOSE AT-A-GLANCE

Strengths: Inexpensive; one good cleanser.

Weaknesses: Bar soap; sunscreen that contains preservatives not recommended for use in leave-on products; claims that are not supported by intelligent formulas.

For more information about Purpose, owned by Johnson & Johnson, call (866) 344-4848 or visit www.purpose.com or www.Beautypedia.com.

☹ **Gentle Cleansing Bar** *($3.99 for 6-ounce bar)* is a standard bar soap and not recommended for any skin type. If your physician advises you to use this product, definitely reconsider—it's not even a little bit gentle.

☺ **Gentle Cleansing Wash** *($6.99 for 6 ounces)* is distinctly preferred to the Gentle Cleansing Bar above, and remains a very good water-soluble cleanser for all skin types except very dry. For the record, this cleanser is identical to Clean & Clear's Foaming Facial Cleanser, Sensitive Skin ($4.39 for 8 ounces). Both companies are owned by Johnson & Johnson.

☹ **Dual Treatment Moisture Lotion with SPF 15** *($9.99 for 4 ounces)* claims to not clog pores (as do many other moisturizers), but the titanium dioxide and thickeners in this product make it easy to refute that claim. You may or may not break out from this in-part titanium dioxide sunscreen, but either way it is not recommended because it contains the skin-sensitizing preservatives methylchloroisothiazolinone and methylisothiazolinone.

😐 **Redness Reducing Moisturizer with SPF 30** *($14.99 for 2.75 ounces)* earns its SPF 30 rating from a combination of three synthetic sunscreen actives along with zinc oxide. The synthetic sunscreens have a higher incidence of causing a sensitizing reaction, so their inclusion in a product for someone with already reddened (presumably sensitive) skin is not wise. A moisturizer with sunscreen that contains only titanium dioxide or zinc oxide as its active ingredients is preferred for anyone dealing with persistent redness or sensitivity issues (Sources: *Cosmetic Dermatology*, March 2004, pages 171–172; and *Cosmetics & Toiletries*, October 2003, pages 73–78). Although this fragrance-free moisturizer is not an ideal choice for those dealing with facial redness, it is still a decent option for normal to dry skin. The formula feels lighter than many SPF 30 products, but unfortunately it doesn't contain a significant amount of antioxidants or other state-of-the-art ingredients. The sunscreen combination is great, but it doesn't warrant a happy face rating because the base formula isn't state-of-the-art. In addition, the redness-reducing claims are misleading, because the formula also contains preservatives that don't have the best track record for someone with sensitive skin.

QUO (MAKEUP ONLY—CANADA ONLY)

QUO AT-A-GLANCE

Strengths: Inexpensive; testers are available for every product; two superb foundations, including one with reliable sunscreen; notable eyeshadows, powder blush, and cream blush; wonderful lipsticks and lipliner; the best makeup brushes available at Canadian drugstores.

Weaknesses: Underachieving concealers and powders; terrible liquid eyeliner; the Faux Glow shimmer powder.

For more information about Quo, visit www.shoppersdrugmart.ca or www.Beautypedia.com. Note: All prices for Quo products are in Canadian dollars; Quo is sold exclusively at Shoppers Drug Mart.

FOUNDATION: ✓☺ **Wet and Dry Foundation** *($18)* is a talc-based, pressed-powder foundation with a suede-like texture that applies smoothly and looks almost like a second skin. This is not a tightly pressed powder, so you need to be careful you don't over-apply, but it blends so readily it's easy to correct mistakes. It has a natural matte finish imbued with a hint of shine and provides light to medium coverage. The selection of six shades features predominantly neutral colors that are best for fair to medium skin.

✓☺ **Optical Illusion Foundation SPF 15** *($20)* is the only Quo foundation that gets the sunscreen right, thanks to its in-part titanium dioxide and zinc oxide active ingredients. This jar-packaged foundation has a slightly thick, mousse-like texture that readily smooths over skin and transforms into a nearly weightless, silky matte finish. Coverage goes from sheer to barely medium, making this a good choice for normal to slightly dry or slightly oily skin types who don't have much to conceal. All six shades are commendable, though it is worth noting that on skin they set lighter (and less pink or peach) than they appear in the jar.

😐 **Light Diffusing Makeup SPF 8** *($15)* not only has an SPF rating that's preposterously low but also lacks the UVA-protecting active ingredients titanium dioxide, zinc oxide, avobenzone, Mexoryl SX, or Tinosorb. What a shame the company left out the sunscreen, because this has a very light texture and a silky foundation that provides light to medium coverage and a satin-matte finish. The six shades are tailored for fair to light skin tones, and all of them are good. Just keep in mind that this is a foundation that must be paired with a sunscreen rated SPF 15 or higher, unless you're only going to use it in the evening.

😐 **Skin Tint SPF 15** *($15)* is a very sheer foundation that imparts more shimmer than color to skin. The sunscreen cannot be relied on for solo use because it lacks sufficient UVA-protecting ingredients. The Light and Medium shades are best used as highlighters, while Dark is a sheer bronze tone. The formula begins slightly thick but blends well to a satin finish.

CONCEALER: 😐 **Illuminating Concealer** *($10)* isn't too illuminating when you consider its slightly chalky matte finish. This is otherwise a standard liquid concealer that has a lightweight texture and blends quite well. The finish isn't a deal-breaker, and three of the four colors are very good (shade 01 is slightly pink), but I wouldn't choose this over L'Oreal's True Match Concealer ($7.89).

😐 **$$$ Bags Away** *($19)* is a creamy compact concealer that features three different tones that can be used alone or blended for a custom shade. I can almost guarantee you will be turned off by the thick texture and the heavy appearance this has on your skin, not to mention that in the three sets of colors, three of four in each compact barely resemble real skin tones, although they can be blended together to get a better approximation. (But why bother, given the number of single-shade neutral concealers available at a nearby L'Oreal or Cover Girl display?)

☹ **Colour Corrector Camouflage** *($17)* comes in a compact and offers four color-correcting shades that do not resemble skin and look incredibly obvious. Even worse is the fairly greasy texture, spotty coverage, and the tendency for this to crease and fade.

POWDER: ☺ **$$$ Satin Face Pressed Powder** *($17)* has a sumptuous, silky texture and a smooth, non-powdery finish that imparts quite a bit of shine. The talc-based formula's seven colors are beautiful, and include options for fair to tan skin tones. This is worth auditioning if you don't mind a shiny powder (and this shine doesn't flake).

😐 **$$$ Mosaic Perfecting Powder** *($18)* is a talc-based pressed powder with multiple colors in a mosaic pattern that come off as a sheer peach shade on skin. It's an OK option to enliven fair to light skin that has a sallow or olive undertone, but for the money there are superior powders at the drugstore. 😐 **$$$ Mosaic Bronzer** *($18)* has the same talc-based formula and multicolored pattern as the Mosaic Perfecting Powder above, only this is a bronze tone whose swirled colors end up looking a bit too peachy orange for most skin tones.

☹ **Tinted Blotting Powder** *($15)* is supposed to minimize shine (oil), yet this dry-textured pressed powder adds shine to skin, and its finish isn't nearly as attractive as the Satin Face Pressed Powder above, or of most other pressed powders for that matter.

BLUSH: The powder ☺ **$$$ Blush** *($17)* is a pleasure to apply because it goes on without a hitch and remains color-true, although the shade selection now features soft colors with at least some degree of shine (most are quite shiny). The Natural shade is a duo blush that provides a brown-based blush color paired with a soft highlighter.

☺ **Cream Blush** *($15)* is better described as a cream-to-powder blush. It has a silky texture and applies evenly (meaning it has just enough slip to allow precise, not sloppy, blending). The two sheer shades have a subtle amount of sparkles, which contribute to this blush's glow-y finish. It is best for normal to dry skin that is fair to light.

😐 **$$$ Two Cheeky Blush** *($19)* features two blush shades in one compact, both shiny and both with a dry, slightly grainy texture and strong pigmentation. Application can be sketchy, but this is nevertheless an option, particularly for women with darker skin tones (who don't mind shiny cheeks). 😐 **$$$ Cheek Tint** *($17)* is a solid, roll-on gel blush that provides a transparent wash of color yet is tricky to blend evenly unless skin is moist. The sheer yet bright shades perk up pale skin, but the waxy finish is not the best.

EYESHADOW: Quo's ✓☺ **Eye Shadow Singles** *($11)* have an astonishingly silky texture that feels almost decadent, making this category a highlight of the Quo line. The selection of ten shades now favors shine, but it absolutely doesn't flake, nor is it glaring. Portrait is the sole matte shade, and Storm is best avoided due to its blueness. ✓☺ **Eyeshadow Quads** *($16)* don't offer a lot of color combinations, but what's available is attractive and the shades are expertly coordinated and include all-matte options (which is not typical for a makeup line). These have the same superlative texture and application characteristics as the Eye Shadow Singles. The Sandbar quad is completely matte, while the sole shiny shade in the other quads should be applied sheer to avoid flaking.

☺ **Eye Shadow Trio** *($15)* has wonderful application and texture traits similar to the Eye Shadow Singles above, but these trios offer less opacity. Unfortunately, three of the four trios are terrible color combinations that favor strong greens and blues. Florentine Pathway is the only workable trio. ☺ **Stay Put Cream Eye Colour** *($13)* is a liquid eyeshadow applied with a sponge tip. It delivers intense, flakeproof shine and has just the right amount of slip to allow for precise blending before setting to a stay-put finish. Four of the six colors are versatile and work well together; avoid Fiji and Riviera.

EYE AND BROW SHAPER: 😐 **Automatic Eye Liner** *($11)* doesn't need sharpening and is retractable. The slick application tends to stay creamy so some smudging is inevitable, though you can use the included pointed sponge tip to soften the line before that happens on its own. 😐 **3-in-1 Brow Pencil** *($10)* is a dual-sided pencil that needs sharpening. One end is a standard, dry-textured brow pencil, and all three colors are workable. The other end of each shade features a clear brow wax in pencil form, used to groom brows and tame unruly hairs. It's OK, but tends to ball up a bit in brow hairs, requiring further smoothing.

☹ **Liquid Eyeliner** *($12)* has too many negatives to make it worth considering over most other liquid eyeliners at the drugstore. The mostly shiny colors have an uneven application that's too wet, which hinders dry time and leads to smearing. In addition, the brush has an awkward point that makes drawing a smooth, flowing line even more difficult.

LIPSTICK, LIP GLOSS, AND LIPLINER: Quo's ✓☺ **Lipstick** *($12)* is a very good, lightweight yet creamy lipstick with a decent stain and an attractive (though not extensive) range of colors. It has a soft gloss finish and opaque coverage, making it a viable option for fans of regular lipstick. ✓☺ **Lip Liner** *($12)* is an automatic, nonretractable lipliner with an agreeable, soft texture that's still firm enough to draw a precise line, and the built-in lip brush is a handy tool for softening things. What's best about this liner is how well it stays in place, though I wish the shade selection were broader. Quo did include a colorless option that works beautifully to stop lipstick from feathering into lines around the mouth.

☺ **Lip Gloss Stick** *($12)* is a sheer-coverage, glossy-finish lipstick that feels comfortable and isn't too slippery. The small shade selection is well edited, making this a good choice if you like sheer lipsticks. ☺ **Lip Gloss** *($12)* is a straightforward wand gloss that's minimally sticky and otherwise everything you'd expect from a basic lip gloss. ☺ **Stay Put Lipstick** *($14)* comes in a slim tube and has a nearly weightless silky texture that glides over lips. It sets quickly to a long-wearing matte finish that transfers minimally and lasts for hours without fading, cracking, or peeling. The only drawback is that it can feel uncomfortable if you're used to any amount of moisture, and not everyone may love the flat finish. Using a gloss with this undermines the formula's tenacity, making this worth trying only if you want a nonemollient, true matte lipstick. ☺ **Lip Balm** *($12)* is a glossy, colorless lip balm in lipstick form. Dry, chapped lips will be happy to meet this rather standard, but effective, product.

MASCARA: ☺ **Lengthening Mascara** *($10)* makes lashes slightly longer than the Major Volume Mascara below, minus much thickness. It doesn't claim to do much more than make lashes longer, and it accomplishes that for those interested in a natural, separated lash look.

😐 **Major Volume Mascara** *($10)* is a mascara that is sure to disappoint if you take its name seriously. Although nothing about its performance is of major consequence, it's a workable lengthening mascara that separates lashes and leaves them soft. Thickness is possible, but only with effort, and it never goes beyond average, which some women may prefer.

FACE AND BODY ILLUMINATING/SHIMMER PRODUCTS: ☺ **$$$ Mosaic Shimmer Bronzer** *($17)* actually has the best mix of shades of all Quo's Mosaic powders. This smooth-textured pressed bronzing powder with a soft shine is recommended for those with light to medium skin who want to create a tan glow without sun exposure.

☹ **Faux Glow** *($17)* has a great name, and does add shine to your skin. You could use it for alluring evening makeup, but I wouldn't recommend that, because with either shade of this iridescent bronzing powder the shine flakes all over and just isn't flattering.

BRUSHES: The brush collection from Quo remains a significant high point. It is doubtful Canadians will find such an admirable collection of professional brushes anywhere else at such reasonable prices (and they're on sale at at least a few times each year). The best ones are the ✓☺ **Large Concealer Brush** *($14)*; ✓☺ **Definer Shadow Brush** *($12)*; the regular ✓☺ **Lip Brush** *($15)*; which is great for medium to full lips, the ✓☺ **Liner/Brow Brush** *($12)*; which is best for eyelining; and the ✓☺ **Retractable Powder Brush** *($20)*.

Also worth considering are the ☺ **Brow/Lash Brush** *($12)*, the synthetic ☺ **Cream Blush Brush** *($16)*, and the regular ☺ **Concealer Brush** *($12)*, which is good for spot application to cover red marks or blemishes.

The 😐 **Powder Brush** *($20)* is a bit too large and floppy for controlled application and the 😐 **Blush Brush** *($16)* is soft and dense, but too full for most women's cheeks. It would make a better powder brush.

SPECIALTY PRODUCTS: ☺ **Eye Primer** *($12)* is meant to be used on eyelids and under the brow prior to eyeshadow application. Essentially a matte-finish concealer, this is housed in a click-pen applicator with an angled sponge-tip applicator. It conceals well and comes in one shade, a nude peach that is best for fair to light skin tones.

😐 **Lip Scrub** *($12)* is packaged to resemble a lipstick, and its emollient, wax base is infused with crushed walnut shells, which will indeed exfoliate but are too abrasive for routine use on lips. Lip Scrub is preferred for exfoliating dry knees, heels, and elbows.

😐 **Lip Winterizer** *($12)* is a water- and glycerin-based tube lip balm that's an OK option for moisturizing lips, but one that (especially for wintertime) isn't nearly as effective as a nonaqueous, emollient lip balm. Plain Vaseline would be a better defense against the elements that cause lips to chap, but if that's not a concern, this is an alternative lightweight lip moisturizer.

RETINOIDS
(INCLUDING AVAGE, AVITA, DIFFERIN, RENOVA, RETIN-A MICRO, RETIN-A, AND TAZORAC)

All of the products in the heading above are prescription-only drugs belonging to a class of active ingredients called "retinoids." Although I do not review these products as I do other products, all of them deserve mention in this book. That's because, depending on your needs and preferences, each has merit for helping skin in numerous ways. Whether your concern is acne, sun damage, wrinkles, loss of firmness, or simply creating and maintaining healthier skin, retinoids are a state-of-the-art, multipurpose treatment. Furthermore, unlike countless cosmetic ingredients and all manner of anti-aging products that make fantastic claims, retinoids are backed by mounds of solid research supporting their mechanism of action, efficacy, and tolerability (Sources: *Cutis*, December 2006, pages 426–432; *Drugs*, 2005, pages 1061–1072; *Dermatologic Therapy*, September–October 2006, pages 297–305; *The Journal of Family Practice*, November 2006, pages 994–996; and *Cutis*, October 2004, pages 4–8).

With regard to the active ingredients in these products, tretinoin (found in Retin-A and Renova) has been around the longest and has the most research behind it. Considered a "first-generation retinoid," tretinoin improves skin-cell function, changing abnormally produced cells into ones that are more normal, which in turn changes the environment of the pore and makes it more difficult for blemishes to form.

Tolerance is a big issue with tretinoin, as its side effects (burning or stinging sensations, peeling, and redness) can be bothersome and visually discouraging, not to mention difficult to camouflage with makeup (Source: *Journal of Drugs in Dermatology*, November–December 2004, pages 641–651). How much (or even if) these side effects will be an issue depends greatly not only on the concentration of tretinoin but also on the vehicle (cream, gel, lotion), frequency of application, and each individual's reaction. Tretinoin in the form of Retin-A Micro seems to be less potentially irritating than "regular" tretinoin (Retin-A cream), which is likely due to Retin-A Micro's controlled delivery system (Source: *Cutis*, July 2003, pages 76–81).

Tazarotene is the active ingredient in Tazorac. It is a synthetic retinoid that works as a cell-communicating ingredient (similar to tretinoin) while normalizing skin-cell production and shedding within the pore lining. Tazarotene also has an anti-inflammatory effect and is frequently used in psoriasis therapy, often with a topical corticosteroid (Sources: *American Journal of Clinical Dermatology*, June 2005, pages 255–272; and *Journal of the American Academy of Dermatology*, August 1997). Side effects of tazarotene are similar to those of tretinoin, including a burning sensation, peeling, and redness. Just as with tretinoin, these side effects typically diminish or resolve with ongoing use as the skin adapts to the active ingredient.

Adapalene is the active ingredient in Differin. Clinical trials have shown that it causes fewer side effects and is thus better tolerated than tretinoin (Sources: *International Journal of Dermatology*, October 2000, pages 784–788; *Journal of Cutaneous Medical Surgery*, October 1999, pages 298–301; and *Skinmed*, September/October 2006, pages 219–223). Adapalene appears to have a particularly precise ability to positively affect the skin-cell lining of the pores, substantially improving exfoliation, which helps prevent blockages that can, in the presence of certain bacteria (*P. acnes*) lead to acne (Sources: *Journal of Drugs in Dermatology*, June 2007, pages 616–622; *Journal of the American Academy of Dermatology*, July 2007, Epublication; and *European Journal of Dermatology*, January–February 2007, pages 45–51).

Regardless of which prescription retinoid you choose, each has documented benefit for skin as well as its share of side effects that, for most patients, resolve with continued (and often modified frequency of) use. Those considering a retinoid for acne should keep in mind that although using a retinoid alone can be very helpful, many dermatologists recommend combination therapy to keep acne under control. This may involve prescription topical antibiotics or over-the-counter disinfectants. Finally, all forms of prescription retinoids increase the skin's sensitivity to sunlight. It is critical for the health of your skin (and even more imperative if you're using a retinoid) that you protect skin every day with a product rated SPF 15 or higher that supplies reliable UVA protection, in order to reduce or forestall the signs of aging.

RETINOIDS AT-A-GLANCE

Strengths: The active ingredient in all but two of the products below is tretinoin, which has mounds of research establishing its multiple anti-aging benefits for skin (particularly sun-damaged skin). Tazorac contains the active ingredient tazarotene, a retinoid that works similarly to tretinoin.

Weaknesses: Some people cannot tolerate tretinoin therapy; all of these products require a prescription; textures of each are not nearly as elegant as using a well-formulated moisturizer.

Rather than review these products and assign the usual face ratings, I present a list of the various options, along with prices based on figures from www.drugstore.com. Note that your actual price for these prescription products will vary based on your health insurance coverage, if any, and whether or not your physician believes that a generic form of tretinoin is an equally effective (and hence less costly) option.

Avage contains 0.1% tazarotene formulated in a bland cream base. It costs approximately $119.50 for a 30-gram tube.

Avita contains 0.025% tretinoin and is available in two sizes in a cream or gel base (the gel base contains 83% alcohol, and is not preferred to the cream). The 45-gram size costs $93.11.

Differin contains Adapalene and is available in cream or gel forms, both with a strength of 0.1%. A 45-gram tube of Differin cream costs $132.93; the same size of alcohol-free gel costs $117.28. Adapalene is not available as a generic. It is owned by Galderma, the company behind the Cetaphil brand.

Renova contains the active ingredient tretinoin and is available in strengths of 0.02% or 0.05%. It is available in cream form, has a more elegant texture than some other types of tretinoin cream, and comes in various sizes. The 40-gram size retails for $126.09.

Retin-A Micro contains tretinoin as the active ingredient, although it is encapsulated in "micro-sponges" for controlled release into skin. It is believed that this delivery system reduces tretinoin's potential to irritate skin. Retin-A Micro is available in two strengths: 0.1% and 0.04%. A 45-gram tube of the 0.04% version costs $120.56; a 45-gram tube of the 0.1% version costs $115.79.

Retin-A contains tretinoin and is available in cream, gel, or liquid textures. The gel is available in 0.025% or 0.01% strengths, but contains 90% alcohol, which significantly increases the potential for irritation. The cream version comes in three strengths: 0.1%, 0.05%, and 0.025%, and is formulated in a bland moisturizing base. The liquid is available only at the 0.05% strength and is in a base of water, alcohol (55%), slip agent, and preservative, and as expected, the alcohol definitely increases the potential for irritating side effects. Costs for the various formats and strengths vary, but are similar to the prices for Renova and Retin-A Micro.

Tazorac is the brand name for the retinoid tazarotene. It is available in 0.1% or 0.05% strengths, in either cream or gel form. The 0.1% strength is approved for acne, while the 0.05% strength is prescribed to manage psoriasis. A 30-gram tube of the cream costs $107.42; a 30-gram tube of the gel costs $101.98. Unlike Retin-A's gel, Tazorac gel is alcohol-free.

REVIVE (SKIN CARE ONLY)

REVIVE AT-A-GLANCE

Strengths: Good cleansers; and, well, that's about it.

Weaknesses: Very expensive; potential unknowns and concerns about how epidermal growth factor (EGF) functions when applied topically on intact skin; EGF is a common ingredient in these products; not all of the sunscreens provide sufficient UVA protection; no products to address the needs of adults with acne.

Note: growth factors do not work alone. Rather, their function is part of an intricate symphony that requires the playing of several "notes" for the "concert" to be a success. Adding a tiny amount of EGF to skin-care products in the hopes that it will work like it does when applied to a wound is sort of like thinking you can frame a house with wood and use nothing to hold the beams together except wishful thinking. Please refer to Chapter Seven, *Cosmetic Ingredient Dictionary*, for detailed information on epidermal growth factor.

For more information about ReVive, call (888) 704-3440 or visit www.reviveskincare.com or ww.Beautypedia.com.

REVIVE INTENSITE PRODUCTS

☹ **$$$ Intensite Creme Lustre** *($375 for 2 ounces)* ups the ante, claiming that this moisturizer can inhibit "the loss of collagen while significantly diminishing visible spider veins, sun damage, and irritation. IGF (Insulin-like Growth Factor) tempers the effects of aging by decreasing wrinkles and thickening the deep structural elements of skin. Vital enzymes offer a non-acid alternative that unveils a vibrant layer of skin without harshness or scaling. Refractory brighteners polish skin with a radiant incandescence for a lustrous complexion that cannot be achieved surgically or chemically." It's amazing how words can create a sense of substance and magnitude when there is so little of that actually to be found.

Perhaps the most important thing for you to know is that while there is definitely research showing IGF has benefit in wound healing (Sources: *Wound Repair and Regeneration*, July 2003, pages 253–260; and *The Journal of Immunology*, June 1, 2003, pages 5583–5589), there is little to no research showing it to have benefit for healthy skin or wrinkles. What research does exist is controversial and meager (Source: *New England Journal of Medicine*, February 27, 2003, pages 777–778). Only one study, observing 12 men older than 60, showed it to have any benefit, but the study had such a short duration that it was questionable whether the safety data could be adequate.

Other than ReVive's founder, Dr. Greg Brown, no one seems to think much of using IGF for wrinkles, and the concern that it may be problematic is not trivial. However, I don't think you need to be worried, because the amount of IGF in this product is minuscule and the type of packaging makes stability practically impossible after the product is opened. As far as the other claims go, there are no vital enzymes in this product that can affect the skin. It does contain some good water-binding agents, but not very much of them, and at this price it should be filled to the brim with state-of-the-art stuff. Oddly disappointing is the paltry amount of rather boring antioxidants. One more point: This does contain palmityl pentapeptide-3 (Matrixyl), which has a good deal of hype about its benefit for skin, although if you are interested in that, Olay uses it and their price ... well, you already know the answer to that one. Oh, and that bit about containing "refractory brighteners"? That merely refers to mica, shiny mineral particles that have nothing to do with skin care.

☺ **$$$ Intensite Fluide Superbe** *($400 for 1 ounce)* is said to be the modern answer to the age-old issues of dryness, and is for anyone who "just can't get enough moisture." I don't know why such people should be so price-gouged for their unresponsive dry skin, but I suppose that comes with the territory for this line and its allegedly "modern" formulas. According to the company, liposomes are used to deliver the olive oil and shea butter that comprise the bulk of this formula. Whether that's true or not, liposomes are not unique to this product, nor do they have to cost this much. Although the price and claims are over the top, there is no denying that this serum contains some truly beneficial ingredients for dry to very dry skin. Olive oil is a brilliant source of antioxidants while being very emollient, and a linoleic acid derivative is used, as are vitamins C and E. This would have been even better with more antioxidants and a broader selection of ingredients that mimic the structure of healthy skin, not to mention if it omitted the fragrant orange oil and volatile fragrant components (all present in amounts unlikely to be problematic for skin).

😐 **$$$ Intensite Les Yeux** *($190 for 0.5 ounce)* is ReVive's answer for dark circles, yet the high-tech ingredients in this product can have no effect on their appearance or reduction. This contains the citrus bioflavonoid hesperidin methyl chalcone, which is present in many products claiming to make dark circles a thing of the past. There is research supporting its use internally as an aid to venous (vein) problems. One study documented that it lowers the filtration rate of capillaries; less blood flowing though capillaries close to the surface of skin potentially means less hemoglobin would oxygenate to cause a dark bluish discoloration under the eyes. However, there is no substantiated research proving that it will have this effect when this ingredient is applied topically. Considering the price, you should expect swift results, but all this will do is make dry skin around the eyes feel better, the same as any moisturizer.

***unrated* Intensite Volumizing Serum** *($600 for 1 ounce)* must have a good story behind it because it costs too much for it not to, right? For $600, you're buying into the following claims: "Intensite Volumizing Serum with KGF (keratinocyte growth factor) augments the subtle loss of facial volume and plumps trouble areas. KGF halts the aging process by turning over dying skin cells 8 times faster and hinders DNA fragmentation. KGF's dynamic activity allows for a molecular dialogue with underlying layers of skin that contributes to increased volume after several weeks. Whitening Tri-Complex depigments the skin, eliminating blemishes and dark spots associated with aging. Powerful anti-radical defense system shields against pollution, stress and damaging UVB rays. Intensite Volumizing Serum is the optimal solution before considering or in preparation for a surgical procedure."

Even if you understand half of that, it sounds like it must be the answer for fighting wrinkles. Phrases such as "halts the aging process" and "shields against pollution" make this sound like (another) fountain of youth. And "depigmenting" skin is not a good thing, because it would leave skin without any color, creating white, albino-like skin. Who wrote this nonsense anyway?

This nonaqueous serum consists mostly of a glycerin ester (an ester is a compound formed by mixing an organic acid and alcohol), several forms of silicone, thickeners, several water-binding agents, antioxidants, and, as the very last ingredient, keratinocyte growth factor (KGF). With the exception of KGF, all of the other ingredients are fairly standard and are used in various products throughout the cosmetics industry, so none of them warrant the price tag (believe me those are cheap ingredients). Combined, they create a serum that will make skin feel soft and smooth, and the water-binding agents will help skin retain moisture. For the amount of money ReVive is asking for this product, you want more than what other companies are offering, because all of them are charging consumers a lot less for the same basic mix of ingredients. That's where KGF comes in.

ReVive defines KGF as "a naturally occurring protein molecule that augments facial volume and fights the aging process by halting DNA fragmentation." They also state that it enhances epidermal regeneration at breakneck speed. Never mind that an ingredient that speeds up the regeneration cycle of cells is a potential recipe for trouble (consider that cancer is the uncontrolled growth of cells). Can KGF add volume to skin and stop DNA fragmentation? No, it can't.

KGF is a cytokine. Simply put, cytokines are chemical messengers secreted by our immune system cells. They stimulate the production of other substances that help the body in some way. Cytokines can have positive effects (like wound healing) or negative effects (like proliferation of unhealthy cells). There is in vitro research showing that KGF plays a role in skin's response to UVB assault, and additional research showing that KGF plays a positive role in wound healing. But it takes a large amount of KGF—not just the little bit present in Intensite Volumizing Serum—to get that result. Plus, wrinkles aren't wounds. Also, when applied topically, KGF has a short biological half-life, meaning that once it gets into the skin, it's not long before it is broken down and becomes ineffective.

Still, there are fascinating studies that look at the application of several growth factors (including KGF) and their roles in wound healing. What's intriguing is that these topically applied growth factors do best when acting on a wound. It's just that wrinkles are not wounds, even if they may feel that way to our ego. There is scant information about how KGF acts on intact skin, and no substantiated information to support ReVive's claims that KGF adds volume to skin the way cosmetic fillers such as collagen do. And the notion that the aging process is halted is as over the top as it gets.

Moreover, KGF and other growth factors do not work alone. Each is part of an intricate, incredibly complex network of chemical processes that signal and transfer cellular information—part of the miracle that is the human body. To imagine that a fractional amount of KGF in a cosmetic product can function as an alternative to cosmetic surgery and somehow have a profound impact on the way skin ages is like trying to drive a car without its engine: it just isn't going to happen, even though everything else is seemingly in place (Sources: *FASEB Journal*, December 14, 2005; *American Journal of Pathology*, volume 167, issue 6, December 2005, pages 1575–1586; *Journal of Anatomy*, July 2005, pages 67–78; and *Journal of Cell Science*, volume 118, part 9, May 1, 2005, pages 1981–1989).

OTHER REVIVE PRODUCTS

☺ **$$$ Cleanser Agressif, for Normal to Oily Skin** *($65 for 6.7 ounces)* is a very standard, but effective, water-soluble cleanser for its intended skin types. It contains a couple of potentially problematic plant extracts, but the amounts are unlikely to create havoc. The real problem is the price, because nothing about this cleanser is superior to a vast number of similar options sold at the drugstore for a fraction of the cost.

☺ **$$$ Cleanser Creme Luxe, for Normal to Dry Skin** *($65 for 6 ounces)* would be rated higher if it did not contain potentially irritating orange oil for fragrance. It is otherwise a very gentle cleanser for its intended skin types, and does a thorough job of removing makeup.

☺ **$$$ Cleanser Gentil, for Normal to Dry Skin** *($65 for 6.7 ounces)* is similar to the Cleanser Agressif above, only with less detergent cleansing agent, which makes it preferred for normal to dry skin. Otherwise, the same comments apply.

☺ **$$$ Cleanser Exfoliante** *($65 for 6 ounces)* is very similar to the Cleanser Creme Luxe above, and the same comments apply, except this version contains jojoba beads for mild exfoliation.

😐 **$$$ Tonique Preparatif** *($52 for 6.7 ounces)* is an amazingly overpriced toner that consists primarily of water, slip agent, aloe, and witch hazel. The chamomile is a nice touch, but its effect is canceled out by the lavender, making this a so-so option for normal to slightly dry skin, but with a price tag that is laughable given the formulary.

☺ **$$$ Arrete Booster C** *($300 for 0.5 ounce)* is a blend of silicones with ascorbic acid (vitamin C), vitamin E, soybean oil, and retinol. The packaging will assuredly keep all of the antioxidants and retinol stable, and this is suitable for all skin types. As for the claims, there is no substantiated research proving that simply mixing vitamin C in a nonaqueous silicone medium will keep it "alive and stable" for up to 12 hours. Vitamin C's stability is improved when such a system (and correct packaging) is used, but whether or not it remains vital for half the day is up for debate (Sources: *International Journal of Pharmaceutics*, October 1999, pages 233–241; and *Drug Delivery*, April 2007, pages 235–245). Although this is a very good antioxidant serum, the astronomical price is such that I cannot in good conscience rate this a Paula's Pick. Offensive pricing does have its limit regardless of the ingredient list. After all, wasting money doesn't have any benefit for skin.

😐 **$$$ Eye Renewal Cream** *($110 for 0.5 ounce)* is a decent moisturizer with some good water-binding agents and a tiny amount of antioxidants. The only reason to consider this product is if you accept the notion that EGF is a good ingredient for skin care. This product cannot reverse sagging or wrinkles; that's a drug claim that the FDA should address with Re Vive. Actually, I'm even more confused as to how the FDA allows these kinds of formulations to even exist.

😐 **$$$ Fermitif Neck Renewal Cream SPF 15** *($115 for 2.5 ounces)* is said to prevent sagging skin that is "defenseless against the pull of gravity from the breasts." This in-part avobenzone sunscreen can help prevent further destruction of the skin's support system, which is a major factor in skin sagging, but any well-formulated sunscreen can do that. Beyond the EGF (which, even if it works as claimed, has nothing to do with lifting skin or firming the neck; it only has to do with skin cells, not collagen production), this is an ordinary moisturizer with sunscreen for dry skin. The inclusion of arnica extract isn't helpful and may cause irritation.

😐 **$$$ Lip and Perioral Renewal Cream** *($115 for 0.5 ounce)* is a nice, silky-soft moisturizer (due to the high content of silicone). The decision about whether or not to spend this kind of money to get the EGF it contains is up to you. There really is no other reason to choose this over many other ordinary lip moisturizers, which is all this ends up being, with its infinitesimally small amount of a controversial ingredient.

😐 **$$$ Moisturizing Renewal Cream** *($150 for 2 ounces)* was the first ReVive product. It contains about 4% to 5% glycolic acid and the pH is 3.3. That makes it a good AHA exfoliant in a very good but bland moisturizing base. However, if you're spending this kind of money on an AHA product, it is only because it contains the showcased EGF. The few antioxidants will not hold up once this jar-packaged product is opened, and it is unknown whether or not light and air exposure hinders the alleged effectiveness of EGF.

☹ **Sensitif Cellular Repair Cream SPF 15** *($195 for 2 ounces)* lacks the UVA-protecting ingredients of titanium dioxide, zinc oxide, avobenzone, Mexoryl SX, or Tinosorb, and is not recommended. Moreover, fragrant orange oil is not a key ingredient for sensitive, fragile skin.

☺ **$$$ Sensitif Oil Free Oil Control Lotion SPF 15** *($195 for 2 ounces)* has the basics right because it includes avobenzone for UVA protection and has an elegant lotion texture that sets to a soft matte finish that those with oily skin will appreciate. It cannot control oil, as the name states, yet does contain some effective water-binding agents. The overriding issue is that any sunscreen requires liberal application if it is to provide the stated level of protection. How liberally do you think you are going to apply a daytime moisturizer that costs this much?

☺ **$$$ Serum Protectif** *($175 for 1 ounce)* contains a lot of state-of-the-art ingredients in small quantities, which all together add up to a fairly good serum for all skin types. Although antioxidant-rich, this product cannot completely shield skin from environmental impurities—no skin-care product can. (For example, how could it protect us from the very air we breathe, or from pollution?) This contains about 3% glycolic acid in a pH-correct base, so some exfoliation will occur, but at this price, you are being taken to the cleaners, and not in a good way.

😐 **$$$ Blanche** *($400 for 1 ounce)* is not named after the character in *The Golden Girls*, but rather refers to bleaching the skin, as in lightening skin discolorations. This water-based serum is suitable for normal to slightly dry skin, but its impact on sun- or hormone-induced discolorations is bound to be minimal. That's because the amount of potentially effective ingredients (Dr. Brown uses *Uva ursi* leaf extract and alpha-arbutin) is very likely too low to work well, although formulary standards have not been established for arbutin. Considering the expense of this product, the potential lack of lightening efficacy is upsetting; you might as well speak to your doctor about a prescription for hydroquinone (such as Tri-Luma), which has been proven to work when used as directed, costs one-fourth this price, and has a large amount of research proving its efficacy.

☹ **Masque De Glaise** *($145 for 5 ounces)* dresses up a standard clay mask by mentioning that it contains a touch of limestone-rich Kentucky mud (probably from Dr. Brown's backyard). How that's supposed to help skin or justify the cost isn't explained, but this is not recommended anyway because it contains the irritating menthol derivative menthoxypropanediol.

unrated **Peau Magnifique Youth Recruit** *($1,500 for 4 0.03-ounce vials)* is said to reset skin's aging clock by at least five years, which, if you think about it for a moment, at this price isn't very impressive. You want to pay $1500 to go from 45 back to 40? What's the difference? The only difference is a clever marketing ploy, nothing more.

What's purportedly in these precious vials is a litany of anti-aging buzz ingredients, including methylsilanol mannuronate (also known as MSM), peptides, growth factors, and telomerase. The latter is what ReVive says is responsible for converting adult stem cells to "newly-mined skin cells, i.e. recruits youth." I suppose we're supposed to think of telomerase as a drill sergeant giving old, malfunctioning cells the boot and gathering new, full-of-life cells to create a younger you. Well, it isn't and it doesn't.

Telomerase is an enzyme that appears to be responsible for creating what are called immortal cells, and immortality sounds like a good thing. The dark side is that telomerase appears to be responsible for the unchecked growth of cells seen in human cancers. Telomerase levels appear to be carefully maintained in normal body tissues, but the enzyme is reactivated in cancer, where immortal cells are likely required to maintain tumor growth (Source: *Science*, 1994, volume 266, pages 2011–2015). Further, the authors of an article published in *Nature* (June 15, 2000) have this to add: "scientists report that using telomerase to extend the life-span of human tissue culture cells … may present some level of cancer risk…." Additionally, other research has revealed that telomerase is capable of maintaining itself if its environment is correct. If that's not the case, however, differentiation can occur and that may negatively affect other cells, such as fibroblasts.

Telomerase may also play a causative role in the formation and development of melanoma, the deadliest form of skin cancer (Sources: *Ontogenez*, March–April 2007, pages 105–119; and *Collegium Antropologicum*, January 2007, pages 17–22). That's not good news for skin, something that Dr. Brown conveniently leaves out of his company's information. Obviously, suggesting that this formula may have concerns about cancer is not so *Magnifique* after all! This contains fragrance in the form of orange peel oil and fragrance components such as limonene and linalool, all of which are potentially irritating, but that seems fairly inconsequential in comparison to the other major issues with this product.

REVLON (MAKEUP ONLY)

REVLON AT-A-GLANCE

Strengths: Superior foundations with sunscreen and each of them provide sufficient UVA protection (though one has a disappointing SPF 6); several outstanding concealers and powders; one of the best cream blushes around; great cream eyeshadow and liquid eyeliner; a beautiful selection of elegant lipsticks, lip gloss, and lipliner; some worthwhile specialty products; earned more Paula's Picks than any other makeup line sold at the drugstore.

Weaknesses: Average eye and brow pencils; several lipsticks with sunscreen lack the right UVA-protecting ingredients; inaccurate claims surrounding their Botafirm complex; mostly average to disappointing mascaras.

For more information about Revlon, call (800) 473-8566 or visit www.revlon.com or www.Beautypedia.com.

FOUNDATION: Revlon seldom has testers for its foundations, but the shade guides provided in most drugstores are fairly accurate. It's still tricky to find your best match without actual testers, but what they provide is better than nothing.

✓☺ **Age Defying Light Makeup with Botafirm SPF 30** *($12.99)* is a brilliant, sheer-coverage foundation that features broad-spectrum sun protection with titanium dioxide, zinc oxide, and octinoxate. This slightly creamy, water-resistant makeup sets to a natural-looking semi-matte finish that is appropriate for someone with normal to slightly oily or slightly dry skin. There are six shades, including Skin Brightener, a very pale peach that softly perks up pale skin and doesn't look all that peachy once it's blended into place. Most of the other shades are great, but watch out for the too-peach Light Medium and Medium Deep. Although this is a sheer makeup, the peachiness of these two shades is hard to blend away. This would be an ideal foundation for casual weekend makeup when you may spend more time outside than usual. Ignore the claims surrounding Revlon's Botafirm ingredient because it doesn't help skin bounce back from expression lines in the least and is a useless ingredient; in fact it's rather a silly claim altogether.

✓☺ **Age Defying Makeup with Botafirm SPF 15** *($13.99)* comes in two formulas, one for dry skin and one for normal/combination skin. Confusingly, the dry-skin formula lists talc as one of the main ingredients, though it provides a soft matte finish. In contrast, the normal/combination skin formula is more emollient, with a finish that's almost matte. Both foundations provide broad-spectrum sun protection; the dry-skin formula has an in-part titanium dioxide sunscreen, while the normal/combination formula contains titanium dioxide and zinc oxide. Texture- and application-wise, both formulas are equally wonderful. Which one you choose depends on the type of finish you prefer, because both provide seamless medium coverage without a heavy feel. Each foundation features 12 shades, and they tend to go on lighter than they appear in the bottle. The best news: With the exception of the too-peach Honey Beige (both formulas), there's not a bad shade in the bunch, and there are options for light to dark (but not very fair or very dark) skin tones. Whether you choose the dry or the normal/combination skin formula, both of these foundations are best for normal to slightly dry or slightly oily skin, but neither firms skin nor reduces the look of expression lines.

✓☺ **ColorStay Makeup with Softflex for Normal to Dry Skin SPF 15** *($12.99)* contains zinc oxide and titanium dioxide for broad-spectrum sun protection, and although it's not emollient enough to please those with dry skin, it has a beautiful satin-matte finish that feels slightly moist and provides medium to nearly full coverage (if layered). Those with dry skin looking for a long-wearing foundation with sunscreen will find that this pairs well with a moisturizer. This isn't nearly as difficult to remove as the original ColorStay Makeup, and it's much easier to blend because it is forgiving of any mistakes rather than setting and refusing to budge. There are 12 shades, and nearly all are praiseworthy. The only shades to avoid are the too-pink Fresh Beige and the slightly orange Cappuccino.

✓☺ **New Complexion One Step Compact Makeup SPF 15** *($12.99)* ranks as the best cream-to-powder foundation at the drugstore, hands down, and it includes titanium dioxide as the only sunscreen active. It applies superbly; has a light, silky texture; and sets to a soft, natural-looking powder finish that is best for normal to slightly oily or slightly dry skin. (Just keep in mind that moisturizer must be applied over any dry spots or this foundation will exaggerate them.) Coverage goes from sheer to medium. This is a must-try if you prefer cream-to-powder foundation. Revlon's 12 shades have been improved, and are a mostly neutral lot. Avoid Natural Beige, Cool Beige, and Warm Beige. Tender Peach is fairly true to its name, but may work for some light skin tones. Regrettably, there are no shades for very light or very dark skin tones.

✓☺ **ColorStay Active Light Makeup SPF 25** *($12.99)* has properties similar to Revlon's former ColorStay Light Makeup SPF 15. It's a worthy successor to that formidable foundation, except in one area: coverage. ColorStay Active Light Makeup SPF 25 offers sheer to medium coverage, and medium coverage is obtainable only if you layer the product. Otherwise, there are more similarities (and improvements) than differences. This version has a slightly fluid texture that applies smoothly, offering enough play time to blend it evenly. As for wearability, ColorStay Active Light Makeup just won't quit. It maintains its finish and appearance on skin almost all day, which is great news for those with oily skin. The tradeoff for such long wear is that this foundation is difficult to remove, so be sure to use a soft washcloth with a gentle, water-soluble cleanser to get it all off. Despite this drawback, it remains an excellent foundation with reliable sunscreen (the actives include in-part titanium dioxide and zinc oxide) for someone with oily to very oily skin. The ten shades do not include options for those with very fair or dark skin; however, those with light to medium skin tones are well served. Avoid True Beige, which is too rose, and the darkest shade, Toast, which is noticeably orange.

☺ **Age Defying Makeup and Concealer SPF 20** *($13.99)* is a creamy, medium- to full-coverage foundation packaged with a coordinating shade of creamy concealer. Both formulas have very smooth textures that are a pleasure to blend, and feel lighter than you'd expect. The foundation sets to a satin finish that feels slightly powdery—but make no mistake: this is meant for those with normal to dry skin. Any oily areas will feel greasier because this formula is emollient. The concealer offers more coverage than the foundation, but is essentially the same formula, and must be set with powder to minimize slippage into lines under the eye. Both products feature titanium dioxide and zinc oxide as active sunscreen ingredients, ensuring broad-spectrum protection. Ignore Revlon's claim that their Botafirm complex minimizes the appearance of lines and wrinkles—it doesn't. The ingredient supposedly responsible for this effect (acetyl hexapeptide-3) has no research to support the antiwrinkle or works-like-Botox claims—even Botox itself doesn't have any effect when rubbed on skin! Among the eight shade combinations offered, Natural Beige's foundation tends to be too pink (the concealer shade is fine), while the concealer shades in Honey Beige and Natural Tan are likely too peach for the intended skin tones. The rest of the shades are commendable, and blend on lighter and a bit more neutral than they appear in the package.

☺ **ColorStay Makeup with Softflex for Combination/Oily Skin SPF 6** *($12.99)* is downgraded from the get-go because of its unusually low SPF rating. This is an area where Revlon typically excels, and the fact that this is a reformulation makes the SPF 6 even more frustrating. Still more perplexing is the fact that this version of ColorStay Makeup has a higher percentage of active ingredients than the Normal to Dry Skin version reviewed above. I thought the SPF 6 (all titanium dioxide) was a mistake, but calls to Revlon confirmed that wasn't the case. If you're willing to pair this with an effective sunscreen rated SPF 15 or higher, it has a superb texture that blends effortlessly and allows enough time to do so before setting to a solid, but not flat-looking, matte finish. It's tricky to get less than medium coverage from this, so if you want something sheer, consider Revlon's ColorStay Active Light Makeup SPF 25 above. In comparison to Revlon's original ColorStay, the improvements found are all around. This version allows you to buff away any blending mistakes, it wears beautifully, and it removes with a water-soluble cleanser. If the sunscreen were rated SPF 15 or higher this would have been a slam-dunk recommendation for normal to very oily skin. Twenty shades are available for fair to dark skin tones, almost all of which are wonderful. Avoid Natural Beige and Golden Caramel. Note: Caramel, Toast, Rich Ginger, Cappuccino, Mahogany, and Mocha shades do not offer any sun protection.

☺ **New Complexion Makeup** *($11.99)* isn't so new anymore, and is actually Revlon's oldest foundation. Although it isn't a terrible choice, it doesn't have the same great qualities of their more recent additions. This remains a very lightweight option for normal to slightly oily skin. It slips nicely over the skin and sets to a natural matte finish that provides light to medium coverage. Its look on skin isn't as seamless as it could be, and you may notice it sinks into lines and large pores, especially in oil-prone areas. Of the nine shades, the only good options are Sand Beige, Medium Beige, and Sun Beige. The rest are too pink, orange, or peach.

CONCEALER: ✓☺ **Age Defying Concealer SPF 20** *($8.99)* is a creamy, compact-style concealer available in three very good yellow-toned shades (but be careful with Neutralizer; it is too peach for fair to light skin tones). The titanium dioxide and zinc oxide sunscreen combination not only ensures excellent UVA/UVB protection, but also contributes to this concealer's medium to full coverage, although it doesn't look too thick or obvious. It has a beautifully smooth application that, given the product's thick texture, blends better than you'd expect. Considering this product's creaminess, it's surprising it has only a slight tendency to crease into lines around the eyes.

☺ **New Complexion Concealer SPF 15** *($9.99)* ranks as a prime choice if you're looking for a slightly creamy, silky-textured concealer that provides outstanding sun protection courtesy of titanium dioxide and zinc oxide. Similar to, but with a thinner texture than, Revlon's Age Defying Concealer SPF 20 above, this provides nearly full coverage without looking artificial. It meshes well with skin, and creases minimally. This compact concealer comes with two shades that must be blended together for best results because one side tends to be too yellow while the other is slightly peach. Getting the correct proportions to match your skin tone is trickier than usual, but with practice you just might be very pleased with this, especially for additional sun protection in the delicate eye area.

☺ **ColorStay Under Eye Concealer SPF 15** *($9.99)* nets its excellent sun protection from a combination of titanium dioxide and zinc oxide, two gentle active ingredients well-suited for use around the eyes. This click-pen concealer has a built-in angled sponge-tip applicator that dispenses a slightly thick but blendable concealer. It smooths over skin, provides decent coverage (this isn't the best choice for very dark circles), and has a satin finish. Overall, this is a great option for normal to dry skin. It poses minimal risk of creasing into lines under the eye, and five of the six shades are superbly neutral. Avoid Light/Medium, which has a peachy cast that doesn't soften enough to look natural.

😐 **ColorStay Blemish Concealer** *($9.99)* contains 0.5% salicylic acid, which is on the low side for handling blemishes, but the pH of this concealer prevents it from working as an exfoliant anyway. This revamped version of the original ColorStay Concealer isn't as winning as its predecessor. It provides uneven, often insufficient, coverage (especially for blemishes), and it never sets to a true matte finish, so slippage and fading will be issues, not to mention that it looks slightly chalky on skin. The six shades are nearly perfect (though Light/Medium is a bit pink), but that's not enough to make this liquid concealer an easy recommendation.

POWDER: ✓☺ **New Complexion Powder** *($11.99)* is a talc- and silicone-based pressed powder with an improved silky texture and soft satin finish suitable for those with normal to dry skin. This is one of the few pressed powders that leaves a soft glow without sparkles. Most of the eight shades are purchase-worthy, but avoid Warm Beige and Natural Beige. Even Out is a color-correcting shade of yellow that may work for some light skin tones, but consider it carefully. ✓☺ **New Complexion Bronzing Powder** *($11.99)* is a talc-based, pressed-powder bronzer that comes in a very natural-looking tan shade with minimal shine. It would work best on light to medium skin tones and has the same texture characteristics and skin type recommendation as the New Complexion Powder above.

✓☺ **ColorStay Pressed Powder** *($9.99)* claims to wear for 16 hours over makeup, and, yes, it can stay that long (assuming you keep your hands off your face and you're not perspiring), but your oily areas will undoubtedly need a touch-up at some point during the day well before 16 hours. This adds up to a wonderful, talc-based powder for normal to very oily skin. The jet-milled powder has a superfine texture that provides a matte finish that doesn't look cakey or chalky, and of the six shades, only Light/Medium and Deep are too peach for their intended skin tones.

☺ **Age Defying Translucent Finishing Powder with Botafirm** *($12.99)* comes in only three shades. That used to be the norm, but take a look at L'Oreal's True Match Pressed Powder for an example of a pressed powder with a shade for almost everyone. There's not a bad option among the three choices Revlon offers, but none of them are suitable for dark skin (I wonder how they explain this to their spokesmodel Halle Berry?). The talc-based formula goes on light, but has a drier, more powdery texture than either the L'Oreal True Match powder or the latest options from Cover Girl.

☺ **Age Defying Skin Smoothing Powder with Botafirm** *($11.99)* is a smooth, talc-based pressed powder that has a more natural (but still powdered-looking) finish than the Age Defying Translucent Finishing Powder with Botafirm above. Two such similar pressed powders could be streamlined into one, and this would be it if for no other reason than the broader shade selection. Among the six shades, the darkest, Early Tan, may be too peach for its intended skin tone. Women of color will find that pressed powders from L'Oreal and Cover Girl offer more skin-true shades. Those with light to medium skin tones and normal to slightly dry skin may want to take a look at this option.

BLUSH: ✓☺ Cream Blush *($9.79)* is misnamed because this is really a cream-to-powder blush. However, if you're looking for a smooth alternative to powder blush and have normal to slightly dry or slightly oily skin (that is, not oily in the cheek area) this is an outstanding option. The color selection is small but well edited, meaning every shade is a winner, though each shade has a touch of shimmer (but it's light enough so it's not distracting). Note that all the shades go on softer than they appear. This blends so easily that it is easy for the color to go "out of bounds" as you apply it, so you may need to practice before you get it to go just where you want it to be. It is best to apply this as a series of dots along the cheekbone and onto the apple of the cheek, then carefully blend each dot together to form one smooth wash of color. The compact features a cleverly concealed mirror that pops out at the touch of a button. Very sleek, and the mirror is just big enough for quick lipstick touch-ups or to check for mascara smudges.

☺ **Bronzer Blush** *($9.79)* has a different and silkier formula than the Powder Blush below, and also imparts more color from both soft tan shades (OK, Natural Bronze is a peachy tan). The shine is discreet and the compact's pop-out mirror is an added convenience. Toss the too-tiny brush Revlon included, unless you want a striped effect.

😐 **Powder Blush** *($9.79)* doesn't impart much color, even with successive applications. It has a silky texture with results that are so soft it's almost like wearing no blush at all, though you are left with sparkles. The sparkles aren't readily visible as you're eyeing the shade in the compact, but don't be fooled—they're part of each shade. This blush is only recommended if you want a hint of color and don't mind sparkly cheeks.

EYESHADOW: ✓☺ Illuminance Creme Eyeshadow *($6.49)* offers four shades of cream-to-powder eyeshadow in a sleek compact. Most cream eyeshadows tend to crease and can be troublesome to blend with other colors, but these hold up quite well and go on softly. Your choices are limited if you prefer neutral tones, but those who enjoy cream eyeshadows should strongly consider these. The best sets are Not Just Nudes, Pink Petals, Seashells, Twilight, and Wild Orchids. Powder eyeshadows may be applied before or after for different effects, and to give the cream shadow greater staying power.

☺ **ColorStay 12 Hour Eye Shadow Quad** *($6.99)* is an impressive eyeshadow whose smooth, slightly thick, but non-powdery texture applies evenly and softly. The color application is on the sheer side, but layering produces more dramatic shading and shaping. Do they last 12 hours without fading or creasing? That's hard to quantify, because so much depends on application, how oily your eyelids are, whether or not you use moisturizer on your eyelids, and what other makeup products you use, such as a matte concealer, foundation, or powder over the eye. The best news is that most of the quads are well coordinated, though all have some degree of shine. The superior quads are Coffee Bean, In the Buff, and Copper Spice. Sandstorm is attractive as well, but the shine is more obvious and not the best for wrinkled eyelids because it will make them more pronounced. Avoid Stonewash Denim and Spring Moss, which are overwhelmingly blue and green.

☺ **ColorStay 12 Hour Eye Shadow Single** *($4.29)* has the same formula as the ColorStay 12 Hour Eye Shadow Quad above, and the same comments apply. Six shades are available, comprising basic highlighter and lid colors. All have either a slight shimmer or a satin finish that feels, but is not, truly matte. These do stay in place and won't smudge, but most powder eyeshadows have this trait.

😐 **EyeGlide Shimmer Shadow** *($6.59)* is a soft-textured cream-to-powder eyeshadow dispensed via a pen with a built-in angled sponge-tip applicator. Each of the shiny colors has the right amount of slip to allow blending without sliding all around the eye area, and they set to a finish that's powdery in feel. The colors are rather soft, and definitely overshadowed by the fairly intense sparkling shine. Although these do tend to stay put and not crease, the particles of shine tend to flake a bit, so don't be surprised if by midday you're noticing shiny specks on your cheeks or under-eye area. If that side effect doesn't bother you, and you are looking for more shine than shadow, give this a try.

EYE AND BROW SHAPER: ✓☺ **ColorStay Liquid Liner** *($7.39)* has an improved brush that enables you to paint a thin or thick line with precision and ease. The formula dries in a flash, so get this on correctly right from the start because once it sets it won't budge all day. This is assuredly worth a look for those who prefer liquid eyeliner or who have trouble getting pencil eyeliners to last. The Black Shimmer shade is infused with obvious silver glitter that doesn't flake, so it's a consideration for evening makeup.

😐 **ColorStay Eyeliner** *($7.39)* is a twist-up, retractable pencil that has almost too much slip and a tip that's soft enough to smush with moderate pressure. Once this sets in place though, it does stay quite well without feeling tacky. If you're willing to acclimate to this pencil's quirks, it is one to consider.

😐 **Luxurious Color Eyeliner** *($8.59)* is a relatively standard eye pencil that needs routine sharpening. The color intensity is strong (Revlon compares it, accurately, to that of a liquid eyeliner), yet the color can be smudged and softened for a smoky effect. It is mildly prone to smearing and some fading, but the rich colors last, making this an option for those who prefer pencils and don't mind sharpening.

😐 **Brow Fantasy Pencil & Gel** *($7.49)* combines a standard brow pencil with a sheer brow gel in one component. The pencil needs sharpening; you get a very small amount (it's roughly a quarter of the length of a standard brow pencil); and the brow gel, while completely non-sticky, imparts almost zero color and does not contain the type of ingredients that keep unruly hairs in place. This is more a blah product than a fantasy, unless your imagination is limited to dreaming in shades of gray!

LIPSTICK, LIP GLOSS, AND LIPLINER: ✓☺ **Super Lustrous Creme** and **Frost Lipsticks** *($7.99)* have an improved formula that is much more subtle in the fragrance department than it used to be. It's a moderately creamy lipstick that feels comfortable without being too slick or greasy and has better-than-average staying power. Revlon claims this is America's #1-selling lipstick, and backs this up with year-long figures from AC Nielsen Scantrak. However, best-selling doesn't mean you should jump on the bandwagon (I can think of a lot of popular items people buy that are not a good idea). In this case, best-seller or not, this is a very good creamy lipstick with a staggering range of 72 shades. If you can't find a color you like, perhaps lipstick just isn't for you!

✓☺ **LipGlide Full Color & Shine** *($8.99)* is an innovative combination of deeply pigmented gloss and packaging. By turning the base at its mid-point, the lip color is slowly fed onto an angled sponge tip, which allows you to easily control how much product comes up. This is actually easier to work with than most of the click-pen or lip-brush products sold by other companies. It applies smoothly and evenly, though the texture is a bit sticky. However, if that doesn't bother you, LipGlide is something you should check out.

✓☺ **LipGlide Sheer Color Gloss** *($8.99)* has packaging and a dispensing method that's identical to Revlon's original LipGlide Full Color & Shine above. The main differences between these two outstanding products are the intensity of the colors (Sheer Color Gloss offers mostly transparent hues) and the level of glossiness. Basically, LipGlide Full Color & Shine has an intensity akin to that of a regular lipstick, while Sheer Color Gloss is more in line with traditional lip gloss, but without the sticky, syrupy feel and ultra-wet look.

✓☺ **ColorStay Lip Liner** *($6.99)* is a retractable, twist-up pencil that really holds up against greasy lipsticks and, true to its name, stays put. The 16 shades do a formidable job of keeping lipstick anchored in place, making this a must-try if you're prone to feathering.

☺ **ColorStay Soft & Smooth Lipstick** *($9.99)* initially feels very smooth and creamy, but lightweight. The lightweight texture remains, but the creaminess dissipates quickly, leaving a slightly moist, semi-matte finish that has notable staying power. Although a far cry from the dry, parched feeling of the original ColorStay lipstick, this isn't for someone who likes their lips to remain emollient and look glossy. In fact, applying a lip gloss on top of this shortens its wear time, although not drastically so. Overall, this is a nice update and good compromise between the dryness of traditional ultra-matte lipsticks and the smoothness of today's best creamy lipsticks. Six of the 36 shades are labeled as **ColorStay Sheer**, and they are indeed softer colors that can be layered for more opacity, but initial application is more translucent. The Sheer formula does not wear as long as the original, but it's impressive compared to many other sheer, glossy lipsticks.

☺ **Colorstay Overtime Lipcolor** *($9.99)* competes nicely with Max Factor's Lipfinity and the identical Cover Girl Outlast Lipcolor. The basic application steps and "rules" are the same as for Lipfinity: you apply a base coat of opaque color using a sponge-tip wand applicator, and wait about one minute for the color to set. Once it has dried (which doesn't feel comfortable, but is integral to the long-wearing part) you can apply the clear, glossy top coat. Unlike Lipfinity and Outlast, Revlon's clever packaging houses both base color and clear topcoat in a single unit. I prefer the fact that Revlon's topcoat comes with a brush applicator rather than a solid, swivel-up stick. Revlon's topcoat also feels thicker than Lipfinity's and provides a glossier finish. It's more tenacious, too—I reapplied the top coat only a few times throughout the day, whereas Lipfinity requires more frequent applications of the top coat to prevent dry lips. Over time, Lipcolor loses points (and a Paula's Pick rating) for not wearing as well as Lipfinity or Outlast. It does stay on, but after testing both formulas over the course of several days, I experienced more flaking and chipping color with Revlon's Overtime Lipcolor. It also tended to feel grainy on the lips after a few hours, and reapplying the topcoat did not ease this feeling. Still, this definitely has its strong points (such as being easy to take off with an oil- or silicone-based remover) and it's certainly worth a test run if you're curious.

☺ **Super Lustrous Lipgloss** *($6.99)* is a standard lip gloss with an angled, sponge-tip applicator and smooth application that finishes glossy and feels slightly sticky. The beguiling shade selection offers sheer and dramatic hues that can be worn alone or to add pizzazz to a lipstick. This reasonably priced gloss competes nicely with more costly options from luxury lines such as Chanel and Yves St. Laurent.

😐 **Renewist Lipcolor SPF 15** *($9.99)* disappoints with its insufficient UVA protection, especially because this would have been a formidable creamy lipstick, since it contains several above-average moisturizing ingredients, including phospholipids, shea butter, and hyaluronic acid. Lips are left with a smooth, slightly slick finish from each of the attractive colors, but the incomplete sun protection is a disappointment, especially from Revlon. The opacity of this lipstick keeps it from earning an unhappy face rating, because that will provide some amount of sun protection.

😐 **Moon Drops Lipstick** *($8.99)* has been around for decades, and even the bright green packaging hasn't changed. Although this is a good, traditional cream lipstick, its fragrance is knock-your-socks-off strong and that also affects how this tastes, which is to say not pleasant. The selection of nearly 30 shades favors bright, bold hues (fans of orange lipstick, take note) rather than the more contemporary palette found in Revlon's Super Lustrous range.

😐 **ColorStay Overtime Sheer Lipcolor** *($9.99)* is Revlon's version of Lipfinity EverLites ($10.29) and Cover Girl Outlast Smoothwear ($9.99). It has the same two-phase concept, with color application followed by a top coat to ensure comfortable wear. Revlon's shades do go on sheer, but their formula tends to dry out too soon, even with regular application of the glitter-infused top coat (which has a thicker, stickier feel than those from competing products and is not the same formula as the top coat in Revlon's ColorStay Overtime Lipcolor above). As such, you don't really get to enjoy the best feature of products like this—namely, long wear without fading, chipping, or leaving telltale marks.

☹ **Super Lustrous Shiny Sheers SPF 15** *($5.95)* have a silky, slick texture and each of the sheer colors produces a lustrous finish, but the sunscreen disappoints by not including the UVA-protecting ingredients of avobenzone, titanium dioxide, zinc oxide, Mexoryl SX, or Tinosorb.

MASCARA: ✓☺ **Fabulash Mascara** *($6.99)* is Revlon's best mascara in years. It promises fuller, clump-free lashes, and it delivers—big-time! You'll get a clean application that defines each lash while lengthening and thickening in the right proportions to produce dramatic but not over-the-top lashes. Add to this the fact that lashes stay soft without flaking or smearing, and Fabulash deserves an enthusiastic round of applause!

✓☺ **3D Extreme Mascara** *($7.99)* promises lashes that are curvier, fuller, and longer, and it really delivers! This proves Revlon's Fabulash Mascara wasn't just a fluke—they are steadily improving their previously average mascaras. 3D Extreme Mascara has a patented brush in which two-thirds of the bristles are short and densely packed, and the other third are longer and wider-spaced. The result is immediate thickness and lengthening that goes on and on, and, yes, a curvy finish that can get quite dramatic with subsequent coats. The formula wears well and removes easily with a water-soluble cleanser. Watch out, L'Oreal!

☺ **3D Extreme Mascara Waterproof** *($8.99)* isn't quite as impressive as the original 3D Extreme Mascara above, but is definitely worth considering if you're looking for a waterproof mascara that provides even length and thickness while lasting all day. This applies with slight clumps that must be combed through for best results, but once it sets you won't see a flake or smear.

☺ **Lash Fantasy Primer & Mascara** *($7.99)* doesn't reach the same peaks of performance as the Fabulash Mascara above, but this two-step mascara is still worth considering. The Primer step is essentially a colorless mascara that's applied first, followed by a regular mascara. Using the Primer versus not using it makes a subtle difference, but whether you do both steps or just apply the mascara, you'll enjoy substantial length and thickness in nearly equal measure. Lashes are perfectly defined without a clump in sight, and this wears beautifully all day.

☹ **Luxurious Lengths Mascara** *($6.99)* isn't a poor mascara, but it isn't nearly as exciting as the Fabulash Mascara, which reigns as Revlon's best. It promises to make lashes look 50% longer and curvier, and almost gets to that point. Lashes are elongated but not to the extent of the best lengthening mascaras from Almay, L'Oreal, Maybelline New York, or Cover Girl. What this mascara does do well is curl lashes, and without clumping along the way. Its dual-sided brush allows you to lengthen with the longer bristles and to add depth and richer color with the shorter, tightly packed ones. However, a comparison of actual performance to the claims means this mascara doesn't earn a top mark.

☹ **Lash Fantasy Waterproof Mascara** *($7.99)* isn't as impressive as the non-waterproof version of Lash Fantasy above, even though here, too, the Primer step makes a slight difference compared to applying the mascara alone. Although this is waterproof, its length and thickness capability are just OK, and if you're not careful during application this smears easily.

☹ **Fabulash Mascara Waterproof** *($6.99)* has the same type of brush as Revlon's original (and amazingly good) Fabulash Mascara, but that's where the similarities start and stop. The waterproof version does hold up when lashes get wet, but the application and wear leave much to be desired. Although this mascara lengthens and provides decent thickness, it clumps as it is applied, goes on unevenly, and flakes throughout the day, not to mention it makes your lashes feel dry and crispy. Almay (owned by Revlon) produces much more reliable waterproof mascaras, particularly their One Coat Nourishing Mascara Triple Effect Waterproof Mascara. Almay, you should tell Revlon what they're doing wrong!

☹ **Luxurious Lengths Waterproof Mascara** *($6.99)* makes the same longer, curvier promises as its non-waterproof counterpart, but the application is terribly uneven, and trying to smooth things out is messy to say the least. It is waterproof and with patience you can build longer, fuller lashes, but so many other mascaras do this without the problematic application, so my strong recommendation is to leave this one on the shelf.

SPECIALTY PRODUCTS: ☹ **Makeup Eraser Pen** *($6.79)* is a pencil designed for "portable perfection and touch-ups on the go." The solvent- and silicone-based formula is dispensed through a felt-tip marker, and does dissolve eyeliner, mascara, or lipstick mistakes. This is convenient for minor mistakes, but you will need a tissue or cotton swab to completely remove signs of the mistake. I was impressed that this works on stubborn makeup, too, and is fragrance-free. Based on the design, this is best for removing or correcting eyeliner or lipliner mistakes, but it doesn't work any better than a cotton swab with makeup remover dabbed on the tip.

☺ **Age Defying Instant Firming Face Primer All Skin Types** *($11.99)* is a silky, silicone-based serum that claims to soften expression lines because it contains Revlon's Botafirm complex (acetyl hexapeptide-8). Although this peptide likely functions as a water-binding agent and, theoretically, a cell-communicating ingredient, it cannot reduce expression lines in any way, shape, or form, and is about as close to Botox injections as a Band-Aid® is to plastic surgery. What this weightless serum does is make skin feel exceptionally smooth, and that helps foundation blend better. The texture and finish of this primer are best for normal to very oily skin.

✓☺ **Age Defying Instant Firming Face Primer for Normal/Combination Skin** *($11.99)* differs from the Age Defying Firming Face Primer All Skin Types above because it has a lotion texture and leaves a slightly moist finish that casts a sheen on skin. It works beautifully under makeup and is fine for its intended skin types. What propels this to Paula's Pick status are the many antioxidants Revlon added, all in impressive amounts. Consider this an elegant, lightweight moisturizer that rivals the best of the best, but keep in mind that you get only 1 ounce of product.

✓☺ **Age Defying Instant Firming Face Primer for Dry Skin** *($11.99)* has a texture that's a cross between the two Age Defying Instant Face Primers above, and is best for normal to slightly dry skin. Those with dry to very dry skin will need something more emollient than this water- and silicone-based lotion, but it's loaded with antioxidants and performs well under makeup, even if your foundation of choice is rich and dewy.

RIMMEL (MAKEUP ONLY)

RIMMEL AT-A-GLANCE

Strengths: Inexpensive; the pressed bronzing powder; some of the best mascaras at the drugstore; respectable powder blush, cream blush, and powder eyeshadows; excellent automatic eye pencil; Lasting Finish Lipstick and Vinyl Lip are must-sees.

Weaknesses: Packaging that isn't very user-friendly; average concealers; several lackluster eyeshadow options; none of the Extra Super Lash mascaras earn their impressive-sounding names; potentially problematic eye-makeup remover.

For more information about Rimmel, owned by Coty, visit www.rimmellondon.com or www.Beautypedia.com. Note: Over a dozen Rimmel products featured on their Web site are not available in the United States; they are exclusive to United Kingdom drugstores. The products reviewed below are those that are consistently found at U.S. stores nationwide, specifically Walgreen's and Wal-Mart. Wal-Mart tends to stock items that Walgreen's doesn't, so expect to visit both stores for a complete selection.

FOUNDATION: ☺ **Recover Illuminating Anti-Fatigue Foundation** *($7.99)* is a silky, slightly moist liquid foundation that spreads easily and sets to a lightweight, satin-matte finish. It does lend a soft glow to the skin, but not to the extent that you'll look well rested or "lit from within." Coverage goes from light to medium, and six shades are available. Among those, half are either too peach or will turn peach on oily areas. Those include Porcelain, Classic Beige, and Sand. This foundation is best for someone with normal to slightly oily or slightly dry skin. One more note: This foundation is highly fragranced.

☺ **Cool Matte Mousse Foundation** *($8.09)* remains true to its name with a soft, mousse-like texture and slight cooling sensation as you blend. I could not find an ingredient list anywhere (it's not on the product itself either, which is a regulatory no-no) to check if the cooling effect was from a menthol derivative, but I doubt it because the effect dissipates quickly as this foundation sets to a silky matte finish. The sheer- to light-coverage formula looks very natural on skin, concealing minor flaws and evening skin tone without looking the least bit masklike. It's best for normal to very oily skin and comes in ten shades, with options for fair but not dark skin tones. The following shades are slightly peach and should be considered carefully: 101 Porcelain, 200 Soft Beige, and 301 Warm Honey. This would earn a Paula's Pick rating if the ingredient list were available (and it should be per FDA and European regulatory mandates).

😐 **Stay Matte Foundation** *($4.99)* is recommended for normal to oily skin, but the moist texture and slightly creamy finish would be more suitable for normal to dry skin, plus it contains enough oil to make its matte finish short-lived. This comes in a tube, provides light to medium coverage, and blends evenly. There are six shades, three of which—Sand, Soft Beige, and Warm Honey—are too pink or peach for most skin tones. Porcelain is slightly pink, but may work for lighter skin tones.

CONCEALER: ☹ **Hide the Blemish Concealer** *($3.99)* is a very greasy, lipstick-style concealer that doesn't cover that well, though it does come in three very good colors. An emollient, wax-based concealer like this is the last thing you want to place over blemishes, at least if the goal is to not make them worse! If you prefer this type of concealer, it would be OK over nonblemished areas, but if you're using it under the eye, creasing is inevitable.

☹ **Clear Complexion Coverstick** *($4.99)* is nearly identical to the Hide the Blemish Concealer above, and the same basic comments apply. This does not contain any ingredients known to promote clear skin, but several of the waxes and the lanolin oil make it a distinct problem for those battling blemishes.

POWDER: ✓ ☺ **Natural Bronzer** *($3.99)* is a talc-based pressed-powder bronzer that has a beautifully smooth texture and application. Shine from each of the three shades is so subtle as to be almost nonexistent, making this a fine choice for daytime wear (though if you have oily skin it probably isn't the best option; those with oily skin need less shine, not more). Speaking of the shades, all have potential, but the orange tinge of Sun Light makes it trickier for fair to light skin tones to pull off, and it's too light for medium skin tones.

☺ **Stay Matte Pressed Powder** *($3.99)* has a smooth texture and non-powdery, but dry matte finish laced with a tiny amount of shine. Those with oily skin will find this doesn't stay matte for long, but it doesn't look thick or cakey, either. While not the most elegant-feeling powder, it's a good, inexpensive option for normal to slightly oily or slightly dry skin. There are three shades, with no options for medium to dark skin tones.

BLUSH: ☺ **Blush** *($2.49)* is a pressed powder that comes in a small compact and features predominantly sheer, warm-toned shades, all with a softly shiny finish. If only these were matte, they would be a steal, as the texture and application are wonderful.

☺ **Soft Cream Blush** *($2.24)* has a luscious texture, though it's definitely cream-to-powder rather than a true cream blush. Still, this is worth a look if you prefer this type of blush and don't mind shine. The sheer colors apply well and fade minimally (unless your skin is very oily, in which case you shouldn't be using this type of blush anyway).

EYESHADOW: ☺ **Special Eyes Mono Eyeshadow** *($2.69)* has a silky, slightly powdery but easy-to-blend texture, and offers mostly shiny to soft shimmer colors. The only matte shades are Matte White (which has limited appeal) and Romance. If you want shiny eyeshadows, this is a good, affordable option. ☺ **Special Eyes Duo Eyeshadow** *($3.99)* has the same formula as the Special Eyes Mono Eyeshadow above, and a surprising number of well-coordinated pairs, each with one matte shade. Take a look at Walnut Pearls and Orchid (both are matte), Metallic Pearls, Desert, Cream Caramel, Biscuit Box, and Spice, where both shades are matte.

☺ **Special Eyes Trio Eye Shadow** *($4.99)* also shares the same formula and application traits as the Special Eyes Mono Eyeshadow above, but unlike the plethora of Duos, the selection of Trios is small. Lynx and Orion are worth considering, though two of the three shades in each are shiny.

☺ **Infinite Waterproof Cream Shadow** *($4.37)* is a cream-to-powder eyeshadow applied with a sponge-tip applicator that's affixed to a wand. Blending is tricky because this has a lot of slip, but with practice it imparts strong, shiny color that stays put and is waterproof (yet removes easily with a water-soluble cleanser).

☹ **Cool Touch Shadow** *($5.99)* is a liquid-to-powder eyeshadow whose metallic shades go on much sheerer than they appear in the tube, though the shine is intense. Each shade sets to a matte (in feel) finish, but they don't hold up well. They aren't prone to creasing but they tend to fade, wear unevenly, and aren't tenacious (you can remove the product with just water, and they definitely come off when you're perspiring). Better, longer-lasting examples of this type of product are M.A.C. Paint ($16) and Maybelline New York's Dream Mousse Shadow ($6.50).

☹ **Stars Glitter Eye Shadow Pencil** *($3.99)* is a needs-sharpening, slightly chunky pencil that imparts minimal, fade-prone color and lots of glitter. What's unusual for pencils like this is that the glitter tends to stay in place quite well. You'll notice some flaking, but much less than with comparable, pricier pencils from NARS or Hard Candy.

☹ **All Over Pencil** *($4.37)* is a chunky, needs-sharpening pencil with colors that are best-suited for eyes rather than cheeks or lips. The application is silky-smooth and the formula sets to a relatively long-lasting finish, putting it a step above the standard creamy pencils that are the norm. This is worth considering if you don't mind routine sharpening, but note that every shade is shiny.

☹ **Metallic Eye Gloss** *($2.97)* comes in two formulas, though they perform identically. One is mineral oil–based while the other is petrolatum-based, meaning these are creamy and leave a moist, crease-prone finish. Shinier than they are metallic, they're an OK option if they're strategically placed and your eye area is perfectly taut, but you can still count on this smearing and slipping fairly quickly.

☹ **Eye Twist Automatic Duo Liner & Shadow** *($4.37)* is a dual-ended, automatic, retractable pencil with a creamy eyeliner on one end and a shiny cream eyeshadow on the other. Although both apply well, they're too creamy to last, and some smearing is inevitable.

EYE AND BROW SHAPER: ✓☺ **Exaggerate Full Colour Eye Definer** *($4.99)* is a superior automatic eye pencil that's also retractable, and includes a built-in sharpener if you desire a finer tip. This applies well, but it takes a few strokes to build intensity. It sets to a soft powder finish that has a low risk of smudging or smearing. The colored tip on the pencil's package is a good indicator of how the color will look on the skin. Avoid the blue and green hues unless you're wearing eyeliner for notice-value.

☹ **Soft Kohl Kajal Eye Pencil** *($2.49)* needs sharpening but is a better pencil in every respect than the Special Eyes Eye Liner Pencil below. Although it is creamy, it has a longer-lasting finish that's less prone to smudging and it glides on with minimal effort. Among the ten shades, Loveable Lilac, Silver, and Jungle Green are shiny. Avoid the latter as well as Cool Blue and Denim Blue. Chianti is an attractive option if you want to move beyond basic brown, black, or gray. ☹ **Professional Eyebrow Pencil** *($2.49)* has a drier, stiffer texture than most standard brow pencils, but its finish really lasts and application is soft and even. This includes a brush built into the cap, which can come in handy.

☹ **Special Eyes Eye Liner Pencil** *($2.49)* is a poor eye pencil choice even if the prospect of sharpening thrills you. It's way too creamy and smears with minimal provocation. Even without provocation you'll notice fading way too soon. ☹ **Professional Liquid Eye Liner** *($5.49)* is a standard liquid liner that comes with a long, skinny brush that can be hard to control over the lash line. Although some may prefer this type of brush, this formula takes too long to dry (even when applied lightly) and it smears easily.

LIPSTICK, LIP GLOSS, AND LIPLINER: ✓☺ **Lasting Finish Lipstick** *($5.99)* is, in short, one of the best creamy lipsticks at the drugstore. It feels wonderful and glides on with a soft, creamy texture and slightly glossy finish, and the color range, while not enormous, is still impressive, each providing a good stain. Check out Balistic if you are a fan of red lipstick that's neither too blue nor too orange.

✓☺ **Vinyl Lip** *($4.99)* is an extremely smooth, decadent-feeling lip gloss that is completely non-sticky and very comfortable to wear. The shade selection is bountiful (a Clear option is available too) and this rates as another gem from Rimmel.

☺ **Cool Shine Lipstick** *($6.25)* adds a lot of sparkling glitter to lips that clings tenaciously but doesn't feel grainy. This is otherwise a light-textured, glossy lipstick with a slightly creamy feel and soft colors revved up by an overdose of sparkles (meaning, be sure you like this effect before purchasing).

☺ **Jelly Gloss Sheer Lipgloss** *($5.49)* comes in a tube and offers smooth-textured, non-sticky results with a wet-look glossy shine. You have to tolerate the fruity scents and flavors, but if you're a fan of Lancome's Juicy Tubes Ultra Shiny Lip Gloss ($16.50) this is comparable, and with the benefit of not being the least bit goopy. The color impact is more ultra-sheer with minimal to no color saturation.

☺ **Exaggerate Full Colour Lip Liner** *($4.99)* is an automatic, retractable lip pencil that is creamy without veering into greasiness. It stays on quite well, and the colors are rich with pigment. It doesn't apply as smoothly as others (you have to apply a fair amount of pressure to get the color to show up), but for the money, this is a safe bet.

😐 **Twist & Shine Lip Polish** *($4.37)* is a cross between a liquid lipstick and a lip gloss, and is housed in a click pen with an angled sponge-tip applicator. It's an OK option that leaves lips looking colored and glossed, but Revlon's Lipglide Full Color and Shine ($8.99) is a superior similar product. 😐 **Twist & Shine Sheers Lip Polish** *($4.37)* has the same packaging and basic qualities as the regular Twist & Shine Lip Polish, except the colors are translucent and the finish slightly glossier. Once again, Revlon trumps Rimmel with their similar but better Lipglide Sheer Color Gloss ($8.99).

😐 **Rich Moisture Cream Lipstick** *($5.79)* has a smooth but overly waxy feel reminiscent of traditional ChapStick. That's not so bad, but what really keeps this lipstick from earning a higher rating is its potent fragrance and greasier-than-it-should-be finish.

😐 **Vinyl Jelly Gloss Lip Liner** *(3.99)* combines the sheerness and fleeting quality of standard lip gloss with a needs-sharpening pencil format. The soft, sheer colors are sure to please, but this product isn't for anyone expecting a long-lasting, defined lip line. What this can be used for is lip gloss. It's almost as shiny, definitely sheer, and all you'd need to do is line and fill in lips with the color of your choice (and take it along, because touch-ups will be frequent). Ultimately, this doesn't substitute for far-easier-to-use glosses in standard gloss containers.

😐 **1000 Kisses Stay On Lip Liner Pencil** *($2.99)* is a standard, needs-sharpening pencil. It has a smooth and comfortably creamy texture and stays on as well as most other pencils, which is to say, well, but not well enough to withstand even one kiss, much less a thousand!

☹ **Volume Boost Liquid Lipcolour** *($6.49)* comes in a brilliant array of ten sheer, glossy colors and has a beautifully smooth application and minimally sticky feel. Why the unhappy face rating, then? This liquid lipstick contains a menthol derivative known as ethyl menthane carboxamide that is ten times cooler than menthol itself (Source: www.leffingwell.com/cooler_than_menthol.htm), which means it also is that much more irritating.

MASCARA: ✓☺ **Volume Flash Instant Thickening Mascara** *($6.49)* ranks as a formidable thickening mascara. It lengthens, too, but is best for creating beautifully separated, really thick lashes. You won't find the thickness is instant, but with some effort (and no clumps) your lashes will be captivatingly dramatic! An added bonus: Lashes stay soft, and this removes easily with a water-soluble cleanser.

✓☺ **Eye Magnifier Eye Opening Mascara** *($6.49)* is said to "lift lashes vertically by 70%" thanks to its Verti-lift brush, but who wants lashes that go vertical when the most attractive look is a panoramic sweep of softly fringed lashes? Luckily this mascara gets very close to that goal and quickly, too. Working the rubber-bristled brush through lashes produces minor clumping, but that's the tradeoff for the dramatic results you get from this mascara. The clumps smooth out quickly and further strokes separate lashes nicely, while increasing thickness and, to a lesser extent, length.

✓☺ **Lash Maxxx 3X Lash Multiplying Effect Mascara** *($4.37)* replaces the familiar round brush applicator with a serrated comb whose variegated teeth allow for creating tremendously long lashes without clumps. Successive coats build some thickness and you can really get to the lash roots for emphasis there, but this is mostly about making lashes very defined and long. Lashes stay soft, the formula doesn't flake, and it comes off easily with a water-soluble cleanser. Not bad for less than five dollars!

☺ **Volume Flash Instant Thickening Waterproof Mascara** *($5.99)* doesn't have the same wow factor as its non-waterproof counterpart above, but it is a slightly thickening waterproof mascara. Application is quick and clean, and unlike the results with many waterproof formulas, lashes aren't left feeling dry and brittle.

😐 **Extreme Definition Ultimate Lash-Separating Mascara** *($6.99)* is a brushless mascara—meaning that it has a miniature comb to sweep on mascara. It does an impressive job of instantly creating long, slightly thick lashes that I wouldn't consider "ultimate," but that are still definitely above average. This can be a time-saving option because lashes are enhanced and separated after just a few strokes. It is prone to minor flaking throughout the day, which is not the best, especially when there are other options that don't flake even a little.

😐 **Extra Super Lash Mascara** *($2.99)* remains a reliable lengthening mascara that applies clump-free and tends to not flake or chip, but thickness is harder to come by. Better than this is Maybelline New York's Unstoppable Full Length Mascara ($6.79). 😐 **Extra Super Lash Curved Brush Mascara** *($2.99)* performs just as well as the straight brush version, but is the one to choose if you want a more defined curl.

😐 **Extra Super Lash Waterproof Mascara** *($6.49)* won't knock your socks off with its lengthening or thickening abilities, but is a very respectable, long-wearing waterproof mascara for those who want slightly longer, separated, and fuller lashes.

😐 **Lycra Lash Extender Mascara** *($6.49)* makes a big deal out of the fact that it contains the synthetic, amazingly stretchable fiber Lycra. Used in mascara, it is supposed to increase lash length by 60% and curl by 50%, all while helping lashes hold their shape for 14 hours. It sounds impressive, but isn't value added because, for all its ballyhoo, Lycra Lash Extender Mascara doesn't produce results anyone would consider "instant" or "dramatic." With several coats you can elongate lashes, and it sets to a soft, eye-opening curl. But thickness is scant, some clumping occurs along the way, and the performance plateaus far too soon to make good on the claims. It's still a valid option if you want a reasonable (but definitely not dramatic) lengthening mascara. Lashes stay soft and the formula is easy to remove.

☹ **Volum' Eyes 5X Volume Comb Mascara** *($6.49)* promises copious volume in one stroke, all without clumping or clogging—and fails miserably. This comb mascara is a mess from the get-go, depositing way too much product and instantly making lashes look clumped and spiky. Trying to smooth things out just causes smearing, and makes this the one Rimmel mascara to absolutely avoid.

SPECIALTY PRODUCTS: 😐 **Gentle Eye Makeup Remover** *($6.49 for 4.2 ounces)* is a relatively standard, non-silicone-based eye-makeup remover whose formula is hindered a bit by the inclusion of sodium lauryl sulfate, a cleansing agent known for being a potent skin irritant. There isn't a lot of it in the product, but this strong detergent cleansing agent is best kept away from the sensitive eye area, so this isn't worth considering over gentler options from Neutrogena, Almay, or L'Oreal.

ROC (SKIN CARE ONLY)

ROC AT-A-GLANCE

Strengths: Some well-packaged products with retinol; one good cleanser; all the sunscreens provide sufficient UVA protection; Facial Peel Kit, though not a peel, is worth auditioning; RoC Canada offers better products than what's sold in the United States.

Weaknesses: Mediocrity reigns supreme—none of the formulas are particularly exciting; antiwrinkle claims tend to go too far; jar packaging.

For more information about RoC, owned by Johnson & Johnson, call (800) 762-1964 or visit www.rocskincare.com or www.Beautypedia.com. And for a better selection of state-of-the-art retinol products from RoC, see the reviews for RoC Canada that follow.

ROC UNITED STATES

😊 **Age Diminishing Facial Cleanser** *($7.99 for 5.1 ounces)* won't make you look younger, but you can count on this gentle, water-soluble formula to leave normal to slightly dry or slightly oily skin clean and refreshed.

☹ **Daily Microdermabrasion Cleansing Disks** *($9.99 for 24 pads)* are dual-sided cleansing discs whose formula is nearly identical to Johnson & Johnson–owned Neutrogena's Illuminating Microderm Cleansing Pads ($6.99 for 24 pads). The RoC disks would be a fine option for manual exfoliation (and the pads slip right over your fingers for convenience) if they didn't contain the irritating menthol derivative menthyl lactate.

😐 **Age Diminishing Daily Moisturizer SPF 15** *($14.79 for 3 ounces)* contains an in-part avobenzone sunscreen, and that can definitely help diminish the appearance of aging. This is otherwise a really boring daytime moisturizer unless you want to ignore current skin-care research and put all your eggs in one basket by betting that soy extract will be the anti-aging miracle. Substantiated research has many positive things to say about soy, and it is a good antioxidant. But the hope that its topical use can diminish wrinkles and discolorations or boost skin's firmness has not yet appeared on the list of proven accomplishments. Regrettably, other than the sunscreen, soy (albeit only a dusting) is the only ingredient of interest here. The mica and titanium dioxide lend a soft shine finish to skin, but that is a cosmetic attribute, not a skin-care benefit.

😐 **Age Diminishing Moisturizing Night Cream** *($15.56 for 1.7 ounces)* contains an impressive amount of antioxidant soybean seed extract, but its potency will be compromised once this jar-packaged moisturizer for normal to dry skin is opened (though even in air-tight packaging, soy isn't going to take even one hour off your age). All told, this isn't worth considering over several other options at the drugstore.

😐 **Protient Fortify Lift and Define Eye Cream** *($19 for 0.5 ounce)* is a lightweight moisturizer for slightly dry skin anywhere on the face. It contains tiny amounts of minerals and a couple of antioxidants. The big-deal ingredient in this eye cream is DMAE, which is technically dimethylaminoethanol. Despite the lack of evidence that DMAE has any effect on skin, there are hundreds of Web sites claiming that it does, only without any accompanying research documentation. It is possible that DMAE can help protect the cell membrane, and keeping cells intact can have benefit, but so far that appears to be only conjecture, not fact, and recent research suggests it can actually have a negative effect on the cell, despite some short-term benefits. There is absolutely no substantiated research proving DMAE can lift the skin around the eyes or reduce puffiness.

😐 **Protient Fortify Lift and Define Night Cream** *($19 for 1.7 ounces)* is nothing more than a blend of water and lots of thickeners with DMAE, described in the review above for Protient Fortify Lift and Define Eye Cream. Unless you're curious to see what DMAE can do for your skin (though there isn't a compelling reason to use it), this is a notably average moisturizer for normal to dry skin positioning itself as a face-lift in a jar.

😐 **Protient Fortify Lift and Define Serum** *($19 for 1.7 ounces)* won't lift or define skin and is actually a really disappointing serum unless you believe the hype about DMAE. Olay and Neutrogena offer much more elegant serums that treat skin to a variety of beneficial ingredients.

😐 **Retinol Actif Pur Anti-Wrinkle Moisturizing Treatment, Day SPF 15** *($17.99 for 1 ounce)* assures UVA protection with its in-part avobenzone sunscreen, and the moisturizing base is suitable for normal to slightly dry skin. But the amount of retinol is paltry, as is the amount of vitamin E. Any improvement in wrinkles would be from the sunscreen alone (keeping wrinkles protected from further sun damage gives skin a chance to repair itself to an extent that, with a smart skin-care routine, wrinkle depth and prominence may indeed be reduced).

😐 **Retinol Actif Pur Anti-Wrinkle Moisturizing Treatment, Night** *($23.35 for 1 ounce)* contains a potentially effective amount of glycolic acid, but the pH is well above 4, not ideal for exfoliation. It can still function as a water-binding agent and, overall, this formula is one of RoC's better options for normal to dry skin (though that's still not saying much). It's an OK option if you're looking for a stably packaged moisturizer with retinol.

😐 **Retinol Correxion Deep Wrinkle Daily Moisturizer SPF 15** *($20 for 1 ounce)* contains an in-part avobenzone sunscreen. The problem is that, even coupled with the other sunscreen ingredients, it's all you'll find here that can help prevent premature aging of skin. RoC claims this product can visibly reduce deep wrinkles, but that is based on hope not fact. Any moisturizer (which is what this is) applied over deep wrinkles can slightly reduce their appearance because moisturizer has a softening effect on skin, and that temporarily makes wrinkles less noticeable.

It would be nice if the price of this product reflected more closely the cost of its contents, because this is a fairly basic moisturizer with more absorbents and dry-feeling ingredients (such as silicone) than emollients. The amount of antioxidants (retinol and vitamin E are present) is too minuscule to matter, which makes this product's inclusion of "retinol" in the name somewhat silly. If you're looking for a good retinol product from RoC, their Retinol Actif Pur Anti-Wrinkle Moisturizing Treatment Night (reviewed above) is preferred, though this is OK as a lightweight broad-spectrum sunscreen for normal to slightly oily skin. Just don't expect any existing wrinkles to be visibly corrected in any significant way.

😐 **Retinol Correxion Deep Wrinkle Night Cream** *($20 for 1 ounce)* makes the same claims as the Retinol Correxion Deep Wrinkle Daily Moisturizer SPF 15 above, only without the sunscreen. This product contains nothing special to fend off or reduce wrinkles, and is quite a standard moisturizer containing mostly water, silicone, slip agent, several thickeners, pH adjusters, glycolic acid (functioning as a water-binding agent in this amount, not an exfoliant), preservative, film-forming agents, emollients, fragrance, retinol, and antioxidants. For the money and the tiny amount of product, you should expect at least more retinol and antioxidants, but with RoC that appears to be just wishful thinking. This is an OK moisturizer for normal to dry skin, but one that's not nearly as impressive as the nighttime options from Dove, Neutrogena, and Olay, most of which cost less than this product.

😐 **Retinol Correxion Deep Wrinkle Serum** *($20 for 1 ounce)* has a silky, silicone-enhanced texture that's suitable for all skin types; it's a shame the fragrance and preservatives carry more weight in this product than retinol or other ingredients of value to aging skin. Neutrogena's Healthy Skin Anti-Wrinkle Cream, Original Formula ($11.99 for 1.4 ounces) is distinctly preferred to this.

😐 **Retinol Correxion Eye Cream** *($19.99 for 0.5 ounce)* contains only a tiny amount of retinol (it's listed after the preservatives) and as such this isn't a top choice if retinol is what you're after. This is otherwise a standard lightweight but hydrating eye cream for slightly dry skin. It does not contain fragrance.

😊 **Resurfacing Facial Peel Kit** *($24.99 for the kit)* should be labeled a facial scrub kit, because that's what this two-step kit really is. The **Resurfacing Facial Peel** is a gel-based scrub that contains polyethylene (plastic) beads as the abrasive agent. It also contains *Mucor meihei* extract, a type of mold whose enzymes are used as a food additive and flavor-enhancer in cheeses. Some cosmetics companies (including Neutrogena) assert that its enzymatic action is akin to exfoliation, but there is no proof of that—and definitely not in comparison to the action of a well-formulated AHA or BHA product. The **Post-Peel Nourisher** is a lightweight moisturizer that happens to be one of RoC's only impressive formulas. It contains a good blend of water-binding agents, emollients, and ingredients that mimic the structure and function of healthy skin. All in all, this kit is worthwhile even though it's not technically a peel, and both products are suitable for normal to slightly dry or slightly oily skin.

ROC CANADA

Note: The following RoC products are available only in Canada. All prices listed below are in Canadian currency. For more information about RoC Canada, call (877) 223-9807 or visit www.rocskincare.ca.

ROC CANADA AT-A-GLANCE

Strengths: Some excellent cleansers; many fragrance-free options; several state-of-the-art moisturizers with retinol; lip balm with sunscreen; packaging that helps keep light- and air-sensitive ingredients stable during use.

Weaknesses: Anti-acne products are irritating and not the least bit helpful for blemish-prone skin; ordinary toners; mostly mediocre moisturizers; no skin-lightening products; pricey for a drugstore line.

ROC CALMANCE PRODUCTS

😊 **Calmance Soothing Cleansing Fluid** *($16 for 200 ml)* is a water- and silicone-based makeup remover that works quickly and easily, but is best used before cleansing to avoid a greasy-feeling residue. The amount of feverfew extract is unlikely to cause irritation.

😐 **Calmance Intolerance Repairing Cream** *($20 for 40 ml)* is a very standard, but good, emollient moisturizer for normal to dry skin. It is designed to soothe skin after laser treatment, but contains only a minor amount of ingredients that can do that, while the feverfew extract can be sensitizing.

😐 **Calmance Soothing Moisturiser** *($20 for 40 ml)* is similar to the Calmance Intolerance Repairing Cream above, except this option contains less feverfew extract and isn't quite as emollient (but that's basically a texture preference). Otherwise, the same review applies.

😐 **Calmance Soothing Regenerating Mask** *($20 for 30 ml)* is a standard moisturizing mask for dry to very dry skin. For a product claiming to soothe redness and irritation, it is surprisingly lacking in ingredients that can do that.

ROC ENYDRIAL PRODUCTS

✓☺ **Enydrial Anti-Drying Cleansing Gel** *($16 for 200 ml)* is a well-formulated, fragrance-free, water-soluble cleanser for normal to oily skin. It removes all but waterproof makeup and rinses completely. The only issue is the targeted skin type; someone with very dry skin will likely find this cleanser too strong.

☺ **Enydrial Dermo-Cleansing Lotion** *($16 for 200 ml)* is a good detergent- and fragrance-free cleansing option for someone with dry skin. Ideally you should use it with a washcloth to ensure complete removal.

☺ **Enydrial Emollient Cream, for Very Dry and Atopic Skin** *($20 for 40 ml)* contains several emollients that are great for very dry skin, and borage has anti-inflammatory properties. Although lacking considerable antioxidants, this moisturizer contains some good anti-irritants. By the way, the ingredient "olus" in this product is the technical name for vegetable oil.

☺ **Enydrial Repairing Lip Care** *($7 for 4.8 grams)* is a good, fragrance-free lip gloss–like lip balm that will prevent lips from ending up in a dry, chapped state.

ROC HYDRA+ PRODUCTS

☺ **Hydra+ 3 in 1 Cleansing Care** *($17 for 200 ml)* is supposed to function as a cleanser, toner, and moisturizer in one, but this is just a standard, fragrance-free cleansing lotion for normal to dry skin not prone to breakouts. It doesn't eliminate the need for a toner and moisturizer.

😐 **Hydra+ Destressant Daily Moisturising Care, Day** *($30 for 40 ml)* is a mediocre fragrance-free moisturizer for normal to slightly dry skin. It's not suitable for daytime use unless you pair it with a product rated SPF 15 or greater. This contains a smattering of antioxidants and a cell-communicating ingredient.

😐 **Hydra+ Destressant Nourishing Moisturiser, Night** *($30 for 40 ml)* is mostly water and a long list of thickeners, plus a bit of vitamin E. It's an OK, fragrance-free moisturizer for dry skin, but contains nothing that will reduce the signs of fatigue—this is not a cup of coffee or a stimulant of any kind.

😐 **Hydra+ Destressant Relaxing Moisturising Care, Day** *($30 for 40 ml)* is similar to the Hydra+ Destressant Nourishing Moisturiser, Night, above, except this contains some silicones for a silkier texture and mineral pigments to add soft shine to skin. Otherwise, the same comments apply.

😐 **Hydra+ Effect Reservoir 24-Hour Moisturisation, Enriched Texture** *($30 for 40 ml)* has merit for normal to dry skin, but is an overall boring formula whose antioxidants are present in amounts too meager to matter.

☹ **Hydra+ Effect Reservoir 24-Hour Moisturisation, Light Texture** *($30 for 40 ml)* has a lighter texture and a slightly better formula than the Hydra+ Effect Reservoir 24-Hour Moisturisation, Enriched Texture, above, but just isn't that exciting for the money. Both moisturizers are fragrance-free.

☹ **Hydra+ Mat 24-Hour Moisturiser, Long Lasting Shine Control** *($25 for 40 ml)*. It would be great if this lightweight lotion for normal to oily skin could keep shine under control for the day, but that won't happen with the tiny amount of absorbent ingredients here. And there isn't anything else in this moisturizer to make it a consideration for any skin type.

☹ **Hydra+ Matifying Re-Sourcing Care, Fresh Hydrating Gel for Combination Skin** *($25 for 40 ml)* is nearly identical to the Hydra+ Mat 24-Hour Moisturiser, for Long Lasting Shine Control, above, and the same review applies.

☹ **Hydra+ Nourishing Re-Sourcing Care, Rich Texture Hydrating Cream for Dry Skin** *($25 for 40 ml)* is a good emollient moisturizer for dry to very dry skin. The rich texture keeps skin pampered, while water-binding agents help dry skin function more normally. This would be rated higher if it contained more than a dusting of its single antioxidant.

RoC Protient Fortify Products

☹ **Protient Fortify Decollete and Neck Firming Balm** *($30 for 40 ml)* is nearly identical to RoC's U.S.-sold Protient Fortify Lift & Define Night Cream above, and the same review applies. Neither product is firming, and nothing about the formula is specific to the needs of the neck and chest area.

☹ **Protient Fortify Eyelid Lift Serum** *($32 for 15 ml)* is identical to RoC's U.S.-sold Protient Fortify Lift and Define Eye Cream above, and the same review applies.

☹ **Protient Fortify Face Contour Firm & Lift Fluid** *($39 for 50 ml)* is very similar to RoC's U.S.-sold Protient Fortify Lift and Define Serum reviewed above, and the same comments apply.

☹ **Protient Fortify Overnight Firming Nourisher** *($42 for 50 ml)* is very similar to RoC's U.S.-sold Protient Fortify Lift and Define Night Cream above, and the same review applies.

☺ **Protient Fortify Lip Contour Definition Balm** *($25 for 15 ml)* is an excellent, Vaseline-based lip balm that contains some thoughtful, helpful ingredients for the money. It would be rated a Paula's Pick if not for the potential risk of products with DMAE (listed on the label as dimethyl MEA).

RoC Purif-AC Products

☹ **Purif-AC Purifying Cleanser** *($16 for 150 ml)* contains the drying, irritating detergent cleansing agent sodium C14-16 olefin sulfonate, and is not recommended. Even if the cleansing agent were gentle, the cinnamon and cedar bark extracts can be irritating.

☹ **Purif-AC Exfoliating Lotion** *($16 for 200 ml)* is an irritating, drying toner because of its alcohol content and the presence of cinnamon and cedar extracts.

☹ **Purif-AC Blemish Correcting Emulsion** *($20 for 40 ml)* fails to impress because the pH is too high for the 1% salicylic acid to work well as an exfoliant, and it contains an appreciable amount of irritating cinnamon and cedar.

☹ **Purif-AC Soothing Reparator** *($21 for 40 ml)* is a moisturizer meant for use if acne medications have made skin dry and sensitive. However, the third ingredient is a synthetic sunscreen agent that someone with sensitized skin would likely not be able to tolerate. In fact, oddly enough, the product is loaded with sunscreen ingredients and contains very few soothing agents, which would have been much more helpful. Note: This product does not have an SPF rating, and so it cannot be relied on for daytime protection.

☹ **Purif-AC Fast Action Gel** *($20 for 15 ml)* the only thing fast about this product is how quickly it will irritate your skin with the witch hazel, alcohol, and fragrant plant extracts it contains. This concoction will not make blemishes retreat.

ROC RETIN-OL PRODUCTS

✓☺ **$$$ Retin-OL Correxion Intensive Nourishing Anti-Wrinkle Care, for Dry Skin** *($44 for 30 ml)* has a formula that adds up to an outstanding moisturizer with retinol for normal to slightly dry skin. It actually contains much more vitamin C than retinol, but the amount of retinol is comparable to that in most competing products. The addition of anti-irritants is icing on the cake!

✓☺ **$$$ Retin-OL Multi-Correxion Multi-Corrective Anti-Ageing Moisturiser, Day/Night** *($42 for 30 ml)* is interchangeable with the Retin-OL Correxion Intensive Nourishing Anti-Wrinkle Care, for Dry Skin, above, and the same review applies.

✓☺ **$$$ Retin-OL Multi-Correxion Multi-Corrective Eye Cream** *($32 for 15 ml)* contains less vitamin C than the two RoC Canada Retin-OL products above, but its overall formula is very similar. It would have been better if it didn't contain fragrance.

✓☺ **$$$ Retin-OL Vitamins A+C+E Triple Action, Day/Night** *($39 for 30 ml)* combines vitamins C and E with retinol in stable packaging and a lightweight lotion formula suitable for normal to oily skin. Best for vitamin C but still supplying a good dose of retinol, this is a prime choice in Canadian drugstores.

☺ **Peel-EX Radiance** *($30 for 40 ml)* bills itself as revolutionary technology, but ends up being all talk and minimal action, at least if you were expecting the claims and results to mesh. This product's formula is nearly identical to that of the Resurfacing Facial Peel in RoC's U.S.-sold Resurfacing Peel Kit reviewed above, and the same comments apply here.

ROC RETIN-OL+ PRODUCTS

Although the "+" symbol may make you think these are RoC Canada's better retinol products, none of them are as well-rounded as the regular Retin-OL products above.

☺ **$$$ Retin-OL+ Day, Intensive Anti-Wrinkle Moisturiser** *($44 for 30 ml)* is a good moisturizer with retinol for normal to dry skin, but for the money, it's not preferred over any of the Retin-OL products above.

☺ **$$$ Retin-OL+ Dry Skin, Intensive Anti-Wrinkle Moisturiser** *($44 for 30 ml)* is a lighter-weight version of the Retin-OL+ Day, Intensive Anti-Wrinkle Moisturiser above, and is better suited for normal to slightly dry skin. The amount of glycolic acid is too low for it to function as an exfoliant.

☺ **$$$ Retin-OL+ Eyes, Intensive Eye Anti-Wrinkle Care** *($34 for 15 ml)* is similar to RoC's U.S.-sold Retinol Correxion Eye Cream reviewed above, but this version is superior because it contains a more generous amount of retinol. It is fragrance-free.

☺ **$$$ Retin-OL+ Max, Intensive Anti-Wrinkle Serum** *($50 for 30 ml)* is similar to RoC's U.S.-sold Retinol Correxion Deep Wrinkle Serum reviewed above, except this contains notably more retinol and less fragrance, which makes it the preferred option (especially for those living in Canada). It would be rated a Paula's Pick if not for the potential risk of using products with DMAE (dimethyl MEA).

☺ **$$$ Retin-OL+ Night, Intensive Anti-Wrinkle Care** *($44 for 30 ml)* is similar to RoC's U.S.-sold Retinol Correxion Deep Wrinkle Night Cream reviewed above, except this version is the better choice because it contains more retinol and a lower concentration of preservatives. The pH is still too high for the glycolic acid to exfoliate skin, but this is still an option for those with normal to dry skin seeking a retinol product.

ROC SOYA PRODUCTS

☺ **$$$ Soya Unify Unifying Cleansing Lotion** *($20 for 150 ml)* is a very standard, but good, cleansing lotion for normal to dry skin not prone to breakouts. It removes makeup easily, but you'll need a washcloth to avoid a residue.

☹ **Soya Unify Unifying Exfoliating Gel** *($20 for 50 ml)* contains menthol, peppermint, rosemary, and balm mint and that makes this topical scrub far too irritating to recommend.

😐 **$$$ Soya Unify Unifying Daily Moisturizer SPF 15** *($39 for 50 ml)* keeps skin shielded from the UVA spectrum with its in-part avobenzone sunscreen, but the base formula contains more shiny mica than soy or other substantial ingredients for normal to dry skin. For the money, this product doesn't add up to good skin care in the least, especially not with this price tag.

😐 **$$$ Soya Unify Unifying Nourishing Cream, Night** *($39 for 50 ml)* ranks as another unexciting formula from RoC, and if you were hoping this moisturizer for normal to slightly dry skin was chockfull of soy, you'd be mistaken. There's enough soy for skin to notice, but the rest of the formula doesn't amount to much, especially considering the price.

OTHER ROC CANADA PRODUCTS

😐 **Demaquillage Actif Cleansing Lotion, for Dry Skin** *($16 for 200 ml)* is a rich, somewhat greasy cleansing lotion that is an OK option for dry to very dry skin, as long as you don't mind using this with a washcloth.

☺ **Demaquillage Actif Cleansing Lotion, for Normal or Combination Skin** *($16 for 200 ml)* is a much lighter but still effective cleansing lotion compared to the version immediately above. It's a simple option for quick makeup removal from normal to dry skin; someone who has combination skin with oily areas will likely prefer a water-soluble cleanser.

✓☺ **Foaming Facial Wash** *($16 for 150 ml)* is a very good, fragrance-free cleanser for normal to oily skin, and it removes makeup easily.

☺ **Eye Makeup Remover Extra Gentle** *($16 for 125 ml)* is a very standard, liquid eye-makeup remover that can be used by all skin types. It is indeed gentle, but would be better without the coloring agents.

☺ **Gentle Exfoliating Scrub** *($16 for 40 ml)* can be a good scrub for dry to very dry or sensitive skin because it contains mild cellulose for exfoliation (cushioned by mineral oil), and is also fragrance-free.

😐 **Demaquillage Actif Skin Toner, for Dry Skin** *($16 for 200 ml)* is a basic toner whose dated formula is an OK option for normal to dry skin that needs hydration. It is fragrance-free.

☹ **Demaquillage Actif Skin Toner, for Normal or Combination Skin** *($16 for 200 ml)* contains a lot of alcohol, which makes it too drying and irritating for all skin types. It also contains a film-forming agent commonly found in hairstyling gels, which is an odd addition to an already-problematic toner.

RoC Canada Sun Products

☺ **Minesol Bronze Moisturising Self Tanning Lotion, for Face and Body** *($19 for 100 ml)* is a self-tanning lotion that works as well as any because it turns skin brown with the same ingredient most self-tanners contain, dihydroxyacetone. The inclusion of three sunscreen ingredients may be appealing, but this product is not SPF-rated and should not be relied on for sun protection.

☺ **Minesol Bronze Self-Tanning Multi-Position Spray** *($21 for 150 ml)* is a good self-tanning mist that tans skin with dihydroxyacetone. The fragrance-free formula is suitable for all skin types.

😐 **Minesol Tan Prolonging Lotion** *($19 for 200 ml)* is a very basic body moisturizer meant to be used after sun exposure to prolong your tan and prevent peeling. Any product that encourages tanning is unethical; ironically, this option doesn't help skin in any way even if it wasn't exposed to the sun.

✓☺ **Minesol High Protection Lipstick SPF 20** *($10 for 3 grams)* is a good, glossy-finish lip balm with sunscreen that features avobenzone for sufficient UVA protection.

Rodan + Fields (Skin Care Only)

Rodan + Fields At-A-Glance

Strengths: Two fantastic skin-lightening products with hydroquinone; a well-packaged retinol product; every sunscreen provides sufficient UVA protection; some fragrance-free options; an effective topical disinfectant for acne; product ingredients are listed on the Web site.

Weaknesses: Expensive; jar packaging hinders effectiveness of several otherwise impressive products; sunscreens should contain more bells and whistles for the money; eyebrow-raising amount of products with irritating ingredients; the Unblemish products are a mixed bag that can cause unnecessary irritation.

For more information about Rodan + Fields, owned by Estee Lauder call (888) 995-5656 or visit www.rodanandfields.com or www.Beautypedia.com.

Rodan + Fields Anti-Age Products

😐 **$$$ Anti-Age Step 1 Wash: Anti-Aging Facial Cleanser** *($35 for 3.4 ounces)* is a thick-textured product that contains granular clay for mild exfoliation and emollients for makeup removal and skin-softening. It's an OK option for normal to dry skin and it rinses surprisingly well. However, it's really more of a topical scrub than a cleanser, and that makes using it twice a day a problem for most skin types, especially someone with dry or sensitive skin. The outlandish price is not reflected in the formula of this rather ordinary scrub, and a scrub in no way, shape, or form has any anti-aging properties whatsoever. What were Rodan + Fields thinking?

☹ **Anti-Age Step 2 Prepare: Anti-Aging Facial Toner** *($40 for 4.2 ounces)* should contain some extraordinary ingredients that have a noticeably positive impact on skin; why else would you spend so much money for a toner? Alas, this water- and alcohol-based product is bound to be problematic for all skin types, causing dryness, irritation, and free-radical damage (Sources: *U.S. Pharmacist*, March 2005, pages 17–23; and http://pubs.niaaa.nih.gov/publications/arh27-4/277-284.htm). There are some very good water-binding agents in this product, but their effect is negated by the alcohol. The hyped ingredient is Melaslow, an extract from the peel of the

Japanese plant *Citrus unshiu*, but there are no studies proving that it improves skin texture and clarity. The only research pertaining to this fruit concerns its anti-inflammatory effect when it's ingested, but consumption is not comparable to topical application (Source: *Cancer Research*, September 15, 2000, pages 5059–5066). Besides, this product contains only trace amounts of the stuff, so the potential, if any, would be nil due to the low concentration.

☹ **$$$ Anti-Age Step 3 Treat: Anti-Aging Facial Cream SPF 15** *($90 for 1.7 ounces)* deserves credit for its in-part avobenzone sunscreen and elegant creamy texture, but such traits are also found in sunscreens that cost considerably less. While this does include a good roster of antioxidants as well as some state-of-the-art water-binding agents, most of them are present only in minor amounts, and for the price that is really disappointing. What's even more disappointing is that this product comes in a jar, which means the ingredients won't remain stable after opening. One other point: Sunscreens need to be used liberally to get the real benefit of any SPF rating, but I can't imagine who is going to use a sunscreen with this price tag that way (Source: *Photochemistry and Photobiology*, July 2001, pages 61–63).

☹ **$$$ Anti-Age Multi-Peptide Treatment Eye Cream with Anti-Oxidants** *($50 for 0.5 ounce)*. Co-founding dermatologist Dr. Kathy Fields says about this particular product "we're thrilled with the clinical results"—but, of course, those results are not available because they aren't published and we were told they weren't available. As for the product itself, it will certainly moisturize skin around the eyes or anywhere on the face, but considering its lackluster main ingredients and the cost, it doesn't measure up. Almost every Lauder-owned company (particularly Clinique and Estee Lauder) has eye-cream formulas that are better than this one (Clinique's is less money, Lauder's more). Among the 66 ingredients in this eye cream are several intriguing water-binding agents and anti-irritants, as well as several antioxidants, but the majority of them are present in amounts too small to be of significance to skin. Besides, the product's jar packaging won't keep any of them stable during use. Peptides are potentially great ingredients, but if you're curious to see what benefit peptides have on your skin, consider Olay's Regenerist products, all of which contain considerably more peptides than this overpriced product. (Current research on peptides and their benefit for skin or ability to stimulate collagen production is best described as conjecture, or guessing; it is not based on definitive published research.)

☺ **$$$ Anti-Age PM Serum Night Treatment Capsules with Retinol Peptide Blend** *($75 for 60 capsules)* is one way to see how a fragrance-free retinol product works for you, and this one, because it's in capsule form, ensures that the retinol remains potent before you apply it. The silicone-based formula will leave all skin types feeling silky-smooth, and a peptide was included to make this more than a one-note product.

☹ **$$$ Anti-Age PM Cream Night Treatment with Skin Recovery Complex** *($90 for 1 ounce)* can take good care of dry to very dry skin, but shortchanges you with the jar packaging, which won't keep the many antioxidants in this moisturizer stable.

RODAN + FIELDS ESSENTIALS PRODUCTS

☹ **Essentials Gentle Wash with Aloe Vera** *($25 for 3.4 ounces)* contains sodium lauryl sulfate as its main detergent cleansing agent, which makes this product too irritating and drying (and definitely not gentle) for all skin types (Source: *Contact Dermatitis*, November–December 2004, pages 259–262). The amount of aloe present is a mere pittance, and aloe is useless in a product that is so quickly rinsed from the skin. I have to say it is a bit shocking to see sodium lauryl sulfate in a product line created by dermatologists, because sodium lauryl sulfate is the benchmark irritating ingredient other cleansers are tested against for dermatologic irritancy.

☺ **$$$ Essentials Moisturize with Melaslow** *($40 for 1.7 ounces)* is a lightweight moisturizer that contains some intriguing ingredients, including arbutin, green tea, and vitamins. It's unfortunate they are present in such meager amounts, but this moisturizer still has merit for someone with normal to slightly oily skin. It contains a high amount of *Citrus unshiu* extract (Melaslow), but as I mentioned above, there is no published research establishing this ingredient's benefit for skin. This product does contain fragrance.

😐 **$$$ Essentials Protect with Avobenzone UVA/UVB Sunscreen SPF 30** *($48 for 4.2 ounces)* contains an in-part avobenzone sunscreen in a lightweight lotion base suitable for normal to oily skin. Water-binding agents are plentiful, while antioxidants are, for the money, lacking. Adding potentially irritating fragrance components doesn't make this an essential choice.

😐 **$$$ Essentials Protect with Avobenzone UVA/UVB SPF 15** *($35 for 1.7 ounces)* is similar to the Essentials Protect with Avobenzone UVA/UVB Sunscreen SPF 30 above, but has a lower percentage of active ingredients, even fewer antioxidants, and almost no water-binding agents. The absence of potentially irritating fragrance components is a plus, but the overall formula isn't too exciting.

RODAN + FIELDS REVERSE PRODUCTS

☹ **Reverse Step 1 Wash: Exfoliant Facial Cleanser** *($35 for 3.4 ounces)* is definitely more of a topical scrub than a cleanser because polyethylene (in synthetic scrub particles) is the second ingredient listed. This is a gritty product that can be too harsh on skin, and the inclusion of peppermint oil only compounds the irritation. (Peppermint oil? What were they thinking?!) For better results with almost zero irritation, try exfoliating with a washcloth and any fragrance-free, water-soluble cleanser.

✓☺ **$$$ Reverse Step 2 Prepare: Skin Lightening Toner** *($35 for 4.2 ounces)* makes its mark (no pun intended) as one of the more intriguing products in this dermatologist-developed line. It's an alcohol-free toner that contains 2% hydroquinone, an excellent, time-proven ingredient to lighten sun- or hormone-induced pigment discolorations. In addition, it comes in opaque packaging that keeps the ingredients stable, and contains antioxidant vitamin C and beneficial plant extracts. Lemon and arnica extracts have no place in a product like this (or any product, for that matter), but the amounts are negligible. The tiny amount of salicylic acid (less than 0.5%) will provide minimal exfoliation, since this product's pH allows it to do so. This is an excellent option to address the skin-lightening needs of those with normal to very oily skin.

✓☺ **$$$ Reverse Step 3 Treat: Skin Lightening Lotion** *($65 for 1.7 ounces)* contains 2% hydroquinone as its active ingredient, so it can have a positive effect on pigment discolorations. Included in this product's lightly creamy base are emollients, film-forming agent, silicone, antioxidants, retinol, and lactic acid (as a water-binding agent, not an exfoliant). This is suitable for someone with normal to slightly dry or slightly oily skin. Interestingly, Rodan and Field's ProActiv brand offers a Skin Lightening Lotion retailing at $21.50 for 1 ounce (though you have to be a ProActiv "member" to buy this product). It is a remarkably similar product that does double duty because it also contains a good amount of glycolic acid (the retinol is absent). Still, that doesn't explain the blatant price discrepancy for essentially the same product—I guess they thought most people wouldn't notice.

☺ **$$$ Reverse Step 4 Protect: UVA/UVB Sunscreen SPF 15** *($35 for 1.7 ounces)* doesn't disappoint in terms of its UVA protection, thanks to an in-part zinc oxide sunscreen, but for the money this is a rather boring formula with tiny amounts of antioxidants and otherwise no truly state-of-the-art ingredients. The zinc oxide is advertised as being the Z-Cote brand, but most other modern sunscreens with zinc oxide use this or another micronized form of the mineral, so it's hardly unique to this product. The happy face rating pertains to this product's sunscreen active ingredients and also to its opaque tube packaging.

😐 **$$$ Reverse Exfoliate: Micro-Dermabrasion Paste** *($65 for 4.2 ounces)* has a price that should give you pause, especially when you consider that the abrasive agents (sugar and baking soda) cost mere pennies. This silicone- and wax-based scrub has an unusual base that can be difficult to rinse from the skin, but it does keep this fragranced scrub gentle. The sugar and baking soda granules will polish the skin, although you can easily achieve this effect for a lot less money by mixing plain cornmeal with your daily cleanser or, better yet, using a clean washcloth. Using regular sugar mixed with your cleanser as a face scrub can be too rough, but it's OK from the neck down (hence the prevalence of emollient sugar scrubs). This paste is a decent option for someone with dry to very dry skin.

RODAN + FIELDS SOOTHE PRODUCTS

😊 **$$$ Soothe Step 1 Wash: Soothing Facial Cleanser** *($35 for 3.4 ounces)* is indeed soothing and, thankfully, fragrance-free. Those with dry to very dry skin (including rosacea sufferers) will appreciate this creamy cleanser's texture and how easily it removes makeup. It rinses fairly well, but you may find you need a washcloth to get everything off. By the way, this is nearly identical to Estee Lauder's Verite LightLotion Cleanser ($23.50 for 6.7 ounces), except here you get less cleanser for more money.

😐 **$$$ Soothe Step 2 Treat: Soothing Facial Cream** *($65 for 1.7 ounces)* is a good, fragrance-free moisturizer for normal to dry skin not prone to breakouts. The emollients and silicone will help improve the look and feel of dry skin, but what a shame jar packaging renders the antioxidants ineffective once you begin using this. The mica and titanium dioxide cast a soft glow on skin, but that is a strictly cosmetic effect and not a skin-care benefit.

✓😊 **$$$ Soothe Step 3 Protect: UVA/UVB Sunscreen SPF 15** *($30 for 1.7 ounces)* would be better for sensitive skin if zinc oxide and/or titanium dioxide were the only active ingredients. The mix of zinc oxide with a synthetic sunscreen may prove problematic for those with delicate complexions, but this is still a good sunscreen for normal to dry skin not prone to blemishes. The fragrance-free formula contains some good antioxidant plant oils and cell-communicating ingredients.

☹ **Soothe As Needed: Soothing Facial Lotion with Hydrocortisone** *($35 for 1 ounce)* is a toner that contains 1% hydrocortisone as the active ingredient. Although this active ingredient works to soothe minor irritation, itching, and inflammation, the amount of alcohol undermines its effectiveness, leaving irritated skin right where it started, and that's not to mention that using hydrocortisone on a regular basis breaks down collagen.

RODAN + FIELDS UNBLEMISH PRODUCTS

Those of you familiar with the Rodan and Fields ProActiv line of skin-care products will find the Unblemish products remarkably similar to the original, except that ProActiv's formulas are actually gentler and cost less. By the way, the Rodan + Fields claim of using "prescription medicine at non-prescription strength" is meaningless. The concentrations of benzoyl peroxide in over-the-counter products do not differ from the concentrations in prescription-only products (several pharmacists I contacted confirmed this). So why mention "prescription strength"? Perhaps they wanted theirs to seem better than others on the market, but they're not. They are the same concentrations and basic formulations as nonprescription or prescription versions.

☹ **Unblemish Step 1 Wash: Acne Medicated Cleanser** *($35 for 3.4 ounces)* contains 3% sulfur as an active ingredient, and although sulfur is a topical disinfectant option for battling blemishes, it is drying and irritating to skin. In a cleanser, you're getting less irritation than with leave-on products, but you'd also need to completely avoid the eye area and mucous membranes, which isn't the most convenient way to wash your face and remove makeup. If a leave-on benzoyl peroxide product (from 2.5% to 10%) doesn't control your acne, sulfur is an option, but given sulfur's side effects, it is best used under a doctor's care and not in a rinse-off product or a cleanser where eye irritation is a daily risk. Labeling this cleanser as gentle is sort of like calling a straitjacket comfortable.

☹ **Unblemish Step 2 Prepare: Facial Toner** *($40 for 4.2 ounces)* is a mixed bag for those with a tendency to break out. This water- and witch hazel–based toner contains about 4% glycolic acid. That isn't the most effective concentration, but the pH is low enough that it will exfoliate skin. However, the witch hazel is potentially irritating, as is the menthyl lactate—a form of menthol. It also contains zinc phenosulfate, which increases the irritation factor, although it does have merit as a topical antimicrobial agent. All told, your skin will likely be more confused than blemish-free.

✓ ☺ **$$$ Unblemish Step 3 Treat: Acne Medicated Lotion** *($40 for 1.7 ounces)* deserves a Paula's Pick rating because it is a well-formulated 2.5% benzoyl peroxide product, but the price is outrageous when you consider that virtually identical treatments are available at one-fourth this price. There is little difference between this product and the Repairing Lotion in the Rodan + Fields ProActiv infomercial product line, which sells for about half the price of this (and was also rated highly). Note: Acne Medicated Lotion will disinfect blemishes, but unless you're inclined to overspend on skin care, you may want to consider more affordable options from Neutrogena, Paula's Choice, Stridex, and Zapzyt before this product.

✓ ☺ **$$$ Unblemish Oil Absorb: Blot Papers with Zincidone** *($19 for 60 sheets)* rank as the most expensive oil-blotting papers around, but are they worth the investment? That depends on whether or not you believe the company's claims for zincidone. Otherwise, these are relatively standard sheets that contain talc, clay, and other absorbents to temper excess shine, and they are indeed an option. Zincidone is a trade name for the ingredient zinc PCA. The company that sells this ingredient makes the claim that zinc "is known to inhibit the enzyme that catalyses the production of dihydroxytestosterone (DHT), the hormone controlling sebaceous gland activity." That claim is possibly true when it's taken orally (though the research shows no strong correlation for this), but there is definitely no substantiated research to support this action when it is applied topically. Furthermore, it is definitely a stretch to blame oily skin on DHT; mainly, this hormone is believed to be responsible for male pattern baldness (androgenetic alopecia). But then why do some men with oily skin still have full heads of hair? And why do some men with dry skin go bald? If DHT is causing oily skin, then I should also be bald by now.

There is research pertaining to zinc's potential anti-acne action when consumed orally and applied topically, but it seems to work best in combination with other acne medications (Source: *Natural Medicines Comprehensive Database*, 8th Edition, 2006, page 1371). A tiny amount of zinc impregnated onto sheets of paper that are lightly pressed onto skin cannot affect the oil glands and signal them to be less productive, but these are very good at removing excess surface oil.

SENSE BY USANA (SKIN CARE ONLY)

According to an article in the May 14, 2007, issue of the cosmetics industry newsletter *The Rose Sheet,* Usana uses "self-preserving technology" in their products. The article mentions that the company relies on ingredients that offer self-preservation benefits, and no longer uses chemical preservatives. However, a quick look at the ingredient lists reveals that they are still using chemical preservatives. Capryoyl glycine and undecylenoyl glycine show up in every Sense product. Without question, both of these ingredients meet the definition of a chemical, and both involve synthetic ingredients and processing in their manufacture (Sources: www.vanwagoner.net/preservatives.htm; www.freepatentsonline.com/20040096528.html; and *International Cosmetic Ingredient Dictionary and Handbook,* 11th Edition, CTFA Publishing, 2006). That doesn't make the products lesser considerations; it just makes Usana's claim misleading. There is no proof that the preservative system they opted to use is any better or safer for skin than more common preservatives such as the parabens.

SENSE BY USANA AT-A-GLANCE

Strengths: A couple of well-formulated moisturizers; good cleanser and scrub; packaging that will keep antioxidants stable.

Weaknesses: Expensive; not much variety; no sunscreens; no products for those with blemishes, oily skin, or skin discolorations; a couple of products contain a potentially irritating amount of alcohol.

For more information about Sense by Usana, call (888) 950-9595 or visit www.usana.com or www.Beautypedia.com.

☺ **$$$ Gentle Daily Cleanser** *($21 for 4 ounces)* would be gentler if it did not contain fragrance and European sage extract, but it's still a good, water-soluble cleanser for all skin types. It's pricey, but certainly works well to remove makeup and not leave skin feeling dry.

☺ **$$$ Rice Bran Polisher** *($18 for 2.5 ounces)* is a topical scrub that contains rice bran wax and rice powder as the abrasive agents. You could consider this a natural scrub, but cornmeal and oatmeal are natural, too, and both cost mere pennies; a washcloth with a gentle water-soluble cleanser is also a "scrub" and cheaper yet. Still, this is an acceptable option for normal to very dry skin. The enzyme papain and salicylic acid do not function as exfoliants in this product; even if they did, their contact with skin is too brief for them to work.

☹ **Hydrating Toner** *($18 for 4 ounces)* is packed with beneficial ingredients for all skin types, but the alcohol that precedes them on the list is a deal-breaker that makes this toner too drying and irritating for all skin types.

😐 **$$$ Daytime Protective Emulsion** *($43.23 for 1.3 ounces)* does not list an SPF rating, yet contains three sunscreen ingredients (including avobenzone) as prime parts of the ingredient list. Without an SPF rating, this cannot be relied on for daytime protection, and because it contains sunscreen ingredients it shouldn't be used at night. However, for what Usana is charging, why not go for a daytime moisturizer with reliable sunscreen that's just as elegant?

✓☺ **$$$ Eye Nourisher** *($30 for 0.4 ounce)* is a terrific, silky-textured moisturizer for normal to dry skin anywhere on the face. The fragrance-free formula contains several antioxidants, notable water-binding agents, and a minimum amount of preservative, which may benefit sensitive skin.

✓☺ **$$$ Night Renewal** *($41 for 1.3 ounces)* is a very good moisturizer for normal to very dry skin. It contains helpful emollients, antioxidants, and several water-binding agents.

✓☺ **$$$ Perfecting Essence** *($58 for 1 ounce)* claims to be a breakthrough in skin-care technology—but, ingredient-wise, this doesn't set a new standard. In fact, most of the bells and whistles in this moisturizer show up in Sense by Usana's other products, and although that's great, it doesn't mean that this product should be placed on a pedestal. Its blend of emollient shea butter with silicone, lots of water-binding agents, and antioxidants makes it an excellent option for those with dry to very dry skin who don't want a moisturizer with a thick texture.

☹ **Serum Intensive** *($50 for 1 ounce)* is only "concentrated" with alcohol, and that can be intensively irritating for all skin types. The glycolic acid content and pH are right-on, but a number of other products offer skin the benefits of AHAs without extraneous irritants.

SEPHORA

SEPHORA AT-A-GLANCE

Strengths: Inexpensive; some good cleansers and makeup removers; the Blotting Papers; good powder foundation; the Light Touch Highlighter; Impressive blush and shiny eyeshadow options; great metallic finish eyeliner; awesome brow kit; bountiful selection of lipsticks and lip glosses; a couple of very good mascaras; several outstanding makeup brushes; the Luminizer shimmer lotion; testers are available in-store for each product, and sales pressure is practically nonexistent.

Weaknesses: Mostly average to below-average toners, moisturizers, and sunscreens; no options for those dealing with acne or skin discolorations; some SPF-rated products (including foundations) lack sufficient UVA-protecting actives; the lip plumper is too irritating; too many disappointing eye-makeup products, including several disappointing eyeliners and brow pencils; unappealing shimmer powders.

For more information about Sephora, call (877) 737-4672 or visit www.sephora.com or www.Beautypedia.com.

SEPHORA SKIN CARE

SEPHORA FACE LINE

☹ **FACE 25 Makeup Removing Wipes, for Face, Eyes & Lips** *($10 for 25 wipes)* are not only expensive for the number of cloths you get, they also don't do a great job of removing makeup, plus the formula contains fragrance components that will be irritating when used around the eyes.

☺ **FACE Deep-Down Cleanser, for Combination to Oily Skin** *($10 for 4.22 ounces)* is a very basic, but good, water-soluble cleanser for its intended skin types.

☺ **FACE Fluid Makeup Remover, for Normal Skin** *($8 for 6.76 ounces)* contains emollients and oils to quickly remove makeup, and is suitable for normal to dry skin not prone to breakouts.

☺ **FACE Foaming Cleanser, for Normal Skin** *($10 for 4.22 ounces)* is a good, water-soluble cleanser for normal to slightly dry skin. The tiny amount of plant extracts does not contribute to this cleanser's performance.

☺ **FACE Milky Makeup Remover** *($8 for 6.76 ounces)* is a standard, detergent-free cleansing lotion for normal to dry skin. It rinses reasonably well, though you may find you need a washcloth for complete removal.

☺ **FACE Purifying Makeup Remover, for Combination to Oily Skin** *($8 for 6.76 ounces)* has a texture that's lighter than the FACE Milky Makeup Remover above, yet works just as well to remove most types of makeup. The thickening agent in this formula is not the best for use by someone with oily skin.

☺ **FACE Soothing Cleansing Cream, for Dry Skin** *($10 for 4.22 ounces)* is a good, water-soluble cleanser with a slight creamy texture. This would work well for normal to dry skin.

😐 **FACE Eye Makeup Remover** *($8 for 4.22 ounces)* has a combination of slip agents and a solvent that do a fairly good job removing most types of makeup, but I wouldn't choose this over a silicone-in-water formula because they do a more thorough job and glide more smoothly over the eye area.

😐 **FACE Hydrating Balancing Cream, for Combination to Oily Skin** *($18 for 1.69 ounces)* doesn't offer skin anything special, but its silky texture sets to a matte finish thanks to the clays it contains. It is a suitable option for oily skin or oily areas, and works well under makeup; it's unfortunate that greater amounts of beneficial ingredients weren't included.

😐 **FACE Moisturizing Cream, for Dry Skin** *($18 for 1.69 ounces)* is an average moisturizer whose blend of glycerin and several thickeners can make dry skin look and feel better. The tiny amount of vitamin E does not make this a "vitamin-enriched moisturizer."

😐 **FACE Moisturizing Gel Cream, for Normal Skin** *($18 for 1.69 ounces)* is a boring moisturizer that will do a moderately effective job of keeping normal skin hydrated; however, without any additional benefits, such as antioxidants (which are barely present), there is no reason to consider this an option. Another shortcoming is that the amount of cornstarch can be a problem for those with blemish-prone skin.

😐 **FACE Repair Balm, for Face, Lips & Hands** *($18 for 1.69 ounces)* is a very thick, emollient moisturizer for dry to very dry skin. The texture of this product limits its appeal, especially for use all over the face, but without question it can keep dry skin protected from further moisture loss, and sometimes dry skin just needs lots of "grease."

😐 **FACE Concealing Blemish Pen, for Combination to Oily Skin** *($14 for 0.085 ounce)* dispenses a thin, tinted fluid from a pen-style component with a brush applicator. The neutral shade is fine for light to almost medium skin tones, but don't count on the salicylic acid to help heal blemishes because the amount is likely too low, while the alcohol that precedes it on the list is potentially drying.

😐 **FACE Exfoliator & Mask, for Dry Skin** *($12 for 1.69 ounces)* claims to work as an exfoliant and moisturizer, but does not contain a single ingredient that can help skin shed dead cells. This is just an emollient moisturizer for dry skin and is pretty much void of anything extra to help skin function in a healthy manner.

✓ ☺ **FACE Exfoliator & Mask, for Normal Skin** *($12 for 1.69 ounces)* cannot relax facial contours, and you wouldn't want it to, because that would mean loose, sagging skin (yet this claim seems to attract women every time). Still this is an option as a gentle scrub/mask for normal to very dry skin. You apply this and let the moisturizing agents go to work, then exfoliate during the rinsing process.

☹ **FACE Peel Off Purifying Mask, for Combination to Oily Skin** *($12 for 1.69 ounces)* is a standard, irritating peel-off mask that contains polyvinyl alcohol and regular denatured alcohol as major ingredients.

OTHER SEPHORA SKIN-CARE PRODUCTS

😐 **Makeup Remover Towelettes** *($10 for 25 towelettes)* are very similar to the FACE 25 Makeup Removing Wipes, for Face, Eyes, and Lips above, except these cloths don't contain the irritating fragrance components.

😐 **Professional Unique Cream Makeup Remover** *($8 for 3.3 ounces)* contains mostly water, mineral oil, thickeners, preservative, and fragrance, which makes it just a rather liquid cold cream. The creamy base and oil will remove makeup, but this type of product is only for dry to very dry skin, and you will need a washcloth to complete the job.

😐 **Express Waterproof Eye Makeup Remover with Vitamin E** *($8.50 for 5 ounces)* works quickly to remove eye makeup thanks to the silicones it contains, but the witch hazel and fragrant rose flower water are unhelpful additives that don't make this worth choosing over superior options from Clinique, Almay, Neutrogena, or Paula's Choice.

😐 **Professional Radical Eye & Lip Makeup Remover** *($8 for 1 ounce)* contains Vaseline, and that's it. That's about as radical as using plain Vaseline, which would perform just as well as this strangely named makeup remover.

😐 **Soothing Eye Makeup Remover** *($8.50 for 4.9 ounces)* is a basic, but good, makeup remover for all skin types, but the couple of fragrant components it contains means you should not use this in the eye area.

😐 **Professional Flawless Toner** *($10 for 4.2 ounces)* is professional in name only because any skin-care professional professing approval for this toner has no idea how basic it is. The rose flower water base is akin to dabbing your face with perfume, and any redeeming ingredients are absent.

☹ **Professional Radiance Flash Spray** *($12 for 1.6 ounces)* is a so-so toner that contains mostly water, slip agents, and preservative. The small amount of glycolic acid likely has no benefit at all, and definitely not as an exfoliant. This also contains a number of fragrance components that don't make it worth considering over many other toners.

😐 **Professional Ultimate Relaxation Cream** *($14 for 1 ounce)* supposedly contains a 3% concentration of Matrixyl, also known as palmitoyl pentapeptide-3, yet it is the last ingredient listed, so that claim cannot possibly be true (or someone at Sephora messed up the ingredient label). Even were it given greater prominence, this peptide has not been shown in substantiated research to improve wrinkles or to have any other benefit for skin. This jar-packaged moisturizer is a basic, not ultimate, option for dry to very dry skin.

😐 **Super Smart Facial Moisturizer SPF 15** *($20 for 1.7 ounces)* provides smart sun protection with its in-part avobenzone sunscreen, but is otherwise a kindergarten-level formula for normal to slightly dry skin and contains few antioxidants. The DNA and RNA here cannot (thankfully) affect building blocks in your skin.

☹ **Super Hydrating Sun Mist SPF 15** *($16 for 4 ounces)* lacks the UVA-protecting ingredients of titanium dioxide, zinc oxide, avobenzone, Tinosorb, or Mexoryl SX, and is not recommended. And alcohol is the first ingredient, making the super-hydrating claim super-bogus.

😐 **Super Shield Skin Saver SPF 30** *($18 for 4 ounces)* includes avobenzone for sufficient UVA protection and is a basic, water-resistant sunscreen for normal to oily skin. It contains more fragrance than antioxidants or other good ingredients for skin, which is always disappointing.

😐 **Super Shield Skin Saver SPF 15** *($20 for 6 ounces)* is identical to the Super Shield Skin Saver SPF 30 above, and the same review applies. Interestingly, both of these sunscreens have the same type and percentage of active ingredients. They're likely the exact same product, but one is labeled SPF 15 to appeal to consumers looking for that level of protection. Based on FDA sunscreen testing requirements, as long as you can prove your sunscreen meets your chosen SPF rating, you can label the product with any SPF that is lower (so a sunscreen that tests as SPF 30 can be labeled SPF 24 or even SPF 2, if desired).

😐 **Super Soothing After-Sun Gel** *($15 for 3.4 ounces)* leaves soothing ingredients by the wayside and instead is a basic concoction of water, film-forming agent (think hairspray), slip agents, aloe, and fragrance. Using fresh juice from an aloe plant would be a much better option than using this nearly do-nothing formulation.

☹ **Super Shield Lip Saver SPF 15** *($5 for 0.5 ounce)* does not provide lips with appropriate UVA protection, instead leaving them vulnerable to damage and making this product one to leave at Sephora.

😐 **Lip Butter** *($6 for 0.2 ounce)* has a Vaseline-based formula that contains waxlike thickeners and mineral oil, so it does its job to keep lips smooth and prevent chapping. Lip Butter is available in several flavors, mostly dessert-themed and all adding a sweet scent. If you don't lick your lips going after the flavor, this could be OK, but it's really just Vaseline, so why bother?

😐 **Matte Blotting Film** *($10 for 50 sheets)* are blotting papers of a synthetic material coated with mineral oil and a polymer blend. They do an average job of absorbing excess oil, but are not as efficient as tissue-paper blotters.

☹ **Professional Flash Lip Plumper** *($12 for 0.07 ounce)* contains a blend of menthol and pepper to plump lips in a flash, but the resulting irritation isn't worth the minor results.

☹ **Professional Most Complete Lip Balm** *($5 for 0.26 ounce)* irritates lips with menthol and a menthol derivative, making this neither professional nor the most complete option for anyone's lips.

✓☺ **Roll-Up Blotting Papers** *($8)* is just a long, rolled sheet of uncoated paper housed in a package that allows the user to tear off however much is needed per application. These are portable and work very well to soak up excess shine and perspiration.

SEPHORA MAKEUP

FOUNDATION: ☺ **$$$ All Over Skin Compact Foundation** *($18)* nearly makes it onto the A-list of highly recommended pressed-powder foundations, but this talc-based version's texture, while smooth, is a bit too dry. It offers a sheer matte finish with a hint of shine, and provides sheer to light coverage. The range of 24 shades is impressive, with mostly neutral shades suitable for fair to dark skin. The only dud is R40, which is too red for most dark shin. This is worth checking out if you have oily skin!

😐 **$$$ Powdered Liquid Foundation SPF 12** *($18)* contains an in-part titanium dioxide sunscreen, but SPF 12 doesn't do skin as much good as SPF 15. This foundation feels silky and dispenses slightly thick, but quickly softens and sets to a powdery finish capable of light to medium coverage. Best for normal to slightly oily skin (the powder finish will exaggerate the slightest bit of dry skin), it is available in 24 mostly gorgeous colors. The following shades are too peach or red: R30, R33, R40, and R45. Shades D60 and D65 are beautiful options for very dark skin.

😐 **$$$ Balancing Liquid Foundation SPF 15** *($20)* leaves skin wanting for sufficient UVA protection, and should not be relied on as your sole source of sunscreen. That's a shame, because this is otherwise a commendable liquid foundation whose water-in-silicone texture glides over skin and sets to an attractive satin-matte finish capable of light to medium coverage. Once again, Sephora's palette of shades wins high marks. Of the 24 options, only D55 is too copper to consider. Shades R33, R40, and R45 should be considered carefully.

☹ **Tinted Moisturizer SPF 15** *($18)* does not contain the UVA-protecting ingredients of titanium dioxide, zinc oxide, avobenzone, Mexoryl SX, or Tinosorb, and is not recommended. Otherwise, this is a very standard, emollient, tinted moisturizer that provides just a hint of color. Given that tinted moisturizers with sunscreen should be a convenient all-in-one product, this misses the mark and should be avoided.

CONCEALER: ☺ **Light Touch Highlighter** *($10)* is aptly named, because this brush-on concealer functions best as a highlighter due to its sheer to light coverage. It has a very smooth texture, just the right amount of slip to make blending easy, and five of the six shades are great. Watch out for Apricot, which is slightly peach, although passable.

😐 **$$$ Concealer Palette** *($18)* presents four creamy concealers in a compact, and comes with a brush that's too small to use unless you like a challenge. This applies well and provides nearly opaque coverage, which results in a heavy look. The creaminess means this is prone to creasing, but setting it with powder minimizes this effect. The flesh-toned palette is neutral, but the color-correcting palette is not. All told, this is an OK option only for those seeking full coverage.

😐 **Cooling Cover Stick** *($12)* is a twist-up concealer that feels cool and slightly wet when applied, but it dries quickly to a matte finish laced with sparkles. Coverage is a bit on the sheer side, and given the lack of slip, blending must be swift. This doesn't feel or look as good on skin as many other concealers, but two of the three shades are suitably neutral.

POWDER: ☺ **$$$ Powder in a Brush** *($18)* brings portability to loose powder. Housed in a self-contained unit, it contains a small amount of sheer, whitish pink, talc-based powder. The powder shakes through a sifter onto a built-in brush (the brush is nicer than expected), allowing for quick touch-ups. The single shade goes on practically colorless and leaves a sheer matte finish, but this is best for fair to medium skin tones.

☺ **All Over Skin Bronzing Powder** *($12)* has a better, smoother feel and softer finish than the All Over Skin Pressed Powder below, and the shine level from each of the two shades is unexpectedly soft. This is a good, affordable choice if you're looking for a pressed-powder bronzer.

😐 **All Over Skin Pressed Powder** *($12)* is a talc- and cornstarch-based powder whose silky, somewhat buttery texture gives way to a dry finish that looks a bit too powdery on skin. Although the price is tempting and most of the shades are appropriate, there are more elegant pressed powders available from L'Oreal, Cover Girl, and Revlon.

BLUSH: This standard pressed-powder ☺ **Blush** *($10)* has a silky texture and sheer, even application. Although all of the colors have shine, there is a workable range of nude, pink, and brighter tones available. ☺ **Cheek Stain** *($12)* is meant for those with normal to dry skin because its moist application and finish will likely prove too intrusive for any other skin type (or anyone with large pores). Those searching for a sheer, balm-like blush whose color impact is akin to the many liquid cheek stains available should check this out. Each translucent color is beautiful and easy to blend, leaving a fresh, dewy finish.

😐 **Sun Cream-to-Powder Bronzing Duo** *($15)* isn't a true cream-to-powder bronzer, but rather a powder that happens to feel slightly creamy. It applies well but does not bronze skin as much as impart a sheer, golden shine.

EYESHADOW: ✓ ☺ **Eye Dew** *($10)* is so shiny—and I'm talking gold lamé here—that you may have to put on sunglasses to choose a color, because these liquid-to-cream eyeshadows are that intense. For fans of such products, this is one to consider because it blends decently and doesn't budge (or crease) once it dries. The Storm and Stone shades are the most workable, while Fog (blue) and Lawn (green) are more clownish than captivating. A little goes a long way, so use restraint when applying it or you'll find yourself starting over! Although I personally am not a fan of this type of product, its long-wear, stay-put capabilities earn it a happy face rating.

☺ **Iridescent Cream Shadow** *($10)* is packaged in a click pen with a built-in synthetic brush. It has an ultra-light, silky texture that feels unusually slick as you blend, but it sets to a powder (in feel) finish loaded with shine. The colors are sheer and most are workable (watch our for the Icy Blue and Dar Green options). Best of all is the fact that, once set, these really stay put and the shine doesn't flake.

😐 **All Over Color Eyeshadow** *($9)* has few good shades to extol and a dry texture that makes smooth application and blending difficult, not to mention slightly flaky. Sephora fared better with their powder blush.

EYE AND BROW SHAPER: ✓☺ **Long Lasting Metallic Eyeliner** *($10)* is Sephora's best liquid eyeliner thanks to its easy-to-use tapered brush that allows for precise, even application of this fast-drying formula. Once set, this wears and wears. The only limitation is that all of the colors have a sparkling metallic finish. If you want a dramatic, shiny effect, this is highly recommended.

✓☺ **$$$ Arch It Brow Kit** *($35)* is just about one of the cutest and most practical brow kits I've ever seen. Packaged in a chic leather case about the size of a change purse are a compact that houses brow powder, brow wax, and two synthetic brushes, a mini clear brow gel, a full-size pair of tweezers, brow stencils, instructions, and a larger (but too scratchy) brow brush. The brow powder is matte, and although the accompanying wax looks too dark to coordinate with the powder, it applies sheer. The instructions indicate how to use the stencils (three shapes are included) to perfect your brows, and although they're brief they're also accurate. If you are new to the practice of brow tweezing and shaping, this kit will get you off to a great start and is highly recommended!

☺ **Lash & Eyebrow Mascara** *($10)* comes in three shades, but only the Clear version is worth considering. The other two shades are metallic, which looks artificial on brows. The dual-sided brush works well and the formula remains non-sticky, though you can find clear brow gels for less money at the drugstore.

😐 **Long Lasting Eye Liner** *($10)* has a very thin brush that can be tough to control, resulting in sketchy application. This also takes longer than it should to dry and, despite the name, its wear time doesn't match that of the prime picks in this category. 😐 **Slim Pencil-Eye** *($4)* comes in a dizzying array of colors, which is really the only reason to consider this otherwise very standard, creamy pencil. At this price, you can afford to experiment with several shades, but I encourage you to look past the many blue, green, and purple choices.

☹ **Sponge Tip Liquid Eye Liner** *($10)* has a pointed sponge tip that you'd think would make application easier, but it tends to lay down color unevenly and too sheer. It dries quickly, but feels sticky, and the result is prone to smearing. ☹ **Eyebrow Palette** *($12)* is a good concept with poor execution. Housed in a round compact are two brow powders, a clear brow wax, and a tiny (mostly useless) applicator. The shades of matte brow powder are too sheer and don't correspond well to their intended brow colors, while the wax keeps things in place, but with an unpleasant feel. For brows, you are far better off with the Arch It Brow Kit above.

☹ **Jumbo Pencil-Eye** *($5)* needs sharpening and applies smoothly, but the texture is too creamy and it stays that way, leading to smearing and fading too soon. ☹ **Eyebrow Pencil** *($8)* comes in two good colors, but this needs-sharpening pencil has a creamy application that is too thick and leads to a smear-prone finish. Almost any brow pencil at the drugstore (or department store) outperforms this one. ☹ **Kohl Pencil** *($8)* is a below-standard pencil that drags and tugs during application yet has a creamy finish that won't stay in place for long. ☹ **Cream Eyeliner Palette** *($15)* may tempt you with its striking, metallic-tinged colors, but be aware that this cream eyeliner is way too emollient and applies unevenly, balling up and smearing as you attempt to smooth things out and build intensity (the colors look rich, but apply sheer), and its wear time is brief and fraught with problems.

LIPSTICK, LIP GLOSS, AND LIPLINER: With over 95 colors available, even the most particular person is bound to find a Sephora ☺ **Lipstick** *($10)* to love. Five types are available, and they are arranged by color, not formula, on the tester unit. The **Creams** feel slick and lightweight rather than traditionally creamy, and have a glossy finish. The shade range is quite good, though not as extensive as it used to be. The **Glitter** formula has been improved and has a texture similar to the Creams, but the colors, while frosted, are softer. They no longer feel grainy. **Metallic** has the same texture as the Creams, but comes in bold, full-coverage colors with a metallic finish. The red shades in this finish are striking. The **Ultra Gloss** is glossier than ever and has a slick, moist feel, a faint stain, and terrific colors, although some of them are a bit too pale.

☺ **Lipgloss Palette** *($8)* ends up being quite a bargain if you like the colors and prefer a sheer, glossy finish. Four shades in one compact allow for a variety of looks and these aren't the least bit sticky. I'd toss the too-tiny brush and use a full-size version or a clean fingertip instead.

☺ **Maniac Long-Wearing Lipstick** *($12)* promises "the satiny radiance of a second skin," and although it doesn't feel quite that light, for a creamy lipstick this is not nearly as thick-textured as many. It applies smoothly and imparts nearly opaque color with a satin finish. The shade selection is well-rounded, but small by Sephora standards, offering mostly shimmer- or glitter-infused colors. As for the long-wearing claims, this doesn't fade within an hour, but it also doesn't make it past lunch without a touch-up either, making it a decent lipstick.

☺ **Round-a-Pout** *($9)* combines four separately divided lip glosses into one orb-like component. The sheer, non-sticky glosses feel and look great, and if you don't mind the larger packaging, give this a try!

☺ **Super Shimmer Lip Gloss** *($10)* has a reasonable price for what amounts to a very good, smooth-textured lip gloss with a barely sticky finish. The shade range is well edited and mostly sheer.

☺ **Ultra Shine Lip Gloss** *($15)* does leave lips ultra-shiny as well as glittery. This showy gloss isn't for the demure, and its slightly thick application feels a bit sticky, but that contributes to its high-gloss finish. Give this a sniff before purchasing to make sure the fruit scent appeals to you.

☺ **Shimmer Gloss** *($5)* is a standard, but good, lip gloss with a lightweight, smooth feel and a non-sticky finish. Color is downplayed in favor of shimmer, just as the name says, which makes this a versatile choice to use over any lipstick.

😐 **Tube Lip Gloss** *($7)* is Sephora's version of the original M.A.C. Lipglass ($12.50), and for the most part you won't be able to tell the difference. Both are colorless, thick, syrupy glosses that provide a wet-look, long-lasting shine that feels sticky. This is worth considering if you're a fan of Lipglass but want to get the same effect for less money.

😐 **Lip Gloss Pencil** *($10)* is meant for those who don't mind constant sharpening and want the look and intensity of a sheer lip gloss in pencil form. This is too emollient for anyone with lines around their mouth.

😐 **Jumbo Pencil-Lip** *($5)* proves Sephora can do pencils right when they try! Although this slightly chunky pencil needs to be sharpened, its silky texture, rich colors, and semi-matte finish are a step above in every sense, and make this a must-try if you prefer lipstick in pencil form. The sharpening aspect keeps this from earning a happy face rating. 😐 **Slim Pencil-Lip** *($4)* is similar to the Slim Pencil-Eye above, and, just like it, the best reason to explore this pencil is the vast shade selection. The creamy formula applies well but doesn't do much to keep lipstick from feathering into lines around the mouth. If that's not an issue, this is a reliable, basic pencil.

☹ **Plumping Lip Gloss** *($10)* has a lot going for it until you realize that the plumping effect comes from the inclusion not only of menthol but also capsicum extract. That's a double-whammy of unhealthy irritation for lips. ☹ **Fresh Gloss** *($7)* contains and is flavored by mint, which makes it not worth considering over countless other tube lip glosses, including several sold by Sephora.

MASCARA: ✓☺ **Lengthening Mascara** *($10)* does just that and quickly, too! It builds beautifully, creating long, fringed lashes without any clumps. This has much more curling impact than the misnamed Curling Mascara below, and lashes stay soft.

✓☺ **Extreme Lash Mascara** *($14)* is a two-step mascara that involves a white base coat followed by a top coat of regular mascara. In most products like this, the primer step doesn't make any difference because you can get the same results by just applying a few coats of the mascara alone. That's not the case here. Using the base coat followed by mascara produces long, thick, lush lashes that are expertly separated. The mascara alone, even with several coats, just doesn't produce equal results.

☺ **Surprising Mascara** *($12)* isn't all that surprising, but while it doesn't have a wow factor, it does provide decent length and thickness without clumping, and it doesn't flake or smear either. Still, you can do better with several mascaras from Maybelline, Rimmel, Almay, or Cover Girl.

😐 **Volume Mascara** *($10)* is lackluster for volume (meaning its ability to thicken and add oomph to lashes), but is fairly impressive if you need a basic lengthening mascara that, with effort, also builds appreciable thickness without clumps. Volume Mascara is easy to remove and makes it through the day without smearing. 😐 **Curling Mascara** *($10)* takes longer to impress than the Volume Mascara above, but with patience it does produce long lashes that have a smidgen of thickness and nice separation, with minimal clumping. This does not curl lashes on its own (but it will if you use an eyelash curler, which is true of all mascaras).

😐 **Triple Action Mascara** *($12)*. If this does three things for lashes, it doesn't do any of them very well! This Sephora-described "best of both worlds" mascara is merely average in all departments, though it is easy to remove with a water-soluble cleanser. 😐 **Mascara Fantastic Color** *($12)* is an acceptable mascara, but in a mascara that's called "fantastic" that is really disappointing. This goes on wetter than most and leaves lashes looking glossy and slightly stuck together. Because of this wetness and slower dry time, smearing can be a problem if you're not careful. 😐 **Waterproof Mascara** *($10)* goes on somewhat thin but cleanly, producing natural-looking, nondramatic length without thickness. It is waterproof and requires a silicone- or oil-based remover.

😐 **Professional Clear Natural Mascara** *($10)* is a very standard, colorless gel mascara that has minimal impact on lashes beyond slightly darkening them and creating a minimal groomed look. This actually works better as a brow gel, but isn't worth the splurge over similar products from Cover Girl or Maybelline New York.

FACE AND BODY ILLUMINATING/SHIMMER PRODUCTS: ✓😊 **Luminizer** *($22)* is a silicone-in-water shimmer lotion housed in a glass bottle with a pump applicator. It has a silky application and a dry finish that leaves skin softly glowing. This is an excellent way to subtly highlight skin, and it mixes well with moisturizer or foundation. All three shades are very good.

😊 **Luminous Trio** *($15)* is a less-expensive copy of Bobbi Brown's popular Shimmer Brick Compact ($38), except that in this instance you get just three stripes of shimmering pressed powder. It feels very smooth and applies well, if a bit heavy. The shine is intense, making this best for highlighting small areas rather than for dusting all over. Both trios are attractive.

☹ **Sparkling Powder In A Brush** *($18)* is similar to the Powder in a Brush above, but for some reason this version doesn't dispense as well. What's even more frustrating is that the loose powder doesn't cling well to skin, and the low-level shine tends to flake.

☹ **Enlightening Shimmer Powder** *($12)* is a letdown. This shiny pressed powder looks thick and chalky on skin and pales in comparison to most shine-infused powders.

BRUSHES: Sephora's **Brushes** *($4–$40)* present some prime choices, especially for applying eyeshadow and powder eyeliner. Over 50 brushes are available, with the best ones being the ✓😊 **Professional Foundation Brush** *($30)*, ✓😊 **Bronzer Brush** *($25)*, ✓😊 **Professional Natural All Over Shadow Brush** *($20)*, ✓😊 **Professional Angle Brush** *($18)*, ✓😊 **Slanted Contour Eyeshadow Brush** *($20)*, ✓😊 **Dome Sable***($15)*, ✓😊 **Eyeshadow Brush** *($15)*, and ✓😊 **Short Handle Crease Eyeshadow Brush** *($15)*. The 😊 **Small Retractable Blush Brush** *($12)* isn't the softest around, but for the money is a good secondary blush or powder brush to stash in your purse.

The 😐 **Powder Brush** *($26)* comes in both a short- and long-handled version and works well, but it isn't as soft and elegant as it could be. Avoid the overpriced ☹ **Fan Brush** *($20)* and the ☹ **Slanted Blush Brush** *($26)*, which are too sparse for precise application.

SPECIALTY PRODUCTS: You will not be disappointed by Sephora's vast selection of 😊 **Makeup Bags** *($4–$35)* and ✓😊 **$$$ Train Cases** *($35–$90)*. The variety is astounding, especially for the makeup bags, and although the train cases are not the sturdiest around, they make elegant, ready-to-travel makeup organizers (unless you'll be carting them around everywhere the way a working makeup artist would). The selection tends to vary by store, so if you want to see everything that's available, check out the Sephora Web site.

😊 **Flirt-It Lash Duo** *($8)* is a kit with pre-cut strips of false eyelashes and adhesive. It's well priced and a basic kit for beginners interested in experimenting with this type of product. The second version features rhinestones at the lash base for a sparkling effect.

😊 **Deluxe Lash Kit** *($18)* is available in classic black or glitter lashes, which have a shiny strip at the base of the lashes. Included is a pair of pre-cut false eyelashes, adhesive, a lash curler, and a storage case. This is worth checking out if you like the look of these lashes and want to experiment, or if you just want to add some drama to your natural lashes for a special occasion.

😊 **Professional Radical Eye & Lip Makeup Remover** *($8)* is a basic, cream-style makeup remover that works well to dissolve eye and lip makeup. Calling it "radical" is radically unprofessional.

☺ **Professional Perfection Makeup Base** *($12)* is positioned as the ultimate pre-makeup base, which it isn't. However, it works well as a lightweight, non-greasy moisturizer for someone with normal to oily skin with dry patches. Just be aware that it leaves a sheer pink opalescent finish.

☺ **Makeup Eraser Pen** *($12)* does come in handy when you need a fast makeup fix for flaking mascara or smeared lipstick. This pen has a wax- and silicone-enriched tip that allows precise application to the trouble spot. Just dab on, blend a bit, and then use a tissue or cotton swab to remove. While not an essential, you may want to consider adding this to your stash of office or evening makeup.

😐 **Skin Smoothing Makeup Base** *($22)* is a very standard silicone-based primer with no extra frills, which doesn't justify the price. Similar to most silicone primers, it will create a silky-smooth surface to enhance foundation application. However, this much silicone doesn't jibe well with every liquid foundation, so be sure to test the combination beforehand.

😐 **Cream All Over Color** *($9)* comes in mostly pale, pastel colors that leave an obvious shine. This product's slightly thick texture and sheer powder finish aren't the most elegant around, but for the money this takes care of adding a glow-y shine to skin. 😐 **Iridescent All Over Color** *($9)* is identical to the Cream All Over Color above except with more obvious shine. The formula allows the shine to cling better than it does in powder form, but it's a shame the application isn't smoother. 😐 **All Over Color Palette** *($24)* functions best as eyeshadow, and bears a strong resemblance to the Eye Shadow Quartets from Hard Candy, which sell for a few dollars more. Packaged as quads, these initially feel creamy but go on dry, dragging over skin and looking too powdery. The mostly tone-on-tone colors are all shiny, just like the selection from Hard Candy. Neither product rises above mediocre.

☹ **Glitter All Over Color** *($9)* has the same average texture and application issues as the Cream and Iridescent All Over Color products above, but the glitter lends an off-putting grainy feel and it tends to flake. None of that is pretty, which makes this product seem juvenile.

☹ **Lipstick Sealant** *($15)* is a clear fluid you brush on to seal lipstick so it's kiss- and budge-proof. It doesn't work that well, and contains enough alcohol to cause lip dryness and irritation.

SHEER COVER

SHEER COVER AT-A-GLANCE

Strengths: One well-formulated toner; the blotting papers; the mineral foundations (particularly the pressed version) are a cut above most others; surprisingly good powder eyeshadow set; Guthy-Renker has an excellent return policy.

Weaknesses: Mostly unimpressive skin care, including a sunscreen that leaves skin vulnerable to UVA damage; poor concealer; average mascara.

For more information about Sheer Cover, call (800) 506-6281 or visit www.sheercover.com or www.Beautypedia.com. Note: Sheer Cover is distributed by Guthy-Renker, and comes with a generous, 60-day return/exchange policy. They'll even take back empty containers if you're unhappy with the products, a rarity in the cosmetics industry. That offer makes it almost irresistible if you're curious to see if mineral makeup will work for you, and Sheer Cover is a cut above its competitors in some key respects.

SHEER COVER SKIN CARE

Sheer Cover's small selection of skin-care products isn't a total letdown, but it's overpriced and not state-of-the-art enough to justify the splurge—not to mention that the sunscreen is truly terrible and the cleanser isn't strong enough to remove the Mineral Foundation.

😐 **$$$ Purifying Cleanser** *($20.95 for 4 ounces; 2-ounce size comes in the kit; $12.95 member price)* is a lightweight, water-soluble cleansing lotion that contains a tiny amount of detergent cleansing agent. The main issue with this cleanser is that it doesn't remove the Sheer Cover Mineral Foundation very well. This fragrance-free cleanser is best for someone with normal to dry skin who wears minimal to no makeup.

☺ **$$$ Refreshing Face Mist** *($22.95 for 2 ounces; $14.95 member price)* is a spray-on, alcohol-free toner that is suitable for normal to dry skin. It contains several good water-binding agents and also has some vitamin-based antioxidants, but the clear bottle packaging won't keep them stable for long. This does contain fragrance. The instructional DVD and how-to guide for Sheer Cover recommends misting this toner over your Mineral Foundation, but doing so encourages streaking and can make the color look a bit blotchy, necessitating more blending.

😐 **$$$ Soothing Mineral Toner** *($22.95 for 4 ounces; $14.95 member price)* does contain minerals, but none of them have substantiated proof that they can encourage collagen production to create firmer skin. Beyond the water and minerals in this toner, there are a few plant extracts and soothing agents, as well as minuscule amounts of witch hazel and alcohol. You're not getting a lot of bang for your buck here, but this fragranced toner is an OK option for all skin types.

😐 **$$$ Base Perfector** *($29.95 for 0.5 ounce; $22.50 member price)* is a mixed bag of positives and negatives. This nonaqueous, silicone-based gel leaves skin feeling very smooth, and it feels nearly weightless. Green tea, vitamin E, and vitamin A are on hand as antioxidants, but the fragrance and fragrant extracts basically cancel out their benefit. This is a decent option if you're looking for a foundation primer, but it is not as matte as many others, so isn't ideal for very oily skin.

☹ **Nourishing Moisturizer SPF 15** *($30.95 for 2 ounces; $18.95 member price; 1 ounce in the kit)* does not contain the UVA-protecting ingredients of titanium dioxide, zinc oxide, avobenzone, Tinosorb, or Mexoryl SX, and has a boring water- and wax-based formula, making it a poor choice all around.

☺ **$$$ Blotting Papers** *($14.95 for 80 sheets; $9.95 member price)* are standard, tissue paper–style blotting sheets that work as well as any, except here you're paying a premium price.

SHEER COVER MAKEUP

Most customers who order Sheer Cover take advantage of the 😐 **$$$ Sheer Cover Intro Kit** *($29.95)*, which allows you to sign up for an automatic replenishment program that bills your credit card the same amount each month. I wouldn't recommend doing that until you're sure you like the products (based on the small sizes, you would need to replenish most of the products monthly anyway). Included in the kit are two shades of the Mineral Foundation, Duo Concealer, Finishing Powder, a sponge applicator, two brushes, and smaller sizes of the Purifying

Cleanser and Nourishing Moisturizer SPF 15 reviewed above. Aside from the skin-care products, the color items in this kit are reviewed below because they are also sold separately, and the kit's overall neutral face rating was based on the mixed-bag nature of the products it contains.

FOUNDATION: ✓☺ $$$ Pressed Mineral Foundation *($29.95; $19.95 member price)* is a smoother, neater way to experiment with mineral makeup, though the composition of this mica-based, talc-free, pressed-powder foundation is not akin to traditional mineral makeup. This has a beautiful soft texture that blends very well and leaves skin with a subtle glow, courtesy of the mica, which is naturally shiny. Coverage goes from sheer (if applied with a brush) to medium (if used with a sponge) and does not look too thick, powdery, or heavy on skin. All five shades are excellent, and there are options for light to dark (but not very dark) skin tones. Unless you need significant camouflage, consider spending your Sheer Cover dollars on this product instead of their Mineral Foundation below.

☺ $$$ Mineral Foundation *($29.95; $19.95 member price)* is the core product of the Sheer Cover line. It's a loose powder whose primary ingredients are titanium dioxide, which lends opacity and allows a small amount of product to provide sufficient coverage, and bismuth oxychloride, a major ingredient in almost all mineral makeups. The latter isn't natural in the least, but it does allow for more opaque coverage than traditional talc-based powders. The good news is that, texture-wise, this is the most finely milled mineral foundation I've reviewed. That makes it look more natural on skin, though it can still look a bit thick and opaque unless applied sheer.

The bad news (though it may not be bad, depending on your preference) is the amount of shine each shade leaves behind. Unlike other mineral makeups whose shine casts an all-over radiant glow, Sheer Cover's version makes skin look sparkly, which is distracting for daytime wear and definitely calls attention to the fact that you're wearing makeup. As for application, if you order the Intro Kit mentioned above, it will come with two brushes: a retractable powder brush and a regular powder brush. The retractable brush has a hollowed-out portion in the handle and when you unscrew the cap at the base, you can pour in some of the Mineral Foundation for touch-ups on the go. Neither one is ideal (both tend to make the process of applying loose powder messier than usual), nor are they as soft and dense as they should be. Therefore, if you decide to try this foundation, you'll also need to invest in a better powder brush.

Eight shades are available, including options for dark (but not very dark) skin tones. The lightest shade (Bisque) is suitable for most fair skin tones. Avoid Almond, which goes on slightly peach, but becomes more peach as it mixes with your skin's oil, and use caution with Nude, which tends to turn pink. The Frost shade is for highlighting only due to its intense shine. Because the Intro Kits come with two shades, the company recommends custom blending unless one of the colors matches your skin exactly. This isn't too difficult, but given the mess mineral makeup can present, it's definitely easier and faster to find one shade of foundation (of any type) that meshes with your skin.

In summary, the Mineral Foundation from Sheer Cover has the same basic traits as most mineral makeup. It can provide full coverage (which will conceal redness from rosacea) and leaves a slightly thick, dry matte finish that is laced with shine. It wears quite well except over very oily areas. Unless the oil-prone areas are set with powder (a step Sheer Cover recommends), you'll notice the color getting darker as the day goes on, or the foundation pooling in pores, neither of which is attractive. Sheer Cover's point of distinction (and the reason to consider it if you can tolerate the clingy sparkles) is a finer texture that blends very well and lends itself to a more natural look—about as natural as this type of foundation can appear on skin, which is a step in the right direction!

CONCEALER: ☹ Duo Concealer *($24.95; $14.95 member price)* has a creamy-slick texture that slips over skin easily, but it just keeps slipping. Because this surprisingly lightweight concealer never sets, creasing and fading are inevitable, even when set with powder. It also doesn't provide much coverage, as is evidenced by watching the women in the Sheer Cover how-to DVD apply it. Most of the shades are quite good (and blend well together), but the aforementioned drawbacks still make this a concealer to ignore.

POWDER: ☺ Finishing Powder *($23.95; $14.95 member price)* is a talc-free loose powder with a weightless texture and a soft, dry finish. This product is included in the Sheer Cover Intro Kit, and is recommended for use after applying the Mineral Foundation (I know, it's odd that you need to set a powder with another powder, but whether this works for you is a personal preference, not a must have). Three shades are available, all of which apply very sheer, leaving skin matte but dusted with a fine layer of sparkles.

☺ $$$ Lip-to-Lid Highlighter *($22.95; $14.95 member price)* is a mica-based, shiny loose powder available in a pink shade for blush or a tan shade for bronzing, contouring, or use as eyeshadow. Both shades leave skin quite shiny, but not ultra-sparkling, making this a good choice for evening glamour. The shine clings well and the effect from either shade is pretty if applied sparingly. Using this on the lips is another story, however, because you have to combine it with a lip balm so it feels comfortable, and doing so isn't as easy or nice looking as just using a regular lipstick or lip gloss.

EYESHADOW: ☺ $$$ Eye Collection *($39.95; $24.99 member price)* provides six pressed-powder eyeshadows in one compact. Each shade has a soft to moderate shimmer, but they apply smoothly, don't flake, and impart soft color that can build to a deeper hue. Only one medium shade is included, leaving you with five colors best for lids or underbrow. With a slightly more thoughtful shade assortment this would have been a Paula's Pick.

EYE AND BROW SHAPER: 😐 $$$ Defining Eye Liner *($19.95; $14.95 member price)* is a standard, needs-sharpening pencil that tends to stay creamy, so some smudging occurs during wear. Considering the number of better eye pencils available at the drugstore for significantly less money, choosing this option doesn't make much sense.

LIPSTICK, LIP GLOSS, AND LIPLINER: ☺ $$$ Lip Collection *($31.95; $22.50 member price)* comes complete with six sheer, sparkling lip glosses in one compact. The tiny brush applicator isn't helpful and should be discarded. Otherwise, as far as lip gloss goes, each shade has a smooth texture, a wet shine finish, and is minimally sticky. This is pricey for what you get, but if you're looking to splurge on sheer lip gloss it won't disappoint.

😐 $$$ Defining Lip Liner *($21.95; $16.95 member price)* needs sharpening and is priced outlandishly, but it happens to be a good, slightly creamy lip pencil that applies well and stays in place. Only one shade is available, but it's a rose brown tone that works with a variety of lipsticks.

MASCARA: 😐 $$$ Extra Length Mascara *($19.95; $14.95 member price)* is a minimalist mascara that does nothing but make lashes look darker and a bit more separated. Yes, it is misnamed, but this may be worth a try if you're pleased with your lashes in their natural state and just want to darken them.

BRUSHES: ☺ $$$ Dual Eye Contour Brush *($27.95; $18.95 member price)* has a soft, full eyeshadow brush on one end and a tapered, domed crease brush on the other. Both sides are practical and facilitate a beautiful application of eye makeup, and the price isn't out of line for the quality.

SHISEIDO

SHISEIDO AT-A-GLANCE

Strengths: Most of the sunscreens provide sufficient UVA protection and present a variety of options, whether you're looking for titanium dioxide, zinc oxide, or avobenzone; a handful of good (but not great) moisturizers; an excellent sunscreen for lips; worthwhile oil-blotting papers; every foundation with sunscreen provides sufficient UVA protection (and there are some wonderful foundations here); pressed powder with sunscreen for oily skin; the unique Hydro Powder Eye Shadow; Perfecting Lipstick is one of the best creamy lipsticks at the department store; mostly good mascaras; all of the Veil products are worth considering.

Weaknesses: Expensive; several drying cleansers; boring toners; a few sunscreens offer insufficient UVA protection; no AHA or BHA products; no products to effectively manage acne; no reliable skin-lightening options despite a preponderance of products claiming to do just that; irritating self-tanners; gimmicky masks; jar packaging; terms like Bio-Regenerine, Phyto-Capsule Emulsification, Optimal Balance Network, and Deacti-Complex are meaningless without significant, proven ingredients to support each technology's alleged function; uneven assortment of concealers (and some terrible colors); the eyeshadow quads; average to disappointing eye and brow shapers; average makeup brushes.

For more information about Shiseido, call (800) 906-7503 or visit www.sca.shiseido.com or www.Beautypedia.com.

SHISEIDO SKIN CARE

SHISEIDO BENEFIANCE PRODUCTS

😐 **$$$ Benefiance Creamy Cleansing Emulsion** *($32 for 6.7 ounces)* is a very standard, water- and oil-based cleansing cream for dry to very dry skin. This is essentially glorified cold cream, and although it removes makeup in a flash, you'll need a washcloth to avoid the greasy residue it leaves behind.

😐 **$$$ Benefiance Creamy Cleansing Foam** *($32 for 4.4 ounces)* is a foaming, creamy-textured, water-soluble cleanser that contains alkaline cleansing agents capable of causing dryness for most skin types.

😐 **$$$ Benefiance Balancing Softener** *($39 for 5 ounces)* won't balance anything and is nothing more than a basic, alcohol-free toner for normal to dry skin. It contains mostly water, glycerin, slip agents, thickeners, a water-binding agent, preservatives, fragrance, a cell-communicating ingredient, and coloring agents.

😐 **$$$ Benefiance Enriched Balancing Softener** *($39 for 5 ounces)* is similar to the Benefiance Balancing Softener above, but is less interesting because most of the helpful ingredients are listed after the preservative. That's really disappointing considering this toner's cost.

😐 **$$$ Benefiance Concentrated Anti-Wrinkle Eye Cream** *($47 for 0.51 ounce)* has a thick, lush texture tailor-made for dry skin anywhere on the face, and contains some tried-and-true emollients. A nice selection of antioxidants is on hand, too, but the jar packaging won't keep them stable during use, which knocks this product's rating down.

😐 **$$$ Benefiance Concentrated Neck Contour Treatment** *($48 for 1.8 ounces)* is primarily a blend of water, silicones, and slip agents along with film-forming agents and some antioxidants, none of which are specific to the neck area. This serum-like product also contains potentially irritating ingredients, although the small amounts means they are likely inconsequential. This product has no hope of making lines on the neck a thing of the past, and there are products from other lines that are better formulated than this gaffe.

☹ **Benefiance Daytime Protective Cream SPF 15** *($44 for 1.3 ounces)* not only leaves skin vulnerable to UVA damage because its sole active ingredient does not cover the full spectrum of UVA light, but the base formula is terribly boring for the money. Plus it is packaged in a jar, so the few antioxidants it does contain won't be around for long.

☹ **Benefiance Daytime Protective Emulsion SPF 15** *($44 for 2.5 ounces)* is an even worse formula compared to the Benefiance Daytime Protective Cream SPF 15 above, and does not deserve even a second's worth of thought.

☹ **Benefiance Energizing Essence** *($53 for 1 ounce)* cannot energize skin, but it contains enough alcohol to cause irritation. Another concern is the inclusion of tranexamic acid. This synthetic ingredient is a drug used to control bleeding during surgical procedures, and it has no purpose or business being in a skin-care product (Sources: www.drugs.com; and *The Journal of Thoracic and Cardiovascular Surgery*, September 2000, pages 520–527).

☹ **Benefiance Facial Lifting Complex** *($53 for 1.7 ounces)* claims to nourish skin and correct sagging, but contains enough alcohol to irritate skin, and the menthol furthers this irritation. This is one of the few products in this book whose claims are over the top and whose formula has no redeeming value for anyone's skin.

😐 **$$$ Benefiance Luminizing Day Essence SPF 24** *($50 for 1.4 ounces)* creates a luminous finish because of the mineral pigments it contains, but other than that cosmetic benefit this is just an ordinary, overpriced, in-part titanium dioxide sunscreen for normal to slightly dry or slightly oily skin. Antioxidants and a cell-communicating ingredient are present, but just barely.

☹ **Benefiance Luminizing Night Essence** *($75 for 1.3 ounces)* lists alcohol as its second ingredient, which damages skin via irritation and generation of free radicals. What a shame, because it does contain enough arbutin to have a positive impact on discolorations.

😐 **$$$ Benefiance Revitalizing Cream** *($47 for 1.3 ounces)* is a relatively standard moisturizer for normal to dry skin, and is definitely overpriced for what you get. The tiny amount of antioxidants will break down shortly after this jar-packaged product is opened.

☺ **$$$ Benefiance Revitalizing Emulsion** *($47 for 2.5 ounces)* is similar to the Benefiance Revitalizing Cream above, but in better packaging and with a greater amount of antioxidants. It is recommended for normal to dry skin.

😐 **$$$ Benefiance Wrinkle Lifting Concentrate** *($62 for 1 ounce)* is sold with the promise of, what else, lifting wrinkles. But Shiseido goes on to claim that this product allows skin to resist future wrinkles, something that's not possible without an effective sunscreen, which is absent here. The showcased ingredient in this product is chlorella extract. According to Shiseido, this reinforces the presence of a protein in skin that's critical to halting the wrinkling process. But none of that is substantiated, and even if it were, there's so little chlorella that your wrinkles wouldn't even notice. Chlorella is an algae and, like almost all species of algae, can act as a water-binding agent and antioxidant on skin. A good question for Shiseido: If this ingredient is that important for stopping wrinkles, why isn't it in every "antiwrinkle" product this line sells?

This product is chiefly a lightweight moisturizer that contains more alcohol than it does beneficial ingredients for skin. Several antioxidants appear, but they're of little use when combined with the potentially drying and irritating effect of the alcohol and the lack of sunscreen.

At best, this is a substandard moisturizer for slightly dry skin that has no positive effect on wrinkles—either past, present, or future.

☺ **$$$ Benefiance Eye Treatment Mask** *($37 for 10 pairs)* seems like a specially targeted product, but it isn't. Although it contains some helpful ingredients for skin, the exciting ones are but a dusting, while the amount of acrylate-based film-forming agent may cause irritation around the eyes. Nothing in this mask solution can treat dark circles.

☹ **Benefiance Firming Massage Mask** *($42 for 1.9 ounces)* contains tranexamic acid, a synthetic drug that has no proven purpose in a skin-care product. One study that involved applying a 2%–3% concentration of the drug to guinea pig skin indicated severely reduced melanin formation resulting from concentrated UV exposure (Source: *Journal of Photochemistry and Photobiology*, December 1998, pages 136–141). In contrast, another study showed that topical applications of vitamin E (as alpha tocopherol) and ferulic acid (another antioxidant) were more effective at inhibiting melanin production than a higher dose of tranexamic acid, and did so while having an added, potent antioxidant benefit (Source: *Anticancer Research*, September/October 1999, pages 3769–3774). Given the precautions and side effects associated with oral administration of tranexamic acid and the unknowns of topical application, it is an ingredient that is best avoided.

☺ **$$$ Benefiance Pure Retinol Instant Treatment Eye Mask** *($60 for 12 pairs)* is basically a gimmicky mask that requires the use of steam to infuse retinol (the very tiny amount Shiseido included) into skin. Steaming your skin, as you might imagine, can cause problems (surfaced capillaries in particular). The bulk of this formula is water, slip agents, silicone, and alcohol, making it an average option that costs far more than it should and has an application recommendation that is a serious blunder.

☺ **$$$ Benefiance Pure Retinol Intensive Revitalizing Face Mask** *($60 for 4 upper and 4 lower face masks)* has a formula very similar to the Benefiance Pure Retinol Instant Treatment Eye Mask above, but this option includes pre-cut mask sheets for the upper and lower eye area. It is not intensive if you are looking for a potent dose of retinol, and won't do much beyond providing mild hydration for slightly dry skin.

☹ **Benefiance Full Correction Lip Treatment** *($35 for 0.5 ounce)* makes claims similar to Olay's Regenerist Anti-Aging Lip Treatment ($19.99 for 0.06 ounce), reviewed in this book, but the Shiseido formula is not nearly as interesting, plus it irritates lips with menthol and has only a scant amount of antioxidants. The waxlike thickeners in this product can help temporarily fill in vertical lip lines, but so can Olay's, for less money and with a much better formula.

SHISEIDO BIO-PERFORMANCE PRODUCTS

☺ **$$$ Bio-Performance Advanced Super Revitalizer (Cream)** *($70 for 1.7 ounces)* isn't advanced when compared to today's state-of-the-art moisturizers, but it does contain several ingredients (including glycerin, squalane, fatty acids, and silicone) that are helpful for dry skin. The tiny amounts of antioxidants will suffer from the jar packaging. The iron oxides produce a slight glow on skin, but don't mistake that for skin being revitalized.

☺ **$$$ Bio-Performance Advanced Super Revitalizer (Cream) Whitening Formula** *($96 for 1.7 ounces)* is similar to the Bio-Performance Advanced Super Revitalizer (Cream) above, except this pricier option contains a selection of plant extracts and vitamin C (as ascorbyl glucoside), which have some research showing them to be effective for skin lightening. However, due to jar packaging, none of these potentially efficacious ingredients will remain stable during use.

😐 **$$$ Bio-Performance Intensive Clarifying Essence** *($70 for 1.3 ounces)* contains nothing that can clarify skin in a manner comparable to a well-formulated AHA or BHA product. This is merely a ho-hum, lightweight moisturizer for normal to slightly dry or slightly oily skin.

✓😊 **$$$ Bio-Performance Super Eye Contour Cream** *($52 for 0.53 ounce)* is an excellent emollient moisturizer suitable for dry to very dry skin anywhere on the face. It is stably packaged, to the benefit of the many vitamin- and plant-based antioxidants it contains.

😐 **$$$ Bio-Performance Super Lifting Formula** *($73 for 1 ounce)* is similar to the Benefiance Concentrated Neck Contour Treatment above, and the same basic comments apply. The addition of a few more water-binding agents in this product doesn't change the fact that it cannot lift skin.

😐 **$$$ Bio-Performance Super Restoring Cream** *($96 for 1.7 ounces)* is sold as an unparalleled age-defying cream, which doesn't explain why Shiseido sells dozens of other moisturizers with this same claim. After all, if this is *the* one, why bother with the rest of them? As it turns out, this is a very good moisturizer for dry skin. Yet it ends up being disappointing because of jar packaging, which hinders the effectiveness of the impressive amount of antioxidants in this product.

Bio-Performance Ultimate Skin Renewal System *(Each product sold individually)* is Shiseido's dual-step exfoliation system, with both products sold separately. The 😐 **$$$ Bio-Performance Super Exfoliating Discs** *($64 for 8 individually wrapped discs)* are said to work like microdermabrasion, and manually exfoliate skin due to their texture and a mixture of talc and rice bran. These discs differ little from those sold in many drugstore lines, including Olay, Neutrogena, and Dove. After using the discs to exfoliate, you are directed to apply the ☹ **Bio-Performance Super Refining Essence** *($75 for 1.8 ounces)*, a water- and glycerin-based serum that contains some good water-binding agents and small amounts of vitamins E and C. The problem is that it also contains numerous fragrance components, which can cause irritation, and that isn't what should be applied to freshly scrubbed skin. Given the potential problems the Refining Essence presents and the fact that the Super Exfoliating Discs are easily replaced by drugstore options (or, for even less money, a washcloth and your favorite cleanser), this pricey system is not recommended.

SHISEIDO ELIXIR PRODUCTS

😐 **$$$ Elixir Cleansing Foam with Collagen Extract I, for Normal to Oily Skin** *($26 for 4.5 ounces)* promises lifted skin as you wash, thanks to the collagen extract it contains. It's a bogus claim because collagen applied topically cannot do a thing to correct sagging. Besides, this is a rather drying cleanser because it contains potassium hydroxide. It is only an option for very oily skin, and even for that skin type it's not a very good option.

😐 **$$$ Elixir Cleansing Foam with Collagen Extract II, for Normal to Dry Skin** *($26 for 4.5 ounces)* is going to be less drying than the Elixir Cleansing Foam with Collagen Extract I above, but it isn't preferred to many other water-soluble cleansers available for a lot less money and without any irritation or dryness.

😐 **$$$ Elixir Perfect Makeup Cleansing Cream** *($30 for 4.9 ounces)* costs a lot of money for what amounts to mostly water, silicone, and oils. However, this will remove makeup and is an OK option for dry to very dry skin.

😐 **$$$ Elixir Perfect Makeup Cleansing Gel** *($30 for 4.9 ounces)* is an average, overpriced liquid makeup remover that loses points for including alcohol (in an amount not too likely to cause irritation, but still, it shouldn't be in such a product) and fragrance.

☺ **$$$ Elixir Perfect Makeup Cleansing Oil** *($30 for 5.7 ounces)* is just mineral oil with thickeners, silicone, emollient, water, preservative, and fragrance. Mineral oil removes makeup quickly and easily, but why spend this much when plain mineral oil costs mere pennies by comparison?

☹ **Elixir Lifting Softener I, for Normal to Oily Skin** *($34 for 5 ounces)* lists alcohol as the second ingredient and also contains peppermint extract, both of which make this toner too drying and irritating for all skin types.

☹ **Elixir Lifting Softener II, for Normal Skin** *($34 for 5 ounces)* contains peppermint and orris root extracts, which makes this boring toner too irritating for all skin types.

☹ **Elixir Lifting Softener III, for Normal to Dry Skin** *($34 for 5 ounces)* would have been an OK toner without the addition of alcohol and peppermint, neither of which are helpful for making skin soft.

☹ **Elixir Lifting Toner** *($34 for 5 ounces)* removes surface oil and "stickiness" due to its alcohol content, but degreasing your skin in this manner is irritating and damaging. The inclusion of menthol makes this even more irritating and a must to avoid. The only thing this product can lift is the money from your wallet.

☺ **$$$ Elixir Collagen Lifting Gel** *($55 for 1.7 ounces)* does contain collagen, but soluble or not, it cannot lift skin to reduce signs of sagging. If anything, because alcohol is the third ingredient, this gel may prove too irritating for most, and that cancels out any positive impact the antioxidants in here could have had.

☺ **$$$ Elixir Concentrated Collagen Lifting Cream** *($50 for 1.4 ounces)* is a very standard, emollient moisturizer for normal to dry skin. The collagen, even though it is encapsulated, cannot provide a lifted appearance to sagging skin; it functions as a water-binding agent only. The wild thyme extract may cause irritation.

☺ **$$$ Elixir Concentrated Night Cream** *($42 for 1 ounce)* is a standard, lighter-weight moisturizing cream for normal to slightly dry skin. The tiny amount of antioxidants won't hold up due to jar packaging, while the orrisroot and thyme extracts are potentially irritating.

☺ **$$$ Elixir Eye Radiance (Eye Cream)** *($38 for 0.7 ounce)* shortchanges skin of antioxidants and other intriguing ingredients, and instead provides it with an average blend of moisturizing agents and thickeners. This is an OK option for dry skin, but it's not worth the price.

☺ **$$$ Elixir Facial Massage Treatment (Cream)** *($35 for 3.5 ounces)* is an incredibly antiquated concoction of mineral oil, water, thickeners, and waxes, and is suitable only for very dry skin. Jar packaging means the meager antioxidants in this product will break down quickly.

☺ **$$$ Elixir Facial Massage Treatment (Emulsion)** *($34 for 2.8 ounces)* is a lightweight moisturizer that is an overall average option for normal to oily skin. Nothing in here can exfoliate skin on its own, but the act of massaging this over skin can result in removal of some superficial dead skin cells. Keep in mind that massaging skin can stretch elastin fibers, and that can end up being unhelpful when done on a regular basis.

☹ **Elixir Facial Massage Treatment (Essence)** *($39 for 1 ounce)* is a lighter version of the Elixir Facial Massage Treatment (Emulsion) above, but this is not recommended due to its alcohol content and the amount of irritating orrisroot extract.

☺ **Elixir Lifting Daytime Protector SPF 25 PA++** *($36.50 for 1.6 ounces)* includes an in-part titanium dioxide sunscreen, but the base formula is mostly water, silicone, and alcohol, which doesn't make it worth considering over several superior sunscreen options. It goes without saying that nothing in this product can lift sagging skin.

😐 **Elixir Lifting Emulsion I, for Normal to Oily Skin** *($36.50 for 4 ounces)* is a very boring, lightweight moisturizer for its intended skin types. The wild thyme and orrisroot extract pose a risk of irritation.

😐 **Elixir Lifting Emulsion II, for Normal Skin** *($36.50 for 4 ounces)* is an overall better formula than the Elixir Lifting Emulsion I above, and is suitable for normal to slightly dry skin. The only concerns are the wild thyme and orrisroot extracts, both present in amounts that may cause irritation.

😐 **Elixir Lifting Emulsion III, for Normal to Dry Skin** *($36.50 for 1.4 ounces)* is an incredibly standard, jar-packaged moisturizer for its intended skin types. It is interesting to notice that while this has a lower price, it contains many of the same ingredients Shiseido uses in their most expensive moisturizers.

😊 **$$$ Elixir Lifting Eye Treatment EX** *($55 for 0.53 ounce)* is a decent moisturizer for dry skin, but a product meant for use around the eyes should be fragrance-free, and this isn't. Still, it contains some good antioxidants and plant oils, and if you're going to devote your cosmetics dollars to Shiseido, this is one of their better products.

☹ **Elixir Moisture Infusion Gel Essence** *($38 for 1.6 ounces)* lists alcohol as the third ingredient, so this is hardly an infusion of moisture for anyone's skin. The alcohol takes precedence over the antioxidants, which are barely present in this formula, and for the money this isn't worth your attention.

😐 **$$$ Elixir Wrinkle Care (Smoothing Essence)** *($47 for 0.67 ounce)* has a very silky texture courtesy of silicones, and the emollients help normal to dry skin stay hydrated. There isn't much else to extol about this product. There's no question it really could have been a much more exciting formula.

☹ **Elixir Clarifying Moisture Mask** *($42 for 6 individually wrapped 2-piece masks)* contains potentially irritating amounts of acrylate-based film-forming agents and also includes peppermint extract. Let me be perfectly clear: This mask is about as moisturizing as a walk in the desert.

☹ **Elixir Pore Minimizing Toning Stick** *($32 for 0.35 ounce)* contains the potent menthol derivative menthoxypropanediol, and as such this is too irritating for all skin types, not to mention minimally effective at making pores appear smaller.

☹ **Elixir Treatment Mask** *($40 for 3.6 ounces)* is a standard, peel-off mask that lists polyvinyl alcohol as its second ingredient, which makes it too irritating for all skin types.

SHISEIDO PURENESS PRODUCTS

☹ **Pureness Foaming Cleansing Fluid** *($19.50 for 5 ounces)* contains potassium myristate as its main cleansing agent. A constituent of soap, it can be drying for most skin types.

😊 **$$$ Pureness Refreshing Cleansing Sheets, Oil-Free, Alcohol-Free** *($15 for 30 sheets)* are cleansing wipes suitable for all skin types, but their cleansing ability isn't such that makeup removal is swift. The *Palo azul* wood extract in this product has no documented benefit for skin.

😊 **$$$ Pureness Refreshing Cleansing Water, Oil-Free, Alcohol-Free** *($19.50 for 5 ounces)* is basically the same formula as the Pureness Refreshing Cleansing Sheets above, only not steeped onto cloths. As such, the same review applies.

☹ **Pureness Deep Cleansing Foam** *($19.50 for 3.6 ounces)* contains potentially drying cleansing agents and irritates skin with menthol, making this a cleanser to avoid.

😊 **$$$ Pureness Pore Purifying Warming Scrub** *($21.50 for 1.7 ounces)* doesn't make much sense as a scrub product designed for someone with oily skin and clogged pores because its main ingredient is mineral oil, followed closely by petrolatum (Vaseline). Although neither of these ingredients poses a risk of clogging pores, both have a thick, greasy texture that won't make someone with oily skin happy. This scrub is actually very good for someone with dry skin. The polyethylene beads (standard for most scrubs) are buffered by the mineral oil base, leaving skin with a soft, smooth feel along with some residual moistness. The warming effect is in the name only, because this scrub contains nothing to warm the skin (although the mechanical action of scrubbing can create a slight sense of warmth). This product does contain fragrance.

😐 **$$$ Pureness Balancing Softener, Alcohol Free** *($21.50 for 5 ounces)* is an OK toner for normal to oily skin, but it absolutely cannot create stronger skin that resists adult acne, as claimed.

☹ **Pureness Anti-Shine Refreshing Lotion** *($21.50 for 5 ounces)* contains a low amount of salicylic acid and has a pH that prevents it from functioning effectively as an exfoliant. This also contains enough alcohol to cause dryness and irritation (and it generates free-radical damage too), all of which won't help treat acne in the least.

😐 **Pureness Matifying Moisturizer, Oil Free** *($30.50 for 1.6 ounces)* is a nearly weightless lotion for normal to oily skin, though its alcohol content may cause problems. Still, this is an option for those who need a bit of hydration with a matte finish.

😐 **Pureness Moisturizing Gel-Cream** *($30.50 for 1.4 ounces)* provides a hint of moisture along with a tiny amount of water-binding agent. It is an average option for normal to oily skin.

☹ **Pureness Pore Minimizing Cooling Essence** *($25.50 for 1 ounce)* lists alcohol as the second ingredient, and that, coupled with the menthol in this product, produces its "cooling essence" on skin. These two ingredients cause needless irritation and won't do a thing to benefit blemish-prone skin, nor will they reduce the appearance of pores, as Shiseido (incorrectly) claims.

☹ **Pureness Blemish Clearing Gel** *($17.50 for 0.5 ounce)* contains a barely effective amount of salicylic acid and the pH of this gel is too high for it to function as an exfoliant. Further, the amount of alcohol this contains makes it too irritating and drying for all skin types.

😐 **$$$ Pureness Matifying Stick, Oil Free** *($24 for 0.14 ounce)* is a silicone-based stick that contains the absorbent ingredient silica, so it does provide a matte finish. However, the waxes that keep this in stick form should not be applied over blemish-prone areas.

😐 **$$$ Pureness Oil-Control Blotting Paper** *($16 for 100 sheets)* consists of blotting papers laced with clay to provide oil absorption and a lasting matte finish. The rosemary extract isn't the best, but without question these work to keep excess shine in check.

SHISEIDO THE SKINCARE PRODUCTS

☺ **$$$ The Skincare Extra Gentle Cleansing Foam** *($28 for 4.7 ounces)* is a standard, glycerin-based foaming cleanser that is an option for all skin types except very dry. It removes makeup completely and rinses well. Shiseido mentions that this is formulated with patent-pending yuzu (*Citrus junos*) seed extract, but it is nowhere to be found on the ingredient list.

☺ **$$$ The Skincare Rinse-Off Cleansing Gel** *($28 for 6.7 ounces)* doesn't rinse completely due to its silicone content, but this is a new twist on standard, water-soluble cleansers and is a consideration for normal to oily skin. The tiny amount of alcohol is not likely to be a problem for skin. This is capable of removing all but the most stubborn types of makeup.

😐 **$$$ The Skincare Instant Eye and Lip Makeup Remover** *($25 for 4.2 ounces)* is a water- and silicone-based makeup remover that is below standard due to its alcohol content.

Several other companies offer a better version of this type of makeup remover for a lot less money, including Almay, Neutrogena, and Paula's Choice.

☹ **The Skincare Purifying Cleansing Foam** *($28 for 4.6 ounces)* contains the drying, alkaline cleansing agent potassium myristate, which makes this cleanser/scrub hybrid a problem for all skin types.

😐 **$$$ The Skincare Hydro-Balancing Softener, Alcohol-Free** *($33 for 5 ounces)* is an OK toner for all skin types. It provides water-binding agents, but that's it, so it's up to you to decide if spending this much for such a basic formula is worthwhile.

☹ **The Skincare Hydro-Nourishing Softener** *($33 for 5 ounces)* costs a lot of money for what amounts to mostly water, slip agent, alcohol, and glycerin. There's enough alcohol to make this a non-softening problem for all skin types, and the peppermint extract only makes matters worse.

☹ **The Skincare Day Moisture Protection SPF 15 PA+, Regular** *($38 for 2.5 ounces)* lacks sufficient UVA-protecting ingredients, which makes this new daytime moisturizer—especially with its lackluster base formula—a resounding disappointment. What is extremely detrimental is that the PA+ is supposed to represent Japan's standard for some level of UVA protection. This system applies only to sunscreens manufactured in Japan, and does not imply superiority, as clearly evidenced here.

☹ **The Skincare Day Moisture Protection SPF 15 PA+, Enriched** *($38 for 1.8 ounces)* is a slightly more emollient version of The Skincare Day Moisture Protection SPF 15 PA+, Regular, above, but other than that the same review applies.

😐 **$$$ The Skincare Eye Revitalizer** *($37 for 0.53 ounce)* is a rather boring moisturizer for dry skin anywhere on the face. The bells and whistles barely make a sound because they are present in such paltry amounts. Meanwhile, the wild thyme extract may cause irritation.

☹ **The Skincare Eye Soother** *($37 for 0.54 ounce)* contains too much alcohol (three forms of the drying, irritating kind) to be soothing, and what precedes the alcohol is as common as a cloudy day in Seattle.

😐 **The Skincare Multi-Energizing Cream** *($40 for 1.7 ounces)* is far from an intensive treatment for dull, dehydrated skin, but is an OK jar-packaged moisturizer for normal to dry skin.

😐 **The Skincare Night Moisture Recharge, Regular** *($40 for 2.5 ounces)* is a lightweight moisturizer that's an average option for normal to slightly dry skin. Shiseido maintains that the yuzu seed extract (present in a next-to-nothing amount in this product) is a "breakthrough ingredient" that encourages the skin to produce more hyaluronic acid. There is no research anywhere to support this claim, but yuzu is a popular citrus fruit in Japan and Korea, and the peel does have considerable antioxidants. However, that's all related to eating the fruit and its skin, not putting it on your skin (Source: *The Journal of Agricultural and Food Chemistry*, September 2004, pages 5907–5913).

😐 **$$$ The Skincare Night Moisture Recharge, Enriched** *($40 for 1.8 ounces)* contains more thickening agents than The Skincare Night Moisture Recharge, Regular above, but is otherwise an equally uninspired moisturizer with a very small amount of the star ingredient, yuzu seed extract.

😐 **The Skincare Night Moisture Recharge, Light** *($40 for 2.5 ounces)* contains mostly water, glycerin, silicone, and alcohol. The few intriguing ingredients are listed after the preservative, making this yet another disappointing, boring, fluid moisturizer.

☺ **$$$ The Skincare Renewing Serum** *($46 for 1 ounce)* makes skin of any age feel silky-smooth due to its silicone content, but it lacks state-of-the-art ingredients and may prove irritating due to the peppermint and wild thyme extracts.

☹ **The Skincare Visible Luminizer Serum, Anti-Dullness** *($46 for 1.6 ounces)* lists alcohol as the second ingredient and also contains peppermint, making this serum (which actually has a lotion texture) too irritating for all skin types. Even without so much alcohol, this is not an impressive formula, and it is incapable of leaving skin energized or taking care of enlarged pores. What a shame, because the packaging is really beautiful.

☺ **The Skincare Moisture Relaxing Mask** *($30 for 1.7 ounces)* contains many of the same ingredients Shiseido uses in all of its moisturizers, which means those would be appropriate for masking, too. This version supplies dry skin with an OK selection of emollients and some water-binding agents, but is a more or less superfluous product.

☹ **The Skincare Purifying Mask** *($28 for 3.2 ounces)* has clay to absorb excess oil, but so do many other masks for oily skin, and most of those don't contain irritating eucalyptus oil.

☹ **The Skincare Protective Lip Conditioner SPF 10** *($21.50 for 0.14 ounce)* lacks the UVA-protecting ingredients of titanium dioxide, zinc oxide, avobenzone, Tinosorb, or Mexoryl SX, and is not recommended.

SHISEIDO UV WHITE PRODUCTS

With no hydroquinone and only a negligible amount of magnesium ascorbyl phosphate to be found in any of these products, there is little reason to accept the notion that your skin will change color one iota if you use Shiseido's UV White line. Even such plant extracts as bearberry, mulberry, or arbutin, which have been shown (in vitro) to inhibit melanin production are missing. As I've discussed previously, hydroquinone, magnesium ascorbyl phosphate, and plant extracts such as bearberry, mulberry, and arbutin all have research (in vitro) showing that they inhibit melanin production (Sources: *Phytotherapy Research*, November 2006, pages 921–934; *Cosmetics & Toiletries*, January 2000, pages 20–25; *Cosmetic Dermatology*, June 1998, pages 16–18, and March 2000, pages 13–18; and *Fourth International Symposium on Cosmetic Efficacy*, 1999, page 26). However, none or only trace amounts of these beneficial ingredients are found in any of these products, so there is little reason to accept the notion that your skin will change color one iota if you use Shiseido UV White line products. It is also interesting to note that two of the ingredients Shiseido bragged about when these products were last reviewed (lempuyang extract and hypotaurine) are no longer present in these products.

☺ **$$$ UV White Clarifying Cleansing Cream** *($32 for 4.7 ounces)* is a very basic, Vaseline-based, wipe-off cleanser that can leave a greasy film on the skin.

☹ **UV White Clarifying Cleansing Foam I** *($27 for 4.5 ounces)* contains alkaline potassium myristate as its main cleansing agent, making this too drying for all skin types.

☺ **$$$ UV White Clarifying Cleansing Foam II** *($27 for 4.5 ounces)* is less drying than the UV White Clarifying Cleansing Foam I above, but not by much, so this is only advisable for those with very oily skin.

☹ **UV White Whitening Softener I** *($43 for 5 ounces)* lists alcohol as its second ingredient, so irritation and free-radical damage are something to worry about from this product. The form of vitamin C used here has minimal research demonstrating its ability to lighten skin.

☹ **UV White Whitening Softener II** *($43 for 5 ounces)* is similar to the UV White Whitening Softener I above, and the same review applies.

☹ **UV White Whitening Toner** *($43 for 5 ounces)* contains several irritating ingredients, including a lot of alcohol, a high amount of potassium hydroxide, and zinc phenosulfate. Although this will not lighten your brown skin discolorations, the irritation it causes might camouflage them by making skin red!

☹ **UV White Control & Protect Base Cream SPF 25 Green** *($35 for 0.88 ounce)* is a tinted sunscreen available in, you guessed it, an unsightly sheer green shade. ☺ **$$$ UV White Control & Protect Base Cream SPF 25 Ivory** *($35 for 0.88 ounce)* is a far more acceptable skin-friendly color. The sole active ingredient here and in the Green version above is titanium dioxide, while the lotion base is suitable for those with normal to oily skin desiring a soft matte finish. The amount of magnesium ascorbyl phosphate is far too low to have even a minor impact on skin discolorations, but daily use of a sunscreen like this can prevent new discolorations from appearing.

😐 **$$$ UV White Whitening Eye Serum** *($45 for 0.6 ounce)* cannot lighten skin discolorations and is barely passable even as a lightweight moisturizer for slightly dry skin.

☹ **UV White Whitening Massage Essence** *($48 for 1.6 ounces)* lists alcohol as the third ingredient and also contains eucalyptus oil, making this the essence of irritation for all skin types.

😐 **$$$ UV White Whitening Moisturizer I, for Normal to Oily Skin** *($43 for 3.3 ounces)* contains more alcohol than potential skin-lightening agents, but the low amount of alcohol is unlikely to be a huge problem for skin. Still, this is a very disappointing formula for the money; at its best, it is an OK moisturizer for normal to slightly oily skin.

😐 **$$$ UV White Whitening Moisturizer II, for Normal to Dry Skin** *($43 for 3.3 ounces)* is, save for the addition of a thickening agent to create a creamy texture, nearly identical to the UV White Whitening Moisturizer I above, and the same basic review applies.

😐 **UV White Whitening Protective Moisturizer I SPF 15** *($35 for 2.5 ounces)* is a blend of pros and cons, with the strong points being an in-part avobenzone sunscreen and a silky texture. The cons include alcohol as the third ingredient, no components with substantiated proof of their skin-lightening ability, and a mere dusting of intriguing ingredients. This adds up to a mediocre option for normal to oily skin.

😐 **UV White Whitening Protective Moisturizer II SPF 15** *($35 for 2.5 ounces)* is similar to the UV White Whitening Protective Moisturizer I SPF 15 above, except with slightly less alcohol and with the silicones replaced by glycols, which leave a more moist finish. Otherwise, the same review applies.

😐 **$$$ UV White Whitening Revitalizer Cream** *($48 for 1 ounce)*. Even assuming that any of the ingredients in here were slam-dunks for diminishing skin discolorations, the jar packaging wouldn't have kept them stable during use, leaving you with an average, overpriced moisturizer for normal to dry skin.

☹ **UV White Intensive Whitening Treatment** *($55 for the kit)* consists of the alcohol-laden **Intensive Whitening Treatment Essence** and six individually wrapped packets of the unimpressive **Intensive Treatment Mask**, which is mostly water, glycerin, acrylate-based film-forming agent (think hairspray), sugar, and starch. It's a gimmicky duo that won't lighten skin discolorations, but will cause irritation and do nothing to improve skin texture or color.

SHISEIDO WHITE LUCENT PRODUCTS

😐 **$$$ White Lucent Brightening Cleansing Foam** *($30 for 4.7 ounces)* is a standard, water-soluble foaming cleanser whose detergent cleansing agents can be slightly drying. This is a decent option for oily skin.

😐 **$$$ White Lucent Brightening Refining Softener, Enriched** *($44 for 5 ounces)*. I don't know what they've "enriched" this misguided toner with, but it has nothing of value for skin. The amount of alcohol poses a slight risk of irritation and likely counteracts the anti-irritant properties of the licorice extract. The inclusion of St. John's wort means this toner should never be applied to skin that's about to be exposed to sunlight.

☹ **White Lucent Brightening Refining Softener, Light** *($44 for 5 ounces)* lists alcohol as the second ingredient, making this overpriced toner too drying and irritating for all skin types.

☹ **White Lucent Brightening Toning Lotion, Cool** *($44 for 5 ounces)* is even more irritating than the White Lucent Brightening Refining Softener, Light, above because it adds menthol to the mix.

😐 **$$$ White Lucent Concentrated Brightening Serum** *($115 for 1 ounce)* is mostly water, slip agents, alcohol, and silicone. It contains vitamin C as ascorbic acid, but not in an amount that can impact skin discolorations. The same goes for the numerous exotic-sounding plant extracts in this product. I imagine most of them were added to make this pricey serum seem unique, but they do not lighten discolorations.

☹ **White Lucent Brightening Massage Cream** *($48 for 2.8 ounces)* is a basic, unimpressive moisturizer that contains more alcohol than ingredients with potential skin-lightening ability (and jar packaging won't keep these ingredients stable anyway). Chalk this up to a huge waste of time and money.

😐 **$$$ White Lucent Brightening Moisturizing Cream** *($50 for 1.4 ounces)* is similar to the White Lucent Brightening Massage Cream above, only with a more emollient base formula. The concern about the alcohol remains, but the emollient helps offset the irritation potential. Still, this is a lot of money for a really basic, jar-packaged moisturizer that cannot lighten discolorations.

☺ **White Lucent Brightening Moisturizing Emulsion** *($50 for 3.3 ounces)* is an OK lightweight lotion for normal to slightly dry or slightly oily skin, but it cannot lighten discolorations, not even a little. The sleek packaging will keep the antioxidants stable during use, but they would be more potent without the alcohol that precedes them on the list.

☹ **White Lucent Brightening Moisturizing Gel** *($50 for 1.4 ounces)* contains enough alcohol to cause dryness and irritation, and there's more salt in here than any potentially helpful skin-lightening agents.

☹ **White Lucent Brightening Protective Moisturizer SPF 16 PA++** *($48 for 2.5 ounces)* offers skin an in-part avobenzone sunscreen, but its lotion base contains enough alcohol to cause irritation and undermine the effectiveness of the antioxidants it contains.

😐 **$$$ White Lucent Brightening Mask** *($66 for 6 masks)* contains a handful of intriguing ingredients, but none of them are present in impressive amounts. That means, for example, that the ascorbic acid (vitamin C) won't fade discolorations or even provide much antioxidant benefit. At $11 per mask, you're getting mostly water, slip agents, alcohol, and the water-binding sugar xylitol. None of this is brightening or whitening, and some of the plant extracts can be irritating, although it's not likely given the small amounts found in this mask. Nevertheless, for this kind of money you should be getting only skin-beneficial ingredients, not this do-nothing mixture.

OTHER SHISEIDO PRODUCTS

☹ **Eudermine Revitalizing Essence** *($55 for 4.2 ounces)* is outrageously priced for what amounts to mostly water, slip agent, and alcohol. It contains a few good water-binding agents, but in amounts too small for skin to notice, especially with the alcohol involved.

☹ **$$$ Future Solution Eye and Lip Contour Cream** *($120 for 0.7 ounce)* comes packaged in a luxurious jar, but no matter how beautiful the container, it can only serve to sabotage the effectiveness of the few antioxidants in this otherwise standard moisturizer. Nothing in this product is exclusive for the eye or lip area, while a couple of the plant extracts can be irritating. A natural constituent of *Ononis spinosa* root (also known as spiny restharrow) is menthol and that makes it potentially irritating (Source: *PDR for Herbal Medicines*, 1st Edition, Montvale, NJ: Medical Economics Company, 1998). Other Japanese plant extracts in this moisturizer have no established benefit for skin, and only sketchy research on their benefits when consumed orally.

😐 **$$$ Future Solution Total Revitalizing Cream** *($225 for 1.8 ounces)* is said to work on every aspect of skin to alleviate all signs of aging, from wrinkles to sagging. But, without a sunscreen, don't bet on this for any future protection against wrinkles and loss of resilience. For the money, this should be brimming with a who's who of today's top ingredients for helping skin function at its best, but it isn't. Even if some of those were included, they'd suffer from the unfortunate choice of (pretty) jar packaging. At best, this is an acceptable moisturizer for normal to dry skin; some of the plant extracts can be irritating, as described above in the review for Future Solution Eye and Lip Contour Cream.

☹ **$$$ Revitalizing Cream** *($138 for 1.4 ounces)* is an incredibly basic, shockingly priced moisturizer for dry to very dry skin. Not a single ingredient in this emollient product is justified by the cost, and jar packaging won't keep the two forms of vitamin E stable during use.

😊 **The Makeup Pre-Makeup Cream SPF 15** *($27 for 1 ounce)* contains an in-part titanium dioxide sunscreen, but that's the only exciting element in this pre-makeup moisturizer for normal to dry skin. The mineral pigments give a slight glow to skin, but that will be concealed after you apply makeup.

😐 **$$$ Whitess Intensive Skin Brightener** *($125 for 1.4 ounces)* is an absurdly overpriced skin-lightening product that contains a high concentration of arbutin to inhibit melanin production. Arbutin is a constituent of cranberries, bearberries, and blueberries, among other fruits. Although arbutin has been shown to have the same skin-lightening capability as hydroquinone, that fact has been established only in animal, human skin model, and in vitro studies, rather than on intact skin (Sources: *Biological and Pharmaceutical Bulletin*, April 2004, pages 510–514; and *Pigment Cell Research*, August 1998, pages 206–212). It is interesting to note that arbutin degrades to become hydroquinone, a change that is related to its efficacy (Source: *Journal of Chemical Ecology*, May 2004, 1067–1082).

Still, it might be worth the price to see if this amount of arbutin, as an alternative to hydroquinone, can have an effect on skin. (Actually, arbutin ends up having more in common with hydroquinone than its natural association would indicate.) Just as an aside, an almost identical product in Shiseido's Cle de Peau line sells for four times as much than this version, though the alcohol and menthol in the more expensive version make it potentially irritating for all skin types.

SHISEIDO SUN PRODUCTS

😐 **Ultimate Cleansing Oil, for Face & Body** *($21 for 5 ounces)* is marketed as a cleanser that will remove long-wearing makeup and water-resistant sunscreens, and although it can do that, the formula is mostly mineral oil, which you can buy for less than a few dollars at any pharmacy around the world.

☺ **$$$ Daily Bronze Moisturizing Emulsion, for Face/Body** *($35 for 5 ounces)* is a self-tanning lotion that works the same way as any self-tanner with dihydroxyacetone. Considering the volatile fragrance components in this product, you're better off trying one of the subtle self-tanners from Jergens, Dove, or Olay available at the drugstore.

☹ **Brilliant Bronze Quick Self-Tanning Gel, for Face/Body** *($28 for 5.2 ounces)* lists alcohol as the second ingredient and isn't really worth the irritation given the number of less expensive self-tanners at the drugstore that have no irritating ingredients.

☹ **Brilliant Bronze Self-Tanning Cream for Face, SPF 17** *($24 for 1.8 ounces)* lacks the UVA-protecting ingredients of titanium dioxide, zinc oxide, avobenzone, Mexoryl SX, or Tinosorb, and is not recommended.

☺ **$$$ Brilliant Bronze Self-Tanning Emulsion, for Face/Body** *($25 for 3.5 ounces)* is a lightweight face and body lotion that works the same as any self-tanner.

😐 **$$$ Brilliant Bronze Tinted Self-Tanning Cream, for Face** *($24 for 1.8 ounces)* comes in your choice of three shades and is a self-tanner with cosmetic pigments to impart instant color. However, the amount of alcohol is potentially irritating.

☹ **Brilliant Bronze Tinted Self-Tanning Gel, for Face/Body** *($28 for 5.4 ounces)* is available in a light or medium tan shade, but both versions list alcohol as the third ingredient, making this tinted self-tanning gel an irritation waiting to happen.

☺ **Extra Smooth Sun Protection Cream SPF 36 PA+++, for Face** *($27 for 1.9 ounces)* deserves a bit of explanation because of its PA+++ designation. This rating system was developed in Japan (where Shiseido is based) as a means to quantify the level of UVA protection a sunscreen can provide. "PA" stands for Protection-Grade of UVA. A PA+ rating signifies some UVA protection (which would apply to most sunscreens today), while a PA++ means moderate UVA protection, and PA+++ symbolizes high UVA protection. Because this particular sunscreen contains over 9% zinc oxide, it qualifies for its PA+++ rating. (This system is not recognized in the United States, Canada, or Australia.) The base formula is suitable for normal to oily skin not prone to blemishes. This would be rated higher if it included greater amounts of antioxidants and did not contain a potentially problematic plant extract.

☺ **Extra Smooth Sun Protection Lotion SPF 33 PA++, for Face/Body** *($28 for 3.3 ounces)* is preferred to the Extra Smooth Sun Protection Cream SPF 36 above because it omits the questionable plant extract and because it provides more product for the same price. It would be rated a Paula's Pick if it contained more than one antioxidant.

☹ **Refreshing Sun Protection Spray SPF 16 PA+, for Body/Hair** *($26 for 5 ounces)* includes avobenzone for UVA protection, but is an alcohol-based product, which makes it a problem for all skin types, as does the orange oil that is present.

😐 **$$$ Sun Protection Eye Cream SPF 32 PA+++** *($30 for 0.6 ounce)* deserves kudos for its in-part zinc oxide sunscreen and silky-cream texture, but it sorely lacks sufficient amounts of state-of-the-art ingredients for skin, and given the price that's an insult. Although the sunscreen is very good, this doesn't compete favorably with similar products from the Lauder-owned lines at the department store (including their relatively inexpensive Good Skin line, which is sold at Kohls). Still, it would work as a good sunscreen.

😐 **Sun Protection Lotion SPF 18 PA+, for Face/Body** *($26 for 5 ounces)* is a standard, in-part titanium dioxide sunscreen suitable for normal to oily skin. Talc contributes to this sunscreen's smooth matte finish. For the money, this should contain more bells and whistles than it does.

☺ **$$$ Ultimate Sun Protection Cream SPF 55 PA+++, for Face** *($33 for 2 ounces)* is an in-part zinc oxide sunscreen for normal to slightly dry skin that definitely covers the broad-spectrum bases and has a silky texture. It's a shame antioxidants are scarce here, because in a sunscreen that costs this much they should be plentiful.

☺ **$$$ Ultimate Sun Protection Lotion SPF 55 PA+++, for Face/Body** *($37 for 3.3 ounces)* is simply a lighter version of the Ultimate Sun Protection Cream SPF 55 PA+++, for Face above, and the same review applies, except this is better for normal to oily skin.

✓☺ **$$$ Sun Protection Lip Treatment SPF 36 PA++** *($18 for 0.14 ounce)* is a very good lip sunscreen that includes an in-part titanium dioxide sunscreen and emollients to keep lips soft and smooth. The added bonus of an antioxidant and anti-irritant make this even better.

SHISEIDO MAKEUP

FOUNDATION: ✓☺ $$$ Dual Balancing Foundation SPF 17 *($35)* is late to the game, as foundations proclaiming they can balance oily areas while providing moisture to dry spots have been around for years, most notably with Clinique's Superbalanced Makeup and Estee Lauder Equalizer Foundation SPF 10. Shiseido's balancing claims are just as out of whack as those of its predecessors, but the foundation itself exceeds them by offering superior sun protection (featuring in-part titanium dioxide) and a fluid, silky texture that applies like a second skin. Once blended, this sets to a natural matte finish that gives skin an attractive dimensional (rather than flat) quality. It's well-suited for combination skin, but not because it is simultaneously controlling oil and maximizing moisture. You'll net light to medium coverage and the selection of ten shades is promising. The following shades are noticeably pink or peach and best avoided: B40, B60, and I60.

✓☺ **$$$ Stick Foundation SPF 15** *($35)* has a wonderfully smooth, light texture and a titanium dioxide sunscreen that blends on with ease, builds from sheer to almost full coverage, and dries to an absorbent powder finish thanks to the amount of clay it contains. It's best for someone with normal to slightly dry or slightly oily skin, since several waxes in it can be problematic for those with breakouts and/or oily skin. Eleven shades are available, including a Color Control shade, which is a greenish yellow tint most often apparent on someone who is seasick! Avoid B20, which is quite pink, and the noticeably peach B60 and I60. The I00 shade is a beautiful option for someone with very fair skin. This is a great choice if you're a fan of Stila's Perfecting Foundation ($30) but want a stick foundation that provides sun protection, too.

✓☺ **$$$ Sun Protection Liquid Foundation SPF 42** *($31)* deserves much praise not only for offering substantial sun protection via its in-part titanium dioxide sunscreen but also for having a silky, lightweight texture that blends easily. It offers a sheer matte finish but can provide medium to nearly full coverage if needed, all without feeling thick or looking heavy. The silicone-enhanced fluid is ideal for normal to very oily skin and an excellent option for outdoor wear when you're active because it stays in place and is water-resistant. That doesn't mean you can apply it once and sit by the pool or play volleyball all day, but it is one of the few foundations that provide sufficient sun protection and keep looking fresh even through strenuous activities. Seven shades are available, with SP40 and SP50 being a bit too peach for most medium skin tones. The other shades are great options for light and dark (but not very dark) skin.

✓☺ **$$$ Sun Protection Compact Foundation SPF 34** *($24 for powder cake; $7 for refillable compact)* is a talc-based pressed-powder foundation that includes an in-part titanium dioxide sunscreen for sufficient UVA protection. It has a smooth texture that's drier than normal, but that's to be expected given the amount of titanium dioxide. What counts beyond sun protection is the natural matte finish this powder leaves while providing sheer to light coverage. All seven shades apply more neutral than they appear in the compact, so don't reject a particular color without trying it first—you may be surprised.

☺ **$$$ Powdery Foundation SPF 14-17** *($28 for powder cake, $7 for compact)* features titanium dioxide as its sole active ingredient, but the SPF rating varies by shade, which explains why Shiseido listed an SPF range rather than settling on one number. (Note that this is not authorized by FDA or Japanese regulations for sunscreens.) This talc-based, pressed-powder foundation has a dry but silky texture that goes on soft and even, providing seamless light to medium coverage. It can function as your only sunscreen if you apply it liberally, but it works best when dusted over a regular sunscreen or foundation with sunscreen. The shade range is beautifully neutral, but lacks options for dark skin. The only color to avoid is the too-peach B60.

✓☺ **$$$ Fluid Foundation SPF 15** *($35)* begins slightly thick but blends superbly and feels lighter than you'd think it would. Medium coverage is the norm because the combination of titanium dioxide (the sole active ingredient) and the foundation's base formula makes it tricky to sheer down. Those with normal to oily skin will appreciate the long-lasting matte finish that doesn't look heavy, and seven of the ten shades are winning options. Avoid B20, B40, and B60; all are too pink or peach to look convincing. Shade O40 may be too yellow for some medium skin tones, but is worth auditioning.

☺ **$$$ The Skincare Essential Tinted Moisturizer SPF 15** *($31)* gets its sun protection completely from titanium dioxide and has a creamy-smooth texture that sets to a lightweight, moist finish suitable for normal to dry skin. Skin receives sheer coverage and appears dewy (this isn't suitable for anyone with combination skin), and although all the shades tend to be peachy, their sheerness makes this a non-issue.

☺ **$$$ Compact Foundation SPF 15** *($28 for powder cake, $7 for compact)* has an application that's more sheer than the Powdery Foundation above due to a reduced level of talc. The sunscreens are titanium dioxide and zinc oxide, which makes this an effective, gentle option for those with sensitive skin. This pressed-powder foundation has an inordinately light texture that applies smoothly and provides a sheer matte finish. It can be difficult to pick up enough powder to obtain meaningful coverage, so this functions best when applied over a sunscreen or foundation with sunscreen rated SPF 15 or higher. The shades have improved considerably since last reviewed; among the ten options, only three should be avoided due to their strong pink tone: B20, B40, and B60. The Ochre range is ideal for those with olive skin.

☺ **$$$ Hydro-Liquid Compact Foundation SPF 17-20** *($28 for foundation; $10 for compact)* isn't liquid at all, but rather a very dry-finish but silky cream-to-powder foundation. The SPF rating varies by shade, but each contains titanium dioxide as the only active ingredient. When carefully blended this can look nearly imperceptible on skin while providing light to medium coverage. Less than perfect blending can result in a heavy appearance because this foundation tends to "grab" over less-than-smooth areas and cannot be easily softened once set. Although 14 shades are available (this is the only Shiseido foundation with colors for dark skin) 5 of them are unacceptably pink or peach. Avoid B20, B40, B60, B80, and I60. The other nine present some attractive options, especially for fair skin.

☺ **$$$ Lifting Foundation SPF 16** *($40)* claims to provide "full coverage as beautiful as bare skin," but that's taking it too far (even though it's fun to imagine). With almost 10% titanium dioxide as the active ingredient, this creamy, thick foundation doesn't provide its complete coverage without looking like makeup. It spreads and blends well yet is very concentrated—a tiny dab covers half the face, yet you'll likely need more than that to ensure sufficient sun protection (unless you're applying this foundation over a regular sunscreen). Lifting Foundation SPF 16 has a silky, matte finish that appears somewhat chalky, something that's more apparent with the darker shades. Still, this formula is a huge step forward from the greasy, full-coverage foundations of years past. Among the ten shades, the only poor choices are B60 (very peach) and the slightly peach shades B20 and I40. Lastly, this foundation won't lift the skin—the real reason to consider it is if you need significant coverage and want a foundation with sunscreen.

CONCEALER: ☺ **$$$ Concealer** *($19)* is Shiseido's best concealer, but given their other lackluster options that's not necessarily saying much. Still, this liquid concealer has its strong points, including a long-lasting matte finish and a formula that's appropriate for use on blemishes. Because talc is the second ingredient it sets quickly, so blending must be deft. On the plus side, this won't crease and it provides significant coverage. It would be worthy of a Paula's Pick rating if only the four shades were better. If you decide to try this, Light and Dark are the best colors; Light Enhancer is sheer and best used for subtle highlighting.

😐 **$$$ Concealer Stick** *($25)* comes in an attractive metal twist-up component and has a creamy texture that glides over skin without being too slippery. It sets to a satin finish and each of the three shades provides considerable coverage, but it has the drawbacks of looking chalky and also being prone to minor creasing. The creasing can be remedied with powder, but the chalky finish keeps this product from earning a higher rating.

☹ **Corrector Pencil** *($16)* is a standard, dry-finish pencil that comes in three average but workable colors. This provides good coverage, but application is an issue, and it looks quite obvious on the skin while also being too stiff to soften.

POWDER: ✓☺ $$$ Pureness Mattifying Compact Oil-Free SPF 16 *($18.50 for powder cake; $7 for compact)* is a slam-dunk recommendation for those with oily to very oily skin looking for an absorbent, matte-finish pressed powder with sun protection. The actives are titanium dioxide and zinc oxide (which are quite absorbent on their own), and the talc-based formula applies well despite feeling too dry. All six shades are recommended.

☺ **$$$ Enriched Loose Powder** *($32)* has an airy texture whose single shade produces a soft, translucent finish on skin. The look is more satiny than powdery, which makes this best for normal to dry skin. If it weren't so sheer the single shade would be very limiting. By the way, the amount of Shiseido's Advanced Nutrient Factor, said to make this powder moisturizing, is negligible. If this powder did not have such a finely milled texture, it would be a mistake to consider. As it is, if you don't mind the shine for daytime, it's an option.

☺ **$$$ Loose Powder** *($32)* isn't too different from the Enriched Loose Powder except that it comes in two colors (white and pale pink) that only work for fair skin tones, and only then because this powder is so sheer. The talc-based formula has a weightless texture and leaves a hint of shine. ☺ **$$$ Pressed Powder** *($21 for powder cake; $7 for compact)* comes in two colors suitable for fair skin and has a talc-based formula that feels smooth but is more powdery than the best options in this category. It's a good option if you have light skin and want a sheer, basic pressed powder, but that's about it.

😐 **$$$ Luminizing Color Powder** *($21 for powder, $10 for compact)* is a talc-based pressed powder that features three colors in one powder cake, one of which is quite shiny. The color selection ranges from pure white shimmer to glittery bronze, and none of them would help set makeup or reduce shine. These are workable as highlighting powders, but the effect depends on careful application so as not to make your foundation look strange.

BLUSH: ☺ **$$$ Accentuating Color Stick** *($30)* has a slick, silicone-based texture that is quick to dry out if you don't replace the cap tightly after each use. Think of this as a hybrid cream-to-powder blush that is best applied over moist skin (applying it over powdered skin assures a spotty, streaked look). Each shade goes on almost as bright as it looks, but blending softens the effect and the product sets to a natural matte finish. This works as lip color, too, though it's best paired with a gloss unless you're comfortable with its matte finish.

EYESHADOW: ☺ **$$$ Hydro-Powder Eye Shadow** *($23)* has an intriguing water-to-powder texture with enough slip to make it easy to blend over small areas. This sets to a matte (in feel) finish and the shades have an iridescent or metallic flake-free shine, depending on which you choose. It's a fun option for evening glamour; the best shades are Goldlights, Whitelights, and Tiger Eye. ☺ **$$$ Silky Eye Shadow Duos** *($28)* must be applied in sheer layers because the formula is pressed so softly that application can be powdery and encourage flaking. If layered, the powder clings well and blends beautifully, with each shade having some degree of shine. Several of the duos are odd or contrasting colors, so unless you're up for a challenge, choose from among the following pairs: S1, S11, S17, S18, S19, or S20.

☹ **Accentuating Color for Eyes** *($21)* may look appealing, but is completely unremarkable. Each color is intensely shiny and densely filled with chunky particles of mica that definitely do reflect light, but also tend to flake all over—bad news for contact lens wearers. In addition, whoever created some of these colors must not realize that bright red and orange eyeshadows don't accent eyes. Rather, sweeping these particular shades over the lid may make others think you've been crying all day or have an eye infection. Still, there are always those with avant-garde tastes, where the intensity of the color, not the flaking, is what really matters.

☹ **Silky Eye Shadow Quad** *($35)* has a formula that's similar to the Accentuating Color for Eyes above, and the same review applies. Even if it had a better formula, the color combinations are poorly done.

EYE AND BROW SHAPER: 😐 **$$$ Eyebrow and Eyeliner Compact** *($28.50)* presents a brow powder and powder eyeliner (either may be used wet or dry) in one compact. The brow tones are good for those with brown or black hair only, yet each applies smoothly considering the dry texture, and the color builds well. Oddly, each duo has a slight amount of shine, which doesn't add much to the result (eyebrows aren't supposed to shine). As for the included applicator, it is best tossed in favor of full-size brushes.

😐 **$$$ Translucent Eyebrow Shaper** *($22)* remains one of the most expensive brow gels around, and let me be the first to tell you how indistinguishable this is from the inexpensive version from Cover Girl, which s also is less sticky than Shiseido's version.

😐 **$$$ Fine Eyeliner** *($27; $13 for refills)* is another liquid eyeliner with a brush that is only capable of applying a thick line. The color seeps into the brush much like ink in a fountain pen, making it hard to control how much comes out at once, but this can be workable once you adapt to its peculiarities. Watch out for Soft Black, which is really olive green.

☹ **Eyeliner Pencil** *($16)* is below average due to its creamy texture, which tends to drag over skin, and its smudge-prone finish. The ☹ **Eyebrow Pencil** *($16)* is also below standard, with stiff, dry application and a waxy/tacky finish that's a far cry from the worry-free result of filling in brows with powder. This is disappointing given how attractive the color choice is. ☹ **Eyeliner Pencil Duo** *($21)* is a needs-sharpening dual-sided pencil with a standard eyeliner color on one end and a shiny pastel or vivid tone on the other. Both ends are too creamy and remain so, which invites smearing and fading.

LIPSTICK, LIP GLOSS, AND LIPLINER: ✓☺ **$$$ Perfecting Lipstick** *($22)* costs more than a lipstick should, but if you're going to spend this much to paint your lips, it might as well be on a superior product like this. Shiseido has created a modern cream lipstick that moisturizes without feeling greasy and affords a soft gloss or shimmer finish from its brilliant, rich colors. There is not a bad shade in the bunch, which may make it hard to choose, but have fun trying! The wand-applied ☺ **$$$ Lip Gloss** *($20)* makes a wonderfully non-sticky, lightweight finishing touch if you aren't put off by the price. The shade selection sizzles and finishes sheer with sparkles that don't feel grainy.

☺ **$$$ Shimmering Lipstick** *($22)* is an emollient, creamy lipstick with a slippery feel that lingers, so count on this making its way into any lines around your mouth. Coverage is moderate while, true to its name, the finish is shimmering. ☺ **$$$ Translucent Gloss Lipstick** *($20)* is a colorless, emollient lip balm that leaves a glossy finish and helps prevent chapping, just like countless other less-expensive lip balms, though this one is glossier than most.

😐 **$$$ Sheer Gloss Lipstick** *($22)* is accurately named! The color selection is certainly worth a look if you prefer this type of lipstick, though it can feel slightly sticky.

😐 **$$$ Lip Liner Pencil** *($16)* is worth considering if you don't mind the price and routine sharpening. It goes on creamy, deposits rich color, and stays in place better than expected given its texture.

MASCARA: Note: Every Shiseido mascara (including Mascara Base) is tenaciously waterproof and you will need an oil- or silicone-based remover to take it off.

☺ **$$$ Distinguish Mascara** *($22)* doesn't distinguish itself from lots of other mascaras that can produce equally impressive length with a hint of fullness. This is a very good mascara, but considering the name and price, upon first use it should give you the impression that it will rise above the rest, and that just doesn't happen. ☺ **$$$ Lasting Lift Mascara** *($22)* has a long, thin spiral brush that allows you to reach every lash and extend it for a defined, separated (and, OK, lifted) result. Length is more prominent than thickness, but successive coats add volume. ☺ **$$$ Extra Length Mascara** *($22)* lengthens quickly and without clumps or smearing. You can build some thickness, but this excels primarily at creating long, perfectly defined lashes.

☺ **$$$ Advanced Volume Mascara** *($22)* promises to thicken lashes for "an intensely dramatic look" and it does that in spades! The tradeoff is a heavy application that requires you to comb through with a clean mascara wand for the most attractive results. The reward is long wear without flaking and very dramatic lashes.

😐 **$$$ Mascara Base** *($22)* is another clear lash primer meant to boost the application and wear of any mascara. Adding Mascara Base before applying most mascaras produced slightly more length, but no extra thickness. The tradeoff was that it's harder to apply mascara evenly over the coating formed on your lashes after you've applied the Base, but, with patience, you can get longer lashes than you can with mascara alone. The difference isn't significant and in the long run, isn't worth the trouble.

FACE AND BODY ILLUMINATING/SHIMMER PRODUCTS: ☺ **$$$ Luminizing Blush Powder** *($45; $30 for powder refills)* wins points for its clever, slim packaging. The cap includes a built-in pressed shimmer powder and the base houses a full, natural-hair powder brush that is concealed with the touch of a button so you can replace the cap without splaying the bristles. Each time you replace the cap, a small amount of powder gets on the tip of the brush, ready for the next application. I wish this weren't so pricey because it is an attractive, convenient way to dust on a sheer layer of shiny powder for special occasions or as evening makeup. The three shades—white, beige, and bronze—are beautiful. The only drawback other than the high price is that the powder doesn't cling to skin as well as it should. If you plan to purchase this product, apply moisturizer or a dry oil spray before powdering so it will cling to your skin more securely.

☹ **$$$ Sheer Enhancer Base SPF 15** *($32)* is a slightly thick liquid base available in two shades: white and a bronze tone that is a bit too coppery for most skin tones. Shiseido maintains that this product "naturally defines facial contours as it minimizes dullness and reflects a translucent brilliance." The slight amount of shimmer in both shades is where the "brilliance" comes into play, but otherwise this isn't a great option for contouring, primarily because it is too sheer and the colors can look strange. The white shade is slightly opaque, and thus provides a bit of camouflage for mild redness or a sallow skin tone. However, the effect is mostly muted once you apply foundation, and you will definitely want to do that because the white shade is not attractive on its own unless you're going for a pasty, pale look. Sheer Enhancer Base has good intentions along with an in-part titanium dioxide sunscreen, but its limitations (and price) should give you pause.

BRUSHES: The straightforward collection of ☹ **$$$ Brushes** *($16–$50)* is supposedly approved by fashion makeup artist Tom Pécheux, and if that's true he must prefer brushes that are mostly too floppy and soft for anything but very sheer application. The only worthwhile brushes are the **Concealer** *($20)* and **Eye Shadow Brush Medium** *($24)*, and even they have drawbacks when compared to the options from most other lines.

SPECIALTY PRODUCTS: ☺ **$$$ Smoothing Veil SPF 16** *($32)* is a silicone-based makeup primer with an in-part titanium dioxide sunscreen. This colorless, solid cream leaves a soft, opalescent finish that feels very silky. It's an extra step whose line- and pore-filling benefit won't be all that noticeable, at least not any more than a foundation can provide. For the most part this is just a great way to get sun protection if your favored foundation does not include sunscreen or lacks effective UVA protection. This can be used by all skin types.

☺ **$$$ Brightening Veil SPF 24** *($32)* features an all titanium dioxide sunscreen in a silicone and nylon-12 base, so you're assured of a silky finish with some good absorbent properties that those with normal to oily skin will enjoy. Those with breakout-prone skin should avoid this product due to its ceresin (a waxlike substance) content. The single shade is a neutral fair beige tone that can function as a lightweight concealer or can be used as a highlighter. The cream-to-powder texture blends right into the skin, and if the shade is a match for you, it can be used as a stand-alone light-coverage foundation. ☺ **$$$ Mattifying Veil SPF 17** *($32)* has an in-part titanium dioxide sunscreen and is composed primarily of various silicones, which leave a solid matte finish on the skin. However, this isn't too far removed from the Smoothing Veil above, and each will have the same basic effect on the skin. You may want to sample both before you decide whether one (or either) of these would make a smart addition to your makeup routine. The Mattifying version is best for normal to very oily skin and does not contain waxes that may clog pores.

☹ **$$$ Eraser Pencil** *($16)* is a wax-based pencil (like almost all other needs-sharpening pencils) that is colorless and designed to remove makeup mistakes, such as those from mascara or eye pencils. You swipe the pencil over the makeup and it wipes off cleanly. This is convenient to have on hand and works quickly, but is not an essential because a bit of foundation, concealer, or a little makeup remover on a cotton swab provides the same results.

SHU UEMURA

SHU UEMURA AT-A-GLANCE

Strengths: Oil-based cleansers for dry to very dry skin; makeup is this line's strong suit; the Pro Spot Concealer provides incredible coverage and comes in a great range of colors; excellent powders, powder blush, and powder eyeshadows; good lipsticks; a brilliant, extremely well-made selection of makeup brushes and all manner of cosmetic applicators.

Weaknesses: Expensive; some sunscreens leave skin vulnerable to UVA damage; no exfoliants; no skin-lightening products; no products to manage acne; mediocre toners and moisturizers; irritating masks; for the money, the pencils and mascaras lack even a mild "wow factor,"; Lip Fix doesn't fix anything; the Brush Cleaner is inferior to using a gentle shampoo to remove makeup residue and oil from your tools.

For more information about Shu Uemura, owned by L'Oreal, call (888) 748-5678 or visit www.shuuemura-usa.com or www.Beautypedia.com.

SHU UEMURA SKIN CARE

The selling point of almost all of the Shu Uemura skin-care products is deep sea water and algae, neither of which is unique to this line or essential for any skin type. Deep sea water does not have any research backing up the claims for its anti-aging benefit for skin. One study examined a species of deep sea urchin whose skin was infected with bacteria present in the water, while another illuminated the fact that deep sea water contains pathogenic bacteria that can cause skin problems, as seen in humans who dive to such depths. So much for deep sea water being helpful.

Other published studies have demonstrated that drinking the stuff had benefits for a sampling of people with atopic eczema/dermatitis syndrome (AEDS). But drinking deep sea water isn't the same as slathering or spraying it on skin, and since this was not a comparison study, who knows if the eczematic patients involved might have had a similar response if they had been drinking green tea, or eating more omega–3 rich foods, such as salmon instead? (Sources: *European Journal of Clinical Nutrition*, September 2005, pages 1093–1096; and *Diseases of Aquatic Organisms*, February 2000, pages 193–199). In short, there is no convincing evidence that seawater, whether bottled near the shore or from leagues below, is superior water for skin.

SHU UEMURA DEPSEA PRODUCTS

😐 **$$$ Depsea Moisture Replenishing Lotion** *($30 for 5 ounces)* is a decent moisturizing toner for normal to dry skin. It would be rated higher if it did not contain so many volatile fragrance components.

😐 **$$$ Depsea Therapy Moisture Recovery Equiwater** *($24 for 5 ounces)* is similar to the B-G Reinforcing Cosmetic Water below, except this replaces the tiny amount of antioxidant beta-glucan with a tiny amount of soy protein and sweet almond oil. What precedes these doesn't add up to a state-of-the-art toner any more than the Replenishing Lotion above does.

☹ **Depsea Water** *($24 for 5 ounces)* presents a collection of facial mists, but whether you choose Bergamot, Chamomile, Hamamelis (witch hazel), Lavender, Rosemary, Rose, or Sage, each one is nothing more than seawater with potentially irritating fragrance components. The Fragrance-Free version is just water and a preservative. Unbelievable! The company maintains that their seawater, taken from great depths, enriches skin with over 60 minerals. Even if that's true, not all minerals are beneficial for skin and even the good ones are neither a panacea nor even that essential for skin when applied topically in a watered-down mist.

☺ **$$$ Depsea Moisture Replenishing Cream** *($38 for 1 ounce)* contains some wonderfully effective ingredients for dry to very dry skin, including standbys such as mineral oil and petrolatum. Water-binding agents and anti-irritants add to the benefits, which is why it's a shame jar packaging was chosen because it won't keep the handful of antioxidants stable during use.

😐 **$$$ Depsea Moisture Replenishing Emulsion** *($55 for 2.5 ounces)* shares many of the same ingredients as the Depsea Moisture Replenishing Cream above, but with a lighter, lotion-like texture. The omissions are enough to knock this moisturizer down to average status, while the many volatile fragrance components increase the odds of this causing irritation.

😐 **$$$ Depsea Moisture Replenishing Essence** *($55 for 1 ounce)* is a basic serum-type moisturizer for normal to oily skin. It is only worth the cost if you firmly believe that Uemura's seawater is an "empowered" ingredient your skin cannot do without (and if you believe that, I'm sure there is some nice swampland you'd be interested in, too).

☹ **Depsea Therapy Moisture Recovery Cream** *($35 for 1 ounce)* contains numerous potentially irritating volatile fragrance components, and is also a lackluster emollient formula that barely supplies what someone with dry to very dry skin needs to recover some softness.

☹ **Depsea Therapy Moisture Recovery Emulsion** *($35 for 1.6 ounces)* lists alcohol as the second ingredient, which won't provide moisture or help skin recover from anything. The rest of the formula is too boring for words. Really.

😐 **Depsea Therapy Moisture Recovery Emulsion SPF 15 Sunscreen** *($38 for 1.6 ounces)* deserves recognition for its in-part titanium dioxide sunscreen and a base formula that those with normal to oily skin will appreciate for its near-weightlessness. However, although the amount of alcohol isn't immense, it offsets the benefit of several other ingredients, and doesn't help this product make the short list of well-formulated daytime moisturizers.

☹ **Depsea Therapy Moisture Recovery Lip Balm SPF 15** *($16 for 0.5 ounce)* lacks the UVA-protecting ingredients of titanium dioxide, zinc oxide, avobenzone, Mexoryl SX (ecamsule), or Tinosorb, and is not recommended.

OTHER SHU UEMURA PRODUCTS

😐 **$$$ Cleansing Beauty Oil Premium A/O** *($32 for 5 ounces)* has the distinction of being the company's best-selling cleanser worldwide, but quite honestly, this mineral oil– and corn oil–based liquid is overwhelmingly standard, and the notion that it is best selling makes me lament how easily taken in women can be by the cosmetics industry. The oils do a great job of dissolving makeup, and the mild surfactants are water-activated, producing a creamy emulsion that rinses better than plain oil would, but it can still leave a residue. This is an OK option for dry to very dry skin. It does contain several volatile fragrance components.

☺ **$$$ Foaming Cleansing Water** *($28 for 5 ounces)* is a gentle, water-soluble cleansing fluid that is a good option for normal to oily skin. It removes most types of makeup, but doesn't work as well on waterproof or long-wearing formulas as the Cleansing Beauty Oil Premium A/O above.

😐 **$$$ High Performance Balancing Cleansing Oil** *($28 for 5 ounces)* is very similar to the Cleansing Beauty Oil Premium A/O above, only with fewer bells and whistles (none of which have much, if any, impact on skin). Otherwise, the same review applies.

☹ **High Performance Balancing Cleansing Oil, Enriched** *($28 for 5 ounces)* is only enriched because the company added some avocado oil, but your skin won't know the difference. The misstep here was including pepper extract, which has no business in a cleanser because it can be very irritating, especially around the eyes and mouth.

☹ **High Performance Balancing Cleansing Oil, Fresh** *($28 for 5 ounces)* creates the illusion of a fresh feeling from the irritating menthol derivative menthoxypropanediol, and is not recommended. Plain mineral oil would work just as well and without hurting skin in the process.

😐 **$$$ B-G Reinforcing Cosmetic Water** *($30 for 5 ounces)* is an incredibly underwhelming toner that is only worth considering if you believe in Shu Uemura's fabled seawater, said to be the purest form of water on earth. There's no proof of this, yet it's no secret that most of the world's seas have become polluted, so the question is, why would you want to apply such water to your skin? Further, once water is purified (as it must be to be used in a skin-care product), it doesn't resemble seawater in the least, which is good news for skin.

☹ **Ace B-G Reinforcing Emulsion** *($65 for 2.5 ounces)* offers a mixed bag of ingredients for normal to slightly dry skin. The glycerin, silicone, plant oil, and several water-binding agents are all pluses, but the amount of jasmine extract is potentially irritating, and this also contains several volatile fragrance components, including linalool and sensitizing eugenol. For the money, this doesn't translate to a wise investment in the quest for healthier skin.

😐 **$$$ Ace B-G Reinforcing Eye Cream** *($47 for 0.5 ounce)* is an OK, lightweight moisturizer for slightly dry skin, but the amount of jasmine extract makes it a potential problem for use around the eyes. It is unfortunate that the many antioxidants in this product are all present in low amounts. This product cannot minimize dark circles or puffiness as claimed.

😐 **$$$ Ace B-G Signs Preventing Essence** *($60 for 1 ounce)* contains more alcohol than helpful ingredients for skin, and that trumps any benefits possible from the many antioxidants in this nonessential Essence. The jasmine extract in here has no anti-aging benefits for skin; it merely adds fragrance.

😐 **$$$ B-G Recharging Night Cream** *($55 for 1 ounce)* has a light yet creamy texture and provides some worthy ingredients to reinforce normal to slightly dry skin's structure, but the jar packaging won't keep the very small amount of antioxidants stable during use.

😐 **$$$ B-G Reinforcing Gel Cream** *($50 for 1 ounce)* is similar to but has a lighter texture than the B-G Recharging Night Cream above, and the same review applies.

😐 **$$$ Principe Eye Zone Complex** *($42 for 0.5 ounce)* is an OK lightweight moisturizer for slightly to moderately dry skin, but the inclusion of tea tree oil and some volatile fragrance components makes it unsuitable for use around the eyes.

😐 **$$$ Principe 21** *($58 for 1 ounce)* is sold as a treatment product to promote renewed, translucent skin, but this blend of mostly water, slip agents, alcohol, and gel-based thickeners won't do much for skin other than feel tacky and be potentially irritating. The water-binding agents and antioxidants show up well after the preservatives, so don't count on them—and don't count on this product to renew anything.

😐 **$$$ B-G Reinforcing Booster** *($95 for 4 of each product)* is a two-step process involving mixing their **Powder** with the **Depsea Water** in this combination system. This is supposed to deliver the maximum dosage of beta-glucan to the inner layers of skin, improving its elasticity and, get this, its immunity. Beta-glucan is a very good antioxidant for skin, but there is no established maximum dosage and the amount Shu Uemura includes barely qualifies as a minimum. The Powder is just a blend of sugars and a slip agent with lecithin, cholesterol, and preservatives; the Depsea Water is just water. Sure, it is said to come from the sea, but that has no special immunity-boosting benefit for skin. At almost $100 for five days' worth of treatments, this counts as one of the most expensive do-nothing products I have reviewed.

☹ **Moisture Eye Zone Mask** *($43 for 12 pairs; 0.06 ounce each)* contains more alcohol than any beneficial ingredients, and alcohol can be drying and irritating, especially in the eye area. The water-binding agents are nice, but this product doesn't benefit the skin in any way over a well-formulated moisturizer, and ends up being a waste of time.

☹ **Moisture Face Mask** *($55 for 8 masks; 0.3 ounce each)* is similar to the Moisture Eye Zone Mask above, and the same review applies. The tiny amount of ceramide cannot overcome the effects of the alcohol and restore skin's moisture balance.

☺ **$$$ Principe Lip Serum** *($22 for 0.33 ounce)* is a good emollient moisturizing fluid with a small amount of water-binding agents and antioxidant. This is a good option for lips, but the claims that it can exfoliate are completely false.

SHU UEMURA MAKEUP

If you'd like to explore all this line has to offer, especially with their brushes and accessories, your best bet is to visit one of their freestanding stores. U.S. locations include San Francisco, Boston, and New York. There are no Shu Uemura stores in Canada. Otherwise, you're most likely to find this line carried at Saks Fifth Avenue, Barneys New York, or Nordstrom.

FOUNDATION: ☺ **$$$ Water Perfect Smoothing Water-in-Fluid Foundation** *($40)* is said to contain "40% deepsea water to perfectly envelop skin in moisture." However, it takes a lot more than water (from the sea or your faucet) to moisturize skin. This lightweight foundation is water- and silicone-based, but also contains a lot of talc, which isn't moisturizing in the least. It has a smooth, fluid texture that blends well and sets to a slightly moist finish with a hint of shine. Coverage goes from sheer to medium, and the formula is best for normal to slightly dry skin. The 16 shades present some impeccable neutrals for fair to light skin, but the following colors are too peach or gold for most skin tones: 345, 535, 554, and 735.

☺ **$$$ Water Perfect Water-in-Cake Foundation SPF 14** *($32.50; $15 for refillable compact)* is a modern interpretation of Shu Uemura's Nobara Cream Foundation, below. Its texture is nearly identical, but it doesn't look as heavy on skin and it offers a less creamy, more powdery finish with medium coverage. The sunscreen is pure titanium dioxide, and it's close enough to the benchmark SPF 15 to deserve a happy face rating. There are ten shades, almost all of which are neutral. Shade 545 is too peach to consider, and there are no shades for dark skin, but those with fair to medium skin will be pleased.

☺ **$$$ Foundation Fluid S** *($34)* is an excellent, nearly weightless sheer-coverage foundation whose natural finish is great for normal to dry skin. All seven shades are beautiful, with shade 393 being particularly suited to those with porcelain skin.

😐 **$$$ Velvet Perfect Adjusting Powdery Foundation SPF 14** *($45; $32.50 for powder refills)* has a silky, almost creamy-feeling powder texture and a smooth application that provides a dry matte finish. This can easily make skin look too powdered, so apply it sparingly. But remember, a sparing application will minimize the sun protection you get from this talc-based powder foundation's titanium dioxide and zinc oxide sunscreen, so it is best to pair it with a regular sunscreen or foundation with sunscreen. Among the eight mostly good shades, avoid the peachy 555 and the ash 734.

☹ **$$$ Nobara Cream Foundation** *($27)* is one of this line's oldest foundations, and the number of shades has been significantly reduced (it probably will be discontinued in the not too distant future). Claiming to be "commonly used on film sets" and "the ideal makeup for photos," it comes in a compact and has a slightly thick, cream-to-powder texture. It blends smoothly and provides medium to full coverage that is difficult to soften (this is not the one to choose if your foundation mantra is "sheer"). The soft cream finish can look slightly heavy in person, so perhaps this would be a workable foundation for film and television makeup (though not for HD close-ups). The six shades are all ideal neutrals, yet there are no options for tan to dark skin tones. All told, this isn't as elegant as the latest cream-to-powder makeups from M.A.C., Clarins, or Prescriptives, but it's worth a look if you need significant coverage.

CONCEALER: ☺ **$$$ Pro Spot Concealer** *($23)* is a thicker liquid concealer whose plastic-tipped applicator is designed for spot application. This offers the most intense camouflage I've ever seen from a liquid concealer, and it blends well over small areas. The finish is opaque and matte, and this absolutely won't crease. Using it around the eyes requires a moisturizer if you have any degree of dryness. Otherwise, five of the six shades have a beautiful soft yellow undertone and are recommended. Avoid 5YR Medium, which is too peach.

☹ **$$$ Eye Pro Concealer** *($23)* has a thick, creamy texture that lacks the necessary amount of slip to allow for seamless blending under the eye. Applying it with a brush is best, but then only if you need full coverage for very dark circles and are willing to trade concealment for a heavier appearance. Three of the four shades are very good; avoid Mauve, for obvious reasons.

☹ **$$$ Pro Concealer** *($23)* is identical to the Eye Pro Concealer above except it comes in a broader range of mostly neutral shades. Avoid 5YR Medium, which is too ash no matter how little you apply. Just as with the Eye Pro Concealer, this version has a heavier finish and is only for those who need full coverage.

☹ **Cover Crayon** *($24)* is a dual-ended pencil concealer with a thick, greasy texture and unappealing colors that look artificial on skin. You've been warned!

POWDER: ✓☺ **$$$ Face Powder Matte** *($33)* has a superfine, talc-based texture that creates a polished, not powdered, matte finish from each of five excellent shades. The jar component is equipped with a helpful sifter screen, making this much less messy than the typical loose powder. Although the finish is matte, this is a superior loose powder for all skin types except very dry.

✓☺ **$$$ Face Powder Sheer** *($33)* has an airy, sheer feel and appearance that's amazingly skinlike, making this a prime choice for normal to dry skin. It would be better if there were more than three shades because the Pearl option is shiny, but Colorless (which goes on translucent) works for fair to medium skin tones. The component has the same helpful sifter screen as the Face Powder Matte above.

BLUSH: ✓☺ **$$$ Glow On** *($21)* has an enviably silky-smooth application and a soft powder texture that imparts color evenly. The shade selection is extensive, though a few of the colors are too pale or orange to work as blush. Still, this product remains one of the highlights of this Japanese line. The best shades include: M Pink 31C, M Pink 33B, M Peach 43B, M Pink 33E, M Pink 31, M Amber 89, M Amber 82, M Amber 85, M Orange 55, M Brown 73, and M Peach 44.

EYESHADOW: ✓☺ **$$$ Pressed Eye Shadow** *($20)* has been reformulated and several readers have written to me complaining that the former true matte shades now have noticeable shine, which in fact they do. The severely limited matte options are a disappointment, but this remains a premier powder eyeshadow with a silky feel and a smooth, flake-free application. The palette is huge, and the medium to dark shades (which aren't as dark as they used to be) apply evenly. The only true mattes are M100 and M200. These are otherwise divided into three different finishes: shades labeled **Pearl** have a standard soft shimmer finish; the **Iridescent** shades have a stronger, more obvious shine than the Pearl; and the **Metallic** colors are just that, and include some beautiful options for evening eye makeup.

EYE AND BROW SHAPER: ☺ **$$$ Liquid Eyeliner** *($33, $15 for refill cartridge)* has a great soft-but-firm brush that allows for one-shot application. The formula dries quickly and wears extraordinarily well (it's actually a bit difficult to remove). Although this is pricey, consider this a must-try if you prefer liquid liner and haven't found one that doesn't smear or fade. Note: This only comes in one shade—black—with a slight iridescent finish.

☺ **$$$ Eyebrow Liner** *($35; $15 for refills)* comes in a durable, sleek metal component and is a very good automatic, retractable brow pencil with a suitably smooth application and a dry finish that stays put. The shade selection is limited, and the built-in brush is too stiff for regular use (it actually hurts a bit to apply), but this is otherwise a winner.

😐 **$$$ Drawing Pencils** *($18)* need sharpening and all of the colors are infused with glitter, but these pencils apply smoothly, their cream finish remains relatively smudgeproof, and the glitter barely flakes. Not bad, but not exceptional, nor is it preferred to lining the eyes with one of Shu Uemura's Pressed Eye Shadows above.

😐 **$$$ Eye Light Pencil White** *($18)* is a dual-ended pencil, with a matte white on one end and a white shimmer on the other. Each end has a creamy but not slippery texture that stays in place surprisingly well. This is workable for highlighting, but keeping it sharpened isn't as convenient as just highlighting with a white or shimmer powder.

😐 **$$$ Eyebrow Manicure** *($25)* is a tinted brow gel whose former "normal" brow colors have been replaced by shimmer-infused shades. OK, the shine has to stop somewhere, and adding it to brows is overkill (who needs shiny eyebrows anyway?). Although this is not a terrible product, the shiny colors limit its appeal and the slightly tacky finish is a step down from the superior tinted brow gels from Bobbi Brown, Paula Dorf, and Paula's Choice.

☹ **Liquid Shimmer Eyeliner** *($25)* is the opposite of the stellar Liquid Eyeliner above. Its brush is too long and thin for controlled application, and the formula tends to go on too heavy, which makes the dry time seem interminable. Once set, this tends to flake, and for $25, that's insulting.

☹ **H9 Formula Eyebrow Pencil** *($22)* is extremely tricky to use, something the counter staff at Shu Uemura's defend because they have a special sharpening/shaving technique they recommend to get this undeniably hard-textured pencil to work. I can't imagine why anyone would want to go through this trouble given the myriad brow pencils available that pose no downside.

LIPSTICK, LIP GLOSS, AND LIPLINER: ☺ **$$$ Lolishine Rouge** *($20)* is a fairly greasy lipstick that offers sheer to light coverage and no stain. The wet, glossy finish is nice, as is the color range, so as long as you don't expect much longevity, these are a soft option. ☺ **$$$ Rouge 4** *($20)* is Shu Uemura's longest-lasting lipstick formula, and it has a traditional creamy texture that provides medium coverage. Color-wise, the selection of pinks, browns, and reds is impressive and the finish each of these offers is attractive. ☺ **$$$ Rouge Unlimited Lipstick** *($23)* has a smooth, creamy feel and a soft, glossy finish that stays slippery, so this won't last for an "unlimited" amount of time. Still, if you're not prone to lipstick bleeding into lines around the mouth it's worth considering, and the range of 48 shades has something for everyone. As an added bonus, every color goes on exactly the way it looks in the tube, and there are some gorgeous red shades.

☺ **$$$ Retractable Lipliner Pencil** *($24, $15 for refill)* is an automatic, retractable lipliner packaged in a black metal component just like the Eyebrow Liner above. It's creamy and easy to apply, but why only two colors?

😐 **$$$ Lolishine Reflects** *($20)* are sheer lipsticks with a glossy, glitter-infused finish. They feel slightly grainy as the glossy feel wears away and the glitter remains, but are an option for those who want glitter with just a hint of color.

😐 **$$$ Sweet Lip Gloss** *($18)* comes in a squeeze tube and is a thick, viscous, and slightly sticky gloss that is very similar to Lancome's Juicy Tubes Ultra Shiny Lip Gloss ($16.50), right down to the bright-looking but sheer rainbow-themed colors and fruity flavors. 😐 **$$$ Lip Pencil** *($16.50)* needs sharpening and drags a bit on application, but the drier finish helps it last longer and resist premature fading. The shade range is small compared to that of all the lipstick colors, but several of the shades are versatile.

😐 **$$$ Drawing Lip Pencil** *($18)* requires routine sharpening so it's not as convenient as automatic lip pencils, but it applies effortlessly and feels comfortably creamy without being prone to smudging. Color-wise, the range favors brown-toned hues and soft pinks, though there are also a few good reds and brighter tones to coordinate with Uemura's vast lipstick palette.

MASCARA: ☺ **$$$ Mascara Length & Waterproof** *($20)* provides exceptional length without a touch of thickness, but it does take patience. The tiny brush makes it easy to reach every lash from root to tip, and, once dry, it is waterproof yet not overly difficult to remove.

😐 **$$$ Mascara Basic** *($27.50)* is a gel-based mascara that supposedly contains the same type of black ink found in Japanese calligraphy pens (which isn't safe for the eye area, so that ends up being a good story and nothing else). This takes lots of effort for minimal payoff and is incredibly difficult to remove because it tends to stain the lashes.

😐 **$$$ Fiber Xtension Lengthening Mascara** *($23)* has been improved and now offers a very smooth, clump-free application. However, for the money, this doesn't do much to impress beyond building modest length, and it leaves lashes feeling slightly dry. By the way, if this has fibers in it, I couldn't find them.

😐 **$$$ Mascara Royal Blue** *($25)* is really royal blue, and bright, too! If you're still exercising to Jane Fonda videos, wearing legwarmers to the grocery store, and the soundtrack to *Flashdance* has never left your CD player, you'll love this. The mascara itself is an average performer and the color doesn't help usability either.

😐 **$$$ Lash Repair** *($22)* won't repair lashes any more than a hair conditioner can repair split ends. This water- and glycerin-based clear gel basically just makes lashes soft and more receptive to curling. It's a lightweight formula that contains several water-binding agents, but it won't strengthen lashes against future damage, at least not any better than wearing regular mascara every day.

☹ **Precise Volume Mascara Waterproof** *($23)* produces sparse results from its uneven application, leading to merely average length and no thickness. The formula is tenaciously waterproof and more difficult than most to remove, making it a poor contender all around.

BRUSHES: Shu Uemura's reputation for superior ✓☺ **$$$ Brushes** *($10–$270)* is well deserved. Few lines offer such an extensive (at times eclectic) assortment of brushes, with all manner of natural hair and synthetic bristles. Although the prices on many of them are out of line, for sheer variety (there are more than 70) this brush collection is hard to beat. The most useful brushes are priced competitively with those from other artistry-driven lines such as M.A.C. and Bobbi Brown. My favorites, due to their shape, density, and overall performance, are the ✓☺ **$$$ Synthetic Brush 10** *($35)*, ✓☺ **$$$ Synthetic Brush 12** *($40)*, and ✓☺ **$$$ Synthetic Brush 14** *($40)*, each of which are great for eyeshadow application; the ✓☺ **$$$ Natural Brush 27** *($60)* for loose powder, ✓☺ **$$$ Natural Brush 14** *($40)*, and ✓☺ **$$$ Natural Brush 14H** *($35)* if you have a large eye area to work with; the ✓☺ **$$$ Natural Brush 20** *($50)* for blush; the ✓☺ **$$$ Natural Brush 10DF** *($45)* for eye contour; and the ✓☺ **$$$ Synthetic Brush 6F** *($22)* and ✓☺ **$$$ Synthetic Brush 6M** *($22)* for lipstick application. If you're feeling indulgent, you won't be disappointed with any of the ✓☺ **$$$ Kolinsky Brushes** *($45–$270)*—they are luxury redefined! There really are no brushes to avoid, though many are not for everyone due to their differing shapes and cuts. The ✓☺ **$$$ Essential Brush Set** *($275)* and ✓☺ **$$$ Portable Brush Set** *($164)* are nicely done, but for this amount of money, it's imperative to make sure you'll regularly use every brush that's in these sets!

SPECIALTY PRODUCTS: Shu Uemura also excels when it comes to accessories. From ☺ **Sponges** and ☺ **Powder Puffs** *($5–$8)* to refillable, customized ☺ **Palettes** *($12–$32)* and expertly designed, durable ☺ **$$$ Makeup Boxes** *($200–$700)*, the professional makeup artist and makeup-savvy consumer looking to organize will appreciate these options. Additionally, those who want to experiment with ☺ **$$$ False Eyelashes** *($15–$25)* will find this line tough to beat, and the boutiques have eyelash bars where experts teach you how to tailor the various lashes to suit your needs. Uemura even sells his own **Eyelash Adhesive** *($8.50)*, and his ☺ **$$$ Eyelash Curlers** *($18)* are a hot commodity because they're well designed and really work.

✓☺ **$$$ Face Paper** *($12 for 40 sheets)* consists of microscopically thin sheets of tissue paper that have a subtle texture that allows them to be a bit more absorbent than regular blotting papers. I don't think the difference is worth the price—not when you consider that many lines sell the same type of product for less than $6 and you get more sheets per package. Still, these non-powdery papers do the job very well and fit in even the tiniest evening bag.

😐 **$$$ UV Under Base SPF 10** *($32)* is a nearly colorless, airy mousse moisturizer with an in-part titanium dioxide sunscreen. It has a unique texture that is incredibly light, but what a shame the SPF value isn't higher so someone with oily skin could take advantage of this product! As is, you'll need to pair it with a foundation, powder, or regular sunscreen rated SPF 15 or higher.

😐 **$$$ Lip Fix** *($18)* is a standard, wax-based lip balm that leaves a slightly stiff, waxy matte finish. It claims to prevent smearing and extend the life of any lip color—but it is no more capable of that than rain is of not feeling wet! Used as plain lip balm, it's not as elegant as most others at the drugstore for a lot less.

☹ **Brush Cleaner** *($13)* is a liquid brush cleanser that contains acetone, the same solvent in many nail-polish removers. It will clean your brushes, but over time it also will break down the hair and make the brush unusable.

SISLEY PARIS

SISLEY PARIS AT-A-GLANCE

Strengths: Most of the sunscreens offer sufficient UVA protection; a unique lip balm; impressive foundations; good loose powder, blush, and eyeshadows; their most expensive mascara provides beautifully defined results.

Weaknesses: Exceedingly expensive, and the prices are not justified; several products contain irritating plant extracts or fragrant oils, most of which have no substantiated proof of benefit for skin; no AHA or BHA products; no products to address acne or oily skin (at least without causing irritation); jar packaging; poor concealer; standard eyeliner and brow options (at Sisley's prices, they should raise the bar); mostly average lipsticks.

For more information about Sisley, call (914) 251-0032 or visit www.sisley-cosmetics.com or www.Beautypedia.com. Note: All Sisley products contain fragrance, and I mean a lot of fragrance, unless otherwise noted.

SISLEY PARIS SKIN CARE

SISLEY PARIS PHYTO-BLANC PRODUCTS

☹ **Phyto-Blanc Buff and Wash Facial Gel** *($105 for 3.4 ounces)* is a cleanser/scrub hybrid that contains a lot of lemon fruit extract and also irritating lavender oil. And the price? Once you know how little the basic ingredients in this product cost, the price is an absolute insult.

☹ **Phyto-Blanc Lightening Toning Lotion** *($105 for 6.7 ounces)* contains a couple of plant extracts with limited research proving their ability to lighten skin discolorations. The amounts are too small to affect pigmentation, plus this toning lotion will irritate skin because it contains alcohol, lavender oil, lemon, and thyme oil.

☹ **Phyto-Blanc White Tensor** *($220 for 1 ounce)* contains a potentially helpful amount of mulberry extract, a plant whose arbutin content can have an effect on melanin synthesis. However, this positive is outweighed by several negatives, including a ridiculous price and irritants such as lemon, lavender oil, and thyme oil, the latter of which can cause contact dermatitis due to its many volatile constituents (Source: www.naturaldatabase.com).

☺ **$$$ Phyto-Blanc Clearing Essence with Vitamin C** *($280 for 8 0.2-ounce vials)* contains enough vitamin C and mulberry extract to be considered an effective alternative skin-lightening product, and each vial is stably packaged. However, the cost is outrageous when you consider the numerous effective skin-lightening options available, including prescription treatments such as Renova or Tri-Luma that sell for less than half the price of Sisley's product, yet have a solid track record for reliable results.

☹ **Phyto-Blanc Ultra-Lightening Mask** *($92 for 2 ounces)* is a below-standard moisturizing mask, a rating that takes account of its incredibly basic formula as well as the lavender and thyme oils it includes, neither of which will lighten skin one iota.

OTHER SISLEY PARIS PRODUCTS

☹ **Botanical Soapless Foaming Cleanser** *($95 for 4 ounces)* lists the drying, irritating detergent cleansing agent sodium lauryl sulfate as a main ingredient, and is not recommended.

😐 **$$$ Cleansing Milk with Sage, for Combination/Oily Skin** *($93 for 8.45 ounces)* is an exceptionally standard detergent-free cleansing lotion that is mostly water, thickeners, and mineral oil. The sage extract and volatile fragrance components can cause irritation, and this is wholly unsuitable for combination or oily skin.

☹ **Creamy Mousse Cleanser Makeup Remover** *($100 for 4.2 ounces)* has a sumptuous texture that feels great on skin, but the rosemary and lavender oils are irritating and make this not worth considering over many other foaming cleansers.

☹ **Soapless Facial Cleansing Bar** *($55 for a 4.4-ounce bar)* is an incredibly drying bar cleanser that contains some irritating plant extracts, including *Styrax benzoin* (what is that doing in a skin-care product?), which can cause contact dermatitis.

😐 **$$$ Lyslait Cleansing Milk with White Lily, for Dry/Sensitive Skin** *($100 for 8.4 ounces)* is a very greasy cleansing lotion for dry to very dry skin. It will remove makeup, but is best used with a washcloth. The many fragrant plants in this milk make it unsuitable for sensitive skin.

☹ **Gentle Eye and Lip Makeup Remover** *($64 for 4.2 ounces)* is not gentle in the least because the major ingredients include orange flower water and gardenia, both of which can be irritating to skin and even more so when used around the eyes. Any, and I do mean *any*, eye-makeup remover at the drugstore bests this product.

😐 **$$$ Buff and Wash Botanical Facial Gel** *($100 for 3.5 ounces)* is a standard scrub with polyethylene (plastic) as the abrasive agent, but for the price such a formula is surprising and definitely not worth the money. The amount of lemon extract in here can be irritating.

😐 **$$$ Gentle Facial Buffing Cream with Botanical Extracts, for All Skin Types** *($78 for 1.7-ounce jar; $72 for a 1.3-ounce tube)* is a water- and wax-based scrub with polyethylene as the abrasive agent. Although it's an OK option for normal to dry skin not prone to blemishes, the price is way out of line for what ends up being a product that is easily replaced with a washcloth!

☹ **Botanical Floral Spray Mist** *($74 for 4.2 ounces)* lists witch hazel as the second ingredient and contains fragrant orange flower water, making it too irritating for all skin types.

😐 **$$$ Botanical Floral Toning Lotion, Alcohol Free, for Dry/Sensitive Skin** *($85 for 8.4 ounces)* is a decent toner for normal to dry skin, but would be better without the witch hazel (present in an amount not likely to cause irritation). The fragrance makes this toner a poor choice for sensitive skin.

☹ **Botanical Grapefruit Toning Lotion, for Combination/Oily Skin** *($74 for 8.4 ounces)* lists alcohol as the second ingredient, followed by irritating grapefruit extract. Nothing in this toner is the least bit helpful for oily skin.

☹ **Lotion with Tropical Resins, for Combination/Oily Skin** *($67 for 4.2 ounces)* contains too much alcohol for any skin type to endure, and most of the plant extracts would be in the Rogues Gallery of Skin Irritants, if there were such a thing.

☹ **All Day All Year, Essential Day Care** *($355 for 1.7 ounces)* is hardly essential and is not recommended for use even one day out of the year. Without sunscreen, this emollient moisturizer for dry skin is a poor choice for daytime, the cost is outrageous, and it contains irritating oils of juniper, sage, and thyme.

☹ **Botanical Eye and Lip Contour Balm** *($115 for 1 ounce)* lists witch hazel distillate (which is mostly alcohol) as the second ingredient, and is not recommended.

😐 **$$$ Botanical Eye and Lip Contour Complex** *($160 for 0.5 ounce)* has moisturizing properties for the eye or lip area, but the overall formula is far from impressive, while the addition of a small amount of rosemary oil and volatile fragrance components may prove irritating.

☹ **Botanical Intensive Day Cream** *($255 for 1.7 ounces)* isn't intensive and is unsuitable for daytime use unless you pair it with another product rated SPF 15 or greater. This is otherwise a plain-Jane emollient moisturizer for dry to very dry skin. The jar packaging won't keep the antioxidants stable during use, while the fragrant oils of juniper, sage, and thyme are irritating.

☺ **$$$ Botanical Intensive Night Cream** *($310 for 1.6 ounces)* is similar to but richer than the Botanical Intensive Day Cream above, and the same skin type and jar-packaging comments apply. For a moisturizer that claims to rebuild skin, this contains a paltry assortment of ingredients that can't even possibly have that function.

☹ **Botanical Moisturizer with Cucumber** *($145 for 1.5 ounces)* is an incredibly basic moisturizer for dry skin, and cucumber alone does not have "everything it takes to reveal the radiance of your complexion." If that were true, wouldn't we be even better off just rubbing pure cucumber on our faces, which would cost only pennies? Due to the price for such an ordinary formula and the inclusion of several volatile fragrance components (including eugenol), this moisturizer is not recommended.

☺ **$$$ Botanical Night Complex, for All Skin Types** *($240 for 1 ounce)* is a very standard moisturizer for dry skin, and it lacks impressive amounts of antioxidants and ingredients that mimic the structure and function of healthy skin. For the price, this product should raise the bar for setting skin-care benefits, but instead it barely gets off the ground.

☹ **Botanical Night Cream with Collagen and Woodmallow, for All Skin Types** *($165 for 1.6 ounce)* is too basic to recommend at any price, and may cause irritation due to the many volatile fragrance components it contains. Using plain Lubriderm from the drugstore would be much better, but that's not saying much.

☹ **Botanical Restorative Facial Cream with Shea Butter, Day and Night for All Skin Types** *($160 for 1.6 ounces)* has a lighter cream texture than most of the Sisley Botanical moisturizers above, but what you're getting for your money is so-o-o standard! Plus, the volatile fragrance components can be irritating, making this even easier to ignore.

☺ **$$$ Botanical Tensor Immediate Lift** *($190 for 1.05 ounces)* is similar to the Phyto-Blanc White Tensor above, only without the lemon, mulberry, or lavender. It contains some good antioxidants, but their benefit is canceled out by volatile fragrance components.

☺ **$$$ Botanical Throat Cream** *($150 for 1.6 ounces)* cannot firm skin, contains nothing that is specific for the throat area, and is mostly mineral oil and thickeners. Who is buying this stuff, and, even worse, believing the inane claims? And in terms of formulators, who are these people? Did they even graduate from junior high? None of the plant extracts in here have any documented benefit for skin of any age.

☹ **Confort Extreme Day Skin Care, for Very Dry and Sensitive Skin** *($180 for 1.6 ounces)* is supposed to be the solution for fragile skin types, but no skin type should have to tolerate such a boring moisturizer that includes irritating thyme and sage oils.

☹ **Confort Extreme Night Skin Care, Very Dry and Sensitive Skin** *($175 for 1.6 ounces)* is an absurdly priced water- and Vaseline-based moisturizer that is not recommended for any skin type because it contains arnica and numerous volatile, irritating fragrance components.

☺ **$$$ Ecological Compound, for Day and Night** *($210 for 4.2 ounces)* contains a mostly small amount of plant extracts, none of which can protect or revitalize skin. This is a basic, water- and mineral oil–based moisturizer that contains an impressive amount of one antioxidant (skin needs more than one beneficial ingredient for it to be healthy and to function optimally), but that doesn't begin to come close to justifying the price.

☺ **$$$ Hydra-Flash Formule Intensive, with Beta-Hydroxy Acid, Essential Oils and Natural Plant Extracts** *($180 for 2.1 ounces)* can be a good moisturizer for normal to slightly dry skin, but it does not contain the beta hydroxy acid indicated on the label. (How bizarre is that?) And the essential oils, if present, are not indicated on the ingredient list. That's actually good news, because the rosemary and marjoram oils that are supposed to be in this product, but aren't on the ingredient label, are irritating. Again, how bizarre is that?

☺ **$$$ Hydra-Global Intense Anti-Aging Hydration** *($230 for 1.4 ounces)* contains lavender and sage oils, and is not recommended. Although the claims for this product's hydrating abilities may sound impressive, it does essentially what any moisturizer can do—but this one misses the mark in more ways than one. And the anti-aging claim—give me a break!

☹ **Sisleya Daily Line Reducer** *($440 for 1 ounce)* claims to restructure skin's framework "spectacularly," and by that they mean stimulate the production of fibroblasts, which are specialized cells responsible for creating connective tissue, including collagen. This product contains a high amount of soy protein, which in vitro research has shown can stimulate basic fibroblast growth factor. However, this research was carried out under carefully controlled conditions not related to the way soy protein is used in a cosmetic product (Source: *Biotechnology Letters*, June 2006, pages 869–875). Furthermore, even if we assume that the soy protein in here could signal fibroblast cells to produce more collagen, the plant extract *Potentilla erecta* (tormentil) has a high tannin content that can be irritating to skin, the thyme oil will produce further skin irritation, and lavender oil causes skin-cell death (Source: *Cell Proliferation*, June 2004, pages 221–229). This ends up being a very expensive gamble to find out if soy protein makes skin look younger while it's being irritated. It's not a bet I would encourage anyone to take. If you are interested in finding out if soy has benefit for your skin, Aveeno has lots of soy in some of their products, as does Neutrogena—for only a fraction of this price, and without any of the negative attributes of this appalling product.

☺ **$$$ Sisleya-Elixer** *($460 for 4 0.17-ounce vials; 0.68 ounce total)* sounds like a youth elixir if there ever was one (there have been thousands over the years since I began reviewing products, and none have ever turned back time by even one day). The main ingredients in this serum are water, glycerin, algae, wax, and potato extract. Who knew such commonplace ingredients could plump up the dermal layer and restart the process and reflexes of young skin? Actually, they cannot do this, and the only reason to invest in these vials is if you thoroughly enjoy wasting your money on empty promises.

☺ **$$$ Sisleya Eye and Lip Contour Cream** *($180 for 0.53 ounce)* is a very emollient moisturizer that would be better for skin around the eyes or for lips if it did not contain so much orange flower water. Nothing in the formula causes the price to make any sense, but this can ease dryness.

☺ **$$$ Sisleya Global Anti-Age** *($410 for 1.7 ounces)*. How many bogus anti-aging moisturizers does one line need? This hyper-expensive option adds nothing new to the mix, and all of the plant ingredients (many of which are antioxidants, a couple of them potentially irritating) will see their effectiveness vanish due to jar packaging. That leaves you with a basic moisturizer for dry skin that is useless as a moisturizer and disturbing as an anti-aging product.

☹ **Sisleya Global Anti-Age, Extra-Rich for Dry Skin** *($410 for 1.7 ounces)* is a more emollient version of the Sisleya Global Anti-Age product above, but this one is not recommended because it contains thyme and lavender oils.

☹ **Tropical Resins Complex, Oil Free, Purifying, for Combination/Oily Skin** *($140 for 1.7 ounces)* contains several plant ingredients that are a problem for all skin types, and none of them can control surface sebum (oil) or make large pores smaller. The amount of *Styrax benzoin* resin is particularly problematic and a serious faux pas in a cosmetic.

😐 **$$$ Botanical Facial Mask with Linden Blossom, for Dry/Sensitive Skin** *($100 for 2.4 ounces)* may confuse skin because the amount of glycerin is enough to hydrate skin, yet the clay that follows absorbs some of the glycerin. Thickening agents and oils make this mask best for normal to slightly dry skin, but you are absolutely not getting anything special for your money.

☹ **Botanical Facial Mask with Tropical Resins, for Combination/Oily Skin** *($80 for 2.1 ounces)* contains several plant irritants, including great plantain, *Styrax benzoin* resin, and myrrh extract, along with several volatile fragrance components. How these are supposed to help oily skin is a good question. Their irritating properties will only make matters worse for this (or any) skin type.

☹ **Express Flower Gel Mask** *($115 for 2.15 ounces)* contains enough iris root extract to cause irritation, and the cabbage rose–water base doesn't help.

😐 **$$$ Radiant Glow Express Mask with Red Clay** *($95 for 2.15 ounces)* is mostly water, wax, and clay, with some thickeners. How's that for wasting your money? The rosemary oil is likely present in too small an amount to be irritating. I'm a bit speechless because this is an overwhelmingly standard clay mask with one of the silliest price tags in this book!

☺ **$$$ Baume Confort Levres, Nutritive Lip Balm** *($62 for 0.3 ounce)* is a unique, emollient lip balm, but that doesn't make it worth the jaw-dropping price compared to several other lip balms.

SISLEY PARIS SUN PRODUCTS

☹ **Botanical Body Sun Cream SPF 10** *($123 for 6.7 ounces)* features avobenzone for UVA protection, but the SPF rating is below standard and the lavender and rose geranium oils are a problem for all skin types.

☹ **Botanical Facial Sun Cream SPF 8** *($185 for 2 ounces)* lacks the UVA-protecting ingredients of titanium dioxide, zinc oxide, avobenzone, Mexoryl SX (ecamsule), or Tinosorb, and is not recommended.

☺ **$$$ Botanical Facial Sun Cream SPF 15** *($195 for 2.1 ounces)* is a good, in-part avobenzone sunscreen for normal to very dry skin. However, at this price, are you really going to apply it liberally, which is essential to achieving the stated level of protection?

☹ **Botanical Sun Oil, Protected Tanning, SPF 4** *($105 for 4.2 ounces)* not only encourages tanning, which is ironic (not to mention unethical) from a company selling dozens of antiwrinkle creams, but it leaves skin vulnerable to UVA damage and has an SPF rating that is one step above doing nothing at all to protect skin.

Broad Spectrum Sunscreen *($127 for 1.4 ounces)* is sold in five versions, and all of them contain an in-part titanium dioxide sunscreen. 😐 **$$$ Colorless SPF 25** is a basic sunscreen for normal to dry skin not prone to breakouts; ☹ **Colorless SPF 30+** contains more titanium dioxide than the SPF 25 version, but is not recommended because it contains irritating sage oil and thymus extract, an ingredient typically derived from slaughtered cows. None of that is helpful for skin. The ☺ **$$$Colorless SPF 40** version is an option for normal to slightly dry or slightly oily skin and is, surprisingly, fragrance-free (save for a tiny amount of cucumber). ☹ **Golden SPF 20** has a light lotion texture and provides a sheer gold tint, but irritates skin with sage oil, as does ☹ **Natural SPF 20.**

☹ **Fluid Body Sun Cream with Botanical Extracts, Spray SPF 20** *($140 for 6.7 ounces)* not only has a price that is bound to discourage liberal application (and liberal application is essential for effective sun protection), but it also contains lavender and geranium oils, which are a problem for all skin types.

☹ **Self Tanning Gel** *($120 for 2.7 ounces)* is a standard, offensively overpriced self-tanner. Enough said, this is just too pathetic for words.

☹ **Self Tanning Lotion for the Body** *($100 for 5 ounces)* contains thymus, sage, and lavender oils in addition to an irritating amount of alcohol and several volatile fragrance components.

☹ **Sunleya Age Minimizing Sun Protection Sunscreen Cream SPF 15** *($215 for 1.7 ounces)* contains thymus and sage oils, making this in-part avobenzone sunscreen impossible to recommend (though the price is reason enough to stay away).

SISLEY PARIS MAKEUP

FOUNDATION: Sisley's foundation shade range does not extend to darker skin tones, but those with fair to light skin are, pardon the pun, well covered.

✓☺ **$$$ Oil-Free Foundation** *($94)* has an elegantly silky, lightweight texture that smooths over skin, setting to a natural-looking satin-matte finish. The natural finish belies the medium coverage you get from this foundation, and although the price is outrageous, it is one of the better options for normal to oily skin. Among the six mostly neutral shades, avoid 5 Golden and 3 Natural.

☺ **$$$ Transmat Foundation** *($84)* is a fluid, but creamy, foundation with a relatively sheer satin-matte finish. It has lots of slip but manages to blend well and provides light to medium coverage. It is best for those with normal to slightly dry skin and a healthy beauty budget. Transmat is offered in eight shades, including some good options for fair skin tones. Avoid Cuivre 5, Naturel 8, and Rose Peche 6, all of which are too pink or peach to look convincing.

☺ **$$$ Compact Foundation** *($75)* is an exceptionally smooth, silicone-based powder foundation. Talc is present in the formula, contributing to its natural matte finish, but it is not a predominant ingredient. That makes this formula best for normal to slightly dry skin seeking light to medium coverage. Application is flawless and the result is very natural, though the price is out of line for what you get. All five shades are neutral. This does contain a tiny amount of rosewood oil, but likely not enough to cause irritation.

CONCEALER: ☹ **Phytocernes Botanical Concealer** *($71)* has a price that is just rude. There must be women buying this stuff, though I can't imagine why. This has a greasy, easy-to-crease texture and three peachy pink colors that are a far cry from neutral. In addition, this product contains irritating rosemary and juniper oils, which should absolutely not be used around the eyes.

POWDER: ☺ **$$$ Transparent Loose Powder** *($69)* has a sheer, weightless feel and offers a smooth, translucent finish that doesn't look the least bit dry or powdery. This talc-based powder comes in four good shades, of which shade 0 is sparkling. Despite my enthusiasm for this product, you should know that equally impressive loose powders are available for one-third the cost.

BLUSH: ☺ **$$$ Phyto Blush** *($70)* is a bargain by Sisley's standards—you get two blush tones (although one is more for highlighting) in one compact. With a very smooth texture and application, this will undoubtedly appeal to women who are somehow convinced that Sisley is a step above the rest. All of the shades have some degree of shine; No. 4 is the most intense.

EYESHADOW: The ☺ **$$$ Eye Shadows** *($26)* are supposedly available in matte, sheer, and shimmering shades, but all of the colors have some amount of shine, and most are noticeably shiny. This is not a smart choice if you have any amount of eye-area wrinkling or sagging (shine only enhances the appearance of wrinkles), but these powder eyeshadows do blend well and are nicely pigmented. Amethyst 9 and Black 16 are almost matte; avoid Transparent Lagoon, which is too blue.

EYE AND BROW SHAPER: 😐 **$$$ Phyto Kohl Perfect Eyeliner** *($38)* is a standard pencil featuring shine-laden shades that will only emphasize a less-than-taut eyelid. The creamy texture glides on and stays put once set, though you can also smudge it for a smoky look. Of course, the same thing can be done with pencils that cost less than $10, too. The 😐 **$$$ Eyebrow Pencil** *($39)* has been improved since it was last reviewed, but remains a standard pencil that needs routine sharpening. The dry but smooth application stays in place and won't make brows look matted or greasy, and there is a spiral brush on the end to groom brows. Suffice it to say this ordinary offering is easily replaced by better options ranging in price from $5 to $10.

LIPSTICK, LIP GLOSS, AND LIPLINER: ☺ **$$$ Metal Velvet Lip Gloss** *($43)* is much nicer than the Glossy Gloss below, though the price should still give you pause. It has a thinner texture with minimal stickiness and a beautiful shimmer-to-metallic finish. The shade selection is impressive, extending from sheer to moderate-intensity colors, including a few vivid hues that make for a striking evening look. ☺ **$$$ Phyto Lip Star** *($49)* is one of the most expensive lip glosses around, but is it one you should invest in? Only if you enjoy spending much more than you should for such a ubiquitous item! This is a very standard, slightly thick lip gloss loaded with sparkles which, combined with the glossiness, provide a very shiny finish. The inclusion of a type of water lily (*Nelumbium speciosum*) has no benefit for lips. It deserves a happy face rating, but there is no need to spend this much on lip gloss.

😐 **$$$ Hydrating Long-Lasting Lipstick** *($46)* is only long-lasting because this full-coverage lipstick is highly pigmented. Otherwise, the creamy-bordering-on-greasy formula remains slippery and is not for anyone with lines around the mouth. Paying this much for what amounts to a below-standard lipstick makes about as much sense as applying false eyelashes to your cheeks (yes, it's that silly!). 😐 **$$$ Glossy Gloss** *($43)* ranks as one of the most expensive lip glosses reviewed in this book. It has a thick, sticky texture and the shimmer-infused shades tend to feel grainy as the gloss wears off. The brush applicator is classy, but it is still absolutely not worth the investment. 😐 **$$$ Lip Liner** *($42)* is a standard pencil with a built-in brush that leans to the greasy side of creamy, but it does have a good stain and nice colors. Contrary to the claim, these won't do much to help stop feathering, nor will the minute amount of plant extracts "soften and protect lips."

MASCARA: ✓☺ **$$$ Phyto Mascara Ultra Volume** *($57)* has a shocking price that may curl your lashes all on its own! At least those who choose to indulge in this mascara will be treated to gorgeous lashes that have magnified thickness, considerable length, and are perfectly defined. Application can be a bit heavy, but combing through lashes separates them nicely and doesn't lead to clumps or flaking. This wears all day without a hitch and removes with a water-soluble cleanser.

😐 **$$$ Ultra Facil Mascara** *($52)* should, for this amount of money, knock your socks off and instantly provide traffic-stopping lashes. It does neither. This is merely an average mascara that leaves lashes soft and provides decent length and thickness with minor clumping that's easily combed through. The formula is not unique in the least, despite the Sisley salesperson's claims to the contrary.

FACE AND BODY ILLUMINATING/SHIMMER PRODUCTS: ☺ **$$$ Magic Touch Highlighter** *($35)* comes in a compact with a sponge-tip applicator that should be tossed out. This cream-to-powder shimmer product is best applied with a brush or fingertip. Both of the colors (pale gold or copper) are extremely shiny and not meant for wrinkled eyes. If that doesn't apply to you, these do blend well and last longer than you might expect.

☺ **$$$ Sun Glow Gel** *($70)* has a ridiculous price tag, but if you're swayed by Sisley at least you won't be disappointed by this silky bronzing lotion's sheer color, easy blending, and soft shimmer finish. It's too shiny to apply over prominent wrinkles, but works well as a mixer product to add more depth (and shimmer) to your foundation.

BRUSHES: Sisley offers a small group of good **Brushes** *($35–$55)* that are nicely shaped and properly sized. There is nothing too exceptional, but if you simply must have Sisley brushes, you won't be disappointed. The 😐 **$$$ Loose Powder Brush** *($55)* is too standard to justify its cost, though the short-handled ☺ **$$$ Sun Glow Duo Brush** *($35)* is compact and dense.

SK-II (SKIN CARE ONLY)

SK-II AT-A-GLANCE

Strengths: Some well-formulated moisturizers and serums; all of the sunscreens provide sufficient UVA protection.

Weaknesses: Shockingly expensive, especially for the wide assortment of mediocre products; unreliable skin-lightening products; AHA/BHA products that contain an ineffective amount of exfoliant; no products to help manage blemishes; jar packaging.

For more information about SK-II, owned by Procter & Gamble, visit www.sk2.com or www.Beautypedia.com.

Note: Pitera is the cornerstone of the SK-II line and is present in every SK-II product. Pitera is the trade name for *Saccharomycopsis* ferment filtrate (SFF), a form of yeast purportedly unique because of the fermenting and filtering process it goes through before being added to these products. As it turns out, many forms of yeast have anti-inflammatory properties and antioxidant properties, including SFF (Source: *Journal of Dermatologic Science*, June 2006, pages 249–257). Other than that, all of the information about Pitera comes from papers presented at medical conferences, not from published studies. Presenting papers at medical conferences is not at all the same thing as publishing the results of studies. I frequently present papers and information at medical conferences, and I wouldn't offer that material as proof of anything because it isn't. The standards for presenting a paper at a medical conference are very different from the requirements for publication of study results in most medical journals.

😐 **$$$ Facial Treatment Cleanser** *($50 for 4 ounces)* is a decent, extremely overpriced, basic, water-soluble, detergent-based cleanser that is an option for normal to oily skin, if only the cost weren't so ludicrous. It does contain Pitera and a few other interesting extras, but in a cleanser they will hardly be on your face before they are rinsed down the drain.

😐 **$$$ Facial Treatment Cleansing Gel** *($50 for 3.5 ounces)* is an extremely standard, mineral oil–based (yes, mineral oil) wipe-off cleanser that, shockingly, comes in a jar! Sticking your fingers into any product is bad news for its stability. This is more reminiscent of a cold cream than anything else, and it's a very expensive cold cream! The only reason to blow $50 on this would be because you actually believed that the Pitera it contains was simply the most important skin-care ingredient ever. It also contains *Crithmum maritimum* extract, from a seaweed commonly known as rock samphire or sea fennel. Some research does show that it has antioxidant properties, but there is also research showing it can be cytotoxic (toxic to cells) (Source: *Journal of Natural Products*, September 1993, pages 1598–1600).

😐 **$$$ Facial Treatment Cleansing Oil** *($50 for 8.4 ounces)* is mostly mineral oil with a few thickening agents, plant extracts, and, of course, Pitera. This is one of the most expensive containers of mineral oil I've ever seen! The few bells and whistles in here aren't nearly enough to make up for the absurd price and the absence of any unique benefit for skin.

😐 **$$$ Facial Treatment Clear Lotion** *($50 for 5 ounces)* is an exceptionally standard toner that is mostly water and Pitera (well, it isn't standard if you think Pitera is the best ingredient ever for skin). There is a tiny, and I mean really tiny, amount of a good water-binding agent, even smaller amounts of salicylic acid, and two alpha hydroxy acids. While the pH is low enough for them to function as exfoliants, the amount of BHA and AHAs is far too low for them to be effective. Spending this much money on what is a basic toner would have to be based only on your faith in Pitera because every other ingredient is easily replaced by better formulations for far less money.

😐 **$$$ Skin Refining Treatment** *($125 for 1.7 ounces)*. I almost fell off my chair when I saw the price of this ordinary salicylic acid (BHA) cream. Other than Pitera—and I have no idea why every product has to have this ingredient—there is no reason to spend this much of your hard-earned money on what amounts to a decent, though basic BHA product. One word of warning: At 2.3, the pH of this product is unusually low, which means there is a high potential for irritation. Also, the jar packaging isn't the best. But given that this fragrance-free product contains the teensiest amount of an antioxidant and some aloe water, even that can't really make a difference.

☹ **Advanced Protect Essence UV, SPF 15** *($80 for 1 ounce)* is problematic because the cost of any expensive sunscreen means you are unlikely to apply it liberally, which means you won't be getting adequate sunscreen protection. Separate from my concerns about application, this product is not recommended even though it contains an in-part zinc oxide sunscreen. That's because, for unknown reasons, SK-II decided to include the irritating menthol derivative menthyl lactate. Any of Olay's sunscreens with zinc oxide or avobenzone are distinctly preferred to this pricey mistake.

😐 **$$$ Advanced Signs Treatment** *($160 for 2.6 ounces)*. Aside from the Pitera and the price tag, there is nothing in or about this product that Olay Regenerist's Daily Regenerating Serum can't do far better. Not to mention that Olay's version is in proper packaging designed to keep its ingredients stable, while Advanced Signs comes in a jar, making it anything but advanced.

☺ **$$$ De-Wrinkle Essence** *($150 for 0.85 ounce)* is an almost identical copy of Olay Regenerist's Targeted Tone Enhancer ($18.99 for 1 ounce), except for the Pitera, of course. The decision about which product to choose seems clear to me, but to be specific, De-Wrinkle is a good, lightweight moisturizer for someone with normal to slightly dry skin. It contains some good antioxidants and a cell-communicating ingredient.

😐 **$$$ Eye Treatment Film** *($80 for 0.5 ounce)* is mostly Pitera, water, slip agents, preservatives, alcohol, and comb extract. The comb extract is from hen or rooster combs, which may mislead you into thinking that it is similar to the hyaluronic acid in some dermal fillers such as Restylane. But it isn't—it's not even close. So, aside from the Pitera, this product comes up a big zero; it's actually one of the most contains-nothing products around. This is all about Pitera, and banking on that is not a reliable investment.

☺ **$$$ Facial Clear Solution** *($100 for 3.3 ounces)* is a good, lightweight, fragrance-free moisturizer for normal to slightly dry skin, but there is nothing in it that will balance skin or change the size of pores. In some ways this is a less impressive product than Olay Regenerist's Daily Regenerating Serum, but if you're interested in Pitera, then this is one more option.

😐 **$$$ Facial Hydrating UV Cream, SPF 15** *($100 for 1.7 ounces)* is almost identical to the Advanced Protect Essence UV, SPF 15 reviewed above, but this version omits the irritant menthyl lactate. However, the jar packaging is disappointing. Although that won't affect the SPF, it will affect the teensy amount of vitamin E, as well as the Pitera.

😐 **$$$ Facial Lift Emulsion** *($110 for 3.3 ounces)*. I'm really getting annoyed at this ingredient, because other than the Pitera (I'm even getting tired of me saying that), this is a decent, though ordinary, fragrance-free, lightweight moisturizer for normal to dry skin that contains too little antioxidants and water-binding agents.

😐 **$$$ Facial Treatment Concentrate** *($300 for 1 ounce)*. Even if you assume that this is a well-formulated moisturizer, its jar packaging leaves much to be desired because antioxidants require airtight packaging for stability. If your skin wanted lots of Pitera, this would be an option. Other than that, this moisturizer has a limited amount of antioxidants and water-binding agents, and for $300 it should have been overflowing with them and in much better packaging.

😐 **$$$ Facial Treatment Essence** *($85 for 2.5 ounces; $130 for 5 ounces)* is supposed to contain "the most concentrated amount of Pitera of all the SK-II skincare products—around 90% pure SK-II Pitera." Indeed, that is all this contains, other than some slip agents, water, and preservatives. What a waste, and what a strange gimmick to thrust on women the world over.

😐 **$$$ Facial Treatment Massage Cream** *($100 for 2.5 ounces)* comes to you in jar packaging that prevents the air-sensitive ingredients from remaining stable. But given that Pitera and a teeny amount of vitamin E are the only ingredients that could be affected, there isn't much to worry about. There is no reason to consider this ordinary water-and-wax basic moisturizer for dry skin.

😐 **$$$ Facial Treatment Repair C** *($135 for 1 ounce)*, despite the name, doesn't contain vitamin C. In fact, all it contains is Pitera, water, slip agents, water-binding agent, and preservatives. The one thing you may be gleaning from this product lineup is that whatever effect Pitera has, P&G must believe it takes a lot of it to provide a benefit. Otherwise, why not just offer one super-Pitera product and call it good, and have this option be something else that is proven to be beneficial for skin?

😐 **$$$ Signs Up-Lifter** *($225 for 1.3 ounces)*. Just when you thought you had had enough of Pitera, this product actually contains an even more concentrated version of this strain of yeast, called Pitera 4. It's there along with many of the same ingredients you find in Olay's Regenerist, and that means this is a good, fragrance-free moisturizer for normal to dry skin. I should mention that there are a few extras in Signs Up-Lifter, like *Padina pavonica* extract, from a form of algae that has some antioxidant properties. But as it turns out, a comparison study (my favorite kind) found that a different form of algae had far more potent antioxidant abilities, namely *Caulerpa racemosa* (Source: *Journal of Experimental Marine Biology and Ecology*, July 2005, pages 35–41). This also contains *Crithmum maritimum* extract, another form of algae that I mentioned in my review of the SK-II Facial Treatment Cleansing Gel above. There is some research that shows *Crithmum maritimum* has some antioxidant properties, but there is also research showing it can be cytotoxic (toxic to cells) (Source: *Journal of Natural Products*, September 1993, pages 1598–1600). In the greater scheme of things, these extras add up to a whole lot of nothing.

☹ **$$$ Whitening Source** *($100 for 1 ounce)* claims it can even out your skin tone and, well, make you whiter. Given that it contains almost exactly the same mix of ingredients that several other SK-II products offer, chances are remote that this will somehow behave differently. There is no research showing that Pitera (the second ingredient) can change skin color. The small amount of vitamin C may have benefit, but no more so than it does in dozens of other products that contain vitamin C. Niacinamide gets prominence here, and although this B vitamin has some research pertaining to its skin-lightening ability, you can test this benefit with Olay's much less expensive Regenerist or Definity products. Whitening Source does contain a very small amount of *Gentiana lutea* root extract, also known as bitterroot or gentian, which has some research showing it has antioxidant properties and can be effective for wound healing. While that may be helpful, those benefits have nothing to do with skin color—and there are thousands of other ingredients with the same attributes that show up in thousands of other products for a lot less money (Sources: www.naturaldatabase.com; and *Phytotherapy Research*, June 2006, pages 91–95).

☹ **$$$ Facial Treatment Mask** *($15 for 1 0.95-ounce mask; $75 for 6 masks)* is just water, Pitera, slip agents, and preservative. It does contain sodium salicylate, but the pH of the product, combined with the characteristics of this type of salicylate, render it a poor choice for exfoliation.

☹ **$$$ Signs Eye Mask** *($95 for 14 dual-mask packettes; 0.02 ounce each)*. If I've done my math right, this mask weighs in at almost $350 for 1 ounce of product, making it the most expensive SK-II item. Oddly, you don't even get the "concentrated" amount of Pitera that's present in several other SK-II products. For the money, even if you were a Pitera adherent, this isn't the way to get the stuff on your skin. It has some interesting ingredients, but again, nothing that would make it rank over and above Olay Regenerist or Definity. The few additional plant extracts in here aren't worth the extra expense or time to apply this mask. For example, it contains *Chrysanthellum indicum* extract (from golden chamomile), which has some research showing it reduces irritation and improves the appearance of rosacea. However, the studies didn't compare the extract with other anti-irritant ingredients or protocols, only with a placebo (Source: *Journal of the European Academy of Dermatology & Venereology*, September 2005, page 564).

☹ **$$$ Whitening Source Intensive Mask** *($85 for 6 0.95-ounce masks)*. The repetitiveness of the formulations in the SK-II line is exhausting. Here, as with most of the SK-II products, you get mostly water, Pitera, slip agents, niacinamide, antioxidant, and preservatives. Overall, this mask isn't worth the money or trouble, and it definitely won't affect skin color.

SKINCEUTICALS (SKIN CARE ONLY)

SKINCEUTICALS AT-A-GLANCE

Strengths: Great line to shop if you're looking for well-formulated vitamin C and retinol products; some outstanding sunscreens, and every one provides sufficient UVA protection; one effective AHA product; good self-tanner; several fragrance-free products.

Weaknesses: Mostly problematic cleansers and toners; fruit and sugar extracts trying to substitute for AHA products when the real deal is much better; ineffective BHA products; jar packaging.

For more information about SkinCeuticals, owned by L'Oreal, call (800) 811-1660 or visit www.skinceuticals.com or www.Beautypedia.com.

☹ **$$$ Clarifying Cleanser** *($22.50 for 5 ounces)* contains 2% salicylic acid along with the AHAs glycolic and mandelic acids. Although the pH of this cleansing scrub would allow chemical exfoliation, the acids are not in contact with skin long enough for that to occur. This is a good, water-soluble option for normal to oily skin, but keep it away from the eye area.

☹ **Cleansing Cream, for Normal to Dry Skin** *($24 for 8 ounces)* contains too much sandalwood extract to make this creamy cleanser worth purchasing. The phellodendron extract has anti-inflammatory properties, but they're canceled out by the sandalwood, not to mention the lesser amount of fragrant orange oil also included.

☹ **Foaming Cleanser** *($24.50 for 5 ounces)* contains several irritating plant extracts, including arnica, ivy, and pellitory, all of which make this otherwise fine water-soluble cleanser not recommended.

☹ **$$$ Gentle Cleanser, for Sensitive Skin** *($26 for 8 ounces)* is a cleansing gel/lotion hybrid that has surprisingly minimal cleansing ability, and the orange oil it contains isn't something that you should apply to sensitive skin. This is an OK option for normal skin when minimal to no makeup needs to be removed.

☹ **$$$ Simply Clean, for Combination or Oily Skin** *($24 for 8 ounces)* does a good job of cleansing and removing makeup for its intended skin types. However, it doesn't deserve a happy face rating due to the problematic plant extracts it includes.

☹ **$$$ Equalizing Toner, for Combination or Oily Skin** *($22 for 8 ounces)* is mostly water and aloe, though the amount of witch hazel is potentially irritating, as are the rosemary and thyme extracts.

☹ **Revitalizing Toner, for Normal or Dry Skin** *($22 for 8 ounces)* lists witch hazel as the second ingredient, while the mixed fruit extracts are not the same as, nor do they perform like, AHAs. The inclusion of irritating plant extracts creates one too many strikes against this toner.

☹ **$$$ C + AHA Exfoliating Antioxidant Treatment** *($115 for 1 ounce)* is a good option if you're looking for a stabilized vitamin C serum that contains approximately 4% glycolic and lactic acids in the correct pH range to exfoliate skin, but that is a limited combination and it isn't worth this price tag. Vitamin C is not the sole answer for skin and there are better-formulated AHA products for far less money.

☺ **$$$ C E Ferulic Combination Antioxidant Treatment** *($122 for 1 ounce)* comes complete with all manner of anti-aging claims, but the only ones you can bank on with this product (based on a significant amount of research) are its abilities to reduce free radicals and to defend skin against oxidative stress. It reportedly contains 15% L-ascorbic acid, a form of vitamin C considered an excellent antioxidant and anti-inflammatory agent (Sources: *Experimental Dermatology*, June 2003, pages 237–244; and *Bioelectrochemistry and Bioenergetics*, May 1999, pages 453–461). Because L-ascorbic acid is stable only in low-pH formulations (Source: *Dermatologic Surgery*, February 2001, pages 137–142), the good news is that this product's pH of 3 is low enough to allow this form of vitamin C to be effective. Also present in this water-based antioxidant serum are vitamin E and ferulic acid. Vitamin E, appearing here as alpha tocopherol, also has a well-established reputation as an effective antioxidant (Sources: *Radiation Research*, July 2005, pages 63–72; *Annals of the New York Academy of Sciences*, December 2004, pages 443–447; and *Journal of Investigative Dermatology*, February 2005, pages 304–307). Ferulic acid is relatively new to the skin-care scene, but earlier research suggests that it provides antioxidant and sun-protective benefits to skin while enhancing the stability of topical applications of vitamin E (Sources: *International Journal of Pharmaceutics*, April 10, 2000, pages 39–47; *Anticancer Research*, September–October 1999, pages 3769–3774; *Nutrition and Cancer*, February 1998, pages 81–85; and *Free Radical Biology and Medicine*, October 1992, pages 435–448). As research into this and similar compounds (such as caffeic and ellagic acid) continues, I suspect we will see more antioxidant-based products enhanced with them, which is great news for keeping skin healthy and protecting it from further damage.

C E Ferulic Combination Antioxidant Treatment is suitable for all skin types. Its brown glass packaging helps keep its high level of antioxidants stable, although an airless pump applicator would have been better than the dropper tip, because that requires you to remove the cover with each use, exposing the oxygen-sensitive antioxidants to air. That is what keeps this product from earning a Paula's Pick rating. After all, who wants to spend this much on one product only to discover that the efficacy is severely diminished after a period of time?

☹ **Daily Moisture Lightweight Pore-Minimizing Moisturizer, for Normal or Oily Combination Skin** *($49.50 for 2 ounces)* begins well with its water-based blend of several species of algae and a light moisturizing agent, but all in all this contains too many potentially problematic plant extracts to make it a slam-dunk for normal to oily skin. Algae extracts cannot make pores smaller, but the cinnamon, ginger, and thyme may make them appear smaller by virtue of the inflammation they cause—yet that's a negative for the long-term health of your skin.

☹ **Emollience Rich, Restorative Moisturizer, for Normal or Dry Skin** *($49.50 for 2 ounces)* not only features jar packaging that undermines the efficacy of its many antioxidants, but this emollient cream also is bound to cause irritation due to the volatile essential oils it contains.

😐 **$$$ Eye Balm Rehabilitative Emollient, for Aging Skin** *($68 for 0.5 ounce)* has a lot going for it, including copious antioxidants and a cell-communicating ingredient, all wrapped up in a lightweight lotion texture for all skin types. What a shame the jar packaging won't keep the state-of-the-art ingredients stable during use.

✓☺ **$$$ Eye Cream Firming Treatment** *($55 for 0.67 ounce)* is an excellent, fragrance-free, antioxidant-rich, lightweight moisturizer for slightly dry skin anywhere on the face. It contains a couple of very good water-binding agents and an efficacious plant oil, along with stabilized vitamin C; however, don't expect it to lighten dark circles as claimed.

😐 **$$$ Eye Gel AOX+** *($45 for 0.5 ounce)* is a good water-based moisturizer for slightly dry skin anywhere on the face. It contains impressive amounts of vitamin C, but a fairly inconsequential amount of ferulic acid and sodium hyaluronate. All in all, this is a one-note product and not nearly as elegant as others in this price category or for even less money.

😐 **Eye Renewal Gel Nighttime Line-Minimizing Treatment** *($27 for 1 ounce)* claims to exfoliate delicate skin around the eyes with a 5% hydroxy acid blend, but the fruit and sugarcane extracts are not the same as AHAs, and the lemon extract can be irritating.

😐 **$$$ Face Cream Rehabilitating Cream, for Aging Skin** *($128 for 1.67 ounces)* offers normal to dry skin several rehabilitating ingredients, including good antioxidants and plant oils. However, the ylang ylang and geranium oils are bad news, and keep this moisturizer from being truly state-of-the-art.

😐 **$$$ Hydrating B5 Gel Moisture Enhancing Gel** *($55 for 1 ounce)* is a simple hydrating mix of a water-binding agent, vitamin B-5 (also known as panthenol), and a preservative. It is suitable for all skin types.

☹ **$$$ Intense Line Defense Potent Nighttime Line-Minimizing Treatment** *($50 for 1 ounce)* is another SkinCeuticals product claiming to exfoliate skin with fruit acids. That's not going to happen, at least not in the same manner and with the same benefits as using a well-formulated AHA or BHA product. Without the reliable exfoliation, you're left with mostly water, an antioxidant, slip agents, and preservatives. Not too intense after all!

☹ **$$$ Phyto Corrective Gel Calming Complexion Gel** *($45 for 1 ounce)* is a water-based serum whose water-binding agents can benefit all skin types, while the *Uva ursi* extract's arbutin content may have a positive impact on skin discolorations. This would be rated higher if not for the thyme extract and the nebulous "herbal fragrance."

☹ **Phyto + Botanical Gel, for Hyperpigmentation** *($65 for 1 ounce)* lists thyme extract as the second ingredient, which makes this arbutin-enhanced skin-lightening gel a problem for all skin types. Chemical components of thyme have been shown to be irritating for skin (Source: www.naturaldatabase.com).

☹ **$$$ Renew Overnight Dry Nighttime Skin-Refining Moisturizer, for Normal to Dry Skin** *($45 for 2 ounces)* provides more fruit acids masquerading as AHAs, while jar packaging ruins the effectiveness of the antioxidants in this moisturizer for normal to dry skin. For the money, you're better off investing in a separate AHA product and a stably packaged moisturizer with state-of-the-art ingredients.

☹ **$$$Renew Overnight Oily Nighttime Skin-Refining Moisturizer, for Normal or Oily Skin** *($45 for 2 ounces)* is a lighter-weight version of the Renew Overnight Dry Nighttime Skin-Refining Moisturizer above, and the same review applies, except that this is indeed better for normal to oily skin.

✓☺ **$$$ Retinol 0.5 Refining Night Cream with 0.5% Pure Retinol** *($42 for 1 ounce)* makes many anti-aging claims, and because it contains a significant amount of retinol the claims you can bank on are building collagen and stimulating cell regeneration. However, since other ingredients can also do that, or at least assist in the process, it's a bit overly optimistic to hang all your hopes on one specialized ingredient such as retinol. Fortunately, this water- and silicone-based serum does contain many other beneficial ingredients for healthy skin, including ceramides, cholesterol, lecithin, antioxidants, and the anti-irritant bisabolol. The opaque bottle with pump applicator helps maintain the stability of the retinol, which is a prerequisite for products with this ingredient. Retinol 0.5 is suitable for all skin types.

Getting back to the claims, SkinCeuticals boasts that this serum will also minimize pore size and correct blemishes. The first claim rests on a subjective judgment. The second claim that retinol is able to correct blemishes is at this point more theoretical than proven. In contrast, tretinoin (the active ingredient in Retin-A) has considerable research supporting its use as a prescription acne treatment. While it's definitely possible that using a retinol serum like this one will result in fewer blemishes, it's not as much of a sure thing as using a tretinoin product. The benefits of retinol versus tretinoin are that retinol has significantly fewer and comparably minor side effects, but the tradeoff is reduced efficacy (Source: *Cosmetic Dermatology*, volume 18, issue 1, supplement 1, January 2005, page 19). This product is not recommended for daytime application because it contains photosensitizing St. John's wort.

✓☺ **$$$ Retinol 1.0 Maximum Strength Refining Night Cream with 1.0% Pure Retinol** *($48 for 1 ounce)* is similar to the Retinol 0.5 product above, except it contains twice as much retinol. The same basic comments apply (including the one about St. John's wort), but a caution is warranted because using retinol at this level (1%) poses a slight risk of side effects that are similar to, but less pronounced than, those caused by topical tretinoin, including redness, flaking/peeling, and possibly stinging. These effects should be short-term as the skin acclimates to retinol, but if they do not dissipate or if they worsen with continued use, stop using the product; retinol at this level may not be right for your skin.

☺ **$$$ Serum 10 AOX+** *($60 for 1 ounce)* is a water-based serum that contains 10% L-ascorbic acid along with penetration-enhancing ingredients, stabilizers, and a couple of water-binding agents. SkinCeuticals added the antioxidant ferulic acid to their vitamin C serums because research has shown it helps boost efficacy, although the only research on topical application of these antioxidants was done in part by Dr. Pinnell (Source: *Journal of Investigative Dermatology*, October 2005, pages 826–832), so it's not exactly impartial. Still, there is enough research on ferulic acid's antioxidant effects when taken internally to rationalize (and further research) its use in skin-care products.

☺ **$$$ Serum 15 AOX+** *($80 for 1 ounce)* is identical to the Serum 10 AOX+ above, except this version provides 15% L-ascorbic acid. Keep in mind that this amount of vitamin C at the pH that's needed for it to be effective may prove more irritating than beneficial for skin (a fact SkinCeuticals mentions on their Web site and in literature for this product). This is not the type of product you'd want to use nightly with other products such as those with retinol, AHAs, BHA, or topical prescription retinoids because such a combination may send skin into irritation overload, so proceed cautiously to see how your skin reacts.

☺ **$$$ Serum 20 AOX+** *($100 for 1 ounce)* is similar to the Serum 10 AOX+ above, except this pricier version increases the vitamin C content to 20%. Otherwise, the same comments and precautions made for the two Serums above apply here, too. Interestingly, the latest research on formulating vitamin C into skin-care products shows that a thickened microemulsion, not a solution as used here, does a better job of keeping the antioxidants stable (Sources: *Drug Delivery*, April 2007, pages 235–245; and *Pharmaceutical Development and Technology*, November 2006, pages 255–261).

☹ **Skin Firming Cream** *($85 for 1.67 ounces)* lists sandalwood extract as the third ingredient, and also contains fragrant juniper oil, which makes this otherwise good but overpriced moisturizer a problem for all skin types.

😐 **$$$ Hydrating B5 Masque** *($45 for 2.5 ounces)* is an exceptionally boring mask that is absolutely not worth the money. The claims make it seem like the ultimate moisture oasis for dry, parched skin, but it is primarily water, glycerin, pH-adjusting agent, and gel-based thickener. Big deal!

😐 **$$$ Blemish Control Gel** *($32 for 1 ounce)* puts 1% salicylic acid in a smooth, gel-based formula that does not contain fragrance or needlessly irritating ingredients. What a letdown to realize the pH range of this product (pH 4.8–5.0, as confirmed by the company and our testing) will not permit the salicylic acid to work its magic effectively on blemishes.

☺ **$$$ Clarifying Clay Masque Deep Pore Cleansing Skin-Refining Masque** *($33 for 2 ounces)* is a standard, but good, clay mask for normal to very oily skin. The fruit and sugar extracts do not exfoliate skin like an AHA product would.

✓☺ **$$$ Antioxidant Lip Repair Restorative Treatment, for Damaged or Aging Lips** *($30 for 0.3 ounce)* has an interesting texture in an overall emollient formula that provides lips with an impressive selection of antioxidants, water-binding agents, and a peptide, which theoretically has cell-communicating ability. If you're going to spend this much for a lip product, it might as well be loaded with extras like this one is! However, this doesn't contain sunscreen, and so should only be used at night.

SKINCEUTICALS SUN PRODUCTS

☺ **$$$ Daily Sun Defense SPF 20** *($28 for 3 ounces)* has an in-part zinc oxide sunscreen and does not contain fragrance, but for all of SkinCeuticals talk about antioxidants (particularly vitamin C), it is disappointing that not a single antioxidant shows up in this sunscreen for normal to dry skin not prone to blemishes.

✓☺ **$$$ Physical UV Defense SPF 30** *($34 for 3 ounces)* improves on the Daily Sun Defense SPF 20 above by including a couple of antioxidants. This creamy sunscreen contains only titanium dioxide and zinc oxide as its active ingredients, making it an excellent choice for sensitive skin, including those with various forms of dermatitis and rosacea. It is fragrance-free.

☺ **$$$ Sans Soleil Moisturizing Sunless Tanner** *($30 for 5 ounces)* is a good self-tanning lotion for normal to dry skin. It combines dihydroxyacetone and the slower-acting erythrulose to turn skin brown, and also includes a tiny amount of antioxidant vitamins. This does contain fragrance.

✓☺ **$$$ Sports UV Defense SPF 45** *($34 for 3 ounces)* is a very good, in-part zinc oxide sunscreen for normal to very dry skin not prone to blemishes. The fragrance-free formula contains antioxidant vitamins that have proven to be positive additions to sunscreens.

☺ **$$$ Ultimate UV Defense SPF 30** *($34 for 3 ounces)* is very similar to the Daily Sun Defense SPF 20 above, except that this one contains the higher percentage of active ingredients necessary to attain an SPF 30 rating. Otherwise, the same comments apply.

SMASHBOX

SMASHBOX AT-A-GLANCE

Strengths: A fragrance-free gentle cleanser; a unique Anti-Shine product that is a must-try if you have very oily skin; mostly good foundations with a neutral range of shades; improved powder eyeshadows; the great Photo Finish Lipstick; a lash primer that really makes a difference; well-constructed makeup brushes that cost less than the department-store competition.

Weaknesses: A small, mostly boring assortment of products priced higher than they should be; a couple of products contain irritants that have no benefit for skin; several lackluster makeup categories, including concealer, blush, eye pencils, and brow shaders; the Cream Eyeliner is a mistake if you expect any amount of longevity; several specialty products that should offer more for the money (and the one with sunscreen leaves skin vulnerable to UVA damage); several products don't offer colors with enough impact to show up well on medium to dark skin tones.

For more information about Smashbox, call (888) 763-1361 or visit www.smashbox.com or www.Beautypedia.com.

SMASHBOX SKIN CARE

☺ **$$$ Cleanser** *($26 for 3 ounces)* is essentially a very expensive version of Cetaphil Gentle Skin Cleanser ($7.99 for 16 ounces). It does an OK job of removing makeup, but the thickening agents make this recommended only for normal to dry skin. It is fragrance-free, again, just like Cetaphil.

😐 **$$$ Eye Makeup Remover** *($14 for 4 ounces)* is a standard, detergent-based eye-makeup remover that would be rated higher if it did not contain fragrance. It works to remove all but waterproof or long-wearing formulas.

☹ **Call Time Skin and Makeup Refresher Spray** *($21 for 5.07 ounces)* offers skin a bevy of antioxidants and some good water-binding agents, but all of these are preceded by irritating witch hazel. This spray-on toner cannot create "melt-proof" makeup. There is no way this mixture can stand up to perspiration, your skin's oil, or humidity.

😐 **Moisturizer** *($34 for 3 ounces)* is an OK option for use under makeup if you have normal to dry skin not prone to breakouts, but this blend of water, thickeners, and glycerin is hardly interesting, though the omission of fragrance was a nice touch.

☹ **Emulsion Lip Exfoliant** *($18 for 0.75 ounce)* works to exfoliate dead, flaky skin on lips with its blend of plant oil and sugar. However, the inclusion of peppermint oil makes this scrub needlessly irritating. Mixing table sugar with a couple of drops of a non-fragrant plant oil would work too, and without the irritation.

SMASHBOX MAKEUP

FOUNDATION: Smashbox's main strengths lie in its foundations. The textures are a bit dated, but the foundations are worth a look, especially if you have fair to light skin (there are some good dark tones, too, just not as many).

☺ **$$$ Conversion Cream to Powder Foundation** *($32)* is a creamier cream-to-powder foundation with a silky-smooth application, yet a somewhat heavy-looking finish. You can achieve medium to full coverage, but the high wax content lends an opacity that tends to camouflage, rather than enhance, skin. Eleven shades are available, with the darker colors being particularly good. Watch out for the slightly pink shade 0 and keep in mind that shade 1 is bound to be too yellow for some fairer skin tones, while shade 4 is slightly peach. This is best for normal to slightly dry or slightly oily skin that's not prone to blemishes.

☺ **$$$ High Definition Healthy F/X Foundation SPF 15** *($38)* is said to be packed with anti-aging and firming ingredients that revitalize skin. The in-part titanium dioxide sunscreen deserves most of the credit for anti-aging (assuming you apply this daily and liberally), but nothing in this product will revitalize or firm skin. The silky, fluid texture is built around no fewer than six forms of silicone, and they ensure a smooth, even application that meshes well with skin, which is this foundation's strongest point. Blending takes longer than usual but is OK, and this sets to a soft satin finish appropriate for normal to slightly dry skin (even if it is prone to blemishes). You'll get medium coverage that looks surprisingly skinlike, and this wears quite well. Among the 12 mostly neutral shades, the only ones to consider carefully are Light L3 and Medium M3. There are no shades for fair or dark skin tones, but everyone in between should find a good match.

☺ **$$$ Wet/Dry Foundation** *($34)* is a talc-based, pressed-powder foundation that is much better used dry than wet. It has a reasonably smooth, slightly dry texture with light to medium coverage and a soft matte finish. There are nine mostly neutral shades that are predominantly best for fair to light skin tones, though Caramel and Cocoa are good, non-ashy shades for lighter African-American skin. The only shade to avoid is Sand, which is too peach for most skin tones.

☹ **Backdrop Cooling Tint SPF 15** *($32)* is a sheer-coverage foundation that contains an in-part avobenzone sunscreen and features eight suitably neutral shades for fair to dark skin. Unfortunately, the cooling effect comes from a significant amount of menthyl lactate, a menthol derivative that makes this foundation too irritating for all skin types, especially for use around the eyes.

😐 **$$$ Studio Seamless Liquid Foundation** *($34)* has become a dated liquid foundation when compared with the qualities of today's best silicone-enhanced foundations. This is the same formula as Smashbox's former generically named Liquid Foundation. The liquidy texture blends on evenly, allowing for light to medium coverage, and it has a satin finish suitable for normal to dry skin. However, it tends to lie on the skin rather than float, a newer and more flattering effect provided by competing products that have set a higher standard of quality. Of the 13 shades (including options for fair and dark skin tones), the colors to avoid are Oak 2.5, Natural 4, and the very peach Warm Beige 5. Ivory and Bisque 1.5 are excellent shades for fair skin, as is Petal 1.25, though its slightly pink cast may not work for some.

CONCEALER: 😐 **$$$ Camera Ready Full Coverage Concealer** *($18)* is a creamy, twist-up stick concealer that applies smoothly and blends well, though it remains moist and quickly settles into lines around the eye. Despite the name, this provides full coverage only if you pile it on—and that causes it to crease even more. This is still worth considering if you want a cream concealer and the eight shades are nearly impeccable (shade 1 is too white for just about anyone), but it must be set with powder to minimize the creasing.

BLUSH: 😐 **$$$ Skin Tint** *($28)* is a water-based stick blush that offers a very soft application of translucent color. I previously came down hard on this product because its texture and finish undermine foundation and powder, but it does have a place for those who go foundation-free, have poreless skin, and just want a hint of juicy color to rev up their complexion. Skin Tint is best for normal to dry skin; using this over even slightly oily cheeks will make your skin look too greasy, and applying this over large pores may make your skin look dotted with color.

😐 **$$$ Blush** *($24)* is a very standard, pressed-powder blush whose price tag is uncalled for. It applies nicely (though a bit too softly to register on darker skin tones or to make an impact under studio lights), but many of the colors are very shiny and the shine tends to flake. Whether you want a sheer or more pigmented powder blush, consider options from M.A.C. or Bobbi Brown before this.

😐 **$$$ O-Glow** *($26)*. Remember mood rings? The jewelry that changed color after being in contact with your skin? Smashbox tries to recapture that idea with a silicone-based clear blush they refer to as "intuitive" because "this clear gel reacts with your personal skin chemistry to turn cheeks the exact color you blush, naturally in just seconds!" Sounds like the perfect "natural blush," but the claim is bogus. Yes, this goes on clear and changes color as it blends—but it turns into the same translucent fuchsia hue on everyone. My office staff has a good range of skin tones, from fair to dark. I asked several women to sample this blush and let me know what color it turned on their skin, and did they think it matches how they blush naturally. All of them had the same color response (fuchsia) and none of them claimed to blush this shade (no one does). I admit, it's cool to watch a clear gel turn into a vibrant pink shade as you blend, and this has a smooth powder finish that lasts, but the color itself isn't personalized and the strong color isn't going to work for everyone.

EYESHADOW: ☺ **$$$ Single Eye Shadow** *($16)* has an impressively smooth texture that applies evenly, and only the shiniest shades are mildly prone to flaking (every color has some amount of shine). The only drawback (and for some this may be a plus) is that even the darkest shades tend to go on sheer, so building intensity takes some effort. The odd hues to avoid include Scan, JPEG, Green Room, Frame, Dream, and Digital.

☺ **$$$ Eye Shadow Trio** *($28)* has the same formula as the Single Eye Shadow above and the same comments apply. All three shades in each set have some degree of shine, though many are soft and suitable for daytime wear (assuming you have smooth, unlined eyelids). The most versatile combinations include Big Screen, Center Stage, and Head Shot. ☺ **$$$ Eyelights Palette** *($34)* presents three creamy-feeling powder eyeshadows in a compact. Each is laden with metallic shine, but they apply amazingly well and offer opaque coverage without flaking. Although not for everyone (and assuredly not for anyone with wrinkles around the eye), this is a dramatic evening eye-makeup option that wears well.

EYE AND BROW SHAPER: 😐 **$$$ Brow Tech** *($24)* is described by Smashbox as "the answer to everyone's prayers," but before you reconsider your pleas for world peace or that new car you've always wanted, consider that this is merely a split-pan compact with a shine-infused brow powder that you mix with the other half, which is a clear, thick wax. But no one needs shiny eyebrows, and the wax can look heavy and thick, not a look everyone will appreciate. 😐 **$$$ Brow Tech Wax** *($20)* is available separately and provides twice the amount of product as the regular Brow Tech, just without the powder brow color.

☹ **Cream Eye Liner** *($22)* is an interesting notion that sounds better than it ends up being. In the "pro" column, these do go on very smoothly and intensely. The "cons" include their tendency to fade, smear, and run with the slightest blink or smile, which makes them not worth the effort, especially at this price. For a superior version of this product, consider the silicone-enhanced Gel Eyeliners available from Bobbi Brown, Stila, M.A.C., Trish McEvoy, and my line. The same review applies to Smashbox's ☹ **Cream Eye Liner Palette** *($32)*, which provides ten shades (tiny amounts of each) in one sleek compact.

LIPSTICK, LIP GLOSS, AND LIPLINER: ☺ **$$$ Photo Finish Lipstick with Sila-Silk Technology** *($22)* is a very emollient, almost greasy cream lipstick with an unusual gloss finish that provides a multidimensional, wet-look shine. The shade selection is well edited yet still manages to offer an impressive range, including some great reds and pinks. The Sila-Silk portion is supposed to lend a unique silky feel to this lipstick, but the ingredients that precede it lend a thicker, moist feel rather than creating a sensation of silkiness.

😐 **$$$ Lip Brilliance** *($28)* is a three-color lip palette that proclaims "the coverage of a lipstick, the smooth feel of a gloss," and this turns out to be partially true. Although this emollient lipstick/gloss hybrid offers full coverage, the texture is thick and sticky, and for the money this is not preferred to using a standard gloss over a good creamy lipstick.

😐 **$$$ Lip Treatment SPF 15** *($16)* does not contain sufficient UVA protection and so cannot be relied on for sun protection. It is otherwise a standard, castor oil–based lip balm in lipstick form that softens dry lips and adds a glossy shine.

😐 **Lip Pencil** *($14)* is a standard pencil with a creamy, but firm, texture and a cream finish that's a bit too short-lived, though the colors are versatile.

MASCARA: ✓☺ **$$$ Layer Lash Primer** *($16)* is one of a handful of lash primers that actually do make a difference, even when used with an already-outstanding mascara. The effect (especially with the best mascaras) isn't night-and-day, but if you're looking to eke a bit more out of your usual mascara, this product is a decent add-on—and that's a refreshing change of pace! One of the reasons it works where others fail is that its conditioning formula keeps lashes soft and flexible while at the same time allowing a regular mascara to adhere evenly to already-pumped-up lashes.

☺ **$$$ That's a Wrap Mascara** *($18)* makes much ado about the "advanced ingredients" and wheat protein it contains to condition and moisturize lashes, but this contains the same roster of ingredients seen in almost every mascara, namely waxes and thickeners. The wheat protein is present in such a tiny amount that your lashes won't notice it's there, but that's OK because several other ingredients do a great job of keeping lashes soft and flexible during wear. Performance-wise, That's a Wrap applies easily, separates lashes well, and lengthens without much thickness. If you prefer mascaras that primarily lengthen without clumping or smudging, this is recommended—but be aware that the same benefit can be had for less money from several drugstore mascaras.

😐 **$$$ Focal Point Lash Building Mascara** *($18)* allows you to gradually build length, but you'll be hard pressed to create thicker lashes, and attempting to do so results in some clumping. Although this is an OK option for making lashes longer, it doesn't compete with the best of what Maybelline New York and L'Oreal have to offer. 😐 **$$$ Limitless Lash** *($22)* is a dual-sided product with one end being a decent lengthening waterproof mascara that isn't as waterproof as it should be and the other being a silicone-based mascara remover applied with a brush. The remover works to dissolve the mascara, but you'll still need to use a regular remover or cleanser to get everything off, and the wand quickly becomes coated with used mascara, which gets kind of gross after a few uses.

FACE AND BODY ILLUMINATING/SHIMMER PRODUCTS: ☺ **$$$ Soft Lights** *($28)* is a smooth-textured pressed shimmer powder that blends beautifully and clings better than expected. The shine ranges from subtle (Glow and Hue) to Las Vegas–caliber glitz. ☺ **$$$ Fusion Soft Lights** *($30)* are nearly identical to the regular Soft Lights, but feature individual strips of color in one unit that can be applied separately or swirled together for a high-shine effect that appears almost glossy (but feels powder dry).

☺ **$$$ Eye Illusion** *($32)* provides four pastel pressed powders in one large component with dividers between each shade. They have a nice, soft texture that applies evenly and leaves a prismatic shine. It is recommended that you use one or more shades over a medium to deep eyeshadow to change the color and light reflection. It does have an interesting effect for evening wear, assuming you want to make your existing eyeshadow a more shiny, pastel shade.

😐 **$$$ Artificial Light Luminizing Lotion** *($30)* has a very silky, fluid feel and produces a shimmer that's softly metallic. It's an OK option for shine, but because this stays moist it is prone to rubbing off and fading. For this amount of money, there should be no drawbacks, and overall this isn't worth considering over better, longer-lasting options from Lorac, Revlon, or Make Up For Ever.

BRUSHES: The assortment of **Brushes** *($18–$52)* is more realistically priced than those of other artistry-based lines, and there are some expert options to consider, all with snazzy red lacquered handles that visually set them apart from the standard black of other lines.

The ones to consider are the ☺ **$$$ #3 Blending** *($32)*, ☺ **$$$ #12 Angle Brow** *($20)*, ✓☺ **$$$ #15 Crease Brush** *($28)*, **#10 Crease Brush** *($28)*, ☺ **$$$ Face & Body Brush** *($52)*, and ☺ **$$$ #9 Cream Eye Liner** *($20)*, the last being one of the better types of this brush around because it's thin enough to use for both upper and lower lashlines and you can make the line as thin or thick as you like using almost any eyeshadow. For those so inclined, Smashbox's synthetic-hair ✓☺ **$$$ #13 Foundation Brush** *($34)* is one of the better brushes of its type available, and the price is comparable to those of most other lines, while the ✓☺ **$$$ #11 Crease Liner Brush** *($30)* is brilliant for detailed shading.

SPECIALTY PRODUCTS: ✓☺ **$$$ Anti-Shine** *($27)* remains an intriguing product. It is mostly water and magnesium with a hint of color (a colorless version is also available). Magnesium (as in Phillips' Milk of Magnesia) absorbs oil very well and does not feel as heavy on the skin as clays do. This formula goes on extremely matte and dry and has great staying power; it is definitely worth trying if you have oily to very oily skin, and it works well with a matte-finish foundation. Anti-Shine may be applied under or over foundation to keep oiliness in check.

☺ **$$$ Compact Anti-Shine** *($28)* has the same oil-absorbing, matte-finish goals as the Anti-Shine above, except this variation mixes silicone and talc with waxes to keep it in solid form. The wax content reduces the amount of time skin stays shine-free, and also isn't the best to use over blemishes. However, this is a workable option if you need only modest shine control and prefer a portable version.

😐 **$$$ Lip & Lid Primer** *($24)* is a dual-sided product with both ends approximating creamy concealers. One end is for the eyelid area while the other is for filling in lines on the lips and creating longer-lasting lip color. Although both sides smooth things out and provide coverage, neither takes the place of a regular concealer (and one that's semi-matte to matte for the eyes, because this one stays too creamy). The lip end has minimal "priming" benefit, and can mix with a lipstick for unattractive results.

😐 **$$$ Photo Finish Foundation Primer** *($36)* is a colorless, silicone-based serum that has little going for it other than being a decent lightweight moisturizer that makes your skin feel smooth, and that can help ensure a semi-matte finish when paired with a matte-finish liquid or powder foundation.

😐 **$$$ Photo Finish Color Correcting Foundation Primer** *($38)* is a pure silicone–based primer that, like others of its ilk, can make skin feel very silky and appear matte. Such an even canvas can facilitate makeup application, but this Smashbox product offers three strangely tinted shades meant to correct uneven skin tones (such as redness, sallowness, and so on). Thankfully, the peach and lavender shades are so sheer the color change is minimal, meaning that your foundation won't look strange when used with them. However, the green shade has too much color, and gives skin an odd, alien hue that substitutes one problem for another. These are not preferred to Smashbox's other Photo Finish primers.

😐 **$$$ Photo Finish Bronzing Foundation Primer** *($38)* is similar to the Photo Finish Foundation Primer above, only with a sheer bronze tint that doesn't leave any shine behind. It's an OK option if you want to try Smashbox's primers and have medium to dark skin.

😐 **$$$ Photo Finish Foundation Primer SPF 15 with Dermaxyl Complex** *($42)* does not contain sufficient UVA protection, so the sun protection claims cannot be relied on, and that's never a good sign for an anti-aging product. This silicone-based primer does contain several antioxidants, but the translucent glass packaging won't help keep them stable, so that's a loss as well. The Dermaxyl complex is a trademark of ingredient manufacturer Sederma. The key ingredient is palmitoyl oligopeptide and although this has potentially intriguing benefits for skin, the amount Smashbox includes doesn't measure up to the quantity Sederma recommends for efficacy. That means, at best, that the peptide functions as a water-binding agent, making this Smashbox primer slightly more hydrating than the ones above—but the price is unwarranted.

😐 **$$$ Filter with Dermaxl Complex** *($28)* has a formula that's similar to the original Photo Finish Foundation Primer above, but contains the peptide found in the Dermaxyl Complex as well as a high amount of film-forming agent. The product is intended for use around the eyes and lips and is dispensed through an angled-tip applicator. It can temporarily smooth and minimally fill in lines around the eyes, but how long the effect lasts depends on how expressive you are. This doesn't fulfill all its promises, but may be worth testing to see if you like the results—just keep in mind that they are temporary.

☹ **$$$ Photo Op Under Eye Brightener** *($18)* is a concealer/highlighter combination product applied with a brush. It imparts sheer to light coverage for minor flaws and leaves obvious sparkles on skin (that's the "brightening" part). Smashbox recommends using this with a concealer, which is a good idea if you need more than meager coverage. In photographs, the amount of shine this leaves behind may prove to be too much, and it's definitely overkill for daytime makeup.

☹ **Brush Cleaner** *($15)* uses primarily water, alcohol, and surfactants to break down built-up makeup and allow it to be rinsed off your brushes. This spray-on product has a low alcohol content, meaning it's mostly water, and that means brushes take some time to dry. I wouldn't choose this method over occasionally shampooing my brushes, toweling them off, and letting them dry overnight, but I suppose some will find this method more convenient.

SONIA KASHUK

SONIA KASHUK AT-A-GLANCE

Strengths: Affordable and widely available (though exclusive to Target stores); impressive skin-care products from a makeup-oriented line; some very good cleansers; good makeup remover; antioxidant-based serum; facial moisturizers with sunscreen provide sufficient UVA protection; great self-tanner; the makeup is still the star attraction, with impressive options for foundation, powder, blush, lip color, and especially makeup brushes.

Weaknesses: No AHA or BHA products or options for those with blemishes; jar packaging; lip balm with sunscreen does not contain the right UVA-protecting ingredients; the concealers, eye pencil, and brow shapers are a letdown; the makeup palettes may seem convenient, but several of the included products are perform poorly.

For more information about Sonia Kashuk, sold exclusively at Target, visit www.target.com or www.Beautypedia.com.

SONIA KASHUK SKIN CARE

✓☺ **Cleanse Tri-Active Cleanser** *($10.99 for 6 ounces)* doesn't really have any toning benefits, but is nevertheless a very good, fragrance-free, water-soluble cleanser for all skin types except very oily. It is adept at removing makeup without leaving skin feeling dry.

☺ **$$$ Wash Facial Cleansing Cloths** *($7.99 for 10 cloths)* work well to remove makeup on all skin types, but you get so few of these detergent-soaked cloths that they end up being the most expensive version of this format at mass-market stores.

✓☺ **Remove Eye Makeup Remover** *($9.99 for 4 ounces)* is a simple, water- and silicone-based makeup remover, but it works beautifully to remove all types of long-wearing makeup and wins extra points for being fragrance-free and including no extraneous ingredients except a tiny amount of coloring agent.

☺ **Polish Exfoliant Face Wash** *($12.99 for 4 ounces)* is a cleanser/scrub hybrid that contains diatomaceous earth as the abrasive agent. As a result, this is a grittier scrub that must be used gently. It's best for normal to oily skin.

☹ **Enhance Firming Eye Cream** *($14.99 for 0.5 ounce)* treats skin to several antioxidants, but they won't hold up for long thanks to jar packaging. This is otherwise a decent emollient moisturizer for dry skin anywhere on the face, and it is fragrance-free.

✓☺ **Repair Vitamin Enriched Serum** *($18.99 for 0.5 ounce)* is a very good, fragrance-free antioxidant serum for normal to dry skin. The salicylic acid will not function as an exfoliant because the pH is too high, but every other aspect makes it deserving of strong consideration.

😐 **Replenish Essential Face Cream SPF 15** *($17.99 for 1.8 ounces)* will provide UVA protection thanks to its in-part avobenzone sunscreen (listed by its chemical name of butyl methoxydibenzoylmethane), but would be a better option for normal to dry skin if it did not use jar packaging. As is, the antioxidant potential will be lost shortly after the product is opened.

😐 **Restore Intense Moisture Creme** *($17.99 for 1.8 ounces)* is a wonderfully rich moisturizer for dry to very dry skin, but the antioxidant oils and vitamins will be compromised due to jar packaging. This does contain fragrance.

😐 **Block SPF 30 Sunscreen** *($14.99 for 4 ounces)* includes avobenzone for sufficient UVA protection, but has a lackluster formula for normal to dry skin. The low alcohol content is only slight cause for concern, but it still diminishes the effectiveness of the tiny amounts of antioxidants.

✓☺ **Bronze Sunless Tanner** *($14.99 for 2.4 ounces)* is an excellent, fragrance-free self-tanning lotion that can be enjoyed by all skin types. It contains dihydroxyacetone and slower-acting erythrulose to turn skin a shade of brown.

☹ **Smooth Lip Balm SPF 15** *($4.99 for 0.10 ounce)* makes lips feel smooth, but leaves them vulnerable to UVA damage because it lacks the UVA-protecting ingredients of titanium dioxide, zinc oxide, avobenzone, Mexoryl SX (ecamsule), or Tinosorb.

SONIA KASHUK MAKEUP

FOUNDATION: ✓☺ **Dual Coverage Powder Foundation** *($10.49)* has a very smooth, talc-based texture that applies sheerer than most pressed-powder foundations and looks natural. The soft, dry finish is best for normal to oily skin, and five shades are available. Linen and Sand tend to turn slightly peach, but are workable, while Ivory is suitable for fair skin and Honey for medium to slightly tan skin tones.

☺ **Radiant Tinted Moisturizer SPF 15** *($11.99)* was formerly known as Hydro-Tint SPF 15, and although the name has changed, the product hasn't. This remains a lightweight tinted moisturizer with an in-part avobenzone sunscreen. It has a cushiony, moist texture on application, but sets to a soft matte finish with the tiniest hint of shine. You'll achieve soft color and very sheer coverage from each of the three shades, all of them outstanding. This formula is best for normal to dry skin. Those with oily or blemish-prone skin will not appreciate the short-lived matte finish, and the thickeners and waxes aren't the best over breakout-prone areas.

☺ **Perfecting Liquid Foundation** *($10.49)* is a very sheer- to light-coverage, dewy finish, liquid foundation for someone with normal to dry skin. It has a great soft texture thanks to the significant amounts of silicone and mineral oil. Six shades are available, and five are nicely neutral and worth considering by light to medium skin tones. Camel is an OK option that may be too orange for some medium skin tones. Note: The color visible through the bottle does not resemble the product after it has dried on skin, which makes choosing the best shade a bit tricky.

CONCEALER: 😐 **Hidden Agenda Concealer Palette** *($9.99)* provides three shades of creamy concealer and one shade of pressed powder in a single compact. The concealer is slightly thick but applies smoothly and covers well. It would be better if it didn't look so heavy with the supplied powder applied over it; a sheerer powder would have worked much better (and the concealer needs to be set with powder to minimize creasing and fading). You'll find only one of the concealer shades is needed, but the range of shades is workable for fair to light/medium skin tones.

😐 **Confidential Concealer with Brightening Pencil** *($6.99)* is a liquid concealer that's so sheer it barely makes a difference if covering dark circles is your goal. It blends well but leaves a shiny finish and is only appropriate for highlighting. The opposite end of this brush-applied concealer is a creamy, retractable pencil that's flesh-toned and loaded with shine. It doesn't so much brighten skin as add sparkles, although they do tend to stay in place.

☹ **Take Cover Concealing Stick** *($7.99)* is a lipstick-style concealer that offers four shades, but you cannot see the color without breaking the product open, and the shade swatches at the Kashuk display aren't that accurate. Not only does this have an unpleasantly thick texture, it also finishes slightly sticky and creases almost instantly. Getting back to the shades, the only acceptable color is Dusk; the others are too pink, peach, or olive to consider.

POWDER: ✓☺ Bare Minimum Pressed Powder *($8.99)* comes in three soft, neutral colors best for fair to light skin tones, and it has a sublimely silky texture and seamless application. This is one of those rare talc-based powders that look very skinlike and enhance the complexion rather than dulling it or making skin look too matte and powdery. Well done!

☺ **Barely There Loose Powder** *($8.99)* remains one of the most elegant and gossamer loose powders you'll find in this price range. Its finely milled, silky texture blends beautifully on skin and it comes in three very good colors, best for fair to light skin tones. Two caveats: This contains cornstarch, which can (in theory) be problematic for those with blemishes, and now features a slightly shiny finish, which isn't ideal if you're using powder to temper shine. This powder is best for normal to dry skin.

✓☺ **Pressed Powder Bronzer** *($8.99)* has the same formula and positive traits as the Bare Minimum Pressed Powder above, save for the addition of a sheer shimmer finish. The golden bronze color is perfect for light to medium skin tones, and this applies softly yet builds well for more intensity.

☺ **Loose Powder Bronzer** *($8.99)* has a more noticeable shine than the Pressed Powder Bronzer above, and the loose format keeps it from clinging to skin as well. This is still an extraordinarily light-textured bronzing powder whose sheer hue is workable for fair to barely medium skin tones.

BLUSH: ✓☺ Beautifying Blush *($7.99)* is a pressed-powder blush with a super-smooth, non-powdery application and a collection of mostly sheer colors. Building intensity with this blush requires effort, but it's a good option for a hint of color. The matte shades include Nude, Flamingo, Spice, and Pink.

☺ **Cheeker Sheers Blush Gelstick** *($7.99)* is more emollient than gel-like, imparting translucent color with a kick (meaning the finish is see-through but the color is readily apparent). Best for normal to very dry skin, this blends well and remains moist to the touch. It is worth considering if your cheeks need a pick-me-up glow and one of the two shades appeals to you.

☺ **Creme Duo Blush** *($8.99)* is definitely creamy, but feels surprisingly light. It smooths over skin without too much slip (which makes blending easier) and sets to a moist, satiny finish suitable for dry to very dry skin. One shade is sans shimmer, while the other has less color and more glow. Used alone or mixed, the result is dewy-fresh cheeks.

☹ **Brush Up On Color** *($12.99)* requires some assembly, as this is a kit that comes with two tiny jars of loose-powder blush and a retractable brush. You're supposed to open one of the containers (the second is a refill) and screw it onto the base of the applicator. It is then dispensed onto the brush, ready to apply. I don't understand why this couldn't come pre-assembled, or at least have been more thoughtfully designed, because it ends up being very messy. Additionally, the loose powder imparts more shine than color, and the shine clings poorly.

EYESHADOW: ☺ **Enhance Eye Color** *($5.99)* represents Kashuk's single eyeshadows and they have a silky, dry application and sheer color deposit that layers well for more intensity. Most of the shades have a slight shimmer, but if you're looking for matte the choices include Opal, Sadeye Pink, and Sable. ☺ **Eye Shadow Duo** *($7.99)* has a slightly different formula than the Enhance Eye Color above; it's less dry and slightly creamy, but still applies smoothly and softly. One shade in each duo is shiny (many duos feature two shiny shades), but it's subtle (more subtle than it appears in the compact) and doesn't flake. ☺ **Eye Shadow Quad** *($12.99)* offers four coordinated eyeshadows in one compact, and the same formula, texture, and application comments mentioned for the Eye Shadow Duo above apply here, too. The colors include options for highlighting, contouring, and eyelining, making these practical kits. Most of the sets have at least one shiny shade, but it's low-key and suitable for daytime makeup.

😐 **Shake & Shimmer Loose Eye Powder** *($4.99)* is packaged in a tiny jar with a sifter and is essentially a way to add lots of glimmering, multicolored shine to the eye area (or elsewhere) if only it clung better to skin! If you decide to try this, it is recommended only for evening glamour.

EYE AND BROW SHAPER: 😐 **Brow Kit** *($9.99)* includes four shades of creamy, sheer brow wax (for blondes, redheads, and brunettes) and two unbelievably small applicators: a wedge brow brush to apply the wax and a mascara-type wand to groom brows. The wax doesn't do much to enhance brows and the colors are too soft for any real definition, while the tools are difficult to work with when compared to full-size brushes. If you try this you'll most likely only need one shade; why these weren't offered as stand-alone colors (without the nearly useless applicators) is a mystery. 😐 **Brow Definer** *($5.99)* is worth considering if you don't mind keeping it sharpened. This dry but not stiff brow pencil supplies soft color and a smooth powder finish that won't smear or run. What a shame the shade selection is so limited!

☹ **Eye Definer** *($5.99)* is a substandard pencil that needs routine sharpening, and the oil-based formula tends to fade and smudge without much provocation. Kashuk's powder eyeshadows (in the brown, black, or gray colors) are much better choices for eyelining.

LIPSTICK, LIP GLOSS, AND LIPLINER: ✓☺ **Tinted Lip Balm** *($5.99)* has a lush, almost creamy texture that is completely non-sticky yet leaves lips with a light wash of glossy color. The shades go on much sheerer than they appear in the compact, so don't let their boldness make you nervous—this is one of the more elegant-feeling lip balms around, and well-suited for handling chapping and dryness.

☺ **Luxury Lip Color** *($7.99)* is a good cross between a gloss and an opaque lipstick. It gives good coverage but has a very slippery, glossy finish. The latest packaging features an improved color swatch that is an accurate representation of how the color will appear on lips. The shades that begin with "Sheer" are indeed softer, more translucent colors.

☺ **Lip Palette** *($11.99)* used to contain shades that had an intensity truer to traditional lipstick, but now four of the five shades are very sheer and resemble a soft-textured, non-sticky lip gloss. One shade, while still glossy, imparts noticeable color, but this palette is only for gloss fans who don't mind routine touch-ups. The included brush is a decent option. ☺ **Lip Gloss** *($7.99)* has a great, smooth feel and a non-sticky finish. The sheer shades are sparkle-filled, yet lips don't feel grainy even after a few hours of wear, which is a plus! Also worth mentioning are the brush applicator and the built-in, almost colorless automatic lipliner. I assume the liner is meant to keep the gloss from feathering into lines around the mouth, but it isn't a formidable border.

☺ **Lip Definer** *($5.99)* has a creamy, oil-based formula that's nearly identical to the Eye Definer above, but the creaminess is not a problem for the lips, unless lipstick feathering into lines around the mouth is an issue. There aren't many colors available, but they cover the basics and are versatile.

MASCARA: ☺ **Lashify Mascara** *($7.99)* loses its Paula's Pick rating because the bar for mascaras has been raised by several mascaras from competing lines with the same price point. However, this is still worth considering if you need a mascara that's better at lengthening than thickening and that wears well without a flake or smear. The packaging now includes a built-in metal lash comb that, while not my personal favorite (plastic combs are safer), works well to add separation to lashes. ☺ **Lashify Mascara with Liner** *($7.99)* is identical to the Lashify Mascara above except, instead of the metal lash comb, the opposite end of the component houses an automatic, retractable pencil eyeliner. The creamy-smooth texture glides on but is meant to be smudged (before that happens on its own). ☺ **Lashify Mascara Waterproof** *($7.99)* performs almost as well as the non-waterproof Lashify Mascara, and offers a bit more oomph than many waterproof mascaras (and this one is definitely waterproof). Consider this if you don't want much lash drama, but foresee tears or a rainstorm.

BRUSHES: Sonia Kashuk offers several professional makeup **Brushes** *($7.99–$19.99)*, with the latest versions having ergonomically designed handles and a polished, futuristic look that's eye-catching. Almost all of them are recommended and a bona fide beauty bargain at these prices. The top choices include ✓☺ **Contoured Large Eye Shadow Brush** *($12.99)*, ✓☺ **Contoured Small Eye Shadow Brush** *($9.99)*, ✓☺ **Contoured Powder Brush** *($19.99)*, and ✓☺ **Contoured/Angled Eye Shadow Brush** *($9.99)*, which also works to fill in and define all but very thin brows. Also recommended is the retractable ✓☺ **Travel Blush Brush** *($9.99)*, which can also be used to apply powder on-the-go.

Avoid the ☹ **Lash and Brow Groomer** *($7.99)* with its sketchy metal lash comb and stiff brow brush.

☺ **Ultimate Brush Set** *($29.99)* includes six full-size brushes plus an eyelash curler in a zippered case. Although randomly available at Target stores, if you locate this set (or purchase it from www.target.com), it's a workable, affordable option with nicely shaped, soft, full brushes. It's not the "ultimate," but it does cover the basics, minus a lip brush.

☺ **Deluxe Travel Brush Set** *($19.99)* is actually nicer than the more expensive Ultimate Brush Set above, except for some odd reason this set lacks a blush brush. There are brushes for powder, shadow, eyelining, or defining brows, as well as a lip brush and mascara comb/brow brush, all in a sleek case with holders for each brush. You could purchase a blush brush separately and squeeze it into this set to make it complete for travel or day-to-day use.

☺ **8-Piece Travel Brush Roll** *($19.99)* is identical to the Deluxe Travel Brush Set except the brushes are housed in a metallic, foldable pouch instead of a hard case. You'll save space for travel, and the zippered side bag is nice for smaller items like pencils and mascara, or even cotton swabs.

The 😐 **Purse Brush Set** *($12.99)* is an OK collection that's about the size of a credit card but thicker. Included are four very small brushes (one for powder, one for eyeshadow, one for concealer, and one for brows or liner). Consider this if you need a very basic set to keep in your desk drawer or weekend travel bag.

SPECIALTY PRODUCTS: ✓☺ **Oil Blotting Papers** *($6.99 for 100 sheets)* are tissue paper–style white blotting papers that work quite well, and they're sized larger than most, which means they aren't the most discrete option to tuck into an evening bag. However, you can mop up more shine with a single sheet, so that may make these more appealing—and the price is right!

If you're looking to curl your lashes, consider Kashuk's well-designed plastic and rubber ☺ **Dramatic Definition Travel Eyelash Curler** *($9.99)* or the traditional metal with rubber pad ☺ **Dramatically Defining Eyelash Curler** *($9.99)*.

😐 **Bronzer** *($8.99)* is a cream-to-powder bronzer with a wonderfully smooth application and a delicate, satin-like finish, but the sole shade is too peachy orange for just about everyone, at least if your intent is to mimic a suntan. It's better as a blush, but you may still need to mix it with a pink or rose tone for proper color balance.

The 😐 **Face Palette** *($15.99)* is smaller and less comprehensive than it used to be, and the product quality has degraded a bit. Housed in a flat, 3 x 5 compact are three eyeshadows, two lip glosses, two shades of cream concealer, a powder blush, and a thin, needs-sharpening brow pencil. The powder eyeshadows tend to apply unevenly and flake a lot, the creamy concealers are crease-prone but cover well, the pencil is just average, and the powder blush is the best product, but it's available separately for less money. The fact that these palettes are named after hair colors is meaningless. For example, all of the nude tones in the Blonde palette would work just as well for a brunette, as would the peachier hues from the Auburn palette.

SOVAGE
(SEE BREMENN RESEARCH LABS)

ST. IVES (SKIN CARE ONLY)

ST. IVES AT-A-GLANCE

Strengths: Inexpensive; a couple of water-soluble cleansers; the eye gel.

Weaknesses: Overly abrasive scrubs; ineffective anti-acne products; no sunscreens; dated moisturizer; overall, the products are substandard, even if they are inexpensive.

For more information about St. Ives, call (800) 333-0005 or visit www.stives.com or www.Beautypedia.com.

☺ **Apricot Face Wash, for Blemish & Blackhead Control** *($3.99 for 6.5 ounces)* cannot control blemishes and blackheads because its 2% salicylic acid will be washed down the drain before it can penetrate the pore and go to work. This cleanser/scrub is still a good, water-soluble option for normal to oily skin, but it won't control blackheads, blemishes, or anything else.

☺ **Apricot Radiance Age-Defying Cream Cleanser Oil-Free, for Younger Looking Skin** *($4.99 for 6.5 ounces)* can be a great water-soluble cleanser for normal to dry skin, but there isn't anything in here to make skin look younger or to defy age in any manner. Oddly, St. Ives includes over a dozen antioxidants in this cleanser; they're of little use to skin in a cleanser, however, because they are just rinsed down the drain.

☹ **Apricot Radiance Blemish-Fighting Cream Cleanser with Salicylic Acid Oil-Free, for Oily/Blemish Prone Skin** *($4.99 for 6.5 ounces)* has much in common with the Apricot

Radiance Age-Defying Cream Cleanser above, except this version contains salicylic acid, tea tree extract, and cornmeal to make it a cleanser/scrub. The salicylic acid won't do a thing to fight blemishes because it is rinsed from the skin too soon and the amount included is too small. This isn't recommended because it contains the irritating menthol derivative menthyl lactate. Tea tree oil in this amount and in a rinse-off product is also not effective.

☹ **Apricot Radiance Deep Cleaning Cream Cleanser Oil-Free, for Combination Skin** *($4.99 for 6.5 ounces)* is nearly identical to the Apricot Radiance Blemish-Fighting Cream Cleanser with Salicylic Acid Oil-Free, for Oily/Blemish Prone Skin above, and the same review applies.

☺ **Apricot Radiance Moisture Rich Cream Cleanser, for Normal to Dry Skin** *($4.99 for 6.5 ounces)* is a good, water-soluble cleanser for normal to very dry skin, but it requires a washcloth for complete removal.

😐 **Apricot Shower Cleanser/Mask, 2-in-1 Formula** *($3.29 for 4.75 ounces)* contains more clay than cleansing agent, and how that is supposed to work with the heat of your shower to deep-clean skin is a mystery. This has merit as an absorbent cleanser for oily skin, but is not ideal for removing makeup.

😐 **Makeup Remover & Facial Cleanser** *($2.50 for 6 ounces)* is a somewhat greasy cleansing lotion that certainly removes makeup, but the residue it leaves behind doesn't make this preferred to a water-soluble cleanser unless you have very dry skin.

☹ **Apricot Scrub Blemish & Blackhead Control with Salicylic Acid, for Oily/Acne Prone Skin** *($3.49 for 6 ounces)* has too many negatives to make it a worthy contender in the facial scrub category. Walnut shells and cornmeal can be too abrasive and tear skin, the amount of sodium lauryl sulfate is drying and irritating, and the volatile fragrance components prompt further irritation. Salicylic acid at 2% is listed as an active ingredient, but it's pointless to include this ingredient in a rinse-off product.

😐 **Apricot Scrub Gentle, for Sensitive Skin** *($3.49 for 6 ounces)* contains the same abrasive agents as the Apricot Scrub above, just less of them. I suppose that makes this the milder choice, but it is still not preferred over gentler facial scrubs or a washcloth with a gentle, water-soluble cleanser. This version omits the sodium lauryl sulfate and does contain a more gentle cleansing agent.

☹ **Apricot Scrub Invigorating, for All Skin Types** *($3.49 for 6 ounces)* is similar to the Apricot Scrub Blemish and Blackhead Control with Salicylic Acid above, except this version does not contain salicylic acid. Otherwise, the same problems exist, so the same review applies.

😐 **Apricot Scrub Renew & Firm Gentle Alpha Hydroxy Complex, for Age-Defying** *($3.29 for 6 ounces)* is a fairly gentle scrub primarily because it contains just a tiny amount of abrasive walnut shell powder and because what's listed before it provides a buffering effect. This can be an OK scrub for normal to dry skin.

😐 **Collagen-Elastin Essential Moisturizers** *($4.69 for 12 ounces)* is about as basic a facial moisturizer for normal to dry skin as you're likely to find at the drugstore. Most cosmetics companies have long since given up claiming that collagen and elastin can reduce wrinkles when applied topically. Why hasn't St. Ives?

☺ **Cucumber & Elastin Eye and Face Stress Gel** *($3.49 for 4 ounces)* is a surprisingly good lightweight moisturizing gel for slightly dry skin. It contains some soothing plant extracts and enough water-binding agents to provide sufficient hydration. The inclusion of fragrance makes this a lesser choice for use around the eyes.

☹ **Peel Off Hydroxy Masque** *($3.29 for 6 ounces)* lists two forms of drying, irritating alcohols as main ingredients, and the BHA and AHA cannot exfoliate skin because the pH of this poorly formulated mask is too high.

STILA

STILA AT-A-GLANCE

Strengths: Two very good sunscreens, each providing sufficient UVA protection, and one of which is fragrance-free; inexpensive for a department-store/boutique line; the foundations are remarkable in most respects, especially shade selection and texture; excellent concealers; bronzing powder with sunscreen; very good options for blush and eyeshadow; Major Lash Mascara really wows; the Brow Polish and Lip Shine are standouts; several attractive, versatile shimmer products; great makeup brushes.

Weaknesses: Everything else in the skin-care selection, because the rest of the products contain irritating fragrant oils in amounts that should not be taken lightly; Convertible Eye Color and Kajal Eye Liner have too many weaknesses; some problematic lip glosses; the lip pencils are average at best.

For more information about Stila, call (866) 415-1332 or visit www.stilacosmetics.com or www.Beautypedia.com.

STILA PETAL INFUSIONS SKIN CARE

☹ **Petal Infusions H2Off** *($18 for 40 cloths)* are below-standard cleansing cloths because they contain several irritating fragrant oils, including bergamot, orange, and lavender. Given that the solution on the cloths is not designed to be rinsed, that's a problem, because you don't want to leave those irritating ingredients on your skin.

☹ **Petal Infusions Eye Make Up Dissolver** *($20 for 90 pads)* may have a lovely floral smell, but because these pads are for your eye area, it doesn't make sense (and isn't a good thing) that they contain lavender and rosewood oils.

☹ **Petal Infusions Retexturizing Scrub** *($22 for 2.5 ounces)* is an abrasive scrub that contains calcium carbonate (chalk) as the main ingredient. Although this is an option if used very gently, the addition of lemon and orange oil makes this an ill-advised scrub for all skin types.

☹ **Petal Infusions Moisturizer, for Dry Skin** *($30 for 1.7 ounces)* contains enough rose flower and lavender oils to make this too irritating for all skin types. The citrus oil is less of an issue, but still has no benefit beyond providing fragrance.

☹ **Petal Infusions Moisturizer, for Normal Skin** *($30 for 1.7 ounces)* contains lavender, grapefruit, and rosewood oils, all with volatile components that can irritate skin—and, in the case of grapefruit oil, cause a phototoxic reaction when skin is exposed to sun.

☹ **Petal Infusions Moisturizer, for Oily Skin** *($30 for 1.7 ounces)* has thickening agents that would be a problem for oily or blemish-prone skin, but the larger problems are the bergamot and lemon oils in this moisturizer.

☹ **Petal Infusions Calming Eye Cream** *($25 for 0.5 ounce)* is a delicately creamy moisturizer for slightly dry to dry skin, but is not recommended for use around the eyes or elsewhere because it contains jasmine and rosewood oils. Linalool is a major constituent of rosewood oil, and has been shown to cause "irritational skin reactions" in the presence of oxygen, which, let's face it, is all around us (Source: *Xenobiotica*, June 2007, pages 604–617).

✓☺ **Petal Infusions Skin Visor SPF 30** *($24 for 2.5 ounces)* is a very good daytime moisturizer with an in-part titanium dioxide sunscreen for UVA protection. Thankfully, there are no irritating essential oils in this product (they finally got it right with their sunscreens). This is recommended for dry skin, and contains some good antioxidants, emollients, and cell-communicating ingredients. The tiny amount of linalool is not cause for concern.

☺ **Petal Infusions Skin Visor SPF 50** *($26 for 2.5 ounces)* provides serious broad-spectrum protection with its in-part zinc oxide sunscreen, which tops out at over 16%. That produces a thicker texture and yet the silicone base helps it apply and finish silky-smooth. Those with medium to dark skin should be aware this sunscreen can leave a slight white cast on skin, despite claims to the contrary. This is best for normal to oily skin, contains a tiny amount of antioxidants (some is better than none), and is fragrance-free.

STILA MAKEUP

FOUNDATION: ✓☺ **$$$ Natural Finish Oil-Free Makeup** *($32)* is an outstanding liquid foundation with an exceedingly silky application that blends beautifully and provides light to medium coverage with a satin-matte finish. The formula is oil-free and an excellent choice for normal to oily skin prone to blemishes. Fourteen shades are available, including options for fair to dark skin tones. Within that range, only shades F, H, and L are too peach to consider.

✓☺ **$$$ Perfecting Foundation** *($30)* launched after most lines had discontinued their stick foundations, as this was a trendy option that, like all trends, was fleeting. However, Stila's option is one that I hope stays in the line, because it is a commendable choice for normal to dry skin not prone to breakouts. Perfecting Foundation has a creamy-soft texture that glides over skin, feeling almost gel-like but leaving a noticeably moist (but not greasy) finish. If not blended well it can look heavy, but smoothing things out with a sponge or, as Stila recommends, applying it with a foundation brush, solves this problem. When it's carefully blended you'll get medium to almost-full coverage—and this doubles as a concealer for trouble spots (though it's not recommended to conceal breakouts). All but one of the nine shades are extraordinary (avoid the slightly orange shade H), and they include options to meet the needs of fair and dark skin tones.

✓☺ **$$$ Illuminating Liquid Foundation** *($35)* is a creamy, mineral oil–based makeup that's very good for dry skin seeking light to medium coverage with a satin-smooth, shimmer finish. The shine is more noticeable than in the Illuminating Powder Foundation reviewed below, but with a sheer powder dusted over it this can lend a radiant glow to the skin. All eight shades are soft and neutral whether skin is fair or dark (but not very dark).

✓☺ **$$$ Sheer Color Tinted Moisturizer SPF 15** *($30)* contains an in-part avobenzone sunscreen for sufficient UVA protection and has a lightweight lotion texture that provides a slight hint of coverage and understated, almost see-through, color. All but one of the ten perfectly neutral shades blends well and sets to a soft matte finish; the Warm shade is bound to be too peach for its intended skin tone. This tinted moisturizer is ideal for those with normal to slightly dry or slightly oily skin who want something less formal than a regular foundation. Note that although it's a bit pricey, it comes in a 1.7-ounce size, whereas similar options typically offer less product.

☺ **$$$ Illuminating Powder Foundation SPF 12** *($24 for powder; $20 for refillable compact)* deserves a happy face rating even though its titanium dioxide–based sunscreen is below the minimum SPF 15. This is recommended with the caveat that it be used over a regular sunscreen or foundation with sunscreen rated SPF 15 or higher. This talc-based powder foundation is extraordinarily silky and applies seamlessly, offering light, non-powdery coverage and a barely there, slightly shiny finish. The eight shades are terrific and not to be missed if you prefer this type of foundation and don't mind the initially high price.

CONCEALER: ✓☺ $$$ Illuminating Concealer *($22)* is not only Stila's best concealer, it's also one of the best liquid concealers around! You'd think something so fluid wouldn't cover well and couldn't last beyond lunch, but this proves itself. It has just enough slip to make blending nearly foolproof, and provides substantial coverage without looking the least bit thick or heavy. Its long-wearing matte finish doesn't crease, and the formula is even aces for use over blemishes because it doesn't have occlusive waxes or thickeners that can make matters worse. Four of the six shades are neutral; Warm is too gold for most medium skin tones, while Bronze is strikingly orange and best avoided. This concealer has a brush applicator, but the brush tends to come out with too much product (definitely more than what's needed—a little goes a long way!), so either remove the excess or dab a bit onto your fingertips and then apply.

☺ $$$ Cover-Up Stick *($18)* is a twist-up stick concealer. Alas, this has a creamy texture that will easily lend itself to creasing under the eye. However, it blends very well and is fine if you need heavier coverage over birthmarks or broken capillaries, and the six colors are uniformly excellent, even if this is not a matte-finish concealer as stated.

😐 $$$ Perfecting Concealer *($20)* has a slightly thick, greasy formula that's a step backward when compared to many other modern concealers. You'll get full coverage with an opacity that camouflages redness and dark circles, but it's tricky to blend and is so emollient it will crease into lines no matter how much powder you use for setting. Substantial coverage without the drawbacks of greasiness and persistent creasing are attainable from M.A.C.'s Select Moisturecover ($15.50), and it costs less, too! If you decide to try Perfecting Concealer, avoid shades H and K, which are too ash and copper for dark skin. The other 12 shades are predominantly neutral and there are some good options for fair skin.

POWDER: ☺ $$$ Sheer Pressed Powder *($25)* goes on quite sheer. This talc-based powder doesn't feel the least bit heavy, nor is it too dry or "powdery." It goes on lightly and has a silky matte finish, yet manages to keep excess oil in check without making skin look flat and dull. The palette of shades is a bit odd: Fair is pure white, while Light and Medium are suitable for fair skin tones only. Dark and Deep are best for light to medium skin tones, while Mocha and Cocoa are meant for darker skin or for use as matte bronzing powders. Sorting through the options to find your best match isn't as easy as it should be, but this pressed powder is still recommended for all skin types except blemish-prone. The cornstarch in this product can be a problem for blemishes.

☺ $$$ Stila Sun SPF 15 Bronzing Powder *($28)* is the latest version of the company's long-standing pressed-powder bronzer, only this trip back to the drawing board resulted in the addition of an in-part titanium dioxide sunscreen. That's great news for those looking to boost their sun protection from foundation or moisturizer with sunscreen, and this talc-based powder has a smooth, lightweight texture and sheer, even application. The only issue is that the colors are more peach than tan-to-bronze, and as such work best as blush for those with fair to light skin tones.

BLUSH: ✓☺ $$$ Rouge Pots *($20)* is aptly described as a "revolutionary air-whipped formula… [that] glides on sheer, blends like a breeze, and leaves cheeks blossoming with color."

This is another surprisingly unique product from Stila, and—aside from the jar packaging (the opening is so narrow it's tricky to remove just a tiny amount of product)—it is hands-down wonderful for those who prefer cream blush to powder blush. A small amount is all you need to produce lively color with a soft glow, and this is deceptively easy to apply and blend. The range of shades is beautiful, each having a translucent effect on the skin that creates a "blushing from within" effect. The best options for those who want softer, muted color are Freesia, Water Lily, and Plumeria. Sweet Pea is a sheer, but bright, pink that would be flattering on light to medium African-American skin tones. Two additional nice features of this blush: It does not make pores look dotted with color and it can be applied over powder without streaking.

✓☺ **$$$ Cheek Color Pan** *($16 for powder tablet; $2 for refillable compact)* is Stila's pressed-powder blush and it has a silky, almost creamy feel that goes on smoothly and offers a shade range that runs from sheer to deep, so there's something for just about every skin color. Most of the shades are nearly matte, and the shiny ones are readily apparent and best for evening makeup. Interestingly, Sephora stores (where Stila is primarily sold) carry only a handful of the available shades. Check out Stila's Web site for the full selection of colors.

☺ **$$$ Convertible Color** *($22)* is a find for dry skin. This is basically a sheer, emollient blush that feels more like a lipstick in compact form. This is intended for use on lips and cheeks for a simple, easy, "finger-painted" look. The texture is creamy bordering on greasy (akin to traditional lipstick), and the large color range is exceptional, with a few eye-catching sheer, but bright, hues. The color of each compact is a very good representation of how the shade appears on skin, though of course the product itself is more translucent.

☺ **$$$ Color Push-Ups** *($20)* is a sheer cream blush that comes in solid form and is housed in a deodorant-style container. It applies and blends reasonably well, and leaves a moist, dewy finish. The colors are beautiful, and this would be an option for those with dry skin who prefer a see-through wash of color. This is not quite as smooth to blend as Stila's Convertible Color, and that product provides a greater color deposit, too.

😐 **Gel Cheek Color** *($16)* has the advantage of being easier to control and blend than liquid cheek tints such as Benefit BeneTint ($28), but this true gel blush from Stila, while offering three very good translucent colors, leaves a slightly tacky finish. It's an OK option for normal to dry skin, but not preferred to a powder blush. If you want to try a gel blush, Clinique's Gel Blush ($12.50) is a better option.

EYESHADOW: Stila's ✓☺ **$$$ Eye Shadow Pan** *($16 for eyeshadow tablet; $2 for refillable compact)* has a gorgeous, smooth, suitably dry texture that blends well. Shine rules the roost here, but at least these apply easily, cling well, and aren't garish. The completely matte options include Bouquet, Chinois, Dune, Eden, Fog, Tone, Storm, Ebony, Java, and Coco.

✓☺ **$$$ Shadow Pots** *($20)* are an intriguing twist on conventional powder or cream eyeshadows. They have an airy, mousse-like texture that does allow enough blending time before setting to a satin-like finish. All of the shades are loaded with shine, but they are options for the under-30 set or for those whose eyelids and underbrow are wrinkle-free. The best thing about Shadow Pots is their versatility. They work well alone (if you want a lot of shine) or they can be mixed together, applied over or under powder eyeshadows, used as eyeliner (the deeper shades, that is), or used as highlighter (the lightest shades) wherever you like. Bobbi Brown's Long-Wear Cream Shadow ($22) is similar to this and includes a couple of matte options.

☹ **Convertible Eye Color** *($20)* is a dual-ended product that gives you an automatic, retractable eye pencil along with an iridescent powder eyeshadow dispensed from a sponge tip.

The pencil is a breeze to work with but the powder eyeshadow tends to apply unevenly and flake no matter how careful you are. For that reason alone, this product isn't recommended.

EYE AND BROW SHAPER: ✓☺ Brow Polish *($12)* comes in a small container, but the price isn't outrageous for what ends up being a very good brow tint that can do double duty to conceal gray hairs between appointments with your colorist. The dual-sided brush allows for easy application, whether you want soft or more dramatically defined (but not overdone) brows. It dries to a soft powdery feel and lasts well without flaking or smearing. Three shades are available: Fair is suitable for blondes, Warm for light brown to auburn hair, and Medium for medium to dark brown brows.

☺ **$$$ Smudge Pots** *($18)* is nearly identical to Bobbi Brown's Long-Wear Gel Eyeliner ($19) and M.A.C.'s Fluidline ($15). These types of gel eyeliners are able to stand up to oily eyelids without fading, smearing, or running. Stila mimicked Brown's basic formulation, offering a slightly moist gel-cream eyeliner that sets to a long-wearing matte finish. It is every bit as tenacious as those from Brown and M.A.C., but the application is not as easy because the color intensity does not build as quickly, going on more sheer and requiring you to layer if you want a solid, more dramatic line. How thin or thick a line you create depends entirely on the type of brush you use; a pointed eyeliner brush produces a thin line, while a wedge brush can easily create a thicker line. The only reason to choose Stila's version over similar products is if you're looking more for a sheer application than for a dramatic one. Basic shades of black, brown, and gray are accompanied by wilder hues, including a bright blue and green that are best avoided.

😐 **$$$ Brow Set** *($18)* offers two slightly shiny brown shades in one pan for defining brows and filling in sparse areas (that's what the lighter shade is intended for). While adding shimmer to brows is just strange, this is an option, though the price is steep for what you get. You can get similar results from a single shade of matte powder eyeshadows.

☹ **Kajal Eye Liner** *($16)* is a rare misstep from Stila, because this is one disappointing, needs-sharpening pencil. It does have a super-soft texture that makes it easy to apply, but it's so creamy (and stays that way) that smearing and fading are inevitable. Yes, you can enhance this pencil's longevity by setting it with a powder eyeshadow, but why not use a pencil (or powder eyeshadow) that lasts well to begin with?

LIPSTICK, LIP GLOSS, AND LIPLINER: ✓☺ $$$ Lip Shine *($17)* is Stila's original lip gloss offering, and it remains superior to what they've done since, although the Lip Glaze remains the more popular choice. Not to discredit Lip Glaze, but Lip Shine has a silkier, lightweight feel and offers a strikingly glossy but non-sticky finish. The squeeze tube includes a built-in brush applicator and the sheer colors are eminently versatile.

☺ **$$$ Lip Color** *($16.50)* is Stila's main lipstick, and it is available in your choice of Creme, Shimmer, or Sheer formulas (thankfully designated on the tester unit so you're not guessing which version you're considering). The Cremes feel thick and are indeed creamy, though they are greasy enough to slip into lines around the mouth. These provide medium coverage and a good stain. The Shimmer formula is smoother and less greasy than the Cremes, and, true to its name, has a shimmer finish. Sheers are glossy and fleeting but the soft colors are beautifully appealing.

☺ **$$$ It Gloss** *($18)* is "It" because the company claims it "takes shine to a whole new level." Make no mistake—this brush-on gloss provides not only a wet-look, glossy finish, but also high-wattage shimmer to spare, all without feeling sticky. Still, lots of glosses have these characteristics, and Stila's attempt, nice as it is, is a reinvention of the wheel. The palette of shades is gorgeous, presenting options that range from sheer nudes to vivid wine tones. If you shop department stores for lip gloss, this product compares favorably with the pricier options from Chanel, Dior, and Lancome (though several drugstore versions excel in this arena as well).

☺ **$$$ Lip Glaze** *($20)* is a moderately thick, smooth lip gloss with a minimally sticky finish and a glaze-like shine. It's packaged in a click-pen component with a built-in brush applicator and the brush itself is nicely cut to fit the contours of the mouth. Lip Glaze is one of Stila's best-selling products, and numerous shades are available, ranging from translucent with shimmer to glossy reds and berry tones.

☺ **$$$ Lip Polish** *($20)* is a lip gloss in a self-dispensing brush applicator, for more money than this clever packaging is really worth ($20 for lip gloss borders on ridiculous). A few clicks at the base release a flow of gloss onto the lip-brush applicator, and you're on your way to semi-rich color with a soft gloss finish. This is similar to Stila's Lip Glaze but the colors are stronger and the finish less sticky.

☺ **$$$ Lip Pots** *($16)* are gloss in a pot, and the larger packaging is what the Rouge Pots above should be using, because it is much easier to swipe a finger across the color and dab it onto skin. This product has a lightweight but moist texture that is unlike traditional gloss. It feels almost like a creamy lipstick that has melted a bit. It is completely non-sticky and provides a moderately glossy finish, and all of the colors are attractive. If you're prone to overspending on lip gloss, this is an above-average way to do it!

😐 **$$$ Hi-Shine Lip Color** *($16.50)* is an incredibly greasy lipstick with a glossy finish that has minimal staying powder. Most of the colors are quite soft, so this is definitely a lipstick that, while great for dry lips, will need frequent reapplication and can bleed into lines around the mouth.

😐 **$$$ Lip Liner** *($14)* needs sharpening, which is inconvenient, but this smooth-textured pencil's slightly dry finish tends to stay put, so the payoff is a long-lasting line that holds up to all but the greasiest lipsticks and glosses. The dozen or so shades consist of mostly nude and neutral tones to complement a variety of lipstick hues.

😐 **$$$ Lip Rouge** *($20)* claims to be a magic marker for the lips. I wouldn't call it indelible, but it has impressive staying power, just not as much as you would expect for the money. Inside a fountain pen–style package, a very pigmented water- and alcohol-based liquid is fed into a brush tip, which is applied to the lips; it then sets into a long-lasting, feels-like-nothing stain. Two cautions: It dries up easily if you don't replace the cap tightly after each use and the hard brush tip makes for less-than-pleasant application.

😐 **Clear Color SPF 8** *($14)* offers a too-low SPF without sufficient UVA protection, which makes this an otherwise completely standard, sheer lipstick with a glossy, slippery finish and decent colors. The only new feature is the incredibly small package, and only half of that is actual product. 😐 **Glaze Lip Liner** *($14)* is a needs-sharpening pencil that is nearly identical to Clinique's Sheer Shaper for Lips ($13.50), though Stila's shade selection is a step above, as is often the case with this line. The pencil imparts sheer (fleeting) color. I asked Stila's makeup artist why sheer lipliners were even needed; couldn't you just apply a regular lipliner softer than usual, or sheer the line with a lip brush? She explained that customers wanted a sheer liner for when they wear lip gloss. When I mentioned that a regular lipliner would help the gloss stay on better than a sheer one, she didn't know what to say. Still, this is worth checking out if the concept intrigues you.

☹ **Lip Glaze Sticks** *($16.50)* need constant sharpening to keep the thick but soft-textured tips workable. But each shade of this sheer lipstick in pencil form is imbued with chunks of glitter, which immediately feels grainy on the lips.

☹ **Plumping Lip Glaze** *($24)* is Stila's worst lip gloss on several counts. The click-pen dispenser with built-in brush is convenient, but on this version it tends to dial up way too much product (and there's no way to put it back), the gloss itself has an unusually thick, syrupy texture that tends to stick lips together, and the formula contains irritating, menthol-based menthoxypropanediol, an ingredient that plumps lips via irritation, and that's not good for lips.

MASCARA: ✓☺ Major Lash Mascara *($12.50)* is a major winner if you're looking for an outstanding thickening mascara! It sweeps on with ease, providing almost instant thickness and enough length so that each lash is well defined but not clumpy. This builds well, too, and wears evenly throughout the day. **✓☺ Fiber Optics Mascara** *($14.50)* must have been changed since its original review, because I wasn't nearly as wowed by my first experience with this mascara. It produces prodigious length and thickness with minimal effort and without a clump in sight. In short, this is an awesome, all-purpose mascara that bests Major Lash Mascara if you need equal parts length and thickness rather than just a thickness boost.

☺ **$$$ Lash Visor Waterproof Mascara** *($12.50)* makes lashes impressively long while also providing more thickness than most waterproof mascaras. Definitely waterproof, Lash Visor provides good lash separation, doesn't clump, and makes it through the day without a smudge or smear.

😐 **$$$ Multi-Effect Mascara** *($20)* purports to be the ultimate formula that does it all, yet using this tells a different story, and its title is Great Expectations, Depressing Results. This curved-brush mascara is marginally adept at building length with minimal thickness, and leaves lashes slightly curled, if you don't mind a careful application that still creates some clumps and is smear-prone for longer than it should be. Stila dares you to try this; I implore you to consider the superior options from the drugstore, or, for Stila fans, the company's truly impressive Major Lash Mascara above.

FACE AND BODY ILLUMINATING/SHIMMER PRODUCTS: ✓☺ $$$ All Over Shimmer Liquid Luminizer *($22)* is an improved version of Stila's original All Over Shimmer ($20). This version is packaged in a glass bottle and includes a brush applicator. It is more fluid, less slick, and less powdery at dry-down than its predecessor, and is overall a significant improvement. Unlike All Over Shimmer, this stays in place, dries quickly after blending, and looks more natural. Its shimmer is more glow-y than shiny, and the shade selection has been whittled down to four (opalescent white, pale pink, light gold, and peachy bronze), all best for fair to medium skin tones. A little goes a long way, so the price is somewhat justified, not to mention that this product is versatile. This is Stila's best shine-enhancing option.

☺ **$$$ Illuminating Tinted Moisturizer SPF 15** *($28)* has an in-part avobenzone sunscreen to ensure sufficient UVA protection, but unless you're willing to apply this all over the face it is best as an adjunct to another product rated SPF 15 or greater. The one-shade-fits-all concept is fine for most skin tones because this moisturizer imparts more soft radiance than color. The lightweight, luminous finish is attractive and suitable for normal to dry skin, but don't expect any coverage (it's really that sheer).

☺/😐 **All Over Shimmer Eyes** *($16)* is an airy loose shimmer that can be used around the eyes or anywhere you want to add shine. The trouble is it doesn't cling well enough—in short order you will find powder on your eyelashes, under your eye, on your cheeks, chin, and, well, just about everywhere else. Loose shimmer powders traditionally don't cling well to skin, so I don't blame this particular product—but this is best used away from the eyes unless you want shiny all over the place. The shade selection is plentiful and the powder can be applied sheer or layered for more intensity. The pearl, tan, gold, and bronze-toned shades are great to mix with a body lotion for adding evening shimmer to shins, calves, or arms. The happy face rating pertains to its use anywhere but the eye area, the neutral face rating for its use over the eye area. ☺ **$$$ All Over Shimmer Powder** *($30)* is silky-smooth and non-powdery, so it applies well and melds with skin rather than looking like it's just sitting on top of it. The shine level is high, but this clings better than you'd expect.

😐 **$$$ All Over Glow** *($28)* provides a shimmery pressed powder blush and coordinating highlighter in one compact. Both have a silky feel and sheer color impact, and the glam, glitter-like shine isn't anyone's definition of subtle. If shiny cheeks are what you're after, this is one (pricey) way to get it.

BRUSHES: Stila provides several great **Brushes** *($18–$52)*, most with a soft but firm feel and excellent shapes. There are even a few unique dual-sided and retractable options, and almost every brush is available in long- or short-handled versions. Stop by and check these out if you are shopping for brushes, especially the following Paula's Picks: ✓☺ **#26 Perfecting Concealer Brush** *($18)*, ✓☺ **#2 Under Eye Concealer Brush** *($18)*, ✓☺ **#9 All Over Blend Brush** *($24)*, ✓☺ **#15 Double Sided Brush** *($32)*, ✓☺ **#17 Retractable Bronzing Brush** *($26)*, and ✓☺ **#20 Eye Enhancer Brush** *($32)*.

The 😐 **$$$ Brush Set** *($75)* is way overpriced for what you get, which isn't even a complete collection of basic brushes, not to mention they're smaller than typical and as such not the best choice for regular use. The 😐 **$$$ #27 Perfecting Foundation Brush** *($20)* is synthetic, but smaller than most, which means application takes more time. Lastly, the 😐 **$$$ #8 Powder Brush** *($50)*, while very soft and expertly cut, is too floppy for controlled application but OK if you want a sheer hint of powder.

SPECIALTY PRODUCTS: ✓☺ **$$$ Sun Gel** *($24)* seems pricey at first, but this small tube of bronzing gel is concentrated—a tiny dab is enough to add a translucent bronze glow to the cheeks and temple area, and the shine is kept to a minimum. The single shade available is a fairly convincing tan color, though it can be too orange for fair skin tones. It blends well, but if you're not used to applying gels it will take some practice to ensure smooth, even application. Bronzing gels are best used over bare skin, or carefully applied over sunscreen (give the sunscreen time to be absorbed before dabbing on the gel). This does not blend well over foundation or powder, and is ideally suited for a natural, sun-kissed look.

STRIDEX (SKIN CARE ONLY)

STRIDEX AT-A-GLANCE

Strengths: A couple of benzoyl peroxide options that are fragrance- and irritant-free.

Weaknesses: All the pads with salicylic acid contain irritants such as menthol, alcohol, or witch hazel; poor cleansers; no oil-absorbing products; no effective AHA or BHA products.

For more information about Stridex, call (888) 784-2472 or visit www.stridex.com or www.Beautypedia.com.

☹ **Cooling Anti-Bacterial Foaming Wash** *($5.29 for 6 ounces)* contains 1% triclosan, an antibacterial agent that has limited effectiveness for combating acne. This could be an option, but, because the bacteria that cause acne are found deep inside the pore, any substance in a rinse-off product won't have a chance to get to the root of the problem. Besides, this cleanser isn't recommended anyway because it contains menthol and spearmint oil.

☹ **Clear Cycle Deep Wash** *($5.16 for 4 ounces)* is a water-soluble cleanser/scrub hybrid with 2% salicylic acid, but it also contains spearmint oil, which makes it too irritating for all skin types, especially near (or, even worse, in) the eyes or on mucous membranes. When will Stridex (and countless other anti-acne lines) learn that clear skin cannot be achieved with senseless irritants?

😐 **Day & Night** *($6.99 for the set; each product is 0.8 ounce)* is sold as a breakthrough approach to clear skin, but the actives (salicylic acid and benzoyl peroxide) have been around for years, and are no more a breakthrough than a bicycle is. The ☹ **Day Gel**, with 2% salicylic acid, contains too much alcohol and witch hazel to make it worth considering, while the ✓☺ **Night Lotion**, with 2.5% benzoyl peroxide, is an excellent topical disinfectant that's free of needless irritants. Considering the price of this duo, it's not so bad that only one of the two products is worthwhile.

☹ **Essential Care Triple Action Pads** *($3.89 for 55 pads)* contain menthol, and as such are too irritating for all skin types. Plus, the detergent cleansing agents are not what you want to leave on skin.

☹ **Facewipes to Go** *($5.29 for 32 wipes)* contain a lot of alcohol and menthol, which makes these on-the-go wipes a problem for all skin types. The amount of salicylic acid is next to useless, too.

☹ **Maximum Strength Triple Action Pads** *($3.99 for 55 pads)* contain menthol and detergent cleansing agents that should not be left on skin.

✓☺ **Power Pads** *($6.99 for 28 pads)* are a unique new option to disinfect blemish-prone skin. Featuring an effective concentration of 2.5% benzoyl peroxide and free of irritating ingredients such as alcohol, witch hazel, or peppermint, these larger-than-usual, nonabrasive pads are recommended for all skin types battling acne. These pads contain a mild detergent cleansing agent, so unless your skin is very oily or you have makeup to remove, they will gently cleanse skin while disinfecting, and they do not need to be rinsed. Nice job, Stridex!

☹ **Sensitive Skin Triple Action Pads** *($3.99 for 55 pads)* are advertised as being alcohol-free, and that's great. (So, if Stridex knows that alcohol is not a good thing to include, then why do they include it in so many of their other products!?) However, although these pads do not contain alcohol, they are still terrible for sensitive skin because they contain menthol and an essentially ineffective amount of salicylic acid.

☹ **Super Scrub Triple Action Pads** *($3.99 for 55 pads)* are textured pads intended to exfoliate skin, but they're merely a great way to really increase the irritation from the menthol in each pad. In other words, don't bother.

STRIVECTIN-SD
(SEE BREMENN RESEARCH LABS)

THREE CUSTOM COLOR SPECIALISTS
(MAKEUP ONLY)

Since 1997, Three Custom Color Specialists have excelled in what they dubbed a Custom Blending Service, of which their lipstick-matching prowess has earned them considerable recognition. Send them a color swatch or the last sliver of a favorite discontinued lipstick and they will duplicate it so accurately you will be stunned. And if you love the results as much as I suspect you will, know that Three Custom keeps everything they did to recreate the shade on file, so reordering is easy. What began as a lipstick color-matching service has expanded over the years to include several other makeup products. In addition to the custom **Lipstick** *($50 for two tubes)*, you may customize **Creme to Powder Blush** *($37.50; $20.50 for additional shades, which must be ordered at the same time as the original price shade)*, **Eyeshadow Singles**, **Brow Powder**, or **Powder Eyeliner** *($36.50; $19.50 for additional shades, which must be ordered at the same time as the original price shade)*, **Creme Concealer** *($36.50; $19.50 for additional shades, which must be ordered at the same time as the original price shade)*, and **Face Powder** *($47.50 for Loose; $28.50 for additional shades, which must be ordered at the same time as the original price shade; $36.50 for Pressed; $19.50 for additional shades, which must be ordered at the same time as the original price shade)*. With the exception of the lipsticks (where they can match any formula), the products above use Three Custom's base formulas and from there create a custom shade and finish per your instructions.

Although these customized options are pricey, the personalization for every product reviewed below is beautifully executed, right down to the postage-paid envelope you receive to send in a remnant or piece of fabric that represents your ideal color. All of the custom items may be further modified with your choice of finish and level or type of shimmer. All told, Three Custom continues to offer a remarkable service. Furthermore, all custom colors are 100% guaranteed, and will be redone (at no additional charge) in the unlikely event that they don't get it just right the first time. In addition to their Custom Color menu, you can also choose from a range of several other makeup essentials, featuring 250 never-to-be-discontinued ready-to-wear colors, reviewed by category below.

THREE CUSTOM COLOR SPECIALISTS AT-A-GLANCE

Strengths: The only company in this book that offers custom color matching for discontinued products; first-rate customer service; the Ready-to-Wear line features several outstanding products; very good makeup brushes; refillable compacts.

Weaknesses: Customization service is expensive; the cream blush goes on too sheer; eye and lip pencils still require routine sharpening.

For more information about Three Custom Color Specialists, call (888) 262-7714 or visit www.threecustom.com or www.Beautypedia.com.

CONCEALER: ☺ **$$$ Creme Concealer Singles** *($19.50; $15 for refills)* is indeed creamy, yet the oil-based formula is also very concentrated and melts into the skin, providing good, even coverage. The range of ten shades (which includes some great options for dark skin tones) is very good, but unless you're certain of which color to purchase it's best to contact the company for assistance rather than guess from the tiny swatches on their Web site. As is true for any creamy concealer, this has a tendency to crease if not set with powder. A strong selling point of this concealer is the significant coverage it provides without looking thick or too heavy.

For makeup artists, a ☺ **$$$ Professional Concealer Palette** *($58)* offers a concealer brush, blending spatula, and all ten shades of the Creme Concealer above to use alone or mix as needed for the ideal shade.

POWDER: ✓☺ **$$$ Loose Powder** *($36.50)* has a texture that's akin to the most finely milled powdered sugar, and produces a beautifully natural-looking polished finish. The shade selection includes five flesh-toned colors along with a sheer white, slightly shiny shade (Translucent) and two bronzing powders (Cool and Warm) that go on sheer and impart a subtle shimmer that isn't the least bit distracting. The glass jar is a bit cumbersome, but this is otherwise a stellar loose powder for those with normal to dry or slightly oily skin.

☺ **$$$ Mini Pressed Powder Single** *($19.50; $15 for refills)* is talc-based and has a silky, lightweight, and dry texture with a natural matte finish that's best for normal to slightly dry or slightly oily skin (those with very oily skin will crave a powder that's more matte than this). The five flesh-toned shades present a good range for fair to dark (but not very dark) skin tones, while the sheer white Translucent tends to work best on pale skin and features a touch of shimmer. Cool and Warm Bronzer shades are also available, and both are believable, accurately named colors that come with a faint hint of shine.

BLUSH: ✓☺ $$$ Creme to Powder Blush *($20.50)* is aluminum starch–based, so although it's initially creamy, it sets quickly to a soft powder finish. If you're adept at the dab-and-blend application this type of blush requires, you will be thrilled by the colors. These are pigment-rich, so use them sparingly for best results, and build color from there.

😐 **$$$ Watercolours for Cheeks** *($20.50)* is a very sheer traditional cream blush whose emollient, lanolin-based texture is best for dry to very dry skin. Each shade imparts a translucent wash of color that can be made slightly more intense with another layer (though this increases the moist finish). Although this is an option if you prefer cream blush, keep in mind that the sheerness of each color and the emollience of the formula don't combine to produce a long-wearing result.

EYESHADOW ✓☺ $$$ Eyeshadow Singles *($19.50; $15 for refills)* remain as impressive as they were when reviewed for the sixth edition of this book. Each shade has a supremely smooth texture that applies evenly, wears well, and doesn't flake (and that includes the shinier shades, too). Although every shade has shine, on most it's very subtle, amounting to a soft, radiant finish that is suitable for daytime. The eyeshadow formula may be used wet or dry, with wet application intensifying the color. Among the 40 shades, the following are best avoided, especially if your goal is a classic, understated eye design: Opal, Cool Sky, Warm Meadow, Cool Meadow, Warm Celery, and Warm Nectar. Note: If you prefer 100% matte eyeshadows, any of Three Custom's brow powders (reviewed below) may also be used as eyeshadows, and all are matte.

EYE AND BROW SHAPER: ✓☺ $$$ Brow Gel *($19.50)* is a standard but effective clear brow gel that grooms brows and keeps unruly hairs in place without feeling too thick or sticky. This also adds a subtle gloss finish to brows, which can be an attractive highlight, especially if your brows are brown or black.

☺ **$$$ Brow Powder** *($19.50; $15 for refills)* is a talc-based brow powder that is a great choice for softly defined brows, and the six colors run the gamut from blonde to raven. This also works as a true matte eyeshadow, but is not as supremely smooth as the Eyeshadow Singles above.

😐 **Eye Pencil** *($14)* needs to be sharpened, but deserves consideration for its smooth application that is just minimally prone to smudging. Three Custom Color Specialists has plenty of powder eyeshadows in shades suitable for eyelining, and although those last longer and won't smudge, this pencil is an option if that's your preferred tool for lining. The Light and Dark Clarifier pencils are peach-toned hues meant for application to the inner rim of the eye. This practice, while theatrical in nature and OK for photographs, is not one to consider on a daily basis due to the risk of smearing and the potential for eye infection (that's true for any pencil used so close to the eye and tear duct).

LIPSTICK, LIP GLOSS, AND LIPLINER: ✓☺ **$$$ Lipstick** *($18.50)* remains a formidable creamy lipstick that applies smoothly and offers full-coverage colors with a good stain. The range of shades is impressive and is conveniently organized into cool and warm tones that range from soft pastels to deep reds and browns. The **Special Shades** *($18.50)* are custom or "themed" colors that have made their way into the line's regular rotation. This collection includes some sheer options (described as such on the Web site) and many of these ready-made shades have matching lip glosses. ✓☺ **$$$ Shimmering Lights Lipstick** *($18.50)* is nearly identical to the regular Lipstick above, except each shade is imbued with varying levels of shimmer.

✓☺ **$$$ Classic Lip Gloss** *($18.50)* comes in a compact that swivels out, and may be applied with a lip brush (recommended) or clean fingertip. This has a supremely smooth yet intensely moisturizing texture that isn't the least bit sticky or syrupy. It finishes to a soft buffed shine and the palette of mostly sheer shades (divided into cool and warm tones) is stunning. Hands down, this is one of the best lip glosses available.

☺ **$$$ Lip Color Palettes** *($45–$53.50; individual palette shades also available separately for $18.50)* come in various combinations and are available for those who cannot get enough of what Three Custom's ready-to-wear lipstick and lip gloss palettes have to offer.

☺ **$$$ Lip Gloss** *($18.50)* is a wand-applicator gloss that has a relatively standard, smooth texture, sheer- to light-coverage colors, and a glossy, completely non-sticky finish. If you love matching lipstick and lip gloss, you'll be pleased to know that all of the main Three Custom Color Specialists ready-to-wear Lipstick shades have a coordinating Lip Gloss color available.

😐 **Lip Liner** *($14)* has been improved, and it shows. This is still a needs-sharpening pencil (the only aspect that keeps it from earning a happy face rating), but it is creamier and applies better than the previous version, all without smearing. The deeper hues are brilliant for women of color.

MASCARA: The simply named ☺ **Mascara** *($19.50)* claims to be a lengthening and thickening formula, and it does deliver both, though not to a dramatic extent. Initial application does little to impress, unless your goal is minimal lash enhancement. However, this mascara definitely improves with successive coats and produces perfectly separated, dark, fringed lashes. The formula wears well all day and removes easily, making it a good choice if you don't want copious length or thickness.

BRUSHES: The Three Custom Color Specialists line is nicely rounded out by a beautiful collection of professional ✓☺ **$$$ Brushes** *($3.50–$55)* that feature elegant, long-handled options for applying color. The only brush that you may want to think twice about is the 😐 **Retractable Lip Brush** *($12.50)*, which is too small for most women's lips. All of the other brushes are highly recommended and will last for years with proper care.

SPECIALTY PRODUCTS: ☺ **$$$ Refillable Trio Compact** *($15)* is sold separately and includes a dual-sided brush. It's a wise investment if you routinely use three colors, and it houses Three Custom's Creme Concealer, Eyeshadows, or Brow Powder.

TRI-LUMA (PRESCRIPTION ONLY)

TRI-LUMA AT-A-GLANCE

Strengths: A very effective option that combines three proven ingredients for lightening sun- or hormone-induced skin discolorations; likely to be more effective for those with melasma than over-the-counter products containing 2% hydroquinone; a much better investment than trying lightening product after product from department store lines, many of which are ineffective; Tri-Luma does not require ongoing use once the discolorations are eliminated (but daily use of a well-formulated sunscreen is essential to keep them from recurring).

Weaknesses: None, other than the expense of seeing a physician for a prescription and the potential risk of irritation with this type of medication.

For more information about Tri-Luma, call (866) 735-4137 or visit www.triluma.com or www.Beautypedia.com.

✓☺ **$$$ Tri-Luma Cream** *($101 for 1.05 ounce)* is discussed in the introduction above. It is available in cream form only, and its base is best for normal to very dry skin (though it can be used by all skin types where stubborn pigment discolorations are a concern).

TRISH MCEVOY

TRISH MCEVOY AT-A-GLANCE

Strengths: Mostly good cleansers; a well-formulated serum; a good absorbent gel for oily skin; the makeup is the crown jewel of this line, with many superb options, particularly the powders, bronzers, eyeshadows, brow gel, Glaze Lip Color, High-Volume Mascara, and Shimmer Pressed Powder; McEvoy's makeup brushes and makeup planners are practically peerless; counter personnel are more often than not very knowledgeable and skilled in the use of these products.

Weaknesses: Expensive; average moisturizers; sunscreens don't provide sufficient UVA protection; no effective AHA or BHA products; jar packaging; the foundations don't have that extra something that raises the bar (yet they should for what they cost); the concealers either crease endlessly or are difficult to work with; disappointing eyeliner options; the lip color with sunscreen leaves lips vulnerable to UVA damage; Double Duty Lip Color is a dud compared to every other long-wearing, two-step lip paint with top coat; tester units make it difficult to identify specific products and finishes.

For more information about Trish McEvoy, call (800) 431-4306 or visit www.trishmcevoy.com or www.Beautypedia.com. Note: McEvoy's Web site has been "under development" since work began on this book. As we go to press, it is still nothing more than a Home page.

TRISH MCEVOY SKIN CARE

☺ **$$$ Even Skin Glycolic Wash** *($42 for 6.5 ounces)* is a good, though absurdly overpriced, standard, water-soluble cleanser for normal to oily skin, but the "scientifically proven AHA blend," which is chiefly glycolic acid, won't exfoliate skin to even out discolorations because it is rinsed down the drain before it has a chance to work. This does contain fragrant plant extracts.

😐 **$$$ Gentle Cleansing Balm** *($55 for 6.8 ounces)* has an extremely rich formula that contains glycerin instead of water and then pairs this skin-friendly ingredient with several plant oils, beeswax, and other emollients. Given the oily formula, makeup removal is quick and simple, but it does not rinse easily and will need to be used with a washcloth. This product is recommended only for someone with very dry skin who prefers a cold cream–style cleanser (although this isn't as thick as traditional cold cream, the way it feels on skin is comparable). It contains fragrance in the form of orange oil.

☺ **$$$ Gentle Cleansing Lotion** *($55 for 6.8 ounces)* is a good, fragrance-free, water-rinsable cleansing lotion that contains considerably less oil than the Gentle Cleansing Balm above, making it a good choice for someone with normal to dry skin. It does not contain detergent cleansing agents, so it doesn't remove makeup very well without the help of a washcloth. Similar, less-expensive options are available from Dove and Neutrogena, which is good to know, since the price of this cleanser is obnoxious for what you get.

☺ **$$$ Gentle Cleansing Wash** *($55 for 6.5 ounces)* is a fairly gentle, water-soluble cleanser for normal to oily or slightly dry skin. The small amounts of balm mint, lavender, and lemongrass extract are unpleasant additions, but should not pose a problem unless you get it in your eyes. In case you're wondering if this cleanser is really worth its brow-raising price—no, it is not. This ordinary formulation doesn't warrant even half the price tag. However, for those with money to burn and an affinity for all things McEvoy, it performs well and does remove makeup.

☺ **$$$ Gentle Eye Makeup Remover** *($24 for 4 ounces)* is a good, but exceptionally standard, water-based fluid makeup remover. It is fragrance- and colorant-free, but is easily replaced by other less expensive options.

😐 **$$$ Even Skin Beta Hydroxy Pads** *($60 for 40 pads)* contain less than 1% beta hydroxy acid (BHA, or salicylic acid) and have a pH of 5.6, which prevents effective exfoliation. So what can these pads do for your skin? A main ingredient in these water-based pads is willow bark extract, and although this is not equivalent to salicylic acid it does function as an anti-inflammatory agent. In addition, these pads contain some great water-binding agents. Therefore, in terms of what to expect, the pads will soften and hydrate your skin, but the only potential for exfoliation is what you'll get from manually massaging the pads over your skin, similar to what you can accomplish with a washcloth.

😐 **$$$ Beauty Booster** *($85 for 1.7 ounces)* has a light texture suitable for normal to slightly dry skin, but overall is a bland formula whose antioxidants (olive oil and vitamin E) will be rendered ineffective due to jar packaging. This also contains potentially irritating fragrant components, and is way too expensive for what you (don't) get.

😐 **$$$ Dry Skin Normalizer** *($60 for 2 ounces)* isn't a poor choice for those needing a fragrance-free moisturizer to remedy dry skin, but for the money, the formula is surprisingly dated and, well ... boring. It contains mostly water, thickeners, emollient, several more thickeners, film-forming agent, paraffin, slip agents, tiny amounts of water-binding agents, silicone, plant oil, a dusting of antioxidants, and preservatives. McEvoy and her team missed an opportunity to offer a state-of-the-art product worthy of its premium price.

☺ **$$$ Beauty Booster Serum** *($125 for 1 ounce)* ends up being a much smarter, though still exorbitantly overpriced, choice compared to the Beauty Booster above. It contains mostly water, acetyl hexapeptide-3, slip agents, another peptide, soothing antioxidant plant extracts, and preservatives. This could have been a much more exciting, well-rounded formula. There is still no substantiated research to support the frequently made claim that acetyl hexapeptide-3 works like Botox by affecting facial muscle contractions; to McEvoy's credit, she does not make such a claim, whereas most companies that sell products containing acetyl hexapeptide-3 do. Considering that peptides have merit as water-binding agents and, theoretically, as cell-communicating ingredients, this serum contains a good amount of them and is an option for all skin types. It's just not as multifaceted as it could have been, owing to the minimal amount of antioxidants or ingredients that mimic the structure of skin, and overall that makes it not worth the price.

☹ **Even Skin Face Corrector** *($42 for 0.88 ounce)* is primarily a blend of silicones with a waxlike thickening agent, but it also contains the ingredient tosylamide, a formaldehyde resin most often seen in nail-hardening products. It is a skin irritant, a cosmetic allergen, and can cause photosensitivity (Sources: *American Journal of Clinical Dermatology*, May 2004, pages 327–337; and *Contact Dermatitis*, May 2000, pages 311–312).

😐 **$$$ Even Skin Vitamin C Cream** *($68 for 1 ounce)* makes normal to dry skin feel amazingly smooth because of its blend of silky silicones and emollient petrolatum. Vitamin C is on board along with a couple of other very good antioxidants, but the choice of jar packaging, while attractive, won't keep these key ingredients stable during use.

😐 **$$$ Intense Eye Treatment** *($48 for 0.5 ounce)* bills itself as a unique formula, but it is a very standard mix of water, aloe, thickeners, and film-forming agents along with minuscule amounts of antioxidants and water-binding agents. It's an OK moisturizer for slightly dry skin around the eyes or elsewhere, but better formulas abound.

😐 **$$$ Line Refiner** *($32 for 0.15 ounce)* provides a small amount of a fragrance-free emollient moisturizer for dry skin, packaged in a portable component. It's just water with lots of thickening agents, some silicone, and wax. That works, but your skin deserves more.

☹ **Luxe Moisture Balm SPF 15** *($28 for 0.28 ounce)* lacks the UVA-protecting ingredients of titanium dioxide, zinc oxide, avobenzone, Mexoryl SX (ecamsule), or Tinosorb, and is not recommended.

😐 **Oil Control Gel** *($28 for 2 ounces)* will definitely help control and absorb excess oil, thanks to magnesium aluminum silicate and cornstarch. This initially thick, peach-tinted, fragrance-free cream morphs into a silky matte finish that leaves skin shine-free, although for how long depends on the other products you use and how active your oil glands are. While this is a good choice for someone with oily skin who wants to control shine, the cornstarch is not the best ingredient to use over blemish-prone skin. Magnesium is an alkaline mineral, giving this product a pH of 8, which can increase the presence of bacteria in the skin, again not great for blemish-prone skin. Despite these drawbacks, this is a workable method for controlling oil breakthrough, and can be a formidable weapon when paired with a matte-finish foundation and powder.

☹ **Protective Shield SPF 15 Moisturizer** *($40 for 2 ounces)* lacks the UVA-protecting ingredients of titanium dioxide, zinc oxide, avobenzone, Mexoryl SX (ecamsule), or Tinosorb, and is not recommended. Shame on Dr. Sherman for not taking the opportunity to address the issue of UVA protection!

TRISH MCEVOY MAKEUP

FOUNDATION: ☺ **$$$ Even Skin Foundation** *($55)* has a liquidy smooth texture and flawless application that looks wonderfully smooth and natural on the skin. It offers a satin finish and sheer to light coverage, and is best for those with normal to dry skin who want a foundation that is moist but lightweight. Eight shades are available, and most are outstanding. Shade 1 is ideal for those with very fair skin, while Shades 2, 3, and 4 rival Stila's best neutral tones. The only slight misstep is Shade 5, which is a bit too peachy. Shade 8 works for dark (but not very dark) skin tones.

☺ **$$$ Even Skin Foundation Moisturizing** *($55)* is similar to the original Even Skin Foundation in most respects, but ups the ante in terms of coverage, so be sure to blend well to avoid a heavy appearance. This isn't much more moisturizing than its predecessor, and both are good options for normal to dry skin. This has a satin finish that imparts a slight shine. Only five shades are offered, with Beige being too peach for most skin tones and Deep Honey having a copper overtone that can be tricky to work with.

☺ **$$$ Cream Powder Makeup** *($35; various compacts sold separately)* has remained the same for years, and is a good foundation for normal to dry skin. Its finish is more creamy than powdery, and it provides light to medium coverage while being easy to blend. Twelve shades are available and most skin tones are well represented. The only shade to be careful with is the slightly pink Shell; Bronze is a decent dark shade.

☺ **$$$ Protective Shield SPF 15 Tinted Moisturizer** *($40)* has an in-part avobenzone sunscreen and a creamy but lightweight texture that slips over skin and provides very sheer coverage. This is best regarded as a sunscreen that adds a hint of color to skin; it won't camouflage redness or other minor flaws. Still, it's definitely worth considering for those with normal to dry skin, and the range of five shades is mostly neutral. Porcelain is an outstanding option for those with very fair skin.

☺ **$$$ Mineral Powder Foundation SPF 15** *($32 for powder tablet; $15 for refillable compact)* is a talc-free, silicone-based, pressed-powder foundation that provides sun protection with titanium dioxide and zinc oxide. The thick but smooth texture doesn't pick up easily on a brush or sponge, but perhaps that was the intent, because applying too much results in a flat, opaque appearance. Applying this with a brush, as an adjunct to your regular sunscreen or foundation with sunscreen, works best. Doing so imparts a natural matte finish and sheer yet even coverage. All three shades are terrific, but are reserved for light to medium skin tones only.

☺ **$$$ Even Skin Perfecting Dual Powder** *($26 for powder tablet; $17 for refillable compact)* is a very good, talc-free, pressed-powder foundation, but it's not in the same league as similar options from Laura Mercier, M.A.C., Clarins, or Lancome. This has a silky, slightly dry texture and an application that is more powdery than usual. It finishes matte yet leaves a bit of shine, too, and provides sheer to light coverage. Among the eight shades, only Golden will be problematic due to its strong yellow tone (although it may work for some medium olive skin tones). Buff is suitable for fair skin, while the darkest shade (Tan) isn't dark enough for most African-American skin tones.

CONCEALER: ☹ **$$$ Protective Shield Concealer** *($21 for concealer tablet; $7.50 for refillable compact)* is a creamy concealer that creases endlessly unless it is set with lots of powder. The castor oil–based formula blends well and provides great coverage with a surprisingly natural finish that's not nearly as difficult to work with as similar concealers from Bobbi Brown and Laura Mercier, among others; however, the creasing keeps it from earning a higher rating. The shade selection has been edited to four; Honey is the only one to avoid because it is blatantly peach.

☹ **$$$ Even Skin Extra Coverage Concealer** *($32)* is an obvious imitation of Laura Mercier's Secret Camouflage ($28), a dual-sided concealer with a thick, almost immovable texture that is tricky to blend. McEvoy's version is creamier than Mercier's, but it's still thick enough so that trying to make it look natural on skin is a time-consuming task, not to mention that blending the two shades together to attain a perfect match isn't particularly easy. If you're up for the challenge and need significant coverage, the best of the three duos is Beige. The Porcelain Duo is slightly pink, and the Honey Duo is too orange to look convincing on its intended range of skin tones.

POWDER: ✓☺ **$$$ Even Skin Finishing Powder** *($30)* has a texture that would make a feather feel heavy, and it leaves a gorgeous sheer finish and a hint of shine. The formula is talc-based, blends imperceptibly, and comes in three beautiful colors. My only complaint is the tiny amount of product you get for the money, though the component is sleek enough to fit in any makeup bag (and maybe that was the point).

✓☺ **$$$ Dual Resort Bronzer** *($28 for powder tablet; $15 for refillable compact)* provides an equal amount of soft copper and golden bronze pressed powders in one compact. Texture and application are exceptionally silky, and although each shade is shiny the effect is more glow than glitter, and it clings well. Both shades work best on fair to light skin tones. ✓☺ **$$$ Matte Bronzer** *($28 for powder tablet; $15 for refillable compact)* doesn't have a true matte finish, but it's close enough to count given the prevailing, here-to-stay shimmer trend (and shimmer done right can be quite attractive). Just like the Dual Resort Bronzer above, this has an amazing silky-smooth feel and applies evenly, allowing you to gradually build color. Two shades are available; Light is warmer thanks to its golden peach tone, while Medium is more realistic if you're trying to fake a tan because it is brown-based with a slight red cast.

☺ **$$$ All Over Face Color** *($28 for powder tablet; $15 for refillable compact)* is another pressed bronzing powder that provides two colors in one tablet. This option isn't as elegant as the ones above due to its slightly grainy texture and very shiny finish (though the shine clings fairly well). If you decide to try this, note that each duo is strongly pigmented, so start sheer unless your skin tone is dark.

BLUSH: ☺ **$$$ Blush** *($20)* is sold as individual powder tablets and it's up to you to decide on a compact or planner page for its placement (the makeup planners are reviewed below). The finely pressed powder feels silky and applies well, depositing more color than you expect. The shade selection presents a good balance of warm and cool tones, and all have some amount of shine. The least shiny shades (suitable for daytime wear) include Nude, Pick Me Up, and Natural.

😐 **$$$ Mineral Loose Powder Blush** *($20)* comes in only one shade (which is a real limitation) and it's a novel, if messy, way to apply blush. The formula is just clay, silicone, and preservative. Clay is indeed a mineral, so the name of this product is accurate; it just doesn't have the same composition as many other "mineral" makeups being sold. When carefully applied, this produces even results with strong color and a soft shine. The component has a clever closure to cover the sifter, which helps minimize mess.

EYESHADOW: Note: All of Trish McEvoy's powder eyeshadows are sold without a compact. Various compacts and cases are available for separate purchase depending on how you want to assemble your eye-makeup wardrobe.

✓☺ **Glaze Eye Shadow** *($15)* has a non-powdery, beautifully smooth texture and seamless application that begins sheer but builds well. Each shade has great cling, and all are shiny, but the effect is a low-key satin sheen. The Glaze shades have a light to medium pigmentation and blend superbly. The regular ✓☺ **Eye Shadow** *($15)* deserves the same comments as the Glaze Shadow above, but these shades have less shine and more coverage. Many of them make effective all-over shades or work for highlighting the underbrow area. ✓☺ **$$$ Deluxe Eye Shadow** *($20)* costs more but provides a greater amount of product. These larger powder tablets have a sumptuous texture and seamless application that make them a pleasure to work with. The mostly matte shades are softer colors that most women would use frequently, making the larger size a wise choice.

☺ **$$$ Eye Definer** *($16)* shadows are dark shades meant for dramatic shading and/or eyelining. Although they're smooth, the level of pigmentation lends a drier feel that can drag a bit. Best applied with a damp brush, every shade is shiny (though on a few dark brown shades it's really subtle). ☺ **$$$ Base Essentials** *($22)* is similar to a liquid concealer and is meant to prep the eyelid area prior to eyeshadow application. It applies evenly and leaves a silky, soft matte finish, but doesn't provide as much camouflage as a traditional concealer. It is waterproof, as claimed, and is worth considering if you find that using concealer or foundation as an eyeshadow base doesn't work for you. ☺ **$$$ Luminizing Eye Base Essentials** *($22)* is identical to the Base Essentials above, except with a soft shine finish. Otherwise, the same comments apply, along with the caveat that this isn't the best look if your eyelid is wrinkled.

😐 **$$$ Cream Definer** *($18)* comes in one shade (Rich Mocha) and has a thick, slightly waxy texture that's malleable for easy application. The question of wear comes into play because although this isn't prone to smearing once set, it doesn't have the longevity of silicone-enhanced gel eyeliners. Those with oily eyelids should avoid this product, and it is not 100% waterproof.

EYE AND BROW SHAPER: ✓☺ $$$ Brow Gel *($20)* has been redone and along with sleek metal packaging comes an improved formula that is different from most brow gels because it keeps hairs in place without feeling the least bit tacky, stiff, or sticky. There is only one clear color, so it works only for those who are just trying to keep their brows in place, not trying to create more definition or fullness. If you're going to spend more than you need to for brow gel, this should be the one you buy.

😐 **$$$ High Definition Gel Eyeliner** *($18)* is similar to the gel eyeliners from Bobbi Brown, M.A.C., and Stila, but doesn't compete as favorably as I was expecting it to. The colors (McEvoy only offers two) go on softer than those from the aforementioned companies, which isn't bad if you want a less intense effect. However, women who use this type of product aren't likely to be meek about eyeliner, and part of the longevity of this type of product is related to its pigment concentration. Even if you did want a softer effect, the formula goes on less smoothly and somewhat powdery, and flakes. All told, it's an OK option that wears reasonably well, but it doesn't equal or outperform the products that preceded it.

😐 **$$$ Classic Eye Pencil** *($20)* is classic in the sense that it's one more creamy pencil that needs routine sharpening and it comes with a pointed smudger to soften the line. The plus with this option is that, for all its creaminess, it is relatively impervious to smudging.

☹ **Eye Brightener** *($22)* is a standard, chunky pencil that needs sharpening. It glides on but remains greasy enough to smudge, so its brightening effect, while attractive, won't last. You can achieve the same effect with one of McEvoy's longer-lasting Glaze Eye Shadows. ☹ **Brow Pencils** *($20)* are very stiff and difficult to apply, plus these dry-finish, too waxy pencils need routine sharpening.

LIPSTICK, LIP GLOSS, AND LIPLINER: ✓☺ $$$ Glaze Lip Color *($21)* is McEvoy's best lipstick. It has a modern, creamy texture and a sexy pearlized finish. It moisturizes lips without feeling thick, and stays on better than her other lipstick options, though it also competes favorably with cream lipsticks from other lines.

☺ **$$$ Cream Lip Color** *($21)* provides full coverage, and features mostly bold and bright colors. More greasy than creamy, this moves easily into lines around the mouth, but if that's not an issue there is no reason to not consider this lipstick, other than its price.

☺ **$$$ Sheer Lip Color** *($21)* has an emollient texture and very glossy finish that's not as sheer as most. There isn't much to choose from color-wise, but the Tres Jolie shade is gorgeous and universally flattering. ☺ **$$$ Maxed Out Pretty Lips** *($21)* packages a selection of McEvoy's lipstick and gloss shades (eight colors altogether) in a slim compact that's slightly larger than a credit card. The palette is pretty and versatile, but you'll need to supply the lip brush.

😐 **$$$ Lip Liner** *($20)* comes in a nice assortment of rich colors, and one end of the pencil has a lip brush. It's a nice touch, but this is too creamy if you're concerned about keeping lipstick in place. If not, and if you don't mind sharpening, it's worth a look.

😐 **$$$ Flawless Lip Sheer Lip Liner** *($20)* looks like a lip pencil (and needs sharpening), but applies like a sheer, slightly greasy lip gloss. The tip is too soft for a defined line and the finish feels slick, so this isn't for anyone with lines around the mouth. 😐 **$$$ Essential Pencil** *($22)* must not be as essential as it once was because less than a handful of shades are available. This thick, needs-sharpening pencil feels slick and slightly greasy while leaving a glossy finish and sheer color. It's an OK, fleeting option, but pricey for what you get. 😐 **$$$ Lipgloss** *($22)* comes with either a sponge-tip or brush applicator, depending on the shade you choose. This is a thick, emollient gloss that imparts a shimmering finish while feeling sticky. If you're going to spend this much money for lip gloss, look to the better options from Chanel, Dior, or Stila, or at the drugstore to options from Neutrogena, Revlon, or L'Oreal before this one.

☹ **Conditioning Lip Color SPF 15** *($21)* is conditioning thanks to emollients, but it lacks the UVA-protecting ingredients of titanium dioxide, zinc oxide, avobenzone, Mexoryl SX, or Tinosorb, and is not recommended. ☹ **Double Duty Lip Color** *($28)* combines a liquid lip stain and a lip gloss in one dual-sided package. The lip stain applies unevenly no matter how patient you are, and it tastes terrible (think saccharin times ten). It also takes too long to set and the gloss affects how well the stain wears. Why anyone would choose this over superior options such as M.A.C.'s Pro Longwear Lipcolour or Cover Girl's Outlast Lipcolor is beyond me.

MASCARA: ✓☺ **$$$ High-Volume Mascara** *($26)* deposits a lot of mascara on lashes, but does so with minimal clumping, and lets you quickly create long, thick lashes. The water-soluble formula removes easily and wears respectably, keeping its dramatic flair without flaking or smearing.

☺ **$$$ Lash Curling Mascara** *($26)* doesn't curl lashes any more than a lot of other mascaras, but it excels at lengthening, though it does take some time to dry (which gives you time to comb out minor clumping). ☺ **$$$ High Volume Waterproof Mascara** *($26)* takes some effort to prove its worth, but the reward is long, lush, and perfectly separated lashes without a clump in sight. The formula is waterproof, and its only drawback (beyond the unreasonable price) is slight flaking.

😐 **$$$ Lash Builder** *($20)* is a pre-mascara product meant to enhance the performance of any mascara. This ends up being just a standard mascara formulation minus the pigment. It makes a slight difference in terms of making lashes longer, but it also makes mascara application less smooth. Lash Builder helps make an average mascara better, but why are you using an average mascara in the first place?

FACE AND BODY ILLUMINATING/SHIMMER PRODUCTS: ✓☺ **$$$ Shimmer Pressed Powder** *($28)* is wonderful. It has a superior smooth texture that blends very well and provides a soft shine that's wearable day or night. All three shades are attractive and the shine doesn't flake. It's an altogether outstanding choice.

☺ **$$$ Highlights** *($32)* add gleaming shine to skin and is recommended for evening makeup because the shine clings surprisingly well. This pressed powder presents two shades in one tablet and applies evenly. Keep it away from wrinkles and large pores and you'll dazzle!

☺ **$$$ Mineral Shimmer Powder** *($20)* is loose powder with a sparkling finish that exhibits slight flaking, but the rich colors make an impact and the airy texture works over any makeup. Considering the type and intensity of shine this powder offers, some flaking is inevitable and isn't a deal-breaker.

☹ **$$$ Even Skin Luminizer** *($35)* is, at first glance, an eye-catching, pale gold shimmer cream. However, its lanolin oil–based texture makes it so thick and greasy it can't help but be difficult to work with, and it's inappropriate for everyone except those with very dry skin. It does make skin look shiny (from the shimmer it contains), but it also makes it look greasy, and that's not the best way to add radiance or luminosity to skin, especially when there are a plethora of other shine-boosting options available in liquid, cream, and powder.

☹ **$$$ Face Shine** *($32)* looks like a pressed powder with shine, but its texture is creamy with a smooth, dry finish (yet it's not a standard cream-to-powder either). It feels heavier than powder and deposits a lot of shine, which rubs off easily. What a shame, because the colors are enticing.

BRUSHES: Trish McEvoy has a well-earned reputation for producing some of the softest, most exquisitely shaped ✓☺ **$$$ Brushes** *($14–$72)* anywhere and, aside from the steep price tag that accompanies many of them, you won't be disappointed with their performance and longevity. McEvoy's brush collection can be considered one-stop shopping for those whose budget extends this far, with the best ones being ✓☺ **$$$ #37 Bronzer** *($62)*, ✓☺ **$$$ #M20 Face Blender** *($52)*, ✓☺ **$$$ #21 Large Laydown** *($53)*, ✓☺ **$$$ #19 Small Laydown** *($20)*, **Retractable Blush Brush** *($58)*, which also works for powder touch-ups, ✓☺ **$$$ #50 Angled Eye Lining** *($25)*, ✓☺ **$$$ #28 Tapered Eyeliner** *($20)*, ✓☺ **$$$ #5 Luxurious Powder Brush** *($72)*, ✓☺ **$$$ #48 Blending Brush** *($46)*, ✓☺ **$$$ #2B Blush Brush** *($46)*, ✓☺ **$$$ #23 Angled Crease Contour Mini Brush** *($32)*, and ✓☺ **$$$ #9 Q-Tip Brush** *($22)*. The ✓☺ **$$$ #10 Eye Shadow Brush** *($28)* isn't for everyone, but is great for sweeping a wash of color over a large eye area.

Note: Trish McEvoy does not offer any brush sets as part of the regular lineup. However, some department stores receive limited-edition sets for promotional events or holidays. Ask a McEvoy salesperson to contact you when such sets arrive at their counter.

SPECIALTY PRODUCTS: ✓☺ **$$$ Face Planners** *($48–$68 for the case, $13–$22 for the pages)* resemble a day planner and remain the most distinguishing element of McEvoy's line. A two- or three-ring binder inside an elegant zippered pouch holds covered plastic "pages" that can be filled (and refilled) with the colors of your choice. It's pricey, but the bags are handsomely made and exceedingly convenient, especially if you're loyal to Trish McEvoy's color line. You can assemble all the products you need for a complete makeup application, from foundation to lip color, and there are interior pockets that can hold several brushes or miscellaneous items that won't fit on the pages.

McEvoy occasionally offers **Limited-Edition Planners** *(prices vary)* that are even sturdier. These sport luxury fabric and have a few extras not found in the mainstay Planners, albeit for a premium price.

☺ **$$$ Finish Line** *($20)* is an alcohol-free, water-based fluid meant to turn any powder eyeshadow into a long-lasting liquid liner. It applies smoothly, dries quickly, and deepens the color payoff of an eyeshadow, making many medium tones suitable for lining. The waterproof claim is accurate, but it's worth noting that even minimal rubbing of your eyes while it's wet causes the product to break down. This is an OK option if you're a fan of eyelining with powders and want to experiment for a different, more intense effect.

☺ **$$$ Makeup Brush Cleaner** *($18)* is a good, spray-on brush cleanser that omits fast-drying solvents like alcohol in favor of water and gentle detergent cleansing agents. It dissolves makeup from brushes without damaging the hair, but with the drawback that the brush cannot be used again immediately. This is a fine option for occasional brush cleansing when you have time to let your brushes dry between uses.

😐 **$$$ Flawless Lip** *($22)* is a clear, silicone-based pre-lipstick base designed to keep lipstick anchored firmly on the lips. It works marginally well, but still can't keep most of McEvoy's lipsticks from their forward march into lines around the mouth. A better version of this product for less money is The Body Shop's Lip Line Fixer ($9).

😐 **$$$ Even Skin Face Primer** *($28)* is a substandard primer whose cream-gel texture belies its basic formula of water, thickeners, and preservative. It's an OK lightweight moisturizer for normal to slightly dry skin, but doesn't make good on its claim of keeping your foundation looking "just applied" all day. A cream-gel moisturizer with silicone (there are countless options available) works much better under foundation.

ULTRACEUTICALS (SKIN CARE ONLY)

ULTRACEUTICALS AT-A-GLANCE

Strengths: Almost all the products are fragrance-free; one very good cleanser and some good vitamin C and retinol moisturizers; an effective AHA product with lactic acid; all the sunscreens provide sufficient UVA protection; stable packaging.

Weaknesses: Expensive; most of the AHA products have pH values too high for exfoliation to occur; irritating skin-lightening products; no effective products for acne-prone skin.

For more information about Ultraceuticals, call (800) 339-5115 or visit www.ultraceuticals.com or www.Beautypedia.com. Note: Ultraceuticals is sold primarily in Australia, but is gradually expanding into the U.S. market.

✓☺ **$$$ Gentle Cleansing Gel** *($33 for 7 ounces)* is an excellent, fragrance-free, water-soluble cleansing gel for all skin types except very dry. The antioxidants are described as "powerful," but their contact with skin is too brief for them to flex any beneficial muscle. Although pricey, this is a prime pick if you prefer cleansing gels.

☺ **$$$ Ultra Milk Cleanser with Soy Extract** *($42 for 7 ounces)* is a good, though exceedingly overpriced, water-soluble cleanser for normal to dry skin. The amount of alcohol is unlikely to be a problem for skin; this cleanser is fragrance-free.

☹ **Ultra Clear Exfoliating Gel** *($42 for 7 ounces)* contains the AHA lactic acid and BHA salicylic acid, but these acids won't exfoliate skin due to this product's pH and its brief contact with skin before the cleanser is rinsed down the drain. Polyethylene beads provide exfoliation, but the inclusion of eucalyptus oil makes this gel-textured scrub too irritating.

☹ **Ultra Green Tea Skin Spritzer** *($32 for 4.2 ounces)* contains a lot more witch hazel (an alcohol-based mixture, meaning it is drying and irritating for skin) than green tea, while the truly state-of-the-art skin-identical substances are present in only minute amounts.

☺ **Antioxidant Daily Moisturiser SPF 30+ Tinted** *($44 for 3.3 ounces)*. Because this line is based in Australia, they are permitted to use combinations of active sunscreen ingredients that are not allowed in the United States. That's why this tinted moisturizer for normal to slightly dry skin not prone to blemishes contains a blend of avobenzone (listed as butyl methoxydibenzoylmethane) with titanium dioxide and zinc oxide. UVA protection is assured, while the sheer tint is an option for light to medium skin tones that want a slight hint of tan. Keep in mind this product provides enough color to interfere with your foundation, so it is best worn alone or simply set with a translucent powder.

☺ **$$$ C-10 Serum** *($65 for 0.88 ounce)* contains 10% ascorbic acid in a water and glycol base (the glycol enhances penetration of the vitamin C). This is a one-note product and very pricey for what you get, but it is an option if you're curious to see what vitamin C can do for your skin. At this price, the M.D. Skincare by Dr. Dennis Gross Hydra-Pure Vitamin C Serum ($90 for 1 ounce) is a much more elegant, varied formula, and your skin deserves more than just a single ingredient, just like your diet is far more healthy if you eat more than just broccoli!

☹ **Dark Circle Eye Cream** *($65 for 0.7 ounce)* contains a nearly insignificant amount of retinol and other antioxidants, although there is no research establishing that retinol is the answer for fading dark circles under the eye. The amount of sodium lauryl sulfate in this moisturizer is cause for concern (it's the fourth ingredient) and makes this not worth considering over hundreds of other eye creams. What is sodium lauryl sulfate, a potent skin irritant and cleansing agent, doing in an eye cream anyway?

☺ **$$$ Protective Daily Moisturiser SPF 30+** *($44 for 3.3 ounces)* came to us with an incomplete ingredient list, and the supplemental information Ultraceuticals provided did not match what was written on the product. Therefore, all I can do is comment on the active ingredients in this sunscreen. The combination of Tinosorb with zinc oxide and octyl methoxycinnamate is a formidable defense against UV rays, and in that sense this sunscreen is recommended, but there is no way to know what else you are putting on your skin and that's a problem (and also not in compliance with FDA or Australian cosmetic/pharmaceutical regulations).

😐 **$$$ Ultra A Treatment Serum** *($60 for 1.5 ounces)* was formerly known as Antioxidant Serum; the new name is designed to spotlight the retinol in this lightweight moisturizer for normal to slightly dry skin. The retinol and other antioxidants are in short supply, while the pH above 5 keeps the salicylic acid from functioning as a truly effective exfoliant. Overall, this isn't worth the money because it doesn't compete well with far superior products for far less money.

☺ **$$$ Ultra ACE Eye and Lip Treatment Serum** *($65 for 0.67 ounce)* contains a good amount of AHAs, but the pH of 4.1 is borderline for allowing them to exfoliate, not to mention that applying AHA products to the lips tends to be more irritating than helpful. This fragrance-free serum deserves consideration for its water-binding agents and antioxidants, including retinol, but is better for the eye area than for the lips.

☺ **$$$ Ultra ACE Facial Treatment Cream** *($59 for 1.66 ounces)* contains an impressive amount of AHAs, but the pH of 4.2 doesn't allow them to work as claimed. This is otherwise a well-formulated, fragrance-free moisturizer that contains antioxidant green tea along with retinol and good water-binding agents. It is an option for normal to dry skin not prone to breakouts.

😐 **$$$ Ultra C Sheer Facial Cream, 20% Pure Vitamin C** *($80 for 1.66 ounces)* is a lightweight moisturizer that contains, at least according to the label, 20% vitamin C as ascorbic acid. This amount may seem impressive, but its acidic component may also prove too irritating for most skin types. The base formula contains far more preservative than state-of-the-art ingredients, but if vitamin C is what you're looking for, this delivers it in stable packaging.

☺ **$$$ Ultra C Treatment Cream, 23% Pure Vitamin C** *($88 for 1.66 ounces)* lists vitamins, the amino acid tyrosine, and antioxidant grape extract as active ingredients. The way the vitamins are quantified (in milligrams per gram) is just bizarre, and there is no research showing that these quantities are sufficient to stimulate collagen production as claimed. So while the numbers might sound like you are getting therapeutic amounts of these substances, they end up being amounts similar to what many other "cosmeceutical" lines boast. Ignoring the actives issue, this is a good, antioxidant-rich moisturizer for normal to dry skin. This product is classified by the Australian Therapeutic Goods Act as a medicine, but because you aren't eating it, and because there is no research showing what kind of medicine it is, for now it is a good moisturizer and not a cure for anything.

✓☺ **$$$ Ultra Hydrating Gel** *($59 for 1.69 ounces)* is an excellent moisturizer for normal to slightly dry or slightly oily skin. It contains the antioxidant beta-glucan along with several water-binding agents and cell-communicating ingredients, and no fragrance. The texture is such that this would work well under makeup, and definitely around the eyes.

☺ **$$$ Ultra Moisturiser Cream with Ceramides, Hyaluronan and Vitamin E** *($55 for 1.7 ounces)* is a good moisturizer for normal to dry skin but the called-out ceramides, hyaluronic acid, and vitamin E incorporated here don't amount to much relative to the amount of waxlike thickeners in this product. This does contain fragrance.

☹ **Even Skintone Serum** *($65 for 0.88 ounce)* lists bearberry extract as an active ingredient, which is not permitted because it isn't an active ingredient. Bearberry has some research showing it can inhibit melanin production due to its arbutin content, but the amount of alcohol in this product makes it too irritating to consider.

☹ **Even Skintone Serum, Gentle Formula** *($65 for 0.88 ounce)* lists alcohol as the second ingredient, so this is hardly a gentle formula. The anti-irritants this contains won't counter the problems this much alcohol will cause for skin.

✓☺ **$$$ Ultra Ace Hydration Booster** *($50 for 2.5 ounces)* is similar to the Ultra ACE Facial Treatment Cream above except you get more for your money and it has a pH of 4, which allows the lactic acid to function as an exfoliant. Other than those pluses, the same comments apply.

☹ **Ultra Clear Treatment Gel** *($42 for 1.5 ounces)* sounds like a slam-dunk for blemishes because of its combination of AHA, BHA, retinol, and tea tree extract. However, the amount of tea tree extract is too low for it to function as a disinfectant and the inclusion of alcohol and eucalyptus oil makes this gel too irritating for all skin types.

URBAN DECAY (MAKEUP ONLY)

URBAN DECAY AT-A-GLANCE

Strengths: Workable options in almost every category; excellent powder blush; bonanza for anyone who wants lots of shiny eyeshadows; several super-smooth lip glosses; makeup brushes; several intriguing specialty products; a much less off-putting marketing strategy.

Weaknesses: Average to poor eye and brow pencils; limited foundation shades; disappointing lash primer/waterproofing product; irritating makeup remover and lip plumper.

For more information about Urban Decay, sold primarily at Sephora boutiques, call (800) 784-URBAN or visit www.urbandecay.com or www.Beautypedia.com.

FOUNDATION: ☺ **$$$ Surreal Skin Liquid Makeup** *($24)* comes in a bottle that looks like it could also house a genie (someone tell Christina Aguilera!), but all that's dispensed is a silky, fluid foundation that blends easily and provides medium coverage. This would have earned a Paula's Pick rating if it looked a bit more natural on skin. As is, the strong matte finish, while great for oily to very oily skin, tends to call attention to itself unless blending is meticulous. If that doesn't deter you (and it's not a deal-breaker) four of the five shades are beautifully neutral; Supernatural has a slight orange cast that won't work for most medium skin tones.

☹ **$$$ Surreal Skin Mineral Makeup** *($28)* marks Urban Decay's attempt to bring their brand of street credibility to the overhyped category of mineral makeup. This loose-powder foundation is packaged in a jar with a sponge affixed to the cap. Once opened, the powder is shaken onto the sponge, where it poofs out and allows you to blend it over your skin. The formula is based on mica and bismuth oxychloride (the same as most mineral foundations and powders), and this product shares the same traits typical for this category of makeup, meaning it offers shine, reliable coverage, and a dry finish that can become uncomfortably dry during the day depending on your skin type. Urban Decay's version has a decidedly light texture, and all five neutral-to-yellow-toned shades are attractive, but you have to accept a slight sparkling effect and the drawbacks of mineral makeup to really enjoy this product. Mineral makeup is not a good choice if you have any degree of dry skin because the ingredients absorb oil (and your moisturizer), making dry skin drier. For someone with very oily skin the makeup typically separates on your skin and pools into pores, which is as unbecoming as it sounds.

CONCEALER: ☺ **$$$ Surreal Skin Creamy Concealer** *($16)* is a liquid concealer with a slightly runny consistency that makes blending tricky and provides coverage that is more sheer than what most people who use concealer want. Still, the two shades (reserved for those with fair to light skin) are good, and this is an OK option if you want sheer coverage and a satin-matte finish. The formula is appropriate for use over blemishes, but don't expect much in the way of camouflage.

POWDER: ☺ **$$$ Baked Bronzing Powder** *($22)* is a talc-based pressed bronzing powder that goes on smoothly and has a sheer, dry finish. The two shades would be more convincing without shine, but if a shiny tan effect is what you want, it clings well. Baked has an unmistakable shine, while Toasted's shine is subtle.

BLUSH: ✓☺ **$$$ Afterglow Blush** *($17)* claims to go beyond blushing to make you glow, and it does that thanks to each shade's pearlescent finish. This creamy-feeling powder blush is excellent, with moderately pigmented shades that go on with more intensity than you may expect. Although each shade has shine that's best for evening glamour, the effect is indeed more of a glow than a sparkle-fest, and it doesn't flake.

EYESHADOW: The classic ☺ **$$$ Eye Shadow** *($16)* features a rainbow of unusual, sometimes shocking colors sold as singles. Most of them have a superior smooth texture that applies and blends wonderfully. Every shade has some degree of shine, but the good news is that except for the colors with glitter (easily identified), the shine clings well. The almost garish shades that you should consider very carefully are Gash, Acid Rain, Mildew, Vert, Shattered, Goddess, Asphyxia, Stalker, and Last Call.

☺ **$$$ Deluxe Eyeshadow** *($17)* has deluxe packaging but formula-wise is quite similar to Urban Decay's regular Eye Shadow, save for an application that's a touch smoother due to the silicone content. The small selection of shades favors strong metallic colors, few of which make for an effective eye design unless you're doing eye makeup for shock value. Still, these apply and blend well and the shine stays put, so they're a consideration.

☹ **$$$ Metal Eye Sheen** *($18)* is packaged in a diamond-shaped clear container, inside which is a silicone-based cream-to-powder eyeshadow that's light on color and heavy on shine. It's an OK option that should have more slip than it does, though it's minimally prone to creasing, so perhaps that was the tradeoff.

EYE AND BROW SHAPER: ☹ **$$$ Smoke Out Eye Pencil** *($14)* needs sharpening, so it doesn't earn higher than a neutral face rating. However, if you don't mind sharpening this is definitely a pencil to check out! It has a smooth texture that glides on and a powder finish that won't smudge or smear once set. The shade selection favors the trendy and odd, but Smoke is a reliable choice that's almost a basic black.

😐 **$$$ Liquid Eye Liner** *($14)* has a long, thin brush that's relatively easy to use and this liquid liner deposits rich color along the entire lash line. Although it wears well once it sets, the dry time is slower than average, which can lead to slight smearing, especially if you blink a lot.

☹ **24/7 Glide-On Eye Pencil** *($15)* does glide on, but this needs-sharpening pencil has a soft tip that's prone to breaking off and a finish that is creamy enough to smudge. It doesn't last all night and isn't the best fit for anyone's "on-the-go" lifestyle, and the colors are mostly clownish. ☹ **Heavy Metal Glitter Liner** *($18)* is a liquid eyeliner that's basically large flecks of colored glitter suspended in a clear fluid. This much shine has its place for those so inclined, but not when the application is as uneven as this, not to mention the slow dry time. ☹ **Brow Beater** *($14)* is a dual-sided, needs-sharpening pencil that includes a brow pencil on one end and a clear wax for grooming on the other. The brow color portion is thick and tricky to apply, while the wax portion is noticeably sticky.

LIPSTICK, LIP GLOSS, AND LIPLINER: ✓☺ **Triple XXX Slick Lip Gloss** *($15)* is a lip gloss whose slick, weightless texture and wet, glossy finish somewhat justify its naughty-sounding name. This pot gloss is adorably packaged, but the contents are also worth getting excited about if you routinely use lip gloss. Few offer such a nice glossy payoff without feeling the least bit sticky or tacky. The petrolatum base means your lips will stay smooth, and the sheer colors (which look much more intense than they actually are) are all goof-proof choices. ✓☺ **$$$ Ultraglide Lip Gloss** *($17)* is one of the best lip glosses around if you prize a smooth application, ultra-glossy finish, and a non-sticky texture that's neither too thin nor thick. The shade selection is pleasingly versatile and, dare I say, more mainstream than what Urban Decay usually offers. Those looking for the same texture and finish, but very sheer, almost transparent color should explore ✓☺ **Lube-in-a-Tube** *($11)*. Why the shades for this group of glosses are named after cities is anyone's guess (who knew Chicago was akin to soft lavender?), but this is nevertheless a terrific gloss. ☺ **$$$ Lip Gunk** *($13)* is a very standard, slightly sticky lip gloss whose main distinction is a handful of unusual colors. It has a thick texture that allows some tenacity while imparting a moderately glossy shine.

☺ **$$$ Ink** *($17)* is packaged like a Magic Marker and has a large felt-tip applicator that imparts a water-based sheer stain to lips. Take the name seriously, because this really does stain like ink and is difficult to remove completely. It is best used as a color base for lipstick or gloss because the product itself does not have a moist or conditioning feel whatsoever. Still, the key selling point is its longevity, and that may be reason enough to try it!

☺ **$$$ Lip Envy** *($17)* is very similar to Ink, but packaged differently, and the formula is slightly thicker, though it's still a water-based stain. The angled applicator makes it easier to be accurate, which is critical with a product like this because mistakes aren't easily wiped away. The three sheer shades (each looks quite dark before applying) are attractive.

😐 **$$$ XXX Shine Lip Gloss** *($16)* has a texture that's syrupy and sticky, quite the opposite of the superior Triple XXX Slick Lip Gloss above. The sheer colors last thanks to this gloss's clingy nature, but the peppermint flavor can be irritating and that isn't good for lips.

😐 **$$$ Sparkler Pen for Lips** *($10)* will likely appeal to teens because this click pen–applied sheer lip gloss has lots of glitter. The formula is sticky but applies smoothly.

☹ **$$$ Lip Pencil** *($14)* has a stiff but still creamy application and a finish that lasts. This needs-sharpening pencil comes in very basic but wearable colors, and is an OK option.

☹ **Commando** *($26)* is an ornately packaged tin of two lip glosses fastened to a silver dog chain as a military chic accessory. The sheer, slightly sticky gloss contains peppermint oil and is not recommended over any of the Urban Decay lip glosses above.

MASCARA: ☺ **$$$ Skyscraper Mascara** *($17)* has an oddly shaped and cut brush that gives you access to average thickness and, with some effort, a good amount of length with clean separation of each lash. Another plus is that the formula keeps lashes very soft, though many other mascaras that cost less can also do that.

😐 **$$$ Big Fatty Mascara** *($18)* purports to thicken and lengthen lashes, and its gigantic brush achieves that, though not to the same impressive extent as mascaras with smaller brushes and more variegated bristles. You may think that a big brush equals big results, but that's not the case here, nor has it been with any other enlarged mascara brush I've ever tried, with one exception: Dior's Mascara Diorshow ($23). If you're curious to see how a large mascara brush will work for you, try Dior's version instead of this average mascara from Urban Decay.

FACE AND BODY ILLUMINATING/SHIMMER PRODUCTS: ☺ **$$$ Heavy Metal Glitter Eye Gel** *($18)* is glitter to the max, but if that's the look you're after for a night of clubbing or a Halloween costume, this is excellent. A clear, clingy gel suspends brilliantly shiny particles of glitter, allowing you to apply it with a brush or a fingertip. It takes a moment to set, but the reward is long wear with negligible flaking.

The **Cocktail Collection** features various sets of cocktail-flavored products, including Pina Colada and Cosmopolitan. This collection features 😐 **$$$ Flavored Body Powder** *($30)*, which has a huge synthetic brush attached to a jar of sparkling powder that clings unevenly but does add head-to-toe gleam. This product is also available in food flavors (such as Marshmallow), which are packaged in cardboard jars and include powder puffs. You'll find that either Powder (food or cocktail-flavored) lasts longer if you apply the ☺ **$$$ Body Balm** *($25)* first, which adds a low-key but still sexy sheen of its own. Last but not least is ☺ **$$$ Shot-O-Gloss** *($15)*, which tastes like the other products it matches (depending on your drink of choice) and imparts much more shimmer than color to lips, while being relatively non-sticky.

😐 **$$$ Baked Body Glow** *($25)* looks like a large roll-on deodorant, but is a sheer, peachy bronze tint for the body. The thick texture must be warmed on the hand or it doesn't glide over skin well, while the result feels a bit too thick and waxy to make it worth considering over numerous bronzing gels, lotions, or self-tanning products—and this one will come off on clothes.

BRUSHES: The synthetic, expertly crafted ☺ **$$$ Good Karma Brushes** *($15–$35)* are a distinct highlight and value of this line. Each one has merit depending on your needs and preferences, but generally speaking the standouts are the ☺ **$$$ Powder Brush** *($35)*, ☺ **$$$ Shadow Brush** *($18)*, ☺ **$$$ Blender Brush** *($24)*, and the ☺ **$$$ Brow Brush** *($15)*, which is also suitable for applying powder eyeliner.

✓☺ **$$$ Big Buddha Brush Set** *($100)* includes all of Urban Decay's well-made brushes in a zippered bag. A brush roll with holders for each tool would be better, but all things considered this set ends up being functionally proficient and a good value.

☺ **$$$ Little Buddha Brush Set** *($65)* includes four brushes, covering options for applying blush, eyeshadow, lipstick, or gloss, and filling in brow color or eyelining. It's an option if you need to augment your existing brush collection, but if you're looking for a comprehensive set, the Big Buddha Brush Set above is the better buy.

SPECIALTY PRODUCTS: ☺ **$$$ Face Case** *($34)* provides tiny amounts of Urban Decay's various eyeshadow and lip gloss formulas, all in a slim but still large (about the size of an evening bag) mirrored cardboard compact. The included applicators aren't the best, but will do in a pinch. If you find an appealing combination of colors and like the products, this is an OK investment. The ☺ **$$$ Urban Arsenal Palette** *($42)* offers a more interesting, convenient assortment of some of the line's best-selling shades. Included are separately packaged lip glosses, mascara, eyeshadow primer, and tablets of eyeshadow plus a powder blush. Again, if you're a fan of these products this is a sensible splurge.

☺ **$$$ Eyeshadow Primer Potion** *($15)* promises to make eyeshadows last longer while keeping them from creasing, and it works. In addition, it facilitates a smoother application and makes blending even easier. The problem is you can get the same results from a good matte-finish concealer that's silicone-based like this one. Because most of today's best concealers follow this format, a product like this, though it works, seems superfluous (unless you don't use a silicone-based type of concealer).

☺ **$$$ Blow Lip Plumper** *($17)* is said to use a high-tech formula to inflate lips to injection-worthy proportions. It doesn't do that in the least, and, as far as I can tell, lacks ingredients capable of causing lips to swell in any manner. It is otherwise a thin-textured, nearly clear lip gloss whose shiny finish can create the illusion of larger lips, though I'll stress again it's not even close to the results possible from lip injections.

☺ **$$$ Eyeshadow Transforming Potion** *($17)* is said to transform eyeshadow into a liquid eye color. This water-based solution is housed in a dual-sided component that provides a synthetic brush meant for drawing wide lines and another for drawing thin, precise lines. Both work well and deepen powder eyeshadow colors, though this requires successive layers because initially the solution causes the color to go on sheer. Once set it wears reasonably well, but it's neither budgeproof nor completely waterproof. The thicker brush tends to dispense too much of the liquid, so be sure to remove some of it before using with a powder eyeshadow.

☹ **Lingerie & Galoshes for Lashes** *($17)* seems like a clever idea: it's a dual-ended product featuring a waterproofing solution on one end and a lash primer on the other. The waterproofing side is designed to be used over a non-waterproof mascara, the idea being that it will make your favorite mascara resistant to tears and water-based activities. Sounds great until you try it—the product doesn't apply easily over lashes and it's not completely waterproof. In fact, mild splashing of the eye area caused smearing and streaking. Adding to this disappointment is that the waterproofing sealer is difficult to remove. The primer's results aren't that great either, but the overall effect is neutral (nearing do-nothing) and it doesn't impede mascara application. All told, there are too many negatives to give this product anything but an unhappy face rating.

☹ **Big Fatty Lip Plumper** *($17)* will make lips look temporarily larger, but does so via several irritating ingredients, including capsicum, ginger root, and benzyl nicotinate. Usually only one of these ingredients is on board, but in this case the triple threat proves too irritating to use regularly.

☹ **Clean & Sober Makeup Remover** *($18 for 3.4 ounces)* begins as a standard, detergent-based liquid makeup remover, but isn't worth considering over many others (price notwithstanding) because it contains potentially irritating plant extracts and volatile fragrance components that should not be used near the eyes.

VANIQA (PRESCRIPTION ONLY)

Vaniqa *($50–60 for 30 grams/1.05 ounce)* is a prescription topical product that is said to reduce unwanted hair growth. Its active ingredient is eflornithine HCl, an ingredient that inhibits the enzyme ornithine decarboxylase within the hair follicle. This effect is believed to be what causes Vaniqa to slow hair growth. The base formula for Vaniqa is a blend of thickeners with silicone, mineral oil, preservatives, and water, so it is suitable for normal to dry skin and not the best for oily or blemish-prone skin. However, if you are restricting its use to a small area (such as the upper lip, where women tend to have the most bothersome issues with unwanted hair), any skin type can use Vaniqa. Vaniqa is also compatible with other skin-care products and may be applied under makeup.

What's important to keep in mind (and it's a fact stated repeatedly in the literature for Vaniqa) is that it does not stop hair growth; it merely slows it down. If you are already using other hair-removal methods on a routine basis, you will need to continue that while using Vaniqa. The difference is that if Vaniqa works for you it is likely that you will be spending less time removing unwanted facial hair, and regrowth will likely not be as resistant to removal as hairs not treated with Vaniqa.

So, how well does Vaniqa work, and what does the research report? A recent double-blind study comparing use of Vaniqa alone with use of Vaniqa combined with laser hair removal showed that the combination had a 93.5% success rate. In contrast, the upper lip area treated with Vaniqa alone had a less impressive success rate of 68% after the six-month study period. Clinical studies for Vaniqa have demonstrated that 60% of women will experience a reduction in hair growth after eight weeks of daily treatment, and the most common side effect is minor skin irritation. Of course, that statistic means that 40% of women won't see a difference with Vaniqa, but that doesn't mean it's not worth trying to see how well (or if) it works for you. If Vaniqa works for you, you must continue to use it, because if you stop, within weeks the rate of regrowth will return to what it was before you started treatment.

(Sources for the above: *Journal of the American Academy of Dermatology*, July 2007, pages 54–59; *Dermatologic Surgery*, October 2006, pages 1237–1243; *Current Medical and Research Opinion*, August 2005, pages 1227–1234; *Skin Therapy Letter*, April 2001, pages 1–3, and December 2005/January 2006, pages 1–4; and *American Journal of Clinical Dermatology*, February 2001, pages 197–201.)

VANIQA AT-A-GLANCE

Strengths: Valid though not slam-dunk option for controlling the growth of unwanted facial hair; minimal side effects.

Weaknesses: Cost and daily compliance; you must continue to use whatever hair-removal method(s) have worked best for you; Vaniqa is available only by prescription and works only for just over half of the women who try it.

For more information about Vaniqa, call (877) 382-6472 or visit www.vaniqa.com or www.Beautypedia.com.

of antioxidants won't help skin due to the unfortunate choice of jar packaging, which allows them to deteriorate after opening.

VICTORIA'S SECRET (MAKEUP ONLY)

VICTORIA'S SECRET AT-A-GLANCE

Strengths: Good concealer, powder blush, brow gel, and mascara; outstanding powder eyeshadow, liquid liner, and long-wearing lip color; good makeup remover; open, well-organized tester unit and a sales staff that encourages playing with color.

Weaknesses: Average foundation (and only one option); the cream and Mosaic eyeshadows; disappointing eye pencil, gel eyeliner, lip balms, and oil-blotting papers.For more information about Very Sexy Makeup by Victoria's Secret, call (800) 411-5116 or visit www2.victoriassecret.com/beauty/ or www.Beautypedia.com.

FOUNDATION: ☹ **Flawless Cream Makeup SPF 30** *($19.50)* is an unusual compact foundation, which makes it even more of a shame that the sunscreen lacks sufficient UVA protection. The texture of this foundation begins slightly creamy, but quickly morphs to a soft powder finish that doesn't look overly dry or powdery. Coverage is sheer to light, but it builds well if you need additional camouflage. Despite the "cream" part of the name, this product is best for normal to slightly oily skin. The range of 13 shades is mostly impressive, but the following colors are too peach or orange to look convincing: M15, M25, and M35. The darkest shades are well-suited for several African-American skin tones, but again, the lack of sufficient sun protection is a disappointment.

CONCEALER: ☺ **Fluid Concealer** *($12)* is applied with a wand applicator and has a beautifully smooth, lightweight texture and soft, even application. The formula sets to a satin-matte finish with just a hint of shine; its only drawback is the layering required to achieve meaningful coverage. All six shades are gorgeous and include options for light to dark skin tones.

POWDER: ☹ **$$$ Finishing Powder Duo** *($18)* provides a slightly shiny and very shiny talc-based pressed powder in one compact with no dividers between the tone-on-tone colors. Although very smooth, this has a waxy feel that is difficult to pick up on a brush and its impact on skin (in terms of coverage, finishing, and especially absorbing oil) is minimal. In addition, the shine clings poorly, so the only reason to consider this is if you want a barely-there application of powder and aren't using it to temper shine. All six compacts have soft, neutral colors for light to dark skin.

BLUSH: ☺ **$$$ Mosaic Blush** *($18)* offers four blocks of pressed-powder color in one sleek compact. Half of these are blush tones, while the others are best for highlighting or, depending on the set, contouring. All of the colors have varying degrees of shine, up to what can only be described as obvious. The good news is the shine clings well despite the powder's smooth but dry texture. This is a good option if you want shiny cheeks.

EYESHADOW: ✓☺ **Silky Eye Shadow** *($12)* has a lavish, silky texture that feels very light and blends on sheer and even. All of the shades have shine, but the nude, tan, and brown colors contain more finely milled shimmer rather than glitter, which makes them more appealing, especially because the shiniest shades tend to flake. This is worth a look if you do not have wrinkles around the eye or will reserve application to the brow bone.

☺ **Dazzling Liquid Shadow** *($12)* is indeed liquid, and surprisingly isn't too slippery, though the texture is best applied over the entire eye area rather than used for detail work. It sets quickly to a sheer, slightly shiny to moderately shiny finish, and is minimally prone to creasing and fading. You'll get more mileage out of a powder eyeshadow, but this is still an OK option if you want something different.

☺ **Beauty Rush Luminous Shadow** *($7)* is a loose-powder eyeshadow packaged in an inkwell-style container with a pointed sponge-tip applicator. It applies surprisingly well (shake before each use) with good color saturation and minimal flaking. The metallic shine of each shade isn't for daytime makeup, but several of the colors are good evening makeup options, and the formula lasts better than you'd expect. Avoid lime-green Money, Baby, and sky-blue Blutopia.

😐 **Long-Wear Cream Shadow** *($12)* isn't as easy to work with as the Dazzling Liquid Shadow above. It has a liquid-to-powder texture and very shiny colors that impart more sparkle than pigment. The main problems involve the long time this takes to set, and that its finish isn't as budgeproof as that of similar products, including Stila's Shadow Pots ($20) or Maybelline New York's Dream Mousse Shadow ($6.50).

😐 **$$$ Mosaic Eye Shadow** *($18)* has almost the same pattern as the Mosaic Blush above, providing four shiny powder eyeshadows in one compact without dividers between the shades. Almost all of the sets are too contrasting to be workable, and the dry texture hinders a seamless, easy-to-blend application. The only well-coordinated quad is Eye Contact.

EYE AND BROW SHAPER: ✓ ☺ **Liquid Liner Pen** *($12)* just may be one of the easiest, most goof-proof liquid eyeliners you'll ever use. Housed in a slim pen-style component, this has a firm yet flexible pointed felt tip that allows you to quickly draw one continuous line. It dries almost instantly, then wears without fading, smearing, or chipping. Classic black and brown shades are the sole options, but both work for just about any eye-makeup design.

☺ **Brow Gel** *($12)* has a great dual-sided brush, but is otherwise an ordinary clear brow gel minus the holding agent (typically PVP—think hairspray) found in most competing products. Although the result here is very light and non-sticky, this isn't a brow gel for anyone whose brow hairs need taming. This is best if your brows could use a soft hold and unruly hairs are absent.

😐 **Sparkling Eye Liner** *($10)* is a standard, needs-sharpening pencil whose two shades are laced with noticeable sparkles. The effect is eye-catching and the application is smooth and even. However, what's particularly noteworthy is that the sparkles tend to stay in place. If the sharpening doesn't bother you and you want a sparkling finish for special occasions, consider this a safe bet.

☹ **Eye Liner** *($10)* requires routine sharpening and always applies a thick line due to the soft texture of the pencil tip. As you may have guessed, the texture of this pencil stays too creamy, and it smudges readily, meaning it won't make it through even the tamest bedroom romp.

☹ **Gel Eye Liner Duo** *($12)* is misnamed because this eyeliner in a compact is very creamy and the colors go on so softly you need lots of layers to build intensity (especially for defining the eye), and that only encourages smearing and smudging. Bobbi Brown, Stila, and M.A.C. got the gel eyeliner concept right, so skip this entry.

LIPSTICK, LIP GLOSS, AND LIPLINER: ✓ ☺ **$$$ Long Wear Lip Shine** *($18)* is the Victoria's Secret version of Max Factor's Lipfinity, and is definitely worth a test run. The dual-sided unit includes a light-coverage color coat (building intensity isn't easy, so this isn't for anyone who wants opaque color) and a glossy top coat that feels smooth rather than sticky. The same application directions apply here as for all other two-step, long-wearing lip products. You'll find this goes on easily, sets quickly (within a minute), and wears very well, with minimal fading and no peeling or chipping. You don't have to spend this much money for long wear, but if price isn't an issue, consider this highly recommended.

☺ **Perfect Lipstick** *($12)* is perfect if you like your lipstick to have sexy names such as Vixen, Love Bite, and Beg Me. Aside from the names, this is a fairly standard cream lipstick with a glossy, glitter-infused finish. Each shade offers moderate coverage, so even the deeper reds and pinks don't overdramatize lips.

☺ **Sheer Moisture Lipstick** *($12)* is a standard, sheer, glossy lipstick available in a selection of well-edited colors, from just-bitten reds to sheer blackberry hues. Although this feels slick, it isn't that greasy—a nice change of pace!

☺ **Lip Gloss** *($12)* comes with a wand applicator and for the most part is a very standard, slightly thick gloss with the appropriately sexy wet-look finish. Fans of shimmer- and glitter-infused lip gloss will appreciate the large selection of shades, from sheer to deep (but even the boldest shades don't apply too strongly).

☺ **$$$ Mosaic Lip Palette** *($18)* presents several stripes of a creamy lipstick with a glossy finish in one compact. Color impact is on the sheer side, but layering makes the shades more intense. The only issue this kit has is the lack of dividers between the colors. The soft texture of the product makes it all too easy to "squish" the shades together, though they're complementary, so the new shade is still attractive.

😐 **Sparkling Lipstick** *($12)* gets its sparkle from large flecks of glitter, and the result on adult lips tends to look more teenage-experimental than sexy. Still, this lipstick has a smooth, lightweight texture and a slightly glossy finish. The shade selection is small and favors sheer hues.

😐 **Lip Liner** *($10)* needs routine sharpening but you may overlook that once you've experienced how smoothly this pencil glides over lips, not to mention its enticing shade range that coordinates beautifully with the lipstick palette. The only drawback is that this pencil's finish is creamy enough to not be for anyone who uses lipliner to keep lipstick from feathering into lines around the mouth.

😐 **Beauty Rush Lip Gloss** *($7)* is one of the more cutesy products in the Victoria's Secret line. This intensely candy-scented, sweet-tasting tube lip gloss is imbued with holographic flecks of glitter that catch light from every direction but look strange once the glossy effect has faded, making frequent touch-ups necessary. It has a thick, syrupy texture and a slightly sticky finish.

☹ **Beauty Rush Soothing Lip Balm** *($7)* isn't soothing in the least because it contains lip-tingling amounts of peppermint oil and menthol. What a shame, because this is otherwise a lightweight but substantially moisturizing glossy lip balm.

☹ **Luxe Lip Balm SPF 15** *($12)* and ☹ **Beauty Rush Lip Conditioner SPF 15** *($7)* lack the UVA-protecting ingredients of titanium dioxide, zinc oxide, avobenzone, Mexoryl SX, or Tinosorb, and neither is recommended for sun protection.

MASCARA: ☺ **Intensifying Mascara** *($12)* works quite nicely in both the lengthening and thickening departments. If you're not looking to create dramatic lashes this fills the bill, and application is swift and clump-free. As for wearability, you'll be impressed that this mascara doesn't flake or smear yet removes with a water-soluble cleanser. ☺ **Lush Lash Primer** *($12)* is one of the few lash primers that make a difference, especially when used with a substandard mascara or a mascara that, for special occasions, you'd like to get more oomph from. The soft, wax-based formula is lighter and more conditioning than standard mascara, keeping lashes flexible and allowing for more mascara to adhere to lashes with each stroke. The results aren't stupendous, but for a slight improvement this is something to consider.

FACE AND BODY ILLUMINATING/SHIMMER PRODUCTS: 😐 **$$$ Loose Shimmer Powder** *($18)* has the most sumptuous texture that feels airy-smooth on skin and imparts a high-shine finish that would get you noticed in even the dimmest room. However, the shine clings poorly and tends to get everywhere in short order. What a shame, because the container includes a sifter cap that allows you to plug the holes, preventing powder from flying where it's not wanted.

BRUSHES: The **Very Sexy Brushes** *($9–$18)* are sexy in name only, and although they're not worth totally dismissing, the new collection isn't as impressive as the previous versions. The best (which is a relative term here) brushes to consider are the ☺ **Blush Brush** *($16)*, which is better for applying contour thanks to its angled cut, and the dense ☺ **Bronzer Brush** *($18)*. The 😐 **Eye Liner Brush** *($12)* has an odd, pointed tip that's almost too dense to work with, but some may find it appealing.

SPECIALTY PRODUCTS: ☺ **Very Sexy Makeup Total Makeup Remover** *($10 for 4 ounces)* is a very standard, but effective and gentle, silicone-based makeup remover. This is fragrance- and colorant-free and must be shaken well before use.

😐 **$$$ Very Sexy Makeup Lip Plumper** *($18 for 0.12 ounce)* seems right at home among the numerous pieces of Victoria's Secret lingerie that promise to make you more voluptuous and to enhance your curves. This has a formula that's remarkably similar to Fusion Beauty's Lip Fusion ($36 for 0.29 ounce); that is, another plumper that works by irritating the lips and causing them to swell temporarily. The "active" ingredient in this product is menthoxypropanediol, which has an effect similar to but twice as intense as menthol, creating a long-lasting cooling, tingling sensation that irritates the lips. The resulting low-grade inflammation makes lips temporarily fuller (or, if you prefer, more plump), but routinely applying this irritant is not a good long-term choice (Source: www.leffingwell.com/cooler_than_menthol.htm). Most lip-plumping products work to an extent, and they're OK for occasional use provided you are realistic about the results. They just don't work remotely like collagen (or any other dermal) injections. This product leaves lips slightly sticky, and has a very sheer pink tint.

☹ **Beauty Rush Oil-Blotting Sheets** *($7 for 50 sheets)* are composed of a thin plastic-like material rather than being the typical tissue-paper variety. Oddly, unlike blotting papers composed of similar materials, these don't absorb oil nearly as well. Chalk this up to a beauty slump.

VINCENT LONGO (MAKEUP ONLY)

VINCENT LONGO AT-A-GLANCE

Strengths: Original Water Canvas foundation; supremely smooth, seamless-finish powders and powder blush; most eyeshadows are great; excellent brow-enhancing options; several great lipsticks with some of the best colors around, whether you want soft nudes or riveting reds; excellent powder highlighter; provides complete product ingredient lists on their Web site.

Weaknesses: Every foundation and lipstick/gloss with sunscreen lacks sufficient UVA-protecting ingredients; terrible concealers; average eye pencils; poor liquid liner and waterproof mascara; makeup brushes should be better considering this line's emphasis on expert application.

For more information about Vincent Longo, call (877) LONGO-99 or visit www.vincent-longo.com or www.Beautypedia.com.

FOUNDATION: ✓☺ **$$$ Water Canvas Creme-to-Powder Foundation** *($52.50, $14 for optional compact)* is Longo's trademark product, and though it has an interesting texture it is not exclusive to Longo's line. For example, Awake's Hydro Manage Makeup ($43, including compact) and Borghese's Molto Bella Makeup ($35.50), like Longo's Water Canvas, are foundations that feel like a spongy liquid powder (Awake and Borghese are not reviewed in this book).

They feel lightweight and have less slip than traditional cream-to-powder makeup, and they dry to a matte, slightly powdery finish that can be a bit tacky. This type of foundation is best for someone with normal to oily or combination skin, or slightly dry skin looking for light to medium coverage. Be aware that this type of foundation can roll and chip out of the container if you aren't meticulous about keeping the compact tightly closed or if you apply too much pressure with your makeup sponge. Longo's version is the most expensive, but also happens to have the most natural-looking result, which may explain its enduring popularity. The selection of 16 shades is mostly outstanding and includes colors for fair to dark skin tones. The only ones to avoid are Sandy Beige, Honey Pecan, and Sienna, all of which are too peach or ash for most skin tones. Note: Literature for this product touts its SPF 6, but the product does not list any active ingredients, so do not rely on it for sun protection.

😐 **$$$ Liquid Canvas Dew Finish SPF 15** *($48.50)* would be another strong foundation from Vincent Longo in every respect if its sunscreen were improved; as it is, it lacks adequate UVA protection. It has a fluid but substantially emollient texture that blends so well and goes on so sheer you'll think you're not wearing foundation—except your skin looks smooth and even-toned. The moist, radiant finish is ideal for those with normal to very dry skin, and the selection of 12 shades presents ample choices for those with porcelain to dark skin tones. The following shades are options, but may be too pink or peach for some skin tones: Porcelain, Medium Beige, and Golden Tan. What a shame the UVA protection is lacking; with it, this foundation would have rated a Paula's Pick.

😐 **$$$ Liquid Canvas Healthy Fluid Foundation SPF 8** *($48.50)* doesn't impress with its embarrassingly low SPF rating, but at least the active ingredient is titanium dioxide. Although not a foundation to consider if you want sufficient sun protection, this has a beautifully silky texture, a seamless application that blends superbly, and a soft matte finish. Coverage is sheer to light, and the result blurs minor imperfections while looking very natural. Twelve shades are available, including great options for fair to light skin. Medium Beige and Golden Tan are slightly peach and should be considered carefully. The darkest shade, Topaz, has a slight tendency to turn ash, while Golden Sienna is too peach for its intended skin tone. This deserves a happy face rating for everything but its low SPF rating, so if you have normal to slightly dry skin it is recommended if you are willing to wear an SPF 15 or greater product underneath.

☹ **Light Canvas Tinted Moisturizer SPF 20** *($38)* not only comes in an assortment of eight mostly peach-toned shades, but the sunscreen also lacks the UVA-protecting ingredients of titanium dioxide, zinc oxide, avobenzone, Mexoryl SX (ecamsule), or Tinosorb. Did I mention that the finish of this poorly formulated tinted moisturizer just sits on the skin's surface, magnifying pores, crevices, and superficial lines? Not a pretty picture, but the insufficient UVA protection is the deal-breaker.

CONCEALER: ☹ **Concealer/Illumina Pencil** *($32.50)* is a dual-sided chunky pencil, with one end a creamy concealer and the other a highlighter with a soft shimmer finish. The shade pairings are better than Longo's other concealers, but the texture is way too greasy to last, and coverage is too sheer. ☹ **Duo Stick Concealer** *($20)* provides two colors in one swivel-up stick, with half of each shade being too pink or peach. Every duo poses a challenge when it comes to blending and wearability because the formula is crease-prone and way too waxy to use over breakouts. ☹ **Cream Concealer** *($26.50)* is an emollient concealer that is among the greasiest you're likely to find. It has way too much slip so it never sets, it creases, and coverage is spotty. Making matters worse is the selection of six shades, almost all of which are too pink, peach, or orange.

POWDER: ✓☺ **$$$ Perfect Canvas Loose Powder** *($40)* has a steep price tag that should give you pause (there are several equally good loose powders that cost half this amount or less), but this talc-based option has a powdered sugar–like texture that looks incredibly natural, refining skin and adding a soft shine without appearing too matte or powdery. It is not absorbent enough for very oily skin, but works well for normal to dry skin. Among the six sheer shades, only Golden Oriental stands out as being a problem due to its peach cast, but it's almost too sheer to matter.

✓☺ **$$$ Pressed Powder** *($26)* is just as impressive as the Perfect Canvas Loose Powder, but has distinct differences. This talc-free formula has an almost creamy texture and a thicker application whose coverage can approach that of a pressed-powder foundation. It provides a shine-free matte finish and comes in six splendid shades. Translucent is a winner for those with very fair skin. Just like Longo's loose powder, this version is best for normal to dry skin.

✓☺ **$$$ Sole Mio Duo Bronzer** *($38.50)* comes in two of the best bronze tones around, with Golden Glow being ideal for fair to light skin and Copper Kiss preferred for medium to tan skin. The silky application should be brushed on sheer due to the pigmentation of the powders, and it leaves a soft shimmer finish that clings well. This is an overall excellent pairing of bronzing and highlighting powder.

BLUSH: ✓☺ **$$$ Day Play Duo Compact Powder Blush** *($35)* is a powder blush that includes two shades in one large compact. The Day shades are soft, sheer colors for use as blush, while the Play shades are deeper and brown-based, ideal for evening makeup or contouring. Used alone or blended together, they have a superior smoothness that practically floats onto the skin and looks naturally flattering. Each duo's shades are well coordinated, and the shine varies from subtle to sparkling. This product is admittedly costly, but if you find a duo where both shades are appealing, it may be worth the expense, and it certainly looks beautiful on skin.

☺ **$$$ Water Canvas Blush** *($42.50)* mimics the concept and application of Longo's Water Canvas Foundation. This blush adaptation comes in standard blush packaging, but it has a spongy, wet-feeling texture. The product's high water content means that you must keep it tightly capped between uses or you'll be left with dry, crumbly color. Application is tricky because this doesn't have as much slip as it should, but once you get the hang of it the payoff is rich, long-lasting color that looks fairly translucent. This applies nicely over a moist-finish foundation, but using it over a matte- or powder-finish foundation leads to streaking and makes blending difficult. It's also an option to use over bare, moisturized skin. All colors have shine, but the shine is extremely subtle for the Swan Lake, Tuscan Spell, and Morning Tender shades.

😐 **$$$ Face Paint Palette** *($32.50)* provides three creamy colors in one sleek compact. The shades in each trio are best as cream blush, but may also be used as eyeshadow—if you don't mind constant creasing. This oil-based formula imparts soft, easy-to-blend color and is best for very dry skin that needs a rich cream blush to add color and glow to skin. This would get a higher rating were it not for superior cream blush options from competitors Bobbi Brown and M.A.C.

EYESHADOW: ✓☺ **$$$ Single Creme Powder Shadow** *($18)* comes in a limited assortment of colors, all with some degree of shine. Each has a smooth texture and even application that deposits strong color yet blends well. Cream Glow and Ima make excellent highlighters for the underbrow area. ✓☺ **$$$ Eyeshadow Trio** *($30)* presents several well-coordinated sets, each packaged in one compact without dividers, so be careful not to intermix shades during application. This eyeshadow has a velvety texture and beautifully even application that stays on (even the shiniest shades don't flake unless you really overdo it). The best sets to consider are Orbit Dusk, Easy Rider, Champagne, Untitled, Topaz DuLux, Vivaldi, Autumn Rhythm (matte), Untitled #3, Evolution (matte), and Timeless. Note that the Trios are divided as follows: Sun Moon Stars encompasses the trendy shade combinations, some good (as noted above) and some too contrasting. All of these have a satin finish. The One Two Three sets are basic colors with a simple gradation of tone-on-tone colors going from light to dark. Although there's not much to choose from, these trios are the easiest for beginners or for those who want a classic eye design. The Sex Lux Pax trios include high-shine colors recommended (wisely) for evening wear or high-fashion makeup. There are some great combinations here, but the pendulum swings toward odd groupings, making this subset the trickiest to work with.

㊀ **$$$ Wet Diamond Eyeshadow** *($24)* feels silky, but each shade is laced with large particles of dimensional, diamond-like shine that clings poorly. The colors tend to fade, too, and each applies more sheer than it appears. If sparkling eyeshadows are your preference, this isn't the product to add to the short list.

EYE AND BROW SHAPER: ✓ ☺ $$$ Bi-Brow Powder Pomade *($22)* combines a matte brow powder and a sheer finishing wax in one component. Almost every other version from numerous other product lines ends up being problematic in one way or another, but not here. Longo's brow powder has a smooth, dry texture and sufficient pigment from each of its three excellent shades (sorry, no options for redheads or auburn brows). The tinted finishing wax grooms brows and adds an attractive sheen without matting hairs or feeling greasy, making this an all-around brilliant brow solution! **✓ ☺ $$$ Brow Pencil/Everbrow Pencil** *($20)* has two names because that is how it is labeled on the box. Forget the indecisive labeling and keep in mind that this is an outstanding automatic, retractable brow pencil that applies easily, doesn't make brow hairs feel tacky, doesn't smear, and comes in a range of workable colors (though the Auburn shade is actually a light charcoal brown).

The regular ㊀ **$$$ Eye Pencil** *($21.50)* and ㊀ **$$$ Duo Eye Pencil** *($26)* are both very standard, creamy eye pencils that need sharpening and come in an array of traditional and trendy colors. Unfortunately, both options stay creamy and smudge in short order, so they are recommended only for smoky eye designs where you intend to smudge the liner or blend with powder eyeshadow to give it more staying power. The Duo Eye Pencil features mostly shiny pairs that are best reserved for evening use, and best avoided by those with eye-area wrinkles. ㊀ **$$$ Eyebrow Micro Pencil** *($20)* is a standard pencil with an oil-based formula that's prone to slight smearing. The pencil tip is purposefully thin, hence the "micro" name. Application is swift and the colors are quite good, but the price is out of line for what amounts to an average brow-enhancing option. If you prefer brow pencils that need sharpening, look for those that have a powdery finish such as options from Dior, or the Retractable Brow Definer from Clarins.

㊀ **$$$ Eye & Lip Pencil** *($21.50)* is a standard, needs-sharpening pencil with a small color range, and all but one of the shades (White Glimmer) are suitable for use as eyeliner or lipliner. The texture is slightly creamy while application glides without being too slick, and it stays in place surprisingly well.

☹ **Liquid Liner** *($17)* excels in some areas but falls flat in others. The thin brush allows for precision and applies color without skipping, but the formula takes way too long to dry and tends to fade before the day is done. At this price, a liquid liner should be perfect!

LIPSTICK, LIP GLOSS, AND LIPLINER: ✓☺ $$$ Lip & Cheek Gel Stain *($22.50)* is a sheer, long-lasting liquid stain that you dot on with a wand applicator and immediately blend. The colors are a step above those of similar products from Benefit, NARS, and Lorac, and that's saying something. The real tiebreaker with this one is how well it blends without streaking. Keep in mind this product has no moisturizing feel, so lip application should be paired with a lipstick or gloss.

☺ **$$$ Gel-X Lipstick Enhanced with Lip-Plumping Moisturizers** *($23)* has a modern feel and goes on slick and opaque and remains slippery, leaving a glossy finish. The strong colors enhance wear, but those prone to lip color feathering into lines around the mouth will notice this occurring almost immediately, so beware. The plumping ingredients include ceramides and vitamins, which have benefit, but not in terms of making lips larger in any way. Still, this is a good lipstick formulation that is worth a try if your budget allows and if you prefer a lightweight but still moisturizing texture.

☺ **$$$ Velvet Riche Lipstick** *($23)* is a classic creamy lipstick. The good news is you get rich, opaque colors that bring to mind the balanced makeup style of the 1940s and 1950s (powdered face, minimal blush, black eyeliner, and ravishing lips). The bad news is that this is a greasy lipstick, and will quickly travel into any lines around the mouth. However, if that is not a concern, this is a fine lipstick to consider, especially if you prefer reds and burgundies (Bruised Cherry, Dakota Red, Ignition, and Five Star are stunners).

☺ **$$$ Wet Pearl Lipstick** *($23)* is likely on its way out given how the shade selection has dwindled, but if you come across it and don't mind the price it's a good lightweight cream lipstick with a glossy, pearlescent finish. ☺ **$$$ Satin Matte Creme Lipstick** *($23)* is one of the basic lipsticks in this line, and although the shade selection is small, this is a good cream lipstick with a semi-matte finish. ☺ **$$$ Creme Frost Lipstick** *($23)* is a standard, but good, creamy lipstick whose colors have a frosted finish. With the exception of Mitzi, all of the shades are pale or very soft. ☺ **$$$ Virgin Lux Lip Gloss** *($22)* adds a sparkling, glossy finish to lips but the colors are almost too sheer to use alone, making this one to pair with a lipstick. The gloss is minimally sticky and you apply it with a sponge tip. A less expensive version of this with more color impact is Revlon's Super Lustrous Gloss ($6.99).

☺ **$$$ Lip Lux** *($22)* is gloss in a compact, and although it feels sticky it has a high level of sparkling shine that gives a heightened dimensional quality to the lips without affecting the color of lipstick worn beneath it. ☺ **$$$ Diamond Lip Gloss** *($22)* has a moderately thick, emollient texture with a sparkling gloss finish that's minimally sticky. Textural attributes aside, the best thing about this pricey gloss is the sheer colors, each of which simply dazzles alone or over lipstick. ☺ **$$$ Perfect Shine Lip Gloss** *($22)* is Longo's most pigmented gloss and also the stickiest, though it's not intolerable. The syrupy texture clings to lips and provides a glass-like shine from each of its intense but still wearable colors.

☹ **$$$ Lipstain Lipstick SPF 15** *($23)* lacks sufficient UVA protection and should not be relied on as a lipstick with ample sunscreen. It has a lightweight texture that doesn't stain but does keep lips moist without being too slick, and the sheer colors are gorgeous. The right sunscreen actives would have made this a slam-dunk recommendation. ☹ **$$$ SPF 12 Baby Balm** *($23)* has a smooth, lip balm–like texture that nurtures dry lips while providing translucent color and a glossy, polished shine. The SPF 12 would have been forgivable (SPF 15 or higher is always preferred) if this provided sufficient UVA protection, but it doesn't. Ugh! The colors are striking and a boon for women who like sheer tones for lips, but the sheerness and lack of sufficient UVA protection mean that your lips are set up for sun damage, and that is not the way to baby them.

😐 **$$$ Wet Pearl Lipstick SPF 20** *($23)* lacks the UVA-protecting ingredients of avobenzone, titanium dioxide, zinc oxide, Mexoryl SX, or Tinosorb, and this is sheer enough to not shield lips on its own. Each of the colors has a strong pearlized finish that alters the way the shade appears on the lips, depending on the lighting. Test this before purchasing to make sure you like the finish—it's nice, but not for everyone, and definitely not for those seeking a lipstick with reliable sunscreen.

😐 **$$$ Gel Crayons** *($22.50)* are chubby pencils that need routine sharpening and have a greasy texture that's short-lived, although the sheer colors are nice. 😐 **$$$ Lip Pencil** *($21.50)* is an extremely standard pencil that needs sharpening. It tends to be on the creamy side, making it more likely to bleed into the lines around the mouth, but it does apply easily. The 😐 **$$$ Duo Lip Pencil** *($26)* has the same formula as the regular Lip Pencil, but you get a bit more for your money with two shades. Still, this is creamy enough that it's not proficient at keeping lipstick from moving into lines around the mouth, and it needs sharpening.

MASCARA: ☺ **$$$ The Curl Mascara** *($23)* claims to be all you need for uplifted lashes. Yet it doesn't do much to enhance or create curl. This does excel at lengthening and absolutely refuses to clump—with several strokes lashes are evenly defined, though they don't get any thicker. The formula wears well all day without flaking or smearing.

☺ **$$$ The Curl Waterproof Mascara** *($23)* has a performance that's nearly identical to the original The Curl Mascara above, only with slightly less length. It is waterproof and—here's the good news—removes easily with a water-soluble cleanser.

☺ **$$$ Volume Riche Mascara** *($23)* has a brush that holds so much mascara you'd swear this would go on as a clumpy mess, but, surprisingly, it doesn't. The brush's short, dense bristles make it tricky to get individual lash separation, but you will get thickened lashes that make for a dramatic look.

Longo's 😐 **$$$ Original Mascara** *($18)* does little to impress, and although it's an OK option for a natural yet defined look, it takes way too much effort for meager results; at this price a mascara should impress instantly. 😐 **$$$ Original Waterproof Mascara** *($20)* performs similarly to the Original Mascara above (they have the same brush), except this formula goes on thinner and is waterproof.

☹ **Waterproof Volume Riche Mascara** *($23)* thickens lashes quite well but takes a lot of effort and patience, and you may not want to deal with the fact that this mascara smears easily before it dries and tends to flake a bit. It is waterproof, but at this price and with the other drawbacks, so what?

FACE AND BODY ILLUMINATING/SHIMMER PRODUCTS: ✓☺ **$$$ Day Play Duo Compact Highlighter** *($38.50)* has the same formula as the Day Play Duo Compact Powder Blush above, which is very good news. This product provides two shades of pressed highlighting powder, each with a soft shine that stays put and adds a glow to skin rather than lots of sparkles. From application to wear, if you're looking for a shiny highlighting powder, this is one of the best.

BRUSHES: The **Brushes** *($10–$85)* available from Longo have gotten better, but they are still not in the same league as those from his competitors. If you're smitten by Longo's products, the best brushes to consider are the ☺ **$$$ Travel Precision Lip Brush #6** *($16)*, ☺ **$$$ Foundation Brush #37** *($30)*, ☺ **$$$ Angle Contour Eyeshadow Brush #31** *($20)*, and ☺ **$$$ Concealer Brush #25** *($22)*, though the latter is larger than usual and so isn't the best for detail work under the eye. The ☺ **$$$ Highlighter Brush #26** *($24)* is an interesting option for applying either a sheer wash or heavier application of powder, shiny or not. The ☺ **Mini Lash Curler** *($16.50)* is worth considering, not only because it is well made and affordably priced but also because it works quite well to curl the outer third of lashes for a wide-eyed look. This is also worth testing by those with small eyes (who may find traditional lash curlers too awkward).

SPECIALTY PRODUCTS: 😐 **$$$ Water Canvas Base Primer** *($39.50)* promises foolproof results regardless of which foundation it's paired with, but ends up being a basic, lightweight, gel-type moisturizer that's mostly water, silicones, and alcohol. It leaves a refined, silky finish, but so do many other gel moisturizers and serums, most supplying skin with a complement of beneficial ingredients. Any of the serums from Olay's Regenerist or Total Effects line best this product, as do silicone-enhanced moisturizers such as Clinique Moisture Surge Extra ($32).

😐 **$$$ Double Swish Makeup Remover** *($23)* is a dual-phase, water-in-silicone remover that is adept at breaking down mascara, long-wearing lipstick, and eyeliner. It would be better without the fragrance and fragrant components (such as amyl cinnamal) because these can irritate the eyes. Although this works, for less money consider similar but fragrance-free options from Almay and Neutrogena.

😐 **$$$ Bang Bang Lip Volume Lotion** *($30)* is said to provide continuous lip plumping with minimal to no irritation, which may entice you to plunk down your credit card for this product. Before you do, know that it works by irritating your lips with benzyl nicotinate. A new twist on standard lip-plumping products is the inclusion of the sulfur compound methylsulfonomethane. This ingredient gained notoriety due to the book *The Miracle of MSM: The Natural Solution for Pain*, although there is little scientific support for its continued use to treat inflammatory conditions such as arthritis. Assuming it has an anti-inflammatory effect when applied to lips, that would make the irritating benzyl nicotinate less potent (which is good), but would also make this plumping product less effective (because it only works via irritation, not some other lip-plumping property). Bottom line: There's little reason to bank on great results, though you may notice a slight increase in the fullness of your lips.

😐 **Hygienic Professional Brush Cleaner** *($12.50)* is a spray-on solution of alcohol, thickener, and fragrance. The alcohol helps remove excess pigment and sanitize brushes, but long-term use will make brush hairs dry and brittle. This is a fast-drying option if you're using the same brushes on multiple subjects, but brushes reserved for personal use are best washed every few months with a gentle shampoo and left to air dry.

☹ **Cushion Lips SPF 20** *($18)* lacks the UVA-protecting ingredients of titanium dioxide, zinc oxide, avobenzone, Mexoryl SX, or Tinosorb, and is not recommended.

WET 'N' WILD

WET 'N' WILD AT-A-GLANCE

Strengths: Inexpensive; reliable, gentle options for cleansers, toner, and scrubs; good tinted moisturizer with sunscreen; one of the best bronzing powders at any price; great powder blush; mostly good eyeshadow and lipstick options; one superior lip gloss; a few great liquid shimmer options.

Weaknesses: No moisturizers without sunscreen (you don't need sunscreen in the evening); no reliable AHA or BHA products or topical disinfectants for those with acne wanting a fresh face; both sunscreens lack sufficient UVA-protecting ingredients; unimpressive concealers; large assortment of average to poor eyelining products; the mascaras do little to impress; some lip products suffer from the inclusion of irritants; the makeup brushes.

For more information about Wet 'n' Wild, visit www.wnwbeauty.com or www.Beautypedia.com. Note: The selection of Wet 'n' Wild products tends to be much better in Canadian drugstores than in the United States.

WET 'N' WILD FRESH FACE SKIN-CARE PRODUCTS

☺ **Fresh Face Skincare Foaming Face Wash** *($4.99 for 5.8 ounces)* is a very standard, but effective and gentle water-soluble cleanser. It contains several water-binding agents, which aren't as critical in a cleanser as they are in a moisturizer, but they nevertheless contribute to this cleanser's performance. This is a good option for all skin types except very dry or very oily. It does contain fragrance.

☺ **Fresh Face Skincare Gentle Cream Cleanser** *($4.99 for 6 ounces)* is a lotion-style cleanser that's close to being water-soluble, though it still isn't the easiest to rinse. This is a good cleanser for someone with normal to dry skin that's not prone to blemishes; just be aware that you may need a washcloth to remove it completely.

😐 **Fresh Face Skincare Clarifying Astringent** *($4.99 for 7.5 ounces)* contains 2% salicylic acid in an alcohol-free, soothing liquid base. What a shame the pH of 5 reduces what the salicylic acid can do as an exfoliant. This would have been an excellent, affordable liquid BHA product, but as it stands, it's just a basic toner for all skin types except very dry.

☺ **Fresh Face Skincare Acne Daily Cleansing Scrub** *($4.99 for 6 ounces)* is a standard but good scrub/cleanser that contains polyethylene beads as the abrasive agent. It also contains 0.5% salicylic acid, an amount that is too low to have any real impact (in a rinse-off product it ends up down the drain anyway). Anti-irritant licorice and green tea extracts, are here too, but also end up in the sink. Still, this is a workable, fairly gentle cleansing scrub for all skin types.

✓☺ **Fresh Face Skincare Exfoliating Scrub** *($4.99 for 6 ounces)* has a formula that is similar to that of the Fresh Face Skincare Gentle Cream Cleanser, reviewed above. The only significant difference is that this one contains the abrasive agent polyethylene rather than a detergent cleansing agent. It is, therefore, a gentle, slightly creamy scrub suitable for normal to dry skin.

😐 **Fresh Face Skincare Refreshing Toner** *($4.99 for 7.5 ounces)* is a standard, alcohol-free toner with a tiny amount of witch hazel—fortunately, too little to be a problem for irritation. It contains a few soothing plant extracts and a mild cleansing agent to help remove leftover traces of makeup or oil, but is really an underwhelming formula, and that doesn't make for great skin care.

☹ **Fresh Face Skincare Clear Skin Oil-Free Moisturizer SPF 15** *($5.99 for 3 ounces)* does not contain the UVA-protecting ingredients of avobenzone, titanium dioxide, zinc oxide, Tinosorb, or Mexoryl SX (ecamsule), and is not recommended.

☹ **Fresh Face Skincare Total Moisturizer SPF 15** *($5.99 for 3 ounces)* does not contain the UVA-protecting ingredients of avobenzone, titanium dioxide, zinc oxide, Tinosorb, or Mexoryl SX (ecamsule), and is not recommended.

😐 **$$$ Fresh Face Skincare Acne Spot Treatment** *($5.99 for 0.75 ounce)* contains 2% salicylic acid in a lightweight gel base, complete with several anti-irritants. What a shame the pH of 4.7 prevents any exfoliation from taking place. The tea tree oil lends a medicinal odor, but the amount of it is unfortunately too low for it to work as a topical disinfectant (a 5% concentration is best). If the pH of this BHA product were in the correct range, it would be a slam-dunk recommendation. As is, there's no compelling reason to purchase it.

WET 'N' WILD MAKEUP

FOUNDATION: ☺ **Ultimate Sheer Tinted Moisturizer SPF 15** *($3.99)* wins instant points for using titanium dioxide as the sole broad-spectrum active sun-protecting ingredient. It has a slightly fluid, thin texture that blends decently and sets to a nearly matte finish suitable for normal to slightly oily skin. True to its name, coverage is sheer and definitely more akin to a tint than a true foundation. All four colors are excellent and there are options for light to tan skin.

☹ **Ultimate Cover Smooth Foundation** *($2.99)* is ultimate only in being irritating for all skin types, because this highly fragranced liquid foundation is loaded with eucalyptus oil, menthol, and camphor. It is not recommended regardless of how much coverage you need (and this foundation doesn't provide significant coverage anyway).

CONCEALER: ☺ **Cover All Liquid Concealer** *($2.99)* has a creamy-smooth texture, but although it provides good coverage it's not a "cover all" solution. This is too emollient for use over blemishes, but is an OK option for under-eye use or concealing minor redness. Among the four shades, Medium, Light, and Beige are strongly pink and should be avoided. Fair is recommended for that respective skin tone.

☹ **Cover All Stick** *($1.99)* is a lipstick-style cream concealer that's very greasy, easily creases under the eye, and offers shades that look nothing like real skin.

POWDER: ✓☺ **Bronzer Ultimate Bronzing Powder** *($2.99)* remains one of Wet 'n' Wild's star products, and for good reason: this inexpensive pressed bronzing powder is one of the best around in terms of smooth application, good intensity, and believable colors. The Light/Medium and Medium/Dark shades are matte, while the others have shine, so you can take your pick (but I suggest saving the shiny ones for evening makeup).

☺ **Ultimate Touch Pressed Powder with Puff** *($2.99)* comes with the cheapest puff imaginable, but that's OK because powder looks best when applied with a brush. This talc-based powder has a smooth, dry texture and silky matte finish. Four shades are available, and only Warm Beige is a dud due to its peachy tone. This pressed powder is best for normal to oily skin.

BLUSH: ✓☺ **Silk Finish Blush** *($2.99)* has been improved and is silkier than ever. For the money, this small collection of powder blushes is among the best at the drugstore. If only the shade selection were more extensive! Heather Silk and Mellow Wine are matte, while Pearlescent Pink has shine. All apply smoothly, have more pigment than you'd expect, and last.

EYESHADOW: ☺ **MegaEyes Eye Shadow** *($2.99)* is sold as trios and at just one dollar per shade deserves mention as a bona fide beauty steal. The creamy-feeling powder texture applies smoothly but sheer, and layered application is recommended to avoid slight flaking. Doing so enhances blending, and every trio has one shade that's dark enough to serve as eyeliner (and these may be applied wet). All of the trios are shiny, which means they're not for wrinkled eyes, but if that doesn't include you the best sets are Belgian Chocolates, Mojave Mauves, Venetian Violets, and Egyptian Sands. This would have rated a Paula's Pick were it not for the minor flaking issue.

☺ **Eye Expressions Eye Shadow/Illuminator** *($3.99)* combines four cream eyeshadows and the MegaGlo Face Illuminator (reviewed below) in one compact. The sheer cream eyeshadows apply and blend well, setting to a soft powder finish that doesn't slip or crease, making these a step above the norm. The eyeshadows and Illuminator are shiny, but the shine on the eyeshadows is softer. This is definitely worth a try if you find a color combination you like.

☺ **MegaEyes Cream Eyeshadow** *($1.99)* isn't creamy so much as gel-like. The water- and glycerin-based formula has good initial slip, allowing for blending over the entire eye area. Spot application is tricky and not this product's forte. The effect is sheer color with intense shine, and flaking is scant once the product has set. These don't crease either, making them a workable alternative to powder eyeshadows if you can handle this much shine. Avoid Blue Heaven and Envy, both of which are too clownish.

😐 **Mega Eyes Shadow Pot** *($1.99)* has a smooth texture and sheer application that make this powder eyeshadow easy to work with and blend. You won't be able to add much depth and there are no shades that are dark enough to serve as eyeliner. All of the shades have some amount of shine; those with visible shiny particles tend to flake while the others do not.

😐 **Ultimate Expressions Eyeshadow Palette** *($4.99)* provides eight powder eyeshadows in one sturdy compact that includes a built-in, pop-out mirror. The set of four shades in the middle is what's needed for shaping, shading, and eyelining; the shades on the periphery are best for highlighting. These shadows have a smooth, minimally flaky texture that applies evenly although they tend to rub off easily, so aren't the best if your goal is long-lasting eye makeup. The darker shades have good pigmentation while the light to medium shades go on sheer, imparting more shine than color (all eight shades have shine). Among the sets, the only one to skip due to an odd assortment of colors is Fantasy Island.

EYE AND BROW SHAPER: ☺ **H2O Proof Liquid Eyeliner** *($3.99)* has a good, firm brush that lays down a continuous line of color and a formula that not only dries quickly but also is tenaciously waterproof. A minor issue is that the color saturation isn't as intense as it could be. This requires layering if you want more definition (and for most of the colors, you will). That's not a deal-breaker, but it's enough to keep this liquid eyeliner from earning a higher rating.

😐 **Ultimate Brow Color & Set** *($2.99)* is a dual-sided product featuring a creamy brow pencil (that needs sharpening) on one end and a sheer, tinted brow gel on the other. The pencil applies smoothly but suffers from some fading, while the brow gel feels slightly tacky (though it does the trick as far as keeping unruly brows in place). The concept is good, but the execution is not as flawless as it could have been.

😐 **Mega Liner Liquid Eyeliner** *($2.99)* dries quickly and doesn't flake, chip, or smear once it has set, but this loses points because its long, thin, somewhat flimsy brush makes drawing an even line unusually tricky. If you're adept at handling this type of brush you may want to consider this—but avoid the green, blue, and purple shades unless it's Halloween.

😐 **H2O Proof Blending Eye Pencils** *($1.99)* need sharpening, but for the money that's not such a bad deal. These pencils apply easily and most of the shades have a metallic or sparkle-infused finish, so this is not the epitome of understated makeup. True to the name, the long-wearing, surprisingly smudge-resistant finish is waterproof. In fact, it takes effort to remove this pencil! How come Wet 'n' Wild can do this for less than $2 and Chanel can't get it right for $25? As you may have guessed, this pencil would be rated higher were it not for the need to routinely sharpen it.

😐 **I-Shimmer Retractable Eye Pencil** *($1.99)* is a very good automatic, retractable eye pencil that suffers from its color choices (only a teal and a blue shade are offered) as well as the fact that the mirror-like shimmer particles tend to flake (but the color remains). What a shame, because this glides on easily and sets to a long-wearing finish.

😐 **Purse Size Twin Eye or Lipliner Pencils** *($1.99)* are standard pencils that need sharpening and are indeed small enough to fit in even a tiny purse or evening bag. These have a different, better formula than the Eyeliner Pencils reviewed below. Although they're still creamy, they have better staying powder and are an OK option for a smoky eye design.

☹ **Eyeliner Pencils** *($0.99)* need sharpening, but even if that doesn't bother you, these extra long pencils are way too creamy and stay that way, which just invites smudging and smearing. I suppose this is one of those cosmetic instances where you get what you pay for.

☹ **Brow Pencils** *($0.99)* are almost as creamy as the Eyeliner Pencils, and tend to ball up and get matted in brow hairs, necessitating more work than filling in and defining the brows should take. These pencils need routine sharpening.

☹ **Idol Eyes Retractable Eye Pencil** *($1.99)* is, without question, one of the worst eye pencils on the market. Yes, it doesn't need sharpening and is retractable, but it tends to drag over skin, deposits color unevenly, and smears with little provocation, plus it is exceedingly difficult to remove. This is a must to avoid.

LIPSTICK, LIP GLOSS, AND LIPLINER: ✓☺ **Glassy Gloss Lip Gel** *($2.99)* comes in a tube and is a very good, super-smooth lip gloss with a slightly liquid texture that slides over lips and produces, yes, a glassy shine. The sheer colors can be worn over any lipstick, and the finish is minimally sticky.

☺ **Wild Shine Lipstick** *($1.99)* is a standard creamy lipstick with medium coverage and an emollient texture that feels moist but that isn't meant for anyone with lines around the mouth. The finish is indeed shiny (glossy) and the shade selection, although rather small, is attractive.

☺ **Precious Metals Lipstick** *($1.99)* has a lightweight, somewhat slick texture and a strong metallic finish. This actually feels more elegant than the price suggests and is worth exploring if this type of finish appeals to you. One caution: The mica particles in this lipstick tend to cling to the lips as the color wears away, creating a whitish shimmer without color.

☺ **Mega Colors Lipstick** *($1.99)* is a traditional cream lipstick that has a lighter feel and less color saturation than most. The finish is creamy with a hint of gloss and the color selection is large enough to offer all the basics and some trendier colors, too.

☺ **Silk Finish Lipstick** *($0.99)* is Wet 'n' Wild's most opaque lipstick, but also its greasiest. The wide shade selection has a nice stain, helping to keep the color around longer, but this is also greasy enough to immediately bleed into any lines around the mouth. If that's not an issue for you and you want full-coverage color, the price is tough to beat!

☺ **Diamond Brilliance Moisturizing Lip Sheen** *($2.99)* should get an audition from anyone who likes a fairly tenacious lip gloss that imparts sheer color and a blatantly glossy finish. This wand-applicator gloss competes favorably with much more expensive options, and doesn't suffer from a cloying fragrance or artificial fruit- or dessert-like flavors. The majority of colors pair well with any lipstick shade, too, though you must be able to tolerate a slightly sticky finish.

☺ **Jumbo Juicy Lip Balm** *($2.99)* is a chunky lip balm whose candy-bright colors may catch your eye. But color isn't what this smooth, slightly glossy lip balm is all about. Every shade applies translucent, but imparts a fruity flavor. Although this will take care of dry lips, the flavor may encourage lip-licking, and that's not a good way to stop dryness.

☺ **MegaSlicks Lip Gloss** *($1.99)* is a good basic lip gloss that feels slightly thick, isn't too slick, and is slightly sticky. All of the sheer shades have soft to moderate shimmer and are applied with a sponge-tip wand. Note: This lip gloss has a strong fragrance.

☺ **Lip Impressions** *($3.99)* comes in a compact with a generous-size mirror and a chintzy dual-sided lip brush. The product comprises four shades of the Wild Shine Lipstick reviewed above and one shade of the MegaGlo Illuminator reviewed below. It's a fine option if you don't mind applying lip color with a brush and find most of the shades appealing.

☺ **MegaLast Long-Lasting Lipcolor** *($3.99)* is Wet 'n' Wild's me-too Lipfinity product, and includes the same two steps (color coat followed by a glossy top coat). The color portion goes on a bit unevenly, requiring more blending before it sets. It's ready for the top coat after a couple of minutes, and even when completely dry, the top coat removes a bit of color (superior options from M.A.C. and Estee Lauder don't do this). Still, this isn't a terrible option for the money, and you'll find that, for the most part, the color wears well and the gloss coat doesn't require frequent touch-ups. This does come off on cups and light kisses, so don't consider it transfer-resistant.

☺ **3-of-a-Kind Twist-Up Sticks for Lips, Eyes, and Cheeks** *($3.99)* has a smooth, slightly slick texture that glides over skin and imparts translucent color and a natural, minimally moist finish. Only one shade (#728) is suitable for use as eyeshadow (though using it as such invites some creasing); the others are best for sheer blush. Applied to lips, the lack of emollients is disappointing, as is the fleeting nature of the sheer colors.

☺ **MegaSlicks Lip Color Retractable Pencil** *($2.99)* looks deceiving because you'd swear it was a pencil that needed to be sharpened. Look closer and it's a cleverly designed automatic pencil whose tip can be wound up or down. This thick pencil has a slightly dry application and semi-matte finish with nearly opaque colors. It wears longer than traditional lipsticks, but you may need to add some gloss for comfort.

😐 **Lipliner Pencil** *($0.99)* is a standard, needs-sharpening pencil that's neither too creamy nor too dry, though the finish is slightly tacky. A few of the colors are excellent versatile shades that you really should check out if you can tolerate the sharpening aspect.

☹ **MegaBrilliance Lip Gloss** *($1.99)* is a lightweight, minimally sticky lip gloss loaded with large flecks of glitter. As you might guess, the glitter feels grainy (almost scratchy) shortly after application, and the effect is far from sophisticated or glamorous.

☹ **Pout Protector with SPF 15** *($2.99)* is a sheer, glossy lipstick/lip balm hybrid with an in-part zinc oxide sunscreen, an unusual trait in lipsticks. The unhappy face rating is due to the flavor of this lipstick, which is of the strong mint variety. You'll feel the tingle as soon you apply this, and it only gets more intense the longer you wear it. How sad, because this would have otherwise been a brilliant, inexpensive way to shield lips from the sun.

☹ **MegaPlump Plumping Lip Gloss** *($3.99)* burns on application and may make you think you've smeared potpourri on your lips given the pervasive cinnamon scent. Two forms of pure cinnamon oil are part of the formula, and although they plump lips, each does so by causing irritation. Most lip-plumping products take the irritation route to inflating the mouth, but few do so with such strong irritants.

MASCARA: 😐 **MegaPlump Mascara** *($3.99)* has a name that makes you think of thick lashes, perhaps? Well, that's what I was hoping would happen with this, but not even successive coats provided any lengthening or thickening. The only thing plump about it is the tube. It wears well, removes easily, and is an OK option if you want minimally enhanced lashes.

😐 **Mega Length Double Action Mascara** *($3.99)* is a two-step product that includes a lash primer and regular mascara. Although the primer does make a slight difference in lash thickness and volume, the mascara portion is lackluster and no match for similar products from L'Oreal (Double Extend), Revlon (Lash Fantasy), or a variety of options from Maybelline.

😐 **H2O Proof Waterproof Mascara** *($2.99)* sells at a price that makes me wish it was a great recommendation, but mascaras have never been one of Wet 'n' Wild's strong suits. This version produces negligible to very modest length and barely any thickness, but it does apply evenly without clumping or smearing, and it is waterproof. If you're OK with an average mascara (perhaps because you already have long, thick lashes or you just want minimal definition), this is an ordinary, but unquestionably affordable, option.

☺ **Mega Lash Lengthening Mascara** *($2.99)* is a reasonably good lengthening mascara if you want something that creates a soft, natural lash look. Performance plateaus quickly, so applying successive coats doesn't produce more dramatic results, but the formula doesn't clump or smear. ☺ **Mega Wink Lash Curling Mascara** *($2.99)* is another OK mascara for a really natural look without a hint of thickness. You'll get soft, separated lashes without clumps and a minimal curled effect. ☺ **MegaProtein Mascara** *($2.99)* contains a tiny, not "mega" amount of soy protein, and protein in and of itself isn't the fast track to gorgeous lashes. This mascara, like most of those from Wet 'n' Wild, does little to impress. Its main accomplishment is average length; you cannot build bigger, longer lashes with this no matter how long you try.

☹ **Mega Volume Thickening Mascara** *($2.99)* is a nearly do-nothing mascara that is seriously misnamed.

FACE AND BODY ILLUMINATING/SHIMMER PRODUCTS: ✓☺ **MegaGlo Face Illuminator** *($2.99)* adds an illuminated gleam to skin thanks to its smooth texture and emollient formula that is suitable only for dry to very dry skin. This has a distinctive moist finish, but tends to stay in place quite well because it doesn't remain slippery once blended. Blushing is best as a highlighter, Toasty is great for a bronze effect, and Rosy is good for a shiny blush.

☺ **MegaPump Shimmer** *($3.99)* is a lightweight shimmer lotion with a smooth texture and opalescent finish on skin. The shimmer effect is subtle but can look more intense depending on the room lighting. ☺ **MegaPump Bronzer** *($3.99)* has the same formula as the MegaPump Shimmer, but produces a sheer bronze tint with a golden shimmer overtone. The shine level is more intense than that of the regular Shimmer above, and looks best on medium to tan skin.

☺ **MegaPump Glitter Gel** *($3.99)* is a clear, water- and alcohol-based gel laced with multicolored glitter particles. The gel base allows the glitter to cling to skin decently, but don't expect this to last all night without some fallout. ☹ **MegaSparkle Loose Confetti** *($2.99)* is loose glitter that has a dimensional, multicolored effect that can be striking in most lighting. The unhappy face rating is because this product has absolutely no ability to cling to skin, meaning the effect is short-lived and glitter gets all over the place. ☹ **MegaShimmer Shimmer Dust** *($2.99)* is a loose shimmer powder that has an unappealingly dry, slightly grainy texture. It imparts subtle to glittery shine depending on the shade, but none of them cling well and they feel terrible on skin when used over large areas (such as the décolletage).

BRUSHES: The too-tiny ☹ **Brush Kit** *($1.99)* gives new meaning to the phrase "Why bother?" and the brushes are all the throwaway variety. ☺ **Plush Brush** *($1.99)* is about as plush as a loofah. Unless your budget is incredibly tight, this isn't worth the savings.

SPECIALTY PRODUCTS: ☺ **Travel Size Eyelash Curler** *($1.99)* is a decent option for a portable, functional eyelash curler, and its plastic and rubber parts tend to be gentler on lashes than those made of metal.

YOUTHFUL ESSENCE BY SUSAN LUCCI (SKIN CARE ONLY)

YOUTHFUL ESSENCE AT-A-GLANCE

Strengths: A few good moisturizers and an eye cream with an in-part avobenzone sunscreen; an excellent mask for dry skin; the company makes complete ingredient lists available on its Web site.

Weaknesses: Needless use of irritating fragrant oils in many products; daytime moisturizer with sunscreen lacks the right UVA-protecting ingredients; no AHA or BHA options, only microdermabrasion-like scrubs; jar packaging.

For more information about Youthful Essence, call (800) 490-2671 or visit www.youthfulessence.com. Youthful Essence is distributed by Guthy-Renker, the same company behind several successful infomercial brands, including Pro-Activ and Sheer Cover.

Note: All prices listed below are regular retail prices. Special reduced pricing is available on all items if you agree to the company's Automatic Delivery Program.

☹ **Cleansing Facial Wash** *($19.50 for 4 ounces)* would have been a good, water-soluble foaming cleanser if it did not contain irritating fragrant oils of thyme, cypress, lavender, rosemary, and geranium. All of these can cause problems for skin and should not get anywhere near the eyes.

😐 **$$$ Vitamin Enriched Resurfacing Cream, Sensitive Skin Formula** *($54.95 for 2.5 ounces)* is a very expensive topical scrub that lists abrasive aluminum oxide as the main ingredient, so it is completely unsuitable for sensitive skin. The emollients and oils make this an OK topical scrub for dry to very dry skin, but the tiny amount of fragrant plant oils isn't going to do your skin any favors.

☹ **Facial Mist & Toner** *($16.70 for 4 ounces)* lists skin cell–damaging lavender oil as the second ingredient, followed by a roster of other irritating fragrant oils. This toner is akin to misting skin with fragrance, and has no benefit whatsoever.

☹ **Daily Protection Moisturizer with SPF 15** *($19.95 for 1 ounce)* lacks the UVA-protecting ingredients of titanium dioxide, zinc oxide, avobenzone, Mexoryl SX, or Tinosorb, and is not recommended.

☺ **$$$ For Eyes Complete Night Treatment** *($28.50 for 0.5 ounce)*, because it is meant for use around the eyes, shouldn't contain fragrance—but at least the amount present here is small. This is more lotion-like than creamy, but will address mild dryness around the eye area, and it does contain several very good water-binding agents along with essential lipids (fatty acids).

☺ **$$$ For Eyes Instant Smoothing Day Treatment SPF 15** *($28.50 for 0.5 ounce)* will keep eye-area skin shielded from sun damage thanks to its in-part avobenzone sunscreen, but this and the other synthetic sunscreen agents included are not the gentlest options for use around the eyes (titanium dioxide and/or zinc oxide are preferred). The base formula is a lightweight cream that contains some good anti-inflammatory ingredients, though none of them have demonstrated an ability to reduce puffy eyes, at least not if the puffiness is caused by the age-related shifting of fat pads beneath the skin. This product also contains the citrus bioflavonoid hesperidin methyl chalcone, the same ingredient touted in Hylexin (reviewed in this book). Youthful Essence does not spotlight this ingredient, but even if they did there is no substantiated proof that topical application of hesperidin methyl chalcone has any effect on dark circles. If you can tolerate using avobenzone and the other sunscreen agents in this product around your eyes, it is a worthwhile fragrance-free consideration.

☹ **$$$ For Night Soothing Treatment** *($34.50 for 1 ounce)* comes packaged in a jar, so even the small amounts of antioxidants that are present in this product won't last long once it's opened. This doesn't contain any particularly soothing ingredients, but it is a well-formulated basic moisturizer to address the needs of normal to dry skin. Aside from the packaging, there isn't anything particularly negative about this product, other than the fact that superior formulations will outperform it and are available in stable packaging.

☺ **$$$ Bright Fix Radiant Pen** *($21.60 for 0.5 ounce)* smooths skin with a silicone-enhanced fluid that is dispensed from a pen-style applicator with brush. The formula contains some very good antioxidants and a helpful amount of skin-identical substances, while the cosmetic pigments help reflect light away from shadowed areas, for a temporary brightening effect. It can be a good option if you need light moisture and smoothing for trouble spots and don't mind the soft-shine finish. This is suitable for all skin types.

☹ **$$$ Personal Microdermabrasion System** *($39.95 for the kit)* was one of the first at-home microdermabrasion kits available (it launched in 2002). What was once unique seems overly familiar today because this type of system is now widely available (and in less-expensive versions, most notably from Neutrogena). The kit includes a **Resurfacing Tool**, with **Sponge Applicators** (1 tool with 2 sponges), that is battery-powered and is used to apply and massage the **Vitamin-Enriched Resurfacing Cream** (2.5 ounces) onto the skin. The vitamin-enriched label is inaccurate because this cream does not contain any "vitamins." Even if it did they aren't necessary because a scrub is rinsed from the skin, though I suppose it looks good to list them on the label and it gives Susan Lucci more to enthuse over during the infomercial for this product.

This somewhat abrasive topical scrub contains aluminum oxide crystals, the same as those found in professional microdermabrasion treatments. However, as I have stated before, I am concerned that these crystals will eventually cause problems if people overdo at-home treatments. Irritation is a concern, and using the hand-held device can result in the crystals becoming lodged in pores, which can cause a host of new problems. When microdermabrasion is performed by a professional with a precision-guided machine, the crystals are suctioned off the skin during treatment, which drastically minimizes their potential for causing problems after the treatment is finished. With at-home systems like this one from Youthful Essence, the likelihood of problems increases because the crystals are not easy to rinse off. Much depends on how zealous consumers are with each use, so you need to keep in mind that it's easy to get carried away while running the device over your face. Moreover, the results obtainable from systems like this are not much better than using other topical scrubs or even a plain washcloth. Even microdermabrasion itself is not proving to be a wonderful way to keep skin smooth and improve collagen production.

An interesting side note is that the developers of Youthful Essence also developed the nearly identical Dermanew Microdermabrasion system, which costs twice as much as Lucci's kit. Dermanew's scrub is principally the same thing as Lucci's, except the Dermanew scrub includes some antioxidants, plant extracts, and several irritating essential oils, which gives Lucci's (and Neutrogena's even less expensive option) the edge all around, assuming you want to give such kits a try.

✓☺ **Repairing Mask** *($30 for 1 ounce)* supplies dry to very dry skin with a wonderfully effective complement of silicone, nonvolatile plant oils, emollients, soothing plant extracts, and cell-communicating ingredients. It's a bit short on antioxidants, but works remarkably well to replenish and soften skin, whether used as an occasional mask or as an overnight treatment. It's pricey for what you get, but that doesn't mean it's not recommended.

YVES ST. LAURENT

YVES ST. LAURENT AT-A-GLANCE

Strengths: Every sunscreen includes avobenzone for sufficient UVA protection; some moisturizers with elegant textures; good makeup removers and toners; good lip balm; one superior pressed-powder and eyeshadow formula; Radiant Touch is a favorite for good reason; Variations Blush is a great way to experiment with cheek color; two fantastic mascaras; very good liquid highlighter; the makeup fares much better than YSL's skin care.

Weaknesses: Expensive; highly fragranced; few sunscreens sport SPF ratings above the benchmark SPF 15; no AHA or BHA products; no products to manage acne or combat skin discolorations; mostly mundane moisturizers and serums; pervasive use of jar packaging; anti-wrinkle claims that epitomize ridiculous, yet cost hundreds of dollars; mostly average foundations, sometimes due to SPF rating below the benchmark SPF 15; eyeshadow quads; mostly average lipstick and gloss options.

For more information about Yves St. Laurent, call (212) 715-7339 or visit www.ysl.com or www.Beautypedia.com.

YVES ST. LAURENT SKIN CARE

YVES ST. LAURENT AGE EXPERT PRODUCTS

☹ **$$$ Age Expert Age Defying Creme SPF 15** *($88 for 1 ounce)* makes some far-fetched turn-back-the-clock claims, all hinged on what they refer to as "The cosmetic alternative to DHEA, Age Expert contains Ganoderic Fraction—an exclusive active ingredient with a structure similar to the famous hormone of youthfulness, capable of reactivating the vital functions of the epidermis." DHEA is the abbreviated name for dehydroepiandrosterone, a male hormone produced in the adrenal glands that contributes to bone density, muscle mass, and skin tone. Its popularity as an oral supplement comes from its reputation for increasing strength, boosting the immune system, enhancing memory and concentration, reducing depression, preventing weight gain, and heightening libido function. What does any of that have to do with skin? Aside from the suggested association between DHEA and male hormone levels, and hormone levels having an effect on skin, there is no research showing that DHEA has any impact on aging skin when applied topically, though it can penetrate into the skin (Source: *Drug Delivery*, September/October 2005, pages 275–280; and *Clinics in Geriatric Medicine*, November 2001, pages 661–672). Besides, it isn't the male hormones that improve the texture and appearance of female skin. The feel and suppleness of a woman's skin are affected by the levels of estrogen and progesterone production (male hormones give men's skin its characteristic appearance). Even more ludicrous, after YSL carries on about this ingredient, it actually doesn't show up in this product (DHEA does appear in other skin-care products). Rather YSL uses a bogus alternative that has nothing to do with DHEA, adding up to a lot of bluster with little substance.

"Ganoderic Fraction" is a fancy term for the ingredient this product does contain, which is the extract of *Ganoderma lucidum*, a mushroom. There is definitely research showing that, when eaten, this fungus can have many potential benefits as an antioxidant and anti-inflammatory, and for liver and blood-pressure support. However, there is no research showing that it has miraculous benefit when applied topically to skin in teeny amounts (which is all this product contains), or even in huge amounts. About all this moisturizer for normal to slightly dry skin has to offer is broad-spectrum sun protection (with avobenzone for UVA screening). All of the intriguing ingredients are listed well after the preservatives, and jar packaging won't keep most of them stable once you open it.

☹ **$$$ Age Expert Age Defying Lotion SPF 15** *($88 for 1 ounce)* is the lotion version of the Age Expert Age Defying Creme SPF 15 above, and aside from having a texture those with normal to oily skin will prefer and not using jar packaging, the same review applies. This is a disappointing product for how much it costs, and how liberally will you apply such an expensive sunscreen, which with daily use you'd be replacing every few weeks?

☹ **$$$ Age Expert Nuit Age Defying Night Creme** *($88 for 1 ounce)* is an emollient blend of mostly water, thickener, film-forming agent, Vaseline, silicone, and more thickeners. It contains a very small amount of water-binding agents and the few antioxidants won't remain stable once this jar-packaged product is opened. Do not expect "ultimate restorative action."

☹ **$$$ Age Expert Yeux Age Defying Eye Creme** *($68 for 0.5 ounce)* contains mostly thickeners, film-forming agents, slip agents, and plant oil. It's an OK moisturizer for dry skin anywhere on the face, but it cannot reduce puffiness or darkness under the eye. If anything, the arnica and cypress can be irritating, though the amount used is likely not cause for concern.

YVES ST. LAURENT CONTOUR EXPERT PRODUCTS

☹ **Contour Expert Intensive Lifting and Reshaping Serum** *($86 for 1 ounce)* promises to restore volume and contour to aging skin, but it absolutely cannot do that. No skin-care product can make sunken features plump and full again, nor can a jawline be redefined. That type of improvement is possible only via cosmetic medical procedures. This serum is primarily water and gum-based thickeners, which have a slight plasticizing effect on skin as they dry. The amount of tansy extract (*Tanacetum vulgare*) is cause for concern because this plant can cause severe contact dermatitis (Source: www.naturaldatabase.com). That alone is reason enough to avoid this product.

☹ **$$$ Contour Expert Reshaping and Lifting Creme SPF 10** *($88 for 1.6 ounces)* contains less tansy extract than the Contour Expert Intensive Lifting and Reshaping Serum above, but still disappoints because of its low SPF rating (though the sunscreen includes avobenzone for UVA protection) and jar packaging. It's an average option for normal to slightly dry skin and does not stand a ghost of a chance of restoring lost facial contours.

☹ **$$$ Contour Expert Yeux Lifting and Anti-Puffiness Eye Care** *($60 for 0.5 ounce)* has a very light texture, and wheat germ extract has water-binding properties for skin. However, several ingredients in this "care" product are cause for concern, including alcohol, tansy, bitter orange, and cypress. All of the other truly beneficial ingredients appear after these problematic ones, making this option a risky proposition.

YVES ST. LAURENT HYDRA FEEL PRODUCTS

☹ **$$$ Hydra Feel Comfort Hydrating Water Creme** *($62 for 1.6 ounces)* has some good emollient ingredients for dry to very dry skin, including macadamia nut oil. However, there's more fragrance here than antioxidants, and what few antioxidants are present won't last long once this jar-packaged moisturizer is opened.

☹ **$$$ Hydra Feel Eye Radiant Hydrating Eye Gel** *($44 for 0.5 ounce)* is said to be enriched with "Baby Skin Complex," which is a scary thought (where did the baby skin come from?) though it certainly is intended to evoke youthful skin. Not to worry, though: Not a single ingredient in this lightweight gel moisturizer is derived from baby skin. Although suitable for normal to slightly dry skin anywhere on the face, this contains few impressive ingredients for the money, and most of the plant extracts have limited to no research concerning their effectiveness for skin of any age.

☹ **Hydra Feel Fresh Hydrating Water Gel** *($62 for 1.6 ounces)* lists alcohol as the second ingredient, and as such is too drying and irritating for all skin types. The amount of alcohol will also make the acrylate-based film-forming agent (think hairspray-type ingredients) that follows it irritating.

☹ **Hydra Feel Soft Hydrating Water Lotion SPF 15** *($62 for 1.6 ounces)* provides sufficient UVA protection with its in-part avobenzone sunscreen, but the second ingredient is alcohol and that makes this non-hydrating product too irritating for all skin types.

😐 **$$$ Hydra Feel Gentle Rehydrating Masque** *($48 for 2.5 ounces)* is a simple but silky blend of water with silicones, slip agents, and a tiny amount of emollient squalane. It's a good mask for normal to dry skin, but doesn't "rehydrate" better than dozens of other moisturizers, many of which offer skin a balanced blend of what YSL includes plus antioxidants and skin-identical ingredients. Sadly, this mask contains more fragrance than anything unique (or worthy of this product's price) for skin.

YVES ST. LAURENT INSTANT PUR PRODUCTS

☺ **$$$ Instant Pur Gentle Milk Cleanser** *($35 for 6.7 ounces)* is a silky, detergent-free cleansing lotion for normal to dry skin. Makeup comes off easily, but you may find you need a washcloth to avoid a residue.

☹ **Instant Pur Self-Foaming Cleanser** *($35 for 5 ounces)* contains the drying, irritating detergent cleansing agent sodium C14-16 olefin sulfonate as a main ingredient, and is not recommended.

☺ **$$$ Instant Pur Instant Eye Make-Up Remover** *($27 for 3.4 ounces)* is a standard, dual-phase eye-makeup remover that works very well to remove all types of makeup. It is fragrance-free and suitable for all skin types, and contains soothing plant extracts. The tiny amount of panthenol this contains will not help make eyelashes stronger.

😐 **$$$ Instant Pur Natural Action Exfoliator, Granule-Free** *($43 for 2.5 ounces)* is sold as an exfoliant that does not contain abrasive particles, instead relying on sugars and oils to remove dead skin cells. Although it is admittedly interesting to watch this gel turn oily and then milky when mixed with water and applied to skin, the tiny amount of sugar won't dissolve a single dead skin cell—though your skin will be smoother and softer after using this due to the moisturizing agents it contains.

☹ **Instant Pur Energising Beauty Toner** *($35 for 6.7 ounces)* contains too much alcohol and too few beneficial ingredients to make it a worthwhile toner for anyone.

😐 **$$$ Instant Pur Hydrating Beauty Toner** *($35 for 6.7 ounces)* is an interesting toner for normal to dry skin. Composed mostly of water, silicones, slip agents, and starch, it has some moisturizing ability and supplies a small amount of antioxidant vitamin E. All of the novel yet effective water-binding agents are listed after the preservative, so they don't count for much.

☺ **$$$ Instant Pur Toning and Cleansing Water, for Face and Eyes** *($35 for 6.7 ounces)* is a good, fairly gentle liquid makeup remover for all skin types except very oily. It is not the best for use around the eyes because it contains fragrance and citrus peel extract.

😐 **$$$ Instant Pur Deep Cleansing Masque** *($37 for 2.5 ounces)* is a very standard clay mask for normal to oily skin, and doesn't contain anything beneficial that is not also found in clay masks sold at the drugstore.

Yves St. Laurent Lisse Expert Products

😐 **$$$ Lisse Expert Advanced Eye and Lip Intensive Anti-Wrinkle Care** *($60 for 0.25 ounce)* is a dual-sided pen: one end dispenses a water- and silicone-based lotion and the other is meant to be used as a massage tool to make the product work better on lines and wrinkles. It is mostly water, silicone, silicone polymer, and salt. You may get some superficial line filling owing to the texture of the silicones, but the effect is short-lived and it's certainly no substitute for what injectable dermal fillers can do.

😐 **$$$ Lisse Expert Advanced Intensive Anti-Wrinkle Creme** *($80 for 1.6 ounces)* is so ordinary it beautifully drives home the point that fashion designers trying to do skin care may have aesthetically pleasing packaging, while the "fabric" of their formulas is much less impressive; they're just hoping to coast by on image alone. If you must have YSL skin care, this is appropriate for normal to dry skin.

😐 **$$$ Lisse Expert Advanced Intensive Anti-Wrinkle Serum** *($90 for 1 ounce)* is an incredibly basic, overpriced, water- and silicone-based serum for all skin types. The styrene film-forming agent can make skin appear smoother and feel slightly taut, but this won't make skin "just like new" any more than wearing Groucho Marx glasses with a moustache is a brilliant disguise.

☹ **Lisse Expert Esthetic Gel-Patch** *($115 for 0.5 ounce)* is one of the biggest wastes of time and money to come along in a long time. Reading the claims for this product might just convince you it's a downright cheap alternative to a face-lift, what with all its talk of signaling the skin's self-repair process and of the diffusion of ingredients precisely where wrinkles need them most. However, the formula tells the true story, and in this case the claims are classic fiction. These supposedly targeted "ultra-technical" patches are mostly water, alcohol, gum-based thickener, and more alcohol. They're very irritating and offer absolutely no hope to anyone concerned about aging skin. At best, the irritants, if left on skin overnight, will cause low-grade inflammation that temporarily makes wrinkled areas look less pronounced. But the long-term cost of assaulting your skin with such irritants (and an accompanying dusting of potentially beneficial ingredients) isn't worth one-quarter of what YSL is charging.

😐 **$$$ Lisse Expert Esthetic Line Eraser Kit** *($225 for the kit)* is composed of a **Peeling Masque**, said to provide a "spectacular cosmetic resurfacing effect," and a **Wrinkle Filler Pen** that supplies a dose of topical hyaluronic acid to plump lines. The Pen is also said to stimulate the skin's own synthesis of hyaluronic acid so it will become plumped from within too, further reducing wrinkles and expression lines. When you're charging a price that approaches the cost of genuine cosmetic corrective procedures, you'd better have a good story. In this case, you can skim the cover and skip to the last page because nothing in this product will resurface skin or plump lines to the same extent as professionally administered treatments.

The Masque contains about 5% glycolic acid and has a pH low enough to exfoliate skin. It is formulated in a simple base of water and slip agents to enhance penetration of the AHA.

The tiny amounts of water-binding and soothing agents are inconsequential compared with the amount of fragrance in this product.

The Wrinkle Filler Pen contains so little hyaluronic acid (used in its salt form, sodium hyaluronate, which is considerably less expensive and less effective than pure hyaluronic acid) that it's barely worth mentioning, particularly since it's minimally capable of exerting any sort of benefit on skin. The product dispensed from this pen is mostly water, film-forming agent, alcohol, and gum-based thickener. The film-forming agent works to temporarily smooth lines, while the alcohol just makes every cell dry and dull.

Using a well-formulated AHA product from another line (almost all cost less than YSL's version) will work far better for skin, and then if you want to see if a "filler"-type product works, consider those from Avon, Estee Lauder, or Prescriptives. They won't make a "Gee, I don't need an injection after all" difference either, but at least they contain far more state-of-the-art ingredients than this version and cost far less!

Yves St. Laurent Temps Majeur Products

☹ **$$$ Temps Majeur Lotion** *($85 for 6.6 ounces)* is a good, alcohol-free toner for normal to dry skin. It contains some good water-binding agents, skin-smoothing silicone, and nonvolatile plant extracts, but for the money it's still fairly ordinary and not worth it.

☹ **$$$ Temps Majeur Creme** *($315 for 1.6 ounces)* has an elegantly silky texture and contains ingredients that help normal to slightly dry or slightly oily skin feel and look better, but the antioxidant activity of the mushroom extract will be lost once this ultra-pricey jar-packaged product is opened. This is prestigious in name only; for the money, it should be loaded with a range of state-of-the-art ingredients.

☹ **$$$ Temps Majeur Elixir De Nuit** *($435 for 0.7 ounce)* is positioned as an amazing elixir whose potency comes from the "treasures of traditional Chinese remedies," an odd association given YSL's haute couture French image. Rest assured: No culture's ancient remedies are the solution for youthful skin. After all, think of how much was unknown about skin hundreds of years ago! This tiny bottle contains mostly safflower oil, a triglyceride, and *Crambe abyssinica* seed oil. The latter's oil content is a source of erucic acid, which is used to manufacture plastic and lighting implements. It is also considered one of the cheaper oils available, which doesn't make the price of this mostly worthless product any more convincing (Source: www.ibiblio.org/pfaf/cgi-bin/arr_html?Crambe+abyssinica&CAN=LATIND). *Crambe abyssinnica* oil contains a fatty acid that can help dry skin, but it isn't nearly as multi-faceted as several other oils are for skin, including olive, evening primrose, and flax seed. This serum-like product is an option for dry skin, but the price is nothing less than ludicrous, and the Chinese remedy claim is just plain hokey.

☹ **$$$ Temps Majeur Nutri-Creme** *($305 for 1.6 ounces)* is a suitable moisturizer for dry to very dry skin, but the workhorse ingredients in this product are found in hundreds of other moisturizers with much more realistic prices. You're not getting anything substantial for your substantial investment; if anything, it's quite a letdown to know that the jar packaging won't keep the efficacious antioxidants in this product stable during use.

☹ **$$$ Temps Majeur Serum** *($300 for 1.6 ounces)* is only worth the price if you believe mushroom stem extract is the fountain of youth. Most species of mushroom have antioxidant capability and other various attributes that can be helpful for skin. But none of these benefits is in line with what YSL claims this serum can do, and the few other potentially intriguing ingredients are barely present. By the way, the gum base of this serum can lend a slightly sticky finish. All told, I wouldn't choose this over serums from Olay, Neutrogena, Clinique, Estee Lauder, or even Clarins.

☹ **$$$ Temps Majeur Yeux** *($115 for 0.5 ounce)* is a good emollient moisturizer for dry skin anywhere on the face. What a shame that the jar packaging won't keep the mushroom extract stable once this product is being used. The mineral pigments create a soft shine effect on skin, and can slightly "brighten" shadowed areas (though a concealer works much better, and if you want shine, you can dust some shimmer powder on top).

☹ **$$$ Temps Majeur Masque** *($145 for 1.6 ounces)* is mostly water and film-forming agent with some thickeners. How this average concoction is supposed to offer skin an "intense burst of energy" is a good question. At best, normal to dry skin will look and feel smoother.

OTHER YVES ST. LAURENT PRODUCTS

☹ **$$$ Ideal Defense Rejuvenating Multi-Protection Creme SPF 8** *($62 for 1.6 ounces)* has an embarrassingly low SPF rating, although avobenzone is included for UVA protection. The base formula is so boring it's tiring to even write about, but suffice it to say you're getting a lot of film-forming agent, which may be irritating, especially in tandem with the sunscreen ingredient.

☹ **$$$ Ideal Defense Rejuvenating Multi-Protection Lotion SPF 8** *($62 for 1.6 ounces)* is a lighter-weight version of the Ideal Defense Rejuvenating Multi-Protection Creme above, and although the formula is a bit more interesting, it's still an overall bust due to the low SPF rating and what you're not getting for your money.

☹ **$$$ Nuit Intense Maximum Replenishing Night Creme** *($74 for 1.6 ounces)* doesn't reach maximum potential on any front, except perhaps for being maximally average for the money. It's an option for normal to slightly dry skin, just not a very good one. You're supposed to believe the common ingredients in this moisturizer can tell time and zero in on regenerating skin at the moment it begins its nighttime repair process, which is just nonsense.

☹ **$$$ Nutri Systeme Intense Nourishing Creme** *($56 for 1.6 ounces)* has merit as a moisturizer for dry to very dry skin, but antioxidants are in short supply, and jar packaging won't keep them stable once you begin using it. If this is YSL's idea of "new generation nourishing skin care," they need to go back to the drawing board!

☺ **$$$ Baume Nourrissant, Moisturizing Lip and Nail Balm** *($23 for 0.5 ounce)* is a standard emollient lip balm that is way overpriced for what you get. However, if you fall for the designer trappings of YSL, at least this product will take good care of dry lips and nails.

YVES ST. LAURENT MAKEUP

FOUNDATION: ☺ **$$$ Perfect Touch Radiant Brush Foundation** *($52)* comes in a unique component that features a built-in synthetic foundation brush. Carefully squeezing the tube pushes a silky liquid foundation onto the brush, allowing you to paint it on. The foundation begins slightly thick but blends very well, providing sheer to light coverage and a luminous finish suitable for normal to dry skin. YSL offers 15 shades, and just over half are remarkably neutral. The following shades are too peach, orange, or copper for most skin tones: #6, #8, #10, #12, #13, and #14. The brush applicator is workable if you prefer this method of applying foundation, though it blends just as well using your fingertips or a makeup sponge. It is worth nothing that this is the only YSL foundation with shades for dark skin tones.

☹ **$$$ Teint de Soie Line Smoothing Foundation** *($51)* has a rich, emollient texture whose first impression makes it eminently suitable for dry to very dry skin seeking medium to full coverage. However, it tends to look heavy on skin and four of the six shades are unabashedly peach or orange (#3, #5BA, #4G1, and #4J1). Given the price and the limited shade options, this is one to skip in favor of Prescriptives' Flawless Skin Total Protection Makeup SPF 15 ($39.50).

☹ **$$$ Teint Singulier Sheer Powder Creme Veil** *($44)* has a slippery texture that dries to a satin-matte finish, providing sheer coverage that would work for someone with normal to dry skin. Most of the four shades are off-color and tend toward pinks and peaches, but this is so sheer it doesn't really matter. Contrary to the vastly inflated claims, this does not "perfectly shape the face" in any way, nor is it capable of concealing blemishes.

☹ **$$$ Teint Eclat de Soie Radiance Smoothing Foundation SPF 8** *($51)* has an SPF rating that's too low for daytime wear, though it is titanium dioxide–based. This liquid foundation has a fluid, silky texture and a very smooth application that sets to a soft, radiant finish. What a shame the sunscreen rating isn't higher! If you decide to pair this with a product rated SPF 15 or greater, it is best for normal to dry skin, and only two of the eight shades (#1 and #3) are a problematic shade of peach.

☹ **$$$ Teint Mat Purete Transfer-Resistant Fluid Foundation SPF 15** *($51)* does not contain the UVA-protecting ingredients of titanium dioxide, zinc oxide, avobenzone, Mexoryl SX (ecamsule), or Tinosorb, and should not be relied on for daily sun protection. That's unfortunate, because this is an otherwise excellent foundation for normal to oily or combination skin. The slightly thick consistency becomes silky and fluid during blending, quickly setting to a dimensional (rather than flat or masklike) matte finish. It provides light to medium coverage and offers good staying power, too. Among the eight shades, #1, #2, and #3 are slightly peach, but may work for some light skin tones. The other shades are flawless.

☹ **$$$ Teint De Jour Tinted Matte Moisturizer** *($38)* starts creamy and then, before you know it, dries to a light-coverage matte finish. Unfortunately, this can look a bit chalky on the skin (titanium dioxide is a prominent ingredient), but at least most of the six sheer shades go on less rose and peach than they look. Avoid shades #3 and #4, which are a bit too peach to soften, despite this product's sheerness.

☹ **$$$ Teint Compact Hydra Feel SPF 10** *($54; $36 for refills)* features an in-part avobenzone sunscreen, yet the SPF rating is frustratingly short of the recommended minimum for daytime protection. This is otherwise an innovative cream-to-powder makeup packaged in an elegant compact complete with a very good sponge applicator. The semi-solid cake doesn't allow you to pick up product as easily as many cream-to-powders, but it smooths onto skin easily and blends to an ultra-light satin finish while providing light to medium coverage. It is best for normal to dry skin looking for a radiant yet natural finish. With the exception of shade #6, all of the colors are impeccable and include options for fair to tan skin tones.

CONCEALER: ☺ **$$$ Touche Eclat Radiant Touch** *($39.50)* is far and away the most popular YSL makeup item and one that is routinely featured in fashion magazine "best of beauty" lists. It's the original brush-on highlighter, cleverly packaged in a pen-style component with a built-in synthetic brush. Although not much for concealing (the coverage isn't too substantial), it functions well as a highlighter or to add a subtle radiance to shadowy areas, particularly under the eyes. It is light enough to layer over a regular concealer (which you'll need if dark circles are apparent), and the best of the four shades are #1 and #2. Shade #3 is slightly peach but likely too sheer to matter, while #4 has an orange cast that limits its appeal. As an option, and I mean a really impressive option, try Maybelline's Instant Age Rewind Double Face Perfector, which works perfectly and for far less money.

☹ **Anti-Cernes Multi-Action Concealer** *($30)*. It takes a lot of chutzpah to charge so much for such a greasy, heavy-looking concealer that creases in no time. If for some reason you prefer this type of product, there are significantly less expensive versions available at the drugstore.

POWDER: ✓ ☺ $$$ Poudre Compact Eclat et Matite *($43)* is a buttery-smooth, talc-based pressed powder that melds with skin to create a very natural non-powdery finish. This is an outstanding pressed-powder option for those with normal to dry skin (those with oily skin or oily areas may find this not absorbent enough). All six shades are neutral and matte.

☺ **$$$ Poudre de Soleil SPF 10** *($44)* is a pressed bronzing powder with a beautifully silky texture and a low-wattage shine finish that doesn't flake. The sunscreen is titanium dioxide, and because this product would be used as an adjunct to a regular sunscreen or foundation with sunscreen, it deserves a happy face rating. There are three shades, with the best being Golden Sun 2. Light Sun 1 is almost too sheer to show even a slight tanned appearance, but may work for very fair skin tones. This applies smoothly and evenly and is definitely a bronzing powder worth considering if your budget is generous.

😐 **$$$ Poudre Sur Mesure Semi-Loose Powder** *($56)* comes in a cake form, but the container shaves off the top layer when you twist it, creating a loose powder. It's less messy than conventional loose powder, but this clever convenience doesn't come cheap. The talc- and aluminum starch–based formula goes on sheer and has a dry finish suitable for normal to very oily skin. Each of the five colors has a bit of shine, so this is not for those who want to use powder to keep shine at bay.

BLUSH: ☺ $$$ Variations Blush *($41)* features four quilted strips of tone-on-tone colors, which is where the "variations" part of the name comes into play (for example, you get subtle variations on pinks or berry tones). All of the shades in each compact have shine and are incredibly silky, while also being strongly pigmented (which is a plus for dark skin tones). Despite the intensity, this applies smoothly and offers a luminous rather than sparkling finish. Compacts 6 and 11 are great for bronzing or contouring.

😐 **$$$ Touche Blush** *($41)* is a loose powder blush whose base component comes with an attached cheek-size sponge for on-the-spot application. The concept is intriguing but the execution tends to place blush-colored powder all over your face instead of just on your cheek area, though you can temper this somewhat if you're extra careful about application. Still, applying blush should be easier than this. Four shades are available (additional, limited-edition shades are often seen in seasonal collections), and although all are sheer and workable, each is infused with large particles of sparkle that tend to go everywhere. If the sparkles don't bother you and you're in the mood for a novel way to apply powder blush, you may want to give this an audition if you happen upon a YSL counter.

EYESHADOW: ✓ ☺ $$$ Ombre Solo Double Effect *($25.50)* presents two tone-on-tone powder eyeshadows in one sleek compact. This is YSL's silkiest eyeshadow formula, and it applies superbly, builds intensity well, and doesn't flake. All of the duos are shiny, but most are not distractingly so (#5 and #6 are the least shiny).

☺ **$$$ Ombres Vibration Eye Shadow Duo** *($36.50)* have better texture and application than the Ombre Solo Smoothing Long-Lasting Eyeshadow below, and are worth considering (price notwithstanding) if you want lots of shine and strong colors. The pairings are much more workable than they used to be, with predominantly brown and gray tones ideal for shadowing and shaping. Avoid duos 13 and 29, whose color combinations are more for shock than allure.

😐 **$$$ Ombre Solo Smoothing Long-Lasting Eyeshadow** *($25.50)* consists of pressed-powder eyeshadows with a silky but dry texture that hinders application a bit and leads to some flaking. The shade selection favors strong shine, with #6 being the only matte option. If the flaking weren't an issue the shine would be tolerable, but at this price an eyeshadow should be nearly perfect in every way.

😐 **$$$ Frozen Eye Shadow** *($24.50)* is a loose-powder eyeshadow packaged in a small, vial-type bottle that includes a sponge-tip wand applicator. Each of the colors lays down intense, opaque shine and must be blended quickly because the consistency causes them to set quickly and then become immovable. The good news about that is the shadow lasts and lasts; the bad news is it's tricky to get such strong, shiny colors blended well. This is one to test at the counter and see if you like the application and the result.

☹ **Ombres Quadralumieres Eye Shadow Quartet** *($50)* is no match for the powder eyeshadows from haute couture fashion competitor Dior, and the prices of the two lines are nearly identical. These YSL quads suffer from a dry texture that makes blending difficult (though they do have some smoothness) and especially from terribly contrasting colors that are for fantasy, not real-world, makeup.

EYE AND BROW SHAPER: ☺ **$$$ Eyeliner Moire Liquid Eyeliner** *($29)* is a liquid liner with a thin, tapered brush that applies evenly, allowing you to lay down a solid line with one swift stroke. All of the colors (except black) are metallic and the formula takes longer than it should to dry, but if you can endure that, it stays on marvelously well.

😐 **$$$ Dessin du Regard Haute Tenue Long-Lasting Eye Pencil** *($24)* would have earned a happy face rating were it not for the required sharpening. It's an above-average pencil whose performance bests many standard pencils due to its smooth application, suitable range of shades, and smudge-proof finish. The following shades may seem like fun, but won't serve to make your eyes the focus: #3, #4, #9, and #12.

😐 **$$$ Dessin de Sourcils Eyebrow Pencil** *($24)* costs a mint and needs routine sharpening, but it's a good, non-greasy eyebrow pencil that won't smudge. It finishes and remains slightly tacky, but that's less of an issue if you apply this softly. Among the standard shades, #4 is puzzlingly shiny.

😐 **$$$ Eyebrow Enhancer Duo** *($25.50)* combines a brow gel and brow color in one dual-sided product. The sheer brow color is applied with a sponge-tip applicator, which is odd but workable if you are really careful, while the brow gel is applied with a regular mascara-like brush. It's an OK option for slightly darkening and grooming brows, but combining the products can feel heavy and give brows a wet look that may or may not be to your liking.

LIPSTICK, LIP GLOSS, AND LIPLINER: ✓ ☺ **$$$ Touche Brilliance Sparkling Touch for Lips** *($29)* is a fantastic lip gloss that is packaged just like the Touche Eclat Radiant Touch highlighter above, meaning the gloss is dispensed onto a synthetic brush applicator. The texture is superb and the finish is a gleaming shine that's not the least bit sticky. As for the colors, they're an enticing mix of sheer, bright, and bold metallic.

☺ **$$$ Fard a Levres Rouge Pur Pure Lipstick SPF 8** *($28)* offers mostly bright shades (including many warm reds and oranges) in a fairly greasy lipstick formula that goes on opaque and has a glossy finish. These are richly pigmented, which is nice, but the glossiness allows them to easily bleed and feather into lines around the mouth. The sunscreen is all titanium dioxide, and although SPF 8 isn't the benchmark to strive for, when it comes to lipsticks, it's better than nothing.

☺ **$$$ Rouge Vibration Magnetic Glow Comfortable Lipstick** *($29)* is a modern, sophisticated lipstick with a highbrow price. It is indeed comfortable and the slim-line case houses a smooth, lightweight cream lipstick that offers medium opacity and a slight stain complete with a high-shine finish.

☺ **$$$ Baume d'Ete Tinted Lip Balm SPF 10** *($23)* has an in-part avobenzone sunscreen and although SPF 10 isn't ideal, it's better than no lip sunscreen at all. This sheer, slightly viscous gloss comes in a tube and has a sticky (but not intolerably so) feel that makes it rather tenacious. It's a good option if you don't mind needlessly splurging on lip gloss.

😐 **$$$ Rouge Personnel Lipstick** *($27.50)* is a creamy lipstick that's said to be unique because the more you apply, the more satiny it becomes. Although this does feel luscious and smooth, almost any creamy lipstick will feel more satiny as it is layered, so the claim isn't too original. This particular lipstick actually requires several layers or it looks uneven, meaning you'll use it up faster than normal, and at this price, well, it's just not worth it.

😐 **$$$ Rouge Pur Shine Sheer Lipstick SPF 15** *($28)* does not contain the UVA-protecting ingredients of titanium dioxide, zinc oxide, avobenzone, Mexoryl SX, or Tinosorb, so it is not recommended as a reliable lipstick with sunscreen. It is otherwise a slick, shimmer-infused lipstick that feels very light and features some gorgeous soft colors. Its neutral face rating is for not including sufficient UVA protection.

😐 **$$$ Golden Gloss Shimmering Lip Gloss** *($27)* gets its shimmer from particles of glitter, and although the multidimensional effect is striking, the glitter tends to feel slightly grainy as the emollience of the gloss wears away. It's not a bad lip gloss, but for the money it should stay smooth and soft longer.

😐 **$$$ Smoothing Lip Gloss** *($27)* is your everyday wand gloss that features sheer, unquestionably glossy colors with a tacky feel. It's an OK option, but if you're all about YSL this isn't preferred to their Touche Brilliance Sparkling Touch for Lips above or a dozen options from the drugstore.

😐 **$$$ Dessin des Levres Lip Liner** *($23)* is a very good standard pencil that feels slightly creamy going on, but ends up having a drier than usual finish, which helps keep it in place. The color range has been toned down and now favors browns, mauves, and reds—so there are clearly some missing links between this and Saint Laurent's lipstick palette.

😐 **$$$ Lip Twins Lip Duo Satin/Shine SPF 8** *($30)* wins points for its unique and very clever packaging. Housed in a cylindrical container just slightly larger than a lipstick tube are a lipstick, lip gloss, and brush applicator. Rotating the bottom of the container reveals pans of lip color, while the brush is pulled out from the top (and although it's small, it's a quality brush). One panel of the component is also a mirror, which you can use to apply or touch up. What's inside is standard fare: a creamy lipstick with reasonable staying powder due to its pigmentation and a sheer, sparkle-infused lip gloss. The sunscreen lacks both a sufficient SPF rating and the right UVA-protecting ingredients, which, beyond the price, is this product's only shortcoming.

MASCARA: ✓ ☺ $$$ Mascara Volume Effet Faux Cils Luxurious Mascara for a False Lash Effect *($26.50)* doesn't quite measure up to the effect obtainable from false eyelashes, but it ranks as YSL's best mascara. That's because it builds beautifully and thickens well without clumps. The result is lashes that are dramatic without being over the top, and all with a soft, fringed curl. This mascara also comes off completely with a water-soluble cleanser.

✓☺ **$$$ Everlong Mascara Lengthening Mascara** *($26.50)* isn't quite as impressive as the Mascara Volume above, but is still worthy of its rating. The short, dense bristles allow you to build prodigious length and enough thickness to satisfy, all with only minor clumps that are easily combed through. This also leaves lashes softly curled, and wears without a smear or flake.

☺ **$$$ Mascara Volume Infini Curl Volumizing Mascara for Infinite Curl** *($26.50)* has a heavy, wet application that leads to smearing if you're not extremely careful, and the effect may not be worth it, depending on your preferences (and budget). This mascara quickly lengthens and uplifts lashes, leading to a sweeping, dramatic effect that begs for shameless flirting. Have a clean mascara wand or lash brush handy because you may need to comb through some minor clumps.

😐 **$$$ Mascara Aquaresistant Mascara Waterproof** *($26.50)* is expertly waterproof, even if lashes get completely soaked. Yet that's about the only exciting aspect of this otherwise ordinary mascara. Lashes get somewhat longer and there are no clumps, but for the money there are much more impressive waterproof mascaras at the drugstore.

😐 **$$$ Mascara Longueur Intense Lengthening Mascara** *($25.50)* does lengthen (and curl), but the effect is far removed from almost anyone's definition of "intense." If anything, applying this mascara will test your patience as it slowly shows you what it isn't capable of. On the plus side, this does not clump, it wears well throughout the day, and it's easy to remove. Still, for the money, I would expect a lot more, and you should too.

FACE AND BODY ILLUMINATING/SHIMMER PRODUCTS: ✓☺ **$$$ Teint Parfait Complexion Enhancer** *($37.50)* is sold as a sheer highlighter for all-over use on the face, and is ideal for this purpose. The easy-to-blend lotion texture imparts a sheer, slight shimmer finish that works under or over foundation. It sets to a matte (in feel) finish and is suitable for all skin types, particularly those with dull complexions. Shade #1 is a pale lilac that may be OK for very fair skin, but test it first; shade #6 has a peachy cast that should also be considered carefully. The four remaining shades are attractive and versatile, and the shimmer stays put. ✓☺ **$$$ Glossy Touch Multi-Purpose Gloss** *($24)* comes in a tube and is a multipurpose gloss that adds a touch of wet shine anywhere it's placed. I am normally skeptical of such products because not only do they undo carefully applied makeup, but they also tend to make skin feel slippery and look too greasy. This product is quite different: it has a thinner consistency and a silky, almost weightless finish, and yet still provides the specified glossy sheen. If this is the type of effect you're after, Glossy Touch is the best way I've found to achieve it without looking or feeling like a goopy mess. It's admittedly pricey, but a little goes a long way.

BRUSHES: The small, workable collection of ☺ **$$$ Brushes** *($27–$52)* has improved nicely, though in terms of overall quality and performance they still lag behind most other lines (many that charge less for similar brushes), including M.A.C., Stila, and Laura Mercier. The 😐 **$$$ Powder Brush** *($52)*, while very soft, is the weakest (but still worthy) option because it's not dense enough to apply more than a sheer dusting of powder. The other brushes are all worth considering and are readily available for testing at the counter.

Z. BIGATTI (SKIN CARE ONLY)

Z. BIGATTI AT-A-GLANCE

Strengths: One antioxidant-rich, silky-textured serum; an expensive but effective lip balm.

Weaknesses: Incredibly expensive and overall disappointing considering these are products from a dermatologist; jar packaging is especially disappointing given the number of antioxidants many products contain; several products contain irritating ingredients with no established benefit for skin; no AHA, BHA, or effective skin-lightening products; no products to manage acne; the sole sunscreen option leaves skin vulnerable to UVA damage; several products contain fragrance ingredients despite the line's claim of being fragrance-free.

For more information about Z. Bigatti, call (888) 430-1529 or visit www.zbigatti.com or www.Beautypedia.com.

☺ **$$$ Re-Storation Champagne Gel Cleanser** *($69 for 4 ounces)* is a good water-soluble cleanser for all skin types except very oily, though the price is ludicrous and the amount of product offered smaller than average. Lots of bells and whistles were added to this cleanser, but they are rinsed down the drain before they can exert a benefit on skin.

☹ **Re-Storation Purify Hydrating Lotion Cleanser** *($70 for 4 ounces)* lists witch hazel extract as its second ingredient and also contains several irritating plant oils, including rosemary, thyme, and grapefruit. It is not recommended.

☹ **Re-Storation Silk Toner** *($60 for 4 ounces)* contains ineffective AHA-like ingredients, some of which are potentially irritating. What is most definitely irritating is the menthol, something a dermatologist should know better than to include in any skin-care product.

☹ **Rescue Intensive Facial Treatment** *($135 for 0.5 ounce)* promises results so dramatic "it's hard to believe it wasn't surgery," but you won't be seeing deep expression lines vanish or any measure of lifting of slackening skin. There is an impressive array of ingredients in this moisturizer for normal to dry skin, though a couple of the more prominent ones (myrrh and saffron) are irritants due to their volatile components. Further down the list but even more troublesome are a trio of irritating plant oils (lime, lavender, and peppermint), which make this antioxidant-rich moisturizer a poor choice for skin in need of rescue.

✓☺ **$$$ Re-Storation Deep Repair Facial Serum** *($198 for 1 ounce)* is a very good, antioxidant-rich serum for all skin types. Yet regardless of the antioxidants present or the amounts included, they cannot prevent further skin damage all by themselves (antioxidants alone cannot protect skin from the ravages of sun exposure). That is one example of the far-fetched claims made for this product, but without question it has benefit for skin if you're looking for a multitude of antioxidants and some intriguing water-binding agents.

😐 **$$$ Re-Storation Delicate Intensive Moisturizing Facial Cream** *($155 for 2 ounces)* is also known as Re-Storation Delicate Moisturizing Facial Treatment, but by any name this needlessly expensive moisturizer for dry to very dry skin sees much of its antioxidant benefit wasted due to the unfortunate choice of jar packaging. That's a shame but less so when you consider that equally good formulas are available in better packaging for less money. This does have most of the elements needed for dry skin to gain an improved barrier function and be better able to protect itself against external causes of dryness. However, for the money, the packaging should be reconsidered.

☹ **Re-Storation Enlighten Skin Tone Provider** *($189 for 2 ounces)* claims to contain several botanical ingredients capable of lightening skin, and references bamboo, licorice, bearberry, and mulberry. Interestingly, however, none of these are on this product's ingredient list, though it does contain *Uva ursi* extract, which is related to bearberry, whose arbutin content has some research demonstrating its skin-lightening ability. The problem is not only jar packaging, which hinders the stability of the plant extracts (some of which are antioxidant), but also the inclusion of an appreciable amount of grapefruit and orange oil, which can cause irritation. Also, these citrus oils can cause phototoxic reactions if skin is exposed to sunlight, potentially leading to further skin discolorations. This obviously is not "the perfect ingredient list" as claimed.

☹ **Re-Storation Eye Return Age-Defying Eye Cream** *($125 for 0.5 ounce)* is also known as Re-Storation Eye Return Anti-Aging Eye Cream, but whichever name you come across, the inclusion of eucalyptus oil is a bad idea for all skin types, and certainly not advised in a product meant for use around the eye. Furthermore, the jar packaging won't keep the antioxidants in this moisturizer stable once it is opened.

😐 **$$$ Re-Storation Goodnight Facial Cream** *($295 for 2 ounces)*. Other than "They've got to be kidding!" there are no words to express how ludicrous the price for this moisturizer is. For almost $300, you're getting primarily water, squalane (an emollient found in hundreds of moisturizers that cost much less than this), thickener, castor oil, silicone, shea butter, mineral oil, and glycerin. You get the idea—these are commonplace (though effective) ingredients that show up in too many moisturizers to count! This contains many excellent water-binding agents and a pleasing array of antioxidants, from vitamin E to superoxide dismutase, but again, so do many other products that wouldn't dare charge this much money for 2 ounces, and Bigatti uses jar packaging! This has potential for dry to very dry skin, but unless you can say to yourself "I enjoy spending a ridiculously high amount of money on a single skin-care product" before purchasing this, I suggest leaving it at the counter. Goodnight Facial Cream contains fragrance in the form of linalool.

😐 **$$$ Re-Storation Illuminate Firming and Brightening Facial Cream** *($175 for 2 ounces)* is also known as Re-Storation Illuminate Exfoliating & Firming Facial Cream. The exfoliation is attributed to the enzyme papain, but it is unreliable at best and the amount of it in this moisturizer is small, not to mention the jar packaging won't keep it or the antioxidants stable during use. This has potential for normal to dry skin, but the only thing causing a brightening effect is the shiny mineral pigment mica.

😐 **$$$ Re-Storation Skin Treatment Facial Cream** *($155 for 2 ounces)* is the original moisturizer from Z. Bigatti that, according to the company, "started a skin-care revolution." Either I (and the media) missed that revolution or the statement is nothing more than the company blowing its own horn. Either way, if this product is supposed to be the ultimate solution and a comprehensive age-fighting formula, why does Z. Bigatti offer so many other moisturizers, all making similar miraculous claims? This is a decent moisturizer for normal to dry skin. It contains some noted cell-communicating ingredients, but the enzymes are too unstable to exfoliate, the fruit extracts don't work like AHAs, and jar packaging will compromise the effectiveness of the antioxidants. That doesn't add up to the ultimate anything, and makes the luxury price tag more of a marketing whim than something that's realistically related to a product that costs a lot to manufacture.

☹ **Re-Storation Skin Treatment Facial Lotion** *($155 for 2 ounces)* is the lotion version of the Re-Storation Skin Treatment Facial Cream above, but although the packaging is better here, the addition of grapefruit and orange oils makes this too problematic for all skin types. If you choose to ignore that issue, at least don't believe the company's advice that this moisturizer is suitable for oily skin because it absolutely is not due to the many emollients and oils it contains.

☹ **Re-Storation Swan Firming Neck Treatment** *($141 for 2 ounces)* contains eucalyptus oil, which has no benefit for the neck or for skin anywhere on the body (and Z. Bigatti recommends this for delicate skin!). The bulk of this formula is ordinary ingredients; the salicylic acid and AHA cannot exfoliate because this product's pH is too high.

☹ **Silk Screen Ultra Light Facial Sunscreen SPF 30** *($68 for 1.7 ounces)* lacks the UVA-protecting ingredients of titanium dioxide, zinc oxide, avobenzone, Mexoryl SX, or Tinosorb, and is not recommended. Not only that, but it's almost shocking that such an expensive, incomplete sunscreen comes from a dermatologist.

☹ **Inception, Total Face Masque** *($149 for a box of 3 individually packaged masques)* consists of pre-packaged fabric masks cut to fit the face. Each mask is soaked in a solution that is primarily a blend of water, soy flour, and several water-binding agents. As the soy flour and water dry, skin begins to feel tighter, similar to what happens when you apply a clay mask. That isn't a distinct advantage and it doesn't excuse the inclusion of irritating grapefruit peel oil, tannic acid (whose astringent quality dehydrates skin cells), and fennel extract. This mask cannot provide an instant lift, though the manner in which the soy flour dries may convince you it is "working." Inception isn't worth even a mildly warm reception.

☹ **Re-Storation Dew Hydrating Facial Mask** *($119 for 2 ounces)* has a ridiculously out-of-line price and only serves to irritate skin because of the eucalyptus oil it contains. I've said it before, but it bears repeating: Not only does expensive not mean better, but also eucalyptus oil contains volatile components that have been proven to be irritating to skin (Sources: *Basic and Clinical Pharmacology and Toxicology*, June 2006, pages 575–581; and www.naturaldatabase.com).

☹ **Re-Storation Impact Fruit Enzyme Facial Mask** *($129 for 2 ounces)* is the most expensive clay mask in this book, and ends up being a problem for all skin types because of the amount of comfrey extract it contains. The rosemary, thyme, juniper, cypress, and eucalyptus oils will cause irritation, as will the arnica extract.

☹ **Lip Envy Lip Treatment Balm** *($55 for 0.3 ounce)* has to be the most expensive jar of lip balm in this book, and yet its main ingredients (mineral oil, beeswax, and Vaseline) are commonplace and not expensive in the least. Although those ingredients will take good care of dry lips, the peppermint oil in this balm will only cause problems.

☺ **$$$ Re-Storation Lip Pout, Lip Treatment Cream** *($55 for 0.17 ounce)* contains ingredients that can hydrate the lips and temporarily fill in lines whose appearance is more pronounced due to dryness or chapping. However, this cannot plump lips and, although it's an option if dryness is a concern, the price is extraordinarily high for what you get.

ZAPZYT (SKIN CARE ONLY)

ZAPZYT AT-A-GLANCE

Strengths: Inexpensive; a couple of good topical disinfectants, though one is packaged in a kit with two other products that won't help acne-prone skin.

Weaknesses: Ineffective BHA options; bar cleanser; no sunscreens (blemish-prone skin still needs sun protection); drying detergent cleansing agent in the "Soothing" cleanser.

For more information about Zapzyt, call (601) 939-0844 or visit www.zapzyt.com or visit www.Beautypedia.com.

☹ **10% Benzoyl Peroxide Treatment Bar** *($6.95 for a 4-ounce bar)* contains a lot of benzoyl peroxide, but its brief contact with skin doesn't give it much chance to disinfect, and the ingredients that keep this detergent-based cleanser in bar form are problematic for blemish-prone skin.

☹ **Acne Wash, with Soothing Aloe & Chamomile** *($5.59 for 6.25 ounces)* violates FDA ingredient disclosure guidelines by listing trade names instead of actual ingredients. Bioterge As-40 is the drying detergent cleansing agent sodium C14-16 olefin sulfonate, while Glucamate Doe-120 is PEG-120 methyl glucose dioleate, which is a thickening agent. The chamomile and aloe won't soothe skin because of the cleansing agent selected here, and the 2% salicylic acid won't keep pores clog-free as claimed.

✓☺ **10% Benzoyl Peroxide Acne Treatment Gel** *($5.29 for 1 ounce)* is a simply formulated but effective topical disinfectant for blemish-prone skin. The gel texture is nearly weightless and the product does not contain needless irritants, including fragrance. The 10% level of benzoyl peroxide can be too potent for some, but this is worth considering if you have not had success with lower-strength versions and aren't ready to consider prescription options to manage acne.

😐 **Pore Treatment Gel** *($5.29 for 0.75 ounce)* is a lightweight gel that contains 2% salicylic acid as the active ingredient. Unfortunately, it cannot exfoliate skin because the pH is 5—and there's little else to make this worth purchasing.

Acne Pack *($14.99 for the kit)* includes three products, two of which are reviewed above but in this kit are packaged under different names (which is just confusing). The ☹ **Acne Cleanser** *(6.25 ounces)* is identical to the Acne Wash with Soothing Aloe and Chamomile above, and the ☹ **Repairing Day Gel** *(0.75 ounce)* is identical to the Pore Treatment Gel above. Because of this, the same reviews apply and neither product is recommended. The only worthwhile product in this kit is the ✓☺ **Repairing Night Gel** *(2 ounces)*, a fragrance-free, water-based gel that contains 5% benzoyl peroxide and no extraneous irritants. It's up to you to decide if the cost of this kit is worth getting only one worthwhile, effective product.

CHAPTER FIVE

The Best Products Summary

END GAME

Well, here we are—the best of the best—the category-by-category lists of products that really impressed me as I was compiling this book. All of the products included in the lists below either met or exceeded the criteria established for their respective categories. As such, all of these products deserve strong consideration, based on your skin type, skin condition, personal preferences, and cosmetics budget. (Speaking of budget, price was not a factor in determining whether a product was included in the lists below or not.)

First of all, if you turned directly to this chapter, figuring that you'd just cut to the chase and start shopping, let me forewarn you that this approach can backfire. Although the streamlined lists below are indeed helpful, you should also read the full review of any product you're considering. In addition, there may be other favorably reviewed options that will work perfectly well for you, although they may not appear on the lists below. Why not? Because unlike in previous editions of this book, I decided to include *only* the products rated as Paula's Picks. The result, in most cases, is that the lists are shorter than ever (in some cases, only one or two products are listed). These shorter lists are in response to frequent requests from my readers and from the media to provide succinct lists of the best of the best—neither group likes too many choices, which I understand completely. To make these shorter lists even easier to navigate, you'll find that the majority of categories are divided according to price as well as to skin type and, in the case of makeup, also according to texture. Interestingly, the lists in some categories include several options that many consumers would consider expensive, while the list of inexpensive products is comparably short. I did not do this intentionally to spotlight the expensive products; rather, it is simply how the reviews turned out as I read through the book one last time to select the products to include on the best-of-the-best lists. You also will notice that certain categories of products that did not receive any Paula's Pick ratings in the last edition of this book now do include Paula's Pick products. For example, the formulary similarities among cleansers, makeup removers, scrubs, toners, and self-tanners were such that rating any one of them as a Paula's Pick meant that all of them should get such an accolade. However, even though the products within each of these categories still have similar formularies, I was able to rate some of them a Paula's Pick, based on them going above and beyond what is standard for that category of products. You will find throughout the book that many cleansers, makeup removes, and self-tanners received a happy face rating. Those are certainly worth considering but simply didn't distinguish themselves from the Paula's Picks in these categories.

As comprehensive as this book is, as it goes to press there are new products being created and launched, and there is ongoing publication and release of new research unveiling the promise of ingredients that may have increased benefits or risks for skin. To keep you up to date on the latest products and corresponding ingredient research, and to make it easy for you to find the best makeup products available, I am pleased to announce the launch of my new Web site, www.Beautypedia.com. This subscriber-based site will replace my longstanding newsletter *Cosmetics Counter Update*. Beautypedia will include the entire contents of this book, and will be updated regularly with new reviews, revisions to existing reviews (e.g., when a product is discontinued), and hundreds of complete line reviews that, for reasons of space and timing, are not included in this book. The number of requests from my readers for such a service has been overwhelming, and I am thrilled that finally it is a reality. In addition to Beautypedia, I will continue to offer my free online Beauty Bulletin (sign up at www.cosmeticscop.com). These two resources provide more extensive in-depth explanations and clarifications about specific topics than I can possibly provide in this book. Beautypedia.com and the Beauty Bulletin also will allow me to provide far more detail about a product's claims and its ingredients. In this book, the goal is to bring more general information together all in one place, giving consumers enough comparative information to find out what works best for them among all the products with great, reliable formulations.

THE QUEST CAN GET CONFUSING

You have heard me say it before: Do not automatically buy a company's group of products just because it is recommended for your skin type. Most cosmetics companies recommend skin-care routines for specific skin types. As helpful as this may seem, it often ends up being a waste of money and may even be problematic for your skin. I strongly suggest that you ignore their categories and the corresponding product names. A person with dry skin who automatically follows a cosmetics company's recommendations could end up using too many products that are too emollient or too heavy, which can cause skin cells to build up and result in dull, rough-feeling skin. Loading up dry skin with too many heavy products can also cause breakouts (particularly whiteheads). Conversely, someone with oily skin may be sold products that contain strong irritants, which cause skin to become dry, irritated, red, and flaky, while still leaving you with oily skin. Someone with blemish-prone skin often ends up purchasing products that are ineffective for that problem. Please make sure you consider each product individually for its quality and its value to your skin, rather than selecting it based on its placement within a series of products, its promotional ads or brochures, or the sales pitches you hear.

Product names are meant to be seductive, not factual. Please keep in mind that a cosmetics company's name for a product does not always correspond with my recommendations. Just because a product label says it "gets rid of wrinkles" or is "good for sensitive skin" or "is a firming and nourishing serum" doesn't mean the formulation itself supports that label or claim. The same is true for eye, chest, or throat creams; despite what the cosmetics industry wants you to believe, these products can be used anywhere on the face, and what counts is what skin type they are good for and whether or not the product contains beneficial ingredients. There is absolutely nothing about any eye cream reviewed in this book that is unique for use in that area. What is most shocking is that eye creams have formulations very similar to those of facial moisturizers; the main differences are that usually the product comes in a smaller container (i.e., you usually get less product) and you usually pay more under the guise that the eye cream is "specially formulated." Of even greater concern is that many specialty eye and face products don't contain sunscreen. So, if you were being diligent about using a sunscreen on your face, but were applying only a designated eye or throat product that didn't contain sunscreen, you would be allowing the sun to harm the skin in those areas.

In addition, you will find many selections in the following lists of recommended products with names that sound like they should be in the dry-skin group, but that I have included in the oily-skin group, and vice versa. That's because ultimately what counts is how the product is formulated, not what the companies want you to believe about the product.

Remember, putting together the best routine for your skin type and your makeup needs is the overall goal.

The sequence of applying products for a particular skin-care regimen for a wide range of skin types is posted on my Web site, www.cosmeticscop.com. As a general rule, the following sequence is a safe, step-by-step guideline, depending on the products that your skin needs: cleanser; scrub; eye-makeup remover (if needed); toner; AHA or BHA product; topical disinfectant (only for blemish-prone skin); topical retinoid (note that with the exception of Differin [adapalene], retinoids cannot be used with benzoyl peroxide), azelaic acid, MetroGel, MetroLotion, MetroCream, or Noritate (one of the latter five if you have been diagnosed with rosacea); serum; skin-lightening product (only if discolorations are an issue); and during the day sunscreen and at night a moisturizer. Sunscreen is always the last item you apply during the day because you must never dilute a sunscreen.

Best Cleansers (Including Cleansing Cloths)

All of the cleansers listed below were chosen for their exceptional formulation, which, in most cases, means that fragrance and fragrant plant extracts have been excluded and that the cleanser is gentle yet effective for removing surface dirt, oil, perspiration, and makeup without making skin feel dry or tight. Those with normal to slightly dry, combination, or very oily skin should use a water soluble cleanser; those with normal to very dry skin can use a water soluble cleanser or, if preferred, a cleansing lotion. Top picks in the cleansing lotion group are included in the list of Best Cleansers for Normal to Dry or Very Dry skin.

Every cleanser on these lists is free of harsh, irritating, or sensitizing ingredients. I never recommend bar soap because the ingredients that keep the bar soap in a bar form can clog pores, and the cleansing agents in them are almost always drying. Emollient wipe-off cleansers may be the only type of cleansers that don't cause dry, sensitive skin to become drier; therefore, I recommend them for that skin type, although such products were not rated Paula's Picks because they are inherently difficult to rinse (and you should never remove a cleanser with tissues—talk about outdated!).

You will notice that I do not specify a group of "medicated" or "anti-acne" cleansers supposedly designed for very oily or blemish-prone skin. This is for two reasons. First, cleansers identified as being good for those skin types generally contain ingredients that are too harsh or irritating, which is not helpful for any skin type. Cleansing must be gentle and thorough, not harsh and drying. Second, cleansers for blemish-prone skin often contain topical disinfectants such as benzoyl peroxide or the exfoliant (and mild antibacterial agent) salicylic acid, but in a cleanser, these effective ingredients are rinsed down the drain before they have a chance to affect your skin for the better.

BEST WATER SOLUBLE CLEANSERS FOR *ALL SKIN TYPES EXCEPT VERY DRY, UNDER $20, ALL SIZES: Dove Cool Moisture Facial Cleansing Cloths ($5.99 for 30 cloths), Cool Moisture Foaming Facial Cleanser ($5.99 for 6.76 ounces), and Daily Hydrating Cleansing Cloths ($6.99 for 30 cloths); **Eucerin** Gentle Hydrating Cleanser ($6.99 for 8 ounces); **Jan Marini** Bioglycolic Bioclean ($20 for 8 ounces); **M.A.C.** Wipes ($16 for 45 sheets); **Neutrogena** One Step Gentle Cleanser ($6.20 for 5.2 ounces); **Olay** Foaming Face Wash, for Sensitive Skin ($4.49 for 6.78 ounces) and Gentle Foaming Face Wash, for Sensitive Skin ($5.99 for 7 ounces).

**All of the cleansers on the list above were either recommended for all skin types or are equally suited for normal to oily or normal to dry skin.*

BEST WATER SOLUBLE CLEANSERS FOR *ALL SKIN TYPES EXCEPT VERY DRY, OVER $20, ALL SIZES: Dior Self-Foaming Cleanser ($28 for 5 ounces); **Lancome** Mousse Clarte, Self-Foaming Mousse Cleanser ($27 for 6.8 ounces); **Ultraceuticals** Gentle Cleansing Gel ($33 for 7 ounces).

**All of the cleansers on the list above were either recommended for all skin types or are equally suited for normal to oily or normal to dry skin.*

BEST WATER SOLUBLE CLEANSERS FOR NORMAL TO OILY/COMBINATION OR BLEMISH-PRONE SKIN, UNDER $20, ALL SIZES: Boots No7 Beautifully Balanced Purifying Cleanser, for Oily/Combination Skin ($7.99 for 6.6 ounces); **Clean & Clear** Foaming Facial Cleanser, Sensitive Skin ($4.39 for 8 ounces); **Clinique** Liquid Facial Soap Mild Formula ($14.50 for 6.7 ounces); **Dove** Sensitive Skin Foaming Facial Cleanser ($5.99 for 6.76 ounces); **Eucerin** Redness Relief Soothing Cleanser ($8.99 for 6.8 ounces); **Good Skin** Perfect Balance Gel Cleanser ($10.50 for 6.7 ounces); **Mary Kay** Deep Cleanser Formula 3 ($10 for 6.5 ounces); **M.D. Formulations** Facial Cleanser Foaming, Non-Glycolic ($18 for 8.3 ounces); **Neutrogena** Fresh Foaming Cleanser ($6.59 for 6.7 ounces); **Patricia Wexler M.D.** Dual Action Foaming Cleanser ($18 for 3.4 ounces); **Paula's Choice** One Step Face Cleanser, for Normal to Oily/Combination Skin ($14.95 for 8 ounces) and Skin Balancing Cleanser, for Normal to Oily/Combination Skin ($14.95 for 8 ounces); **pHisoDerm** Deep Cleaning Cleanser, for Normal to Oily Skin ($4.49 for 6 ounces) and pH_2O Daily Replenishing Wash ($6.29 for 6 ounces); **Physicians Formula** Deep Pore Cleansing Gel, for Normal to Oily Skin ($6.95 for 8 ounces); **RoC Canada** Enydrial Anti-Drying Cleansing Gel ($16 for 200 ml) and Foaming Facial Wash ($16 for 150 ml); **Sonia Kashuk** Cleanse Tri-Active Cleanser ($10.99 for 6 ounces).

BEST WATER SOLUBLE CLEANSERS FOR NORMAL TO OILY/COMBINATION OR BLEMISH-PRONE SKIN, OVER $20, ALL SIZES: Cellex-C Betaplex Gentle Foaming Cleanser ($29 for 6 ounces); **Laura Mercier** Oil-Free Gel Cleanser ($35 for 8 ounces).

BEST CLEANSERS FOR NORMAL TO DRY OR VERY DRY SKIN, UNDER $20, ALL SIZES: The Body Shop Aloe Gentle Facial Wash, for Sensitive Skin ($14 for 4.2 ounces); **Boots** No7 Soft & Soothed Gentle Cleanser, for Normal/Dry Skin ($7.99 for 6.6 ounces) and Time Dimensions Conditioning Cleansing Cream ($8.99 for 6.7 ounces); **Clinique** Liquid Facial Soap Extra Mild ($14.50 for 6.7 ounces); **Good Skin** All Calm Creamy Cleanser ($15 for 6.7 ounces) and Soft Skin Creamy Cleanser ($10.50 for 6.7 ounces); **L'Oreal Paris** Nutri-Pure Self Foaming Cleanser, for Normal to Dry Skin ($5.86 for 5 ounces); **M.D. Formulations** Facial Cleanser Basic, Non-Glycolic ($18 for 8.3 ounces); **Neutrogena** Extra Gentle Cleanser ($7.19 for 6.7 ounces); **Nu Skin** Nutricentials Creamy Cleansing Lotion, for Normal to Dry Skin ($14.92 for 5 ounces); **Olay** Daily Facials Skin Soothing Cleansing Cloths, for Sensitive Skin ($5.99 for 30 cloths); **Paula's Choice** One Step Face Cleanser, for Normal to Dry Skin ($14.95 for 8 ounces) and Skin Recovery Cleanser, for Normal to Very Dry Skin ($14.95 for 8 ounces); **pHisoDerm** Deep Cleaning Cleanser, for Sensitive Skin ($4.89 for 6 ounces); **Physicians Formula** Gentle Cleansing Lotion, for Normal to Dry Skin ($7.25 for 8 ounces); **Sonia Kashuk** Cleanse Tri-Active Cleanser ($10.99 for 6 ounces).

BEST CLEANSERS FOR NORMAL TO DRY OR VERY DRY SKIN, OVER $20, ALL SIZES: La Roche-Posay Toleriane Purifying Foaming Cream ($20 for 4.22 ounces); **Laura Mercier** Foaming One-Step Cleaner ($35 for 5 ounces) and One-Step Cleanser ($35 for 8 ounces); **M.D. Formulations** Facial Cleanser, Sensitive Skin Formula ($32 for 8.3 ounces); **Peter Thomas Roth** Gentle Cleansing Lotion, with Azulene for Sensitive, Dry, Mature or Normal Skin Types ($32 for 8 ounces).

BEST TONERS

There are far more similarities than differences among toners. Almost without exception, the majority of toners either are boring concoctions of water and glycerin or contain irritating ingredients such as alcohol, witch hazel, and menthol. The small selection of toners in the lists below are those with truly state-of-the-art formulations. The companies that make these products endeavored to create toners that go beyond just softening skin and/or removing the last traces of makeup. Recognizing that a well-formulated toner can be an integral part of one's skin-care routine, the options below supply skin with antioxidants, sophisticated water-binding agents, and/or cell-communicating ingredients—all essential elements for creating and maintaining healthy, radiant skin.

BEST TONERS FOR NORMAL TO OILY/COMBINATION SKIN, UNDER $20, ALL SIZES: Jane Iredale Pom Mist ($17.50 for 2 ounces, *recommended for all skin types*); **Nu Skin** NaPCA Moisture Mist ($10.74 for 8.4 ounces); **Paula's Choice** Healthy Skin Refreshing Toner, for Normal to Oily/Combination Skin ($14.95 for 6 ounces) and Skin Balancing Toner, for Normal to Oily/Combination Skin ($14.95 for 6 ounces).

BEST TONERS FOR NORMAL TO OILY/COMBINATION SKIN, OVER $20, ALL SIZES: M.D. Formulations Moisture Defense Antioxidant Spray ($28 for 8.3 ounces); **Prescriptives** Immediate Smooth Skin Conditioning Exfoliator ($19.50 for 3.4 ounces).

BEST TONERS FOR NORMAL TO VERY DRY SKIN, UNDER $20, ALL SIZES: Jane Iredale Pom Mist ($17.50 for 2 ounces, *recommended for all skin types*); **Nu Skin** NaPCA Moisture Mist ($10.74 for 8.4 ounces); **Paula's Choice** Moisture Boost Hydrating Toner, for Normal to Dry Skin ($14.95 for 6 ounces) and Skin Recovery Toner, for Normal to Very Dry Skin ($14.95 for 6 ounces).

BEST TONERS FOR NORMAL TO VERY DRY SKIN, OVER $20, ALL SIZES: Estee Lauder Re-Nutriv Intensive Softening Lotion ($40 for 8.4 ounces); **M.A.C.** Lightful Softening Lotion ($28 for 5 ounces); **Prescriptives** Immediate Smooth Skin Conditioning Exfoliator ($19.50 for 3.4 ounces).

BEST SCRUBS

Exfoliating the skin (i.e., getting rid of unwanted, dead, or built-up layers of sun-damaged skin cells and improving skin-cell turnover) is beneficial for almost all skin types, especially for those with sun-damaged skin or a tendency toward breakouts or clogged pores; however, even those with dry skin can benefit for many reasons. Despite the fact that most beauty experts, as well as dermatologists and plastic surgeons, agree that exfoliating the skin is a wonderful way to take care of both oily and dry skin, the method of exfoliating remains a point of contention. Today's assortment of scrubs is, almost without exception, far removed from the 1980s' versions that abraded skin with walnut shells, almond pits, and other harsh additives; irritation, dryness, and redness were typical problems for people who used such scrubs. In some respects, that irritation (or at least the potential for it) came back to the forefront in a number of scrubs claiming to be microdermabrasion-in-a-jar. Although these scrubs often contain the same aluminum oxide crystals that are used in professional microdermabrasion treatments, their use at home is not equivalent to a real microdermabrasion session. However, as it turns out, professionally administered microdermabrasion is not all that great either, at least not if your goal is to stave off wrinkles and encourage collagen production to a noticeable degree. I would encourage anyone considering microdermabrasion to keep their expectations low; greater benefits can be obtained from a series of Intense Pulsed Light (IPL) treatments in conjunction with an exfoliation routine done at home.

Although there are some very good scrubs available, I encourage you to consider using a well-formulated AHA or BHA product instead because the benefits of the latter products far outweigh those that you can get from a topical scrub, and they will provide greater visible results all around. I acknowledge that many people like to use scrubs, and that's why I chose the ones below. Those listed as best for normal to oily skin are typically gel-based and rinse completely; those listed as best for normal to dry skin provide an exfoliating benefit while also cushioning skin with emollients or other moisturizing ingredients. In addition, none of the scrubs below contain common irritants such as menthol, and most are fragrance-free.

Note: Fans of topical scrubs should consider instead just using a washcloth with their normal cleanser. I can almost guarantee you'll get equal results and with less potential for irritation (depending on how zealously you use a scrub); plus, you won't have to add another product to your skin-care routine.

Second Note: I no longer recommend mixing baking soda with your cleanser because of its alkaline pH and the potential issues that may have for skin. And again, using a washcloth with your regular cleanser will be just as effective.

BEST SCRUBS FOR NORMAL TO OILY/COMBINATION SKIN, UNDER $20, ALL SIZES: Good Skin Polished Skin Gentle Exfoliator ($14 for 3.4 ounces); **Neutrogena** Fresh Foaming Scrub ($5.69 for 4.2 ounces); **Olay** Definity Pore Redefining Scrub ($9.99 for 5 ounces).

BEST SCRUBS FOR NORMAL TO DRY SKIN, UNDER $20, ALL SIZES: Kiehl's Ultra Moisturizing Buffing Cream with Scrub Particles ($14.50 for 4 ounces); **Neutrogena** Pore Refining Cleanser ($7.49 for 6.7 ounces); **Paula's Choice** Silky Start Sugar Scrub for the Body, for All Skin Types ($10.95 for 4 ounces); **Wet 'n' Wild** Fresh Face Skincare Exfoliating Scrub ($4.99 for 6 ounces).

BEST SCRUBS FOR NORMAL TO OILY/COMBINATION OR NORMAL TO DRY SKIN, OVER $20, ALL SIZES: *There were no scrubs above $20 rated Paula's Pick because paying extra for a facial scrub doesn't make sense when there are plenty of less expensive options. Moreover, using a washcloth with your favorite cleanser is just as effective; the only reason to use a facial scrub is personal preference (and the pricey options are not better than what you'll find at the drugstore).*

BEST MAKEUP REMOVERS

Recently, I was asked to participate in a medical advisory group meeting attended by some of the most prominent dermatologists in the field. Among the fascinating topics discussed there was a brief discussion about makeup removal. I mentioned that a basic remedy for puffy, irritated, crepey skin around the eyes was to be sure to remove every last trace of eye makeup before you go to bed. One of the dermatologists echoed my concern, mentioning that when she looks at some of her patients' skin under a magnifying glass she is always surprised at how much makeup is crusted into the lines around their eyes. Not a pretty picture. That got me thinking about the need for makeup removers. In the past, I would have recommended using only a gentle, water-soluble cleanser for cleaning your face and removing makeup, and for some women who wear minimal makeup, that works great. But for those who apply foundation, concealer, eyeshadows, eyeliner, and mascara, a simple routine like that isn't going to do the trick, and a dedicated makeup remover needs to be part of your nightly routine. I still feel it is important to begin by washing your face with a gentle, water-soluble cleanser and removing as much makeup as you can that way. Gently massaging a cleanser over the face and eyes prevents tugging and pulling, which is far better for skin. Then, to make sure you remove the last traces of makeup use a gentle makeup remover and a soft pad of cotton, pulling and tugging as little as possible. A cotton swab soaked in makeup remover works great for taking off stubborn eyeliner or waterproof mascara at lash roots.

The makeup removers below are all fragrance-free and do not contain ingredients known to be irritating when used around the eyes. Whether you choose a detergent- or silicone-based product, all of the options below work quickly and efficiently with minimal effort.

BEST MAKEUP REMOVERS THAT USE GENTLE DETERGENT CLEANSING AGENTS FOR ALL SKIN TYPES, UNDER $15, ALL SIZES: Neutrogena Make-Up Remover Cleansing Towelettes ($7.99 for 25 towelettes); **Nivea** Visage Eye Make-Up Remover ($6.13 for 2.5 ounces).

BEST MAKEUP REMOVERS THAT USE GENTLE DETERGENT CLEANSING AGENTS FOR ALL SKIN TYPES, OVER $15, ALL SIZES: Dr. Brandt D-Face Makeup Remover ($35 for 4 ounces); **Peter Thomas Roth** Gentle Eye & Face Make-Up Remover ($22 for 4 ounces).

BEST MAKEUP REMOVERS THAT USE SILICONE FOR ALL SKIN TYPES, UNDER $15, ALL SIZES: Artistry Eye & Lip Makeup Remover ($13.95 for 4 ounces); **Mary Kay** Oil-Free Eye Makeup Remover ($14 for 3.75 ounces); **Paula's Choice** Gentle Touch Makeup Remover ($12.95 for 4 ounces); **Pond's** Bare & Repair, Conditioning Eye Make-Up Remover ($6.09 for 4 ounces); **Sonia Kashuk** Remove Eye Makeup Remover ($9.99 for 4 ounces).

BEST MAKEUP REMOVERS THAT USE SILICONE FOR ALL SKIN TYPES, OVER $15, ALL SIZES: Clinique Take the Day Off Makeup Remover for Lids, Lashes & Lips ($16.50 for 4.2 ounces); **Dior** Duo-Phase Eye Make-Up Remover ($25 for 4.2 ounces); **Elizabeth Arden** All Gone Eye and Lip Makeup Remover ($16 for 3.4 ounces); **Laura Mercier** Waterproof Eye Makeup Remover ($18 for 4 ounces); **Prescriptives** Better Off, Fast-Acting Waterproof Eye Makeup Remover ($18 for 4.2 ounces).

BEST LOTION-STYLE MAKEUP REMOVERS THAT WORK BEST FOR DRY TO VERY DRY SKIN, ALL PRICES, ALL SIZES: The Body Shop Camomile Waterproof Eye Make-Up Remover ($12.50 for 3.3 ounces); **Physicians Choice** Eye Makeup Remover

Lotion, for Normal to Dry Skin ($4.75 for 2 ounces). *Note: There are limited options in this category because so few lotion-style makeup removers do their job without leaving a greasy residue that ideally should be removed. Several lotion-style makeup removers received a happy face rating, and are worth considering in addition to those above if you prefer this type of product.*

BEST TOPICAL DISINFECTANTS

For someone who struggles with blemishes, a topical disinfectant is a fundamental way to effectively treat this condition. One of the primary causes of blemishes is the presence of a bacterium, and killing this bacterium can be of great help to many of those suffering with varying degrees of acne. Benzoyl peroxide is considered the most effective topical disinfectant for the treatment of blemishes. Generally, benzoyl peroxide products come in concentrations of 2.5%, 5%, and 10%, and as a general rule, it's best to start with a lower concentration to see if that works for you. If not, you can then try the next higher concentration. If you find that the higher concentrations don't work, then it may be time for you to consult a dermatologist or health care provider for a prescription topical disinfectant and/or for other topical acne treatments (e.g., Retin-A, Avita, Tazorac, or generic versions of these [active ingredient tretinoin, and, in the case of Tazorac, tazarotene]).

All of the following benzoyl peroxide products are Paula's Picks because they contain appropriate concentrations with no other irritating or harsh ingredients. Surprisingly, most of the benzoyl peroxide products available from drugstores contain the maximum amount (10%) of benzoyl peroxide. Although this can be effective, this high concentration also increases the chance of side effects, while likely not providing a significantly greater anti-acne benefit relative to that of the lower concentrations.

BEST TOPICAL DISINFECTANTS FOR BLEMISH-PRONE SKIN, UNDER $15, ALL SIZES: Clean & Clear Persa-Gel 10, Maximum Strength ($4.99 for 1 ounce); **Clearasil** Tinted Acne Treatment Cream ($5.99 for 1 ounce) and Vanishing Acne Treatment Cream ($5.99 for 1 ounce); **Clinique** Acne Solutions Emergency Gel Lotion ($13.50 for 0.5 ounce); **Mary Kay** Acne Treatment Gel ($7 for 1 ounce); **Oxy** Oxy Lotion, Vanishing Acne Medication ($5.69 for 1 ounce) and Oxy Spot Treatment ($5.49 for 0.65 ounces); **Stridex** Power Pads ($6.99 for 28 pads); **Zapzyt** 10% Benzoyl Peroxide Acne Treatment Gel ($5.29 for 1 ounce) and Repairing Night Gel (2 ounces, sold as part of Zapzyt's Acne Pack, $14.99).

BEST TOPICAL DISINFECTANTS FOR BLEMISH-PRONE SKIN, OVER $15, ALL SIZES: N.V. Perricone Outpatient Therapy Acne Treatment Gel Cream ($55 for 2 ounces); **Paula's Choice** Blemish Fighting Solution, for All Skin Types ($15.95 for 2.25 ounces) and Extra Strength Blemish Fighting Solution ($15.95 for 2.25 ounces); **Peter Thomas Roth** BPO Gel 5% ($24 for 3 ounces) and BPO Gel 10% ($26 for 3 ounces); **ProActiv Solution** Repairing Lotion ($21.75 for 2 ounces); **Rodan + Fields** Unblemish Step 3 Treat: Acne Medicated Lotion ($40 for 1.7 ounces).

BEST AHA & BHA PRODUCTS

Alpha hydroxy acids (AHA, such as glycolic acid and lactic acid) and beta hydroxy acid (BHA, which is salicylic acid) work by exfoliating the skin chemically instead of mechanically via abrasion. For many reasons, these can be less irritating and can create results that are more even and smoother than scrubs, which is why facial scrubs have become less and less a part of most daily skin-care routines (though they do have their proponents). There is also research showing that AHAs and BHA can improve skin thickness and cell turnover, increase collagen content, reduce skin discolorations, and improve pore function (i.e., by reducing the number of clogged pores and breakouts). Similar impressive research simply does not exist for scrubs.

If you decide to use an AHA or BHA product, particularly one from my list of recommendations, you may be wondering if you still need to use a mechanical scrub. The answer is not absolute, so you will have to judge that for yourself. Most people with normal to dry and/or sensitive skin should probably use only the AHA or BHA product and no other exfoliating process (except perhaps once in awhile). Someone with normal to oily or breakout-prone skin should use a good BHA product, but may also find benefit from using a mechanical scrub once a day or once every other day (but never use a scrub over acne lesions; acne cannot be scrubbed away).

The goal with chemical exfoliants is to use one effective AHA (between 5% and 10% concentration) or one BHA (1% to 2% concentration) product, and only as needed—which may be twice a day, once a day, or once every other day, depending on your skin type and its response. The AHA and BHA products recommended below not only have formulations with the appropriate concentrations but also have a pH between 3 and 4, which is critical if those ingredients are to be effective as exfoliants. Unlike in the sixth edition of this book, AHA and BHA products rated as Paula's Picks not only meet the basic formulary requirements that allow exfoliation to occur, but also do so without added fragrance or needlessly irritating ingredients. In addition, all of the AHA and BHA options below contain beneficial ingredients such as water-binding agents, antioxidants, and/or anti-irritants. You will find AHA (but no BHA) products reviewed throughout this book with a happy face rating (although not necessarily a Paula's Pick), and these are options if your goal is exfoliation. However, the choices below are preferred.

AHAs are best for those with normal to dry skin, and BHA is best for those with normal to oily or blemish-prone skin. This is because AHAs cannot penetrate oil and, therefore, cannot get into the pore lining. BHA can penetrate oil and, therefore, can get into the pore where it can improve and repair pore function while dissolving blockages of dead skin cells and oil that contribute to blackheads and acne. Whichever you choose, always monitor your skin's response, and remember, irritation is never the goal.

BEST ALPHA HYDROXY ACID PRODUCTS FOR NORMAL TO OILY/COMBINATION SKIN, UNDER $20, ALL SIZES, ALL STRENGTHS: Neutrogena Pore Refining Cream SPF 15 ($14.99 for 1 ounce); **Paula's Choice** 8% Alpha Hydroxy Acid Gel, for All Skin Types ($17.95 for 4 ounces).

BEST ALPHA HYDROXY ACID PRODUCTS FOR NORMAL TO OILY/COMBINATION SKIN, OVER $20, ALL SIZES, ALL STRENGTHS: M.D. Formulations Vit-A-Plus Night Recovery ($50 for 1 ounce, *contains AHA and BHA*); **Murad** Night Reform Treatment ($65 for 1 ounce); **Peter Thomas Roth** AHA 12% Ceramide Hydrating Repair Gel ($48 for 2 ounces) and Glycolic Acid 10% Hydrating Gel ($48 for 2 ounces).

BEST ALPHA HYDROXY ACID PRODUCTS FOR NORMAL TO DRY SKIN, UNDER $20, ALL SIZES, ALL STRENGTHS: Neutrogena Healthy Skin Face Lotion, Night ($12.59 for 2.5 ounces); **Paula's Choice** 8% Alpha Hydroxy Acid Gel, for All Skin Types ($17.95 for 4 ounces) and Skin Revealing Body Lotion with 10% Alpha Hydroxy Acid, for All Skin Types ($19.95 for 8 ounces).

BEST ALPHA HYDROXY ACID PRODUCTS FOR NORMAL TO DRY SKIN, OVER $20, ALL SIZES, ALL STRENGTHS: Jan Marini Bioglycolic Facial Lotion SPF 15 ($36 for 2 ounces); **M.D. Formulations** Moisture Defense Antioxidant Lotion ($50 for 1 ounce) and Vit-A-Plus Illuminating Serum ($65 for 1 ounce); **Neostrata** Exuviance Professional Rejuvenating Complex ($42 for 1 ounce), Bionic Eye Cream, PHA 4 ($50 for 0.5 ounce), Daytime Protection Cream SPF 15, PHA 10 ($33 for 1.75 ounces), and Renewal Cream, PHA 12 ($43 for 1.05 ounces); **Peter Thomas Roth** AHA 12% Ceramide Hydrating Repair Gel ($48 for 2 ounces), Glycolic Acid 10% Hydrating Gel ($48 for 2 ounces), and Glycolic Acid 10% Moisturizer ($45 for 2 ounces); **Ultraceuticals** Ultra Ace Hydration Booster ($50 for 2.5 ounces).

BEST BETA HYDROXY ACID PRODUCTS FOR NORMAL TO OILY/COMBINATION SKIN, UNDER $20, ALL SIZES, ALL STRENGTHS: Clearasil Daily Blackhead Control Pads with Natural Sea Salt ($7.99 for 80 pads); **Neutrogena** Oil-Free Acne Stress Control 3-in-1 Hydrating Acne Treatment ($7.99 for 2 ounces); **Paula's Choice** 1% Beta Hydroxy Acid Gel, for All Skin Types ($17.95 for 4 ounces), 1% Beta Hydroxy Acid Lotion, for All Skin Types ($17.95 for 4 ounces), 2% Beta Hydroxy Acid Gel, for All Skin Types ($17.95 for 4 ounces), 2% Beta Hydroxy Acid Liquid, for All Skin Types ($17.95 for 4 ounces), and Weightless Body Treatment with 2% Beta Hydroxy Acid, for All Skin Types ($19.95 for 8 ounces).

BEST BETA HYDROXY ACID PRODUCTS FOR NORMAL TO OILY/COMBINATION SKIN, OVER $20, ALL SIZES, ALL STRENGTHS: bare escentuals bareVitamins Skin Rev-er Upper ($21 for 2.3 ounces); **Jan Marini** Factor-A Plus Mask ($60 for 2 ounces); **M.D. Formulations** Vit-A-Plus Night Recovery ($50 for 1 ounce, *contains AHA and BHA*).

BEST BETA HYDROXY ACID PRODUCTS FOR NORMAL TO DRY SKIN, UNDER $20, ALL SIZES, ALL STRENGTHS: Paula's Choice 2% Beta Hydroxy Acid Lotion, for All Skin Types ($17.95 for 4 ounces) and Weightless Body Treatment with 2% Beta Hydroxy Acid, for All Skin Types ($19.95 for 8 ounces).

BEST BETA HYDROXY ACID PRODUCT FOR NORMAL TO DRY SKIN, OVER $20, ALL SIZES, ALL STRENGTHS: ProActiv Solution Clarifying Night Cream ($28.75 for 1 ounce).

BEST MOISTURIZERS (INCLUDING EYE CREAMS)

I have written extensively about (and mention throughout this book) ingredients that have substantiated research proving they are necessary (if not integral) to creating a truly state-of-the-art moisturizer. Regardless of your skin type (more on that below) or texture preference, all of the moisturizers listed below meet that goal of substantiated research brilliantly. What remains offensive, however, is that most of the moisturizer formulations don't warrant their outlandish claims, ridiculous prices, or your belief that you've finally found the fountain of youth. None of the options below will "eliminate wrinkles," "lift sagging skin," "restore youthful contours," or "make you look years younger." What each will do, to some degree, is restore a healthy barrier (essential for allowing skin to repair itself and generate new collagen), reduce inflammation, help prevent (although not completely eliminate) free-radical damage, restore vital elements needed to maintain healthy skin, and create a feeling of smoothness and softness that most will find aesthetically pleasing.

Moisturizers for oily skin are difficult to evaluate. As a rule, if oily skin is not being irritated or assaulted with harsh skin-care products, it does not need a moisturizer. Lotions and creams in general can be problematic for oily skin; even gels and serum-type moisturizers can feel heavy on oily skin. For this reason, I rate moisturizers, regardless of their designation as gels, lotions, antiwrinkle, anti-aging, or otherwise, on the basis of their value for normal to dry or dry to slightly dry or slightly oily skin. As a result, there is no group of moisturizers for oily skin. Even when a product is labeled as being for someone with oily or combination skin, it is meant to be used only over dry areas, not over oily areas.

If you are not using harsh or irritating skin-care products and are not undergoing potentially irritating procedures such as microdermabrasion or facial peels, but still have dry, red patches of skin in areas that are oily, it can be indicative of a skin disorder such as rosacea, dermatitis, psoriasis, or seborrhea. That does not require a moisturizer, but rather a change in how you are taking care of your skin or an appointment with a dermatologist for a medical diagnosis. If you have oily skin but also have dry areas (and you are certain you have no skin disorders, you are not using irritating skin-care products, and you are not subjecting yourself to irritating non-invasive procedures), consider using the moisturizers in the slightly dry or dry skin group below, but use them only over dry areas, not all over.

Because many of you have written me asking about moisturizers with retinol, and because this vitamin A ingredient has more than proven its worth for all skin types, I have also included lists of the best moisturizers with efficacious amounts of retinol. All of these products are packaged to ensure that the retinol remains stable during use, which is absolutely essential for this light- and air-sensitive ingredient.

Packaging is a big deal for state-of-the-art moisturizers, and I'm not talking about visual appeal (though this entices many a consumer and fashion magazine editor). Rather, I am referring to the need for opaque, non-jar packaging that demonstrates the manufacturer has made efforts to ensure the continuing potency of the bells and whistles, particularly antioxidants, after you start using the product. Almost without exception, antioxidants are prone to degradation when repeatedly exposed to light and air (the manner in which they work to protect our skin bears this out). It is thus very disappointing to report that hundreds of the moisturizers reviewed in this book did not make the lists below and were not rated a Paula's Pick solely because of clear or jar packaging. The Lauder companies are the biggest offenders in this regard. Although their packaging for moisturizers has improved in some respects, they still package the majority of their outstanding moisturizer formulations in jars. Also, using a product that repeatedly requires you to dip your fingers into a jar isn't the most hygienic way to take care of your skin.

Please refer to each moisturizer's individual review for an assessment of claims and information on formulary specifics, such as whether or not it is fragrance-free (many on the lists below are) and, in some cases, comparisons with less expensive options.

BEST LIGHTWEIGHT MOISTURIZERS FOR NORMAL TO SLIGHTLY DRY, OILY, OR COMBINATION SKIN, UNDER $30, ALL SIZES: Aveda Tourmaline Charged Eye Creme ($30 for 0.5 ounce); **Good Skin** All Firm Rebuilding Serum ($25 for 1 ounce); **Olay** Regenerist Perfecting Cream ($18.99 for 1.7 ounces); **Paula's Choice** HydraLight Moisture-Infusing Lotion, for Normal to Oily/Combination Skin ($18.95 for 2 ounces), Skin Balancing Moisture Gel, for Normal to Oily/Combination Skin ($16.95 for 2 ounces), and Silk Mist Moisturizing Body Spray, for All Skin Types ($14.95 for 4 ounces); **Peter Thomas Roth** Moisturizing Multi-Tasking After Shave Balm ($24 for 3.4 ounces).

BEST LIGHTWEIGHT MOISTURIZERS FOR NORMAL TO SLIGHTLY DRY, OILY, OR COMBINATION SKIN, OVER $30, ALL SIZES: Clinique Repairwear Intensive Night Lotion ($47.50 for 1.7 ounces), Turnaround Concentrate Visible Skin Renewer ($36.50 for 1 ounce), Continuous Rescue Antioxidant Moisturizer Combination/Oily to Oily ($39.50 for 1.7 ounces), Moisture In-Control Oil-Free Lotion ($35 for 1.7 ounces), and Moisture Surge Extra Refreshing Eye Gel ($26 for 0.5 ounce); **Cosmedicine** Opti-mologist Eye Cream with Light Diffusers ($45 for 0.5 ounce) and Opti-mologist PM Intensive Eye Cream ($48 for 0.5 ounce); **DDF** Nourishing Eye Cream ($45 for 0.5 ounce); **Dr. Denese New York** Pro-Peptide Makeup Primer ($39 for 1 ounce); **Estee Lauder** Hydra Complete Multi-Level Moisture Lotion, for Normal/Combination Skin ($40 for 1.7 ounces), Idealist Refinishing Eye Serum ($48 for 0.5 ounce), and Fruition Extra Multi-Action Complex ($46.50 for 1 ounce); **Glymed Plus** Living Cell Clarifier ($38.50 for 2 ounces); **M.D. Formulations** Moisture Defense Antioxidant Hydrating Gel ($45 for 1 ounce) and Critical Care Calming Gel ($39 for 1 ounce); **MD Skincare by Dr. Dennis Gross** Continuous Eye Hydration ($42 for 0.5 ounce) and Hydra-Pure Oil-Free Moisture ($75 for 1 ounce); **N.V. Perricone** Vitamin C Ester Eye Therapy ($50 for 0.5 ounce) and Advanced Eye Area Therapy ($95 for 0.5 ounce); **Peter Thomas Roth** Environmental Repair Hydrating Gel ($40 for 2 ounces); **Prescriptives** Intensive Rebuilding Lotion ($80 for 1.7 ounces); **SkinCeuticals** Eye Cream Firming Treatment ($55 for 0.67 ounce); **Ultraceuticals** Ultra Hydrating Gel ($59 for 1.69 ounces).

BEST MOISTURIZERS FOR NORMAL TO DRY SKIN, UNDER $30, ALL SIZES: Artistry Delicate Care Calming Moisturizer ($28.65 for 2.5 ounces); **Good Skin** All Bright Moisture Cream ($23.50 for 1.7 ounces); **M.A.C.** Strobe Cream ($29.50 for 1.7 ounces); **Olay** Total Effects 7-in-1 Anti-Aging Moisturizer, Mature Skin Therapy ($17.49 for 1.7 ounces); **Paula's Choice** Hydrating Treatment Cream, for Normal to Dry Skin ($16.95 for 2 ounces) and Slip Into Silk Body Lotion, for All Skin Types ($15.95 for 8 ounces).

BEST MOISTURIZERS FOR NORMAL TO DRY SKIN, OVER $30, ALL SIZES: Clinique Continuous Rescue Antioxidant Moisturizer Dry/Combination ($39.50 for 1.7 ounces); **Cosmedicine** MegaDose PM Skin Fortifying Serum ($85 for 1 ounce) and MegaDose Skin Fortifying Serum ($80 for 1 ounce); **Dr. Denese New York** Triple Strength Wrinkle Smoother ($54 for 2 ounces); **Kinerase** Pro+ Therapy Ultra Rich Eye Repair ($85 for 0.5 ounce); **MD Skincare by Dr. Dennis Gross** Hydra-Pure Antioxidant Firming Serum ($95 for 1 ounce); **Nu Skin** Tru Face IdealEyes Eye Refining Cream ($42.75 for 0.5 ounce); **N.V. Perricone** Alpha Lipoic Acid Eye Area Therapy ($50 for 0.5 ounce); **Sense by Usana** Eye Nourisher ($30 for 0.4 ounce).

BEST MOISTURIZERS FOR DRY TO VERY DRY SKIN, UNDER $30, ALL SIZES: Osmotics TriCeram ($30 for 3.4 ounces); **Paula's Choice** Skin Recovery Moisturizer, for Normal to Very Dry Skin ($16.95 for 2 ounces) and Beautiful Body Butter, for Dry to Extra Dry Skin ($14.95 for 4 ounces).

BEST MOISTURIZERS FOR DRY TO VERY DRY SKIN, OVER $30, ALL SIZES: Babor HSR Lifting Decollete Cream ($84 for 1 ounce); **Clinique** CX Rapid Recovery Cream ($75 for 1.7 ounces) and Continuous Rescue Antioxidant Moisturizer Very Dry to Dry ($39.50 for 1.7 ounces); **Estee Lauder** Verite Special EyeCare ($37.50 for 0.5 ounce); **Glymed Plus** Cell Science Eye Calm ($36 for 0.3 ounce); **Sense by Usana** Night Renewal

($41 for 1.3 ounces) and Perfecting Essence ($58 for 1 ounce); **Shiseido** Bio-Performance Super Eye Contour Cream ($52 for 0.53 ounce).

BEST MOISTURIZERS CONTAINING RETINOL, UNDER $30, ALL SIZES: Alpha Hydrox Retinol Night ResQ ($14.99 for 1.05 ounces); **Neutrogena** Healthy Skin Anti-Wrinkle Cream, Original Formula ($11.99 for 1.4 ounces), Healthy Skin Anti-Wrinkle Intensive Eye Cream ($17.69 for 0.5 ounce), Healthy Skin Anti-Wrinkle Intensive Night Cream ($17.39 for 1.4 ounces), Pore Refining Cream SPF 15 ($14.99 for 1 ounce), and Healthy Skin Enhancer SPF 20 ($10.99).

BEST MOISTURIZERS CONTAINING RETINOL, OVER $30, ALL SIZES: DDF Retinol Energizing Moisturizer ($85 for 1.7 ounces); **Estee Lauder** Diminish Anti-Wrinkle Retinol Treatment ($80 for 1.7 ounces); **Lancome** Re-Surface Eye, Retinol Concentrate Wrinkle Corrector for Eyes ($47 for 0.5 ounce); **M.D. Formulations** Vit-A-Plus Illuminating Serum ($65 for 1 ounce); **Prescriptives** Skin Renewal Cream ($60 for 1 ounce); **RoC Canada** Retin-OL Correxion Intensive Nourishing Anti-Wrinkle Care, for Dry Skin ($44 for 30 ml), Retin-OL Multi-Correxion Multi-Corrective Anti-Ageing Moisturiser, Day/Night ($42 for 30 ml), Retin-OL Multi-Correxion Multi-Corrective Eye Cream ($32 for 15 ml), and Retin-OL Vitamins A+C+E Triple Action, Day/Night ($39 for 30 ml); **Ultraceuticals** Ultra Ace Hydration Booster ($50 for 2.5 ounces).

BEST SERUMS

At one point, I would have lumped serums into the same category as moisturizers because, for the most part, that is what many of them are—moisturizers—albeit with a thinner consistency than traditional creams and lotions. However, as I was reviewing serums for this book, I couldn't help but notice the great strides many of them have made in terms of the bevy of sophisticated ingredients they contain. Most of these ingredients have substantiated research proving their benefit for skin of all ages. And many serums have a texture that is suitable for oily or breakout-prone skin. As such, serums can be a brilliant way for those with this skin type and/or condition to obtain the benefits of antioxidants and cell-communicating ingredients, including retinol (serums containing an impressive amount of retinol in stable packaging are listed separately).

You will notice that the longer list of serums is on the expensive side. I wish this weren't the case, but it is. There are two reasons. One is that most cosmetics companies position serums as specialty or targeted products, almost always with an anti-aging angle. Therefore, as the perceived (or the claimed) benefits increase, so does the price. Second, and the more real-world reason for the high prices, is that it is expensive to create serums (most are non-aqueous, and water is the least expensive yet most pervasive skin-care ingredient around) that contain the level and range of state-of-the-art ingredients noted in the products below. The cost of several of the ingredients in these serums is, on a pound-for-pound basis, staggering when compared to the cost of ubiquitous ingredients such as triglycerides, glycerin, or mineral oil. Although most of the best serums are costly, at least you know you're getting an intelligently formulated product whose ingredients have a proven track record of improving skin's health and appearance. Just as with the moisturizers listed above, please refer to each serum's individual review for an assessment of the claims and information on formulary specifics, such as whether or not it is fragrance-free (many on the lists below are) and, in some cases, comparisons with less expensive options.

Note: The ultra-light and mattifying serums recommended for oily to very oily skin were included primarily due to their absorbent matte finish and weightless texture. Please refer to each product's individual review to see how they compare in terms of antioxidant content and other extras. All such serums work well under foundations that have a matte or powdery finish.

BEST SERUMS FOR ALL SKIN TYPES EXCEPT VERY OILY SKIN, UNDER $30, ALL SIZES: Patricia Wexler M.D. Advanced No-Injection Wrinkle Smoother ($29.50 for 0.5 ounce); **Paula's Choice** Skin Recovery Super Antioxidant Concentrate, for Normal to Very Dry Skin ($22.95 for 1 ounce) and Super Antioxidant Concentrate, for All Skin Types ($22.95 for 1 ounce); **Sonia Kashuk** Repair Vitamin Enriched Serum ($18.99 for 0.5 ounce).

BEST SERUMS FOR ALL SKIN TYPES EXCEPT VERY OILY SKIN, OVER $30, ALL SIZES: Artistry Time Defiance Derma Erase ($45.55 for 0.14 ounce) and Skin Refinishing Lotion ($48.85 for 1 ounce); **Bobbi Brown** Intensive Skin Supplement ($55 for 1 ounce); **Chanel** Age Delay Rejuvenation Serum ($68.50 for 1 ounce); **Clinique** CX Antioxidant Rescue Serum ($125 for 1 ounce), Repairwear Deep Wrinkle Concentrate for Face and Eye ($55 for 1.4 ounces), and Advanced Stop Signs ($38.50 for 1.7 ounces); **DDF** C3 Plus Serum ($62 for 0.5 ounce) and Mesojection Healthy Cell Serum ($80 for 1 ounce); **Elizabeth Arden** Ceramide Advanced Time Complex Capsules Intensive Treatment for Face and Throat ($65 for 60 capsules; 0.95 ounce), Ceramide Gold Ultra Restorative Capsules ($68 for 60 capsules; 0.95 ounce), and Prevage Eye Anti-Aging Moisturizing Treatment ($95 for 0.5 ounce); **Estee Lauder** Advanced Night Repair Concentrate Recovery Boosting Treatment ($85 for 1 ounce), Perfectionist [CP+] with Poly-Collagen Peptides Correcting Serum for Line/Wrinkles/Age Spots ($55 for 1 ounce), and Re-Nutriv Ultimate Lifting Serum ($200 for 1.7 ounces); **Good Skin** Tri-Aktiline Instant Deep Wrinkle Filler ($39.50 for 1 ounce); **La Mer** The Lifting Face Serum ($210 for 1 ounce); **Mary Kay** TimeWise Even Complexion Essence ($35 for 1 ounce) and TimeWise Targeted-Action Line Reducer ($40 for 0.13 ounce); **MD Skincare by Dr. Dennis Gross** Hydra-Pure Redness Soothing Serum ($85 for 1 ounce) and Hydra-Pure Vitamin C Serum ($90 for 1 ounce); **Nu Skin** 180° Night Complex ($64.60 for 1 ounce), Clear Action Acne Medication Night Treatment ($36.58 for 1 ounce), and Celltrex CoQ10 Complete ($47.50 for 0.5 ounce); **Prescriptives** Super Line Preventor Xtreme ($47.50 for 1 ounce) and Redness Relief Gel ($50 for 1 ounce); **Z. Bigatti** Re-Storation Deep Repair Facial Serum ($198 for 1 ounce).

BEST ULTRA-LIGHT OR MATTIFYING SERUMS FOR VERY OILY SKIN, UNDER $30, ALL SIZES: Clinique Pore Minimizer Instant Perfector ($16.50 for 0.5 ounce); **Olay** Regenerist Daily Regenerating Serum ($18.99 for 1.7 ounces), Regenerist Daily Regenerating Serum, Fragrance-Free ($18.99 for 1.7 ounces), Regenerist Eye Lifting Serum ($18.99 for 0.5 ounce); **Paula's Choice** Skin Balancing Super Antioxidant Mattifying Concentrate, for Normal to Very Oily Skin ($22.95 for 1 ounce); **Smashbox** Anti-Shine ($27).

BEST ULTRA-LIGHT OR MATTIFYING SERUM FOR VERY OILY SKIN, OVER $30, ALL SIZES: La Roche-Posay Biomedic C-Recovery Treatment ($50 for 1 ounce).

BEST SERUMS WITH RETINOL FOR ALL SKIN TYPES, UNDER $30, ALL SIZES: Paula's Choice Skin Balancing Super Antioxidant Mattifying Concentrate, for Normal to Very Oily Skin ($22.95 for 1 ounce) and Skin Recovery Super Antioxidant Concentrate, for Normal to Very Dry Skin ($22.95 for 1 ounce); **philosophy** eye believe, deep wrinkle peptide gel ($30 for 0.5 ounce).

BEST SERUMS WITH RETINOL FOR ALL SKIN TYPES, OVER $30, ALL SIZES: DDF Silky C Serum ($72 for 1 ounce); **Dr. Denese New York** HydroShield Eye Serum ($44 for 0.5 ounce), HydroShield Ultra Moisturizing Face Serum ($49 for 0.5 ounce), Neck Saver Serum ($34 for 1 ounce), and HydroSeal Hand & Decollete Serum ($35 for 3 ounces); **Estee Lauder** Re-Nutriv Intensive Lifting Serum ($175 for 1 ounce); **Jan Marini** Factor-A Eyes for Dark Circles ($60 for 60 capsules); **M.D. Formulations** Vit-A-Plus Illumination Spot Treatment, for All Skin Types ($38 for 0.11 ounce); **SkinCeuticals** Retinol 0.5 Refining Night Cream with 0.5% Pure Retinol ($42 for 1 ounce) and Retinol 1.0 Maximum Strength Refining Night Cream with 1.0% Pure Retinol ($48 for 1 ounce).

BEST SUNSCREENS AND DAYTIME MOISTURIZERS WITH SUNSCREEN (SPF 15 OR GREATER, INCLUDING EYE CREAMS)

Many, if not most, of the changes that take place on our skin over the years, such as wrinkles, skin discolorations, loss of elasticity, texture problems, and dryness, are the result of sun damage from exposure to the sun without appropriate or adequate sun protection. Sunscreens are essential for skin care day in and day out, 365 days a year. If applied correctly (meaning liberally and reapplied as often as needed), *they are the only true antiwrinkle product.* They can also potentially help prevent some forms of skin cancer and are an absolute must if you have already been treated for any type of skin cancer (or have a family history of it). If you are not using a sunscreen of some kind (lotion, cream, gel, serum, or foundation with sunscreen) with SPF 15 or greater and that contains the UVA-protecting ingredients of avobenzone, zinc oxide, titanium dioxide, Mexoryl SX, or, outside the United States, Tinosorb, then you are doing nothing of value for the long-term health of your skin. Really, all of the antiwrinkle, firming, anti-aging, or rejuvenating products in the world are completely and totally useless if you are not protecting your skin from the sun every day. It is of vital importance to the health of your skin to include a well-formulated sunscreen in your daily skin-care routine. Arguably, the most unethical thing the cosmetics industry does is sell women a plethora of antiwrinkle products that more often than not do not include reliable sun protection.

As you look over the lists in this category, you will notice that there are nearly equal numbers of sunscreens for normal to dry skin as for normal to oily skin. I am pleased that in the last few years many cosmetics chemists have created lightweight sunscreens whose texture and typically smooth matte finish are just what someone struggling with oily skin or oily areas needs. Still, for the face, someone with oily skin may prefer to use a foundation with sunscreen rated SPF 15 or greater, and apply a well-formulated sunscreen from the neck down. This is one area of skin care that is becoming less difficult for someone with oily skin, but it still takes experimentation to figure out what product with sunscreen works best for you. Those dealing with breakout-prone skin should consider sunscreens from the list of options for normal to slightly dry or oily/combination skin. Keep in mind that despite non-comedogenic or non-acnegenic claims made on labels, no sunscreen is guaranteed to be problem-free for someone struggling with acne.

All of the following sunscreens were rated Paula's Picks for two important reasons. One, each has an SPF 15 or greater and includes avobenzone, titanium dioxide, zinc oxide, Mexoryl

SX, or Tinosorb (the latter approved for use outside the United States) as one or more of the **active ingredients** (if these are listed someplace else on the ingredient list, it does not count toward reliable sun protection). Avobenzone may be listed on an ingredient label by its chemical name, butyl methoxydibenzoylmethane, and Mexoryl SX may be listed as ecamsule. Two, every sunscreen on the lists below contains a range of antioxidants and also includes other skin-beneficial ingredients such as those that mimic healthy skin's structural components. Antioxidants are proving to be an incredibly helpful addition to sunscreens because they not only boost the efficacy of the active ingredients, but also help offset free-radical damage from sun exposure. Selecting a daytime moisturizer with sunscreen or "regular" sunscreen without antioxidants isn't giving your skin as much of a fighting chance against the cascade of damage that sun exposure can cause (and that can be severely minimized with diligent, liberal application and, when needed, reapplication, of sunscreen rated SPF 15 or greater).

BEST SUNSCREENS AND DAYTIME MOISTURIZERS WITH SUNSCREEN FOR NORMAL TO SLIGHTLY DRY OR OILY/COMBINATION SKIN, UNDER $30, ALL SIZES: Almay Daily Moisturizer for Normal/Combo Skin with Grape Seed SPF 15 ($11.99 for 4 ounces); **Aveeno** Skin Brightening Daily Treatment SPF 15 ($19 for 1 ounce); **Avon** Anew Advanced All-in-One Max SPF 15 Lotion ($16.50 for 1.7 ounces), Anew Retroactive+ Day Defense SPF 15 ($25 for 1.7 ounces), Ageless Results Renewing Day Cream SPF 15 ($14.50 for 1.7 ounces), and Hydra-Radiance Moisturizing Day Lotion SPF 15 ($12 for 4 ounces); **Clinique** Sun-Care UV-Response Face SPF 30 ($17.50 for 1.7 ounces) and Sun-Care UV-Response Face Cream SPF 50 ($15.50 for 1.7 ounces); **Coppertone** Ultra Sheer Faces Sunscreen Lotion SPF 30 ($9.69 for 3 ounces); **DDF** Moisturizing Photo-Age Protection SPF 30 ($28 for 4 ounces); **Dove** Energy Glow Brightening Moisturizer SPF 15 ($10.99 for 1.7 ounces) and Essential Nutrients Day Lotion ($6.59 for 4.05 ounces); **Good Skin** All Right Oil-Free Sunscreen SPF 30 ($12 for 1.7 ounces) and Clean Skin Oil-Free Lotion SPF 15 ($15 for 1.7 ounces); **M.A.C.** Studio Moisture Fix SPF 15 ($28 for 1.7 ounces); **Mary Kay** SPF 30 Sunscreen ($14 for 4 ounces); **Neutrogena** Healthy Skin Visibly Even Daily SPF 15 Moisturizer ($13.09 for 1.7 ounces), Healthy Defense SPF 30 Daily Eye Cream, Light Tint ($11.99 for 0.5 ounce), Pore Refining Cream SPF 15 ($14.99 for 1 ounce), Active Breathable Sunblock SPF 30 ($9.99 for 4 ounces), Active Breathable Sunblock SPF 45 ($9.99 for 4 ounces), Age Shield Sunblock SPF 30 ($9.99 for 4 ounces), Age Shield Sunblock SPF 45 ($9.99 for 4 ounces), Ultra Sheer Dry-Touch Sunblock SPF 30 ($9.99 for 3 ounces), Ultra Sheer Dry-Touch Sunblock SPF 45 ($9.99 for 3 ounces), and UVA/UVB Sunblock Lotion SPF 45 ($8.99 for 4 ounces); **Olay** Regenerist Enhancing Lotion with UV Protection SPF 15 ($18.99 for 2.5 ounces) and Regenerist UV Defense Regenerating Lotion SPF 15 ($18.99 for 2.5 ounces); **Paula's Choice** Skin Balancing Daily Mattifying Lotion SPF 15, for Normal to Oily/Combination Skin ($18.95 for 2 ounces), Essential Non-Greasy Sunscreen SPF 15, for Normal to Oily/Combination Skin ($12.95 for 6 ounces), and Ultra-Light Weightless Finish SPF 30 Sunscreen Spray, for All Skin Types ($15.95 for 4 ounces); **philosophy** a pigment of your imagination SPF 18 ($30 for 2 ounces); **Pond's** Mend & Defend, Intensive Protection SPF 15 Moisturizer ($9.39 for 3.3 ounces).

BEST SUNSCREENS AND DAYTIME MOISTURIZERS WITH SUNSCREEN FOR NORMAL TO SLIGHTLY DRY OR OILY/COMBINATION SKIN, OVER $30, ALL SIZES: Clinique Repairwear Day SPF 15 Intensive Lotion ($47.50 for 1.7 ounces); **DDF** Daily Protective Moisturizer SPF 15 ($36 for 1.7 ounces); **Estee Lauder** DayWear Plus Multi

Protection Anti-Oxidant Lotion SPF 15, for Oily Skin ($38 for 1.7 ounces), Future Perfect Anti-Wrinkle Radiance Lotion SPF 15, for Normal/Combination Skin ($65 for 1.7 ounces), and Re-Nutriv Intensive Protective Base SPF 30 ($65 for 1.7 ounces); **MD Skincare by Dr. Dennis Gross** Powerful Sun Protection SPF 30 Sunscreen Lotion ($42 for 5 ounces) and Powerful Sun Protection SPF 30 Sunscreen Packettes ($42 for 60 packettes); **Peter Thomas Roth** Oil-Free Sunblock SPF 30 ($26 for 4 ounces), Ultra-Lite Oil-Free Sunblock SPF 20 ($26 for 4 ounces), and Ultra-Lite Oil-Free Sunblock SPF 30 ($26 for 4 ounces); **Prescriptives** All You Need+ Broad Spectrum Oil Absorbing Lotion SPF 15 ($40 for 1.7 ounces).

BEST SUNSCREENS AND DAYTIME MOISTURIZERS WITH SUNSCREEN FOR NORMAL TO DRY OR VERY DRY SKIN, UNDER $30, ALL SIZES: Almay Sun Protector for Body SPF 30 ($8.99 for 4.2 ounces) and Sun Protector for Face SPF 30 ($8.99 for 4.2 ounces); **Artistry** Moisture Rich Protective Moisturizer SPF 15 ($28.65 for 2.5 ounces); **Estee Lauder** Multi-Protection Sun Lotion for Face SPF 30 ($22 for 1.7 ounces); **Good Skin** All Bright Moisturizing Sunscreen SPF 30 ($12 for 1.7 ounces) and All Bright Hand Cream SPF 15 ($16 for 1.7 ounces); **Kiss My Face** Face Factor Face + Neck SPF 30 ($10 for 2 ounces); **Mary Kay** TimeWise Day Solution Sunscreen SPF 25 ($30 for 1 ounce); **Nu Skin** Sunright Body Block SPF 30 ($13.97 for 3.4 ounces) and Sunright Body Block SPF 15 ($13.97 for 3.4 ounces); **Paula's Choice** Skin Recovery Daily Moisturizing Lotion with SPF 15, Normal to Dry Skin ($18.95 for 2 ounces) and Extra Care Moisturizing Sunscreen SPF 30+, for Normal to Dry Skin ($12.95 for 6 ounces); **Pond's** Radiance Restore, Age-Defying Skin-Brightening SPF 15 Moisturizer ($12.99 for 1.7 ounces); **Rodan + Fields** Soothe Step 3 Protect: UVA/UVB Sunscreen SPF 15 ($30 for 1.7 ounces); **Stila** Petal Infusions Skin Visor SPF 30 ($24 for 2.5 ounces).

BEST SUNSCREENS AND DAYTIME MOISTURIZERS WITH SUNSCREEN FOR NORMAL TO DRY OR VERY DRY SKIN, OVER $30, ALL SIZES: Cellex-C Sunshade SPF 30+ ($45 for 2 ounces); **Cosmedicine** Primary Care Multi-Tasking Moisturizer SPF 20 ($48 for 1.35 ounces); **Elizabeth Arden** Extreme Conditioning Cream SPF 15 ($36 for 1.7 ounces); **Estee Lauder** Re-Nutriv Intensive Lifting Hand Creme SPF 15 ($45 for 3.4 ounces) and Resilience Lift Extreme Ultra Firming Lotion SPF 15, for Normal/Combination Skin ($70 for 1.7 ounces); **Jan Marini** Bioglycolic Facial Lotion SPF 15 ($36 for 2 ounces); **Neostrata** Daytime Protection Cream SPF 15, PHA 10 ($33 for 1.75 ounces) and Oil Free Lotion SPF 15, PHA 4 ($30 for 1.75 ounces); **Prescriptives** Anti-Age Advanced Protection Lotion SPF 25 ($60 for 1.7 ounces) and Intensive Rebuilding Hand Treatment SPF 15 ($38 for 3.4 ounces); **SkinCeuticals** Sports UV Defense SPF 45 ($34 for 3 ounces).

BEST "MINERAL" SUNSCREENS AND DAYTIME MOISTURIZERS WITH SUNSCREEN WHOSE ONLY ACTIVES ARE TITANIUM DIOXIDE AND/OR ZINC OXIDE, WHICH ARE BEST FOR NORMAL TO DRY OR SENSITIVE SKIN, UNDER $30, ALL SIZES: Clinique Super City Block Oil-Free Daily Face Protector SPF 25 ($16.50 for 1.4 ounces); **Good Skin** All Calm Gentle Sunscreen SPF 25 ($12 for 1.7 ounces); **Neutrogena** Healthy Defense SPF 30 Daily Eye Cream, Light Tint ($11.99 for 0.5 ounce); **Paula's Choice** Pure Mineral Sunscreen SPF 15, for Normal to Very Dry Skin ($14.95 for 6 ounces).

BEST "MINERAL" SUNSCREENS AND DAYTIME MOISTURIZERS WITH SUNSCREEN WHOSE ONLY ACTIVES ARE TITANIUM DIOXIDE AND/OR ZINC OXIDE, WHICH ARE BEST FOR NORMAL TO DRY OR SENSITIVE SKIN, OVER $30, ALL

SIZES: Obagi Nu-Derm Physical UV Block SPF 32 ($40 for 2 ounces); **SkinCeuticals** Physical UV Defense SPF 30 ($34 for 3 ounces).

BEST SELF-TANNERS

By and large, almost all self-tanners will work as indicated, because 99% of them contain the same "active" ingredient, dihydroxyacetone (DHA). DHA reacts with amino acids found in the top layers of skin to create a shade of brown; the effect takes place within two to six hours, and color depth can be built with every reapplication. DHA has a long history of safe use, but it is critical to keep in mind that the "tan" you get from DHA does not provide any sun protection. If you decide to use a self-tanner, be sure you continue to protect exposed skin every day with a well-formulated sunscreen rated SPF 15 or greater and that contains the UVA-protecting ingredients of avobenzone, titanium dioxide, zinc oxide, Mexoryl SX (ecamsule), or Tinosorb.

Self-tanners with sunscreen tend to be a problem if used as your sole source of sun protection. The reason is that ideally a self-tanner should be applied sparingly, while a sunscreen requires liberal application. If you apply a self-tanner with sunscreen liberally, you risk a blotchy or too-dark result. Conversely, applying a self-tanner with sunscreen sparingly will not get you to the level of protection stated on the label, and that puts your skin at risk for damage.

If all self-tanners are similar, how did I decide which ones to rate as Paula's Picks? Good question! Although I have no doubt you will have success with any self-tanner rated with a happy face in this book (for best results, be sure to follow the application instructions exactly), the handful of options below are the self-tanners that, for the most part, are also state-of-the-art moisturizers or gels that just happen to turn skin a beautiful shade of tan. I'd recommend starting with any of the options below before others because what each contains will prove helpful for skin (especially normal to dry skin) while imparting a sunless tan, which is the only kind I (and any dermatologist informed on the dangers of tanning in the sun) recommend.

BEST SELF-TANNERS FOR ALL SKIN TYPES, UNDER $15, ALL SIZES: Almay Sunless Tanning Gel for Body ($9.99 for 4.2 ounces) and Sunless Tanning Gel for Face ($9.99 for 1.7 ounces); **Paula's Choice** Almost the Real Thing Self-Tanning Gel, for All Skin Types ($12.95 for 5 ounces); **Sonia Kashuk** Bronze Sunless Tanner ($14.99 for 2.4 ounces).

BEST SELF-TANNERS FOR ALL SKIN TYPES, OVER $15, ALL SIZES: Clarins Self Tanning Instant Gel ($29.50 for 4.4 ounces) and Liquid Bronze Self Tanning, for Face and Decollete ($28 for 4.2 ounces); **Clinique** Self-Sun Body Quick Bronze Self-Tanner ($17 for 4.2 ounces) and Self-Sun Face Quick Bronze Tinted Self-Tanner ($17 for 1.7 ounces); **Estee Lauder** Go Bronze Plus Tinted Self-Tanner for Face ($22.50 for 1.7 ounces), Body Performance Naturally Radiant Moisturizer ($35 for 6.7 ounces), and Sunless SuperTan, for Face ($22.50 for 1.7 ounces); **Lancome** Flash Bronzer Tinted Self-Tanning Moisturizing Mousse with Pure Vitamin E ($29.50 for 5.3 ounces).

BEST FACIAL MASKS

Although I am rarely a woman of few words, I'm not one to get too excited about facial masks. First, as you will see from the limited options below, there are not many exciting, interesting, or particularly helpful facial masks. Many facial masks for normal to oily skin contain clay as their main ingredient, along with some thickening agents, and although that can be a benefit because it absorbs oil, the improvement is short-lived. Other masks contain clay as well, but also include water-binding agents and plant oils, and that can make them better for normal to combination or slightly dry skin. Masks for normal to dry skin are often just moisturizers and nothing more, and don't necessarily warrant the extra time it takes to apply them. They aren't bad for skin, they just aren't a necessary step.

There are also masks that contain a plasticizing agent that you subsequently pull or peel off your skin. These do impart a temporary soft feeling to the skin because what you're doing is pulling off a layer of skin, but that is hardly beneficial or lasting (and I did not rate this type of mask favorably).

Facial masks can be a pampering, relaxing interval for women, but for good skin care, what you do daily is vastly more important than what you do once a week or once a month. The Paula's Picks in this category are the masks that either have a unique, beneficial twist (such as a clay mask that absorbs excess oil and imparts soothing agents without stripping skin) or, as is the case for every facial mask for normal to dry or very dry skin, feature outstanding formulas that supply skin with helpful ingredients. Any of the moisturizing masks for normal to very dry skin will work even better if left on overnight, and there are no ingredients in the masks listed below that are harmful or irritating if left on skin longer than the directions indicate.

BEST MASK FOR NORMAL TO OILY/COMBINATION AND/OR BLEMISH-PRONE SKIN, UNDER $15, ALL SIZES: Noxzema Continuous Clean Clay Mask ($5 for 4 ounces); **Paula's Choice** Skin Balancing Carbon Mask, for Normal to Oily/Combination Skin ($12.95 for 4 ounces).

BEST MASKS FOR NORMAL TO OILY/COMBINATION AND/OR BLEMISH-PRONE SKIN, OVER $15, ALL SIZES: Estee Lauder So Clean Deep Pore Mask ($22 for 3.4 ounces); **Jan Marini** Factor-A Plus Mask ($60 for 2 ounces); **Nu Skin** Epoch Glacial Marine Mud ($23.51 for 7 ounces).

BEST MASKS FOR NORMAL TO DRY OR VERY DRY SKIN, UNDER $15, ALL SIZES: Paula's Choice Skin Recovery Hydrating Treatment Mask, for Normal to Very Dry Skin ($12.95 for 4 ounces); **Sephora** FACE Exfoliator & Mask, for Normal Skin ($12 for 1.69 ounces).

BEST MASKS FOR NORMAL TO DRY OR VERY DRY SKIN, OVER $15, ALL SIZES: Aveda Tourmaline Charged Radiance Masque ($26 for 4.2 ounces); **Babor** Fruitaction Mask ($21 for 1.7 ounces); **Estee Lauder** Resilience Lift Extreme Ultra Firming Mask ($40 for 2.5 ounces); **Laura Mercier** Intensive Moisture Mask ($32 for 3.7 ounces); **N.V. Perricone** Olive Oil Polyphenols Hydrating Nutrient Mask ($65 for 2 ounces); **Prescriptives** Intensive Rebuilding Deep Hydrating Mask ($28 for 3.4 ounces); **Youthful Essence by Susan Lucci** Repairing Mask ($30 for 1 ounce).

BEST SKIN-LIGHTENING PRODUCTS

The products listed below either contain the time-proven, safe skin-lightening agent hydroquinone or they contain ingredients related to it, such as arbutin or other agents that research (however limited) has shown hold some promise for lightening sun- or hormone-induced brown skin discolorations. Some of these skin-lightening products also contain an

AHA or BHA at the correct pH for exfoliation to occur. The synergistic combination of hydroquinone and a chemical exfoliant not only allows the hydroquinone to work better but also helps remove layers of uneven, sun-damaged skin (and those with BHA can help keep breakouts and blackheads at bay).

Hydroquinone has become a controversial ingredient, despite considerable research demonstrating its safety when properly formulated (meaning following over-the-counter guidelines rather than adulterating products with compounds that can cause skin problems). For detailed information about this "gold standard" skin-lightening agent, please refer to Chapter Seven, *Cosmetic Ingredient Dictionary*. Over-the-counter hydroquinone products are available in strengths of 1% to 2%; higher concentrations are available from dermatologists and plastic surgeons (e.g., Tri-Luma, listed below). Keep in mind that no skin-lightening product will work if you don't use an effective sunscreen daily. Also, if you're using any over-the-counter product with hydroquinone and you haven't noticed any skin-lightening results after three months of daily use (plus daily use of a well-formulated sunscreen rated SPF 15 or greater), you should discontinue use. If this occurs, it is very likely that, for whatever reason, over-the-counter strengths of hydroquinone are not going to be effective for you.

BEST SKIN-LIGHTENING PRODUCTS THAT CONTAIN HYDROQUINONE FOR ALL SKIN TYPES, UNDER $20, ALL SIZES: Alpha Hydrox Spot Light Targeted Skin Lightener ($15 for 0.85 ounce); **Paula's Choice** Clearly Remarkable Skin Lightening Gel, for All Skin Types ($16.95 for 2 ounces) and Remarkable Skin Lightening Lotion, for All Skin Types ($16.95 for 2 ounces).

BEST SKIN-LIGHTENING PRODUCTS THAT CONTAIN HYDROQUINONE FOR ALL SKIN TYPES, OVER $20, ALL SIZES: Glymed Plus Derma Pigment Bleaching Fluid ($37 for 2 ounces); **Peter Thomas Roth** Ultra Gentle Skin Lightening Gel Complex ($55 for 2 ounces); **ProActiv Solution** Skin Lightening Lotion ($21.50 for 1 ounce); **Rodan + Fields** Reverse Step 2 Prepare: Skin Lightening Toner ($35 for 4.2 ounces) and Reverse Step 3 Treat: Skin Lightening Lotion ($65 for 1.7 ounces); **Tri-Luma** (prescription only).

BEST SKIN-LIGHTENING PRODUCTS THAT DO NOT CONTAIN HYDROQUINONE FOR ALL SKIN TYPES, UNDER $20: *Note: There were no products that met this prerequisite; please refer to the list below for Paula's Pick options of skin-lightening products that do not contain hydroquinone.*

BEST SKIN-LIGHTENING PRODUCTS THAT DO NOT CONTAIN HYDROQUINONE FOR ALL SKIN TYPES, OVER $20, ALL SIZES: M.D. Formulations Vit-A-Plus Illumination Spot Treatment, for All Skin Types ($38 for 0.11 ounce); **MD Skincare by Dr. Dennis Gross** Hydra-Pure Radiance Renewal Serum ($95 for 1 ounce); **Peter Thomas Roth** Potent Botanical Skin Brightening Gel Complex ($50 for 2 ounces); **philosophy** a pigment of your imagination SPF 18 ($30 for 2 ounces).

BEST OIL-ABSORBING PAPERS

This is another category for which it was difficult to pick the top options due to the basic and similar nature of the products in this category. The ones that made the cut did so because they had a nifty convenience feature, were noticeably more absorbent than the competition, or proved to be a very cost-effective option. Keep in mind that the many oil-absorbing papers reviewed throughout this book are options as well, though those with added oil, powders, or clays tend to be more troublesome than oil-absorbing papers without these ingredients.

BEST OIL-ABSORBING/BLOTTING PAPERS FOR NORMAL TO VERY OILY SKIN, ALL PRICES, ALL SHEET COUNTS: E.L.F. Professional Shine Eraser ($1 for 50 sheets); **Paula's Choice** Oil-Blotting Papers ($6.95 for 100 sheets); **Rodan + Fields** Unblemish Oil Absorb: Blot Papers with Zincidone ($19 for 60 sheets); **Sephora** Roll-Up Blotting Papers ($8 per roll); **Shu Uemura** Face Paper ($12 for 40 sheets); **Sonia Kashuk** Oil Blotting Papers ($6.99 for 100 sheets).

BEST LIP PRODUCTS (INCLUDING LIP EXFOLIATORS)

Lips are certainly a focal point of the face, and an area that should not be ignored when it comes to sun protection and moisturizing. All of the products below are excellent options to remove dry, flaky skin from chapped lips, protect lips from daily sun exposure, or provide broad-spectrum sun protection. Unless you apply an opaque lipstick every day, it is important to use a lip balm or lipstick with sunscreen rated SPF 15 or greater (recommended lipsticks with sunscreen appear elsewhere in this chapter). Taking the time to protect your skin from sun exposure should always include your delicate, sun-vulnerable lips, too.

BEST LIP BALMS WITH SUNSCREEN (SPF 15 OR GREATER), UNDER $10, ALL SIZES: Blistex Clear Advance SPF 30 ($1.89 for 0.15 ounce) and Pro Care SPF 30 ($2.49 for 0.16 ounce); **Kiss My Face** Cranberry Orange Organic Lip Balm SPF 15 ($3.50 for 0.15 ounce), Sliced Peach Organic Lip Balm SPF 15 ($3.50 for 0.15 ounce), Strawberry Organic Lip Balm SPF 15 ($3.50 for 0.15 ounce), and Vanilla Honey Organic Lip Balm SPF 15 ($3.50 for 0.15 ounce); **Mary Kay** Lip Protector Sunscreen SPF 15 ($7.50 for 0.16 ounce); **Paula's Choice** Moisturizing Lipscreen SPF 15 ($7.95 for 0.16 ounce); **RoC Canada** Minesol High Protection Lipstick SPF 20 ($10 for 3 grams).

BEST LIP BALMS WITH SUNSCREEN (SPF 15 OR GREATER), OVER $10, ALL SIZES: BlissLabs Super Balm Lip Conditioner with SPF 15 ($10 for 0.5 ounce); **Jane Iredale** Lip Drink SPF 15 ($10.50 for 0.18 ounce); **Shiseido** Sun Protection Lip Treatment SPF 36 PA++ ($18 for 0.14 ounce).

BEST LIP BALMS WITHOUT SUNSCREEN, UNDER $10, ALL SIZES: The Body Shop Cocoa Butter Lip Care Stick ($5 for 0.15 ounce) and Hemp Lip Care Stick ($5 for 0.15 ounce); **La Roche-Posay** Ceralip Lip Repair Cream ($10 for 0.5 ounce); **Paula's Choice** Lip & Body Treatment Balm ($9.95 for 0.5 ounce); **philosophy** kiss me clear tube ($10) and kiss me red tube ($10); **Sonia Kashuk** Tinted Lip Balm ($5.99).

BEST LIP BALMS WITHOUT SUNSCREEN, OVER $10, ALL SIZES: Babor B. Young Lip Balm ($11 for 0.5 ounce); **La Prairie** Cellular Lip Line Plumper ($75 for 0.075 ounce); **M.A.C.** Lip Conditioner ($12 for 0.5 ounce); **Prescriptives** Lip Specialist, Triple Action Therapy ($15 for 0.21 ounce); **SkinCeuticals** Antioxidant Lip Repair Restorative Treatment, for Damaged or Aging Lips ($30 for 0.3 ounce).

BEST MANUAL LIP EXFOLIATORS, ALL PRICES, ALL SIZES: Benefit Lipscription ($32 for two-piece set); **The Body Shop** Lipscuff ($10); **Paula's Choice** Exfoliating Treatment ($9.95 for 0.5 ounce).

BEST FOUNDATIONS (INCLUDES LIQUID, CREAM, PRESSED-POWDER, CREAM-TO-POWDER, AND STICK FOUNDATIONS)

Choosing the right foundation color is not only time-consuming, but also exceedingly frustrating. The only way to discover your ideal match is to apply the foundation on your facial skin, perhaps two different colors on either side of your face, and then to check it in daylight. If the color isn't an exact match, you have to go back in and try again. Another hurdle is to find a foundation with a pleasing texture, one that feels soft and silky, but doesn't streak, cake, or look thick, and that takes experimentation, too. Determining how much coverage you want is another factor, and then there's what type of foundation (liquids or creams or stick formulas). Now tell me that isn't a challenge!

Money-wise, if you can splurge on only one cosmetic product, foundation is it. This is the one category where spending a little bit more is the best option, not because expensive means better, but because it's just way too risky to buy a foundation you can't try on first, either with a tester at the cosmetics counter or with samples you can take home or, in some cases, order online. Still, many mass-market outlets and drugstores have very good hassle-free return policies for used makeup, and it's wise to inquire about that before purchasing makeup in these environments (note: all of them require you to keep your receipt as proof of purchase). Do not keep a foundation that ends up being the wrong color—return it and keep trying until you get it right.

Remember that most cream-to-powder foundations or stick foundations are best for those with normal to slightly dry or slightly oily skin because the ingredients that keep these types of foundations in their cream or stick form can be problematic for oily or blemish-prone skin, and the often-powdery finish isn't flattering on dry skin.

I cannot emphasize enough how much foundation has improved over the last few years. Companies such as Estee Lauder, Lancome, L'Oreal, Revlon, and more continue to raise the bar, which only means better foundations for consumers. The foundations on the list below, whether cream, liquid, cream-to-powder, or powder, all have exemplary, class-leading textures, beautiful finishes, reliable coverage, and a selection of neutral shades that match real skin tones (rather than masking skin with an odd shade of pink, rose, or peach). If you have stayed away from foundation because of a previous misstep or negative experience, there has never been a safer time to try it again; the right one can make a huge difference in the appearance of your skin. And if you have oily to very oily skin, choosing a foundation with sunscreen is a great idea because it will help keep excess shine in check while eliminating the need for you to apply two products (when it comes to very oily skin, fewer products is better).

Note: Several foundations with sunscreen reviewed in this book would have earned a Paula's Pick rating had their SPF value been higher. Because it is widely accepted that SPF 15 is the minimum amount of daytime protection needed, I made the decision (with occasional exceptions) to not give foundations with sunscreen below SPF 15 a rating above a neutral face. However, if you are willing to pair such a foundation with another product rated SPF 15 or greater, then you may in fact want to consider those foundations as well. This is one more reason why, depending on your needs and preferences, shopping from the Best Products list alone may not be the best approach.

Second Note: Due to requests from readers, I have divided the Best Foundations list not only by skin type and price, but also by foundations *with* sunscreen and *without* sunscreen. For several reasons, women expressed an interest in separate lists of my favorite foundations that do not contain sunscreen. Please note that, for the health of your skin, using a foundation without sunscreen during daylight hours means that you must pair it with a separate product rated SPF 15 or greater and applied to all areas of exposed skin.

BEST FOUNDATIONS WITH SUNSCREEN (SPF 15 OR GREATER) FOR VERY OILY SKIN, UNDER $20: Boots No7 Stay Perfect Foundation SPF 15 ($15.99); **L'Oreal Paris** True Match Super Blendable Makeup SPF 17 ($9.99) and H-I-P Flawless Liquid Makeup SPF 15 ($13); **Revlon** ColorStay Active Light Makeup SPF 25 ($12.99).

BEST FOUNDATIONS WITH SUNSCREEN (SPF 15 OR GREATER) FOR VERY OILY SKIN, OVER $20: Clarins Truly Matte Foundation SPF 15 ($34); **Illuminare** Ultimate All Day Foundation/Concealer Matte Finish Sunscreen Makeup SPF 21 ($27); **Laura Mercier** Mineral Powder SPF 15 ($35); **Shiseido** Sun Protection Liquid Foundation SPF 42 ($31).

BEST FOUNDATIONS WITH SUNSCREEN (SPF 15 OR GREATER) FOR NORMAL TO OILY/COMBINATION SKIN, UNDER $20: Almay Nearly Naked Liquid Makeup SPF 15 ($12.49); **Cover Girl** TruBlend Powder Foundation SPF 15 ($9.49) and AquaSmooth Makeup SPF 15 ($8.50); **L'Oreal Paris** True Match Super Blendable Makeup SPF 17 ($9.99) and H-I-P Flawless Liquid Makeup SPF 15 ($13); **M.A.C. Studio Stick Foundation SPF 15** ($28.50); **Paula's Choice** Best Face Forward Foundation SPF 15 ($14.95) and Natural Finish Oil-Absorbing Makeup SPF 15 ($14.95); **Quo** Optical Illusion Foundation SPF 15 ($20); **Revlon** Age Defying Makeup with Botafirm SPF 15, Dry Skin ($13.99) and New Complexion One Step Compact Makeup SPF 15 ($12.99).

BEST FOUNDATIONS WITH SUNSCREEN (SPF 15 OR GREATER) FOR NORMAL TO OILY/COMBINATION SKIN, OVER $20: Chanel Double Perfection Fluide Matte Reflecting Makeup SPF 15 ($42.50); **Clinique** Superbalanced Compact Makeup SPF 20 ($26.50; $19.50 for refills); **Shiseido** Dual Balancing Foundation SPF 17 ($35), Stick Foundation SPF 15 ($35), Sun Protection Compact Foundation SPF 34 ($24 for powder cake; $7 for refillable compact), and Fluid Foundation SPF 15 ($35).

BEST FOUNDATIONS WITH SUNSCREEN (SPF 15 OR GREATER) FOR NORMAL TO DRY SKIN, UNDER $20: Paula's Choice All Bases Covered Foundation SPF 15 ($14.95); **Revlon** Age Defying Makeup with Botafirm SPF 15, Normal/Combination Skin ($13.99) and ColorStay Makeup with Softflex for Normal to Dry Skin SPF 15 ($12.99).

BEST FOUNDATIONS WITH SUNSCREEN (SPF 15 OR GREATER) FOR NORMAL TO DRY SKIN, OVER $20: Clinique Dewy Smooth Antiaging Makeup SPF 15 ($21.50); **Prescriptives** Flawless Skin Total Protection Makeup SPF 15 ($39.50).

BEST FOUNDATIONS WITH SUNSCREEN (SPF 15 OR GREATER) FOR DRY TO VERY DRY SKIN, UNDER $20: *Regrettably, there were no Paula's Picks in this category. It is exceedingly difficult to find a truly emollient foundation for very dry skin, primarily because the rich ingredients that people with this skin type need don't lend themselves to a long-lasting makeup application (they tend to interfere with color cosmetics applied afterward). Finding such a foundation that includes sunscreen with the right UVA-protecting ingredients is even more of a challenge. My recommendation for those with this skin type is to choose any of the foundations for normal to dry skin and apply an emollient moisturizer underneath or consider the two pricier options listed below.*

BEST FOUNDATIONS WITH SUNSCREEN (SPF 15 OR GREATER) FOR DRY TO VERY DRY SKIN, OVER $20: Chanel Vitalumiere Satin Smoothing Creme Compact SPF 15 ($55); **Giorgio Armani** Designer Shaping Cream Foundation SPF 20 ($65).

BEST SHEER FOUNDATIONS/TINTED MOISTURIZERS WITH SUNSCREEN (SPF 15 OR GREATER) FOR ALL SKIN TYPES EXCEPT VERY OILY, UNDER $20: Avon Visual Perfection Tint Releasing Moisturizer SPF 20 UVA/UVB ($12.50); **Boots** No7 Soft & Sheer Tinted Moisturiser SPF 15 ($11.99); **Clinique** Almost Makeup SPF 15 ($19.50); **Neutrogena** Healthy Skin Enhancer SPF 20 ($10.99) and Healthy Skin GlowSheers SPF 30 ($12.25); **Paula's Choice** Barely There Sheer Matte Tint SPF 20 ($14.95); **Revlon** Age Defying Light Makeup with Botafirm SPF 30 ($12.99).

BEST SHEER FOUNDATIONS/TINTED MOISTURIZERS WITH SUNSCREEN (SPF 15 OR GREATER) FOR ALL SKIN TYPES EXCEPT VERY OILY, OVER $20: Aveda Inner Light Tinted Moisture SPF 15 ($25); **Bobbi Brown** SPF 15 Tinted Moisturizer ($40); **Estee Lauder** DayWear Plus Multi Protection Anti-Oxidant Moisturizer Sheer Tint Release Formula SPF 15, for All Skin Types ($38 for 1.7 ounces) and DayWear Plus Multi Protection Tinted Moisturizer SPF 15 ($35); **N.V. Perricone** Active Tinted Moisturizer SPF 15 ($65 for 1.7 ounces); **Stila** Sheer Color Tinted Moisturizer SPF 15 ($30).

BEST FOUNDATIONS *WITHOUT* SUNSCREEN FOR VERY OILY SKIN, UNDER $20: Almay Clear Complexion Liquid Makeup ($12.49); **Avon** Beyond Color Line Softening Mousse Foundation ($12); **Clinique** Superfit Makeup ($19.50).

BEST FOUNDATIONS *WITHOUT* SUNSCREEN FOR VERY OILY SKIN, OVER $20: Lancome Teint Idole Ultra Enduringly Divine and Comfortable Makeup ($36); **Make Up For Ever** Powder Foundation ($40), Duo Mat Powder Foundation ($32), and Mat Velvet + Mattifying Foundation ($34).

BEST FOUNDATIONS *WITHOUT* SUNSCREEN FOR NORMAL TO OILY/COMBINATION SKIN, UNDER $20: The Body Shop All in One Face Base ($16.50); **Cover Girl** TruBlend Whipped Foundation ($7.89) and TruBlend Liquid Makeup ($9.49); **Good Skin** All Firm Makeup ($15); **Quo** Wet and Dry Foundation ($18); **Sonia Kashuk** Dual Coverage Powder Foundation ($10.49).

BEST FOUNDATIONS *WITHOUT* SUNSCREEN FOR NORMAL TO OILY/COMBINATION SKIN, OVER $20: Clarins Express Compact Foundation Wet/Dry ($36) and Colour Tint ($34); **Clinique** Perfectly Real Makeup ($22.50) and Perfectly Real Compact Makeup ($22.50); **Estee Lauder** Individualist Natural Finish Makeup ($32.50); **Giorgio Armani** Luminous Silk Foundation ($55) and Silk Foundation Powder ($48); **Laura Mercier** Flawless Face Silk Creme Foundation ($40) and Foundation Powder ($40); **Lorac** Oil-Free Wet/Dry Powder Makeup ($35); **M.A.C.** Studio Fix ($25); **Make Up For Ever** Powder Foundation ($40) and Duo Mat Powder Foundation ($32); **Sheer Cover** Pressed Mineral Foundation ($29.95; $19.95 *member price*); **Sisley Paris** Oil-Free Foundation ($94); **Stila** Natural Finish Oil-Free Makeup ($32), **Vincent Longo** Water Canvas Creme-to-Powder Foundation ($52.50, $14 for optional compact).

BEST FOUNDATIONS *WITHOUT* SUNSCREEN FOR NORMAL TO DRY SKIN, UNDER $20: *For numerous reasons (primarily the fact that the best foundation options for normal to dry skin tend to be those with sunscreen, and that the preferred options tend to be from the department store), there were no foundations in this category that received a Paula's Pick* *rating. However, throughout the book are several inexpensive foundations for normal to dry skin that received a happy face rating and as such are worth considering.*

BEST FOUNDATIONS *WITHOUT* SUNSCREEN FOR NORMAL TO DRY SKIN, OVER $20: Bobbi Brown Oil-Free Even Finish Compact Foundation ($40); **Clarins** Soft Touch Rich Compact Foundation ($36) and Extra Firming Foundation ($37.50); **Lancome** Dual Finish Versatile Powder Makeup ($34.50) and Dual Finish Fragrance Free Versatile Powder Makeup ($34.50); **Laura Mercier** Moisturizing Foundation ($40); **Lorac** Satin Makeup ($35); **Make Up For Ever** Powder Foundation ($40); **Prescriptives** Virtual Youth Lifting Moisture Makeup ($32.50); **Stila** Perfecting Foundation ($30).

BEST FOUNDATIONS *WITHOUT* SUNSCREEN FOR DRY TO VERY DRY SKIN, UNDER $20: *Note: Regrettably, there were no Paula's Picks in this category. It is exceedingly difficult to find a truly emollient foundation for very dry skin, primarily because the rich ingredients people with this skin type need don't lend themselves to a long-lasting makeup application (they tend to interfere with color cosmetics applied afterward). My recommendation to those with this skin type is to choose any of the foundations for normal to dry skin and apply an emollient moisturizer underneath, or consider the two pricier options listed below).*

BEST FOUNDATIONS *WITHOUT* SUNSCREEN FOR DRY TO VERY DRY SKIN, OVER $20: M.A.C. Select SPF 15 Moistureblend ($28.50); **Stila** Illuminating Liquid Foundation ($35).

BEST FOUNDATIONS WITH MAXIMUM COVERAGE, REGARDLESS OF SKIN TYPE, WITH AND WITHOUT SUNSCREEN, ALL PRICES: *No maximum coverage foundations received a Paula's Pick rating because all of them had aesthetic or shade issues that make them difficult to work with or wear without looking obvious and heavy. However, for those who need intense camouflage (such as for birthmarks, vitiligo, or bruising), the best options (which I encourage you to test before purchasing) include:* **Cle de Peau Beaute** Teint Naturel Cream Foundation ($110); **Dermablend** Cover Creme SPF 30 ($27.50); **Elizabeth Arden** Flawless Finish Sponge-On Cream Makeup ($32); **Estee Lauder** Maximum Cover Camouflage Makeup for Face & Body SPF 15 ($28.50); **Exuviance by Neostrata** CoverBlend Concealing Treatment Makeup SPF 20 ($22.50); **Illuminare** Extra Coverage Foundation/Concealer Semi-Matte Finish Sunscreen Makeup SPF 21 ($27); **M.A.C.** Full Coverage Foundation ($27); **Mary Kay** Full Coverage Foundation ($14); **Shu Uemura** Nobara Cream Foundation ($27).

BEST CONCEALERS

Although there are lots of good concealers available in all price ranges, the options below represent the elite, whether you prefer a liquid formula (generally best for normal to oily skin or for use on blemishes) or cream formula (generally best for normal to dry skin not prone to blemishes or for under-eye use). Each concealer below has a beautiful texture, provides moderate to significant coverage without looking thick or cakey, and has an impressive wear time with minimal to no risk of creasing into lines around the eye. I have no doubt you will be pleased with almost any concealer on this list, but please refer to each individual review for details before making your final decision.

I do not recommend color-correcting concealers because they rarely (if ever) look convincing in natural light, and they often substitute one visible discoloration for another. Concealers in the list below that are marked with an asterisk provide effective sun protection with an SPF 15 or higher that includes UVA-protecting ingredients.

BEST LIQUID CONCEALERS, UNDER $15: L'Oreal Paris True Match Concealer ($7.89) and AirWear Long-Wearing Concealer ($10.19); **M.A.C.** Select Cover-Up ($14.50); **Mary Kay** MK Signature Concealer ($9.50); **Maybelline New York** Instant Age Rewind Under Eye Concealer ($5.39) and Instant Age Rewind Double Face Perfector ($8.99); **Origins** Quick, Hide! Easy Blend Concealer ($13.50); **Paula's Choice** No Slip Concealer ($9.95).

BEST LIQUID CONCEALERS, OVER $15: Benefit Lyin' Eyes ($18); **Chanel** Quick Cover ($35); **Clinique** All About Eyes Concealer ($15.50); **Dior** DiorSkin Sculpt Lifting Smoothing Concealer ($29); **Elizabeth Arden** Flawless Finish Concealer ($16); **Stila** Illuminating Concealer ($22).

BEST CREAM, CREAM-TO-POWDER, AND STICK CONCEALERS, UNDER $15: Paula's Choice Soft Cream Concealer ($9.95); **Revlon** *Age Defying Concealer SPF 20 ($8.99).

BEST CREAM, CREAM-TO-POWDER, AND STICK CONCEALERS, OVER $15: Becca Compact Concealer ($35); **Benefit** Galactic Shield! ($20); **Cle de Peau Beaute** Concealer ($68); **Lancome** Absolue Concealer Radiant Smoothing Concealer ($30) and *Photogenic Skin-Illuminating Concealer SPF 15 ($25.50); **Prescriptives** Camouflage Cream ($17.50) and *Flawless Skin Total Protection Concealer SPF 25 ($22).

BEST POWDERS

Quite honestly (well, I'm always honest in these books, but it deserves mention here), it is getting more and more difficult to find a bad loose or pressed powder. For the most part, all of them have an appreciable degree of silkiness and do their jobs of setting makeup, absorbing excess oil, and helping made-up skin look finished. The powders below are those whose qualities surpass the norm, set new benchmarks, and perform beautifully, with most setting to a finish that resembles a second skin (albeit a better looking one). Those who find the lists below too limiting should know that any powder rated with a happy face is also worth considering (but, for various reasons, isn't in the same league as the powders below). Depending on your preferences and expectations, the powder field is mostly wide open (and the shade options for women of color continue to improve; ashy powders were few and far between for this edition of the book).

Expense does not distinguish powders one from the other; there are equally beautiful options at the drugstore as there are at the department store. For example, L'Oreal and Lancome (owned by L'Oreal) each have equally impressive loose powders for normal to dry skin. Lancome's has more elegant packaging, but that doesn't affect the outcome on your face.

A separate category of pressed powders are those that contain sunscreen with an SPF 15 and the mineral-based UVA-protecting ingredients of titanium dioxide or zinc oxide. These are excellent options as a way to touch up makeup and add sunscreen protection over your foundation to be sure you have all-day coverage. Because of their thicker texture, these can also double as powder foundation, though they are best used over a regular sunscreen or over a foundation with sunscreen to ensure sun protection.

Note: The recommendations for skin type that follow are more interchangeable than you might expect. Choosing a powder truly has more to do with your preference (what kind of finish you like), how much of the product you use, and what kind of foundation you wear. However, powders listed as best for dry skin typically have a satiny (as opposed to dry matte) finish, which is a more attractive choice for women with dry skin who use powder.

Conversely, powders recommended for normal to oily skin have a drier, noticeably matte finish (though none of the matte-finish powders below make skin look flat or dull).

BEST LOOSE POWDERS FOR NORMAL TO OILY/COMBINATION OR VERY OILY SKIN, UNDER $15: Boots No7 Perfect Light Loose Powder ($12.99) and No7 Perfect Light Portable Loose Powder ($12.99).

BEST LOOSE POWDERS FOR NORMAL TO OILY/COMBINATION OR VERY OILY SKIN, OVER $15: Bobbi Brown Sheer Finish Loose Powder ($32); **Chanel** Natural Finish Loose Powder ($47.50); **Jane Iredale** Amazing Matte Loose Powder ($31); **Laura Mercier** Loose Setting Powder ($32); **M.A.C.** Select Sheer Loose Powder ($20); **Make Up For Ever** Super Mat Loose Powder ($24); **Shu Uemura** Face Powder Matte ($33).

BEST LOOSE POWDERS FOR NORMAL TO DRY SKIN, UNDER $15: Almay Nearly Naked Loose Powder $12.49; **Jane** Translucent Loose Staying Powder ($3.79); **L'Oreal Paris** Translucide Naturally Luminous Powder ($10.59); **Paula's Choice** Skin Perfecting Loose Powder ($12.95); **Physicians Formula** Loose-to-Go Multi-Colored Loose Powder ($11.95).

BEST LOOSE POWDERS FOR NORMAL TO DRY SKIN, OVER $15: Clarins Loose Powder ($34); **Clinique** Blended Face Powder & Brush ($18.50); **Giorgio Armani** Micro-fil Loose Powder ($47); **Good Skin** Totally Natural Loose Powder ($16); **La Mer** The Powder ($65); **Lancome** Absolue Powder Radiant Smoothing Powder ($50); **Lauren Hutton's Good Stuff** Texture-Light Loose Powder ($25); **Shu Uemura** Face Powder Sheer ($33); **Three Custom Color Specialists** Loose Powder ($36.50); **Vincent Longo** Perfect Canvas Loose Powder ($40).

BEST PRESSED POWDERS FOR NORMAL TO OILY/COMBINATION OR VERY OILY SKIN, UNDER $15: Avon Personal Match Pressed Powder ($9); **Cover Girl** TruBlend Pressed Powder ($7.49) and Advanced Radiance Age-Defying Pressed Powder ($6.99); **Maybelline New York** Dream Matte Face Powder ($7.99); **Paula's Choice** Sheer Perfection Pressed Powder ($12.95); **Revlon** ColorStay Pressed Powder ($9.99); **Sonia Kashuk** Bare Minimum Pressed Powder ($8.99).

BEST PRESSED POWDERS FOR NORMAL TO OILY/COMBINATION OR VERY OILY SKIN, OVER $15: Bobbi Brown Sheer Finish Pressed Powder ($30); **Giorgio Armani** Sheer Powder ($44); **Laura Mercier** Pressed Setting Powder ($30); **Lorac** Translucent Touch Up Powder ($32); **M.A.C.** Select Sheer Pressed Powder ($20); **Prescriptives** Virtual Matte Oil-Control Pressed Powder ($28).

BEST PRESSED POWDERS FOR NORMAL TO DRY SKIN, UNDER $15: Almay Line Smoothing Pressed Powder ($13.99); **The Body Shop** Pressed Face Powder ($14); **Cover Girl** TruBlend Pressed Powder ($7.49) and Advanced Radiance Age-Defying Pressed Powder ($6.99); **L'Oreal Paris** True Match Super-Blendable Powder ($9.99); **Maybelline New York** Finish Matte Pressed Powder ($5.59); **Paula's Choice** Sheer Perfection Pressed Powder ($12.95); **Revlon** New Complexion Powder ($11.99).

BEST PRESSED POWDERS FOR NORMAL TO DRY SKIN, OVER $15: Estee Lauder AeroMatte Ultralucent Pressed Powder ($26); **M.A.C.** Mineralized Skinfinish ($24.50); **Trish McEvoy** Even Skin Finishing Powder ($30); **Vincent Longo** Pressed Powder ($26); **Yves St. Laurent** Poudre Compact Eclat et Matite ($43).

BEST PRESSED POWDERS WITH SUNSCREEN FOR ALL SKIN TYPES, UNDER $15: Neutrogena Healthy Defense Protective Powder SPF 30 ($10.99); **Paula's Choice** Healthy Finish Pressed Powder SPF 15 ($14.95).

BEST PRESSED POWDERS WITH SUNSCREEN FOR ALL SKIN TYPES, OVER $15: Chanel Purete Mat Shine Control Powder SPF 15 ($42.50); **Dior** DiorSkin Compact SPF 20 ($41); **Prescriptives** Flawless Skin Total Protection Powder SPF 15 ($30); **Shiseido** Pureness Mattifying Compact Oil-Free SPF 16 ($18.50 for powder cake; $7 for compact).

BEST BRONZING POWDERS, GELS, AND LIQUIDS

The short lists below represent what I found to be the top-performing bronzing products, whether you prefer powder (the predominant form) or a gel-type product. Each bronzing product not only is easy to apply and blend, but also produces a convincing, real-tan color and is suitable for a range of skin tones. Those looking for a bronzing powder or liquid with noticeable shine should refer to the list of Best Face/Body Illuminating/Shimmer Products below. The bronzing powders on this list have a matte or semi-matte finish, which is far more natural (at least for daytime) than trying to create a fake tan that glistens.

BEST PRESSED BRONZING POWDERS, UNDER $15: Paula's Choice Healthy Finish Pressed Bronzing Powder SPF 15 ($14.95); **Revlon** New Complexion Bronzing Powder ($11.99); **Rimmel** Natural Bronzer ($3.99); **Sonia Kashuk** Pressed Powder Bronzer ($8.99); **Wet 'n' Wild** Bronzer Ultimate Bronzing Powder ($2.99).

BEST PRESSED BRONZING POWDERS, OVER $15: M.A.C. Bronzing Powder ($20); **Trish McEvoy** Dual Resort Bronzer ($28 for powder tablet; $15 for refillable compact), and Matte Bronzer ($28 for powder tablet; $15 for refillable compact); **Vincent Longo** Sole Mio Duo Bronzer ($38.50).

BEST BRONZING GELS, ALL PRICES: Becca Translucent Bronzing Gel ($34); **Bobbi Brown** All Over Bronzing Gel SPF 15 ($25); **Stila** Sun Gel ($24).

BEST BRONZING CREAMS AND LIQUIDS, ALL PRICES: Maybelline New York Dream Mousse Bronzer ($6.99); **Benefit** Glamazon ($26).

BEST BLUSHES

Today's best powder blushes have silky-smooth textures, apply evenly, don't fade, and come in a range of pigment density (so you can create either a dramatic or soft appearance with little effort). For the most part, blush is probably one of the easiest cosmetics to get right because it is nearly impossible to buy a bad blush. Not that there aren't some real losers out there, but there are far more winners. The problem with blush is usually in application, and that is where good brushes come into play. Using the proper brush is essential for getting blush to go on correctly. With very few exceptions, you should just discard the mini-brushes that come packaged with a powder blush in favor of an elegant, professional-size blush brush.

Powder blush is by far the most popular form of this makeup staple, but for variety's sake many lines offer cream, cream-to-powder, and liquid or gel blushes. Those that proved particularly impressive (or easier than usual to work with) earned my top rating and are on the lists below. Because most blushes in all forms have some degree of shine (clearly, many women must want shiny cheeks), I did not take a matte finish into consideration as strongly as I have in the past. There are some terrific matte blushes on the lists below, but, for the most part, what passes for matte still has a hint of shine. Any noticeably shiny blush on the lists below was included because the shine does not flake or interfere with a smooth application. Please refer to each blush's individual review for comments on its finish (matte, almost matte, or level of shine).

Note: The cream blushes on the lists below are recommended only for dry to very dry skin that is not prone to blemishes.

BEST POWDER BLUSHES, UNDER $15: Good Skin Naturally Cheeky Powder Blush ($15); **Jane** Blushing Cheeks Blush ($3.79); **L'Oreal Paris** Feel Naturale Light Softening Blush ($11.99), True Match Super-Blendable Blush ($9.99), and Bare Naturale Gentle Mineral Blush ($14.49); **Paula's Choice** Soft Matte Blush ($8.95) and Barely There Sheer Matte Blush ($9.95); **Sonia Kashuk** Beautifying Blush ($7.99); **Wet 'n' Wild** Silk Finish Blush ($2.99).

BEST POWDER BLUSHES, OVER $15: American Beauty Blush Perfect Cheek Color ($15); **Clarins** Compact Powder Blush ($26); **Dior** DiorBlush ($32.50); **Estee Lauder** Tender Blush ($25); **Jane Iredale** PurePressed Blush ($26); **Lorac** Blush ($16); **M.A.C.** Powder Blush Sheertone ($17.50) and Powder Blush Sheertone Shimmer ($17.50); **Make Up For Ever** Sculpting Blush Powder Blush ($24); **NARS** Blush ($25); **Shu Uemura** Glow On ($21); **Stila** Cheek Color Pan ($16 for powder tablet; $2 for refillable compact); **Urban Decay** Afterglow Blush ($17); **Vincent Longo** Day Play Duo Compact Powder Blush ($35).

BEST CREAM-TO-POWDER OR STICK BLUSHES, UNDER $15: Avon Split Second Blush Stick ($8) and Beyond Color Mousse Blush ($9); **Maybelline New York** Dream Mousse Blush ($6.99); **Revlon** Cream Blush ($9.79).

BEST CREAM-TO-POWDER OR STICK BLUSHES, OVER $15: Clarins Multi Blush ($26); **Dior** Pro Cheeks Ultra-Radiant Blush ($30); **Stila** Rouge Pots ($20); **Three Custom Color Specialists** Creme to Powder Blush ($20.50).

BEST LIQUID OR GEL BLUSHES, UNDER $15: *There were no Liquid or Gel Blushes priced $15 or less and reviewed in this book that earned a Paula's Pick rating.*

BEST LIQUID OR GEL BLUSHES, OVER $15: Benefit BeneTint ($28); **BlissLabs** Ink Pink Blushing Balm ($22); **Illuminare** Perfect Color Blush Ultimate SPF 21 ($18); **Lorac** Sheer Wash ($17.50); **NARS** Color Wash ($25); **Vincent Longo** Lip & Cheek Gel Stain ($22.50).

BEST TRADITIONAL CREAM BLUSHES, UNDER $15: *There were no traditional Cream Blushes priced $15 or less and reviewed in this book that earned a Paula's Pick rating.*

BEST TRADITIONAL CREAM BLUSHES, OVER $15: Bobbi Brown Pot Rouge for Lips and Cheeks ($22); **Laura Mercier** Creme Cheek Colour ($22); **M.A.C.** Blushcreme ($17.50).

BEST EYESHADOWS

In much the same way loose and pressed powders continue to improve for the better, so do eyeshadows. Those listed below have enviable silky textures, apply seamlessly, blend and build well, and have staying power. You can shop the cosmetics counters in both the drugstores and the department stores and find wonderful textures and colors, although when it comes to variety of matte shades, the scales remain tipped in favor of the department stores (primarily in the makeup artist–driven lines such as M.A.C., Stila, and Bobbi Brown). Those of you who love eyeshadow with some shine will find these options almost limitless, regardless of where you shop. The good news is that today's best shiny eyeshadows add more glow than glitter to your eyes, and the shine clings much better than in the past (though there are still plenty of shiny eyeshadows that flake, none of which are on the lists below).

BEST POWDER EYESHADOWS (INCLUDING SINGLES, DUOS, TRIOS, AND QUADS), UNDER $15: Clinique Colour Surge Eye Shadow Velvet ($13.50) and Colour Surge Eye Shadow Soft Shimmer ($13.50); **Elizabeth Arden** Color Intrigue Eyeshadow ($14.50); **M.A.C.** Eye Shadow Veluxe ($14); **Paula's Choice** Soft Matte Eyeshadow ($8.95) and Soft Matte Eyeshadow Trios ($10.95); **Physicians Formula** Matte Collection Quad Eye Shadow ($6.75) and Bright Collection Shimmery Quads Eye Shadow ($6.75); **Quo** Eye Shadow Singles ($11); **Trish McEvoy** Eye Shadow ($15) and Glaze Eye Shadow ($15); **Victoria's Secret** Silky Eye Shadow ($12).

BEST POWDER EYESHADOWS (INCLUDING SINGLES, DUOS, TRIOS, AND QUADS), OVER $15: Becca Eye Color Powder ($20); **Clinique** Colour Surge Eye Shadow Duo ($17.50) and Colour Surge Eye Shadow Quad ($25); **Dior** 5-Color Eyeshadow Compact ($52), 1-Colour Eyeshadow ($23.50), and 2-Colour Eyeshadow ($32); **Estee Lauder** Pure Color EyeShadow ($17.50); **Jane Iredale** PurePressed Eye Shadows ($17.50) and Duo Eye Shadows ($27); **Lorac** Glam Rocks Loose Metallic Eye Shadow ($16); **Quo** Eyeshadow Quads ($16); **Shu Uemura** Pressed Eye Shadow ($20); **Stila** Eye Shadow Pan ($16 for eyeshadow tablet; $2 for refillable compact); **Three Custom Color Specialists** Eyeshadow Singles ($19.50; $15 for refills); **Trish McEvoy** Deluxe Eye Shadow ($20); **Vincent Longo** Eyeshadow Trio ($30); **Yves St. Laurent** Ombre Solo Double Effect ($25.50).

BEST CREAM-TO-POWDER, STICK, GEL, LIQUID, AND CREAM EYESHADOWS, UNDER $15: Revlon Illuminance Creme Eyeshadow ($6.49); **Sephora** Eye Dew ($10).

BEST CREAM-TO-POWDER, STICK, GEL, LIQUID, AND CREAM EYESHADOWS, OVER $15: Bobbi Brown Long-Wear Cream Shadow ($22); **Illuminare** All Day Eye Colors SPF 15 ($18); **Stila** Shadow Pots ($20); **Vincent Longo** Single Creme Powder Shadow ($18).

BEST EYE AND BROW SHAPERS

There are numerous options to line eyes and define the brows, depending on your mood, makeup style, and the amount of time you have to apply such products.

I am still a fan of lining eyes with a matte-powder eyeshadow, used wet or dry (with wet application producing a more intense effect). However, in the past couple of years I have abandoned my powder eyeshadow in favor of the various gel-type eyeliners available. The ones below apply easily, allow me to create any kind of line I'd like (depending on the brush I use), and last all day without smearing, flaking, or fading. In some respects, these are similar to liquid eyeliners, but they tend to dry faster, are easier to apply, the effect is softer, and they last longer. There are, however, some incredible liquid eyeliners to consider if that is your preference.

When it comes to eye and brow pencils, those rated as standard tend to have more similarities than differences. I did not rate any pencil that needed routine sharpening a Paula's Pick because there are enough excellent automatic (no sharpening required) pencils available; I just can't understand why anyone would bother with the other kind, though this is still the dominant version both at drugstores and department stores. The eye and brow pencils on the lists below have quick, smooth applications and a long-wearing finish. The eye pencils tend to be creamier but don't smear, while the brow pencils have a drier texture and powder-like finish (much better for brows than wax-laden, greasy brow pencils).

Several companies sell tinted eyebrow gels as a way to fill, groom, and define the brow. There are also a few companies that make a clear brow gel that isn't much different from using hairspray on a toothbrush and brushing it through the brow. For the most part, the natural-colored brow gels are great, and I strongly recommend them as another way to make eyebrows look fuller but not artificial. If you can learn how to use the eyebrow "mascaras," they are a great alternative (or adjunct) to brow pencils. The brow gels listed below are those that keep brows groomed while not feeling sticky or making brow hairs feel stiff or look obviously coated.

BEST LIQUID, CAKE, OR GEL EYELINERS, UNDER $15: Almay Liquid Eyeliner ($6.49); **The Body Shop** Liquid Eyeliner ($11.50); **Clinique** Brush-On Cream Liner ($14.50); **Cover Girl** Liquid Pencil Felt Tip Eyeliner ($5.69); **L'Oreal Paris** Lineur Intense Felt Tip Liquid Eyeliner ($8.29), Voluminous Eyeliner ($7.49), and H-I-P Color Truth Cream Eyeliner ($11); **M.A.C.** Fluidline ($14.50); **Paula's Choice** Constant Color Gel Eyeliner ($12.95); **Physicians Formula** Eye Definer Felt-Tip Eye Marker ($6.95); **Revlon** ColorStay Liquid Liner ($7.39); **Sephora** Long Lasting Metallic Eyeliner ($10); **Victoria's Secret** Liquid Liner Pen ($12).

BEST LIQUID, CAKE, OR GEL EYELINERS, OVER $15: Artistry Control Eyeliner ($19.90); **Bobbi Brown** Long Wear Gel Eyeliner ($19); **Lancome** Artliner Precision Point EyeLiner ($27); **Prescriptives** Perfect Every Line Gel Eyeliner ($17.50).

BEST AUTOMATIC EYE PENCILS, UNDER $15: Cover Girl Outlast Smoothwear All-Day Eyeliner ($6.99); **M.A.C.** Technakohl Liner ($14.50); **Maybelline New York** Expertwear Defining Liner ($5.79), Unstoppable Smudge-Proof Waterproof Eyeliner ($6.59), and Line Stylist Eyeliner ($6.95); **Paula's Choice** Ultra-Thin Eye & Brow Pencil ($7.95); **Rimmel** Exaggerate Full Colour Eye Definer ($4.99).

BEST AUTOMATIC EYE PENCIL, OVER $15: *There were no Paula's Picks in the book for this category. You will find a small assortment of pricier eye pencils rated Paula's Pick on www.Beautypedia.com; however, spending over $15 for an eye pencil doesn't make much sense.*

BEST AUTOMATIC EYEBROW PENCILS, UNDER $15: M.A.C. Eye Brow Pencils ($13.50); **Origins** Fill in the Blanks Eyebrow Enhancer ($13.50); **Paula's Choice** Ultra-Thin Eye & Brow Pencil ($7.95); **Physicians Formula** Brow Definer Automatic Brow Pencil ($5.95).

BEST AUTOMATIC EYEBROW PENCILS, OVER $15: Clarins Retractable Brow Definer ($22.50; $10 for pencil refills); **Prescriptives** Groom Stick for Brows ($18.50); **Vincent Longo** Brow Pencil/Everbrow Pencil ($20).

BEST EYEBROW POWDERS, UNDER $15: *Note: Although there were no products specifically labeled as "brow powders" that earned a Paula's Pick rating in this price range, please refer to the list of Best Powder Eyeshadows above. Most of those have shades that can be used with a brush to fill in and define eyebrows.*

BEST EYEBROW POWDERS, OVER $15: Sephora Arch It Brow Kit ($35); **Three Custom Color Specialists** Brow Powder ($19.50; $15 for refills); **Vincent Longo** Bi-Brow Powder Pomade ($22).

BEST EYEBROW GELS AND BROW TINTS, UNDER $15: E.L.F. Wet Gloss Lash & Brow Clear Mascara ($1); **Paula's Choice** Brow/Hair Tint ($9.95); **Stila** Brow Polish ($12).

BEST EYEBROW GELS AND BROW TINTS, OVER $15: Bobbi Brown Natural Brow Shaper ($17); **Dior** Brow Gel ($17); **Jane Iredale** PureBrow Colours ($16); **Three Custom Color Specialists** Brow Gel ($19.50); **Trish McEvoy** Brow Gel ($20).

BEST LIPSTICKS

How does one decide what constitutes a "best" lipstick? Given the number of lipsticks available and women's wide range of preferences for this essential cosmetic (some like sheer with a glossy finish, others want moderate coverage with a satin finish, or semi-matte textures with shimmer, and on and on and on…). The top picks listed below include all of that and more, with the widest range of choice being the cream lipsticks. Cream lipsticks are middle-of-the-road options that balance what most women want from a lipstick (comfort, moisture, and long-wearing color) with what they don't like but are willing to tolerate (slippery feel, routine touch-ups, and lipstick coming off on coffee cups and significant others). The cream lipsticks rated Paula's Picks have remarkably smooth yet non-greasy textures that provide lots of moisture without slip-sliding all over your mouth. The color range for each was taken into consideration as well, and almost without exception (such as the case with a couple of matte-finish options), the shade range includes soft pink, rose, and nude tones along with deeper reds, burgundies, and plum tones. That being said, it must be noted that the numerous lipsticks rated with a happy face are also worth considering. It all depends on your preferences; that's why it was so difficult to narrow down the list of the best options in this category. Despite the struggle, I feel confident that after all the lipsticks I tested at counters (not on my lips, nor did I show a bias for lipsticks whose colors looked great on me) those listed below are exemplary in their category and worthy of must-see status.

I am thrilled that there are so many wonderful options in the long-wearing lip color category. Max Factor created a new category with the launch of their Lipfinity product, and the copycatting has resulted in some truly remarkable products that, in some ways, best the progenitor.

BEST MATTE OR SEMI-MATTE LIPSTICKS, ALL PRICES: Avon My Lip Miracle Lipcolor ($8); **Clinique** Long Last Soft Matte Lipstick ($14); **M.A.C.** Matte Lipstick ($14); **Paula's Choice** Smooth Matte Lipstick ($9.95).

BEST CREAM LIPSTICKS, UNDER $15: Clinique Colour Surge Lipstick ($14) and Long Last Soft Shine Lipstick ($14); **Jane** Lipkick Rich Color Lipstick [also known as Moisture Rich Color Lipstick] ($4.49); **L'Oreal Paris** H-I-P Intensely Moisturizing Lipcolor ($10); **M.A.C.** Amplified Crème Lipstick ($14); **Paula's Choice** Soft Cream Lipstick ($9.95); **Quo** Lipstick ($12); **Revlon** Super Lustrous Lipsticks, Creme or Frost ($7.99); **Rimmel** Lasting Finish Lipstick ($5.99).

BEST CREAM LIPSTICKS, OVER $15: Clarins Le Rouge Lipstick ($21.50); **Elizabeth Arden** Color Intrigue Lipstick ($18.50) and Ceramide Plump Perfect Lipstick ($21.50); **Estee Lauder** Electric Intense LipCreme ($22); **Giorgio Armani** Lipstick Mania ($25); **Lancome** Color Design Sensational Effects Lipcolor Smooth Hold ($21); **NARS** Semi-Mattes ($23); **Shiseido** Perfecting Lipstick ($22); **Three Custom Color Specialists** Lipstick ($18.50) and Shimmering Lights Lipstick ($18.50); **Trish McEvoy** Glaze Lip Color ($21).

BEST SHEER LIPSTICKS, ALL PRICES: Avon Glazewear Lipstick ($8); **Boots No7** Sheer Temptation Lipstick ($9.99); **Estee Lauder** Electric Intense Liquid LipCreme ($22).

BEST LIPSTICKS OR LIP GLOSS WITH SUNSCREEN RATED SPF 15 OR GREATER, ALL PRICES: Aveda Lip Tint SPF 15 ($11); **Chanel** Aqualumiere Sheer Colour Lipshine SPF 15 ($24.50); **E.L.F.** Super Glossy Lip Shine SPF 15 ($1); **Paula's Choice** Sheer Cream Lipstick SPF 15 ($10.95).

BEST LIP PAINTS/STAINS AND LONG-WEARING LIPCOLOR

BEST LIP PAINTS/STAINS AND LONG-WEARING LIPCOLOR, UNDER $15: Cover Girl Outlast All-Day Lipcolor ($9.99) and Outlast Smoothwear All-Day Lipcolor ($9.99); **Max Factor** Lipfinity ($10.89) and Lipfinity EverLites ($10.89); **Maybelline New York** Superstay Lipcolor ($9.99); **Paula's Choice** Constant Color Lip Paint ($10.95).

BEST LIP PAINTS/STAINS AND LONG-WEARING LIPCOLOR, OVER $15: American Beauty Super Plush 10-Hour Lipcolor ($16.50); **Bobbi Brown** Matte Stain for Lips ($20); **Estee Lauder** Double Wear Stay-in-Place Lip Duo ($24); **Lorac** Co-Stars ($19); **M.A.C.** Pro Longwear Lipcolour ($20) and Pro Longwear Lustre Lipcolour ($20); **Victoria's Secret** Long Wear Lip Shine ($18); **Vincent Longo** Lip & Cheek Gel Stain ($22.50).

BEST LIP GLOSSES

Lip gloss deserves its own header because it is so popular and in such high demand. Regardless of where I went or what line I was looking at, if there was one makeup item that made women of all ages gleeful, it was lip gloss. I don't know whether it's the low-commitment sheer colors or the glossy finish reminiscent of youth and sex appeal (ads for lip gloss have become quite racy of late, and it's often associated with lingerie). Sephora can be a veritable madhouse of women trying on lip glosses, and several colors were out of stock (necessitating several return trips), further testament to the popularity of this type of lip makeup. The lip glosses below are divided by price and by color saturation. Sheer lip glosses may be worn alone or over a lipstick; opaque or nearly opaque lip glosses (also known as liquid lipsticks) may be worn alone or over a bold lipstick for added depth and color impact. Each option below comes in a gorgeous range of shades and does not have a sticky, gooey, or syrup-like finish. Of course, spending a lot on lip gloss isn't the best idea because it is fleeting, but for those so inclined, there are some great expensive options, too.

BEST SHEER (COLOR) LIP GLOSSES, UNDER $15: Boots Botanics Lip Gloss ($8.99); **Clinique** Superbalm Moisturizing Gloss ($13.50); **L'Oreal Paris** Colour Riche Lip Gloss ($5.49); **M.A.C.** Lipgelee ($14); **Max Factor** Colour Perfection Luxe Gloss ($5.89) and Maxalicious Glaze ($5.99); **Neutrogena** MoistureShine Gloss ($6.79); **Paula's Choice** Soft Shine Moisturizing Lip Gloss ($9.95) and Liquid Diamonds High Shine Lip Gloss ($9.95); **Revlon** LipGlide Sheer Color Gloss ($8.99); **Rimmel** Vinyl Lip ($4.99); **Urban Decay** Triple XXX Slick Lip Gloss ($15) and Lube-in-a-Tube ($11); **Wet 'n' Wild** Glassy Gloss Lip Gel ($2.99).

BEST SHEER (COLOR) LIP GLOSSES, OVER $15: Clarins Colour Quench Lip Balm ($19); **Giorgio Armani** Lip Shimmer ($26); **Hard Candy** Bon Bon Lip Gloss Set ($18); **Laura Mercier** Liquid Crystal Lip Glace ($22); **Make Up For Ever** Super Lip Gloss ($16) and Fascinating Lip Gloss ($18); **Stila** Lip Shine ($17); **Three Custom Color Specialists**

Classic Lip Gloss ($18.50); **Urban Decay** Ultraglide Lip Gloss ($17); **Yves St. Laurent** Touche Brilliance Sparkling Touch for Lips ($29).

BEST PIGMENTED/OPAQUE LIP GLOSSES, UNDER $15: Avon Glazewear Liquid Lip Color ($6) and Glazewear Metallics Lip Gloss ($6); **Clinique** Colour Surge Impossibly Glossy ($14.50); **L'Oreal Paris** Glam Shine Dazzling Plumping Lipcolour ($8.99); **Revlon** LipGlide Full Color & Shine ($8.99).

BEST PIGMENTED/OPAQUE LIP GLOSSES, OVER $15: Giorgio Armani Midnight Lip Shimmer ($26); **Lorac** Lip Intensity Lip Gloss ($16); **Make Up For Ever** Liquid Lip Color ($18); **Prescriptives** Moonbeam Extreme Chromatic Lipcolor ($17.50).

BEST LIP PENCILS

Automatic lip pencils (i.e., do *not* need sharpening) are the only ones that earned a Paula's Pick rating. If you don't mind routinely sharpening pencils, there are some good ones to consider outside of the short list presented here. Otherwise, the pencils below come in a superb range of shades, glide on easily, and have a long-wearing finish that doesn't fade easily.

BEST AUTOMATIC LIP PENCILS, UNDER $15: Almay Ideal Lipliner Pencil ($7.49); **Clinique** Quickliner for Lips ($13.50); **Origins** Automagically Lip Lining Pencil ($13.50); **Paula's Choice** Long-Lasting Anti-Feather Lipliner ($7.95); **Quo** Lip Liner ($12).

BEST AUTOMATIC LIP PENCILS, OVER $15: Clarins Retractable Lip Definer ($22); **Lancome** Le Crayon Lip Contour ($21).

Note: For even the best lip pencils, spending more than $15 doesn't make much sense.

BEST MASCARAS

I must hand it to the cosmetics chemists involved in formulating mascaras, because the wealth of superior choices is expanding almost monthly! I should also mention the wide variety of mascara brushes that are available, from a thin comb with serrated edges to a tightly packed full row of nylon bristles, each providing different effects and each deserving of experimentation to see if you prefer the results from one type of brush over another. Performance of any mascara comes down to the perfect marriage of brush and formula, with packaging components (such as the wiper) coming in a close second. The rest is preference-related depending on the lash look you want. I am ecstatic to report there are excellent mascaras in all price ranges, and obviously it is not logical to buy the most expensive mascara when reasonably priced ones are equally good. Given that this is one product you can't readily test at the counters, try a few of the inexpensive ones listed below and see if that isn't the most sensible and beautiful decision.

Because the mascaras listed below are only those rated Paula's Pick, you'll find that each has its own "wow factor"; that is, they offer impressive results quickly and go the distance when it comes to superior application and wear. Although there are plenty of formidable options here, you should also know that any mascara rated with a happy face in this book is worth considering, again, depending on your preferences.

BEST MASCARAS, UNDER $15: Almay One Coat Nourishing Mascara Triple Effect ($7.99), Intense i-Color Mascara Volumizing Lash Color ($7.49), and One Coat Nourishing Mascara Lengthening ($5.99); **Clinique** Lash Doubling Mascara ($13.50) and High Impact Mascara ($13.50); **L'Oreal Paris** DoubleExtend Lash Extender & Magnifier Mascara ($10.49), Full Definition Voluminous Volume Building Mascara, Lash Architect 3-D Dramatic Mascara ($8.29, straight or curved brush), and H-I-P High Drama Volumizing Mascara ($10); **M.A.C.** Pro Lash Mascara ($11) and Zoom Lash Mascara ($11); **Max Factor** Volume Couture Mascara ($6.99); **Maybelline New York** Full 'n Soft Mascara ($6.79), Lash Discovery Mascara ($6.79), Sky High Curves Extreme Length and Curl Mascara ($6.79), Volum' Express Mascara 3X ($6.79; regular or curved brush), Volum' Express Turbo Boost Mascara 7X ($6.99), XXL Volume + Length Microfiber Mascara ($7.59), and Intense XXL Volume + Length Microfiber Mascara ($7.59); **Paula's Choice** Lush Mascara ($9.95) and Epic Lengths Mascara ($9.95); **Revlon** Fabulash Mascara ($6.99) and 3D Extreme Mascara ($7.99); **Rimmel** Volume Flash Instant Thickening Mascara ($6.49), Eye Magnifier Eye Opening Mascara ($6.49), and Lash Maxxx 3X Lash Multiplying Effect Mascara ($4.37); **Sephora** Lengthening Mascara ($10) and Extreme Lash Mascara ($14); **Stila** Fiber Optics Mascara ($14.50) and Major Lash Mascara ($12.50).

BEST MASCARAS, OVER $15: Chanel Sculpte Cils Sculpting Mascara Extreme Length Fine Lashes ($25); **Clarins** Pure Volume Mascara ($22), Pure Curl Mascara ($22), and Wonder Volume Mascara ($22); **Elizabeth Arden** Defining Mascara ($17); **Giorgio Armani** Soft Lash Mascara ($25); **Lancome** Fatale Exceptional Volume Sculpting 3D Comb Mascara ($23), L'Extreme Instant Extensions Lengthening Mascara ($23), Definicils High Definition Mascara ($23), and Cils Design Pro Custom Design Double Mascara ($35); **Laura Mercier** Thickening and Building Mascara ($19); **Make Up For Ever** Lengthening Mascara ($19); **Sisley Paris** Phyto Mascara Ultra Volume ($57); **Trish McEvoy** High-Volume Mascara ($26); **Yves St. Laurent** Mascara Volume Effet Faux Cils Luxurious Mascara for a False Lash Effect ($26.50) and Everlong Mascara Lengthening Mascara ($26.50).

BEST WATERPROOF MASCARAS, UNDER $15: Almay One Coat Nourishing Mascara Triple Effect Waterproof ($7.99); **Max Factor** Lash Perfection Mascara Waterproof ($6.99); **Maybelline New York** Lash Discovery Waterproof Mascara ($6.79) and Sky High Curves Extreme Length and Curl Mascara Waterproof ($6.79).

BEST WATERPROOF MASCARAS, OVER $15: Bobbi Brown No Smudge Mascara ($20); **Chanel** Inimitable Waterproof Mascara ($27); **Dior** DiorShow Waterproof Mascara ($23); **Estee Lauder** Illusionist Waterproof Maximum Curling Mascara ($21); **Lancome** Definicils Waterproof High Definition Mascara ($23); **Make Up For Ever** Waterproof Lengthening Mascara ($20).

BEST FACE AND BODY ILLUMINATING/SHIMMER PRODUCTS

Given that most cosmetics lines offer at least a few shine-enhancing options, it made sense for this growing, seemingly here-to-stay group of products to have its own category of Paula's Picks. The options below favor liquid shimmer products because they not only tend to be the most versatile but also tend to have the most flattering finishes and shine that clings well to skin. These products are recommended for evening or special-occasion makeup (except weddings if you're the bride; shimmer and shine tend to register as greasy, glossy skin in photographs).

BEST LIQUID, CREAM, CREAM-TO-POWDER, OR GEL SHIMMER PRODUCTS, UNDER $20: Almay Face Brightener Sheer Shimmer SPF 15 ($12.49); **Wet 'n' Wild** MegaGlo Face Illuminator ($2.99).

BEST LIQUID, CREAM, CREAM-TO-POWDER, OR GEL SHIMMER PRODUCTS, OVER $20: Chanel Sheer Brilliance ($42) and Bronze Universel de Chanel Sun Illuminator ($42.50); **Giorgio Armani** Fluid Sheer ($55); **Lorac** Oil Free Luminizer ($28) and TANtalizer Body Bronzing Luminizer ($30); **Prescriptives** Magic Illuminating Potion Foundation Primer ($30); **Sephora** Luminizer ($22); **Stila** All Over Shimmer Liquid Luminizer ($22); **Yves St. Laurent** Teint Parfait Complexion Enhancer ($37.50) and Glossy Touch Multi-Purpose Gloss ($24).

BEST PRESSED POWDER WITH SHIMMER, UNDER $15: Jane Shimmering Bronzer ($5.99).

BEST PRESSED POWDERS WITH SHIMMER, OVER $15: Becca Pressed Shimmer Powder ($34); **Benefit** 10 ($26); **Laura Mercier** Shimmer Bloc ($38); **Trish McEvoy** Shimmer Pressed Powder ($28); **Vincent Longo** Day Play Duo Compact Highlighter ($38.50).

BEST MAKEUP BRUSHES

Professional-size brushes are available in all price ranges. Keep in mind that the density, shape, and cut of the brush is more important than the source of the bristles. Although many cosmetics companies love to brag about the type and grade of animal hair used for their brushes, remember, you are not buying a mink coat. Hair softness, brush shape, and firmness (which affect application) are what matters the most, no matter the source. A few companies offer synthetic brushes that are often exquisite replications of natural-hair brushes that must be felt to be believed. These synthetic brushes are perfectly worthwhile options, and an easy solution for anyone conflicted about using animal-hair brushes for applying makeup. Companies that offer a good selection of excellent synthetic brushes are indicated with an asterisk. Please note that not every single brush in the lines listed below is rated a Paula's Pick. For comments on individual brushes and individual Paula's Pick brushes, please refer to the cosmetics company reviews in Chapter Four, *Product-by-Product Reviews*. A brush collection that rates a Paula's Pick represents a superior combination of performance, craftsmanship, and value.

BEST MAKEUP BRUSHES (INCLUDING INDIVIDUAL BRUSHES AND BRUSH SETS), ALL PRICE RANGES: ***Aveda** ($11-$32.50); ***Becca** ($19-$64); **Bobbi Brown** ($20–$55 for single brushes; $85–$225 for brush sets); ***The Body Shop** ($8.50–$24.50); **Chanel** ($25–$48.50); **Illuminare** ($10–$25 for single brushes; $50 for the Application Tools Kit); **Jane Iredale** ($9–$39); **Laura Mercier** ($10–$52; $45–$250 for Travel, Mini, or Master Sets with portfolio); **Lorac** ($9–$35); **M.A.C.** ($10–$71); ***Make Up for Ever** ($13–$54); **NARS** ($21–$55); ***Origins** ($17.50–$32.50); **Paula's Choice** ($9.95–$17.95 for single brushes; $34.95–$79.65 for brush sets); **Prescriptives** ($16–$50); **Quo** ($12–$20); **Sephora** ($4–$40); ***Shu Uemura** ($10–$270); **Smashbox** ($18–$52); **Sonia Kashuk** ($7.99–$19.99); **Stila** ($18–$52); **Three Custom Color Specialists** ($3.50–$55); **Trish McEvoy** ($14–$72); and ***Urban Decay** ($15–$35).

BEST SPECIALTY PRODUCTS

Following is a list of miscellaneous products that have interesting effects, are available by prescription only (yet definitely worth considering if their pharmacologic action applies to your needs), or have an intriguing premise that just doesn't fit squarely into the above categories. For details about these products, please refer to the reviews in Chapter Four, *Product-by-Product Reviews*.

BEST SPECIALTY PRODUCTS, ALL TYPES, ALL PRICES: The Body Shop Lip Line Fixer ($9); **Botox Cosmetic** (price varies depending on geographical location and amount used per treatment); **Avage, Avita, Differin, Retin-A, Retin-A Micro, Renova**, and **Tazorac** (all *prescription-only* retinoids that offer numerous benefits for skin); **Dr. Denese New York** Perfect Pucker Line Filler with Pro-Peptide Factor ($36.50 for 0.3 ounce); **Jan Marini** Age Intervention Eyelash Conditioner ($160 for 0.23 ounce); **M.A.C.** Prep + Prime Lip ($14.50); **Mary Kay** TimeWise Age-Fighting Lip Primer ($22 for 0.5 ounce); **Obagi** Tretinoin Cream 0.05% and 0.1% ($65–$75 for 20 grams); **Paula's Choice** Skin Relief Treatment, for All Skin Types ($14.95 for 4 ounces) and Cuticle & Nail Treatment ($10.95 for 0.06 ounce); **Revlon** Age Defying Instant Firming Face Primer for Normal/Combination Skin ($11.99) and Age Defying Instant Firming Face Primer for Dry Skin ($11.99); **Sephora** Train Cases ($35–$90); **Smashbox** Layer Lash Primer ($16); **Tri-Luma** Tri-Luma Cream ($101 for 1.05 ounces, *prescription only*); **Trish McEvoy** Face Planners ($48–$68 for the case, $13–$22 for the pages); **Vaniqa** Vaniqa ($50–60 for 30 g/1.05 ounce, *prescription only*).

LINES WITH THE MOST PAULA'S PICK PRODUCTS

The product lines that have the most Paula's Pick products are listed below, in descending order; that is, Clinique has the most, M.A.C. the next most, and so on. Every product line listed has at least ten products that received a Paula's Pick rating. As such, these lines are smart choices as starting points for assembling a state-of-the-art skin-care routine or, where applicable, assembling a reliable makeup wardrobe, including outstanding brushes. This list does NOT mean, however, that the lines below are the only ones reviewed in this book that are worth shopping, or that the number of Paula's Picks corresponds to my agreeing with any of the claims made for the products.

Clinique, M.A.C., Estee Lauder, Neutrogena, Prescriptives, Trish McEvoy, L'Oreal Paris, Maybelline New York, Revlon, Stila, Shu Uemura, Lancome, Almay, Clarins, Good Skin, Laura Mercier, Bobbi Brown, Peter Thomas Roth, Sephora, Sonia Kashuk, Avon, Chanel, Lorac, Dior, Make Up For Ever, Olay, Quo, Vincent Longo, Becca, Cover Girl, Elizabeth Arden (including Prevage), Giorgio Armani, Mary Kay, and **M.D. Formulations**

LINES WHOSE PRODUCTS DID NOT EARN A SINGLE PAULA'S PICK

Although none of the companies listed below has a single product that was rated a Paula's Pick, several of them do offer good options that may be worth considering depending on your needs and preferences. Please do not let these companies' inclusion on this list dissuade you from reading reviews of their products because you may in fact find that you disagree with my assessment of their products. As a consumer, the final choice about what to purchase and use is up to you. Lines indicated with an asterisk are flagged because it is especially disappointing that, given the number of products available, not a single product received a Paula's Pick rating.

***Arbonne, *Aubrey Organics, Banana Boat, Biore, Bremenn Research Labs, Burt's Bees, CeraVe, Cetaphil, *Darphin, *Decleor Paris, Dermablend, *Dermalogica, Erno Laszlo, Freeze 24-7, Garnier Nutritioniste, Hydroderm, *Jurlique International, *Lumene, Lush, Mederma, *Natura Bisse, Noxzema, Purpose, ReVive, SK-II,** and **St. Ives.**

CHAPTER SIX

Animal Testing

Without question, the very topic of this chapter is one many consumers are passionate about, and rightly so. Animals, particularly domesticated pets, are an integral part of life that bring great joy, contentment, and meaning to our existence. I cannot imagine my life without animals, and am reminded of this every time I enter my dog-friendly (and dog-populated) office. Yet in the grand, evolutionary scheme of things, there comes a time when we must consider the pros and cons of using animals for researching the effects of substances, products, and procedures in order to determine their relative effectiveness, toxicity, or safety for human use. I am familiar with both sides of the argument, and as you will see from the information below, I have opted to take a bipartisan approach to this topic.

The National Anti-Vivisection Society (NAVS) is a nonprofit educational group that opposes the use of animals for any purpose, whether in product testing, research, or education. Although I find some of their policies and agendas to be one-sided and radical, I still support many of their efforts to stop unnecessary animal testing and prevent animal cruelty in all forms. NAVS and I differ in that I do not oppose the use of animal testing for health-care research when it concerns afflictions such as breast cancer, Alzheimer's, and heart disease, and I am not vegan (NAVS and PETA, People for the Ethical Treatment of Animals, are both opposed to the use of animals for any medical or food use). However, I do oppose the inhumane treatment of animals (no animal should suffer needlessly in the effort to help humankind), as well as the testing of standard cosmetic formulations and ingredients on animals. In this regard, NAVS and I agree. And it is a fact that hundreds of cosmetic ingredients have a history of safe use by humans, thus negating the need for further animal testing.

The definitive book on the issue of animal testing and the cosmetics, household, and personal care industry is NAVS *Personal Care for People Who Care,* now in its thirteenth edition. It provides lists that show which companies do and do not test on animals, and includes a symbolic rating system that helps illuminate the shades of gray existing between an otherwise straightforward "yes" or "no" response. For example, the latest edition of this book provides information on cosmetics companies that do not conduct animal testing themselves, yet also do not have a formal agreement on testing concerns with the companies from whom they purchase ingredients for their products. Some consumers will undoubtedly find this extra effort from NAVS helpful, and overall this is a must-read source for any consumer interested in purchasing products that have not been tested on animals. You can obtain the book by calling NAVS at (800) 888-6287, by communicating via e-mail at navs@navs.org, or by writing them at The National Anti-Vivisection Society, 53 W. Jackson Blvd., Suite 1552, Chicago, IL 60604.

This 200-page guide is available for $13.50 per book, plus shipping and handling. For more information, visit their Web site at www.navs.org.

Please note: When a product's label states that the company that made it doesn't test on animals, and the company reports this information to NAVS for the listing they ultimately use in their book *Personal Care for People Who Care*, there is every reason to believe that information is correct. However, it is naive to assume that this general information means animal testing information was not an integral part of creating the product. For example, all sunscreen ingredients and almost all the antioxidants, plant extracts, vitamins, cell-communicating ingredients, and on and on, that are currently used in cosmetics, have all been tested on animals at some point. In reality, what we know about the efficacy and toxicity (if any) of these ingredients was first obtained from animal testing. I have broached this apparent double standard with NAVS several times but they refuse to acknowledge this challenge to their criteria, preferring to take an all-or-nothing approach despite a historical perspective. Therefore, while the label on a skin-care product may indeed be accurate in regard to the particular product and the company's policy of animal testing, what it does not represent is the vast group of ingredient manufacturers and university research facilities that use animal testing to determine the basic efficacy of cosmetic ingredients that every company in the industry uses to determine what ingredients they will use in their products.

A Personal Note: I am pleased to say that my skin-care company, Paula's Choice, does not test any aspect of its products on animals, during any stage of development. I also do not ask any other lab or company to conduct animal testing on my behalf. I donate a portion of my company's earnings to The Humane Society of the United States (HSUS) every year (particularly during the month of April, which is officially Prevention of Cruelty to Animals month). I am also dedicated to many other charities that protect animals but HSUS is one of those I donate to regularly. Please check out the HSUS Web site at www.hsus.org. Their mailing address is The Humane Society of the United States, 2100 L Street NW, Washington, DC 20037. They can use your financial help as well. HSUS's approach to the issue of animal rights and animal testing is one I agree with most strongly.

By the way, animal rights groups such as NAVS and PETA have lots of information on their Web sites concerning alternatives to animal testing. Although there are some viable options to some types of animal testing (which I wholeheartedly support), most of the non-animal research that is available does not approximate what can be learned from testing an ingredient, product, or drug on a living creature. For example, there is no way an in vitro test or even human skin-cell samples grown in a lab can replicate what happens to major systems in the body when an ingredient (including a drug) is ingested, or what happens to a heart during surgery, or how breast cancer might be cured. Animal testing is not the perfect or ideal solution; but despite the profound moral and ethical dilemmas it presents, it is the best option researchers in the medical and pharmaceutical fields have right now in their efforts to advance the area of hope for human health.

COMPANIES THAT CONDUCT ANIMAL TESTING ON THEIR FINISHED PRODUCTS:

Aveeno (Johnson & Johnson)
*Avita
Banana Boat (Energizer)
Botox Cosmetic (Allergan)
Clean & Clear (J&J)
Clearasil
Coppertone (Schering–Plough)
Cover Girl (Procter & Gamble)
Dove (Unilever)
Eucerin (Beiersdorf, Inc.)
La Prairie (Beiersdorf, Inc.)
Max Factor (P&G)
Neutrogena (J&J)
Nivea (Beiersdorf, Inc.)
Noxzema (P&G)
Olay (P&G)
Pond's (Unilever)
Purpose (J&J)
*Retin-A, *Renova (J&J)
RoC & RoC Canada (J&J)
SK-II (P&G)
*Tazorac

COMPANIES THAT *DO NOT* USE ANIMAL TESTING ON THEIR FINISHED PRODUCTS

Almay (Revlon)
American Beauty (Estee Lauder)
Arbonne International
Aubrey Organics
Aveda (Estee Lauder)
Avon
Becca
Benefit
Biore
Bobbi Brown (Estee Lauder)
The Body Shop (L'Oreal)
Boots
Burt's Bees
Chanel
Clarins
Clinique (Estee Lauder)
Darphin Paris (Estee Lauder)
DDF (Doctor's Dermatologic Formula; P&G)
Decleor
Dermablend (L'Oreal)
Dermalogica
Dr. Brandt
E.L.F.
Elizabeth Arden
Erno Laszlo
Estee Lauder
Garnier Nutritioniste (L'Oreal)
Giorgio Armani (L'Oreal)
Good Skin (Estee Lauder)
Hard Candy
Illuminare
Jane
Jurlique
Kiehl's (L'Oreal)
Kiss My Face
La Mer (Estee Lauder)
La Roche-Posay (L'Oreal)
Lancome (L'Oreal)
Laura Mercier
Lauren Hutton's Good Stuff
L'Oreal
Lush
M.A.C. (Estee Lauder)
Mary Kay
Maybelline New York (L'Oreal)
M.D. Formulations
Natura Bisse
Neostrata (including Exuviance)
N.V. Perricone, M.D.
Origins (Estee Lauder)
Osmotics
Paula's Choice
Peter Thomas Roth

philosophy
Prescriptives (Estee Lauder)
Proactiv Solution
Revlon
Rodan + Fields
Sense by Usana
Shiseido
Shu Uemura (L'Oreal)
Smashbox
St. Ives (Alberto-Culver)
Stila
Three Custom Color Specialists
Ultraceuticals
Urban Decay

COMPANIES WITH UNKNOWN OR UNREPORTED ANIMAL TESTING STATUS

Alpha Hydrox (Neoteric Cosmetics, Inc.)
Amatokin (Bremenn Research Labs)
Artistry (Amway/Quixtar)
Babor
bare escentuals
Blistex
Cellex-C
CeraVe
Cetaphil
Cle de Peau
Cosmedicine
*Differin (Galderma)
Dior (LVMH)
Dr. Denese New York
Freeze 24-7
Glymed Plus
Hydroderm
Hylexin (Bremenn Research Labs [Klein-Becker])
Idebenol (Bremenn Research Labs)
Jan Marini Skin Research, Inc.
Jane Iredale
Kinerase (Valeant Pharmaceuticals)
Lorac
Lumedia (Bremenn Research Labs)
Lumene
Make Up For Ever
MD Skincare by Dr. Dennis Gross
Mederma (Merz Pharmaceuticals)
*MetroGel, MetroLotion & MetroCream (Galderma Laboratories)
Murad
NARS (Shiseido)
Nu Skin
Obagi
Oxy
Patricia Wexler, M.D.
pHisoDerm
Physicians Formula
Prestige Cosmetics
Prevage (Allergan)
Quo
ReVive
Sephora (LVMH)
Sheer Cover
Sisley Paris
SkinCeuticals (L'Oreal)
Sonia Kashuk
Sovage (Bremenn Research Labs)
Stridex
StriVectin-SD (Klein-Becker)
Tri-Luma (Galderma Laboratories)
Trish McEvoy
*Vaniqa (SkinMedica Inc.)
Victoria's Secret
Vincent Longo
Wet 'n' Wild
Youthful Essence by Susan Lucci
Yves St. Laurent
Z. Bigatti
ZAPZYT

* = prescription only

CHAPTER SEVEN

Cosmetic Ingredient Dictionary

Over the past several years, the amount of research that has taken place on cosmetic ingredients of all kinds, especially on plants and their components, is nothing less than astounding. Given this additional research, I have completely revised and updated this chapter so that it contains the latest information on all of the newest ingredients and updates on ingredients that have been used in cosmetics for years.

All of my comments about the efficacy of the plant extracts included in products throughout this edition and in the following list are based on published research, as indicated in the sources shown in parentheses. Anecdotal experience or ancient folklore history did not play a role in my evaluation of any natural ingredient because this type of information is unreliable at best and at worst farfetched and potentially dangerous.

Please keep some basic things in mind. First, regarding research or studies on plant extracts, their efficacy depends on the part of the plant being used (for example, stems may have components and benefits [or problems] that are very different from those of the leaves or roots), the time of year (and day) the plants are collected, the type of extraction or preservation methods used, and the amount of the extract contained in the product. Second, because the cosmetics industry has no standards for any of these issues, even a general comment about the effectiveness of an extract cannot be translated with any certainty into how effective that extract will be when it is included as an ingredient in a cosmetic product. So, what the research provides is basically a collective or overall approach to understanding something about the benefit you may be gaining from an ingredient, but it is by no means an absolute certainty.

When valid studies and research do exist for various plant extracts, it is important to realize that most of the comments about efficacy are the result of research that examined a pure concentrate or a pure tincture (a plant substance in a simple solution with a single base ingredient). There are very few studies on any plant extract with respect to its effectiveness when mixed into a cosmetic at low concentrations or in combination with a host of other ingredients. That's not to say plant extracts in cosmetics are without benefit. Rather, in many cases the amounts used may be questionable in terms of potential efficacy (but they look good on the label for consumers seeking natural ingredients).

All of the following comments relate primarily to external (topical) application only. Benefits listed as obtainable when the plant extracts or vitamins are taken into the system orally as supplements do not necessarily relate to and/or can be very different from those obtainable from topical application. For oral and systemic benefits, please refer to www.naturaldatabase.com (note that this is a subscription-based Web site, but an incredibly valuable one) or www.pubmed.com for a comprehensive free database of abstracts and published research from thousands of scientific journals (including alternative medicine).

My strong suggestion is that you use this dictionary to gain an understanding of the significance of an ingredient in terms of its claims and its potential for irritation, and then use that information to make comparisons among products before you make your purchase.

It is also difficult to accurately assess a product's effects for specific skin conditions. For example, it is difficult to determine whether a cosmetic will clog pores or trigger breakouts because formulations vary so widely and the exact amount of the ingredient is not disclosed. Plus, there are no regulatory guidelines for the use of cosmetic ingredients for specific skin disorders. (There are a few exceptions to this, including sunscreens, benzoyl peroxide for blemishes, and salicylic acid, which are pharmaceuticals not cosmetics.) If you are prone to breakouts, then the best approach for determining a product's chance of causing problems is to determine how thick it is and how emollient (rich) it feels. The thicker a product, the more likely that the thickening/emollient ingredients it contains could find their way into a pore and cause a reaction. The lighter in weight a product is (as long as it does not contain irritating ingredients), the far less likely it is to cause problems.

The A–Z list in this chapter is by no means exhaustive. Books can (and have) been written on this topic alone! The ingredients chosen for inclusion in this dictionary were selected based on how often they appear in cosmetic products, how well-known they are, and/or whether there are unique claims surrounding their alleged benefits. You will find entries for a wide selection of ingredients, from emollients to slip agents and preservatives, that will provide you with a greater understanding of how these ingredients function and what they can and cannot do.

***Acacia senegal*.** Herb that can have anti-inflammatory properties, but that is used primarily as a thickening agent. *See* gums.

Accutane. Trade name of prescription-only anti-acne drug that is taken orally. Active ingredient is isotretinoin, which is derived from vitamin A. This drug works by essentially stopping oil production in sebaceous glands (the oil-producing structures of the skin) and literally shrinking these glands to the size of a baby's (Source: *Dermatology*, 1997; volume 195, Supplemental 1:1–3, pages 38–40). This prevents sebum (oil) from clogging the hair follicle, mixing with dead skin cells, and rupturing the follicle wall to create an environment where the bacterium (*Propionibacterium acnes*) can thrive, which can result in pimples or cysts. Relatively normal oil production resumes when treatment is completed; although the sebaceous glands may slowly begin to enlarge again, they rarely become as large as they were before treatment. "Because of its relatively rapid onset of action and its high efficacy with reducing more than 90% of the most severe [acne] inflammatory lesions, Accutane has a role as an effective treatment in patients with severe acne that is recalcitrant to other therapies" (Source: *Journal of the American Academy of Dermatology*, November 2001, Supplemental, pages 188–194).

Accutane is controversial, however, for several reasons, but principally because of its most insidious side effect—it has been proven to cause severe birth defects in nearly 90% of the babies born to women who were pregnant while taking it. Other commonly reported, although temporary, side effects of Accutane include dry skin and lips, mild nosebleeds (the inside of your nose can get really dry for the first few days), hair loss, aches and pains, itching, rash, fragile skin, increased sensitivity to the sun, headaches, and peeling palms and hands. More serious, although much less common, side effects include severe headaches, nausea, vomiting, blurred vision, changes in mood, depression, severe stomach pain, diarrhea, decreased night vision, bowel problems, persistent dryness of eyes, calcium deposits in tendons, an increase in cholesterol levels, and yellowing of the skin. However, there is current research indicating that depression does not occur during the course of taking Accutane (Sources: *Canadian Journal of Clinical Pharmacology*, June 2007, pages 277–233; *Psychological Reports*, December 2006, pages 897–906; *European Journal of Dermatology*, September–October, 2006, pages 565–571; and *Journal of Drugs in Dermatology*, May 2006, pages 467–468).

acetone. Strong solvent used in nail polish removers.

acetyl carnitine HCL. *See* L-carnitine.

acetyl glucosamine. Amino acid sugar and primary constituent of mucopolysaccharides and hyaluronic acid that has good water-binding properties for skin. In large concentrations it can be effective for wound healing. There is research showing that chitosan (which is composed of acetyl glucosamine) can help wound healing in a complex physiological process (Sources: *Cellular-Molecular-Life-Science*, February 1997, pages 131–140; and *Biomaterials*, June 2001, pages 1667–1673). However, the amount used in those studies was significantly greater than the amount used in cosmetics. In terms of exfoliation, the research that does exist was done by Proctor & Gamble (Source: *Journal of the American Academy of Derma*tology, February 2007, Supplement 2, page AB169). Further, there is no research demonstrating that wrinkles are related to wounds.

acetyl hexapeptide-3. Synthetically derived peptide used in a wide range of skin-care and makeup products, especially those claiming to have a muscle-relaxing effect similar to Botox injections. These claims typically have to do with relaxing muscle contractions when making facial expressions, thus reducing the appearance of expression lines. The company that sells acetyl hexapeptide-3 (trade name Argireline), Centerchem (www.centerchem.com), is based in Spain. According to their Web site, "Argireline works through a unique mechanism which relaxes facial tension leading to a reduction in superficial facial lines and wrinkles with regular use. Argireline has been shown to moderate excessive catecholamines release." The truth of this claim about the effects of topical application of Argireline is based only on information from Centerchem; there is no published research substantiating any use of Argireline topically on skin.

Catecholamines are compounds in the body that serve as neurotransmitters such as epinephrine, adrenaline, and dopamine. Epinephrine prepares the body to handle emergencies such as cold, fatigue, and shock. A deficiency of dopamine in the brain is responsible for the symptoms of Parkinson's disease. These actions are not something you want a cosmetic to inhibit or reduce.

If acetyl hexapeptide-3 really worked to relax facial muscles, it would work all over the face (assuming you're using the products as directed). If all the muscles in your face were relaxed you'd have sagging, not youthful, skin, not to mention that it also would affect your hand (you apply it with your fingers), which would prevent you from picking up a cup or holding the steering wheel of your car. Despite all the fear about Botox that is espoused by companies featuring this peptide in their "works like Botox" products, there is considerably more efficacy, usage, and safety documentation available for Botox.

Despite the claims made for acetyl hexapeptide-3 (Argireline), there is a clinical study that shows that this ingredient is not even remotely as effective as Botox in reducing wrinkles (Sources: www.cremedevie.com/clinical_details.htm; and *International Journal of Cosmetic Science*, October 2002). It is also interesting to note that even Botox when applied topically on skin has no impact on the skin or muscles in any way shape or form! (Source: *Cosmetic Dermatology*, July 2005, pages 521–524.) *See* peptide.

acetylated castor oil. Used as an emollient and thickening agent in cosmetics. *See* glyceryl ester.

acetylated lanolin. Emollient derived from lanolin. *See* lanolin.

acetylated lanolin alcohol. Ester of lanolin alcohol used as an emollient and occlusive agent. Esters are compounds formed from an alcohol and an acid with the elimination of water, and are common cosmetic ingredients.

acetylated palm kernel glycerides. Emollient and thickening agents used in cosmetics. *See* glyceryl ester.

Achillea millefolium. *See* yarrow extract.

acid. Anything with a pH lower than 7 is acidic; a pH above 7 is alkaline. Water has a pH of 7. Skin has an average pH of 5.5.

acne soap. Soaps that often contain antibacterial ingredients, and that are often overly drying and irritating to skin due to the cleansing agents they contain. A study reported in *Infection* (March–April 1995, pages 89–93) demonstrated that "in the group using soap the mean number of inflammatory [acne] lesions increased.... Symptoms or signs of irritation were seen in 40.4% of individuals...." Furthermore, if the antibacterial agents are in a cleanser, any benefit is washed down the drain.

acrylate. *See* film-forming agent.

acrylate copolymer. *See* film-forming agent.

acrylates/C10-30 alkyl acrylate crosspolymer. *See* film-forming agent.

Actaea racemosa. *See* black cohosh.

active ingredient. The active ingredients list is the part of a cosmetic, drug, or pharmaceutical ingredient label that must adhere to specific FDA-mandated regulations. Active ingredients must be listed first on an ingredient label. The amount and exact function of each active ingredient is controlled and must be approved by the FDA. Active ingredients are considered to have a pharmacological altering effect on skin, and these effects must be documented by scientific evaluation and approved by the FDA. Active ingredients include such substances as sunscreen ingredients, skin-lightening agents, and benzoyl peroxide. *See* inactive ingredient.

adenosine triphosphate. Organic compound of adenosine that is formed by hydrolysis of yeast nucleic acids. All living things need a continual supply of energy to function. Animals obtain energy by oxidizing foods, plants obtain energy by chlorophyll's interaction with sunlight. However, before the energy can be used, it must first be changed into a form that the organism can readily use. This special form, or carrier, of energy is the molecule adenosine triphosphate (ATP). In humans, ATP is the major energy source within the cell that drives a number of biological processes such as protein synthesis. The cell breaks down ATP by hydrolysis to yield adenosine diphosphate (ADP), which is then further broken down to yield adenosine monophosphate (AMP). Research into topically applied adenosine triphosphate is just beginning, but it appears to have strong potential as a cell-communicating ingredient and as an inflammation modulator (Sources: *The Journal of Investigative Dermatology*, volume 124, issue 4, April 2005, pages 756–763; and *Journal of Cutaneous Medicine and Surgery*, volume 8, issue 2, March–April 2004, pages 90–96). *See* cell-communicating ingredients.

advanced glycation endproduct. Advanced glycation endproducts (AGEs) are formed by the body's major fuel source, namely glucose. This simple sugar is essential for energy, but also can bind strongly to proteins (the body's fundamental building blocks), forming abnormal structures—AGEs—that progressively damage tissue elasticity. Once AGEs are generated, they begin a process that prevents many systems from behaving normally by literally causing tissue to cross-link and become hardened (Source: *Proceedings of the National Academy of Sciences*, March 14, 2000, pages 2809–2813). The theory is that by breaking these AGE bonds you can undo or stop the damage they cause. There are studies showing that aminoguanidine and carnosine are AGE inhibitors that can prevent glucose cross-linking of proteins and the loss of elasticity associated with aging and diabetes; however, many other substances are potential candidates as AGE inhibitors as well. One study examined over 92 substances, and 29 of them showed some degree of inhibitory activity, with 9 compounds proving to be 30 to 40 times stronger than aminoguanidine (Source: *Molecular Cell Biology Research Communications*, June 2000, pages 360–366). AGEs and free-radical damage may be inextricably linked (Sources: *European Journal of Neuroscience*, December 2001, page 1961; and *Neuroscience Letters*, October 2001, pages 29–32), but none of the studies show that there is any relevance when it comes to topical application of these substances as they are included in cosmetics.

Aerocarpus santalinus. *See* red sandalwood.

Aesculus hippocastanum. *See* horse chestnut extract.

agar. An extract from seaweed used as an emulsifier and thickening agent. *See* algae.

***Agaricus bisporus* extract**. Extract of mushroom that is thought to help regulate skin cell production by inhibiting cell growth, particularly for use in psoriasis, but research in this regard is mixed (Sources: *Free Radical Research*, January 2006, pages 31–39; and *British Journal of Dermatology*, January 1999, pages 56–60). Internally, there is research showing it can inhibit the growth of breast cancer cells and colon cancer cells (Source: *Cancer Research*, October 1993, pages 4627–4632).

AGE. *See* advanced glycation endproduct.

***Agrimonia eupatoria* leaf extract**. Plant extract that research shows inhibits the hepatitis B virus and has antioxidant properties. Whether or not it has benefit when applied topically is not known. There is no research showing it to be effective for cellulite (Sources: *Phytotherapy Research*, April 2005, pages 355–358; and *Journal of Ethnopharmacology*, January 2005, pages 145–150).

AHA. Acronym for alpha hydroxy acid. AHAs are derived from various plant sources or from milk. However, 99% of the AHAs included in cosmetics are synthetic. In low concentrations (less than 3%) AHAs work as water-binding agents. At concentrations over 4% and in a base with an acid pH of 3 to 4, these can exfoliate skin cells by breaking down the substance in skin that holds skin cells together. The most effective and well-researched AHAs are glycolic acid and lactic acid. Malic acid, citric acid, and tartaric acid may also be effective, but are less stable and less skin-friendly; there is little research showing that they have any benefit for skin.

AHAs may irritate mucous membranes and cause irritation. However, AHAs are widely used for therapy of photodamaged skin, and also have been reported to normalize hyperkeratinization (over-thickened skin) and to increase viable epidermal thickness and dermal glycosaminoglycans content. A vast amount of research has substantially described how the aging process affects the skin and has demonstrated that many of the unwanted changes can be improved by topical application of AHAs, including glycolic and lactic acid (Sources: *Plastic and Reconstructive Surgery*, April 2005, pages 1156–1162; *Cutis*, August 2001, pages 135–142; *Journal of the European Academy of Dermatology and Venereology*, July 2000, pages 280–284; *American Journal of Clinical Dermatology*, March-April 2000, pages 81–88; *Skin Pharmacology and Applied Skin Physiology*, May-June 1999, pages 111–119; *Dermatologic Surgery*, August 1997, pages 689–694 and May 2001 pages 1–5; *Journal of Cell Physiology*, October 1999, pages 14–23; and *British Journal of Dermatology*, December 1996, pages 867–875).

Because AHAs exfoliate sun-damaged skin from the surface of the skin, and because this layer imparts some (albeit minimal) sun protection for skin, there is a risk of increased sun sensitivity after using an AHA (Source: *Photodermatology, Photoimmunology, and Photomedicine*, February 2003, pages 21–27). However, wearing a sunscreen eliminates this risk.

***Ahnfeltia concinna* extract**. *See* algae.

***Ajuga turkestanica* extract**. Asian plant extract that limited in vitro research has shown is an effective ingredient to increase aquaporin activity in skin cells (Sources: *Journal of Drugs in Dermatology*, June 2007, Supplement, pages 20-24; and *European Journal of Dermatology*, November/December 2002, pages 25-26). *See* aquaporin.

alanine. *See* amino acid.

albumin. Found in egg white, and can leave a film over skin. It can constrict skin temporarily, making it look smoother for a brief period, but it can also cause irritation and is not helpful for skin.

Alchemilla vulgaris. Plant with antimicrobial properties. Its high tannin content can cause skin irritation (Source: *Journal of Ethnopharmacology*, July 2000, pages 307–313).

alcloxa. Technically known as **al**uminum **chl**orhydr**ox**y **a**llantoinate, alcloxa has constricting properties that can be irritating for skin.

alcohol. Group of organic compounds that have a vast range of forms and uses in cosmetics. In benign form they are glycols used as humectants that help deliver ingredients into skin. When fats and oils (*see* fatty acid) are chemically reduced, they become a group of less-dense alcohols called fatty alcohols that can have emollient properties or can become detergent cleansing agents. When alcohols have low molecular weights they can be drying and irritating. The alcohols to be concerned about in skin-care products are ethanol, denatured alcohol, ethyl alcohol, methanol, benzyl alcohol, isopropyl alcohol, and sd alcohol, which not only can be extremely drying and irritating to skin, but also can generate free-radical damage (Sources: "Skin Care—From the Inside Out and Outside In," *Tufts Daily*, April 1, 2002; *eMedicine Journal*, May 8, 2002, volume 3, number 5, www.emedicine.com; *Cutis*, February 2001, pages 25–27; *Contact Dermatitis*, January 1996, pages 12–16; and http://pubs.niaaa.nih.gov/publications/arh27-4/277-284.htm). In a product where these ingredients are at the top of the ingredient list, they will be problematic for all skin types; when they are at the bottom of an ingredient list, there most likely is not enough present to be a problem for skin.

***Aleurites fordii* oil**. Oil from the Polynesian tung tree, which may have antimicrobial properties for skin (Source: *Journal of Ethnopharmacology*, November 1995, pages 23–32).

alfalfa extract. Can be an antioxidant in skin-care products (Source: *Journal of Agricultural Food Chemistry*, January 2001, pages 308–314).

algae. Algae are very simple, chlorophyll-containing organisms in a family that includes more than 20,000 different known species. A number of species have been used for drugs, where they work as anticoagulants, antibiotics, antihypertensive agents, blood cholesterol reducers, dilatory agents, insecticides, and anti-tumorigenic agents. In cosmetics, algae act as thickening agents, water-binding agents, and antioxidants. Some algae are also potential skin irritants. For example, the phycocyanin present in blue-green algae has been suspected of allergenicity and of causing dermatitis on the basis of patch tests (Source: *Current Issues in Molecular Biology*, January 2002, pages 1–11). Other forms of algae, such as Irish moss and carrageenan, contain proteins, vitamin A, sugar, starch, vitamin B1, iron, sodium, phosphorus, magnesium, copper, and calcium. These are all beneficial for skin, either as emollients or antioxidants (Source: *Journal of Agricultural Food Chemistry*, February 2002, pages 840–845). However, the claims that algae can stop or eliminate wrinkling, heal skin, or provide other elaborate benefits are unsubstantiated.

algin. Brown algae. *See* algae.

aliphatic hydrocarbon. Hydrocarbon contained in natural gas and mineral oils. It is a synthetic fluid with varying properties that range from solvent to slip agent. *See* slip agent and solvent.

alkaline. Anything with a pH higher than 7 is alkaline; a pH below 7 is acidic. Water has a pH of 7; skin has an average pH of 5.5. Skin irritation can be caused by products with a pH of 8 or higher (Sources: *eMedicine Journal*, January 7, 2002, volume 3, number 1, www.emedicine.com; *Cutis*, December 2001, Supplemental, pages 12–19; and *Contact Dermatitis*, April 1996, pages 237–242). Also, research indicates that the bacterium that causes acne, *Proprionibacterium acnes*, proliferates when the skin is more alkaline (Sources: *Infection*, March–April 1995, pages 89–93; and *Journal of Antimicrobial Chemotherapy*, September 1994, pages 321–330).

alkyloamides. Identified on skin-care product labels as DEA (*See* diethanolamine), triethanolamine (TEA), and monoethanolamine (MEA), these are used primarily for their foaming ability in shampoos, but can also be used as thickening or binding agents. They can be skin irritants. In addition, alkyloamides contain a free amine that can combine with formaldehyde-releasing preservatives in cosmetics, and there is concern that they may form carcinogens.

allantoin. By-product of uric acid extracted from urea and considered an effective anti-irritant.

all-trans retinoic acid. Active ingredient in Retin-A and Renova. *See* tretinoin.

almond oil. Non-volatile oil extracted from the seeds of almonds and used as an emollient. *See* natural moisturizing factor (NMF).

Aloe barbadensis. *See* aloe vera.

aloe extract. *See* aloe vera.

aloe juice. *See* aloe vera.

aloe vera. There is no real evidence that aloe vera (*Aloe barbadenis*) helps the skin in any significant way. An article in the *British Journal of General Practice* (October 1999, pages 823–828) stated that "Topical application of aloe vera is not an effective preventative for radiation-induced injuries.... Whether it promotes wound healing is unclear.... Even though there are some promising results, clinical effectiveness of oral or topical aloe vera is not sufficiently defined at present." There is research indicating that isolated components of aloe vera, such as glycoprotein, can have some effectiveness for wound healing and as an anti-irritant (Sources: *Journal of Ethnopharmacology*, December 1999, pages 3–37; *Free-Radical Biology and Medicine*, January 2000, pages 261–265; and *British Journal of Dermatology*, October 2001, pages 535–545). However, when mixed into a cosmetic product, it is doubtful those qualities remain, although it may still play a role in binding moisture to skin (Source: *Skin Research and Technology*, November 2006, pages 241–246).

In pure form, aloe vera's benefits on skin are probably its lack of occlusion and the refreshing sensation it provides. Aloe serves as a water-binding agent for skin due to its polysaccharide (complex carbohydrate) and sterol content. (An example of a sterol that's beneficial for skin is cholesterol) Although research has shown aloe also has anti-inflammatory, antioxidant, and antibacterial qualities, no study has proven it to be superior to other ingredients with similar properties, including vitamin C, green tea, pomegranate, and many other antioxidants (Source: www.naturaldatabase.com).

alpha bisabolol. *See* bisabolol.

alpha glucan oligosaccharide. Emollient used in cosmetics that also has water-binding properties. *See* mucopolysaccharide.

alpha hydroxy acid. *See* AHA.

alpha lipoic acid. Enzyme that, when applied topically on skin, can be a very good antioxidant. While studies of alpha lipoic acid do exist, none of them were carried out on people, and none were double-blind or placebo-controlled to evaluate effects on wrinkling (Source: *Clinical & Experimental Dermatology*, October 2001, pages 578–582). Most of the research was done on human dermal fibroblasts in vitro (test tube) in cell-culture systems. In vitro results are interesting, but it's not known if the results translate to human skin. These models do mimic human skin, but something that mimics human skin is not the same as living skin. There is research showing that alpha lipoic acid, when taken orally, can help prevent cellular damage via its antioxidant properties (Source: *Annals of the New York Academy of Sciences*, April 2002, pages 133–166). Again, whether or how that translates into an effect on skin is unclear. It is clear from the research that alpha lipoic acid is a potent antioxidant, but this isn't the only one and, to date, there are lots of great antioxidants, whether in the form of food, supplements, or applied topically to skin. *See* antioxidant.

alpha-tocopherol. *See* vitamin E.

***Alteromonas* ferment extract**. *Alteromonas* is a gram-negative bacteria found in seawater. It may have water-binding properties for skin, but there is scant research supporting this or any other benefit for skin.

Althaea rosea. *See* mallow.

Althea officinalis. Latin name for the marshmallow plant. *See* mallow.

alumina. Aluminum oxide, which is used as an abrasive, a thickening agent, and an absorbent in cosmetics.

aluminum chlorohydrate. Chemically a salt, and used in antiperspirants, it can be extremely irritating on abraded skin. In terms of a risk of breast cancer related to underarm deodorant, in October 2002, a study conducted at the Seattle-based Fred Hutchinson Cancer Research Center, published in the *Journal of the National Cancer Institute*, looked at the issue of underarm deodorant use and breast cancer. The study compared the use of underarm deodorant in 810 women who had been diagnosed with breast cancer, and 793 women who were not affected by the disease. When the two groups were compared, researchers found no evidence of an increased risk of breast cancer linked to using an antiperspirant or deodorant, or using an antiperspirant or deodorant after shaving with a traditional razor blade. In short, the researchers believed their study proved there was no link between underarm deodorants and breast cancer risk.

aluminum magnesium silicate. Salt that has absorbent properties.

aluminum powder. Metallic element used as a coloring agent. It is composed of finely ground particles of aluminum. Permanently listed (since 1977) by the FDA as a safe coloring additive.

aluminum silicate. Salt that has absorbent and abrasive properties.

aluminum starch octenylsuccinate. Powdery thickening agent, absorbent, and anticaking agent used in cosmetics.

aluminum sulfate. Topical disinfectant and typical ingredient in deodorants. It can be a skin irritant.

amino acid. Fundamental constituents of all proteins found in the body, such as: alanine, arginine, asparagine, aspartic acid, cysteine, cystine, glutamic acid, glutamine, glycine, histidine, isoleucine, leucine, lysine, methionine, phenylalanine, proline, serine, threonine, tryptophan, tyrosine, and valine. Some of these amino acids can be synthesized by the body; others, the essential amino acids must be obtained from protein in the diet. In skin-care products, these types of ingredients act primarily as water-binding agents, and some have antioxidant properties and wound-healing abilities as well. However, these substances cannot affect, change, or rebuild wrinkles. Whether the protein in a skin-care product is derived from an animal or a plant, the skin can't tell the difference. *See* protein and natural moisturizing factor (NMF).

aminobutyric acid. Amino acid that has water-binding properties for skin and may be an anti-inflammatory. It supposedly also increases growth hormone when taken orally, but the only support for this is a single obscure study that was conducted more than two decades ago on fewer than 20 subjects, and the results have yet to be replicated by other scientists.

aminomethyl propanediol. Used to adjust pH in cosmetics.

aminomethyl propanol. Used in cosmetics at concentrations of 1% or less to adjust pH.

aminophylline. Pharmaceutical ingredient present in prescription bronchodilators (medications designed to open blocked air passageways in the lungs) and present in some cellulite lotions and creams. Aminophylline gained notoriety as an ingredient in cellulite creams as a result of a study published in *Obesity Research* (November 1995, Supplemental, pages 561S–568S). The validity of this research was called into question because one of its authors was marketing an aminophylline cream being sold at the time, and thus was not considered an objective investigator. Also, the number of participants in the study was small, and most of them also were dieting and exercising at the same time that they were applying the aminophylline cream (Source: *Annals of Pharmacotherapy*, March 1996, pages 292–293).

Doubt about aminophylline's value also was revealed in research published in *Plastic and Reconstructive Surgery* (September 1999, pages 1110–1114), which described a double-blind study that compared the effectiveness of three different treatments for cellulite on three separate groups of women. One investigated twice-daily application of aminophylline cream compared with a placebo; another twice-weekly treatment using endermologie (a machine rolled over the skin's surface, which has been claimed to get rid of cellulite) on one leg and nothing on the other; and a third combining endermologie on both legs with the same cream regimen used by the first group. "No statistical difference existed in measurements between legs for any of the treatment groups.... [Even] the best subjective assessment, by the patients themselves, revealed that only 3 of 35 aminophylline-treated legs and 10 of 35 [e]ndermologie-treated legs [felt] their cellulite appearance improved." There is no other research showing this to be helpful, and the risk of absorption and bronchial involvement when applied topically remains unclear.

ammonium chloride. Alkaline salt used as a pH balancer in skin-care products; it is not used in concentrations that would be problematic for skin.

ammonium glycolate. Synthetic form of glycolic acid used as a pH adjuster and exfoliant. It is sometimes paired with regular glycolic acid to maintain the pH in a range that allows exfoliation.

ammonium laureth sulfate. Can be derived from coconut; used primarily as a detergent cleansing agent and is considered gentle and effective. *See* surfactant.

ammonium lauryl sulfate. Can be derived from coconut; used primarily as a detergent cleansing agent and is considered gentle and effective. *See* surfactant.

amniotic extract or fluid. There is research showing that pure concentrations of amniotic fluid (human) have some benefit for wound healing (Sources: *Journal of Hand Surgery*, March 2001, pages 332–339; and *Cornea*, September 1996, pages 517–524). However, there is no research showing that amniotic fluid is effective for wrinkles or other skin-care needs, or when diluted in cosmetic formulations.

amodimethicone. *See* silicone.

amygdalic acid. *See* mandelic acid.

amyl cinnamate. Fragrant component.

amyl salicylate. Fragrant component.

amyris oil. Fragrant oil. It has no other known benefit for skin.

Anacyclus pyrethrum. *See* pellitory.

***Anacystis nidulans* extract**. *See* algae.

***Ananas sativus* fruit extract**. *See* pineapple extract.

andiroba oil. Extracted from the Brazilian mahogany tree; it has anti-inflammatory properties (Source: www.rain-tree.com/andiroba.htm).

***Angelica archangelica* root oil**. Volatile oil obtained from the angelica plant. The oil contains chemical constituents that can be phototoxic, including bergapten, imperatorin, and xanthotoxin. Although some components of angelica oil have antioxidant ability, it is a risky ingredient to use on skin if it is exposed to sunlight (Sources: www.naturaldatabase.com; and *Journal of Agricultural and Food Chemistry*, March 2007, pages 1737–1742).

***Angelica polymorpha sinensis* root extract**. *See* dong quai.

anisaldehyde. Synthetic fragrance used in cosmetics.

anise. Also known as aniseed, it can have potent antioxidant and antibacterial properties (Source: *Phytotherapy Research*, February 2002, pages 94–95), but its fragrant component makes this a potential skin irritant, and it can cause photosensitivity (Source: www.naturaldatabase.com).

annato extract. Natural plant colorant derived from the flesh surrounding the seed of *Bixa orellana*, a shrub native to South America. It produces a deep yellow-orange to red color.

***Anthemis nobilis* flower extract**. *See* chamomile.

anthocyanin. Group of naturally occurring substances found in plants that give fruits, vegetables, and plants their unique color. Derived from two Greek words meaning plant and blue, anthocyanins are the pigments that make blueberries blue, raspberries red, and so on. Anthocyanins are potent antioxidants, and there is research showing that plants rich in anthocyanins (e.g., pomegranates and grapes) have anti-tumor properties. More than 300 different anthocyanins have been identified (Sources: *Journal of Agricultural Food Chemistry*, January 2006, pages 319–327; and *International Journal of Cancer*, January 2005, pages 423–433).

antibacterial. Any ingredient that destroys or inhibits the growth of bacteria; in the case of skin-care products, particularly the bacteria that cause blemishes.

anti-inflammatory. Any ingredient that reduces certain signs of inflammation, such as swelling, tenderness, pain, irritation, or redness.

anti-irritant. Any ingredient that reduces certain signs of inflammation, such as swelling, tenderness, pain, itching, or redness. For more information, refer to Chapter Two, *Healthy Skin: Rules to Live By.*

antioxidant. For a detailed explanation of antioxidants, please refer to Chapter Two, *Healthy Skin: Rules to Live By. See* free-radical damage.

apricot kernel. Seed that, especially when finely ground, is a natural exfoliant.

apricot kernel oil. Emollient plant oil pressed from the seeds of apricots, and similar to other nonfragrant plant oils. *See* natural moisturizing factor (NMF).

aquaporin. Group of ten different proteins that form water channels in living things to regulate the water content of skin and other organs. Aquaporin 3 is abundant in the skin of humans and animals. In relation to aquaporin 3, glycerol absorption and transportation through these "water channels" is fundamental to preventing water loss and increasing skin's elasticity (Sources: *Proceedings of the National Academy of Sciences of the United States*, June 10, 2003, pages 7360–7365; and *The Journal of Experimental Biology*, October 2003, page 3).

arachidic acid. Derived from peanut oil and used as an emollient and thickening agent in cosmetics.

arachidonic acid. Produced from phospholipids and fatty acids. There is research showing that this is potentially unsafe and mutagenic when used topically, though more study is needed to decide this conclusively (Sources: *Journal of Cellular and Molecular Life Sciences*, May 2002, pages 799–807; and *Journal of Environmental Pathology, Toxicology, and Oncology*, 2002, volume 21, number 2, pages 183–191).

arachidyl alcohol. Waxy substance used as a thickening agent and emollient in cosmetics.

arachidyl propionate. Waxy substance used as a thickening agent and emollient in cosmetics.

***Arachis hypogaea* extract**. Extract of the plant commonly known as the peanut. It can have emollient and anti-inflammatory properties for skin, although peanut allergy is one of the five most frequent food allergies in children and adults (Source: *Allergy*, 2002, volume 57, Supplemental 72, pages 88–93).

arbutin. Hydroquinone derivative isolated from the leaves of the bearberry shrub, cranberry, blueberry, some mushrooms, and most types of pears. Because of arbutin's hydroquinone content, it can have melanin-inhibiting properties. Although the research describing arbutin's effectiveness is persuasive (even though most of the research has been performed on animals or in vitro), concentration protocols have not been established. That means we just don't know how much arbutin it takes to have an effect in lightening the skin. Many cosmetics companies use plant extracts that contain arbutin, such as bearberry and mulberry leaf extract, but again, there is limited research, mostly animal studies or in vitro, showing that the arbutin-containing plant extracts used in skin-care products have any impact on skin. Whether or not these extracts are effective in the small amounts present in cosmetics has not been established (Sources: *Phytotherapy Research*, July 2004, pages 475–479; *Biological & Pharmaceutical Bulletin*, April 2004, pages 510–524; *Clinical and Experimental Dermatology*, September 2002, pages 513–515; *Analytical Biochemistry*, June 2002, pages 260–268, and June 1999, pages 207–219; *Pigment Cell Research*, August 1998, pages 206–212; and *Journal of Pharmacology and Experimental Therapeutics*, February 1996, pages 765–769). *See* hydroquinone.

Arctium lappa. *See* burdock root.

***Arctostaphylos uva ursi* leaf**. *See* bearberry.

arginine. Amino acid that has antioxidant properties and can be helpful for wound healing (Sources: *Journal of Surgical Research*, June 2002, pages 35–42; *Nitric Oxide*, May 2002, pages 313–318; and *European Surgical Research*, January–April 2002, pages 53–60). *See* amino acid.

Argireline. *See* acetyl hexapeptide-3.

arnica extract. Extract from the plant *Arnica montana*. There is research showing that when arnica is taken orally before surgery it reduces inflammation and reduces bruising (Source: *Archives of Facial and Plastic Surgery*, January–February 2006, pages 54–59). However, it is repeatedly stated in all herbal journals used for the compilation of this dictionary that arnica should not be applied to abraded skin because it is a significant skin irritant. *The PDR Family Guide to Natural Medicines & Healing Therapies* says: "Repeated contact with cosmetics containing arnica can cause itching, blisters, ulcers, and dead skin." (Other Sources: IFA—International Federation of Aromatherapists; and www.int-fed-aromatherapy.co.uk). Arnica also is associated with a high incidence of skin sensitization (Source: *American Journal of Contact Dermatitis*, June 1996, pages 94–99).

arrowroot. Thickening agent; it has no known benefit for skin.

artemia extract. *See* algae.

***Artemisia absinthium* extract**. *See* mugwort extract.

Artemisia vulgaris. *See* mugwort extract.

Ascophyllum nodosum. Species of seaweed. *See* algae.

ascorbic acid. Form of vitamin C that has antioxidant properties (Sources: *Advances in Experimental Medicine and Biology*, 2002, number 505, pages 113–122; and *Journal of Investigative Dermatology*, February 2002, pages 372–379) and anticancer properties when taken orally (Source: *Cancer Detection and Prevention*, 2000, volume 24, number 6, pages 508–523). Ascorbic acid is difficult to stabilize in formulations (Source: *International Journal of Pharmaceutics*, October 1999, pages 233–241). Its acid component is a skin irritant.

ascorbyl glucosamine. Form of vitamin C that has little research showing it has the antioxidant or skin-lightening properties of other forms of vitamin C, although one study did show it to be ineffective for skin lightening (Source: *Dermatology*, 2002, volume 204, number 4, pages 281–286).

ascorbyl glucoside. Form of vitamin C combined with glucose. It can function as an antioxidant, but only minimal research substantiates this. The research that does exist combined ascorbyl glucoside with niacinamide (Source: *Skin Research and Technology*, May 2006, pages 105–113). It is possible the benefit resulted from only the niacinamide, and not the combination.

ascorbyl methylsilanol pectinate. Form of vitamin C that is considered stable and that functions as an antioxidant and thickening agent. *See* vitamin C.

ascorbyl palmitate. Stable and nonacidic form of vitamin C that is effective as an antioxidant (Source: *Biochemical and Biophysical Research Communications*, September 1999, pages 661–665).

asparagine. *See* amino acid.

***Asparagopsis armata* extract**. Extract derived from seaweed. *See* algae.

aspartic acid. *See* amino acid.

astaxanthin. *See* astaxanthin extract.

astaxanthin extract. Carotenoid (carotene pigment) found in plants, algae, and fish, particularly salmon, that functions as a potent antioxidant (Source: *General Physiology and* Biophysics, June 2007, pages 97-103; and *International Journal for Vitamin and Nutrition Research*, 1995, volume 65, issue 2, pages 79–86). Preliminary research suggests that astaxanthin may be able to prevent the oxidative damage to skin after exposure to UVA radiation (Source: www.naturaldatabase.com). *See* antioxidant.

Astragalus membranaceus. Latin name for the Chinese herb Huang-Qi, also known as milk vetch. *See* milk vetch root.

Astragalus sinicus. *See* milk vetch root.

ATP. *See* adenosine triphosphate.

***Atractyloydes lancea* root extract**. Also known as Chinese Thistle Daisy, this root extract is used in Chinese and Japanese alternative medicine for angiogenesis (the formation of new blood vessels) in type-2 diabetes because it contains beta-eudesmol. Some of its other components have been shown to have anti-inflammatory properties as well. Whether or not this can be of benefit when the entire extract is applied topically is unknown (Sources: *Yajugaku Zasshi, The Pharmaceutical Society of Japan*, March 2006, pages 133–143; *European Journal of Pharmacology*, April 2005, pages 105–115; and *Planta Medica*, July 2001, pages 437–442).

Avena sativa. Oat plant. Oat extract can have anti-irritant and anti-inflammatory properties (Source: *Skin Pharmacology and Applied Skin Physiology*, March–April 2002, pages 120–124).

avobenzone. Synthetic sunscreen ingredient (also known as Parsol 1789 and butyl methoxydibenzoylmethane) that can protect against the entire range of the sun's UVA rays (Sources: *Photodermatology, Photoimmunology, and Photomedicine*, August 2000, pages 147–155; and *International Journal of Pharmaceutics*, June 2002, pages 85–94). *See* UVA.

avocado oil. Emollient oil similar to other nonfragrant plant oils. It has antioxidant properties. *See* natural moisturizing factor (NMF).

awapuhi. English name for wild ginger. *See* ginger extract.

Azadirachta indica. *See* neem extract.

azelaic acid. Trade name Azelex and available by prescription; a component of grains such as wheat, rye, and barley. It is effective for a number of skin conditions when applied topically in a cream formulation at 15% and 20% concentrations. In 2002 the FDA approved azelaic acid for the treatment of acne.

For the most part, azelaic acid is recommended as an option for acne treatment (Source: *International Journal of Dermatology*, May 2007, pages 533–538), but there is also some research showing it to be effective for treatment of skin discolorations. For example, "The efficacy of 20% azelaic acid cream and 4% hydroquinone cream, both used in conjunction with a broad-spectrum sunscreen, against melasma was investigated in a 24-week, double-blind study with 329 women. Over the treatment period the azelaic acid cream yielded 65% good or excellent results.... Severe side effects such as allergic sensitization or exogenous ochronosis were not observed with azelaic acid" (Source: *International Journal of Dermatology*, December 1991, pages 893–895). However, other research suggests that azelaic acid is more irritating than hydroquinone mixed with glycolic acid or kojic acid (Source: *eMedicine Journal*, www.emedicine.com, November 5, 2001). If you have had problems using hydroquinone along with tretinoin for skin lightening, then azelaic acid may be a consideration. *See* hydroquinone, tretinoin.

Azelex. *See* azelaic acid.

azuki beans. Legumes that are often ground up for use in skin-care scrub products.

azulene. Chamomile extract used primarily as a coloring agent in cosmetics. It can have antioxidant and anti-inflammatory properties (Sources: *Journal of the European Academy of Dermatology and Venereology*, September 2001, pages 486–487; and *Biochemical and Biophysical Research Communications*, 1996, volume 92, number 3, pages 361–364). However, there is research showing that azulene can cause cellular mutation when exposed to UVA light so it best to not use this in leave-on products (Source: *Mutation Research*, September 2003, pages 19–26). *See* chamomile.

babassu oil. Plant oil that can have emollient properties for skin. There is no research showing it has special properties for skin.

Bacillus subtilis. Naturally occurring bacterium that is widespread and can be used to control plant diseases, fungal plant infestation, and several types of mildew. Based on available information, the bacterium appears to have no adverse effects on humans or the environment (Source: U.S. Environmental Protection Agency, /www.epa.gov/pesticides/biopesticides/factsheets/fs006479e.htm). It has no known benefit when applied to skin.

balm mint extract. Extract derived from a fragrant plant; it poses some risk of skin irritation. It also has some reported antiviral properties (Source: *Phytomedicine*, 1999, volume 6, pages 225–230). Claims that it can help heal wounds are not substantiated.

balsam peru. Fatty resin that when applied topically can cause allergic skin reactions and contact dermatitis. It also has the potential to cause photodermatitis and phototoxicity. Balsam peru is also a standard used in patch tests for skin sensitivity due to its high incidence of causing reactions (Sources: www.naturaldatabase.com; and *Journal of the American Academy of Dermatology*, December 2001, pages 836–839). Among 3,000 known allergens, balsam peru is ranked in the top ten for most frequent offenders (Source: *Deutsche Medizinische Wochenschrift*, July 2006, pages 1584–1589).

banana extract. Extract from banana fruit that has some weak antioxidant properties (Source: *Free Radical Research*, February 2002, pages 217–233).

barberry. Plant whose primary component, berberine, is an alkaloid that can have antibacterial properties and some cellular anti-inflammatory response. However, it can also be a skin irritant because of its effect on cells (Sources: *Alternative Medicine Review*, April 2000, pages 175–177; and *Healthnotes Review of Complementary and Integrative Medicine*, www.healthwell.com/healthnotes/herb).

barium sulfate. Mineral used as a whitening agent in cosmetics. It can be a skin irritant.

barley extract. Extract from barley plants. Can have antioxidant properties when ingested, but there is no research showing this to be the case when applied topically (Source: *Journal of Agricultural Food and Chemistry*, March 2001, pages 1455–1463).

batyl alcohol. Derived from glycerin and used as a stabilizing ingredient and skin-conditioning agent.

bay leaf oil. Can be a potent antioxidant (Source: *Biological and Pharmaceutical Bulletin*, January 2002, pages 102–108), but also can be a potent skin irritant due to its fragrant component.

bearberry extract. Latin name *Arctostaphylos uva ursi*, there is research showing that this extract has antibacterial and antioxidant properties (Sources: *Food Microbiology*, April 2003, pages 211–216; and *Pharmaceutical Biology*, June–July 2004, pages 289–291), and there is a small amount of research showing it can have skin-lightening properties (Source: *International Journal of Dermatology*, February 2003, pages 153–156). Bearberry extract's potential efficacy is derived from its active components: hydroquinone and arbutin (Sources: *Phytochemical Analysis*, September–October 2001, pages 336–339; and http://supplementwatch.com/suplib/supplement.asp?DocId=1306). Hydroquinone is well established as a melanin-inhibiting agent; arbutin has far less quantitative information available, but in high concentrations it has shown it can inhibit melanin production (Source: *Biological & Pharmaceutical Bulletin*, January 1996, pages 153–156). However, the small amount of bearberry extract present in skin-care products makes it unlikely that these products can affect melanin production. *See* arbutin and hydroquinone.

bee pollen. Can have antioxidant properties (Source: *Journal of Agricultural Food Chemistry*, April 2001, pages 1848–1853), but there is no research showing this to be the case when applied topically. Bee pollen can also be a potent skin irritant and allergen (Source: *International Archives of Allergy and Immunology*, June 2001, pages 96–111).

beeswax. Substance made by bees to build the walls of their honeycomb. It is a thickening agent that has some emollient properties.

behenic acid. Fatty acid used as a thickening agent and surfactant. *See* fatty acid.

behentrimonium chloride. Skin-conditioning agent and emulsifier.

behenyl alcohol. Thickening agent used in cosmetics. It is not related to irritating forms of alcohol.

Bellis perennis. *See* daisy flower extract.

bentonite. Type of clay that is used as an absorbent in cosmetics. It can be drying for skin, though its absorbent properties are helpful for those with oily skin.

benzalkonium chloride. Antimicrobial agent used as a preservative in skin-care products. There is no research showing it has any effect against the acne bacterium *Propionibacterium acnes*. It can be a skin irritant (Source: *SKINmed*, May–June 2005, pages 183–185).

benzephenone-3. Also called oxybenzone, a sunscreen agent that protects skin primarily from the sun's UVB rays and some, but not all, UVA rays (Sources: www.photodermatology.com/sunprotection.htm; and *Skin Therapy Letter*, 1997, volume 2, number 5). *See* UVA.

benzocaine. Topical anesthetic (Sources: *Dermatol Surgery*, December 2001, pages 1010–1018; and *Pediatric Dentistry*, January–February 2001, pages 19–23).

benzoic acid. Preservative used in skin-care products; it is considered less irritating than some other forms of preservatives.

benzoin extract. Balsam resin that has some disinfecting and fragrant properties; it may also be a skin irritant (Source: www.naturaldatabase.com).

benzophenone. Group of compounds used in cosmetics as sunscreen agents to protect mostly from UVB radiation and from some, but not all, UVA radiation (Sources: www.photodermatology.com/sunprotection.htm; and *Skin Therapy Letter*, 1997, volume 2, number 5). *See* UVA.

benzothonium chloride. Compound used as a preservative in cosmetics. It is generally considered less irritating than some other forms of preservatives.

benzoyl peroxide. Considered the most effective over-the-counter choice for a topical antibacterial agent in the treatment of blemishes (Source: *Skin Pharmacology and Applied Skin Physiology*, September–October 2000, pages 292–296). The amount of research demonstrating the effectiveness of benzoyl peroxide is exhaustive and conclusive (Source: *Journal of the American Academy of Dermatology*, November 1999, pages 710–716). Among benzoyl peroxide's attributes is its ability to penetrate into the hair follicle to reach the bacteria that cause the problem, and then kill them—with a low risk of irritation. It also doesn't pose the problem of bacterial resistance that some prescription topical antibacterials (antibiotics) do (Source: *Dermatology*, 1998, volume 196, issue 1, pages 119–125). Current research shows benzoyl peroxide is more effective than some other prescription treatments for acne, such as oral antibiotics or topical antibiotics (Source: *Lancet*, December 2004, pages 2188–2195).

Benzoyl peroxide solutions range in strength from 2.5% to 10%. It is best to start with lower concentrations because a 2.5% benzoyl peroxide product is much less irritating than a 5% or 10% concentration, and it can be just as effective. The concentration that is required depends entirely on how stubborn the strain of bacteria in your pores happens to be.

benzyl alcohol. *See* alcohol.

Berberis aristata. *See* barberry.

bergamot oil. A volatile citrus oil that, when used topically, is a photosensitizer and has photomutagenic properties, meaning it can induce malignant changes to cells (Sources: www.naturaldatabase.com; *Journal of the American Academy of Dermatology*, September 2001, pages 458–461; and *Journal of Dermatology*, May 1994, pages 319–322).

***Bertholletia excelsa* extract**. *See* Brazil nut extract.

beta hydroxy acid. *See* salicylic acid.

beta sitosterol. Plant extract, similar to cholesterol, that can have antimicrobial properties (Source: *Journal of Ethnopharmacology*, January 2002, pages 129–132) and, therefore, may be a problem for healthy skin cells. There is a small amount of research showing it has anti-inflammatory properties (Source: *Biological & Pharmaceutical Bulletin*, May 2001, pages 470–473).

beta-carotene. Member of the carotenoid family. There are hundreds of carotenoids, including lycopene and lutein. Beta-carotene is a precursor that helps form retinol (vitamin A). It is converted to vitamin A in the liver as needed. Topically, beta-carotene is potentially a good antioxidant and can reduce the effects of sun damage, although this benefit is dose dependent. There is research showing that too much beta-carotene can generate oxidative damage (Sources: *Photochemistry and Photobiology*, May 2002, pages 503–506; *The Federation of American Societies for Experimental Biology Journal*, August 2002, pages 1289–1291; and *Berkeley Wellness Newsletter*, www.berkeleywellness.com/html/ds/dsBetaCarotene.php).

beta-glucan. Polysaccharide, meaning that it is a sugar (e.g., starch and cellulose) that can be derived from yeast. It has some antioxidant properties and is a strong anti-inflammatory agent (Source: *Free Radical Biology and Medicine*, February 2001, pages 393–402). *See* mucopolysaccharide.

Betula alba. *See* birch bark extract.

BHA. Acronym for butylated hydroxyanisole, a potent synthetic antioxidant (Sources: *Journal of Agricultural Food Chemistry*, May 2002, pages 3322–3327; and *Free Radical Biology and Medicine*, 1996, volume 20, number 2, pages 225–236), but also a suspected carcinogen (Source: *Mutation Research and Genetic Toxicology and Environmental Mutagenesis*, July 2002, pages 123–133). The acronym BHA should not be confused with beta hydroxy acid (salicylic acid), which is an exfoliant. Salicylic acid is abbreviated in discussions as BHA, but it would never be listed that way on a cosmetic ingredient list.

BHA (beta hydroxy acid). *See* salicylic acid.

BHT. Butylated hydroxytoluene, a potent synthetic antioxidant that also has carcinogenic properties (Sources: *Mechanisms of Ageing and Development*, May 2002, pages 1203–1210; and *Free Radical Biology and Medicine*, February 2000, pages 330–336). *See* BHA.

bifida ferment lysate. Type of gram-positive bacteria found in the digestive system. It has no known effect on skin when applied topically.

bifidus extract. Carbohydrate in human milk that stimulates the growth of *Lactobacillus bifidus* in the intestine. In turn, the *Lactobacillus bifidus* lowers the pH of the intestinal contents and suppresses the growth of *Escherischia coli* and other pathogenic bacteria. Whether or not bifidus extract can have benefit for skin is unknown.

bilberry extract. Some research shows bilberry (*vaccinium myrtillis*) to be effective as an antioxidant when ingested due to its antocyanin content. This effect has not been demonstrated on skin (Source: *Journal of Agricultural Food Chemistry*, September 2001, pages 4183–4187).

bioflavonoid. Diverse range of substances that are components of many fruits and vegetables. Many have been shown to have potent antioxidant and gene-regulatory activity (Sources: *Annals of the New York Academy of Science*, May 2002, pages 70–77; *Planta Medica*, August 2001, pages 515–519; and *Free Radical Biology and Medicine*, June 1998, pages 1355–1363).

biotin. Also known as vitamin H, a water-soluble vitamin produced in the body by certain types of intestinal bacteria and obtained from food. Considered part of the B complex group of vitamins, biotin is necessary for the metabolism of carbohydrates, fats, and amino acids (the building blocks of protein). However, it has no reported benefit for skin when applied topically.

birch bark extract. Extract derived from the plant *Betula alba* (common name white birch). It can have potent antioxidant properties (Source: *Journal of Agricultural Food Chemistry*, October 1999, pages 3954–3962), but can also have astringent properties, which makes it a potential irritant for skin if it is one of the main ingredients in a product.

birch leaf extract. *See* birch bark.

bisabolol. Can be extracted from chamomile or derived synthetically. It is an anti-irritant.

bis-diglyceryl polyacyladipate. Used as an emollient and thickening agent in cosmetics. *See* glyceryl ester.

bismuth oxychloride. The standard primary ingredient included in most powders that are referred to as "mineral makeup." The claim for bismuth oxychloride is that it is all-natural and better for skin than talc. In fact, in many ways talc is a more natural, unadulterated, pure ingredient than bismuth oxychloride. Bismuth oxychloride, which seldom occurs in nature, is manufactured by combining bismuth, a by-product of lead and copper metal refining, with chloride (chlorine compound) and water. It's used in cosmetics because it has a distinct shimmery, pearlescent appearance and a fine white powder texture that adheres well to skin. Bismuth oxychloride is heavier than talc. Pure bismuth is a naturally occurring, grayish-white powder. It and its derivatives are used as skin protectives, thickeners, and absorbent agents. Bismuth oxychloride was permanently listed by the FDA as a coloring agent in 1977 and as a synthetic ingredient (Source: *The International Cosmetic Ingredient Dictionary and Handbook*, Eleventh Edition, 2006).

bitter orange flower. *See* orange blossom.

black cohosh. There is research showing that black cohosh when taken orally can have an effect on menopausal and pre-menopausal symptoms (Source: *Journal of the American Pharmaceutical Association*, March–April 2000, pages 327–329). However, there is no research showing that black cohosh can have this or any effect when applied topically on skin (Source: www.herbmed.org).

black currant oil. Non-volatile plant oil. *See* gamma linolenic acid.

black elderberry. When taken orally, this has potent antioxidant properties (Source: *Journal of Agricultural Food Chemistry*, May 2000, pages 1588–1592), but it is not known if it has benefit when applied topically.

black locust extract. Extract that can have antioxidant properties, although it also may have toxic components (Source: FDA, Center for Food Safety & Applied Nutrition, "Poisonous Plant Bibliography," www.fda.gov).

black mulberry. There is no research showing this has any benefit when applied topically to skin.

black pepper extract and oil. Used topically as a counter-irritant, which means it can cause significant skin irritation (Source: www.naturaldatabase.com). *See* counter-irritant.

black raspberry. Fruit that has potent antioxidant properties (Source: *Journal of Agricultural Food Chemistry*, June 5, 2002, pages 3495–3500).

black tea. *See* green tea.

blackberry. Berries that have potent antioxidant properties (Source: *Journal of Agricultural Food Chemistry*, June 5, 2002, pages 3495–3500).

bladderwrack extract. Extract derived from seaweed; it can be an effective antioxidant and has water-binding properties for skin (Sources: *Journal of Cosmetic Science*, January-February 2002, pages 1–9; and *Journal of Agricultural Food Chemistry*, February 2002, pages 840–845).

bloodwort. Also known as yarrow. *See* yarrow extract.

bois oil. Fragrant oil that has no research showing it has benefit for skin (Source: www.naturaldatabase.com).

borage seed extract. Extract of the plant *Borago officinalis*, it can have anti-irritant and anti-inflammatory properties (Source: *Biofactors*, 2000, volume 13, pages 179–185).

borage seed oil. Contains gamma linolenic acid (Source: www.naturaldatabase.com). *See* gamma linolenic acid.

***Borago officinalis* seed oil**. *See* borage seed oil.

borate. Group of compounds used in cosmetics in small quantities primarily as pH adjusters (they have a pH of 9 to 11) or as antimicrobial agents (Source: *Biological Trace Element Research*, winter 1998, pages 343–357). In larger amounts, due to their high pH, they can be significant skin irritants.

borax. Also known as sodium borate decahydrate, borax is a mineral composed of sodium, boron, oxygen, and water. It has fungicide, preservative, insecticide, herbicide, and disinfectant properties. Borax functions as a bleaching agent by converting some water molecules into hydrogen peroxide (H_2O_2), which generates free-radical damage and is a problem for skin. The pH range of borax is about 9 to 11; therefore, it can be a significant skin irritant when used in cosmetics.

boric acid. May have wound-healing benefits (Source: *Journal of Trace Elements in Medicine and Biology*, October 14, 2000, pages 168–173), but in cosmetics is used primarily as an antimicrobial agent.

boron nitride. Synthetic, inorganic powder, which in cosmetics has absorbent properties similar to those of natural powders such as talc.

Boswellia carterii. *See* frankincense extract.

bovine spongiform encephalopathy. *See* Mad Cow Disease.

boysenberry. Berry that can have potent antioxidant properties (Source: *Journal of Agricultural Food Chemistry*, June 5, 2002, pages 3495–3500).

Brassica campestris. *See* rapeseed oil.

Brazil nut extract. Extract for which there is a small amount of research showing it can have antioxidant properties (Source: *Chemosphere*, February 1995, pages 801–802).

broad spectrum. Term that, when applied to sunscreen, refers to a sunscreen's ability to protect the skin from both UVA and UVB rays from the sun. As this book goes to press, this term is not regulated by the FDA; thus, a cosmetics company can make this claim about a product even when it does not actually provide complete UVA or UVB broad-spectrum protection. *See* UVA and UVB.

bromelain. Bromelain is a crude extract from the pineapple that contains, among other components, various closely related proteinases, demonstrating, in vitro and in vivo, anti-edematous, anti-inflammatory, antithrombotic, and fibrinolytic activities. The active factors involved are biochemically characterized only in part. Due to its efficacy after oral administration, its safety, and lack of undesired side effects, bromelain has earned growing acceptance and compliance among patients as a phytotherapeutical drug. Recent results from preclinical and pharmacological studies recommend bromelain as an oral drug for complementary tumor therapy: "Bromelain acts as an immunomodulator by raising the impaired immunocytotoxicity of monocytes against tumor cells … modulation of immune functions, its potential to eliminate burn debris and to accelerate wound healing. Topical bromelain (35% in a lipid base) has achieved complete debridement on experimental burns in rats" (Source: *Cellular and Molecular Life Sciences*, August 2001). There is a good deal of research supporting oral use of bromelain, particularly to reduce edema and inflammation (Source: *Phytomedicine*, December 2002, pages 681–686).

The research about bromelain is related to oral consumption and animal studies. Theoretically, bromelain breaks down the connecting structure that holds surface skin cells together, which causes exfoliation but can also cause irritation. However, exactly how much bromelain is needed (the amount used in skin-care products is typically less than 1%), whether it is stable as used in cosmetics, and in what bases and pH it works best have not been established. There is little to no research demonstrating how bromelain reacts on skin.

bronopol. Technical name 2-bromo-2-nitropropane-1,3-diol, a formaldehyde-releasing preservative (Source: *Contact Dermatitis*, December 2000, pages 339–343). When combined with an amine in cosmetics it may release nitrosamines. *See* formaldehyde-releasing preservative.

bronze powder. Mineral coloring agent derived from copper. Permanently listed (since 1977) by the FDA as a safe coloring additive.

bumetrizole. Sunscreen ingredient that absorbs primarily UVB light.

***Bupleurum falcatum* extract**. There is no research showing extracts of this plant have any benefit for skin, though it may have some wound-healing properties for peptic ulcers. It does contain glucoside and polysaccharide, but whether these can affect skin through topical application of the extract is unknown (Source: *Phytotherapy Research*, February 2002, pages 91–93). *See* mucopolysaccharide.

burdock root. Small amount of research shows that this plant may be effective as an anti-inflammatory agent and antioxidant (Source: www.herbmed.org).

butcher's broom extract. There is evidence showing that this extract can reduce edema and venous problems when taken orally (Source: *Journal of Alternative Complementary Medicine*, December 2000, pages 539–549). It may also have anti-inflammatory properties for skin, but there is little evidence for that.

butyl acetate. Solvent used in nail polish and many other products.

butyl methoxydibenzoylmethane. *See* avobenzone.

butylene glycol. *See* propylene glycol.

butylparaben. *See* parabens.

***Butyrospermum* fruit**. Fruit from the karite tree, scientific name *Butyrospermum parkii*, from which the fat is obtained to make shea butter. *See* shea butter.

Buxus chinensis. *See* jojoba oil.

C12-15 alkyl benzoate. Used as an emollient and thickening agent in cosmetics. *See* glyceryl ester.

C12-18 acid triglyceride. Used as an emollient and thickening agent in cosmetics. *See* glyceryl ester.

C18-36 acid triglyceride. Used as an emollient and thickening agent in cosmetics. *See* glyceryl ester.

C20-40 pareth-40. Mixture of polyethylene glycols of various molecular weight that can function as stabilizing agents, solubolizers, and surfactants.

caffeic acid. Potent antioxidant that may have some anticarcinogenic properties (Sources: *Toxicology*, January 2006, pages 213-220; and *Bioorganic & Medicinal Chemistry Letters*, June 2002, pages 1567–1570.).

caffeine. Alkaloid found in coffee, tea, and kola nuts. It's often included in skin-care products with claims that it will reduce cellulite or puffy eyes. Given the prevalence of Starbucks stores all over the world, it would be great news for women's thighs and eyes if that were the case, but, unfortunately, that is far from the case.

Caffeine's popularity in products related to cellulite is due to its distant relationship to aminophylline (a pharmaceutical once thought to reduce cellulite), which is a modified form of theophylline (Source: *Yale New Haven Health Library, Alternative/Complementary Medicine*, www.yalenewhavenhealth.org), and caffeine contains theophylline (Source: *Progress in Neurobiology*, December 2002, pages 377–392). There is no substantiated research proving theophylline can affect cellulite, but researchers have disproved aminophyilline's claimed impact on cellulite. The second reason caffeine may show up in cellulite products stems from research showing it to have benefit for weight loss, but that's only when you drink it, not when you rub it on your thighs.

There are only two studies showing caffeine to have benefit for reducing cellulite. One was conducted by Johnson & Johnson, which owns the RoC and Neutrogena brands, both of which sell cellulite creams that contain caffeine. The other was conducted by cosmetics ingredients manufacturers that sell anti-cellulite compounds (Source: *Journal of Cosmetic Science*, July–August 2002, pages 209–218). There is no independent research showing that caffeine can provide any benefit for treating cellulite.

When it comes to puffy eyes, there is no research indicating caffeine can have this benefit when applied topically. However, caffeine does have potential as an antioxidant, so it isn't a wasted ingredient in skin-care products (Sources: *BMC Complementary and Alternative Medicine*, March 2006, http://www.biomedcentral.com/1472-6882/6/9; *Bioscience, Biotechnology, and Biochemistry*, November, 2005, pages 2219–2223; *Obesity Research*, July 2005, pages 1195–1204; and *Sports Medicine*, November 2001, pages 785–807).

***cajeputi* oil**. *See Melaleuca cajeputi* oil.

calamine. Preparation of zinc carbonate, colored with ferric oxide (a form of rust). Zinc carbonate is a counter-irritant used to reduce itching. It is still an irritant when applied to skin so it should be used only as needed. *See* counter-irritant.

calcium ascorbate. Form of vitamin C; other forms include ascorbic acid, L-ascorbic acid, ascorbyl palmitate, and magnesium ascorbyl phosphate. Calcium ascorbate, often referred to as Ester-C, is considered a stable form of vitamin C and an antioxidant (Sources: *Medical Science Monitor*, October 2007, pages 205–210; and *Journal of Cosmetic Science*, November–December 2006, pages 465–473). *See* Ester-C.

calcium carbonate. Chalk; used as an absorbent in cosmetics.

calcium d-pantetheine-s-sulfonate. *See* calcium pantetheine sulfonate.

calcium gluconate. Calcium is an essential mineral for the body. A small amount of research shows calcium gluconate may be a good anti-inflammatory and healing agent when applied topically (Source: *Annals of Emergency Medicine*, July 1994, pages 9–13).

calcium pantetheine sulfonate. There is a small amount of in vitro research showing that this may have melanin-inhibiting properties (Source: *Pigment Cell Research*, June 2000, pages 165–171).

calcium pantothenate. Also known as pantothenic acid. *See* pantothenic acid.

calendula extract. Extract derived from the plant commonly known as pot marigold, there is little research showing that it has any effect on skin, though it may have antibacterial, anti-inflammatory, and antioxidant properties. Note: If you have ragweed (or similar plant) allergies, topical application of calendula is not recommended because of the risk of an eczematous allergic reaction (Source: www.naturaldatabase.com).

***Calophyllum inophyllum* seed oil**. *See* tamanu oil.

Camellia japonica. The leaf has been shown in vitro to be potent antioxidant and also able to inhibit the expression of collagen-depleting MMP-1 when applied to human fibroblast cells (Source: *Journal of Cosmetic Science*, January/February 2007, pages 19-32). *See* matrix metalloproteinases.

Camellia oleifera. *See* green tea.

Camellia sinensis. *See* green tea.

camphor. Aromatic substance obtained from the wood of a tree common to Southeast Asia, *Cinnamomum camphora*, or manufactured synthetically. When applied to the skin camphor produces a cooling effect and dilates blood vessels, which can cause skin irritation and dermatitis with repeated use (Sources: *British Journal of Dermatology*, November 2000, pages 923–929; and *Clinical Toxicology*, December 1981, pages 1485–1498). *See* counter-irritant.

cananga extract. Fragrance used in cosmetics; it can be a skin irritant, much like ylang ylang.

Cananga odorata. *See* ylang ylang.

candelilla wax. Extract derived from candelilla plants; used as a thickening agent and emollient to give products such as lipsticks or stick foundations their form.

***Cannabis sativa* L. oil**. *See* hemp seed oil.

canola oil. Plant lipid that has barrier-repair and anti-inflammatory properties (Source: *British Journal of Dermatology*, February 1996, pages 215–220). *See* natural moisturizing factor (NMF).

caprylic/capric triglyceride. Extract derived from coconut and considered a good emollient and thickening agent in cosmetics.

caprylyl glycol. Skin-conditioning agent that may be plant-derived or synthetic. Often used as part of a preservative blend with phenoxyethanol and chloroxylenol, two preservatives that meet current global regulations.

capsaicin. Component of capsicum. When used topically, capsaicin can prevent the transmission of pain. It is also a potent topical irritant and can trigger dermatitis. *See* capsicum.

capsicum. Large group of plants consisting primarily of the pepper family, including chili peppers and paprika. These are used as counter-irritants to relieve muscle aches. Capsicum and substances derived from it can cause allergic reactions or skin irritation and should never be applied to abraded skin (Source: www.naturaldatabase.com). *See* counter-irritant.

capsicum oleoresin. Fatty resin derived from capsicum plants. It can be a skin irritant and should not be applied to abraded skin. *See* capsicum.

caramel. Natural coloring agent.

carbomer. Group of thickening agents used primarily to create gel-like formulations.

carbopol. *See* carbomer.

carboxylic acid. *See* L-carnitine.

cardamom. Plant of the ginger family, used as fragrance in cosmetics. Terpene, one of its major constituents, can be a skin irritant and sensitizer.

carmine. Natural red color that comes from the dried female cochineal beetle. It is sometimes used to color lip gloss, lipsticks, and other cosmetics. The FDA approved carmine for food use in 1977.

carnauba wax. Natural, hard wax obtained from the leaves of palm trees. Used primarily as a thickening agent, but also has film-forming and absorbent properties.

carnitine. Naturally occurring amino acid. Deficiencies of this small but essential component can result in muscle loss and a multitude of other problems. Research abounds for carnitine, especially acetyl-L-carnitine, which is considered to have more bioavailability in terms of its effect on aging and brain function. Research into how this amino acid affects skin when applied topically is limited, though a few studies indicate it can be an antioxidant (Sources: *Medical Science Monitor*, June 2005, pages 176–180; and *International Journal of Biochemistry and Cell Biology*, February 2003, pages 149–156).

carnosic acid. Component of rosemary that is a potent antioxidant (Sources: *Free Radical Biology and Medicine*, June 2002, pages 1293–1303; and *Journal of Agricultural Food Chemistry*, March 2002, pages 1845–1851).

carnosine. Composed of amino acids, it has anti-inflammatory and antioxidant properties. There is some research showing it has antiglycation properties (Source: *Life Sciences*, March 2002, pages 1789–1799).

carnosol acid. *See* carnosic acid.

carrageenan. Seaweed gum used in cosmetics as a thickening agent with water-binding properties.

carrot oil. Emollient plant oil similar to other nonfragrant plant oils. *See* natural moisturizing factor (NMF).

***Carthamus tinctorius* oil**. *See* safflower oil.

carvone. Essential oil used as a flavoring agent and fragrance component in cosmetics. It can be a significant skin sensitizer or allergen (Sources: *Planta Medica*, August 2001, pages 564–566; and *Contact Dermatitis*, June 2001, pages 347–356).

***Carya illinoensis* oil**. *See* pecan oil.

casein. Substance derived from milk protein that may have some antioxidant properties when applied topically, although the research for this is limited (Source: *International Journal of Food Science and Nutrition*, July 1999, pages 291–296).

***Castanea sativa* seed extract**. *See* chestnut seed extract.

castor oil. Vegetable oil derived from the castor bean. It is used in cosmetics as an emollient, though its unique property is that when dry it forms a solid film that can have water-binding properties. It is rarely associated with skin irritation or allergic reactions, but can have a slightly sticky feel on skin.

catalase. Enzyme that decomposes hydrogen peroxide into water and oxygen and that has significant antioxidant properties (Source: *Journal of Investigative Dermatology*, April 2002, pages 618–625).

***Caulerpa taxifolia* extract**. *See* algae.

cedarwood. Fragrant plant extract. There is evidence that cedarwood oil is allergenic and can cause skin irritation. There is also a small amount of research showing it produces tumors on mouse skin (Source: www.naturaldatabase.com).

***Cedrus atlantica* bark extract**. Fragrant oil that can be a skin irritant.

celandine. Extract from the plant *Chelidonium majus* that has some research showing it has antiviral properties. There is no research showing it has benefit when applied topically.

cell-communicating ingredients. Cell-communicating ingredients, theoretically, have the ability to tell a skin cell to look, act, and behave better, more like a normal healthy skin cell would, or to stop other substances from telling the cell to behave badly or abnormally. They do this by either direct communication with the skin cell or by blocking damaging cellular pathways or other cell-communicating substances. Cell-communicating ingredients complement antioxidants to improve skin-cell function.

Examples of cell-communicating ingredients include niacinamide, adenosine triphosphate, vitamin A (retinol), tretinoin (all-trans-retinoic acid—the active ingredient in prescription products such as Renova and Retin-A), and possibly peptides. Assorted plant extracts and growth factors may play a role in blocking damaging cell communication or enhancing healthy cell communication.

(Sources: *Journal of Biological Chemistry*, August 2007, pages 22964, 22976; *Seminars in Immunopathology*, April 2007, pages 15–26; *Journal of Investigative Dermatology*, December 2006, pages 2697–2706; *Microscopy Research and Technique*, January 2003, pages 107–114; *Nature Medicine*, February 2003, pages 225–229; *Journal of Investigative Dermatology*, March 2002, pages 402–408; *International Journal of Biochemistry and Cell Biology*, July 2004, pages 1141–1146; *Experimental Cell Research*, March 2002, pages 130–137; *Skin Pharmacology and Applied Skin Physiology*, September–October 2002, pages 316–320; and www.signaling-gateway.org). *See* antioxidant and peptide.

cellulose. Primary fiber component of plants. Used in cosmetics as a thickening agent and to bind other ingredients together.

Centaurea cyanus. *See* cornflower.

Centella asiatica. Extract of herb that may be listed on labels as asiatic acid, hydrocotyl, or gotu kola. It has antibacterial, anti-psoriatic, and wound-healing properties (Sources: *International Journal of Lower Extremity Wounds*, September 2006, pages 137–143; *Aesthetic Plastic Surgery*, May–June 2000, pages 227–234; *Phytomedicine*, May 2001, pages 230–235; and *Contact Dermatitis*, October 1993, pages 175–179).

cephalin. Phospholipid. *See* fatty acid and natural moisturizing factor (NMF).

cera alba. Beeswax; used as a thickening agent in cosmetics.

cera microcristallina. *See* petrolatum.

Ceramide 1. *See* ceramides.

Ceramide 3. *See* ceramides.

Ceramide 6-II. *See* ceramides.

ceramides. Naturally occurring skin lipids (fats) that are major structural components of the skin's outer structure. Skin as a barrier system inhibits water movement via its extracellular matrix, which has a unique composition of 50% ceramides, 25% cholesterol, and 15% free fatty acids (Sources: *Journal of Lipid Research*, September 2007; *Journal of Investigative Dermatology*, November 2001, pages 1126–1136; and *Experimental Dermatology*, October 2005, pages 719–726). Ceramides are necessary for the skin's water-retention capacity as well as for cell regulation. Adding ceramides to skin-care products can help to restore the skin's barrier system (Sources: *American Journal of Clinical Dermatology*, June 2005, pages 215–223; *Journal of Dermatological Science*, September 2006, pages 159–169; *Skin Pharmacology and Applied Skin Physiology*, September–October 2001, pages 261–271; and *Cutis*, December 2005, Supplemental, pages 7–12).

ceresin. Derived from clay, ceresin is a waxy ingredient used as a thickening agent in cosmetics. It can be sensitizing for some skin types.

ceteareth-20. Fatty alcohol that is used to thicken cosmetics and keep ingredients mixed together and stable.

cetearyl alcohol. Fatty alcohol used as an emollient, emulsifier, thickener, and carrying agent for other ingredients. Can be derived naturally, as in coconut fatty alcohol, or synthetically.

cetearyl ethylhexanoate. *See* cetearyl alcohol.

cetyl acetate. A mixture of cetyl alcohol and acetic acid used as a skin-conditioning agent and emollient.

cetyl alcohol. Fatty alcohol used as an emollient, emulsifier, thickener, and carrying agent for other ingredients. Can be derived naturally, as in coconut fatty alcohol, or synthetically. It is not an irritant and is not related to sd alcohol or ethyl alcohol.

cetyl dimethicone. Silicone polymer that functions as skin-conditioning agent. *See* silicone.

cetyl esters. Synthetic wax used in cosmetics as a thickening agent and emollient.

cetyl PEG/PPG-10/1-dimethicone. Silicone that functions as a skin-conditioning agent and emulsifier. *See* silicone.

chamomile. Plant species include *Matricaria recutita*, *Chamomilla recutita*, and *Matricaria chamomilla*. Chamomile tea, brewed from dried flower heads, has been used traditionally for medicinal purposes. The main constituents of the flowers include phenolic compounds, primarily the flavonoids apigenin, quercetin, patuletin, luteolin, and their glucosides. The principal components of the essential oil extracted from the flowers are the terpenoids α-bisabolol and its oxides and azulenes, including chamazulene. Chamomile has moderate antioxidant and antimicrobial activities, and significant anti-platelet activity in vitro. Animal model studies indicate it may have potent anti-inflammatory action, some antimutagenic and cholesterol-lowering activities, as well as antispasmodic and anxiolytic effects. However, human studies are limited, and clinical trials examining the purported sedative properties of chamomile tea are absent. Adverse reactions to chamomile, consumed as a tisane or applied topically, have been reported among those with allergies to other plants in the daisy family (Sources: *Phytotherapy Research*, July 2006, pages 519–618; www.herbmed.org; *European Journal of Drug Metabolism and Pharmacokinetics*, October–December 1999, pages 303–308; and *Planta Medica*, October 1994, pages 410–413).

chaparral extract. There is conflicting research about its efficacy as an anticancer agent, though it does contain a component that has antioxidant properties (Source: *Society for Experimental Biology and Medicine*, January 1995, pages 6–12; and www.healthwell.com/healthnotes/). When ingested, it may cause liver toxicity (Sources: *Molecular and Cellular Biochemistry*, June 1999, pages 157–161; *Archives of Internal Medicine*, April 1997, pages 913–919; and www.quackwatch.com/01QuackeryRelatedTopics/OTA/ota04.html). Topically it can have antimicrobial properties (Source: *Journal of Ethnopharmacology*, June 1996, pages 175–177).

charcoal. Primarily carbon substance formed by charring organic material in absence of oxygen. One teaspoonful of Activated Charcoal USP has a surface area of more than 10,000 square feet, which gives charcoal unique absorption properties. It also can disinfect wounds.

chaulmoogra oil. Once the treatment for leprosy worldwide due to its antimicrobial properties (Source: *Proceedings of the National Academy of Sciences*, February 2000, pages 1433–1437). It can be a skin irritant.

chelating agent. Any of numerous ingredients that bind with metal ions or metallic compounds, preventing them from adhering to a surface (such as skin, hair, or clothing) or causing contamination or discoloration, such as in the case of trace amounts of iron. Examples are tetrasodium EDTA and tetrahydroxypropyl ethylenediamine. The EDTA complex is most common because of its broad effectiveness and compatibility with most cosmetic ingredients.

chestnut seed extract. Also known as European chestnut, the extract has a high tannin content, which has astringent and drying properties on skin (Source: *American Herbal Products Association's Botanical Safety Handbook*, CRC Press, LLC, 1997). Chestnut seed has no documented beneficial effect on skin.

China clay. *See* kaolin.

chitosan. Derived from chitin, a polysaccharide found in the exoskeletons of shrimp, lobster, and crabs. It is used widely in pharmaceuticals as a base in formulations. There is also extensive research showing it can be effective in wound healing, as well as having antibacterial and anti-inflammatory properties (Sources: *Journal of Pharmacy and Pharmacology*, November 2002, pages 1453–1459; *Biomaterials*, November 2001, pages 2959–2966; *International Journal of Food Microbiology*, March 2002, pages 65–72; *Journal of Pharmacy and Pharmacology*, August 2001, pages 1047–1067; and *British Journal of Plastic Surgery*, October 2000, pages 601–606). *See* mucopolysaccharide.

chlorella. *See* algae.

chlorhexidine. Topical antiseptic, it can cause irritation (Source: *Toxicology in Vitro*, August–October 2001, pages 271–276).

chlorophene. Used as a preservative in cosmetics.

chlorphenesin. Alcohol used as a preservative in cosmetics.

chloroxylenol. Chemical compound used as a disinfectant and preservative due to its action against certain types of bacteria and fungi.

cholecalciferol. Technical name for vitamin D. *See* vitamin D.

cholesterol. The barrier function of skin depends on the stratum corneum extracellular lipid matrix, which includes ceramides, cholesterol, and free fatty acids. Smaller amounts of cholesterol sulfate and cholesteryl oleate may be present. Cholesterol in cosmetics can help maintain the skin's normal function. It is also a stabilizer, emollient, and water-binding agent (Source: *Journal of Structural Biology*, June 2007, pages 386–400). *See* natural moisturizing factor (NMF).

choline. Part of the vitamin B complex and a constituent of many other biologically important molecules, such as acetylcholine (a neurotransmitter) and lecithin.

chondroitin sulfate. *See* glycosaminoglycans.

Chondrus crispus. Form of red seaweed. *See* algae and carrageenan.

chromium hydroxide green. Earth mineral used as a coloring agent/additive and permanently listed (as of 1977) by the FDA for use in cosmetic products.

chromium oxide green. *See* chromium hydroxide green.

chrysanthemum extract. Can have anti-inflammatory benefit for skin.

***Chrysanthemum parthenium* extract**. *See* feverfew extract.

Cichorium intybus. Source of a plant extract with antioxidant properties (Source: *Archives of Pharmaceutical Research*, October 2001, pages 431–436).

***Cimicifuga racemosa* root extract**. *See* black cohosh.

***Cinnamomum camphora*.** *See* camphor.

***Cinnamomum*.** *See* cinnamon.

cinnamon. Can have antimicrobial and antioxidant properties (Sources: *Cutaneous and Ocular Toxicology*, March 2007, pages 227–233; and *Letters in Applied Microbiology*, January 2002, pages 27–31), but it can also be a skin irritant (Source: *Contact Dermatitis*, October 1993, pages 202–205).

citric acid. Extract derived from citrus and used primarily to adjust the pH of products to prevent them from being too alkaline.

Citrullus colocynthis. Bitter apple; considered a skin irritant.

Citrus amara. *See* orange blossom.

Citrus aurantifolia. *See* lime.

Citrus aurantium. *See* orange blossom.

***Citrus aurantium* extract.** Bitter orange extract. It can have antioxidant properties when eaten (Source: *Journal of Agricultural Food Chemistry*, December 1999, pages 5239–5244); however, used topically its methanol content makes it potentially irritating for skin (Source: *Contact Dermatitis*, January 1992, pages 9–11).

Citrus medica limonium. *See* lemon.

clary oil. Used as fragrance; can be a skin irritant or sensitizer.

clay. *See* bentonite and kaolin.

clove leaf. *See* clove oil.

clove oil. Potent skin irritant and inflammatory when used repeatedly (Sources: IFA—International Federation of Aromatherapists, www.int-fed-aromatherapy.co.uk; www.naturaldatabase.com; and *Contact Dermatitis*, March 2002, pages 141–144). Clove oil contains 73% eugenol, a volatile substance that research has shown causes skin-cell death (Source: *Cell Proliferation*, August 2006, pages 241–248).

clover blossom. Contains eugenol, which can be a skin sensitizer and cause photosensitivity.

clover leaf oil. *See* clover blossom.

cocamide DEA and MEA. *See* alkyloamides and diethanolamine.

cocamidopropyl betaine. One of the more gentle surfactants used in skin-care products. *See* surfactant.

cocamidopropyl hydroxysultaine. Mild surfactant. *See* surfactant.

cocoa butter. Oil extracted from cocoa beans, used as an emollient and with properties similar to those of other nonfragrant plant oils. *See* natural moisturizing factor (NMF).

cocoa extract. Can have potent antioxidant properties (Sources: *Experimental Biology and Medicine*, May 2002, pages 321–329; and *Journal of Agricultural Food Chemistry*, July 2001, pages 3438–3442).

cocoglycerides. Used as an emollient and thickening agent in cosmetics. *See* glyceryl ester.

coconut. Has degreasing and cleansing properties, which is why detergent cleansing agents are frequently derived from coconut oil. *See* surfactant.

coconut oil. Non-volatile plant kernel oil that has emollient properties for skin.

Cocus nucifera. *See* coconut oil.

***Codium tomentosum* extract**. *See* algae.

coenzyme Q10. Also known as ubiquinone, it is a vitamin-like substance present in all human cells and responsible for cell protection and production of the body's energy.

A handful of studies have shown that coenzyme Q10 (CoQ10) may have an effect on skin and the appearance of wrinkles (Sources: *Biofactors*, November 2005, pages 179–185; and *Journal of Cosmetic Dermatology*, March 2006, pages 30–38). However, one study was performed in vitro and the other was not placebo-controlled, so there is no way to tell whether other formulations could net the same results.

There is also research showing that sun exposure depletes the presence of CoQ10 in the skin (Sources: *Journal of Investigative Dermatology*, 2005, volume 125, number 4, pages 12–13; and *Journal of Dermatological Science*, August 2001, Supplement, pages 1–4). This is not surprising because many of the skin's components become diminished on exposure to the sun. The latest research suggests that topical application of CoQ10 has antioxidant and anti-inflammatory effects. As such, it is one of many helpful antioxidants for skin, but it is not the only one or the "best" (Sources: *Journal of Cosmetic Dermatology*, March 2006, pages 30–38; and *Biofactors*, 2003, pages 289–297).

***Coffea arabica* extract**. *Coffea arabica* is the coffee plant, and there is research showing that coffee extract has antioxidant properties (Source: *Journal of Agricultural and Food Chemistry*, June 2002, pages 3751–3756).

***Cola acuminata* seed extract**. *See* kola nut.

Coleus barbatus. Member of the mint family and also known as forskolin; can be a skin irritant. *See* counter-irritant.

collagen. Collagen is a type of protein found extensively throughout the body. It supports skin, internal organs, muscles, bone, and cartilage. There are more than 25 types of collagen that occur naturally in the body. Collagen works in tandem with elastin to give skin its texture, structure, and appearance. Sun damage (extrinsic aging) and aging (intrinsic aging) causes collagen in the skin to deteriorate. As a cosmetic ingredient, collagen is derived from animal sources, but plant derivatives that act like collagen (pseudo-collagen) are also used. In any form, collagen is a good water-binding agent. Collagen in cosmetics, regardless of the source, has never been shown to have a direct effect on producing or building collagen in skin.

collagen amino acid. Amino acids hydrolyzed from collagen. These have good water-binding properties for skin. *See* amino acid and natural moisturizing factor (NMF).

colloidal oatmeal. *See* oatmeal.

colloidal silver. Refers to ground-up silver suspended in solution. *See* silver.

colostrum. The thick, yellowish fluid secreted by the mammary glands prior to and during the first few days after birth, before actual milk is produced by the breast. Colostrum is a highly nutritive substance, loaded with proteins, immune-building substances, and growth factors. Colostrum's primary purpose is to supply antibodies and growth factors to help newborns fight viruses and bacteria and to jump-start the growth of muscle, bone, and tissue. There is some research showing it has benefits when applied topically for wound healing, but there is also research showing that it was not helpful. The source of colostrum in supplements and skin-care products is bovine (Sources: *Journal of Reproductive Immunology*, July 1998, pages 155–167; *Indian Journal of Pediatrics*, July 2005, pages 579–581; *Cells Tissues Organs*, January 2000, pages 92–100; *Australasian Biotechnology*, July–August 1997, pages 223–228; and *Journal of Dermatologic Surgery Oncology*, June 1985, pages 617–622).

coltsfoot. According to *The PDR Family Guide to Natural Medicines & Healing Therapies*, 1998 and a *German Commission E Monograph*, 1998 coltsfoot is potentially carcinogenic due to its pyrrolizidine alkaloid content, and it is not recommended for repeated use on skin.

comfrey extract. Several studies have shown that comfrey extract can have carcinogenic or toxic properties when taken orally. It is a major problem for the body when consumed orally because of pyrrolizidine alkaloids. These compounds occur naturally in every part of the comfrey plant, and are absorbed through the skin, where they cause problems when the liver attempts to metabolize them. It is these metabolites (referred to as pyrroles) that are highly toxic (Sources: www.naturaldatabase.com; *International Journal of Molecular Sciences,* 2002, pages 948–964; and http://www.ansci.cornell.edu/plants/toxicagents/alkaloids/pyrrolizidine.html).

Topical application of comfrey has anti-inflammatory properties, but is recommended only for short-term use and only then if you can be sure the amount of pyrrolizidine alkaloids is less than 100 micrograms per application—something that would be impossible to determine without sophisticated testing equipment, making comfrey an ingredient to avoid. The alkaloid content makes it a potential skin irritant (Sources: *Chemical Research in Toxicology,* November 2001, pages 1546–1551; and *Public Health Nutrition,* December 2000, pages 501–508).

***Commiphora myrrha* extract**. *See* myrrh.

coneflower. Another name for echinacea; has soothing properties.

Copaifera officinalis. *See* balsam peru.

copper gluconate. Copper is an important trace element for human nutrition. The body needs copper to absorb and utilize iron, and copper is also a component of the powerful antioxidant enzyme superoxide dismutase. Copper supplements have been shown to increase superoxide dismutase levels in humans (Source: *Healthnotes Review of Complementary and Integrative Medicine,* www.healthnotes.com). The synthesis of collagen and elastin is in part related to the presence of copper in the body, and copper is also important for many other processes. For example, there is research showing that copper is effective for wound healing and as an antioxidant (Sources: *British Journal of Dermatology,* January 1999, pages 26–34; *Journal of Clinical Investigation,* November 1993, pages 2368–2376; *Biomedical Research on Trace Elements,* 2005, volume 16, number 4, pages 302–305; and *Federation of European Biochemical Sciences Letter,* October 1988, pages 343–346). *See* superoxide dismutase.

copper peptides. *See* copper gluconate.

copper sulfate. Effective for topical wound healing, but there is no research showing it has any impact when used in skin-care products (Source: *American Journal of Physiology Heart Circulation and Physiology,* May 2002, pages 1821–1827).

***Corallina officinalis* extract**. *See* algae.

coriander. Herb and spice plant, the source of a fragrant component; it can be a potential skin irritant (Source: www.naturaldatabase.com). It also may have some antibacterial and antifungal properties, but these properties have not been established for topical use on skin (Source: *Journal of Food Protection,* July 2001, pages 1019–1024).

corn oil. Emollient oil with properties similar to those of other nonfragrant plant oils (Source: *British Journal of Dermatology,* June 1994, pages 757–764).

cornflower. Can have anti-inflammatory properties (Source: *Journal of Ethnopharmacology,* December 1999, pages 235–241).

cornmint. Also known as wild mint; it can be a skin irritant. *See* counter-irritant.

cornstarch. Starch obtained from corn and sometimes used as an absorbent in cosmetics instead of talc. However, when cornstarch becomes moist, it can promote fungal and bacterial growth (Source: www.radiation-oncology.com/homecare/html/skin_13.htm).

***Cornus* extract**. *See* dogwood.

Corylus americana. *See* hazelnut oil.

Corylus avellana. *See* hazelnut oil.

coumarin. Organic compound found in plants and derived from the amino acid phenylalanine. It creates the fragrance in fresh-mowed hay. More than 300 coumarins have been identified from natural sources, especially green plants. These varying substances have disparate pharmacological, biochemical, and therapeutic applications. However, simple coumarins are potent antioxidants (Sources: *Journal of Natural Products*, September 2001, pages 1238–1240; *Chemistry and Physics of Lipids*, December 1999, pages 125–135; and *General Pharmacology*, June 1996, pages 713–722).

counter-irritant. Ingredients such as menthol, peppermint, camphor, and mint are counter-irritants (Sources: *Archives of Dermatologic Research*, May 1996, pages 245–248; and Code of Federal Regulations Title 21—Food and Drugs, revised April 1, 2001, CITE: 21CFR310.545, www.fda.gov). Counter-irritants are used to induce local inflammation for the purpose of relieving inflammation in deeper or adjacent tissues. In other words, they substitute one kind of inflammation for another, which is never good for skin. Irritation or inflammation, no matter what causes it or how it happens, impairs the skin's immune and healing response (Source: *Skin Pharmacology and Applied Skin Physiology*, November–December 2000, pages 358–371). And although your skin may not show it or doesn't react in an irritated fashion, if you apply irritants to your skin the damage is still taking place and is ongoing, so it adds up over time (Source: *Skin Research and Technology*, November 2001, pages 227–237).

cranberry seed extract. Extract of the cranberry fruit. Natural components known as proanthocyanidins are responsible for this extract's antioxidant and anti-inflammatory properties (Source: www.naturaldatabase.com).

cranberry seed oil. Extract derived from the seed of this red berry; the oil (which is not red) has potent antioxidant ability because it is a rich source of polyphenols (Source: *Journal of Agricultural and Food Chemistry*, November 2, 2005, pages 8485—8491). *See* antioxidant.

***Crataegus monogina* extract**. *See* hawthorn extract.

creatinine. Compound formed by the metabolism of the amino acid creatine. Creatine resides primarily in muscle tissue and blood and is normally excreted in the urine as creatinine. Both creatine and creatinine are cell-signaling ingredients in the body. Theoretically, they should perform a similar function when applied topically, but there is no research to support this. Research on oral supplementation with creatinine has had mixed or unimpressive results, particularly for those who take it to build lean muscle mass (Source: www.naturaldatabase.com).

cucumber extract. Claims of cucumber having anti-inflammatory or soothing properties are anecdotal, as there is no research to support this contention.

***Cucumis sativus* extract**. *See* cucumber extract.

***Curcuma longa* root**. *See* turmeric.

curcumin. Potent antioxidant and anti-inflammatory spice that can be effective in wound healing (Sources: *Biochemical Pharmacology*, August 2007; *Journal of Trauma*, November 2001, pages 927–931; and *Advances in Experimental Medicine and Biology*, 2007, pages 1–595). *See* turmeric.

Cyamopsis tetragonoloba. *See* guar gum.

cyanocobalamin. *See* vitamin B12.

cyclamen aldehyde. Synthetic fragrant component in products; it can be a skin irritant.

cyclohexasiloxane. *See* silicone.

cyclomethicone. Silicone with a drier finish than dimethicone. *See* silicone.
cyclopentasiloxane. *See* silicone.
Cymbopogon citrates. *See* lemongrass extract.
Cymbopogon martini. *See* geranium extract.
cysteine. *See* amino acid.
cystine. *See* amino acid.
cytochrome. Protein found in blood cells that, with the aid of enzymes, serves a vital function in the transfer of energy within cells. There are three types of cytochromes, indicated by A, B, or C, with cytochrome C being the most stable. However, because cytochromes require a complex process that is triggered by a sequence of other components to be effective in their function of cellular respiration, they serve no function alone when applied topically on skin.
cytokines. Diverse, potent, and extremely complex chemical messengers secreted by the cells of the immune system. They stimulate the production of other substances to help protect the body. Cytokines encourage cell growth, promote cell activation, direct cellular traffic, and destroy target cells—including cancer cells. Interleukins, transforming growth factor, and interferon are types of cytokines. It is also important to note that cytokines can also have unwanted, potentially serious side effects (Sources: www.medlineplus.com; and the National Cancer Institute, www.nci.nih.gov or www.cancer.gov).
D&C. According to the FDA, D&C is an identification that indicates a coloring agent has been approved as safe in drug and cosmetics products, but it does not apply to food.
daisy flower extract. There is no research showing this extract has any benefit for skin. Also known as tansy, it can cause severe contact dermatitis and is considered unsafe for topical application (Source: www.naturaldatabase.com).
dandelion extract. Can be a potent allergen (Source: *Archives of Dermatology*, January 1999, pages 67–70).
Daucus carota. Also known as wild carrot. It can have antioxidant properties, but applied topically it can cause dermatitis (Source: www.naturaldatabase.com).
DEA. *See* diethanolamine.
DEA oleth-10 phosphate. Used as an emulsifying agent, which is a group of ingredients essential to most cosmetic formulations because they can keep unlike ingredients mixed together smoothly (a prime example is oil and water).
Dead Sea minerals. Several studies demonstrate that Dead Sea minerals can have a positive effect on psoriatic skin (Sources: *Israel Journal of Medical Sciences*, November 2001, pages 828–832; *British Journal of Dermatology*, June 2001, pages 1154–1160; *International Journal of Dermatology*, February 2001, pages 158–159; and *Journal of the American Academy of Dermatology*, August 2000, pages 325–326). Psoriasis is a skin condition characterized by rapidly dividing, overactive skin cells. No one is quite sure how the Dead Sea minerals and salts affect psoriasis. One of the more popular theories regarding their benefit is that the mineral content of the water slows down the out-of-control cell division. Some research indicates that the benefit is cumulative and that the results can last for up to five months. However, there is no research showing that these minerals have any effect on wrinkles, dry skin, or acne.
decyl glucoside. Used as a gentle detergent cleansing agent. *See* surfactant.
dehydroepiandrosterone. *See* DHEA.

deionized/demineralized water. Filtered water used in cosmetics. All water used in cosmetic formulations goes through this process to remove components that could interfere with a product's stability and performance.

denatured alcohol. *See* alcohol.

deoxyribonucleic acid. *See* DNA.

detergent cleansing agent. *See* surfactant.

deuterium oxide. *See* heavy water.

dextran. Polysaccharide that has water-binding properties for skin. *See* also mucopolysaccharide.

dextrin. Carbohydrate that is classified as a polysaccharide. It is used as an adhesive when mixed with water. For skin it can have water-binding properties.

DHA. *See* dihydroxyacetone.

DHEA. Also called prasterone and dehydroepiandrosterone, DHEA is a naturally occurring prohormone that is converted in the body primarily to androgens (male hormones), and to a lesser degree to estrogens. It is controversial as an oral supplement because long-term use has been associated with women developing secondary masculine traits, liver damage, disrupted menstrual cycles, and defects in fetuses. More superficial risks include hair loss, acne, and weight gain. Topically, it is possible that DHEA can increase collagen production and prevent collagen destruction by decreasing matrix metalloproteinases (MMP), but the research about this is extremely limited and the studies that do exist were performed only on a handful of people (Sources: *Drug Delivery*, September–October 2005, pages 275–280; *Journal of Endocrinology*, November 2005, pages 169–196; *Journal of Investigative Dermatology*, November 2005, pages 1053–1062, and February 2004, pages 315–323; *Gynecological Endocrinology*, December 2002, pages 431–441; www.fda.gov; and www.mayoclinic.com/health/dhea/NS_patient-dhea).

diatomaceous earth. Light-colored porous rock composed of the skeletons of minute sea creatures called diatoms. Typically used as an abrasive material in scrub products.

diazolidinyl urea. Formaldehyde-releasing preservative (Source: *Contact Dermatitis*, December 2000, pages 339–343). *See* formaldehyde-releasing preservative.

dibutyl phthalate. Very common ingredient in almost every nail polish and synthetic fragrance sold today. It is used as a plasticizer and is a key component in giving nail polish its unique properties. The Centers for Disease Control and Prevention (CDC, www.cdc.gov) published the *National Report on Human Exposure to Environmental Chemicals—Results for Mono-butyl phthalate* [which is] *(metabolized from Dibutyl phthalate)*. The report noted that measurable levels of phthalate were found in the urine of the participants in the study. However, the CDC also stated that "Finding a measurable amount of one or more phthalate metabolites in urine does not mean that the level of one or more phthalates causes an adverse health effect. Whether phthalates at the levels of metabolites reported here are a cause for health concern is not yet known; more research is needed" (Sources: Centers for Disease Control and Prevention, www.cdc.gov/nceh/dls/report/results/Mono-butylPhthalate.htm; and *Environmental Health Perspectives*, December 2000, volume 108, issue 12). In animal tests, dibutyl phthalate has been shown to produce detrimental effects. The Environmental Working Group (EWG, www.ewg.org), an environmental research organization, found that "DBP is a developmental and reproductive toxin that in lab animals causes a broad range of birth defects and lifelong reproductive impairment in males [when] exposed in utero and shortly after birth. DBP damages the testes, prostate gland, epididymis, penis, and seminal vesicles. These effects persist throughout the animal's life." At this time, there is no conclusive or agreed-upon research pointing to phthalates being a problem for humans.

diethanolamine. Colorless liquid used as a solvent and pH adjuster. Also used as a lather agent in skin- and hair-care products when coupled with a foaming or detergent cleansing agent. In 1999 the National Toxicology Program (NTP) completed a study that found an association between cancer and tumors in laboratory animals and the application of diethanolamine (DEA) and certain DEA-related ingredients to their skin (Sources: Study #TR-478, Toxicology and Carcinogenesis Studies of Diethanolamine, CAS No. 111-42-2, July 1999—http://ntp-server.niehs.nih.gov/; and *Food Chemistry and Toxicology*, January 2004, pages 127–134). For the DEA-related ingredients, the NTP study suggested that the carcinogenic response is linked to possible residual levels of DEA. However, the NTP study did not establish a link between DEA and the risk of cancer in humans. According to the FDA (Source: *Office of Cosmetics and Colors Fact Sheet*, December 9, 1999), "Although DEA itself is used in very few cosmetics, DEA-related ingredients (e.g., oleamide DEA, lauramide DEA, cocamide DEA) are widely used in a variety of cosmetic products. These ingredients function as emulsifiers or foaming agents and are generally used at levels of 1% to 5%. The FDA takes these NTP findings very seriously and is in the process of carefully evaluating the studies and test data to determine the real risk, if any, to consumers. The Agency believes that at the present time there is no reason for consumers to be alarmed based on the usage of these ingredients in cosmetics. Consumers wishing to avoid cosmetics containing DEA or its conjugates may do so by reviewing the ingredient statement required to appear on the outer container label of cosmetics offered for retail sale to consumers." A study from 1999 on the potential effects of DEA involved applying a pure concentration of this ingredient directly to mouse skin for a period of 14 weeks (minimum) and 2 years (maximum). The study reported no evidence of carcinogenicity when low doses (50–100 mg per kilogram of body weight) were used. Internal changes to organs (liver, kidneys) and external signs (inflammation, ulcers) were found as the dosages of DEA increased (up to 800 mg was used) (Source: *National Toxicology Program Technical Report Service*, volume 478, July 1999, pages 134–212). Although the results of this study are interesting, it is still unrelated to how DEA is used in cosmetics products and how consumers use them. In most instances, our contact with DEA in any form is brief, and most likely is not cause for alarm.

diethylhexyl malate. Emollient and skin-conditioning agent derived from the solvent ethyl hexanediol.

dihydroxyacetone. Ingredient present in all self-tanners that affects the color of skin. Derived from sugar, it reacts with amino acids found in the top layers of skin to create a shade of brown; the effect takes place within two to six hours and it can build color depth with every reapplication. It has a long history of safe use.

diisopropyl adipate. Used as a film-forming agent, emollient, and skin-conditioning agent.

diisostearoyl trimethylolpropane siloxy silicate. Skin-conditioning agent in the silicone family. *See* silicone.

dimethicone. *See* silicone.

dimethicone copolyol. *See* silicone.

dimethicone crosspolymer. Silicone derivative used as a stabilizing or suspending agent or as a thickener. *See* silicone.

dimethiconol. *See* silicone.

dimethyl capramide. Functions as a stabilizer and solvent in cosmetics.

dimethyl ether. Colorless gas used as a propellant in aerosol products. It is toxic if inhaled and can be irritating to skin (Source: *Handbook of Cosmetic and Personal Care Additives*, Second Edition, volume 2, 2002, Synapse Information Resources, Inc.).

dimethyl MEA. *See* dimethylaminoethanol (DMAE).

dimethylaminoethanol (DMAE). What little research there is about DMAE relates to its effect as an oral supplement, and the findings are mixed. DMAE, known chemically as 2-dimethyl-amino-ethanol, has been available in Europe under the product name Deanol for over 30 years. As an oral supplement it is popularly known for improving mental alertness, much like *Ginkgo biloba* and coenzyme Q10. However, the research about DMAE does not show the same positive results found with the other two supplements. Because DMAE is chemically similar to choline, it is thought to stimulate production of acetylcholine, and because acetylcholine is a brain neurotransmitter, it's easy to see how it could be associated with brain function. However, only a handful of studies have looked at DMAE for that purpose and they have not been conclusive in the least, while some have shown that DMAE may be problematic or not very effective (Sources: *Mechanisms of Aging and Development*, February 1988, pages 129–138; *Neuropharmacology*, June 1989, pages, 557–561; and *European Neurology*, 1991, pages 423–425). Despite the lack of evidence supporting any claim that DMAE has any effect on skin, there are hundreds of Web sites claiming that it does. It is possible that DMAE can help protect the cell membrane, and keeping cells intact can have benefit, but so far that appears to be only conjecture, not fact.

A study published in *The British Journal of Dermatology* (May 2007) has shown contrary evidence that it may actually pose risks for the skin. In vitro tests of the pure substance, as well as tests of creams that contain DMAE, demonstrated a fairly fast and significant increase in protective elements around the skin cell. However, a short time later the researchers observed a significant decrease in cell growth and in some cases they found that it had halted cell growth altogether.

Dioscorea villosa **extract**. *See* wild yam extract.

dipentaerythrityl hexacaprylate/hexacaprate. Mixture of fatty acids used as an emollient and thickening agent.

dipotassium glycyrrhizinate. *See* anti-irritant and licorice extract.

di-PPG-3 myristyl ether adipate. Derivative of myristyl alcohol (a fatty alcohol) and adipic acid (a buffering and neutralizing ingredient). It is used as a skin-conditioning agent and solvent in cosmetics.

disodium cocoamphodiacetate. Mild detergent cleansing agent. *See* surfactant.

disodium diglyceryl phosphate. Used as an emollient and thickening agent in cosmetics. *See* glyceryl ester.

disodium EDTA. *See* EDTA.

disodium glyceryl phosphate. Used as an emollient and thickening agent in cosmetics. *See* glyceryl ester.

disodium lauraminopropionate. A mild surfactant. *See* surfactant.

disodium rutinyl disulfate. No research shows this antioxidant has any impact on cellulite.

disteardimonium hectorite. Used as a suspending agent, often with pigments.

DMAE. *See* dimethylaminoethanol (DMAE).

DMDM hydantoin. Formaldehyde-releasing preservative (Source: Household and Personal Products Industry, May 2001, "Preserving Personal Care and Household Products"). *See* formaldehyde-releasing preservative.

DNA. Abbreviation for deoxyribonucleic acid. DNA is found in all cells. It is the primary component of genes—and genes are the means by which cells transmit hereditary characteristics. DNA is the basis for all genetic structure; its components include adenine (A), guanine (G), thymine (T), and cytosine (C). It is the mapping of these substances that makes up the genetic code of all human traits and cellular functions. DNA is also the genetic material that is required for all cellular division and growth. Including DNA in a skin-care product is pointless because it cannot in and of itself affect a cell's genetic elements. The formation of DNA is a complex process within the cell that requires a multitude of proteins and enzymes for it to have an effect on the body's genetic material. It is also doubtful that you would want to ever put anything on your skin that could affect genetic material, particularly via a cosmetic for which there are no safety or efficacy regulations. Beyond that, any successful attempt to affect what DNA does would potentially create a significant risk of cancer.

docosahexaenoic acid. *See* fatty acid.

dog rose. *See* rose hip.

dogwood. There is a small amount of research showing that dogwood has antioxidant and anti-inflammatory properties (Source: *Journal of Agricultural Food Chemistry*, April 2002, pages 2519–2523).

dong quai. Latin name *Angelica polymorpha sinensis*, is an herb that has been shown in some studies to have estrogenic activity and a positive effect in mitigating menopausal and pre-menopausal symptoms, although several other studies disprove this (Sources: *Archives of Gynecology and Obsterics*, November 2007, pages 463–469; *Journal of the American Pharmaceutical Association*, March–April 2000, pages 327–329; and *Fertility and Sterility*, December 1997, pages 981–986). There is also research showing that it can stimulate the growth of breast cancer cells (Source: *Menopause*, March–April 2002, pages 145–150) and research indicating it has antioxidant properties (Source: *Journal of Agricultural Food Chemistry*, May 2007, pages 3358–3362). There are no studies showing that dong quai has any effect topically on skin.

***Dromiceius* oil.** *See* emu oil.

dulse. *See* algae.

***Durvillaea antarctica* extract**. Extract derived from a species of algae (*Durvillea antarctica*). *See* algae.

ecamsule. *See* Mexoryl SX.

ectoin. Skin-conditioning agent that also functions in cosmetics as a stabilizer. There is limited research demonstrating that ectoin helps protect skin from UVA damage and has efficacy and application characteristics that women tend to prefer in moisturizers. However, the research did not reveal to what the effects of ectoin were compared, or whether or not other ingredients (such as green tea or pomegranate extracts) may provide even better protection from environmental damage (Sources: *Skin Pharmacology and Physiology*, May 2007, pages 211–218, and September/October 2004, pages 232–237).

EDTA. Acronym for ethylenediaminetetraacetic acid, a stabilizer used in cosmetics to prevent ingredients in a given formula from binding with trace elements (particularly minerals) that can exist in water and with other ingredients to cause unwanted product changes to the texture, the odor, and the consistency. The technical term for ingredients that perform this function is chelating agent.

egg yolk. Egg yolk is mostly water and lipids (fats), especially cholesterol, which makes it a good emollient and water-binding agent for skin.

eicosapentaenoic acid. Fatty acid derived from salmon oil; it is a good emollient for skin. It has also been shown to inhibit collagen breakdown and improve cell function (Sources: *European Journal of Dermatology*, July-August 2007, pages 284–291; and *Journal of Lipid Research*, May 2006, pages 921–930). *See* fatty acid.

Elaeis guineensis. *See* palm oil.

elastin. Major component of skin that gives it flexibility. Sun damage causes elastin in skin to deteriorate. Elastin can be derived from both plant and animal sources and is used in cosmetics as a good water-binding agent. Elastin in cosmetics has never been shown to affect the elastin in skin or to have any other benefit, although it most likely functions as a water-binding agent.

elderberry. Has potent antioxidant properties (Source: *Free Radical Biology and Medicine*, July 2000, pages 51–60).

elecampane. Latin name *Inula helenium*; it is a plant that can be very irritating to the skin and can trigger allergic reactions (Source: *Contact Dermatitis*, October 2001, pages 197–204).

emollient. Supple, waxlike, lubricating, thickening agents that prevent water loss and have a softening and soothing effect on the skin. Please refer to Chapter Two, *Healthy Skin: Rules to Live By*, for additional information.

emu oil. The emu is a large, flightless bird indigenous to Australia, and emu oil has become an important component of the Australian economy. As a result there is research from that part of the world showing it to be a good emollient that can help heal skin; however, there is no research showing it has any anti-aging or anti-wrinkling effects. Emu oil's reputation is driven mostly by cosmetics company claims and not by any real proof that emu oil is an essential requirement for skin.

English ivy extract. Can be a skin irritant due to its stimulant and astringent (skin-constricting) properties (Source: www.naturaldatabase.com).

ensulizole. Sunscreen agent, formerly known as phenylbenzimidazole sulfonic acid. Ensulizole is the established name that must be used on sunscreen labels (Source: www.fda.gov). It is primarily a UVB-protecting sunscreen agent, providing only minimal UVA protection. Ensulizole protects the skin from wavelengths of UV light in the range 290 to 340 nanometers, whereas the UVA range is 320 to 400 nanometers (Source: United States Pharmacopeia (USP), http://www.uspdqi.org/pubs/monographs/sunscreen_agents.pdf). For complete protection, this ingredient (as well as many other UVB-protecting sunscreen ingredients) must be paired with the UVA-protecting ingredients avobenzone (also called Parsol 1789 and butyl methoxydibenzoylmethane), titanium dioxide, zinc oxide, or Mexoryl SX; outside the United States it can also be paired with Tinosorb. Because ensulizole is water-soluble, it has the unique characteristic of feeling lighter on skin. As such, it is often used in sunscreen lotions or moisturizers whose aesthetic goal is a non-greasy finish (Source: www.emedicine.com/derm/topic510.htm).

***Enteromorpha compressa* extract**. Extract from green algae. *See* algae.

enzymes. Vast group of protein molecules, produced by all living things, that act as catalysts in chemical and biological reactions, including photosynthesis, helping cells communicate, inhibiting free-radical damage, and much more. Enzymes are used in skin-care products to facilitate exfoliation, to help overall biological processes in skin that have slowed down because of age or sun damage, and to inhibit free-radical damage. Enzymes accelerate biochemical reactions in a cell that would proceed minimally or not at all if the enzymes weren't present. Most enzymes are finicky about how and under what conditions they will act. Sometimes several enzymes are required to carry out a particular chemical reaction, and their actions are affected by temperature and pH. Some enzymes depend on the presence of other enzymes, called coenzymes, to function, or they depend on a specific body temperature. It would require an exceptionally complicated process to stimulate enzyme activity via topical application to the skin. Enzymes are divided into six main categories, including oxidoreductases, transferases, hydrolases, lyases, isomerases, and ligases. The names of most individual enzymes end in –ase. *See* bromelain, papain, and oxidoreductases.

epidermal growth factor (EGF). Stimulates cell division of many different cell types. There is research showing it to be helpful for wound and burn healing (Sources: *Journal of Controlled Release*, April 2007, pages 169–176; *Journal of Burn Care and Rehabilitation*, March–April 2002, pages 116–125; and *Journal of Dermatologic Surgery and Oncology*, July 1992, pages 604–606). There is also research showing that its effect is no different from that of a placebo and that it may not be effective at all (Sources: *The British Journal of Surgery*, February 2003, pages 133–146; *Wounds*, 2001, volume 13, number 2, pages 53–58; and *Plastic and Reconstructive Surgery*, August 1995, pages 251–254). It can have anti-inflammatory properties when applied to skin (Source: *Skin Pharmacology and Applied Skin Physiology*, January-April 1999, pages 79–84), although it also can promote tumor growth (Source: *Journal of Surgical Research*, April 2002, pages 175–182). In general, the potentially frightening consequences of growth factors can come into play when they are taken internally, as in certain cancer treatments (interleukin and interferon are growth factors), because they can be highly mitogenic (causing cell division), and at certain concentrations and lengths of application can cause cells to overproliferate. This overabundance of cells causes problems, one result of which is cancer. No one is exactly certain what happens when EGFs are applied to healthy, intact skin, but there is concern that with repeated use EGFs can cause skin cells to overproduce, and that's not good (psoriasis is an example of what happens when skin cells overproduce).

All of the research that does exist on EGFs has primarily studied their short-term use for wound healing. *See* human growth factor.

***Epilobium angustifolium* extract.** Extract derived from a plant commonly known as fireweed or willow herb. Can have antimicrobial (Source: *Il Farmaco*, May–July 2001, pages 345–348) and anti-irritant properties for skin (Source: *Journal of Agricultural Food Chemistry*, October 1999, pages 3954–3962).

epigallocatechin-3-gallate. *See* green tea.

***Equisetum arvense*.** *See* horsetail extract.

ergocalciferol. Technical name for vitamin D. *See* vitamin D.

ergothioneine. Component of animal tissue that has potent antioxidant properties (Sources: *Journal of Cosmetic Dermatology*, September 2007, pages 183–188; *Biomedicine and Pharmacotherapy*, September 2006, pages 453–457; and *Food and Chemical Toxicology*, November 1999, pages 1043–1053).

***Eriobotrya japonica*.** *See* loquat extract.

erythropoietin (Epo). Stimulates the growth of cells that carry oxygen throughout the body (Source: *Melanoma Research*, August 2006, pages 275–283). *See* human growth factor.

erythrulose. Substance chemically similar to the self-tanning agent dihydroxyacetone. Depending on your skin color, there can be a difference in the color effect with erythrulose. However, dihydroxyacetone completely changes the color of skin within two to six hours, while erythrulose needs about two to three days for the skin to show a color change.

escin. Extract derived from horse chestnut (*Aesculus hippocastanum*), this ingredient has been prescribed as an oral supplement to reduce some symptoms of chronic vein insufficiency, such as varicose veins, pain, tiredness, tension, swelling in the legs, itching, and edema. However, because horse chestnut contains significant amounts of the toxin esculin, it can be lethal, and some experts recommend not using it. When applied topically, however, there is research showing that a gel containing 2% escin can improve circulation. Results from another study showed a reduction in inflammation in sports injuries when escin was combined with heparin (a mucopolysaccharide used as an anti-clotting medication) and a form of salicylic acid (diethylammonium salicylate). Escin is also a potent antioxidant. As a skin-care ingredient escin clearly has a place, but as for improving cellulite that's an entirely different story. While it may seem logical that blood flow and cellulite are related, the research just isn't there to support the notion (or your thighs). Plus, cellulite products contain far less of this ingredient than the amount used in the studies (Sources: *British Journal of Sports Medicine*, 36 June 2002, pages 183–188; *Angiology*, March 2000, pages 197–205; www.naturaldatabase.com; *Archives of Dermatology*, November 1998, pages 1356–1360; and *International Journal of Cosmetic Science*, December 1999, page 437).

esculin. Component of horse chestnut, it is considered a toxin and is not recommended for skin (Source: *Clinical Pharmacology*, 2002, http://cponline.hitchcock.org/).

essential oil. *See* volatile oils.

ester. A compound formed from the reaction between an alcohol and an acid via the elimination of water. Triesters (groups of three esters) form the backbone of many fats, waxes, and oils that have emollient and skin-conditioning properties (Source: *A Dictionary of Chemistry*, Third Edition, Oxford Paperback, 1996). Almost all of the esters used in cosmetic products are non-irritating and in most cases are quite beneficial for dry skin.

Ester-C. Trade name for a combination form of vitamin C that contains mainly calcium ascorbate, but in addition contains small amounts of the vitamin C metabolites dehydroascorbic acid (oxidized ascorbic acid), calcium threonate, and trace levels of xylonate and lyxonate. The manufacturer of this ingredient states that the metabolites, especially threonate, increase the bioavailability of the vitamin C in the product, and that they performed a study in humans demonstrating the increased bioavailability of vitamin C in Ester-C. However, this study has not been published in a peer-reviewed journal. There is a small, in vitro study that supports the notion that Ester-C is more potent than ascorbic acid by itself (Source: *Medical Science Monitor*, October 2007, pages 205–210). A small published study of vitamin C bioavailability in eight women and one man found no difference between Ester-C and commercially available ascorbic acid tablets with respect to the absorption and excretion of vitamin C (Source: *The Bioavailability of Different Forms of Vitamin C*, The Linus Pauling Institute, Oregon State University, www.orst.edu/dept/lpi/ss01/bioavailability.html). There also are studies that show no difference when comparing the effects of Ester-C with those of ascorbic acid (Source: *Biochemical Pharmacology*, June 1996, pages 1719–1725).

estradiol. One of the three main forms of estrogen produced by the body; the other two are estrone and estriol. Estradiol is the most physiologically active form of estrogen. Many hormone replacement therapy (HRT) and birth-control prescription drugs contain estradiol. One study revealed that topical application of estradiol has photoprotective properties due to its anti-inflammatory nature, while another small-scale study showed that topical application of 0.01% estradiol had collagen-stimulating effects on postmenopausal skin (Sources: *Proceedings of the National Academy of Sciences of the United States of America*, August 22, 2006, pages 12837–12842; and *European Journal of Obstetrics, Gynecology, and Reproductive Biology*, February 2007, pages 202–205). However, as a component of estrogen, it is not without its risks and unknowns.

Decreased production of estrogen by the ovaries can lead to symptoms such as hot flashes, night sweats, vaginal dryness, urinary tract infections, depression, and irritability. With a physician's prescription, licensed pharmacists may make a combination of natural estrogens. Whether or not natural estrogens are safe has not been well-researched.

Although HRT can prevent associated problems with loss of estrogen in perimenopausal and menopausal women, it is no longer being prescribed without caution because of studies that show there is an increased risk of breast cancer, heart attacks, strokes, gall bladder disease, and blood clots (Source: *Annals of Internal Medicine*, www.acponline.org/journals/annals/hrt.htm).

Topically, according to the FDA (www.fda.gov), "The estrogen content of an OTC product, be it a drug or a drug as well as cosmetic, may not exceed 10,000 IU per ounce, and users must be directed to limit the amount of product applied daily so that no more than 20,000 IU of estrogen or equivalent be used per month. Some estrogen-containing products have been claiming to prevent or reduce wrinkles, treat seborrhea, or stimulate hair growth. The Advisory Review Panel on OTC Miscellaneous External Drug Products has concluded that there are inadequate data to establish the safety of these products and that they are ineffective and may therefore be misbranded, even if marketed as cosmetics without making medicinal claims ... In a Final Rule, published in the *Federal Register* of September 9, 1993, 58 FR 47608, the FDA accepted this panel's recommendation and determined that all topically-applied hormone containing drug products for OTC human use are not generally recognized as safe and effective and are misbranded."

ethanol. *See* alcohol.

ethoxydiglycol. *See* solvent.

ethyl alcohol. *See* alcohol.

ethyl macadamiate. Mixture of fatty acids from macadamia nut oil. *See* fatty acid and macadamia nut oil.

ethyl vanillin. Flavoring agent derived from vanilla. It has antioxidant properties (Source: *Journal of Agricultural and Food Chemistry*, April 2004, pages 1872–1881).

ethylhexyl stearate. *See* stearic acid.

ethylparaben. *See* parabens.

eucalyptus extract. Extract that may have antibacterial, antifungal, and antiviral properties on the skin (Source: *Skin Pharmacology and Applied Skin Physiology*, January–February 2000, pages 60–64). It also may be a skin irritant, particularly on abraded skin (Sources: *Clinical Experimental Dermatology*, March 1995, pages 143–145; and www.alternativedr.com/conditions/ConsHerbs/Eucalyptusch.html). *See* counter-irritant.

eucalyptus oil. *See* eucalyptus extract.

Eugenia aromatica. *See* clove oil.

Eugenia caryophyllus. *See* clove oil.

eugenol. *See* clove oil and methyleugenol.

Euphrasia officinalis. *See* eyebright.

evening primrose oil. Can have significant anti-inflammatory and emollient benefits for skin (Sources: *Surgeon*, February 2005, pages 7–10; *Skin Pharmacology and Applied Skin Physiology*, January–February 2002, pages 20–25; and *Journal of Agricultural Food Chemistry*, September 2001, pages 4502–4507). However, whether or not evening primrose oil can mitigate certain symptoms of premenstrual syndrome (PMS) is unknown. "Trials of evening primrose oil have also had conflicting results; the two most rigorous studies showed no evidence of benefit" (Source: *Journal of the American College of Nutrition*, February 2000, pages 3–12). *See* gamma linolenic acid.

Ext. D&C. Type of coloring agent. According to the FDA (www.fda.gov), when Ext. D&C is followed by a color, it means that the color is certified as safe for use only in drugs and cosmetics to be used externally, but not around the eyes or mouth. It is not safe for foods.

eyebright. A plant; although the name sounds like it would be beneficial for the eye area, there are no studies demonstrating it has any benefit for the eye area or skin. The information about this plant's effect on the skin or the eye is strictly anecdotal and ophthalmic use may be harmful (Source: www.naturaldatabase.com).

faex. A type of yeast. *See* yeast.

***Fagus sylvatica* extract**. *See* yeast.

farnesol. Extract of plants that is used in cosmetics primarily for fragrance. A few animal studies and some in vitro research investigated farnesol's antibacterial properties (Source: *Chemotherapy*, July 2002, pages 122–128), and it may also have some antioxidant properties (Source: *Journal of Bacteriology*, September 1998, pages 4460–4465), but there is no research showing it has any benefit on skin.

farnesyl acetate. *See* farnesol.

fatty acid. Substance typically found in plant and animal lipids (fat). Fatty acids include compounds such as glycerides, sterols, and phospholipids. They are used in cosmetics as emollients, thickening agents, and, when mixed with glycerin, cleansing agents. Fatty acids are natural components of skin and are components of a complex mixture that makes up the outermost layer that protects the body against oxidative damage (Sources: *Free Radical Research*, April 2002, pages 471–477; and *Journal of Lipid Research*, May 2002, pages 794–804). Fatty acids can help supplement the skin's intercellular matrix. *See* natural moisturizing factor (NMF).

fatty alcohol. Made from fatty acids; fatty alcohols are used in cosmetics as thickening agents and emollients. They are not drying or irritating forms of alcohol. *See* fatty acid.

FD&C. Type of coloring agent. According to the FDA, when FD&C is followed by a color, the color is certified as safe for use in food, drugs, and cosmetics.

fennel oil. Volatile, fragrant oil that can cause skin irritation and sensitivity. *See* fennel seed extract.

fennel seed extract. Can have antioxidant properties, but on skin it can be a skin irritant and photosensitizer (Source: www.naturaldatabase.com).

ferric ammonium ferrocyanide. Inorganic salt of ferric ferrocyanide. *See* ferric ferrocyanide.

ferric ferrocyanide. Also known as Iron Blue, a coloring agent used in cosmetic products, including those designed for use around the eye. Permanently listed (since 1978) by the FDA as safe, although the EPA considers it toxic when found in water systems.

Ferula galbaniflua. *See* galbanum.

feverfew extract. Can be very irritating to the skin and can trigger allergic reactions (Source: *Contact Dermatitis*, October 2001, pages 197–204). However, when taken orally it has been shown to relieve migraines and have anti-inflammatory properties (Source: www.naturaldatabase.com).

fibroblast growth factor (FGF). Within the body, stimulates growth of the nervous system and bone formation. *See* human growth factor.

fibronectin. Type of protein found in the skin's intercellular matrix, similar to collagen and elastin. Fibronectin's deterioration from sun damage and other factors is an element in skin aging and wrinkling. As is true for all proteins, regardless of their origin, it is probably a good water-binding agent for skin. However, applying fibronectin topically on skin doesn't help reinforce or rebuild the fibronectin in your skin.

***Ficus carica* fruit extract**. *See* fig.

fig. Fruit that contains psoralens, which are compounds that may cause photodermatitis. Topical application can cause contact dermatitis. Latex from the fruit is used topically to treat skin tumors and warts, which has nothing to do with anti-aging (Source: www.naturaldatabase.com).

Filipendula glaberrima. Also known as Nakai, the root of this plant extract has been shown in vitro to be not only a potent antioxidant but also able to inhibit the expression of collagen-depleting MMP-1 when applied to human fibroblast cells (Source: *Journal of Cosmetic Science*, January/February 2007, pages 19-32). *See* matrix metalloproteinases.

Filipendula rubra. *See* meadowsweet extract.

film-forming agent. Large group of ingredients that are typically found in hair-care products, but that are also widely used in skin-care products, particularly moisturizers. Film-forming agents include PVP, acrylates, acrylamides, and copolymers. When applied they leave a pliable, cohesive, and continuous covering over the hair or skin. This film has water-binding properties and leaves a smooth feel on skin. Film-forming agents can be weak skin sensitizers (Source: *Contact Dermatitis*, October 2007, pages 242–247).

fir needle oil. Volatile, fragrant oil that can cause skin irritation and sensitivity.

fireweed extract. Extract from the *Epilobium angustifolium* plant; also known as willow herb. *See Epilobium angustifolium* extract.

fish cartilage extract. May have water-binding properties, but there is no research showing that this has any benefit for skin.

flavonoid. *See* bioflavonoid.

flax. Plant source of linen and edible seeds. Flax seeds and seed oil have antioxidant properties (Source: *Biofactors*, 2000; volume 13, pages 179–185). The seeds are also a source of linolenic acid. *See* linolenic acid.

flaxseed oil. From seeds of the flax plant; a source of fatty acids, particularly omega-3. *See* flax.

floralozone. One of a number of synthetic fragrant components.

***Foeniculum vulgare* extract**. *See* fennel oil and fennel seed extract.

folic acid. Part of the B-vitamin complex; when taken orally, it is a good antioxidant. That benefit has not been demonstrated when it is applied topically on skin.

formaldehyde-releasing preservative. Common type of preservative found in cosmetics (Source: *Contact Dermatitis*, December 2000, pages 339–343). Despite some claims, there is no higher level of skin reaction to formaldehyde-releasing preservatives than to other preservatives (Source: *British Journal of Dermatology*, March 1998, pages 467–476). In fact, there is a far greater risk to skin from a product without preservatives, because of the contamination and unchecked growth of bacteria, fungus, and mold that can result if no preservatives are used. However, there is concern that when formaldehyde-releasing preservatives are present in a formulation that also includes amines, such as triethanolamine (TEA), diethanolamine (DEA), or monoethanolamine (MEA), nitrosamines can be formed, and nitrosamines are carcinogenic substances that can potentially penetrate skin (Source: *Fundamentals and Applied Toxicology*, August 1993, pages 213–221). Whether or not that poses a health risk of any kind has not been established. *See* preservatives.

fragrance. One or a blend of volatile and/or fragrant plant oils (or synthetically derived oils) that impart aroma and odor to products. These are often skin irritants (Sources: *Dermatology*, 2002, volume 205, number 1, pages 98–102; *Contact Dermatitis*, December 2001, pages 333–340; and *Toxicology and Applied Pharmacology*, May 2001, pages 172–178). *See* volatile oil.

frankincense extract. Fragrant component used in skin-care products; it can be a skin irritant. There is no research showing frankincense has any benefit for skin (Sources: www.herbmed.com; and www.naturaldatabase.com).

free-radical damage. Occurrence that takes place at an atomic level and is a complex physiological process. Molecules are comprised of atoms. Atoms comprise all matter in the universe. Atoms are made up of protons, neutrons, and electrons. Electrons occur in pairs, and when an element only has a few paired electrons it can easily become unstable. Oxygen and oxides are primary examples of potential unstable elements in our environment. When oxygen interacts with skin (and because the air we breathe is 20% oxygen, that happens all the time), it almost always loses one of its electrons. This oxygen molecule, which now is minus one electron, is a free radical. Because it is now unstable the oxygen molecule quickly finds another electron, and it does this by taking an electron from another molecule in the skin, which is usually a healthy substance such as collagen, skin-identical substances, or antioxidants in the skin which have lots of electrons to spare. Once those substances are robbed of all their electrons they break down and are destroyed. Oxygen molecules (or other potential free radical substances) attempting to repair themselves in this way trigger a cascading event termed free-radical damage. The reactions that cause free-radical damage take place in mere fractions of a second. Antioxidants are substances that prevent oxidative damage from being triggered. *See* antioxidant.

The primary causes of free-radical damage on skin are sunlight, pollution, air, cigarette smoke, herbicides, and solvents (such as alcohol). Antioxidants are a way to reduce and potentially neutralize free-radical damage (Sources: *Journal of Clinical Pathology*, March 2001, pages 176–186; and *Drugs and Aging*, 2001, volume 18, number 9, pages 685–716).

fructose. Often called fruit sugar, fructose is a type of sugar composed of glucose. It has water-binding properties for skin. *See* water-binding agent.

fruit acid. *See* sugarcane extract.

Fu ling. *See Poria cocos* extract.

***Fucus vesiculosus* extract**. *See* bladderwrack extract.

fuller's earth. Mineral substance that is similar to kaolin (a clay). Composed mainly of alumina, silica, iron oxides, lime, magnesia, and water, it is used as an absorbent and thickening agent in cosmetics.

fumaric acid. Naturally occurring acid that has been proven effective for systemic and topical treatment of severe psoriasis vulgaris (Source: *Journal of Investigative Dermatology*, February 2001, pages 203–208); however, it can also cause serious skin irritation (Source: *Dermatology*, 1994, volume 188, number 2, pages 126–130). In small amounts it can be used as a pH adjuster in cosmetics.

GABA. GABA (gamma aminobutyric acid/gamma amino-butyric acid) is an amino acid synthesized in the brain that acts as a neurotransmitter inhibitor and is associated with reducing the incidence of seizures and depression (Sources: *Advances in Experimental Medicines and Biology*, 2004, volume 548, pages 92–103; and *Archives of General Psychiatry*, July 2004, pages 705–713). Cosmetics companies include GABA in products and then claim that topical application relaxes muscles, thus sparing consumers from going through Botox injections. However, GABA has not been proven to relax muscles and reduce the appearance of wrinkles or expression lines when applied topically. Cosmetics companies are hoping that consumers will associate the topical application of products containing GABA with its internal function of controlling the manner in which nerve impulses fire. There is no substantiated research proving GABA works in this manner when applied topically, and if it did, it would be cause for alarm. Because if GABA worked as stated and you applied it to your entire face, what's to stop it from affecting the muscles around your mouth, jaw, or neck? If it really relaxed muscles upon application, consumers would see more skin sagging, not to mention problems controlling the (relaxed) muscles in your fingers (assuming they come in contact with the product).

Lastly, the whole nonsense of using GABA in cosmetic products is refuted by the fact that GABA does not work alone to exert its effect internally on nerves. It requires many other substances (substances that are not present in the skin-care products containing GABA) for it to prevent nerves from being triggered and causing muscles to relax (Sources: www.emedicine.com; www.naturaldatabase.com).

galactoarabinan. Polysaccharide extracted from the western larch tree. *See* polysaccharide.

galbanum. Fragrant substance that, because of its resin and volatile oil content, can be extremely irritating and sensitizing on abraded skin. There is no research showing it has any benefit on skin.

gamma linolenic acid (GLA). Fatty acid used in cosmetics as an emollient, antioxidant, and cell regulator. GLA is considered to promote healthy skin growth and is an anti-inflammatory agent. GLA is found in black currant oil or seeds, evening primrose oil, and borage oil (Source: *Biochemical and Biophysical Research Communications*, March 17, 1998, pages 414–420). However, there is no research showing GLA to be effective in the treatment of wrinkles (Sources: *British Journal of Dermatology*, April 1999, pages 685–688; and *Dermatology*, 2000, volume 201, number 3, pages 191–195). When taken orally, GLA has been shown to have some anticancer properties, but there is no research showing that that effect translates to skin. *See* fatty acid.

***Ganoderma lucidum* extract**. Mushroom stem extract. There is no research showing it to be effective when used topically on skin (Source: www.naturaldatabase.com), although it does have antioxidant properties (Source: *Journal of Agricultural and Food Chemistry*, October 2002, pages 6072–6077).

***Gardenia florida* extract**. Flower extract used in cosmetics to impart fragrance; also functions as an antioxidant (Source: *Natural Product Research*, February 2007, pages 121–125). There is limited research proving its benefit for skin, and its fragrance component may be irritating, thus canceling out the antioxidant benefit.

gelatin. Protein obtained from plants or animals and used in cosmetics as a thickening agent.

***Gellidiela acerosa* extract**. Extract derived from a type of algae. *See* algae.

***Gentiana lutea* (Gentian) root extract**. Active part of the gentian plant, constituents of which are anti-inflammatory and antibacterial (Sources: www.naturaldatabase.com; and *Phytomedicine*, February 2007, epublication).

geranium extract. Extract that can have potent antioxidant properties (Source: *Phytomedicine*, June 2000, pages 221–229).

geranium oil. Fragrant oil that can have antimicrobial properties but also can be a skin sensitizer or irritant (Sources: *Contact Dermatitis*, June 2001, pages 344–346; and *Journal of Applied Microbiology*, February 2000, pages 308–316).

Geranium pretense. Geranium plant. *See* geranium extract and geranium oil.

Germaben II. Trade name for diazolidinyl urea. *See* diazolidinyl urea.

ginger extract. Extract from a plant in the *Zingiberacae* family that has research showing it has anti-inflammatory and anti-carcinogenic activity when taken orally (Sources: *Carcinogenesis*, May 2002, pages 795–802; and *Food and Chemical Toxicology*, August 2002, pages 1091–1097). However, topically it can be a skin irritant (Source: IFA—International Federation of Aromatherapists, www.int-fed-aromatherapy.co.uk).

ginger oil. *See* ginger extract.

***Ginkgo biloba* leaf extract**. Research shows this potent antioxidant helps improve blood flow. It is often used in anti-cellulite products because of its relation to circulation. However, there is no research showing that improved circulation affects cellulite (Sources: *Medical Hypotheses*, March 2006, pages 1152–1156; *Journal of Burn Care and Rehabilitation*, November–December 2005, pages 515–524; *Journal of Pharmaceutical and Biomedical Analysis*, February 2005, pages 287–295; and *Planta Medica*, November 2004, pages 1052–1057).

ginseng. Herb in the family *Araliaceae*, native to Asia. A small number of studies carried out on animals have shown that ginseng may have anti-tumor, anti-cancer, and wound-healing properties (Sources: *Journal of Korean Medical Science*, December 2001, Supplemental, pages 38–41; and *Cancer Letter*, March 2000, pages 41–48), although there is also research showing that it can stimulate the growth of breast cancer cells (Source: *Menopause*, March–April 2002, pages 145–150). There is also in vitro research showing it can stimulate collagen production (Source: *Journal of Ethnopharmacology*, January 2007, pages 29–34). There is no evidence indicating that it has any benefit or risk when applied topically in skin-care products.

GLA. *See* gamma linolenic acid.

glabridin. Main ingredient in licorice extract. It has anti-inflammatory properties. There is research showing it to be effective in reducing skin discolorations (Source: *Pigment Cell Research*, December 1998, pages 355–361).

gluconolactone. *See* polyhydroxy acid.
glucose. Monosaccharide that has water-binding properties for skin. *See* mucopolysaccharide and water-binding agent.
glucose tyrosinate. *See* tyrosine.
glutamic acid. Amino acid derived from wheat gluten. It can have water-binding properties for skin. There is no research showing glutamic acid has any special properties when used in topical cosmetic formulations. *See* amino acid.
glutamine. Can help improve the barrier function of skin (Source: *Journal of Biological Chemistry*, July 1998, pages 1763–1770). *See* amino acid.
glutathione. Potent antioxidant (Source: *Free Radical Research*, March 2002, pages 329–340). *See* antioxidant.
glycereth-26. Used as an emollient and thickening agent in cosmetics. *See* glyceryl ester.
glycereth-26 phosphate. Used as an emollient and thickening agent in cosmetics. *See* glyceryl ester.
glycereth-6 laurate. Used as an emollient and thickening agent in cosmetics. *See* glyceryl ester.
glycerin. Also called glycerol; it is present in all natural lipids (fats), whether animal or vegetable. It can be derived from natural substances by hydrolysis of fats and by fermentation of sugars. It can also be synthetically manufactured. For some time it was thought that too much glycerin in a moisturizer could pull water out of the skin instead of drawing it into the skin, but that theory now seems to be completely unfounded. What appears to be true is that glycerin shores up the skin's natural protection by filling in the area known as the intercellular matrix and by attracting just the right amount of water to maintain the skin's homeostasis. There is also research indicating that the presence of glycerin in the intercellular layer helps other skin lipids do their jobs better (Sources: *American Journal of Contact Dermatitis*, September 2000, pages 165–169; and *Acta Dermato-Venereologica*, November 1999, pages 418–421). *See* intercellular matrix and natural moisturizing factor (NMF).
glycerine. *See* glycerin.
glycerol. *See* glycerin.
glycerol monostearate. Used as an emollient and thickening agent in cosmetics. *See* glyceryl ester.
glycerol triacetate. Used as an emollient and thickening agent in cosmetics. *See* glyceryl ester.
glycerol trioleate. Used as an emollient and thickening agent in cosmetics. *See* glyceryl ester.
glyceryl cocoate. Used as an emollient and thickening agent in cosmetics. *See* glyceryl ester.
glyceryl dipalmitate. Used as an emollient and thickening agent in cosmetics. *See* glyceryl ester.
glyceryl distearate. Used as an emollient and thickening agent in cosmetics. *See* glyceryl ester.
glyceryl ester. Large group of ingredients that are composed of fats and oils. At room temperature, the fats are usually solid and the oils are generally liquid. Some tropical oils are liquids in their sites of origin and become solids in cooler or different applications. These multitudinous fats and oils are used in cosmetics as emollients and lubricants as well as water-binding and thickening agents.

glyceryl isopalmitate. Used as an emollient and thickening agent in cosmetics. *See* glyceryl ester.

glyceryl isostearate. Used as an emollient and thickening agent in cosmetics. *See* glyceryl ester.

glyceryl myristate. Used as an emollient and thickening agent in cosmetics. *See* glyceryl ester.

glyceryl oleate. Used as an emollient and thickening agent in cosmetics. *See* glyceryl ester.

glyceryl palmitate. Used as an emollient and thickening agent in cosmetics. *See* glyceryl ester.

glyceryl stearate. Used as an emollient and thickening agent in cosmetics. *See* glyceryl ester.

glycine. *See* amino acid.

***Glycine soja* oil**. Oil derived from wild soybeans; it has emollient properties. *See* natural moisturizing factor (NMF).

glycogen. Polysaccharide that has water-binding properties for skin. *See* polysaccharide.

glycol stearate. Used as an emollient and thickening agent. *See* glyceryl ester.

glycolic acid. *See* AHA.

glycolipid. Type of lipid composed of sugar (monosaccharide) and fat (lipid) that forms an important component of cell membranes and ceramides. Glycolipids coat cell walls, forming a barrier that holds skin and water content in place. *See* ceramides, lipid, and mucopolysaccharide.

glycoproteins. Cell-to-cell communicating ingredients created when a protein links with a carbohydrate. Glycoproteins play a critical role in the body in relation to how various systems recover from internal and external stresses. They also are fundamentally involved in cellular repair, among other functions. However, there is no evidence that they can affect wrinkles in any way when applied topically (Sources: www.glycoscience.com; www.anatomyatlases.org; and *The Journal of Immunology*, November 1, 2000, pages 5295–5303, and September 1991, pages 1614–1620). In addition, when glycoproteins are combined with saccharides they form substances that compose the skin's intercellular matrix. This matrix keeps skin cells and the skin's structure intact, with glycoprotein derivatives such as polysaccharides and glycosaminoglycans such as hyaluronic acid. *See* mucopolysaccharide, natural moisturizing factor (NMF), and protein.

glycosaminoglycans. Also known as mucopolysaccharides; these are a fundamental component of skin tissue, and are essentially a group of complex proteins. Chondroitin sulfate and hyaluronic acid are part of this ingredient group. *See* chondroitin sulfate, hyaluronic acid, mucopolysaccharide, and natural moisturizing factor (NMF).

glycosphingolipid. *See* glycolipid and natural moisturizing factor (NMF).

glycyrrhetic acid. Extract from licorice that has anti-inflammatory properties (Sources: *American Journal of Respiratory and Cellular Molecular Biology*, November 1998, pages 836–841; and *Planta Medica*, August 1996, pages 326–328). *See* licorice extract.

Glycyrrhiza glabra. Licorice plant. *See* glycyrrhetic acid and licorice extract.

gold. Relatively common allergen that can induce dermatitis about the face and eyelids (Source: *Cutis*, May 2000, pages 323–326). There is no research showing it has any benefit when applied topically to skin.

goldenseal. A plant that may have antibacterial or antiviral properties when taken orally. There is no evidence that such an effect occurs when applied topically on skin; however, it can be a skin irritant.

gotu kola. *See Centella asiatica.*

grape seed extract. Contains proanthocyanidins, which are very potent antioxidants, helpful for diminishing the sun's damaging effects and lessening free-radical damage (Sources: *Current Pharmaceutical Biotechnology*, June 2001, pages 187–200; and *Toxicology*, August 2000, pages 187–197). It has also been shown to have wound-healing properties (Source: *Free Radical Biology and Medicine*, July 2001, pages 38–42). There is no difference in the antioxidant potential among different types of grapes (Source: *Journal of Agricultural Food Chemistry*, April 2000, pages 1076–1080).

grape seed oil. Emollient oil that also has good antioxidant properties. *See* grape seed extract and linoleic acid.

grapefruit oil. Citrus oil whose volatile components (chiefly substances known as furocoumarins) are irritating to skin. Topical application of grapefruit oil may cause contact dermatitis or a phototoxic reaction when skin is exposed to sunlight (Source: www.naturaldatabase.com).

green tea. Significant amounts of research have established that tea, including black, green, and white tea, has many intriguing health benefits. Dozens of studies point to tea's potent antioxidant as well as anticarcinogenic properties. However, a good deal of this research is on animal models, which do not directly relate to effects on human skin (Source: *Skin Pharmacology and Applied Skin Physiology*, 2001, pages 69–76). There is only limited information about tea's effect on skin (Source: *Photodermatology, Photoimmunology, and Photomedicine*, February 2007, pages 48–56).

The *Journal of Photochemistry and Photobiology* (December 31, 2001) stated that the polyphenols "are the active ingredients in green tea and possess antioxidant, anti-inflammatory and anticarcinogenic properties. Studies conducted by our group on human skin have demonstrated that green tea polyphenols (GTP) prevent ultraviolet (UV)-B...-induced immune suppression and skin cancer induction." Green tea and the other teas (e.g., white tea, which is what green tea begins as) show a good deal of promise for skin, but they are not the miracle that cosmetics and health food companies make them out to be. As the *Annual Review of Pharmacology and Toxicology* (January 2002, pages 25–54) put it, "Tea has received a great deal of attention because tea polyphenols are strong antioxidants, and tea preparations have inhibitory activity against tumorigenesis. The bioavailability and biotransformation of tea polyphenols, however, are key factors limiting these activities in vivo [in humans]. Epidemiological studies ... have not yielded clear conclusions concerning the protective effects of tea consumption against cancer formation in humans."

Most researchers agree that tea (black, green, or white) has potent anti-inflammatory properties and that it is a potent antioxidant. Current research also indicates that epigallocatechin-3-gallate (EGCG), an extract of tea, can prevent collagen breakdown and reduce UV damage to skin (Source: *Journal of Dermatological Science*, December 2005, pages 195–204).

guaiac wood. Used as a fragrant extract in cosmetics; it is a potent skin irritant.

Guaiacum officinale. *See* guaiac wood.

guar gum. Plant-derived thickening agent.

guarana. Herb that contains two and a half times more caffeine than coffee. It can have constricting properties on skin and can therefore be a skin irritant. *See* caffeine and *Paullinia cupana* seed extract.

gums. Substances that have water-binding properties, but that are used primarily as thickening agents in cosmetics. Some gums have a sticky feel and are used as film-forming agents in hairsprays, while others can constrict skin and have irritancy potential. Natural thickeners such as acacia, tragacanth, and locust bean are types of gums.

Hamamelis virginiana. *See* witch hazel.

hamamelitannin. Tannin that is found in witch hazel. It can be a skin irritant, but it also has potent antioxidant properties. *See* tannin.

***Haslea ostrearia* extract**. Extract derived from a water plant also known as blue algae. In pure concentrations this extract can have antiviral properties on skin. *See* algae.

hawthorn extract. Extract that when taken orally may improve circulation (Source: *Phytomedicine*, 1994, volume 1, pages 17–24). The bioflavonoids in hawthorn are potent antioxidants. (Source: *Planta Medica*, 1994, volume 60, pages 323–328), but there is no research showing that this extract has any benefit for skin.

hayflower extract. Plant extract that, due to its constricting effect on skin, can be an irritant. There is no research supporting the claim that it has any effect on skin.

hazelnut oil. Oil extracted from the hazelnut and that is used as an emollient. *See* natural moisturizing factor (NMF).

heavy water. Water in which hydrogen atoms have been replaced by deuterium; it is used chiefly as a coolant in nuclear reactors.

Hedera helix. *See* English ivy extract.

hedione. Synthetic fragrant component in products, which also can be a skin irritant.

helianthus oil. *See* sunflower oil.

hemp seed oil. From the hemp plant, *Cannabis sativa*. Because both hemp and marijuana are from the genus Cannabis, they are often thought (erroneously) to have similar properties. However, because hemp contains virtually no THC (delta-9-tetrahydrocannabinol), the active ingredient in marijuana, it is not used as a drug of any kind. In cosmetics, hemp seed oil is used as an emollient. Other claims about its effect on skin are not substantiated. *See* fatty acid.

hepatocyte growth factor (HGF). Stimulates division in cells lining the liver, skin cells, and cells that produce skin color. *See* human growth factor.

hesperidin. Flavonoid found in various plants such as citrus and evening primrose oil. It has potential as a potent antioxidant—reducing the effects of sun damage and preventing some cancers. It is also taken orally to improve circulation and to strengthen capillaries. There is no published research showing it combats cellulite (Sources: *Photochemistry and Photobiology*, September 2003, pages 256–261; *Phytotherapy Research*, December 2001, pages 655–669; and *Anticancer Research*, July-August 1999, pages 3237–3241).

hesperidin methyl chalcone. Citrus bioflavonoid often seen in products claiming to banish dark undereye circles. There is research supporting its internal use as an aid to venous (vein) problems. One study documented that it lowers the filtration rate of capillaries, and less blood flowing though capillaries close to the surface of the skin potentially means that less hemoglobin would be oxygenated to cause the dark bluish discoloration under the eyes.

However, there is no substantiated research proving that it will have this effect when this ingredient is applied topically.

Another study detailed this ingredient's use when combined with the root of the *Ruscus aculeatus* plant and vitamin C, but again it was about oral consumption for alleviating symptoms of varicose veins and helping prevent them from becoming a chronic disease (Source: *International Angiology*, September 2003, pages 250–262). It is clear from published research that hesperidin methyl chalcone does have various benefits for the body, but diminishing severe dark circles via topical application is not one of them (Source: www.pdrhealth.com/drug_info/nmdrugprofiles/nutsupdrugs/hes_0295.shtml).

hexyl laurate. Skin-conditioning agent and emollient that is a mixture of hexyl alcohol and lauric acid.

hexylene glycol. *See* propylene glycol.

***Himanthalia elongate* extract**. Extract of a species of algae. *See* algae.

Hippophae rhamnoides. *See* sea buckthorn.

histidine. *See* amino acid.

hoelen. A mushroom that grows underground on the roots of pines and other trees around the world. It has antibacterial, preservative, wound-healing, and water-binding properties when applied topically (Sources: *BioMed Central (BMC) Complementary and Alternative Medicine*, 2001, volume 1, issue 1, page 2; and *Burns*, March 1998, pages 157–161).

hops. There is no research showing that hops have any benefit for skin. However, components in hops may have antioxidant and antibacterial properties. The plant may also have estrogenic properties.

***Hordeum vulgare* extract**. *See* barley extract.

horse chestnut extract. May have anti-inflammatory properties for skin. Orally it has been shown to reduce edema in the lower leg by improving the elastic tissue surrounding the vein (Sources: *Pharmacological Research*, September 2001, pages 183–193; *Phytotherapy Research*, March 2002, number S1, pages 1–5; and *American Journal of Clinical Dermatology*, 2002, volume 3, number 5, pages 341–348). *See* escin.

horse elder. *See* elecampane.

horseradish. Plant that can irritate skin and should never be applied to abraded skin.

horsetail extract. Plant extract that has a high tannin, alkaloid, and nicotine content, which can have skin-constricting properties and be irritating to skin (Source: www.herbmed.org). It also has antioxidant properties, but there are many other potent antioxidants that can be used that do not cause skin irritation.

Huang qi. *See* milk vetch root.

human growth factor. The topic of human growth factor (HGF) is exceedingly complicated. The physiological intricacies of the varying HGFs and their actions challenge any layperson's comprehension. Nonetheless, because the use of HGF seems to be the direction some skin-care companies are taking, and because there is a large body of research showing its efficacy for wound healing (but not for wrinkles), it does deserve comment.

HGFs make up a complex family of hormones that are produced by the body to control cell growth and cell division in skin, blood, bone, and nerve tissue. Most significantly, HGFs regulate the division and reproduction of cells, and they also can influence the growth rate of some cancers. HGFs occur naturally in the body, but they also are synthesized and used in medicine for a range of applications, including wound healing and immune-system stimulation. HGFs are chemical messages that bind to receptor sites on the cell surface (receptor sites are places where cells communicate with a substance to let them know what or what not to do). HGFs must communicate with cells to instruct them to activate the production of new cells, or to instruct a cell to create new cells that have different functions. Another way to think of HGFs is that they are messengers designed to be received or "heard" by specific receptor sites or "ears" on the cell. HGFs, such as transforming growth factor (TGF, stimulates collagen production) or epidermal growth factor (EGF, stimulates skin-cell production), play a significant role in healing surgical wounds. The main task of HGFs is to cause cell division, which is helpful; however, at certain concentrations and over certain durations of application they can cause cells to over-proliferate, which can cause cancer or other health problems.

But what happens when you put HGFs on skin, particularly TGF and EGF, which some companies claim their products contain? The risk is that they could accelerate the growth of skin cancer by stimulating the overproduction of skin cells. In the case of TGF, which stimulates collagen production, it can encourage scarring, because scars are the result of excessive collagen production, and if you make too much collagen you get a scar or a knot on the skin such as a keloidal scar. Most of the research on the issue of HGFs for skin has looked primarily at the issue of wound healing, and at short-term use of HGFs. In skin-care products, however, they would be used repeatedly, and possibly over long periods of time. A shortcoming of HGFs, according to an article by Dr. Donald R. Owen in *Global Cosmetic Industry* (March 1999), is that "The body produces these [HGFs] in exquisitely small concentrations at just the right location and time .... Actual growth factors such as [EGF and TGF-B] are [large] configurations, which do not penetrate the skin .... They [also] lose their activity within days in water or even as solids at normal temperatures .... [Yet], even after all these complications, the siren's song is too strong. We [the cosmetics chemists] will use them."

(Sources: *Journal of Burn Care and Rehabilitation*, March–April 2002, pages 116–125; *Journal of Dermatologic Surgery and Oncology*, July 1992, pages 604–606; *Journal of Anatomy*, July 2005, pages 67–78; *International Wound Journal*, June 2006, pages 123–130; *Tissue Engineering*, January 2007, pages 21–28; *Wounds*, 2001, volume 13, number 2, pages 53–58; *Plastic and Reconstructive Surgery*, August 1995, pages 251–254, and September 1997, pages 657–664; *Skin Pharmacology and Applied Skin Physiology*, January–April 1999, pages 79–84; and *Journal of Surgical Research*, April 2002, pages 175–182).

The research into HGFs is without question intriguing, but much remains unknown at this time, especially in terms of long-term risk or stability when they are used in cosmetics and applied to skin. In this arena, if cosmetics companies continue to use HGFs, it is the consumer who will be the guinea pig.

humectant. *See* water-binding agent.

***Humulus lupulus* extract**. *See* hops.

hyaluronic acid. Component of skin tissue that is used in skin-care products as a good water-binding agent. *See* natural moisturizing factor (NMF).

Hydnocarpus anthelmintica. *See* chaulmoogra oil.

Hydrastis canadenis. *See* goldenseal.

hydrocortisone. Hormone from the adrenal gland that can also be created synthetically. It has potent anti-inflammatory properties for skin, but prolonged use can destroy collagen in the skin and cause skin fragility (Sources: American Academy of Dermatology Guidelines of Care for the Use of Topical Glucocorticosteroids, www.aadassociation.org/Guidelines/topicalglu.html; *Journal of the American Academy of Dermatology*, 1996, volume 35, pages 615–619; and *Cosmetic Dermatology*, July 2002, pages 59–62).

hydrocotyl extract. *See Centella asiatica*.

hydrogen peroxide. There is a great deal of current research showing that hydrogen peroxide is problematic as a topical disinfectant because it can greatly reduce the production of healthy new skin cells (Source: *Plastic and Reconstructive Surgery*, September 2001, pages 675–687). Hydrogen peroxide is also a strong oxidizing agent, meaning that it generates free-radical damage. While it can function as a disinfectant, the cumulative problems that can stem from impacting the skin with a substance that is known to generate free-radical damage, impair the skin's healing process, cause cellular destruction, and reduce optimal cell functioning are serious enough that it is better to avoid its use (Sources: *Carcinogenesis*, March 2002, pages 469–475; *Anticancer Research*, July–August 2001, pages 2719–2724; and *Cellular and Molecular Biology*, April 2007, pages 1–2). *See* free-radical damage.

hydrogenated coco-glyceride. Used as an emollient and thickening agent in cosmetics. *See* glyceryl ester.

hydrogenated didecene. Skin-conditioning agent derived from didecene, which is a hydrocarbon. Hydrocarbons are organic compounds that contain only carbon and hydrogen. Examples of common hydrocarbons include mineral oil, petroleum, and paraffin wax.

hydrogenated lecithin. *See* lecithin.

hydrogenated palm glyceride. Used as an emollient and thickening agent in cosmetics. *See* glyceryl ester.

hydrogenated polydecene. Synthetic polymer that functions as an emollient and skin-conditioning agent.

hydrogenated polyisobutene. Synthetic polymer used as a skin-conditioning agent and emollient.

hydrolyzed jojoba esters. Essential fatty acids from the jojoba plant, broken down by water to form a new complex with properties different from the original source. An analogy of this process is the manner in which humans digest food to turn it into energy. Jojoba esters function as skin-conditioning agents.

hydrolyzed silk. *See* silk.

hydrolyzed vegetable protein. Composed of various protein substances derived from vegetables and broken down by water to form a new complex with properties different from the original source. Used as a water-binding agent.

hydroquinone. Strong inhibitor of melanin production that has long been established as the most effective ingredient for reducing and potentially eliminating melasma (Source: *Journal of Dermatological Science*, August, 2001, Supplemental, pages 68–75), meaning that it prevents skin from making the substance responsible for skin color. Hydroquinone does not bleach the skin, which is why "bleaching agent" is a misnomer; it can't remove pigment from the skin cell. Over-the-counter hydroquinone products can contain 0.5% to 2% concentrations of hydroquinone; 4% (and sometimes higher) concentrations are available only from physicians.

In medical literature, hydroquinone is considered the primary topical ingredient for inhibiting melanin production. Using it in combination with some other ingredients—especially tretinoin—can greatly reduce and even eliminate skin discolorations (Sources: *Cutis*, March 2006, pages 177–184; *Journal of Drugs in Dermatology*, September–October 2005, pages 592–597; *Journal of Cosmetic Science*, May–June 1998, pages 208–290; and *Dermatological Surgery*, May 1996, pages 443–447). Interestingly, hydroquinone also is a potent antioxidant (Source: *Journal of Natural Products*, November 2002, pages 1605–1611).

Some concerns about hydroquinone's safety on skin have been expressed, but the research when it comes to topical application indicates that negative reactions are minor, are a result of using extremely high concentrations, or result from the use of other skin-lightening agents such as glucocorticoids or mercury iodine. This is particularly true in Africa, where adulterated skin-lightening products are commonplace (Sources: *British Journal of Dermatology*, March 2003, pages 493–500; and *Critical Reviews in Toxicology*, May 1999, pages 283–330).

According to Howard I. Maibach, M.D., professor of dermatology at the University of California School of Medicine, San Francisco, "Overall, adverse events reported with the use of hydroquinone ... have been relatively few and minor in nature.... To date there is no evidence of adverse systemic reactions following the use of hydroquinone, and it has been around for over 30 years in skin-care products." Maibach also stated that "hydroquinone is undoubtedly the most active and safest skin-depigmenting substance...." Research supporting Maibach's contentions was published in the *Journal of Toxicology and Environmental Health* (1998, pages 301–317). Concern about hydroquinone having carcinogenic properties is mostly related to industrial-grade materials and uses. For cosmetic use there appears to be no similar evidence.

Despite hydroquinone's impressive track record and efficacy, the FDA, in September 2006, recommended that products containing hydroquinone be sold only with a prescription due to their opinion that it posed certain health risks. The FDA asserts there are animal studies showing it may be a possible carcinogen, and studies from Africa showing there is a risk of a skin disorder called ochronosis (Source: http://www.fda.gov/OHRMS/DOCKETS/98fr/E6-14263.htm).

However, there is abundant research from reputable sources that shows hydroquinone to be safe and extremely effective (Sources: *Cutis*, August 2006, Supplemental, pages 6–19; *Journal of Cosmetic Laser Therapy*, September 2006, pages 121–127; *American Journal of Clinical Dermatology*, July 2006, pages 223–230; and *Journal of the American Academy of Dermatology*, May 2006, Supplemental, pages 272–281). Surprisingly, there is even research showing that workers who handle pure hydroquinone actually have lower incidences of cancer than the population as a whole (Source: *Critical Reviews in Toxicology*, May 1999, pages 283–330).

Hydroquinone can be an unstable ingredient in cosmetic formulations. When exposed to air or sunlight, it oxidizes and will turn brown. Therefore, when you are considering buying and using a hydroquinone product, make sure that it is packaged in a non-transparent container that does not let in light and that minimizes exposure to air. Hydroquinone products packaged in jars are not recommended because they become ineffective shortly after opening.

For continued and increased effectiveness, hydroquinone must be used long term. Unprotected sun exposure should be avoided, because it reverses the effect of hydroquinone by increasing melanin production. Occasionally, at higher concentrations, persons with darker skin will experience increased pigmentation, but this is rare. It also can cause mild skin irritation and there is the possibility of an allergic reaction. Hydroquinone in 1% to 2% concentrations is available in over-the-counter products; 4% concentrations are available by prescription only (Source: *American Journal of Clinical Dermatology*, September–October 2000, pages 261–268).

hydroxyethylcellulose. Plant-derived thickening agent typically used as a binding agent or emulsifier. Also used (most often in styling products) as a film-forming agent.

hydroxylated lecithin. *See* lecithin.

hydroxyproline. Derived from the amino acid proline, hydroxyproline is a fundamental component of collagen and other structural proteins. Skin's ability to heal is partly determined by the presence of hydroxyproline within it. Whether topical application of hydroxyproline to the skin can help with wound healing has not been substantiated. However, it does have water-binding properties similar to those of collagen.

hydroxypropyl guar. *See* guar gum.

***Hypericum* extract**. *See* St. John's wort.

hypoallergenic. Term used by the cosmetics industry to lead consumers to believe they are using a product that will not cause them to have an allergic or sensitizing skin reaction to a product. However, the word *hypoallergenic* is not regulated in any manner by the FDA and therefore it is used indiscriminately by cosmetics companies without any substantiation or need to show proof of the claim.

hyssop. Fragrant plant extract that may have some antibacterial properties (Source: *International Journal of Food Microbiology*, August 2001, pages 187–195). It may also be a skin irritant.

Ilex paraguariensis. *See* yerba mate extract.

Illicium vernum. *See* anise.

imidazolidinyl urea. Formaldehyde-releasing preservative (Source: *Contact Dermatitis*, December 2000, pages 339–343). *See* formaldehyde-releasing preservative.

inactive ingredient. The list of inactive ingredients is the part of an ingredient label that is not regulated by the FDA other than the requirement that it be a complete list of the contents in descending order of concentration; that is, the ingredient with the largest concentration is listed first, then the next largest, and so forth. Thousands and thousands of inactive ingredients are used in cosmetics, and there is controversy about how truly inactive these substances are in regard to safety as well as about their long-term or short-term effects on skin or the human body.

inositol. Major component of lecithin that may have water-binding properties for skin. It is not a vitamin, although it is sometimes mistakenly thought of as a B vitamin.

insulinlike growth factor (IGF). Stimulates fat cells and connective tissue cells. *See* human growth factor.

intercellular matrix. "Mortar" that holds layers of skin cells together, creating a contiguous natural, external barrier. Preserving the intercellular layer intact keeps bacteria out, moisture in, and the skin's surface smooth. Skin's intercellular matrix (also referred to in this book as skin-identical ingredients) includes ceramides, hyaluronic acid, vitamin C, glycerin, cholesterol, and free fatty acids. *See* natural moisturizing factor (NMF).

interleukin (IL). Stimulates growth of white blood cells. *See* human growth factor.

Inula helenium. *See* elecampane.

iodopropynyl butylcarbamate. Used as a preservative in cosmetics. *See* preservatives.

***Iris florentina* extract**. *See* orris root.

Irish moss extract. Type of red algae. *See* algae.

iron oxides. Compounds of iron that are used as colorings in some cosmetics. They also are used as a metal polish called jewelers' rouge, and are well-known in their crude form as rust.

isobutyl acetate. *See* solvent.

isobutylparaben. *See* parabens.

isocetyl salicylate. *See* sodium salicylate.

isododecane. Hydrocarbon ingredient used as a solvent. Isododecane enhances the spreadability of products and has a weightless feel on skin. All hydrocarbons used in cosmetics help prevent the evaporation of water from the skin.

isoflavone. Plant estrogen with potent antioxidant properties (Source: *Free Radical Biology and Medicine*, December 2001, pages 1570–1581).

isohexadecane. Used as a detergent cleansing agent, emulsifier, and thickening agent in cosmetics.

isoleucine. *See* amino acid.

isoparaffin. *See* paraffin.

isopropyl alcohol. *See* alcohol.

isopropyl lanolate. Derived from lanolin, it is used in cosmetics as a thickening agent and emollient.

isopropyl myristate. Used in cosmetics as a thickening agent and emollient. Historically, animal testing has shown it causes clogged pores (Source: *Archives of Dermatology*, June 1986, pages 660–665). Results derived from animal testing were eventually considered unreliable, however, and there is no subsequent research showing this ingredient is any more of a problem for skin than other emollient, waxy, thickening ingredients used in cosmetics.

isopropyl palmitate. Used in cosmetics as a thickening agent and emollient. As is true for any emollient or thickening agents, it can potentially clog pores, depending on the amount in the product and your skin's response.

isostearamide DEA. Used as a surfactant, water-binding agent, and thickening agent. *See* surfactant, water-binding agent, and thickening agent.

isostearic acid. Fatty acid used as a binding agent and thickener. *See* fatty acid.

isotretinoin. *See* Accutane.

ivy extract. *See* English ivy extract.

Japan wax. Vegetable wax obtained from sumac berries, and used as a thickening agent and emollient in cosmetics.

jasmine oil. Fragrant oil, often used as a source of perfume, that can be a skin irritant or sensitizer (Sources: www.naturaldatabase.com; *Contact Dermatitis*, June 2001, pages 344–346; and *Cutis*, January 2000, pages 39–41). It may have antifungal properties (Source: *Mycoses*, April 2002, pages 88–90).

Jasminium grandiflorum. *See* jasmine oil.

jewelweed. Has antifungal properties (Sources: www.naturaldatabase.com; and *Plant Physiology*, April 2002, pages 1346–1358). There is one animal study showing that, when taken orally, it can stop itching associated with dermatitis (Source: *Phytotherapy Research*, September 2001, pages 506–510); however, when applied topically there is no benefit when compared to a placebo in cases using jewelweed to reduce itching related to dermatitis or poison ivy

(Source: *American Journal of Contact Dermatitis*, September 1997, pages 150–153).

jojoba oil. Emollient oil similar to other nonfragrant plant oils. *See* natural moisturizing factor (NMF).

jojoba wax. Semi-solid portion of jojoba oil. *See* natural moisturizing factor (NMF).

jonquil extract. Fragrant plant extract that poses a strong risk of skin irritation.

Ju hua. *See* chrysanthemum extract.

juniper berry. Can have anti-inflammatory properties for skin (Source: *Pharmacology and Toxicology*, February 1998, pages 108–112), although the methanol content, with repeated application, can cause skin irritation.

Juniperus communis. *See* juniper berry.

kaolin. Naturally occurring clay mineral (silicate of aluminum) that is used in cosmetics for its absorbent properties.

Kathon CG. *See* methylchloroisothiazolinone.

kava-kava extract. Extract of the *Piper methysticum* plant that has analgesic (anti-inflammatory) properties, but can also cause skin irritation and dermatitis (Sources: *Alternative Medicine Review*, December 1998, pages 458–460; and *Clinical Experimental Pharmacology and Physiology*, July 1990, pages 495–507).

kawa extract. *See* kava-kava extract.

kelp extract. *See* algae.

***Kigelia africana* extract**. Extract of African plant commonly known as the sausage tree. The African lore about this extract is that it can firm breast tissue, but there is no supporting research for this myth. The research on this ingredient is limited and mostly in vitro, but it does appear to have anti-inflammatory and antioxidant properties (Sources: *Experimental and Toxicologic Pathology*, August 2007, pages 433–438; and *Journal of Natural Products*, November 2005, pages 1610–1614).

kinetin. Trade name N6-furfuryladenine, a plant hormone responsible for cell division. As a "natural" skin-care ingredient, it is promoted primarily as having been clinically proven to reduce the signs of aging, improve sun damage, reduce surfaced capillaries, and offer many other skin benefits of particular interest to aging baby boomers. There is a good deal of research on kinetin when it comes to plants or in test tubes (in vitro), with cells, and even on flies, but there is no published research on kinetin's topical effect, either on animal or human skin (Source: *Dermatologic Clinics*, October 2000, pages 609–615).

Although there are two unpublished clinical studies responsible for much of the attention kinetin is getting, both were sponsored by Senetek, the company that licenses the use of kinetin. On a closer look, according to MedFaq.com (a now-defunct Internet source that evaluated the legitimacy of medical research), the data are far less convincing than Senetek wants you to know. These studies, paid for by Senetek, were both performed by Dr. Jerry L. McCullough, Professor of Dermatology, University of California, Irvine. According to MedFaq, "The first study was well-designed—there was a control group and [it was done] double-blind.... After 24 weeks, a good response was noted in 30% of the subjects treated with kinetin ... [but] there was no statistically significant difference between the people taking kinetin and the people just getting the placebo." Another study was then performed that did not use a placebo control group, but in which everyone was using a product that contained some amount of kinetin. Not surprisingly, in this protocol the results for skin were much better. "Essentially all of the subjects reported improvement after 24 weeks ..."

regardless of how much kinetin the product contained. As MedFaq states, "This outcome could also have a variety of causes unrelated to kinetin: It could reflect an improvement over time, a change across seasons, the subjects' enthusiasm, or it could have been caused by the cream or lotion the kinetin is in. In the first study, all of the subjects followed 'a standard skin-care regimen consisting of a gentle-skin cleanser and daily use of sunscreen.' If that regimen was followed in the second experiment, it too might explain the improvement."

Recent studies indicate that kinetin can help increase cell differentiation (turnover rate) and that it works best in the presence of calcium as an inducing agent, but that combination is not what is being used in skin-care products that contain kinetin (Source: *Annals of the New York Academy of Sciences*, May 2006, pages 332–336). Kinetin may have benefit as a cell-communicating ingredient, but this has been demonstrated only in vitro (Source: *Proteonomics*, February 2006, pages 1351–1361).

kiwi fruit extract. As a food, kiwi has significant antioxidant properties that may even be greater than those of vitamin C (Source: *Nutrition and Cancer*, 2001, volume 39, number 1, pages 148–153). Whether that benefit translates into its use on skin has not been demonstrated. The acid component of the kiwi can be a skin irritant.

kojic acid. By-product of the fermentation process of malting rice for use in the manufacture of sake, Japanese rice wine. There is definitely convincing research, both in vitro and in vivo and in animal studies, showing that kojic acid is effective for inhibiting melanin production (Sources: *Biological and Pharmaceutical Bulletin*, August 2002, pages 1045–1048; *Analytical Biochemistry*, June 2002, pages 260–268; *Cellular Signaling*, September 2002, pages 779–785; *American Journal of Clinical Dermatology*, September–October 2000, pages 261–268; and *Archives of Pharmacal Research*, August 2001, pages 307–311). Both glycolic acid and kojic acid, as well as glycolic acid with hydroquinone, are highly effective in reducing the pigment in melasma patients (Source: *Dermatological Surgery*, May 1996, pages 443–447). So why aren't there more products available containing kojic acid? Kojic acid is an extremely unstable ingredient in cosmetic formulations. Upon exposure to air or sunlight it turns a strange shade of brown and loses its efficacy. Many cosmetics companies use kojic dipalmitate as an alternative because it is far more stable in formulations. However, there is no research showing that kojic dipalmitate is as effective as kojic acid, though it is a good antioxidant. There is a small amount of research showing that kojic acid is a skin irritant (Source: www.emedicine.com, "Skin Lightening/Depigmenting Agents," November 5, 2001).

kola nut. One of the major components of the kola nut is caffeine, which can be a skin irritant. However, kola nut also has a primary amine content that can form nitrosamines, which are potential carcinogens (Source: *Food and Chemical Toxicology*, August 1995, pages 625–630). *See* caffeine.

kudzu root. Source of isoflavone, genistein, and daidzein, all plant estrogens (Sources: *Phytochemistry*, June 2002, pages 205–211; and *Journal of Alternative Complementary Medicine*, spring 1997, pages 7–12). It can be a potent antioxidant.

kukui nut oil. Non-volatile oil from a plant native to Hawaii; it has emollient properties for skin (Source: *Journal of the Society of Cosmetic Chemists*, September–October 1993).

lactic acid. Alpha hydroxy acid extracted from milk, although most forms used in cosmetics are synthetic. It exfoliates cells on the surface of skin by breaking down the material that holds skin cells together. It may irritate mucous membranes and cause irritation. *See* AHA.

Lactobacillus bifidus. Type of "friendly" bacteria found in the intestine that helps maintain a healthy natural flora in the large intestine by creating an environment that prevents potentially harmful bacteria from growing. Whether or not this has benefit when applied topically on skin is unknown. *See* bifidus extract.

lactobionate. Polysaccharide that has water-binding properties for skin.

lactobionic acid. *See* polyhydroxy acid.

lactoperoxidase. Enzyme derived from milk; it has antibacterial properties for skin and may be helpful for eliminating acne-causing bacteria (Sources: *Journal of Experimental Therapeutics and Oncology*, 2007, volume 6, issue 2, pages 89–106; and *Journal of Applied Microbiology*, May 2006, pages 1034–1042).

lady's mantle extract. *See Alchemilla vulgaris.*

lady's thistle extract. Extracts for which there is a great deal of research showing it has many medical health applications when taken orally. There is no research showing it to be beneficial for skin, though it may cause allergic reactions (Source: www.naturaldatabase.com).

Laminaria digitata. *See* algae.

Laminaria japonica. *See* algae.

Laminaria longicruris. *See* algae.

Laminaria saccharine. *See* algae.

lanolin. Emollient, very thick substance derived from the sebaceous glands of sheep. Lanolin has long been burdened with a reputation for being an allergen or sensitizing agent, which has always been a disappointment to formulators because lanolin is such an effective moisturizing agent for skin. A study in the *British Journal of Dermatology* (July 2001, pages 28–31) may change all that. The study concluded "that lanolin sensitization has remained at a relatively low and constant rate even in a high-risk population (i.e., patients with recent or active eczema)." Based on a review of 24,449 patients who were tested with varying forms of lanolin, it turned out that "The mean annual rate of sensitivity to this allergen was 1.7%"—and it was lower than that for a 50% concentration of lanolin. It looks like it's time to restore lanolin's good reputation. That's a very good thing for someone with dry skin, though it can be a problem for someone with oily skin, because lanolin closely resembles the oil from human oil glands.

lanolin alcohol. Emollient derived from lanolin. *See* lanolin.

lappa extract. *See* burdock root.

***Larrea divaricata* extract**. *See* chaparral extract.

Larrea tridentata. *See* chaparral extract.

L-ascorbic acid. Form of vitamin C that is a potent antioxidant and anti-inflammatory agent (Sources: *Bioelectrochemistry and Bioenergetics*, May 1999, pages 453–461; and *International Journal of Radiation Biology*, June 1999, pages 747–755). However, claims that it can eliminate or prevent wrinkles when applied topically are not substantiated in any published studies. In addition, it is stable only in a formulation with a low pH, and that is potentially irritating for skin (Source: *Dermatologic Surgery*, February 2001, pages 137–142).

lauramphocarboxyglycinate. Mild detergent cleansing agent. *See* surfactant.

laureth-23. Derived from lauryl alcohol and used either as a surfactant or emulsifier (or, in many cases, as both). *See* surfactant.

laureth-4. Derived from lauryl alcohol and used either as a surfactant or emulsifier (or, in many cases, as both). *See* surfactant.

laureths. Substances that in various combinations create a wide range of mild detergent cleansing agents called surfactants. *See* surfactant.

lauroyl lysine. Amino acid derivative that functions as a skin- and hair-conditioning agent. It also contributes to a product's texture by helping to gel solvents, while also remaining stable under high heat conditions (Source: *Organic and Molecular Biochemistry*, November 2003, pages 4124–4131).

Laurus nobilis. *See* bay leaf oil.

lauryl alcohol. *See* surfactant.

lauryl glucoside. *See* surfactant.

lauryl lactate. Mixture of lauryl alcohol and lactic acid that functions as a skin-conditioning agent and emollient; also used to impart fragrance.

lavandin oil. Essential oil of the hybrid lavender plant *Lavandula hybrida* and used in cosmetics as a fragrance ingredient. Its irritant potential for skin is similar to that of lavender oil and camphor. Lavandin yields four times more oil per volume of plants than true lavender, but it is of inferior quality and has a distinct camphor scent. It is not used in perfumery, but instead to scent soaps, air fresheners, and similar items.

Lavandula angustifolia. *See* lavender extract and oil.

Lavandula officinalis. *See* lavender extract and oil.

lavender extract and oil. Primarily a fragrance ingredient, although it may have antibacterial properties. There is no research showing it has any benefit for skin (Sources: *Phytotherapy Research*, June 2002, pages 301–308; and *Healthnotes Review of Complementary and Integrative Medicine*, www.healthwell.com/healthnotes/Herb/). It can be a skin irritant (Source: *Contact Dermatitis*, August 1999, page 111) and a photosensitizer (Source: *Family Practice Notebook*, www.fpnotebook.com/DER188.htm). Research also indicates that components of lavender, specifically linalool, can be cytotoxic, meaning that topical application causes skin-cell death (Source: *Cell Proliferation*, June 2004, pages 1365–2184).

L-carnitine. Also known as carboxylic acid, it is often erroneously labeled an amino acid (which it is not). It has been claimed to have miraculous (albeit unsubstantiated) properties for enhancing the metabolization of fat when taken orally. There is research in animal studies showing it has anti-aging benefits when taken orally (Source: *Annals of the New York Academy of Sciences*, April 2002, pages 133–166). However, there is no known benefit for skin when it is applied topically in skin-care products, though it may have antioxidant properties. *See* antioxidant.

L-cysteine. *See* antioxidant.

lecithin. Phospholipid found in egg yolks and the membranes of plant and animal cells. It is widely used in cosmetics as an emollient and water-binding agent. *See* natural moisturizing factor (NMF).

lemon. Potent skin sensitizer and irritant. Though it can have antibacterial properties, the irritation can hurt the skin's immune response (Source: www.naturaldatabase.com).

lemon balm. *See* balm mint extract.

lemon oil. Can be a skin irritant, especially on abraded skin (Source: www.naturaldatabase.com).

lemongrass extract. Extract that can have antibacterial properties (Source: *Journal of Applied Microbiology*, 2000, volume 88, pages 308–316), but it also may be a skin irritant.

lemongrass oil. Also known as Oil of Verbena; can be effective as a mosquito repellent (Source: *Phytomedicine*, April 2002, pages 259–262). As a volatile fragrant oil, it contains compounds (including limonene and citral) that can cause irritation.

***Lentinus edodes* extract**. Extract from the shiitake mushroom that may have antimicrobial and antibacterial properties, although it could be a potential skin irritant (Source: *International Journal of Antimicrobial Agents*, February 1999, pages 151–157). There is research showing it also has antitumor activity when taken orally (Source: *Mutation Research*, September 2001, pages 23–32).

***Leptospermum scoparium* oil**. *See* manuka oil.

leucine. Amino acid. *See* amino acid and natural moisturizing factor (NMF).

***Levisticum officinale* root extract**. *See* lovage root extract.

licorice extract. Extract that has anti-inflammatory properties (Source: *Healthnotes Review of Complementary and Integrative Medicine*, www.healthwell.com/healthnotes/Herb/). *See* glycyrrhetic acid.

licorice root. *See* licorice extract.

***Lilium candidum* bulb extract**. Extract derived from the white lily bulb. There is no research showing this has any benefit for skin.

lime (oil or extract). Citrus fruit whose volatile compounds are skin irritants and photosensitizing (Source: www.naturaldatabase.com).

Limnanthes alba. Plant commonly known as meadowfoam; its seed oil is a non-volatile plant oil used as a skin-conditioning agent.

limonene. Chemical constituent of many fragrant natural ingredients, notably citrus oils (d-limonene) and pine trees or species of the mint family (l-limonene). Early research suggests that limonene may be a potential anti-cancer ingredient and immune stimulant when consumed orally, but other research suggests that limonene may promote the growth of tumors. Topically, limonene can cause contact dermatitis and is best avoided unless its presence in skin-care products is minuscule (Sources: www.naturaldatabase.com; and *Journal of Occupational Health*, November 2006, pages 480–486).

linalool. Fragrant component of lavender and coriander that can be a potent skin irritant, allergen, or sensitizer once it is exposed to air (Sources: *Contact Dermatitis*, May 2002, pages 267–272, and June 2005, pages 320–328). Current research indicates that this component of lavender can be cytotoxic (meaning toxic to skin cells) (Source: *Cell Proliferation*, June 2004, pages 1365–2184).

linden flower extract. Major active constituents in linden are flavonoids and glycosides. Flavonoids are potent antioxidants and glycosides are monosaccharides that have water-binding properties (Source: *Healthnotes Review of Complementary and Integrative Medicine*, www.healthwell.com/healthnotes/Herb/).

linoleic acid. Unsaturated fatty acid used as an emollient and thickening agent in cosmetics. There is some research showing it to be effective in cell regulation and skin-barrier repair, as well as an antioxidant and an anti-inflammatory (Sources: *Archives of Dermatological Research*, July 1998, pages 375–381; *Clinical and Experimental Dermatology*, March 1998, pages 56–58; *Journal of Investigative Dermatology*, May 1996, pages 1096–1101; and *Seminars in Dermatology*, June 1992, pages 169–175). *See* fatty acid and natural moisturizing factor (NMF).

linseed oil. Non-volatile plant oil. Linoleic acid is a component of linseed oil. *See* linoleic acid.

***Linum usitatissimum* extract**. *See* linseed oil.

lipid. Wide range of ingredients found in plants, animals, and human skin. Lipids include fatty acids, sebum, and fats. In skin-care products, these are emollients and thickening agents. *See* fatty acid and natural moisturizing factor (NMF).

liposomes. Delivery system (not an ingredient) capable of holding other ingredients and releasing them after the liposome is absorbed into the skin. Liposomes are microscopic lipid (fat) sacs that are widely used as a way to deliver other ingredients into skin (Source: *Journal of Pharmaceutical Sciences*, March 2002, pages 615–622).

lithium magnesium sodium silicate. Synthetic silica-based clay composed of lithium, sodium, and magnesium. Used as a thickening agent and an absorbent.

Litsea cubeba. *See* lemongrass oil.

locust bean. *See* gums.

Lonicera japonica. Honeysuckle extract. A plant with soothing properties for skin.

loquat extract. Extract derived from a subtropical flower that has antioxidant and antitumor properties similar to those of green tea (Sources: *Journal of Agricultural Food Chemistry*, April 2002, pages 2400–2403; and *Phytochemistry*, February 2002, pages 315–323).

lotus seed extract. Extract that can have anti-inflammatory and antioxidant properties (Sources: *Planta Medica*, August 1997, pages 367–369; and *Journal of Plant Physiology*, May 2001, pages 39–46).

lovage root extract. Extract that is administered orally as a diuretic. In cosmetics, it is used as a fragrance. Theoretically, it can cause phototoxic reactions, including photosensitivity dermatitis (Source: www.naturaldatabase.com).

***Luffa cylindrica* seed oil or extract**. Components of a plant that have antifungal properties (Source: *Peptides*, June 2002, pages 1019–1024) and antitumor properties, by preventing synthesis of certain proteins (Source: *Life Sciences*, January 2002, pages 899–906). They also have anti-inflammatory properties (Source: www.naturaldatabase.com). They may also be toxic to skin-cancer cells (Source: *Melanoma Research*, October 1998, pages 465–467). When the fruit from the luffa plant is dried it is used as an abrasive sponge.

lupine. Legume that is a source of isoflavones, a form of plant estrogen that has antioxidant properties (Sources: *Phytochemistry*, January 2001, pages 77–85; and *Bioscience, Biotechnology, and Biochemistry*, June 2000, pages 1118–1125). *See* isoflavone.

lupine oil. Extract of *Lupinus albus*, a legume; it has emollient and antioxidant properties, though it may also have significant allergen or skin-sensitizing potential. *See* lupine.

***Lupinus albus* extract**. Species of legume. *See* lupine and lupine oil.

lutein. Carotenoid that has potent antioxidant properties (Source: *Photochemistry and Photobiology*, May 2002, pages 503–596).

lycopene. Carotenoid pigment that has potent antioxidant properties (Source: *Photochemistry and Photobiology*, May 2002, pages 503–596).

lye. *See* potassium hydroxide and sodium hydroxide.

lysine. Amino acid. *See* amino acid.

macadamia nut oil. Used in cosmetics as an emollient for dry skin.

Mad cow disease. Technically known as bovine spongiform encephalopathy, or BSE, mad cow disease is a chronic degenerative disease affecting the central nervous system of cattle. The concern for humans is the risk of eating meat or meat products that contain the BSE pathogen. Whether bovine-derived ingredients used in cosmetics can harbor the disease and cause health risks is unknown, but theoretically there is a remote possible risk. Some researchers believe that there is no evidence BSE can be contracted through the skin (Source: *Cosmetic Dermatology*, December 2001, pages 43–47); however, neither cooking nor preserving nor any of the other processing that most cosmetics go through can eliminate BSE pathogens. That means that if animal by-products are used in cosmetics (in particular bovine placenta and spleen extracts), they can pose a risk, albeit remote, to the user. The British BSE Committee (www.bse.org.uk/), in various reports, has mentioned a concern that people could become infected if the creams are used on broken skin.

It is important to realize that very few products contain those kinds of ingredients. If you are thinking of buying cosmetics that contain animal organ extracts of any kind, you may want to reconsider, or discard them if you have already made a purchase.

magnesium. Earth mineral that has strong absorbent properties and some disinfecting properties. Magnesium obtained via diet or oral supplements is essential for maintaining health.

magnesium aluminum silicate. Powdery, dry-feeling, white solid that is used as a thickening agent and powder in cosmetics.

magnesium ascorbyl palmitate. Stable derivative of vitamin C that can be an effective antioxidant. *See* vitamin C.

magnesium ascorbyl phosphate. Form of vitamin C that is considered stable and an effective antioxidant for skin (Sources: *Photochemistry and Photobiology*, June 1998, pages 669–675; and *Journal of Pharmaceutical and Biomedical Analysis*, March 1997, pages 795–801). For skin lightening, there is only a single study showing it to be effective for inhibiting melanin production (Source: *Journal of the American Academy of Dermatology*, January 1996, pages 29–33). The study concluded that a moisturizer with a 10% concentration of magnesium ascorbyl phosphate "suppressed melanin formation.... The lightening effect was significant in 19 of 34 patients with chloasma or senile freckles and in 3 of 25 patients with normal skin." One study is not exactly anything to write home about, not to mention that at present there are no products on the market that contain 10% magnesium ascorbyl phosphate.

magnesium carbonate. Inorganic mineral salt used as an absorbent, opacifying agent, coloring agent, or to adjust the pH of cosmetic products.

magnesium gluconate. Magnesium is an essential mineral the body uses to maintain circulatory and nervous system function. There is a small amount of research showing that it has antibacterial properties (Sources: *Bulletin of Experimental Biology and Medicine*, February 2001, pages 132–135; and *Journal of Pharmacy and Pharmacology*, May 1998, pages 445–452). There is also research showing it may be helpful for healing burns.

magnesium hydroxide. Active ingredient in milk of magnesia. It is an absorbent and has antibacterial properties for skin.

magnesium laureth sulfate. Mild detergent cleansing agent. *See* surfactant.

magnesium oleth sulfate. Mild detergent cleansing agent. *See* surfactant.

magnesium stearate. Used as a thickening agent in cosmetics.

magnesium sulfate. Commonly known as Epsom salt, a magnesium salt used as a thickening agent.

malic acid. *See* AHA.

mallow. Can be used as a thickening agent in cosmetics and may have anti-inflammatory and soothing properties for skin due to its content of mucilage, flavonoids, and anthocyanidins

(Source: *Healthnotes Review of Complementary and Integrative Medicine*, www.healthwell.com/healthnotes/Herb/Mallow.cfm).

***Malva sylvestris* extract**. Extract from the blue mallow flower, it may have some anti-inflammatory and soothing properties for the skin, as well as some potential antioxidant benefits (Sources: www.naturaldatebase.com; *International Journal of Food Sciences and Nutrition*, February 2004, pages 67–74; and *Journal of Ethnopharmacology*, January 2004, pages 135–143).

Malvaceae extract. Extract from plants of the Malvaceae family, which includes over 1,000 species, found in tropical and temperate regions the world over. Their varying benefits and problems are diverse. Consequently, if "Malvaceae" is present on a cosmetic ingredient label, it is misleading, because each of the 1,000 species has its own pros and cons.

mandarin orange oil or extract. Primarily used as a fragrance; it can be a skin irritant. There is no research showing it has any benefit when applied topically.

mandelic acid. Alpha hydroxy acid, also known as amygdalic acid. There is scant research showing this to be an effective alternative to other AHAs, though it does have germicidal activity. Unlike glycolic acid, mandelic acid is light-sensitive and should be packaged in an opaque container (Source: *Handbook of Cosmetic and Personal Care Additives*, Second Edition, volume 2, Synapse Information Resources, 2002).

manganese gluconate. Mineral found in trace amounts in tissues of the body. While manganese plays a vital role in the processes of many body systems, there is no evidence it serves any purpose topically on skin, though it may act as an antioxidant.

manganese violet. Coloring agent/additive permanently listed (as of 1976) by the FDA for use in cosmetic products, including those designed for use around the eye.

***Mangifera indica* root**. Extract derived from the mango tree; it can have antioxidant properties (Source: *Journal of Agricultural Food Chemistry*, February 2002, pages 762–766).

manuka oil. Extract derived from the New Zealand tea tree; the oil is similar to that of the Australian tea tree, *Melaleuca alternifolia*. Manuka oil has antifungal and antibacterial properties (Sources: *Phytotherapy Research*, December 2000, pages 623–629; and *Pharmazie International Journal of Pharmaceutical Sciences*, June 1999, pages 460–463). *See* tea tree oil.

marigold. *See* calendula extract.

marionberry. Fruit that has potent antioxidant properties (Source: *Journal of Agricultural Food Chemistry*, June 5, 2002, pages 3495–3500).

marjoram. Herb with a fragrant component used in cosmetics; can be a skin irritant.

marshmallow. *See* mallow.

Mastocarpus stellatus. *See* algae.

mate extract. *See* yerba mate extract.

***Matricaria* oil**. *See* chamomile.

matrix metalloproteinases. Also called MMPs, a group of 23 different enzymes that cause substances in the body to break down. Of the 23 types, MMP-1, also known as collagenase, is responsible for the destruction of collagen. Generated primarily by unprotected sun exposure and the aging process, it is also present in sebum (which may be a cause of acne) (Sources: *Journal of Investigative Dermatology*, October 2005, pages 673–684; *Photochemistry and Photobiology*, October 2003, pages 355–360; and *Photodermatology, Photoimmunology, and Photomedicine*, April 2001, pages 178–183).

One of the primary ways to decrease MMPs in skin, particularly MMP-1 is smart sun behavior and use of well-formulated sunscreens. There is also research showing that epigallocatechin-3-gallate (a derivative of green tea), retinoic acid (RA), eicosapentaenoic acid (an omega-3 fatty acid), beta-carotene, DHEA (though this is controversial), polysaccharides, vitamin E, and vitamin C, and flavonoids, to name a few, can inhibit MMPs and increase TIMPs (tissue inhibitors of metalloproteinases; when TIMPs increase in skin, MMPs decrease).

MEA. Abbreviation for monoethanolamine. *See* alkyloamides and triethanolamine.

meadowsweet extract. Extract that can have anti-inflammatory properties (Source: *Journal of Agricultural Food Chemistry*, October 1999, pages 3954–3962).

Medicago sativa. *See* alfalfa extract.

Melaleuca alternifolia. *See* tea tree oil.

***Melaleuca cajeputi* oil**. There is no research showing that this oil, which is derived from a plant in the same family as the plant that is the source of tea tree oil, has any antibacterial properties. It may cause skin irritation (Source: *The Illustrated Encyclopedia of Essential Oils*, Rockport, MA, Element Books, 1995, page 170).

melasma. Melasma or chloasma are brownish discolorations of the face, hands, chest, and neck. Pregnancy is a common cause of melasma, as well as taking oral contraceptives. However, unprotected exposure to sunlight is also a major cause.

Melia azadirachta. *See* neem extract or oil.

melibiose. Saccharide that can have good water-binding properties. *See* mucopolysaccharide and natural moisturizing factor (NMF).

Melissa officinalis. *See* balm mint extract and counter-irritant.

Mentha arvensis. *See* cornmint.

Mentha piperita. *See* counter-irritant and peppermint.

Mentha spicata. *See* counter-irritant and spearmint oil.

Mentha viridis. *See* counter-irritant and spearmint oil.

menthol. Derived from peppermint; menthol can have the same irritating effect as peppermint on skin (Source: *Archives of Dermatologic Research*, May 1996, pages 245–248). *See* counter-irritant and peppermint.

menthone. Major constituent of peppermint. *See* peppermint.

menthoxypropanediol. Synthetic derivative of menthol. It is known to produce effects that are twice as strong as menthol, which makes it doubly irritating for skin or lips. Menthoxypropanediol is most often used in lip-plumping products (Source: http://www.leffingwell.com/cooler_than_menthol.htm). *See* menthol.

menthyl lactate. Used as a cooling agent and fragrance in cosmetics. It is a derivative of menthol and is supposed to be less irritating than menthol. *See* counter-irritant and menthol.

methanol. *See* alcohol.

methionine. *See* amino acid and antioxidant.

methyl gluceth-20. Liquid that functions as a water-binding and skin-conditioning agent.

methylchloroisothiazolinone. In combination with methylisothiazolinone, it goes by the trade name Kathon CG. Introduced into cosmetics in the mid-1970s, it elicited a great number of sensitizations in consumers. This led to it not being included in cosmetics other than rinse-off products (Sources: *Contact Dermatitis*, November 2001, pages 257–264; and *European Journal of Dermatology*, March 1999, pages 144–160).

methyldibromo glutaronitrile. Formaldehyde-releasing preservative (Source: *Contact Dermatitis*, December 2000, pages 339–343). *See* formaldehyde-releasing preservative.

methyldihydrojasmonate. Synthetic fragrant component.

methyleugenol. Natural constituent of plant oils such as those from rose, basil, blackberry, cinnamon, and anise. According to the November 9, 1998, issue of *The Rose Sheet* (an insider cosmetics industry newsletter), the National Toxicology Program Board of Scientific Counselors concluded that "methyleugenol, a component of a number of essential oils, has shown clear evidence of carcinogenic activity in male and female rats and mice." The study is an animal model and so the results may or may not be applicable to humans.

methylisothiazolinone. Preservative that should be used only in rinse-off products because it can be too irritating when left on skin. *See* methylchloroisothiazolinone and preservatives.

methylparaben. *See* parabens.

methylpropanediol. Glycol that functions as a solvent. Methylpropanediol can enhance the penetration of ingredients (such as salicylic acid) into the skin.

methylsilanol mannuronate. *See* silicone.

methylsilanol PEG-7 glyceryl cocoate. A glyceryl ester used as an emollient and thickening agent in cosmetics. *See* glyceryl ester and silicone.

methylsufonylsulfate. *See* antioxidant.

methylsulfonylmethane. Also known as MSM. There is no published research to back up claims made about any benefit this sulfur compound may have for arthritis or other physical ailments. There is no research about its effect when applied topically. Sulfur is stored in every cell of the body, particularly in the hair, nails, and connective tissue of joints and skin, where it is an important structural protein component. An MSM manufacturer sponsored two very small trials, but the results have not been published. Until additional research is published, MSM enthusiasm should be tempered. MSM is available in capsules and powder for oral intake or in creams for topical use. To date, there have been no reports of toxicity (Sources: *Harvard Health Letter*, August 2000, www.health.harvard.edu; *Healthnotes Review of Complementary and Integrative Medicine*, www.healthwell.com/healthnotes/herb; and www.drweil.com).

Mexoryl SX. Also called ecamsule (technical name terephthalylidine dicamphor sulfonic acid), Mexoryl SX is a synthetic sunscreen agent developed and patented by L'Oreal and used in the company's sunscreen products sold outside the United States since 1993 (first approved for use in Europe in 1991). In July 2006, the FDA approved the use of Mexoryl SX in the United States, but only in a single sunscreen product, La Roche-Posay's Anthelios SX SPF 15 (L'Oreal owns La Roche-Posay). The FDA did not approve Mexoryl SX for use in any other sunscreen; only in that one specific product. Anthelios SX will list Mexoryl SX as ecamsule on the label along with the other actives avobenzone and octocrylene (both of these sunscreen ingredients have been approved for use in the United States for years).

L'Oreal blitzed the media with press releases about this approval, touting Mexoryl SX's improved stability when compared with avobenzone, or intimating that it is the best UVA sunscreen available. According to sunscreen expert Ken Klein, president of Cosmetech Labs, who also teaches sunscreen formulation classes for the Society of Cosmetic Chemists, although Mexoryl SX does not degrade after hours of sun exposure at the same rate as avobenzone, it does indeed break down, losing 40% of its protective properties. Studies have shown that after controlled doses of UV exposure, avobenzone breaks down at a rate of 65%, so Mexoryl SX does have a slight stability edge. However, avobenzone can be made more stable by combining it with other active ingredients, specifically octocrylene (Source: *International Journal of Pharmaceutics*, January 13, 2006, pages 123–128). Outside the United States, Tinosorb (another sunscreen active) is often used to enhance the stability of avobenzone (Source: *Photochemistry and Photobiology*, September 2001, pages 401–406). It is also important to note that all sunscreen ingredients break down to some extent when exposed to sunlight, which is why reapplication of sunscreen is critical to maintaining protection.

Interestingly, the press releases touting Mexoryl SX's superiority as a UVA-protecting sunscreen ingredient don't mention the active ingredients titanium dioxide and zinc oxide, which have long been available worldwide in sunscreen formulations, and that offer protection across a greater range of wavelengths with almost no possible risk of irritation, which is a pervasive problem with synthetic sunscreen agents such as Mexoryl SX. Regarding protection, UVA rays have a range of 320–400 nanometers. Although Mexoryl SX protects within this range, titanium dioxide and zinc oxide protect across the entire UVA and UVB spectrum, from 230 to 700 nanometers. Mexoryl SX is an effective UVA sunscreen agent, but it is by no means the only or absolute best one to look for.

mica. Earth mineral included in products to give them sparkle and shine.

microcrystalline wax. Plastic-type, highly refined wax derived from petroleum. Used as a thickener and to give products a semi-solid to solid smooth texture.

Microcystis aeruginosa. Latin name for spirulina. *See* algae.

milk protein. *See* protein.

milk vetch root. There is a good deal of research showing this root has antioxidant properties (Source: www.naturaldatabase.com), but there is little evidence that it functions that way when applied topically.

millet seed extract. Extract from a cereal grain that has no established benefit for skin, but is added to cosmetic formularies as a skin-conditioning agent.

mimosa oil or extract. Extract used as a fragrance in cosmetics.

mineral oil. Clear, odorless oil derived from petroleum that is widely used in cosmetics because it rarely causes allergic reactions and it cannot become a solid and clog pores. Despite mineral oil's association with petroleum and the hype that it is bad for skin, keep in mind that petroleum is a natural ingredient derived from the earth and that once it becomes mineral oil USP (cosmetics- and pharmaceutical-grade mineral oil), it has no resemblance to the original petroleum. Cosmetics-grade mineral oil and petrolatum are considered the safest, most nonirritating moisturizing ingredients ever found (Sources: *Cosmetics & Toiletries*, January 2001, page 79; and *Cosmetic Dermatology*, September 2000, pages 44–46). Yes, they can keep air off the skin to some extent, but that's what a good antioxidant is supposed to do; they don't suffocate skin! Moreover, mineral oil and petrolatum are known to be efficacious in wound healing, and are also among the most effective moisturizing ingredients available (Source: *Cosmetics & Toiletries*, February 1998, pages 33–40).

mint. Can be a skin irritant and cause contact dermatitis. *See* counter-irritant.

***Mitracarpe scaber* extract.** Extract from a plant native to West Africa, it has been shown to have some antimicrobial properties (Source: *Letters in Applied Microbiology*, February 2000, pages 105–108).

mixed fruit extracts. *See* sugarcane extract.

montmorillonite. *See* bentonite.

***Morus bombycis* root extract.** *See* mulberry extract.

***Morus nigra* root extract.** *See* black mulberry.

mucopolysaccharide. Also known as glycosaminoglycans. This is a large class of ingredients that includes hyaluronic acid, which is found universally in skin tissue. These substances, in association with protein, bind water and other cellular elements so they remain intact, forming a matrix that holds skin cells together. See natural moisturizing factor (NMF) and intercellular matrix.

***Mucor miehei* extract.** Extract of a type of mold whose enzymes are used as a food additive and flavor enhancer in cheeses. It has no established benefit for skin, though companies using this ingredient often describe its enzymatic action as being akin to exfoliation. If that is the case, there is no proof to support the claims.

mugwort extract. There is no research showing this extract has any benefit for skin (Sources: www.naturaldatabase.com; and www.pubmed.com).

mulberry extract. Due to its arbutin content, this extract can have some value in preventing melanin production. Although there is limited research showing this to be the case, the research has been done only in vitro (Sources: eMedicine Journal, November 5, 2001, volume 2, number 11, www.emedicine.com; and *Biophysical Research Communications*, volume 243, number 3, pages 801–803). *See* arbutin.

myristic acid. Detergent cleansing agent that also creates foam and can be drying. See surfactant.

myristyl myristate. Used in cosmetics as a thickening agent and emollient.

myrrh. Fragrant gum resin that can be a skin irritant. There is little research showing it has any benefit for skin (Source: *Healthnotes Review of Complementary and Integrative Medicine*, www.healthwell.com/healthnotes/), although there is a small amount of research showing it may have antifungal and antibacterial properties (Source: *Planta Medica*, May 2000, pages 356–358).

myrtle extract. Contains volatile oil and tannins, and can have fungicidal, disinfectant, and antibacterial properties. It contains 1,8-cineole, a constituent responsible for toxicity. It is recommended that this not come in contact with skin (Sources: *Journal of Natural Products*, March 2002, pages 334–338; and www.naturaldatabase.com).

***Myrtus communis* extract.** *See* myrtle extract.

N6-furfuryladenine. Technical name for kinetin. *See* kinetin.

N-acetyl-L tyrosine. *See* tyrosine.

NaPCA. *See* natural moisturizing factor (NMF) and sodium PCA.

***Narcissus poeticus* wax**. Fragrant flower extract that can cause irritation and dermatitis (Source: www.naturaldatabase.com).

Nardostachys jatamansi. *See* spikenard.

***Nasturtium officinale* extract**. *See* watercress extract.

natto gum. Fermentation product of soy protein. It may be a potent antioxidant (Source: *Journal of Agricultural Food Chemistry*, June 2002, pages 3592–3596).

natural ingredient. The FDA has tried to establish official definitions and guidelines for the use of certain terms such as *natural* and *hypoallergenic*, but its regulations were overturned in court. That means that cosmetics companies can use these terms on ingredient labels to mean anything they want, with the result that they almost always mean nothing at all. The term *all-natural* has considerable market value in promoting cosmetic products to consumers, but a close look at an ingredient label reveals that plant extracts make up only a small percentage of the product. Plus, when a plant is added to a cosmetic, preserved, and stabilized with other ingredients, it loses its natural qualities (Source: *FDA Consumer Magazine*, May–June 1998, revised May 1998 and August 2000).

natural moisturizing factor (NMF). One of the primary elements in keeping skin healthy is making sure the structure of the epidermis (outer layer of skin) is intact. The components that do this are often called natural moisturizing factor (NMF) or ingredients that mimic the structure and function of healthy skin. While the oil and fat components of skin prevent evaporation and provide lubrication to the surface of skin, it is actually the intercellular matrix, along with the skin's lipid content, that gives skin a good deal of its surface texture and feel.

The intercellular matrix is the skin's first line of defense against water loss. When the lipid and NMF content of skin is reduced, we experience surface roughness, flaking, fine lines, and a tight, uncomfortable feeling. The longer the skin's surface layer (stratum corneum) is impaired, the less effective the skin's intercellular matrix becomes (Sources: *Skin Research and Technology*, August 2000, pages 128–134; and *Dermatologic Therapy*, 2004, volume 17, Supplement 1, pages 43–48). Moreover, the skin's healing process is impaired. NMFs make up an expansive group of ingredients that include amino acids, ceramides, hyaluronic acid, cholesterol, fatty acids, triglycerides, phospholipids, glycosphingolipids, urea, linoleic acid, glycosaminoglycans, glycerin, mucopolysaccharide, and sodium PCA (pyrrolidone carboxylic acid). Ingredients that mimic the lipid content of skin include apricot oil, canola oil, coconut oil, corn oil, jojoba oil, jojoba wax, lanolin, lecithin, olive oil, safflower oil, sesame oil, shea butter, soybean oil, squalane, and sweet almond oil, all of which can be extremely helpful in making dry skin look and feel better.

All of the skin's supporting NMFs and lipids are present in the intercellular structure of the epidermis, both between skin cells and in the lipid content on the surface of skin. When any of these ingredients are included in skin-care products, they appear to help stabilize and maintain this complex intercellular-skin matrix. More important, all of these ingredients, and many more, help support the intercellular area of the skin by keeping it intact. This support helps prevent surface irritation from penetrating deeper into the skin, helps keep bacteria out, and aids the skin's immune/healing system. Using moisturizers of any kind that contain NMFs (whether they are labeled as anti-aging, antiwrinkle, serums, lotions, or sunscreens) allows your skin to do its job of repairing and regenerating itself without the impedances brought on when skin is suffering from dryness, environmental distress, or excess irritation (Sources: *Clinical Geriatric Medicine*, February 2002, pages 103–120; *Progressive Lipid Research*, January 2003, pages 1–36; *Journal of the European Academy of Dermatology and Venereology*, November 2002, pages 587–594; *Contact Dermatitis*, June 2002, pages 331–338; *Journal of Investigative Dermatology*, May 1996, pages 1096–1101; *British Journal of Dermatology*, November 1995, pages 679–685; *Skin Pharmacology and Physiology*, September–October 2004, pages 207–213; *Free Radical Research*, April 2002, pages 471–477; and *Journal of Lipid Research*, May 2002, pages 794–804).

neem extract or oil. Extract from leaves of the neem tree, it has potential toxic effects, although it also has been shown to have antimicrobial properties (Sources: *Life Sciences*, January

2001, pages 1153–1160; *Journal of Ethnopharmacology*, August 2000, pages 377–382; *Phytotherapy Research*, February 1999, pages 81–83; and *Mutation Research*, June 1998, pages 247–258).

neopentyl glycol dicaprylate/dicaprate. Used as an emollient and thickening agent.

neopentyl glycol diheptanoate. Mixture of neopentyl glycol (film-forming agent and solvent) and heptanoic acid (fatty acid made from grapes), the compound functions as a non-aqueous skin-conditioning agent and thickener.

neroli. *See* orange blossom.

neroli oil. Fragrant plant oil that can be a skin irritant and sensitizer.

nettle extract. Extract that may have anti-inflammatory properties (Source: *Healthnotes Review of Complementary and Integrative Medicine*, www.healthwell.com/healthnotes/Herb/Nettle.cfm).

niacin. *See* niacinamide.

niacinamide. Also called vitamin B3, niacin, and nicotinic acid, this water-soluble ingredient is stable in the presence of heat and light. Topical application of niacinamide has been shown to increase ceramide and free fatty acid levels in skin, prevent skin from losing water content, and stimulate microcirculation in the dermis (Sources: *British Journal of Dermatology*, September 2000, pages 524–531; and *Journal of Cosmetic Dermatology*, April 2004, page 88). One small study showed that 2% niacinamide was more effective than petrolatum (Vaseline) at reducing water loss from skin and increasing its hydration levels (Source: *International Journal of Dermatology*, March 2005, pages 197–202). Procter & Gamble, whose Olay skin-care line sells several products with niacinamide, published a double-blind study involving 50 women. The subjects used a product containing 5% niacinamide (whether that amount is included in Olay's niacinamide products was not mentioned) for a period of 12 weeks. Results included an improvement in the appearance of wrinkles, a decrease in skin discolorations, less redness, a reduction in sallowness, and improved elasticity (Source: *Dermatologic Surgery*, July 2005, pages 860–865). Another study seconded P&G's findings that niacinamide is a helpful ingredient for addressing skin discolorations. It appears that topical niacinamide has an inhibitory effect on the transfer of melanosomes to skin cells, thus it interrupts the process that causes irregular pigmentation to form (Source: *Experimental Dermatology*, July 2005, pages 498–508).

In addition to niacinamide's growing reputation as an excellent barrier-repair and skin-lightening agent, some animal studies and in vitro studies on human fibroblasts (cells that produce connective tissue such as collagen) demonstrated that niacinamide may have a mitigating effect on skin tumors (Source: *Nutrition and Cancer*, February 1997, pages 157–162). There are fewer studies that examined niacinamide's anti-acne properties. An older study that compared a gel containing 4% niacinamide with the prescription acne medicine Clindamycin found that niacinimide works just as well as the prescription, but without the risk of antibiotic resistance (Source: *International Journal of Dermatology*, June 1995, pages 434–437).

Perhaps even more important is niacinamide's potential as a cell-communicating ingredient (Sources: *Journal of Radiation Research*, December 2004, pages 491–495; *British Journal of Dermatology*, October 2003, page 681; and *Journal of Dermatological Science*, volume 31, 2003, pages 193–201). *See* cell-communicating ingredients.

nicotinamide. *See* niacinamide.

nicotinic acid. *See* niacinamide.

nitrogen. Used as a propellant in cosmetic products; as nitric oxide, it can generate free-radical damage and cause cell death (Source: *Mechanisms of Ageing and Development*, April 2002, pages 1007–1019). Topically applied nitrogen in the amounts present in skin-care products has minimal research (and no third-party, substantiated research) establishing its benefit for skin, but it does not appear to be harmful in its pure form.

nonoxynols. Used as mild surfactants. *See* surfactant.

nordihydroguaiaretic acid. Component of some plants that has been shown to have anti-cancer properties for skin and that may also protect skin from sun damage; also a potent antioxidant (Sources: *British Journal of Cancer*, April 2002, pages 1188–1196; *Molecular Carcinogenesis*, June 2002, pages 102–111; and *Biochemical Pharmacology*, March 2002, pages 1165–1176).

nylon-12. Powder substance that is used as an absorbent and thickening agent.

Nymphaea tetragona. Also known as pygmy waterlily. The stem has been shown in vitro to be not only a potent antioxidant but also able to inhibit the expression of collagen-depleting MMP-1 when applied to human fibroblast cells (Source: *Journal of Cosmetic Science*, January/February 2007, pages 19-32). *See* matrix metalloproteinases.

oak root extract. Extract that may have antibacterial properties on skin, but that also can be a skin irritant.

oatmeal. Can have anti-irritant and anti-inflammatory properties (Source: *Skin Pharmacology and Applied Skin Physiology*, March–April 2002, pages 120–124).

octinoxate. *See* octyl methoxycinnamate.

octisalate. Technical name for the active sunscreen ingredient octyl salicylate (also known as ethylhexyl salicylate). *See* octyl salicylate.

octocrylene. Sunscreen agent that protects skin from the UVB range of sunlight (Sources: www.photodermatology.com/sunprotection.htm; and *Skin Therapy Letter*, 1997, volume 2, number 5, www.dermatology.org/skintherapy).

octyl methoxycinnamate. Sunscreen agent used to protect skin primarily from the sun's UVB rays (Sources: www.photodermatology.com/sunprotection.htm; and *Skin Therapy Letter*, 1997, volume 2, number 5, www.dermatology.org/skintherapy).

octyl palmitate. Used in cosmetics as a thickening agent and emollient.

octyl salicylate. Sunscreen agent used to protect skin primarily from the sun's UVB rays (Sources: www.photodermatology.com/sunprotection.htm; and *Skin Therapy Letter*, 1997, volume 2, number 5, volume 2, number 5, www.dermatology.org/skintherapy).

octyl stearate. Used in cosmetics as a thickening agent and emollient.

octyldodecanol. Emulsifier and opacifying agent, used primarily as a thickener in moisturizers because of its lubricating and emollient properties.

octyldodecyl myristate. Mixture of octyldodecanol (thickener) and myristic acid that forms a new compound used as a skin-conditioning agent and emollient. *See* myristic acid.

octyldodecyl neopentanoate. Skin-conditioning agent and emollient.

o-cymen-5-ol. Preservative used in cosmetics. *See* preservatives.

***Oenothera biennis* oil**. *See* evening primrose oil.

oleic acid. Fatty acid used as a surfactant and thickening agent. *See* fatty acid, surfactant, and thickening agent.

oleths. Mild surfactants. *See* surfactant.

oleyl erucate. Skin-conditioning agent derived from oleyl alcohol, which is obtained chiefly from fish oil.

olibanum extract. *See* frankincense extract.

olive oil. Emollient plant oil similar to all nonfragrant plant oils. The concept of olive oil having anti-aging properties stems from some evidence that diets high in olive oil may help prevent heart disease (Sources: *European Journal of Clinical Nutrition*, January 2002, pages 72–81; and *Lipids*, November 2001, pages 1195–1202, and Supplemental, pages S49–S52). There are also a small number of animal tests showing that topically applied olive oil can protect against UVB damage (Sources: *Carcinogenesis*, November 2000, pages 2085–2090; and *Journal of Dermatological Science*, March 2000, Supplemental, pages S45–S50). It does seem that olive oil is a good antioxidant and assuredly it's a good moisturizing ingredient, but research shows similar results for other oils as well. *See* natural moisturizing factor (NMF).

opium poppy seed. Potent analgesic (Source: *Phytotherapy Research*, September 2000, pages 401–418), although there is no research showing this to be effective when applied topically to skin.

orange blossom. Fragrant extract that can also be a skin irritant.

Orbignya martiana. *See* babassu oil.

Orbignya oleifera. *See* babassu oil.

orchid. Fragrant flower that can be a skin irritant.

oregano. Has potent antibacterial and antifungal properties, but can also be a skin irritant (Source: *Journal of Food Protection*, July 2001, pages 1019–1024).

Origanum majorana. *See* marjoram.

***Origanum vulgare* flower extract**. *See* oregano.

orris root. Used primarily as a fragrant component due to its violet-like scent (Source: www.botanical.com/botanical/mgmh/i/irises08.html). It can cause allergic or sensitizing skin reactions and there is no research showing it has any benefit for skin (Source: *Botanical Dermatology Database*, http://bodd.cf.ac.uk/BotDermFolder/BotDermC/CACT.html).

Ortho Tri-Cyclen. Low-dosage birth-control pills (generic norgestimate/ethinyl estradiol) approved for use in the United States for the treatment of acne. In Canada, the birth control pill Diane-35, a combination of cyproterone acetate and ethinyl estradiol, is approved for treatment of acne (Source: *Skin Therapy Letter*, 1999, volume 4, number 4, www.dermatology.org/skintherapy). According to a double-blind, placebo-controlled study published in *Fertility and Sterility* (September 2001, pages 461–468), other "low-dose birth-control pills can be an effective and safe treatment for moderate acne." The double-blind, placebo-controlled, randomized clinical trial found that the birth-control pill containing levonorgestrel (Alesse) reduced the appearance of acne.

***Oryza sativa* oil**. *See* rice oil.

oryzanol. Component of plants and their products, such as rice bran, that has potent antioxidant properties.

oxidoreductase. Large group of enzymes that reduce or block oxygen in different forms from generating free-radical damage.

oxybenzone. Sunscreen agent that protects primarily from the sun's UVB rays, and some, but not all, UVA rays (Sources: www.photodermatology.com/sunprotection.htm; and *Skin Therapy Letter*, 1997, volume 2, number 5, www.dermatology.org/skintherapy). *See* UVA.

oxygen. Many cosmetic products contain antioxidants, ingredients that reduce the negative effect of oxygen or oxidative substances on skin. At the same time, the cosmetics industry also sells products that contain hydrogen peroxide (H_2O_2) or other oxygen-releasing ingredients, which supposedly deliver an oxygen molecule when they come in contact with skin, although that generates free-radical damage (Source: *Human and Experimental Toxicology*, February 2002, pages 61–62). Why the concern about supplying oxygen to the skin? Oxygen depletion is one of the things that happen to older skin, regardless of whether it's been affected by sun damage or any other health-related factor. Why or how that happens is completely unknown, though it is thought to have something to do with blood flow and a reduction in lung capacity as we age. It is also believed that, with age, the issue isn't so much the amount of oxygen but rather a change in the blood's ability to use the oxygen it has.

However, when wound healing is a problem, regenerating the tissue often demands, in addition to other factors, increased topical oxygen, because wound repair can be facilitated by oxygen therapy. Yet this method of treating wounds lacks research showing it to be effective or to be the best option for skin (Source: *Annals of the New York Academy of Sciences*, May 2002, pages 239–249).

Oxidative stress is an unavoidable consequence of life in an oxygen-rich atmosphere. The "Oxygen Paradox" is that oxygen is dangerous to the very life forms for which it has become an essential component of energy production. The first defense against oxygen toxicity is the sharp reduction in the amount of oxygen present in cells, from the level present in air of 20% to a tissue concentration of only 3% to 4% oxygen. These relatively low tissue levels of oxygen mean that most oxidative damage never occurs. Cells, tissues, organs, and organisms have multiple layers of antioxidant defenses, plus damage replacement and repair systems to cope with the stress and damage that oxygen engenders (Source: *Journal of the International Union of Biochemistry and Molecular Biology*, October–November 2000, pages 279–289). *See* free-radical damage.

ozokerite. Mineral that is used as a thickening agent in cosmetics, especially in lipsticks and stick foundations.

P. elisabethae. The "P." is short for the genus *Pseudopterogorgia*. *See* sea whip extract.

PABA. *See* para-aminobenzoic acid (PABA).

padimate O. Sunscreen agent that protects skin primarily from the sun's UVB rays (Sources: www.photodermatology.com/sunprotection.htm; and *Skin Therapy Letter*, 1997, volume 2, number 5, www.dermatology.org/skintherapy).

***Padina pavonica* extract**. *See* algae.

***Paeonia albiflora* extract**. *See* peony flower.

***Paeonia suffruticosa* extract**. *See* peony root extract.

palm oil. Has emollient and antioxidant properties for skin (Source: *Free Radical Biology and Medicine*, 1997, volume 22, number 5, pages 761–769). *See* antioxidant and natural moisturizing factor (NMF).

***Palmaria palmata* extract**. Extract from a type of algae whose common name is dulse. *See* algae.

palmarosa oil. *See* geranium oil.

palmitic acid. Detergent cleansing agent that also creates foam and can be drying. *See* surfactant.

palmitoyl pentapeptide 3. Trade name Matrixyl, a fatty acid mixed with amino acids. The only research showing this has any significance for skin was carried out by the ingredient manufacturer, Sederma. In their research, three different "half-face" studies with a total of about 45 participants showed it to be better than a retinol or vitamin C product (Source: *Journal of Cosmetic Science,* January–February 2001, pages 77–78). Without independent substantiation, however, there is no way to know how accurate this company-funded research is. Further, according to Sederma's research, the recommended concentration for this ingredient is 3% to 5% and there are few, if any, lines that include more than just a trace amount in their products. *See* amino acid and fatty acid.

***Panax* ginseng root extract**. Root extract that may have potent antioxidant properties (potentially anti-cancer) and may promote wound healing. Whether or not it can have an impact on cellulite is unknown (Sources: *Journal of Agricultural and Food Chemistry,* April 2006, pages 2558–2562; *Phytotherapy Research,* January 2005, pages 65–71; *Archives of Pharmacal Research,* February 2002, pages 71–76; and *Cancer Letters,* March 2000, pages 41–48).

Panicum miliaceum. *See* millet seed extract.

pansy extract. Extract for which there is a small amount of research showing it has anti-inflammatory and antioxidant properties (Source: www.naturaldatabase.com).

pantethine. Also known as pantothenic acid. *See* pantothenic acid.

panthenol. Alcohol form of vitamin B. *See* pantothenic acid.

pantothenic acid. Also called vitamin B5, and often touted as being effective for acne. However, there is only one study supporting this notion and it dates from the early 1980s (Source: *International Journal of Dermatology,* 1981, volume 20, pages 278–285). There is no current research showing this to be an effective treatment for acne, but there is a small amount of research showing that it can be effective for hydration and wound healing (Source: *American Journal of Clinical Dermatology,* 2002, volume 3, number 6, pages 427–433).

papain. Enzyme extracted from papaya. Applied topically, papain can cause severe irritation, itching, and allergic reactions (Source: www.naturaldatabase.com). There is one study showing it may be effective for exfoliation, but only in a pure concentration (Source: *Archives of Dermatological Research,* November 2001, pages 500–507). *See* enzymes.

***Papaver somniferum* seed**. Latin name for the opium poppy seed. *See* opium poppy seed.

papaya extract. Extract that is the source of papain, which theoretically can have exfoliating properties on skin, although the majority of the research was not performed on skin. Papaya can be a skin irritant. *See* enzymes.

para-aminobenzoic acid (PABA). Sunscreen ingredient rarely used since the 1990s because of strong potential for allergic reactions.

parabens. Group of preservatives, including butylparaben, propylparaben, methylparaben, and ethylparaben, that are the most widely used group of preservatives in cosmetics. It is estimated that more than 90% of all cosmetic products contain some form of paraben. Parabens are believed to cause less irritation than some preservatives. There is research showing that in animal models (and in vitro) parabens can have weak estrogenic activity. Whether that poses any health risk for humans who are using cosmetics is unknown. The technical findings of the study, which involved both oral administration and injection into rat skin, did show evidence of a weak estrogen effect on cells in a way that could be problematic for binding to receptor sites that may cause proliferation of MCF-7 breast cancer cells. The study concluded that "future work will need to address the extent to which parabens can accumulate in hormonally sensitive tissues and also the extent to which their weak oestrogenic activity can add to the more general environmental oestrogen problem" (Source: *Journal of Steroid Biochemistry and Molecular Biology*, January 2002, pages 49–60).

Does this mean you should stop buying products that contain parabens? That's a good question, but the answer is neither simple nor conclusive, even by the standards of the study itself. This is a potentially serious issue and the FDA is conducting its own research to determine what this means for human health (Source: *The Endocrine Disruptor Knowledge Base* (EDKB), http://edkb.fda.gov/index.html). To keep the concern in perspective, it is important to realize that parabens are hardly the only substances that may have estrogenic effects on the body.

Any estrogen, including the estrogen our bodies produce, may bind to receptor sites on cells either strongly or weakly. So, parabens can either stimulate the receptor to imitate the effect of our own estrogen in a positive way, or they can generate an abnormal estrogen response. Ironically, plant estrogens, or phytoestrogens (such as those found in soy), also produce chemicals that mimic estrogen. It is possible that a weak plant estrogen can help the body, but it can also be possible that a strong plant estrogen can make matters worse. For example, there is research that shows coffee to be a problem for fibrocystic breast disease. The reason for this is thought to be because coffee exerts estrogenic effects on breast cells (Sources: *American Journal of Epidemiology*, October 1996, pages 642–644; *Journal of the American Medical Women's Association*, spring 2002, pages 85–90; and www.som.tulane.edu/ecme/eehome/newsviews/whatsnew/archive/jan_dec2002.html).

A study in the *Journal of Applied Toxicology* (volume 24, issue 1, January-February 2004, pages 5–13) mentioned that "although recent reports of the oestrogenic properties of parabens have challenged current concepts of their toxicity in these consumer products, the question remains as to whether any of the parabens can accumulate intact in the body from the long-term, low-dose levels to which humans are exposed." The study discussed the fact that traces of parabens have indeed been found in human breast tumors, but was quick to point out that it is unknown if this would be the same in healthy breast tissue. Parabens present in tumors may not be the causative factor, but rather a result, of finding parabens when cancer cells are examined. It is also important to realize that parabens are used in food products as well (Source: *Food Chemistry and Toxicology*, October 2002, pages 1335–1373), which could very well be the source. As yet, no one has any idea (or has evaluated) whether it is the consumption of parabens or their application to the skin that is responsible for their presence in human tissue. And no one knows what the presence of parabens in human tissue means. *See* preservatives.

paraffin. Waxy, petroleum-based substance used as a thickener in cosmetics.

Paraffinum liquidum. *See* mineral oil.

Parsol 1789. *See* avobenzone.

***Passiflora edulis* extract**. *See* passion fruit extract.

passion fruit extract. There is no research showing this has any benefit for skin.

patchouli. Fragrant oil derived from mint. It contains eugenol and can be a skin sensitizer and irritant. *See* counter-irritant.

***Paullinia cupana* seed extract**. Also called guarana, this extract is used primarily in herbal supplements and beverages as a stimulant. In animal studies (mice), it has been shown to affect fat metabolism. There is also research showing that repeated use of guarana can result in persistent increases in heart rate and blood pressure as well as in unfavorable actions on glucose and potassium homeostasis. Such effects could be detrimental in persons with hypertension, atherosclerosis, or glucose intolerance—conditions that are strongly associated with obesity. Guarana is sometimes used in cellulite products because of its theophylline and caffeine components. Research has shown it can be absorbed into the skin. Whether or not topical application can affect fat metabolism or have other associated health risks in humans is not known (Sources: *International Journal of Pharmaceutics*, April 2006, www.sciencedirect.com/; *Food and Chemical Toxicology*, June 2006, pages 862–867; *Clinical Nutrition*, December 20005, pages 1019–1028; and *Clinical Pharmacology & Therapeutics*, June 2005, pages 560–571).

pawpaw extract. *See* papaya extract.

peanut oil. Emollient plant oil similar to all nonfragrant plant oils.

pecan oil. Emollient plant oil similar to all nonfragrant plant oils.

pectin. Natural substance found in plants, especially apples, and used in cosmetics as an emulsifier and thickening agent.

PEG compound. PEG is the acronym for polyethylene glycol. Various forms of PEG compounds are mixed with fatty acids and fatty alcohols to create a variety of substances that have diverse functions in cosmetics, including acting as surfactants, binding agents (to keep ingredients blended), stabilizers, and emollients. *See* polyethylene glycol.

PEG-100 stearate. *See* PEG compound and thickening agent.

PEG-120 methyl glucose dioleate. *See* surfactant.

PEG-150 distearate. *See* thickening agent.

PEG-40 hydrogenated castor oil. Emollient ingredient that is a mixture of polyethylene glycol (PEG) with castor oil. *See* polyethylene glycol (PEG) and castor oil.

PEG-80 sorbitan laurate. Mild surfactant. *See* surfactant.

***Pelargonium graveolens* oil**. *See* geranium oil.

pellitory. Plant whose root extract can cause skin irritation; its safety is unknown.

pentadecalactone. Synthetic fragrance used in cosmetics.

pentasodium pentetate. Used as a chelating agent in cosmetics to prevent various mineral components from binding together and negatively affecting the formulation.

pentaerythrityl tetraoctanoate. Synthetic compound as an emollient and thickening agent. *See* thickening agent.

peony flower. European flower used topically for treating a variety of skin diseases, including skin fissures (painful cracks in skin). Evidence of its effectiveness for these purposes is anecdotal. There is not enough known about the effects of peony flower to substantiate its use or safety in cosmetic products (Source: www.naturaldatabase.com).

peony root extract. There is research showing that the root of the peony plant can have anticancer properties as well as antioxidant properties (Sources: *Cancer Letters*, December 2001, pages 17–24; *Archives of Pharmaceutical Research*, April 2001, pages 105–108; and *Chemical and Pharmaceutical Bulletin*, January 2001, pages 69–72). However, there is no research showing that it has that benefit for skin (Source: www.naturaldatabase.com).

peppermint. Both the oil and the extract can have antimicrobial properties (Source: *Journal of Agricultural and Food Chemistry*, July 2002, pages 3943–3946), but they can also have an irritating, sensitizing effect on skin (Source: www.naturaldatabase.com). *See* counter-irritant.

peptide. Peptides are portions of proteins, which are long chains of amino acids. In the body, peptides regulate the activity of many systems by interacting with target cells. Enzymatic action breaks proteins into peptides so they can exert their influence on the body. Some peptides have hormonal activity, others have immune activity, some are cell-communicating ingredients that tell cells how to react and what to do, some are believed to play a role in wound healing, and still others are believed to affect the pathology of skin conditions such as atopic dermatitis and eczema.

Whether peptides have benefit when applied topically to skin for wound healing, skin-barrier repair, or as disinfectants is difficult to ascertain because they generally cannot penetrate skin and at the same time remain stable because they are too hydrophilic, or water-loving. Ironically, peptides can become unstable in water-based formulas (Sources: *Biotechniques*, July 2002, pages 190–192; and *IFSCC Magazine*, July 2004, page 153). Further, because peptides are vulnerable to the presence of enzymes, when peptides are absorbed, the abundant enzymes present in skin can break the peptides down to the point where they have no effect at all. However, the latest research is examining how different types of synthesized peptides can enter the living membrane of cells and, more interesting, transport biologically active ingredients to these cells. Some of these peptides have demonstrated a remarkable anti-inflammatory effect. Creating specific peptide chains in the lab and then attaching a fatty acid component to them allows peptides to overcome their inherent limitations: being absorbed and remaining stable. Lab-engineered peptides appear to have the kind of efficacy and benefit that go beyond the skin's surface, but more conclusive, long-term research is essential to gain an understanding of what, if anything, is really taking place (Sources: *Cosmetics & Toiletries*, June 2004, page 30; *Pharmaceutical Research*, March 2004, pages 389–393; and *The Journal of Investigative Dermatology*, September 2005, pages 473–481). It is reasonable to assume that as synthetic peptide technology broadens, we will see more options for use in skin-care products promoting anti-aging properties, specifically, tissue regeneration (Source: *Cosmetics & Toiletries*, March 2003, pages 43–52).

For these specialized peptides to exert a benefit beyond that of a water-binding agent, three criteria must be met: the peptides must be stable in their base formula, they must be paired with a carrier that enhances absorption into the skin, and they must be able to reach their target cell groups without breaking down. Achieving this goal is no easy feat, but one that cosmetics scientists are predicting will have significant potential in the realm of anti-aging skin-care ingredients.

Persicaria hydropiper. Also known as water pepper. All parts of this plant extract have been shown in vitro to be not only a potent antioxidant but also able to inhibit the expression of collagen-depleting MMP-1 when applied to human fibroblast cells (Source: *Journal of Cosmetic Science*, January/February 2007, pages 19-32). *See* matrix metalloproteinases.

***Persea gratissima* oil**. *See* avocado oil.

petitgrain mandarin. *See* mandarin orange oil or extract.

petrolatum. Vaseline is pure petrolatum. For some unknown and unsubstantiated reason, petrolatum has attained a negative image in regard to skin care, despite solid research to the contrary. Topical application of petrolatum can help the skin's outer layer recover from damage, reduce inflammation, and generally heal the skin (Source: *Acta Dermato-Venereologica*, November–December 2000, pages 412–415). *See* also mineral oil.

PHA. *See* polyhydroxy acid.

phenoxyethanol. Common cosmetic preservative that is considered one of the less irritating ones to use in formulations. It does not release formaldehyde. *See* preservatives.

phenoxyisopropanol. Alcohol used as a solvent and preservative. *See* solvent and preservative.

phenyl trimethicone. Silicone with a drier finish than dimethicone. *See* silicone.

phenylalanine. *See* amino acid.

phosphatidylcholine. Active ingredient in lecithin. Every cell membrane in the body requires phosphatidylcholine (PC). It is also a major source of the neurotransmitter acetylcholine. Acetylcholine is used by the brain in areas that are involved in long-term planning, concentration, and focus, but all of that information is associated with ingesting PC, not putting it on the skin. PC is considered a very good water-binding agent and aids in the penetration of other ingredients into the skin. It absorbs well without feeling greasy or heavy (although other ingredients can perform similarly, including glycerin, ceramides, and hyaluronic acid) (Sources: *Skin Pharmacology and Applied Skin Physiology*, September–October 1999, pages 235–246; and *Journal of Controlled Release*, March 29, 1999, pages 207–214.) *See* lecithin and water-binding agent.

phosphatidylethanolamine. *See* phospholipid.

phospholipid. Type of lipid (fat) composed of glycerol, fatty acids, and phosphate. Phospholipids are essential to the function of cell membranes by providing a stable surrounding structure. Lecithin is an example of a phosopholipid. *See* glyceryl ester and natural moisturizing factor (NMF).

phosphoric acid. Used as a pH adjuster in cosmetics and skin-care products.

photosensitizer. Ingredient that can cause the skin to have an irritated or inflamed reaction when exposed to sunlight.

***Phyllanthus emblica* fruit extract**. Extract that has antioxidant and anti-inflammatory properties (Sources: *Journal of Ethnopharmacology*, May 2000, pages 171–176; and *Planta Medica*, December 1997, pages 518–524).

phytantriol. Hair- and skin-conditioning agent that also has water-binding properties.

phytic acid. Component of plants that has antioxidant properties.

phytoestrogen. *See* plant estrogen.

phytonadione. One form of vitamin K. *See* vitamin K.

phytosphingosine. Long-chain, complex fatty alcohol that functions as a water-binding agent and also has preservative qualities. Its name is derived from the term *sphingoid*, coined in 1884 by chemist J. L. W. Thudichum because the way the molecules of this substance lined up reminded him of the riddle of the Sphinx. Research shows it is effective in regulating damaged or diseased epithelial cells. It seems this ingredient can also be a cell-communicating ingredient, albeit one that is best for compromised skin (Source: *Journal of Investigative Dermatology*, October 2003, pages 1135–1137).

phytosterol. Cholesterol-like molecules found in all plant foods; the highest concentrations are found in vegetable oils. Phytosterols in the natural diet may lower cholesterol (Sources: *Annual Reviews of Nutrition*, 2002, volume 22, pages 533–549; and *Metabolism*, May 2002, pages 652–656). However, regarding topical application, there is research showing that the high lipid content of phytosterols can make the skin extremely sensitive to light (Source: *Photochemistry and Photobiology*, September 1997, pages 316–325).

pinecone extract. Components of this extract, specifically linolenic and linoleic acids, can have antioxidant properties (Source: *Tree Physiology*, June 2002, pages 661–666) and antibacterial properties for skin (Source: *International Journal of Food Microbiology*, May 2000, pages 3–12).

pine oil. Can have disinfectant properties (Source: *Antimicrobial Agents and Chemotherapy*, December 1997, pages 2770–2772), but it can also be a potent skin irritant and should never be used on abraded or chafed skin. May be used as an extract or oil.

pineapple extract. Contains the enzyme bromelain, which can break down the connecting layers between skin cells to exfoliate skin. However, bromelain used alone is a more effective source of exfoliation, and does not have the irritating properties of the pineapple. *See* bromelain.

***Pinus lambertiana* wood extract**. Pine extract that may have skin-sensitizing properties (Source: Botanical Dermatology Database, http://bodd.cf.ac.uk/index.html).

***Pinus sylvestris* extract**. *See* pinecone extract.

Piper nigrum. *See* black pepper.

pistachio seed oil. Emollient plant oil with uses similar to peanut oil in cosmetics. *See* peanut oil.

***Pistacia vera* seed oil**. *See* pistachio seed oil.

Pisum sativum. Latin name for the garden pea. It does have antioxidant activity, but there is no research showing that it can reduce cellulite (Source: *Phytotherapy Research*, October 2003, pages 987–1000).

plasticizing agents. Ingredients that place a thin layer of plastic over the skin. Typically these are used in facial masks so they can be peeled off the skin. *See* film-forming agent.

plum extract. Extract of *Prunus americana* that may have antioxidant activity when applied topically (Source: *Phytotherapy Research*, February 2002, pages 63–65).

Pogostemon cablin. *See* patchouli.

poloxamers. *See* surfactant.

polyacrylamide. *See* film-forming agent.

polyaminopropyl biguanide. Synthetic polymer that functions as a preservative.

polybutene. Polymer derived from mineral oil and used as a thickener and lubricant.

polycaprolactone. Biodegradable thermoplastic polymer derived from the chemical synthesis of crude oil. It may have application in supporting skin-tissue growth for the purposes of skin grafts (Source: *Tissue Engineering*, August 2001, pages 441–455).

polyethylene glycol. Also listed as PEG on ingredient labels, polyethylene glycol is an ingredient that self-proclaimed "natural" Web sites have attempted to make notoriously evil. They gain a great deal of attention by attributing horror stories to PEG, associating it with antifreeze (however, antifreeze is **ethylene** glycol, not **polyethylene** glycol), and there is no research indicating that PEG compounds pose any problem for skin. Quite the contrary: PEGs have no known skin toxicity and can be used on skin with great results (Sources: *Advanced Drug Delivery Reviews*, June 2002, pages 587–606; and *Cancer Research*, June 2002, pages 3138–3143). The only negative research for this ingredient indicates that large quantities given orally to rats can cause tumors, but that is unrelated to topical application.

Polyethylene, when it is not combined with glycol, is the most common form of plastic used in the world. It is flexible and has a smooth, waxy feel. When ground up, the small particles are included in scrubs as a gentle abrasive. When mixed with glycol, it becomes a viscous liquid. In the minuscule amounts used in cosmetics, it helps keep products stable and performs functions similar to those of glycerin. Because polyethylene glycol can penetrate skin, it is also a vehicle that helps deliver other ingredients deeper into the skin. It is also used internally in medical procedures to flush and clean the intestinal tract. *See* propylene glycol.

polyglucuronic acid. *See* film-forming agent.

polyglycerol monostearate. Used as an emollient and thickening agent in cosmetics. *See* glyceryl ester.

polyglycerol polyricinoleate. Used as an emollient and thickening agent in cosmetics. *See* glyceryl ester.

polyglyceryl methacrylate. *See* film-forming agent.

polyglyceryl-3 methylglucose distearate. *See* glyceryl ester.

***Polygonum cuspidatum* root extract**. Extract of the Japanese knotweed plant. When eaten it may have weak estrogenic activity (Source: *Bioorganic and Medicinal Chemistry Letters*, July 2001, pages 1839–1842) and antitumor activity (Source: *Journal of Nutrition*, June 2001, pages 1844–1849). It also has antioxidant properties (Source: *Biological & Pharmaceutical Bulletin*, January 1995, pages 162–166).

polyhydroxy acid. Ingredients such as gluconolactone and lactobionic acid are types of polyhydroxy acid (PHA). They are supposed to be as effective as AHAs but less irritating (NeoStrata is the company that holds a patent on glycolic acid as an antiwrinkle agent, as well as a patent for gluconolactone for reducing the appearance of wrinkles). Gluconolactone and lactobionic acid are chemically and functionally similar to AHAs. The significant difference between them and AHAs is that gluconolactone and lactobionic acid have larger molecular structures, which limits their ability to penetrate into the skin, resulting in a reduction of irritating side-effects. Supposedly, this reduced absorption into the skin does not hamper their effectiveness. Does that mean gluconolactone and lactobionic acid are better for your skin than AHAs in the form of glycolic acid or lactic acid? According to an Internet-published class lecture by Dr. Mark G. Rubin (Source: http://128.11.40.183/laser-news/rubin_lecture/21.html), a board-certified dermatologist and assistant clinical professor of dermatology at the University of California, San Diego, research on gluconolactone demonstrated only a "6% decrease in dermal penetration" in comparison to glycolic acid, which "isn't a dramatic improvement." Gluconolactone may be slightly less irritating for some skin types, but this isn't the magic bullet for exfoliation that beauty magazines and some cosmetics companies have been extolling. There is no independent research information available about lactobionic acid.

polyhydroxysteatic acid. Synthetic polymer related to stearic acid. It functions as a suspending agent.

polyquaterniums. Group of ingredients used primarily in hair-care products for their antistatic and film-forming properties. They can have water-binding properties for skin due to the sheer "plastic" film layer they create on skin.

polysaccharide. Natural component of skin that can be a good water-binding agent and potentially have antioxidant properties. *See* mucopolysaccharide and natural moisturizing factor (NMF).

polysorbate-20. *See* polysorbates.

polysorbates. Fatty acids that are used as emollients and thickening agents in cosmetics. *See* fatty acid.

polyvinyl alcohol. *See* plasticizing agents.

polyvinylpyrrolidone. Usually listed on ingredient labels as PVP or PVP copolymer, it is one of the primary ingredients used in hairstyling products to hold hair in place. When present in minuscule amounts in skin-care products, it places an imperceptible film over the skin that is considered to be water-binding and that helps give the appearance of firmer skin. It can be a skin sensitizer for some individuals. *See* film-forming agent.

pomegranate extract. Extract that contains ellagic acid, and is considered effective as an anticarcinogen and antioxidant when taken orally. There is no research showing what effect, if any, this extract can have on skin (Sources: *Journal of Agricultural Food Chemistry*, January 2002, pages 81–86, and 166–171; and *International Journal of Oncology*, May 2002, pages 983–986).

***Poria cocos* extract**. Also known as Hoelen and Fu ling. Extract derived from a mushroom, which has antioxidant and anti-inflammatory properties (Sources: *Life Sciences*, January 2002, pages 1023–1033; and *Journal of Ethnopharmacology*, November 2000, pages 61–69).

***Porphyridium cruentum* extract**. Extract derived from a type of red algae. There is research showing components of red algae contain the omega-3 fatty acid eicosapentaenoic acid, the omega-6 fatty acid arachidonic acid, and other skin-friendly ingredients such as polysaccharides. Whether or not the entire red algae extract provides benefit when applied topically on skin is not known (Sources: *Bioseparation*, September 2000, pages 299–306; and *Free Radical Biology and Medicine*, February 1996, pages 241–249).

***Portulaca oleracea* extract**. Extract that may have anti-inflammatory or analgesic properties (Sources: *Journal of Ethnopharmacology*, July 2001, pages 171–176, and December 2000, pages 445–451).

potassium. Important element in diet that is present in such fruits as bananas and citrus. It is also an earth mineral that has absorbent properties and some disinfecting properties, but can also be a skin irritant.

potassium ascorbyl tocopheryl phosphate. Blend of vitamins C and E with phosphorus that functions as an antioxidant. *See* antioxidant.

potassium cetyl phosphate. Used as a detergent cleansing agent. *See* surfactant.

potassium hydroxide. Also known as lye, a highly alkaline ingredient used in small amounts in cosmetics to modulate the pH of a product. It is also used as a cleansing agent in some cleansers. In higher concentrations it is a significant skin irritant.

potassium myristate. Detergent cleansing agent that is a constituent of soap; it can be drying and sensitizing for some skin types. *See* surfactant.

PPG-2-myristyl ether propionate. Skin-conditioning agent that may be plant-derived or synthetic. Composed from derivatives of polypropylene glycol and myristyl alcohol.

PPG-12 buteth-16. Versatile ingredient composed of several non-volatile alcohols. Functions as a skin-conditioning agent, emulsifier, solvent, and surfactant.

PPG-14 butyl ether. Used as a hair- and skin-conditioning agent.

PPG-2 myristyl ether propionate. Mixture of glycols and fatty alcohols used as a skin-conditioning agent and, in some cases, as a thickening agent.

pregnenolone acetate. Precursor to other hormones, it can affect levels of progesterone and estrogen in the body when taken orally. When applied to skin it may work as a water-binding agent. There is no information about whether absorption through the skin is possible.

preservatives. Substances used in cosmetics to prevent bacterial and microbial contamination of products. While there is definitely a risk of irritation from these types of ingredients, the risk to skin and eyes from using a contaminated product is considered by many scientists to be even greater.

progesterone USP. A study published in the *American Journal of Obstetrics and Gynecology* (June 1999, pages 1504–1511) states that "In order to obtain the proper (effective) serum levels with use of a progesterone cream, the cream needs to have an adequate amount of progesterone in it [at least 30 milligrams per gram]. Many over the counter creams have little [for example, 5 milligrams per ounce] or none at all. The creams that are made from Mexican yams are not metabolized to progesterone by women. The cream used in the above study (Pro-Gest) contains pure United States Pharmacopoeia [USP] progesterone." Dr. John Lee, author and longtime proponent of topically applied progesterone, explains that "The USP progesterone used for hormone replacement comes from plant fats and oils, usually a substance called diosgenin, which is extracted from a very specific type of wild yam that grows in Mexico, or from soybeans. In the laboratory, diosgenin is chemically synthesized into real human progesterone. Some companies are trying to sell … 'wild yam extract' [or other plant extracts] … claiming that the body will then convert it into hormones as needed. While we know this can be done in the laboratory, there is no evidence that this conversion takes place in the human body." Dr. Lee is quick to explain that he doesn't sell any of these products and receives no profit from their sale. He also does not recommend the use of natural progesterone creams with any other active hormones or herbs. *See* Paula's article "Progesterone" at www.cosmeticscop.com.

proline. *See* amino acid.

propolis. Brownish, resinous material that is collected by bees and used to construct the hive. It has antibacterial and anti-inflammatory properties for skin (Source: *Antimicrobial Agents and Chemotherapy*, May 2002, pages 1302–1309).

propylene carbonate. Liquid used as a solvent and film-forming agent. *See* film-forming agent.

propylene glycol. Along with other glycols and glycerol, this is a humectant or humidifying and delivery ingredient used in cosmetics. There are Web sites and spam e-mails stating that propylene glycol is really industrial antifreeze and that it is the major ingredient in brake and hydraulic fluids. These sites also state that tests show it is a strong skin irritant. They further point out that the Material Safety Data Sheet (MSDS) on propylene glycol warns users to avoid skin contact because systemically (in the body) it can cause liver abnormalities and kidney damage. As ominous as this sounds, it is so far from the reality of cosmetic formulations that almost none of it holds any water or poses real concern. It is important to realize that the MSDS sheets are talking about 100% concentrations of a substance. Even water and salt have frightening comments regarding their safety according to their MSDSs. In cosmetics, propylene glycol is used only in the smallest amounts to keep products from melting in high heat or freezing when it is cold. It also helps active ingredients penetrate the skin. In the minute amounts used in cosmetics, it is not a concern in the least. Women are not suffering from liver problems because of propylene glycol in cosmetics. And finally, according to the U.S. Department of Health and Human Services, within the Public Health Services Agency for Toxic Substances and Disease Registry, "studies have not shown these chemicals [propylene or the other glycols as used in cosmetics] to be carcinogens" (Source: www.atsdr.cdc.gov). See Paula's article, "Propylene Glycol" at www.cosmeticscop.com.

www.atsdr.cdc.gov). See Paula's article, "Propylene Glycol" at www.cosmeticscop.com.

propylene glycol stearate. Mixture of propylene glycol and stearic acid used as a skin-conditioning agent and emulsifier. *See* propylene glycol and stearic acid.

propylparaben. *See* parabens.

proteases. Enzymes that are part of a process that causes the breakdown of amino acids and proteins in skin (Source: www.chemistry-info.net/). There is research showing that proteases, when applied topically to skin, can reduce the visible scaling associated with dry, flaky skin (Source: *Archives of Dermatological Research*, November 2001, pages 500–507). Whether proteases can be of benefit for wound healing when applied topically is unclear (Source: *Experimental Dermatology*, October 2001, pages 337–348).

protein. Proteins are the fundamental components of all living cells and include a diverse range of biological substances, such as enzymes, hormones, and antibodies, that are necessary for the proper functioning of any organism, plant or animal. The human body contains perhaps 100,000 different proteins, each composed of an assortment of 20 or so amino acids. The sequence of these amino acids determines the unique properties of each protein, such as, for example, its role as an enzyme acting as a catalyst for a specific biochemical reaction. If even one of the essential amino acids is missing, the protein cannot be formed. This fact is well known to nutritionists because ensuring an adequate supply of essential amino acids is important in determining the nutritional value of proteins in the diet. Components of proteins can have varying benefits for skin, but overall they are used for their water-binding and emollient properties.

Prunella vulgaris. *See* self-heal.

Prunus americana. *See* plum extract.

***Prunus domestica* seed extract**. *See* plum extract.

Prunus dulcis. *See* almond oil.

Pseudopterogorgia elisabethae. *See* sea whip extract.

Pueraria lobata. *See* kudzu root.

pullulan. Glucan gum produced by black yeast that contains polysaccharides, which makes it a good water-binding agent, thickening agent, and antioxidant. *See* beta-glucan and mucopolysaccharide.

***Punica granatum* extract.** *See* pomegranate extract.

purified water. *See* deionized water.

PVM/MA decadiene crosspolymer. Synthetic polymer used as a film-forming and thickening agent.

PVP. *See* polyvinylpyrrolidone.

PVP copolymer. *See* polyvinylpyrrolidone.

PVP/dimethylaminoethylmethacrylate. Polymer formed from PVP (polyvinylpyrrolidone) and the film-forming agent dimethylaminomethacrylate. *See* film-forming agent and polyvinylpyrrolidone.

pycnogenol. Antioxidant derived from the bark of the French Maritime pine tree. The term pycnogenol was previously used generically, but is now a U.S.-registered trademark. Only one company (Horphag Research, Ltd.) has access to this ingredient, and it is patent-protected.

There is a great deal of research on pycnogenol. However, most of the research dates back to 1990 and earlier (Source: U.S. Patent No. 4,698,360 entitled "Plant Extract with a Proanthocyanidins Content as Therapeutic Agent Having Radical Scavenging Effect and

Use Thereof"). Prior to and even after pycnogenol was trademarked, it was used freely as a generic term for procyanidins. Procyanidins (also known as proanthocyanidins) are pigments belonging to the flavonoid family of ingredients. In addition to being derived from pine bark, procyanidins occur naturally in grape seeds (so red wine is a good source), peanut skins, unripe strawberries, apples, and cocoa beans.

There are studies supporting the notion that pycnogenol is a potent antioxidant with strong free-radical-scavenging properties (Source: Free Radical Biology and Medicine, September 1999, pages 704–724). The most recent studies examined the effect of pycnogenol when taken as an oral supplement for various conditions, most often circulation problems (Sources: *Angiology*, October–November 2006, pages 569–576; and *Clinical and Applied Thrombosis/Hemostasis*, April 2006, pages 205–212). However, there is no research showing that it can have any effect on wrinkles (Source: *Dermatologic Surgery*, July 2005, pages 873–880). *See* antioxidant and bioflavonoid.

pyridoxine hydrochloride (HCL). Scientific name for vitamin B6; may have antibacterial and antioxidant benefits for skin when applied topically.

Pyrus cydonia. *See* quince seed.

Pyrus malus. Species of apple; the pectin derived from it is used as a thickener in cosmetics.

quaternium-15. Formaldehyde-releasing preservative used in cosmetics. It can be a skin sensitizer, as can all preservatives.

quaternium-18 hectorite. Used as a suspending agent and also has emulsifying properties.

quercetin. Flavonoid pigment that has antioxidant and anti-inflammatory properties. Quercetin has antihistamine properties when taken internally via foods (e.g., apples, red wine, and buckwheat natural sources) or supplement form (Source: www.naturaldatabase.com). *See* bioflavonoid.

quercus. *See* oak root extract.

***Quercus infectoria* extract**. *See* oak root extract.

quillaja extract. Extract of the Chilean soap bark tree. It contains a good amount of saponins, which have cleansing, antimicrobial, and water-binding properties for skin. *See* saponin.

quince seed. Used as a thickening agent in cosmetics, but also has skin-constricting properties (Source: www.naturaldatabase.com) and may cause skin irritation.

quinoa oil. Derived from quinoa grain, it may have antifungal properties (Source: *Journal of Agricultural Food Chemistry*, May 2001, pages 2327–2332). It may also have emollient properties for skin, but there is little research showing this to be the case.

***Ranunculus ficaria* extract**. Extract that may have antibacterial and antifungal properties and that is used in the treatment of hemorrhoids. However, applied topically it can cause skin irritation and may also cause photodermatitis (Source: www.naturaldatabase.com).

rapeseed oil. Nonfragrant oil that has emollient and potential antioxidant properties for skin (Source: *British Journal of Nutrition*, May 2002, pages 489–499).

raspberry seed extract. *See* red raspberry extract.

raspberry seed oil. *See* red raspberry extract.

red algae. *See* algae.

red clover. Can have antioxidant and anti-inflammatory properties (Source: *Photochemistry and Photobiology*, September 2001, pages 465–470). It is sold as an herbal supplement for relief of menopausal symptoms such as hot flashes and vaginal dryness. Red clover does contain high concentrations of four major isoflavones that have been shown to have estrogenic properties.

However, in studies, red clover was found to be no better than a placebo for menopausal symptoms (Sources: *Harvard Women's Health Watch*, December 2001, www.health.harvard.edu/medline/Women/W1201e.html; and www.naturaldatabase.com).

red raspberry extract. Fruit extract that has potent antioxidant properties (Source: *Journal of Agricultural Food Chemistry*, June 5, 2002, pages 3495–3500) and antibacterial properties (Source: *International Journal of Food Microbiology*, May 2000, pages 3–12). It also can cause irritation due to its tannin content.

red sandalwood. Has a phytoestrogen component (Source: *Phytochemistry*, March 2000, pages 605–606), but can also be a skin irritant (Source: *Contact Dermatitis*, January 1996, page 69).

reducing agent. In cosmetics, substance that has the ability to split or break down the disulfide bonds of hair. Therefore, reducing agents are typically used in hair-straightening or hair-waving products and in depilatories. The chemical reaction they generate has antioxidant properties, but they can also be strong skin irritants.

Renova. *See* Retin-A and tretinoin.

resorcinol. Considered an effective topical disinfectant in concentrations of 1% to 3% (Source: www.fda.gov). However, there is also research showing it to be overly irritating for skin (Source: *Journal of the European Academy of Dermatology and Venereology*, July 1999, pages 14–23). As a result it is rarely used nowadays for treating blemishes.

resveratrol. Potent polyphenolic antioxidant that is abundant in red grapes and, therefore, in red wine (unfortunately for some of us, not in white wine). Resveratrol has been reported in numerous studies to be one of the most potent natural chemopreventive agents inhibiting the cellular processes associated with tumor development, including initiation, promotion, and progression. It also has significant anti-inflammatory properties. Conversely, there is research showing it to be associated with cell death when applied topically if skin is exposed to sunlight (Sources: *Anticancer Research*, September–October 2004, pages 2783–2840; *Medicinal Chemistry*, November 2005, pages 629–633; *Molecular Nutrition and Food Research*, May 2005, pages 405–430; *Antioxidant Redox Signal*, December 2001, pages 1041–1064; and *Mutation Research, Genetic Toxicology and Environmental Mutagenesis*, September 2001, pages 171–180).

Retin-A. One of several prescription-only drugs (others include Renova, Retin-A Micro, and Avita) that contain tretinoin (technical name: all-trans retinoic acid), which is the acid form of vitamin A, as the active ingredient. In skin, tretinoin is the form of vitamin A that can actually affect cell production by binding to the tretinoin receptor sites on the cell. There is a great deal of research establishing that tretinoin is effective in improving cell production in skin that has been damaged (often by exposure to sunlight). Tretinoin is a valid method for addressing wrinkles and, overall, for improving cell production. Applying tretinoin does not produce miraculous results, but the positive outcome in terms of skin health is indisputable. However, it is highly possible that applying tretinoin to the skin will cause irritation, which is a major drawback of this drug. *See* tretinoin.

retinol. If the layers of connective tissue beneath the skin on the thighs are indeed the main cause of cellulite (along with excess or poorly formed fat deposits), then improving skin structure should, theoretically, make a difference, and there is growing evidence that this is the case. Retinol (the entire vitamin A molecule) is one of the ingredients known to help improve skin structure. Of all the ingredients to look for in a cellulite product, this should be at the top of the list. However, most cellulite products contain only teeny amounts of retinol (at best) and are often in packaging that won't keep this air-sensitive ingredient stable. One other point: Johnson & Johnson has a study showing that a combination of retinol, caffeine, and ruscogenine can reduce the appearance of cellulite. Of course, J&J-owned companies RoC and Neutrogena both sell cellulite products with that combination of ingredients (Sources: *Journal of Cosmetic Science*, July–August 2001, pages 199–210; *Journal of the European Academy of Dermatology & Venereology*, July 2000, page 251; and *American Journal of Clinical Dermatology*, November–December 2000, pages 369–374).

retinyl palmitate. Form of vitamin A. It is a combination of retinol (pure vitamin A) and palmitic acid. There is research showing it to be effective as an antioxidant and skin-cell regulator (Sources: *European Journal of Medical Research*, September 2001, pages 391–398; and *Journal of Investigative Dermatology*, September 1997, pages 301–305). *See* retinol.

riboflavin. *See* vitamin B2.

rice bran oil. Emollient oil similar to other nonfragrant plant oils. There is no research showing this has any superior benefit for skin.

rice oil. Emollient similar to other nonfragrant plant oils. There is no research showing this has any superior benefit for skin.

rice starch. Absorbent substance sometimes included in products rather than talc. It can cause allergic reactions and, because it is a food derivative (as opposed to a mineral derivative like talc), it can support bacterial growth in pores.

ricinoleate. Glyceryl triester used in cosmetics as a thickening agent and emollient.

Ricinus communis. *See* castor oil.

RNA. Ribonucleic acid is a single strand of molecules, copied exactly from the DNA in the cell nucleus, that is required for the body's production of protein. This single strand is a linear, ladder-like sequence of nucleotide bases (chemicals that form its structure) that corresponds precisely to the sequence of bases in the DNA strand (the core of the body's genetic makeup). RNA in a skin-care product is useless because it cannot affect a cell's genetic elements. The production of DNA and RNA is an extremely complex process that requires a multitude of proteins and enzymes to have its effect on the body's genetic material. And let me say that it is doubtful that you would ever want to put anything on your skin that could affect your genetic material, and particularly not via a cosmetic, for which there are no safety or efficacy regulations.

***Robinia pseudacacia* extract**. *See* black locust extract.

Rosa canina. *See* rose hip oil.

Rosa centifolia. *See* rose hip oil.

***Rosa damascena* oil**. Oil of a very fragrant pink rose used as fragrance in cosmetics.

Rosa eglanteria. *See* rose hip oil.

***Rosa gallica* flower extract**. Fragrant extract.

Rosa mosqueta. *See* rose hip oil.

Rosa centifolia flower. *See* rose hip.

***Rosa roxburghii* extract**. Extract from the chestnut rose; can be a source of antioxidants for skin, and does not impart fragrance (Source: *International Journal of Clinical Chemistry and Applied Molecular Biology*, November 2001, pages 37–43).

Rosa rubiginosa. *See* rose hip oil.

rose flower. Highly fragrant substance that can be a skin irritant.

rose flower oil. Fragrant, volatile oil that can be a skin irritant and sensitizer. There is no research showing this has any benefit for skin.

rose hip. Seed-containing part of a rose. *See* rose hip oil and vitamin C.

rose hip oil. Good emollient oil that has antioxidant properties (Sources: *Journal of Agricultural Food Chemistry*, March 2000, pages 825–828; and *Journal of Nutrition*, March 2002, pages 461–471).

rose oil. Fragrant, volatile oil that can be a skin irritant and sensitizer.

rosemary extract. Extract that can have antioxidant benefit for skin (Source: *Journal of Agricultural Food Chemistry*, October 1999, pages 3954–3962), but its aromatic components can cause irritation or sensitizing or toxic reactions on skin (Source: *Chemical Research in Toxicology*, November 2001, pages 1546–1551).

rosemary oil. *See* rosemary extract.

***Rosmarinus officinalis* extract**. *See* rosemary extract.

royal jelly. Milky white, thick substance secreted by worker bees that has been shown to have some immune-modulating benefits (Source: *Comparative Immunology, Microbiology and Infectious Diseases*, January 1996, pages 31–38). The myriad other claims about royal jelly, such as being able to prevent wrinkles and heal acne, are all anecdotal and have no research to substantiate them.

Rubus idaeus. *See* red raspberry extract.

Rubus occidentalis. *See* black raspberry.

Rubus ursinus x idaeus. *See* boysenberry.

Rubus ursinus. *See* marionberry.

Ruscus aculeatus. *See* butcher's broom extract.

rutin. Bioflavonoid that is extracted from various plants and used in cosmetics as an antioxidant and emollient (Sources: *Cell Biology and Toxicology*, 2000, volume 16, number 2, pages 91–98; and *Life Sciences*, January 14, 2000, pages 709–723). *See* bioflavonoid.

saccharide isomerate. Good water-binding agent and emollient for skin. *See* mucopolysaccharide.

saccharides. *See* mucopolysaccharide.

Saccharomyces cerevisiae. *Saccharomyces*, from the Latin, literally means "sugar fungus," and is the scientific name for the yeasts used in fermentation, specifically baker's yeast. It is the simplest single-cell organism that operates in a manner similar to human cells and is, therefore, an important organism used in genetic and molecular biology research. The *Saccharomyces cerevisiae* genome has been sequenced. There are many versions of this fungus fermented with various compounds. Cosmetic ingredient manufacturers extol this yeast as having significant properties for skin, but there is little independent research supporting its use on skin. However, some extracts of yeast, such as beta-glucan (a potent antioxidant) are derived from yeast (Sources: *Proceedings of the National Academy of Sciences*, August 15, 1989, pages 6018–6022; and http://www.in-cosmetics.com/ExhibitorLibrary/3/BiodynesO3.pdf).

Saccharomyces lysate. *See* yeast.

***Saccharomyces* calcium ferment**. Extract of yeast fermented in the presence of calcium ions. It has no known benefit for skin.

***Saccharomyces* copper ferment**. Extract of yeast fermented in the presence of copper ions. There is no known benefit for skin, though it may have antioxidant properties.

***Saccharomyces* iron ferment**. Extract of yeast fermented in the presence of iron ions. *See Saccharomyces* copper ferment.

***Saccharomyces* magnesium ferment**. Extract of yeast fermented in the presence of magnesium ions. *See Saccharomyces* copper ferment.

***Saccharomyces* manganese ferment**. Extract of yeast fermented in the presence of manganese ions. *See Saccharomyces* copper ferment.

***Saccharomyces officinarum* ferment**. Derived from the sugarcane plant. Glycolic acid is also derived from sugarcane, but sugarcane extract does not have the same exfoliating properties as glycolic acid. There is no research showing that sugarcane extract has any benefit for skin. *See* AHA.

***Saccharomyces* potassium ferment**. Extract of yeast fermented in the presence of potassium ions. *See Saccharomyces* copper ferment.

***Saccharomyces* silicon ferment**. Extract of yeast fermented in the presence of silicon ions. *See Saccharomyces* copper ferment.

***Saccharomyces* zinc ferment**. Extract of yeast fermented in the presence of zinc ions. *See Saccharomyces* copper ferment.

safflower oil. Emollient plant oil similar to all nonfragrant plant oils. Safflower oil can be an antioxidant when consumed in the diet, but whether it retains this benefit when applied topically to skin is unknown. *See* natural moisturizing factor (NMF).

sage extract. Extract that can be a potent antioxidant (Source: *Journal of Agricultural Food Chemistry*, March 2002, pages 1845–1851). However, its fragrant camphor and phenol components can also cause skin irritation (Source: *Clinical Toxicology*, December 1981, pages 1485–1498).

salicin. *See* willow bark.

salicylic acid. Referred to as beta hydroxy acid (BHA), it is a multifunctional ingredient that addresses many of the systemic causes of blemishes (Source: *Seminars in Dermatology*, December 1990, pages 305–308). For decades dermatologists have been prescribing salicylic acid as an exceedingly effective keratolytic (exfoliant), but it also is an anti-irritant This is because salicylic acid is a derivative of aspirin (both are salicylates—aspirin's technical name is acetylsalicylic acid), and so it also functions as an anti-inflammatory (Sources: *Archives of Internal Medicine*, July 2002, pages 1531–1532; *Annals of Dermatology and Venereology*, January 2002, pages 137–142; *Archives of Dermatology*, November 2000, pages 1390–1395; and *Pain*, January 1996, pages 71–82). Another notable aspect of salicylic acid for treating breakouts is that it has antimicrobial properties (Sources: *Preservatives for Cosmetics*, 1996, by David Steinberg, Allured Publishing; and *Health Canada Monograph Category IV, Antiseptic Cleansers*, www.hc-sc.gc.ca/english/). It is also well documented that salicylic acid can improve skin thickness, barrier functions, and collagen production (Sources: *Dermatology*, 1999, volume 199, number 1, pages 50–53; and *Toxicology and Applied Pharmacology*, volume 175, issue 1, pages 76–82). As an exfoliant, in concentrations of 8% to 12%, it is effective in wart-remover medications. In concentrations of 0.5% to 2%, it is far more gentle, and, much like AHAs (*See* AHA), can exfoliate the surface of skin. In addition, BHA has the ability to penetrate into the pore (AHAs do not), and thus can exfoliate inside the pore as well as on the surface of the skin, which makes it effective for reducing blemishes, including blackheads and whiteheads.

***Salix alba* extract**. *See* willow bark.

Salvia officinalis. *See* sage extract.

Sambucus canadensis. *See* elderberry.

Sambucus cerulea. Blue elderberry. May have antioxidant properties for skin (Source: *Phytotherapy Research*, February 2002, pages 63–65). *See* elderberry.

Sambucus nigra. *See* black elderberry.

sandalwood oil. Fragrant oil that can cause skin irritation or allergic reactions (Source: *American Journal of Contact Dermatitis*, June 1996, pages 77–83). There is one animal study showing it to have antitumor properties (Source: *European Journal of Cancer Prevention*, October 1999, pages 449–455).

***Santalum album* seed extract**. Latin name for sandalwood extract, which is used in cosmetics as a fragrance. It can have antioxidant properties and there is research showing it minimizes herpes breakouts. It also can be a skin irritant or sensitizer (Sources: *Journal of Ethnopharmacology*, July 2000, pages 23–43; and *European Journal of Cancer Prevention*, August 1997, pages 399–401).

***Saponaria officinalis* extract**. *See* soapwort.

saponin. Group of natural carbohydrates, found in plants, that have considerable potential as pharmaceutical and/or nutraceutical agents in natural or synthetic form. Saponins, from a variety of sources, have been shown to have anti-inflammatory and antioxidant properties (Sources: *Fitoterapia*, July 2002, page 336; *Phytotherapy Research*, March 2001, pages 174–176; and *Drug Metabolism and Drug Interaction*, 2000, volume 17, issue 1-4, pages 211–235).

***Sargassum filipendula* extract**. *See* algae.

sausurrea oil. Also called costus oil. Volatile oil and fragrant component used in cosmetics; it can be a skin irritant. It is known to cause contact dermatitis (Source: www.naturaldatabase.com).

saw palmetto extract. Plant extract that, when taken orally, has been shown in short-term trials to be efficacious in reducing the symptoms of benign prostatic hyperplasia (Source: *Annals of Internal Medicine*, January 2002, pages 42–53). It may have an anti-inflammatory effect on skin, but there is little research to support this. Saw palmetto's reputation is based primarily on the fact that it can reduce the presence of the male hormone dihydrotestosterone, and so it could theoretically reduce hair loss, but this effect has not been proven. There is anecdotal information that it can also have estrogenic effects; but not only is that unlikely, it is also highly improbable that it could have such effects when applied topically (Source: *Healthnotes Review of Complementary and Integrative Medicine*, www.healthwell.com/healthnotes/Herb/Saw_Palmetto.cfm).

***Saxifraga sarmentosa* extract**. *See* strawberry begonia.

sclareolide. Fermented from clary sage and used as a fragrant component in cosmetics.

sclerotium gum. Used as a thickening agent in cosmetics.

***Scutellaria baicalensis* extract**. *See* skullcap extract.

sd alcohol. *See* alcohol.

sd alcohol 40-2. Denatured alcohol used as a solvent. It can be drying and irritating to skin when one of the main ingredients in a cosmetic product. Lesser amounts are not cause for concern. *See* alcohol.

Sea buckthorn. Berry extract that grows on a shrub-like tree. Sea buckthorn is believed to have several topical benefits, but the research to support such claims is lacking (Source:

www.naturaldatabase.com). More convincing is the research pertaining to sea buckthorn's ability to help skin heal when administered to wound sites, and it does appear to have some antioxidant ability (Sources: *The International Journal of Lower Extremity Wounds*, June 2005, pages 88–92; and *Indian Journal of Experimental Biology*, October 2006, pages 821–831).

sea salt. Can be effective as a topical scrub, but if left on skin it can increase skin sensitivity to UVB radiation (Source: *Der Hautarzt*, June 1998, pages 482–486).

sea whip extract. Extract from a creature that inhabits coral reefs, known for its anti-inflammatory properties (Source: *Life Sciences*, May 22, 1998, pages 401–407) and antibacterial properties (Source: *Journal of Natural Products*, January 2001, pages 100–102).

Seamollient. Trade name for an algae extract. *See* algae.

seaweed. Group of sea plants (scientific name: algae) of all sizes and shapes, and having a gelatin-like consistency. Many seaweeds have antioxidant and anti-inflammatory properties, but many other claims of benefits are not proven. *See* algae.

sebacic acid. Used as a pH adjuster.

selenium. Mineral considered to be a potent antioxidant (Source: *Biomedicine and Pharmacotherapy*, June 2002, pages 173–178). *See* antioxidant.

self-heal. Plant that has antihistamine, anti-inflammatory, antiviral, and antioxidant properties when taken orally (Sources: *Life Sciences*, January 2000, pages 725–735; *Planta Medica*, May 2000, pages 358–360; and *Immunopharmacology and Immunotoxicology*, August 2001, pages 423–435). However, there is no research demonstrating this has any benefit for skin when applied topically.

***Serenoa serrulata* extract**. *See* saw palmetto.

sericin. Scientific name for silk protein. *See* silk protein.

serine. *See* amino acid.

sesame oil. Emollient oil similar to other nonfragrant plant oils. *See* natural moisturizing factor (NMF).

Sesamum indicum. *See* sesame oil.

sesquioleate. Used in cosmetics as a thickening agent and emollient.

Shao-yao. *See* peony root extract.

shea butter. A plant lipid that is used as an emollient in cosmetics. *See* natural moisturizing factor (NMF).

Siegesbeckia orientalis. Chinese herb (also known as St. Paul's wort) for which there is no research showing that it has any benefit for skin.

silica. Mineral found abundantly in sandstone, clay, and granite, as well as in parts of plants and animals. It is the principal ingredient of glass. In cosmetics it is used as an absorbent powder and thickening agent.

silica dimethyl silylate. Used as a slip and suspending agent. *See* silica and silicone.

silicate. Inorganic salt that has potent absorbing and thickening properties.

silicone. Substance derived from silica (sand is a silica). The unique fluid properties of silicone give it a great deal of slip, and in its various forms it can feel like silk on the skin, impart emolliency, and be a water-binding agent that holds up well, even when skin becomes wet. In other forms, it is also used extensively for wound healing and for improving the appearance of scars (Source: *Journal of Wound Care*, July 2000, pages 319–324).

silk. *See* silk protein.

silk powder. Synthetically derived powder used as an absorbent and slip agent. *See* slip agent.

silk protein. Protein substance (also called sericin) formed by converting silk, which is the soft, lustrous thread obtained from the cocoon of the silkworm. Silk protein can have water-binding properties for skin. However, whether the protein applied to skin is derived from animals or plants, the skin can't tell the difference. There is a small amount of research showing silk protein may have topical antioxidant properties (Source: *Bioscience, Biotechnology, and Biochemistry*, January 1998, pages 145–147).

siloxane. *See* silicone.

silver. Metallic element that in cosmetics can have disinfecting properties; however, prolonged contact can turn skin grayish blue. Silver can be irritating to skin, and can cause silver toxicity (Sources: *Annals of Dermatology and Venereology*, February 2002, pages 217–219; and *Critical Reviews in Toxicology*, May 1996, pages 255–260). *See* silver sulfadiazine.

silver chloride. *See* silver sulfadiazine.

silver sulfadiazine. Can be effective for wound healing (Source: *Journal of Vascular Surgery*, August 1992, pages 251–257). However, it is safe for skin only for short-term use because silver can penetrate abraded skin and cause silver toxicity (Source: *Clinical Chemistry*, February 1997, pages 290–301).

silver tip white tea leaf extract. *See* green tea and white tea leaf extract.

***Silybum marianum* extract**. *See* lady's thistle extract.

simethicone. Mixture of dimethicone with silica; related to silicones, but used as an antifoaming agent.

Skin-identical ingredient. *See* intercellular matrix and Chapter Two, *Healthy Skin: Rules to Live By*.

skin respiratory factor. *See* tissue respiratory factor.

skullcap extract. Herbal extract from *Scutellaria baicalensis* that has antioxidant and anti-inflammatory properties for skin (Source: *Life Sciences*, January 2002, pages 1023–1033).

slip agent. Term used to describe a range of ingredients that help other ingredients spread over the skin and penetrate into the skin. Slip agents also have humectant properties. Slip agents include propylene glycol, butylene glycol, polysorbates, and glycerin, to name a few. They are as basic to the world of skin care as water.

slippery elm bark. Can be an anti-irritant and anti-inflammatory.

soap. True "soaps" are regulated by the Consumer Product Safety Commission and are not required to list their ingredients on the label. They are made up solely of fats and alkali. Many bar cleansers are not soaps, but contain synthetic detergent cleansing agents and various thickening agents that keep the bar in its bar form. Most soaps are considered very drying and potentially irritating for skin due to their alkaline base (i.e., a pH over 8). Bar cleansers can be more gentle than bar soaps, but are more often than not still drying, depending on their composition (Sources: *Cutis*, December 2001, pages 12–19; *Archives of Dermatologic Research*, June 2001, pages 308–318; and *Dermatologic Clinics*, October 2000, pages 561–575).

soapwort. Plant from which is derived an extract with detergent cleansing properties. There is some research showing it has antiviral and antibacterial properties (Sources: *Biochemical and Biophysical Research Communications*, May 1997, pages 129–132; and *Phytotherapy Research*, 1990, volume 4, pages 97–100).

sodium acrylate/acryloydimethyl taurate copolymer. Synthetic polymer used as a stabilizing and suspending agent and as a thickening agent.

sodium ascorbate. *See* ascorbic acid.

sodium benzoate. Salt of benzoic acid used as a preservative. *See* preservatives.

sodium bisulfite. Used in acid-type permanent waves to alter the shape of hair. It is less damaging than alkaline permanent waves, but also has limitations regarding how much change it can effect in hair. It can be a skin irritant.

sodium borate. *See* borate.

sodium C14-16 olefin sulfate. Can be derived from coconut. Used primarily as a detergent cleansing agent, but is potentially drying and irritating for skin. *See* surfactant.

sodium carbonate. Absorbent salt used in cosmetics; it can also be a skin irritant.

sodium chloride. More popularly known as common table salt. Used primarily as a binding agent in skin-care products and occasionally as an abrasive in scrub products.

sodium chondroitin sulfate. Derived from natural mucopolysaccharides, it functions as a skin-conditioning agent and helps reinforce skin's intercellular matrix.

sodium citrate. Used primarily to control the pH level of a product, this ingredient also has antioxidant and preservative properties.

sodium cocoate. Used as a cleansing agent primarily in soaps. It can be drying and irritating for skin.

sodium cocoyl isethionate. Derived from coconut, it is a mild detergent cleansing agent. *See* surfactant.

sodium dehydroacetate. Organic salt used as a preservative. *See* preservatives.

sodium hexametaphosphate. Salt with multiple functions in cosmetics. It can act as a detergent, an emulsifier, a texturizer, and a preservative that prevents metallic compounds from negatively affecting a product.

sodium hyaluronate. *See* hyaluronic acid.

sodium hydroxide. Also known as lye, it is a highly alkaline ingredient used in small amounts in cosmetics to modulate the pH of a product. It is also used as a cleansing agent in some cleansers. In higher concentrations it is a significant skin irritant.

sodium hydroxymethylglycinate. Derived from amino acids and used as a skin- and hair-conditioning agent, and to a lesser extent as a preservative.

sodium lactate. Sodium salt of lactic acid. Used primarily as a water-binding and buffering agent (to adjust a product's pH value).

sodium lactobionate. White, crystalline powder used to synthesize other chemicals. May function as a preservative in skin-care products. There is no research proving this ingredient exfoliates skin.

sodium laureth sulfate. Can be derived from coconut; it is used primarily as a detergent cleansing agent. It is considered gentle and effective. *See* surfactant and Paula's article, "Sodium Lauryl Sulfate and Sodium Laureth Sulfate," at www.cosmeticscop.com.

sodium laureth-13 carboxylate. Used primarily as a detergent cleansing agent. *See* surfactant.

sodium lauroamphoacetate. Mild surfactant also used as a lather agent. *See* surfactant.

sodium lauroyl lactylate. Used as an emulsifier and mild thickening agent in cosmetics. In higher concentrations, it functions as a surfactant. *See* surfactant.

sodium lauroyl sarcosinate. Surfactant known (and used) for its foam-boosting properties. *See* surfactant.

sodium lauryl sulfate. There has been a great deal of misinformation circulated on the Internet about sodium lauryl sulfate (SLS). Used primarily as a detergent cleansing agent, SLS can be derived from coconut. Although it is a potent skin irritant it is not toxic or dangerous for skin. In concentrations of 2% to 5%, SLS can cause allergic or sensitizing reactions for many people. It is used as a standard in scientific studies to establish irritancy or sensitizing properties of other ingredients (Sources: *European Journal of Dermatology*, September–October 2001, pages 416–419; *American Journal of Contact Dermatitis*, March 2001, pages 28–32; and *Skin Pharmacology and Applied Skin Physiology*, September–October 2000, pages 246–257). Being a skin irritant, however, is not the same as a link to cancer, which is what erroneous warnings on the Internet are falsely claiming about this ingredient!

According to a Health Canada press release (February 12, 1999, www.hc-sc.gc.ca/), "A letter has been circulating [on] the Internet which claims that there is a link between cancer and sodium laureth (or lauryl) sulfate (SLS), an ingredient used in [cosmetics]. Health Canada has looked into the matter and has found no scientific evidence to suggest that SLS causes cancer. It has a history of safe use in Canada. Upon further investigation, it was discovered that this e-mail warning is a hoax. The letter is signed by a person at the University of Pennsylvania Health System and includes a phone number. Health Canada contacted the University of Pennsylvania Health System and found that it is not the author of the sodium laureth sulfate warning and does not endorse any link between SLS and cancer. Health Canada considers SLS safe for use in cosmetics. Therefore, you can continue to use cosmetics containing SLS without worry." Further, according to the American Cancer Society's Web site (www.cancer.org), "Contrary to popular rumors on the Internet, Sodium Lauryl Sulfate (SLS) and Sodium Laureth Sulfate (SLES) do not cause cancer. E-mails have been flying through cyberspace claiming SLS [and SLES] causes cancer ... and is proven to cause cancer.... [Yet] A search of recognized medical journals yielded no published articles relating this substance to cancer in humans." *See* surfactant and Paula's article, "Sodium Lauryl Sulfate and Sodium Laureth Sulfate," at www.cosmeticscop.com.

sodium metabisulfite. Reducing agent that alters the structure of hair. It can also be used as a preservative in formulations, and can be a skin irritant. However, it can also be an antioxidant (Source: *Journal of Pharmaceutical Science and Technology*, September–October 1999, pages 252–259).

sodium methyl cocoyl taurate. Mild surfactant. *See* surfactant.

sodium methyl taurate. Mild surfactant. *See* surfactant.

sodium PCA. PCA (pyrrolidone carboxylic acid) is a natural component of skin that is also a very good water-binding agent. *See* natural moisturizing factor (NMF).

sodium salicylate. Salt form of salicylic acid (BHA). Because it is not the acid form of salicylate (i.e., salicylic acid), it does not have exfoliating properties.

sodium silicate. Highly alkaline and potentially irritating antiseptic and mineral used in cosmetics (Source: *American Journal of Contact Dermatitis*, September 2002, pages 133–139).

sodium sulfite. Reducing agent that alters the structure of hair. It can also be used as a preservative in cosmetic formulations, and can be a skin irritant. *See* reducing agent.

sodium tallowate. Sodium salt of tallow. *See* tallow.

sodium thioglycolate. *See* thioglycolate.

sodium trideceth sulfate. *See* surfactant.

Solanum lycopersicum **extract**. *See* tomato extract.

Solanum tuberosum **extract**. Extract that is potato starch. Used as a thickening agent in cosmetics.

soluble fish collagen. *See* collagen.

solvent. Describes a large group of ingredients, including water, that are used to dissolve or break down other ingredients. Solvents are also used to degrease skin and to remove sebum.

Sonojell. Trade name for petrolatum. *See* petrolatum.

sorbic acid. Preservative derived from mountain ash berries or manufactured synthetically. Sorbic acid is used in many products, including several foods and even in contact lens solutions. A study of contact sensitization to preservatives among 514 volunteers with eczema showed that sorbic acid caused a reaction in only 0.6% of participants. In contrast, many other preservatives had much higher rates of negative reactions, upwards of 13.6% (Source: *Ceska a Slovenska Farmacie*, May 2004, pages 151–156).

sorbitan stearate. Used to thicken and stabilize cosmetic formulations.

sorbitol. Can be created synthetically or derived from natural sources. Similar to glycerin, it is a humectant, thickening agent, and slip agent.

soy extract. Potent antioxidant and anti-inflammatory agent for skin (Sources: *Cancer Investigation*, 1996, volume 14, number 6, pages 597–608; *Skin Pharmacology and Applied Skin Physiology*, May–June 2002, pages 175–183; and *Journal of the American Academy of Dermatology*, June 2005, pages 1049–1059). Soy is one of many phyto (i.e., plant) chemicals that are biologically active against free radicals. Polyphenol compounds, such as the catechins found in green tea, also fit this profile. Soy extract's increased use in anti-aging products is largely due to studies showing that genistein (a component of soy) has a collagen-stimulating effect and that various compounds in soy influence skin thickness and elasticity (Sources: *Cosmetics & Toiletries*, June 2002, pages 45–50; and *Journal of Cosmetic Science*, September–October 2004, pages 473–479). Researchers have also looked at Bifidobacterium-fermented soy milk extracts. On mouse skin and in human skin fibroblasts (lab cultured), this bacteria-modified form of soy was shown to stimulate production of hyaluronic acid in skin. This was due to the amount of genistein released during the fermentation process (Sources: *Skin Pharmacology and Physiology*, 2003, pages 108–116; and *Photochemistry and Photobiology*, May-June 2005, pages 581–587).

Studies performed on mouse skin have shown that topical application of soy milk and other soy compounds has a protective effect against UVB light damage. It is theorized that these benefits will translate to human skin as well, but conclusive evidence has not yet materialized (Sources: *Oncology Research*, volume 14, numbers 7/8, 2004, pages 387–397; and *Photodermatology, Photoimmunology, & Photomedicine*, April 2003, page 56).

There is no research showing that soy extract or soy oil has estrogenic effects when applied to skin, as it can when taken orally (Source: *International Journal of Toxicology*, 2004, volume 23, Supplement 2, pages 23–47). Some companies have asserted that soy can affect hair growth and lighten skin color when applied topically. The single study citing this was done by Johnson & Johnson, the company that sells products claiming to have this effect (Source: *Experimental Dermatology*, December 2001, pages 405–413).

soy isoflavones. *See* soy extract.

soy oil. Emollient oil similar to all nonfragrant plant oils. *See* natural moisturizing factor (NMF) and soy extract.

soy protein. *See* soy extract.

soya sterol. Form of phytosterol. There is no research showing soy sterols have any estrogenic or antioxidant benefit for skin. *See* phytosterol.

spearmint oil. Fragrant, volatile oil that can cause skin irritation and allergic reactions. *See* counter-irritant.

SPF. *See* sun protection factor.

spikenard. Plant that has antibacterial properties for skin.

Spiraea ulmaria. *See* meadowsweet extract.

spirulina. *See* algae.

squalane. *See* natural moisturizing factor (NMF) and squalene.

squalene. Oil derived from shark liver or from plants (usually olives) and sebum. It is a natural component of skin and is a good emollient that has antioxidant and immune-stimulating properties (Sources: *Lancet Oncology*, October 2000, pages 107–112; and *Free Radical Research*, April 2002, pages 471–477). *See* natural moisturizing factor (NMF).

St. John's wort. Contains several components that are toxic on skin in the presence of sunlight (Sources: *Planta Medica*, February 2002, pages 171–173; and *International Journal of Biochemistry and Cell Biology*, March 2002, pages 221–241). St. John's wort's association with improving depression when taken as an oral supplement is unrelated to its topical impact on skin. However, it also has potent antioxidant properties (Source: *Journal of Agricultural Food Chemistry*, November 2001, pages 5165–5170).

star anise. *See* anise.

steapyrium chloride. Antistatic agent used in hair-care products.

stearalkonium chloride. Antistatic ingredient used in hair-care products to control flyaways and aid in helping a brush or comb get through hair.

stearalkonium hectorite. Used as a suspending agent.

stearates. *See* stearic acid.

stearic acid. Fatty acid used as an emollient and as an agent to help keep other ingredients intact in a formulation. *See* fatty acid and thickening agent.

stearyl alcohol. Fatty alcohol used as an emollient and to help keep other ingredients intact in a formulation. *See* fatty alcohol.

stearyl methicone. Silicone polymer used as a skin-conditioning or occlusive agent. *See* silicone.

strawberry begonia. There is no research showing this has any benefit for skin.

styrax benzoin. *See* benzoin extract.

styrene/acrylates copolymer. Synthetic polymer. *See* film-forming agent.

subtilisin. Protease enzyme obtained from the fermentation of *Bacillus subtilis*. *See* proteases.

sucrose. Monosaccharide that has water-binding properties for skin. *See* mucopolysaccharide and water-binding agent.

sugarcane extract. Ingredients like sugarcane extract, fruit extracts, mixed fruit extracts, and milk solids may claim an association with AHAs, but they are not the same thing nor do they have the same beneficial effect on skin. While glycolic acid can indeed be derived from sugarcane, if you assume that sugarcane will net you the same result as glycolic acid, that would be like assuming you could write on a tree the way you can write on paper. Wood is certainly where paper begins, but paper wouldn't exist if the wood didn't undergo complex mechanical and chemical processes. Similarly, the original forms of these extracts do not have the same effect as the ingredients that are derived from them. The same is true for lactic acid, derived from milk. If milk were as acidic as lactic acid, you would not be able to drink it without serious complications. There is a vast difference between the extracted, pure ingredient and the original form of the source material. *See* AHA.

sulfur. Antibacterial agent (Source: *Applied Microbiology and Biotechnology*, October 2001, pages 282–286) that can be a potent skin irritant and sensitizer. Sulfur also has a high pH, which can encourage the growth of bacteria on skin.

sun protection factor. Most commonly seen as SPF, it is a number that is assigned to a product that identifies its ability to protect the skin from sunburn or to protect the skin from turning pink or red when exposed to sun. SPF numbering is regulated by the FDA, and is a measure of the amount of time a person can stay in the sun without getting burned if a sunscreen is applied. Because sunburn results from UVB radiation, not UVA radiation, SPF is primarily a measure of UVB protection. At this time, there is no numbering system to indicate the level of protection a sunscreen can provide from UVA radiation, which affects the deeper layers of skin. *See* sunscreens and UVA.

sunflower oil. Non-volatile plant oil used as an emollient in cosmetics.

sunscreens. Products considered over-the-counter drugs in the United States and as such are strictly regulated by the FDA. Sunscreens provide protection from sunburn and some amount of sun damage. There is a great deal of confusion regarding the efficacy and use of sunscreens. The FDA instituted new regulations that were supposed to take effect in 2002, but most of them did not come into play because the FDA's Final Sunscreen Monograph was, for various reasons, never officially updated. According to the FDA's July–August 2002 issue of *Consumer* magazine, "Under the new regulations manufacturers will no longer be allowed to [use] ... confusing terms such as 'sunblock,' 'waterproof,' 'all-day protection,' and 'visible and/or infrared light protection' on these [sunscreen] products. In addition to these changes ... tanning preparations that do not contain a sunscreen ingredient [are required] to display the following warning: 'Warning: This product does not contain a sunscreen and does not protect against sunburn. Repeated exposure of unprotected skin while tanning may increase the risk of skin aging, skin cancer, and other harmful effects to the skin even if you do not burn.

"To figure out how much protection a sunscreen provides, most consumers turn to a simple number: the SPF, or sun protection factor, listed on the label. Studies show that most consumers understand that the higher the number, the more the product protects the skin."

The FDA then goes on to say: "Unfortunately, studies also show that people often have the mistaken notion that the higher the SPF number of the sunscreen they use, the longer they can stay—and will stay—in the sun.... Sunscreen should not be used to prolong time spent in the sun. Even with a sunscreen, you are not going to prevent all the possible damage from the sun. Some of the newer research in the last several years shows that [for] the sub-erythemal doses [exposure to the sun that does not cause reddening of the skin], as little as one-tenth the energy needed to get a sunburn, starts the process of skin damage of one sort or another.

"The public under-applies sunscreens by as much as half of the recommended amount, concluded a study published in the *Archives of Dermatology*. Consequently, the study argued, consumers are receiving only half of the SPF protection they believe the product provides." The issue of liberal application has been confirmed in other research as well (Source: *Photochemistry and Photobiology*, July 2001, pages 61–63). *See* sun protection factor and UVA.

superoxide dismutase. Enzyme considered to be a potent antioxidant in humans (Sources: *Journal of Investigative Dermatology*, April 2002, pages 618–625; *Journal of Photochemistry and Photobiology B*, October 2001, pages 61–69; and *European Journal of Pharmaceutical Sciences*, August 2001, pages 63–67). *See* antioxidant.

surfactant. Shortened term for **surf**ace **act**ive **agent**. Surfactants degrease and emulsify oils and fats and suspend soil, allowing them to be washed away, as laundry products do. I refer to these substances throughout my writing as "detergent cleansing agents." Surfactants and detergent cleansing agents are often used interchangeably by chemists and researchers (Sources: Food and Drug Administration, *Office of Cosmetics and Colors Fact Sheet*, February 3, 1995, www.fda.gov; *Dermatology*, 1995, volume 191, number 4, pages 276–280; *Tenside, Surfactants, Detergents*, 1997, volume 34, number 3, pages 156–168; and http://surfactants.net). Surfactants are used in most forms of cleansers and many of them are considered gentle and effective for most skin types. There are several types of surfactants that can be sensitizing, drying, and irritating for skin.

sweet almond oil. Emollient oil. *See* natural moisturizing factor (NMF).

***Symphytum officinale* extract.** *See* comfrey extract.

Szechuan peppercorn. From a plant native to Szechuan Province in China. It grows on trees, and so differs from black pepper, which grows on climbing vines. Used extensively in Szechuan cooking, Szechuan pepper is known for the "numbing" sensation it produces on the tongue. It is considered a counter-irritant. *See* black pepper extract and oil and counter-irritant.

talc. Naturally occurring silicate mineral (any group of substances containing negative ions composed of silicon and oxygen) of magnesium. Current, extensive research indicates there is no increased risk of lung cancer when using talc-based products or for those involved in the manufacture of talc products (Source: *Occupational and Environmental Medicine*, January 2006, pages 4–9), although there is epidemiological evidence that frequent use of pure talc over the female genital area may increase the risk of ovarian cancer (Sources: *International Journal of Cancer*, November 2004, pages 458–464; and *Anticancer Research*, March-April 2003, pages 1955–1960). However, a study review in *Regulatory Toxicology and Pharmacology* (August 2002, pages 40–50) stated that "Talc is not genotoxic, [it] is not carcinogenic when injected into ovaries of rats.... There is no credible evidence of a cancer risk from inhalation of cosmetic talc by humans."

tallow. Substance extracted from the fatty deposits of animals, especially from suet (the fat of cattle and sheep). Tallow is often used to make soap and candles. In soap, because of its fat content, it can be a problem for breakouts.

tamanu oil. From a tree native to Polynesia. It is reputed to have wondrous wound-healing properties, as well as being a cure-all for almost every skin ailment you can think of, from acne to eczema to psoriasis, but all of the miraculous claims are hinged on anecdotal, not scientific, evidence. There's no harm in using this oil in skin care—like most oils, it is composed of phospholipids and glycolipids, and these are natural constituents of healthy skin and are good water-binding agents. Tamanu oil may have anti-inflammatory properties and there is some research showing it has anti-tumor properties, though this has not been proven in any direct research on skin.

Tanacetum parthenium. *See* feverfew extract.

tangerine oil. Fragrant, volatile citrus oil that can be a skin irritant.

tannic acid. Potent antioxidant; it may have some anticarcinogenic properties (Sources: *Bioorganic & Medicinal Chemistry Letters*, June 2002, pages 1567–1570; and *Nutrition and Cancer*, 1998, volume 32, number 2, pages 81–85).

tannin. Component of many plants. It can have an anti-tumor benefit when consumed in tea or foods (Source: *Nutrition and Cancer*, 1998, volume 32, number 2, pages 81–85). There is some research on animals showing that this benefit may translate to skin (Source: *Photochemistry and Photobiology*, June 1998, pages 663–668). Tannins can also have constricting properties on skin, and may cause irritation with repeated use.

Taraktogenos kurzii. *See* chaulmoogra oil.

Taraxacum officinale. *See* dandelion extract.

tartaric acid. *See* AHA.

Tazorac. Chemically known as tazarotene, it is a synthetically derived retinoid with properties similar to those of tretinoin (active ingredient in Retin-A and Renova). Tazorac is a brand-name prescription drug, owned by Allergan, that is available in gel and cream textures and is prescribed for managing acne. Tazarotene is also sold under the brand name Avage (also from Allergan), and this version is marketed for treating wrinkles and sun-induced skin discolorations. Tazarotene works similarly to tretinoin by modulating cell differentiation and proliferation. It also has anti-inflammatory and immune-modifying properties, which is why it is used (often successfully) as a topical prescription for managing psoriasis (Sources: www.emedicine.com; and *American Journal of Clinical Dermatology*, June 2005, pages 255–272).

TEA. *See* triethanolamine.

tea tree oil. Also known as melaleuca, from the name of its plant source, *Melaleuca alternifolia*. It can have disinfecting properties that have been shown to be effective against the bacteria that cause blemishes. According to *Healthnotes Review of Complementary and Integrative Medicine* (www.healthwell.com/healthnotes/Herb/Tea_Tree.cfm) and the *Medical Journal of Australia* (October 1990, pages 455–458), 5% tea tree oil and 2.5% benzoyl peroxide are effective in reducing the number of blemishes, with a significantly better result for benzoyl peroxide when compared to the tea tree oil. Skin oiliness was lessened significantly in the benzoyl peroxide group versus the tea tree oil group. However, the tea tree oil had somewhat less irritating side effects. Concentrations of 5% to 10% are recommended. However, the amount present in most skin-care products is usually less than 1% and, therefore, considered not effective for disinfecting. *See* Paula's article "Tea Tree Oil—Melaleuca," at www.cosmeticscop.com.

TEA-lauryl sulfate. While there is abundant research showing sodium lauryl sulfate is a sensitizing cleansing agent, there is no similar supporting research for TEA-lauryl sulfate. However, because the relationship between the two is so close, I decided to recommend against using either of them. The basis for this is a judgment call, made from a desire to protect skin from sensitization; however, there are no specific studies I can cite for this recommendation, although there are those who will understandably disagree with my conclusion. *See* sodium lauryl sulfate.

terephthalylidine dicamphor sulfonic acid. *See* Mexoryl SX.

Terminalia catappa. Can be a potent antioxidant (Source: *Anticancer Research*, January-February 2001, pages 237–243).

Terminalia sericea. Herb that is effective against some forms of gram-positive and gram-negative bacteria when used in pure form, but is not effective against acne-causing bacteria. It also has anti-inflammatory and antifungal properties (Sources: *Journal of Ethnopharmacology*, January 2006, pages 135–138, and June 2005, pages 301–308).

***Terminalia sericea* extract**. Extract that has anti-inflammatory and antibacterial properties, but there is no research showing it has any effect on the appearance of cellulite (Sources: *Journal of Ethnopharmacology*, February 2005, pages 43–47; and *European Journal of Pharmaceutics and Biopharmaceutics*, March 2003, Pages 191–198).

tetradibutyl pentaerithrityl hydroxyhydrocinnamate. *See* antioxidant.

tetrahexyldecyl ascorbate. Stable form of vitamin C. *See* vitamin C.

tetrahydrobisdemethoxycurcumin. Antioxidant and anti-inflammatory plant extract. *See* curcumin.

tetrahydrodemethoxycurcumin. *See* curcumin and turmeric.

tetrahydrodiferuloylmethane. Antioxidant and anti-inflammatory plant extract. *See* curcumin.

tetrahydromethoxycurcumin. Antioxidant and anti-inflammatory plant extract. *See* curcumin.

tetrahydroxypropyl ethylenediamine. *See* chelating agent.

tetrasodium EDTA. Chelating agent used to prevent minerals present in formulations from bonding to other ingredients.

tetrasodium etidronate. Used as a chelating agent in cosmetics to prevent varying mineral components from binding together and negatively affecting the formulation.

thiamine HCL. Vitamin B1. There is no research showing this to be effective when applied topically on skin.

thickening agent. Substances that can have a soft to hard waxlike texture or a creamy, emollient feel, and that can be great lubricants. There are literally thousands of ingredients in this category that give each and every lotion, cream, lipstick, foundation, and mascara, as well as other cosmetic products, their distinctive feel and form.

thiodipropionic acid. Acid-based synthetic antioxidant. There is no research pertaining to its benefit for skin, but in theory, and when stably packaged, it should exert an antioxidant effect when applied topically.

thioglycolate. Compound used in permanent waves and depilatories either to alter the structure of hair or to dissolve it. These are potent skin irritants.

thiotaurine. Amino acid. Potentially, it can have antioxidant properties for skin (Source: Shiseido Corporation, www.shiseido.co.jp/e/e9608let/html/let00027.htm). *See* amino acid.

threonine. *See* amino acid.

thyme extract. Extract derived from the thyme plant. It can have potent antioxidant properties (Source: *Journal of Agricultural Food Chemistry*, March 2002, pages 1845–1851). Its fragrant component can also cause skin irritation.

thyme oil. *See* thyme extract.

thymus hydrolysate. Form of animal thymus derived by acid, enzyme, or other methods of hydrolysis. It can have water-binding properties for skin, but has no other special or unique benefit.

***Thymus serpillum* extract**. Extract of wild thyme. *See* thyme extract.

Thymus vulgaris. *See* thyme extract.

Tilia cordata. *See* linden flower extract.

Tinosorb M. *See* Tinosorb S.

Tinosorb S. In Europe there are two sunscreen ingredients—Tinosorb S (bis-ethylhexyloxyphenol methoxyphenyl triazine) and Tinosorb M (methylene bis-benzotriazolyl tetramethylbutylphenol)—that are approved for sun protection across the entire range of UVA radiation (Sources: *Photochemistry and Photobiology*, September 2001, pages 401–406; and Ciba Specialty Chemicals Corporation, North America, www.cibasc.com). Whether they are preferred over the other UVA-protecting ingredients used in sunscreens has not been established. At this time, neither Tinosorb M nor Tinosorb S has been approved for use in the United States or Canada. *See* UVA.

tissue respiratory factor (TRF). Trade name for a form of yeast suspended in alcohol. There is only one independent study, performed on animals, that showed it to have some wound-healing benefits (Source: *Journal of Burn Care Rehabilitation*, March–April 1999, pages 155–162).

titanium dioxide. Inert earth mineral used as a thickening, whitening, lubricating, and sunscreen ingredient in cosmetics. It protects skin from UVA and UVB radiation and is considered to have no risk of skin irritation (Sources: www.photodermatology.com/sunprotection.htm; and *Skin Therapy Letter*, 1997, volume 2, number 5). *See* UVA.

Tocopherol. *See* vitamin E.

tocopherol acetate. *See* vitamin E.

tocopheryl acetate. *See* vitamin E.

tocopheryl lineolate. *See* vitamin E.

tocotrienols. Superpotent forms of vitamin E that are considered stable and powerful antioxidants. There is some research showing that tocotrienols are more potent than other forms of vitamin E for antioxidant activity (Source: *Journal of Nutrition*, February 2001, pages 369S–373S), but the studies cited in this review were all performed on animal models or in vitro. According to the University of California at Berkeley's *Wellness Guide to Dietary Supplements* (October 1999), "[Tocotrienol] research in humans is very limited, and the results conflicting." The research that has been done has centered on large doses of oral tocotrienols, animal studies, or test-tube trials. Companies that want you to believe that tocotrienols are now the answer for your skin are only guessing whether or not the laboratory evidence translates to human skin as it exists in the real world (Source: *Healthnotes Review of Complementary and Integrative Medicine*, www.healthnotes.com). Full-scale clinical studies on humans to assess the benefits of topical tocotrienols have not yet been performed, so for now (as is true for all antioxidants), choosing it as the "best" one is a leap of faith. *See* vitamin E.

tomato extract. Extract that has weak antioxidant properties (Source: *Free Radical Research*, February 2002, pages 217–233). Tomatoes contain lycopene, which is a significant antioxidant, but it is more bioavailable from tomato paste than from fresh tomatoes (Source: *American Journal of Clinical Nutrition*, 1997, volume 66, number 1, pages 116–122). It can also be a potential skin irritant depending on what part of the tomato is used, but there is no way to know that from an ingredient label. *See* lycopene.

tormentil extract. Plant that can be irritating due to its tannin content, which causes skin constriction.

tourmaline. Inert, though complex, mineral. One of its unique properties is that it is piezoelectric, meaning that it generates an electrical charge when under pressure, which is why it's typically used in pressure gauges. Tourmaline is also pyroelectric, which means that it generates an electrical charge during a temperature change (either increase or decrease). One of the results of generating such an electric charge is that dust particles will become attached to one end of a tourmaline crystal. However, none of that can take place in a cosmetic. There is no published research showing tourmaline has any proven effect on skin whatsoever. *See* Paula's article "Tourmaline," at www.cosmeticscop.com.

tragacanth. Natural gum used as a thickener in cosmetics.

transforming growth factor (TGF). Stimulates wound healing and collagen growth. *See* human growth factor.

trehalose. Plant sugar that has water-binding properties for skin.

tretinoin. Topical, prescription-only medication that can improve skin cell production after skin has been damaged. It is the active ingredient in Retin-A, Renova, Tazorac, and Avita. One of the more significant problems of sun damage is abnormal and mutated cell growth. An article in *Clinics in Geriatric Medicine* (November 2001, pages 643–659) stated that "Studies that have elucidated photoaging pathophysiology have produced significant evidence that topical tretinoin (all-trans retinoic acid), the only agent approved so far for the treatment of photoaging, also works to prevent it" (Sources: *Cosmetic Dermatology*, December 2001, page 38; and *Journal of Investigative Dermatology*, 2001, volume 111, pages 778–784). Tretinoin affects and improves actual cell production deep in the dermis, far away from the surface of skin (Sources: *Clinical and Experimental Dermatology*, October 2001, pages 613–618; *Clinics in Geriatric Medicine*, November 2001, pages 643–659; and *Photochemistry and Photobiology*, February 1999, pages 154–157).

tribehenin. Also known as glyceryl tribehenate, a skin-conditioning agent that is a mixture of glycerin and behenic acid. See glycerin and fatty acid.

tricaprylin. Mixture of glycerin and caprylic acid. Has emollient properties and is used as a skin-conditioning agent. *See* glycerin.

triclosan. Good antibacterial agent used in many products, from those for oral hygiene to cleansers (Sources: *Federation of European Microbiological Societies Microbiology Letter*, August 2001, pages 1–7; and *American Journal of Infection Control*, April 2000, pages 184–196). However, whether triclosan is effective for treatment of acne has not been researched. There is also controversy over whether or not triclosan may contribute to creating strains of bacteria that are resistant to antibiotics due to its overuse in cosmetic products. There also is concern about whether, in practical use, it can in fact impart the benefits of disinfection indicated on the label (Source: *Journal of Hospital Infection*, August 2001, Supplement A, pages S4–S8).

tridecyl salicylate. Salt form of salicylic acid (BHA). When it is no longer an acid (as in this case), salicylic acid no longer has exfoliating properties.

tridecyl stearate. Used in cosmetics as a thickening agent and emollient.

tridecyl trimellitate. Used as a skin-conditioning agent and thickening agent. *See* thickening agent.

triethanolamine. Used in cosmetics as a pH balancer. Like all amines, it has the potential for creating nitrosamines. There is controversy as to whether this poses a real problem for skin, given the low concentrations used in cosmetics and the theory that nitrosamines cannot penetrate skin.

triethoxycaprylylsilane. Silicone that functions as a binding agent and emulsifier. *See* silicone.

Trifolium pratense. *See* red clover.

triglyceride. Used as an emollient and thickening agent in cosmetics. *See* glyceryl ester and natural moisturizing factor (NMF).

trihydroxystearin. Mixture of glycerin and fatty acids used as an emollient and thickening agent. *See* fatty acid.

trilaurin. Group of ingredients that are triesters of glycerin and aliphatic acids, and known generically as glyceryl triesters. These are used in cosmetic products as thickening agents and emollients (Source: *International Journal of Toxicology*, 2001, volume 20, Supplement 4, pages 61–94).

trimethylsiloxysilicate. Used as a skin-conditioning and occlusive agent. *See* silicone.

trioclanolin. Derived from lanolin and used as a texture enhancer, most commonly in powder-based products such as eyeshadows and powder blush.

trioctanoin. Used as an emollient and thickening agent in cosmetics. *See* trilaurin.

trioctyldodecyl citrate. Mixture of octyldodecanol and citric acid used as a skin-conditioning agent and emollient. *See* octyldodecanol and citric acid.

trisodium EDTA. Similar to tetrasodium EDTA. Used as a water-softening and chelating agent (a compound that binds and separates metals, keeping them from bonding to other ingredients). *See* tetrasodium EDTA.

***Triticum vulgare* oil**. *See* wheat germ oil.

tryptophan. *See* amino acid.

turmeric. Spice made from the dried, ground root of a plant; its extract is called curcumin. A natural yellow food coloring that has potent antioxidant properties (Sources: *Food Chemistry and Toxicology*, August 2002, pages 1091–1097; and *Planta Medica*, December 2001, pages 876–877). Because it is a potent spice, it also may have irritating properties for skin.

Tussilago farfara. *See* coltsfoot.

tyrosinase. Enzyme that stimulates melanin production. *See* tyrosine.

tyrosine. Amino acid in skin that initiates the production of melanin (melanin is the component of skin that gives it "color"). According to information on the FDA's Web site (www.fda.gov), tyrosine's "use is based on the assumption that it penetrates the skin, increases the tyrosine content of the melanocytes, and thus enhances melanin formation. This effect has not been documented in the scientific literature. In fact, an animal study reported a few years ago demonstrated that ingestion or topical application of tyrosine has no effect on melanogenesis [the creation of melanin]." Tyrosine is important to the structure of almost all proteins in the body. However, the chemical pathway needed for tyrosine to function is complex, and this pathway cannot be duplicated by including tyrosine in a skin-care product or by applying it topically.

ubiquinone. *See* coenzyme Q10.

ultramarines. Inorganic pigments (of various colors) permanently listed by the FDA for external use only, including around the eye area.

***Ulva lactuca* extract**. Extract from the plant known as sea lettuce, it has some anti-inflammatory and antioxidant properties for skin (Source: *Phytotherapy Research*, December 2000, pages 641–643). However, there is no research showing that it has any benefit for cellulite reduction.

Undaria pinnatifida. Form of brown algae. *See* algae.

urea. Component of urine, although synthetic versions are used in cosmetics. In small amounts urea has good water-binding and exfoliating properties for skin; in larger concentrations it can cause inflammation (Source: *Skin Pharmacology and Applied Skin Physiology*, January-February 2002, pages 44–54).

Urtica dioica. *See* nettle extract.

UVA. Ultra-violet **A** radiation. The sun produces a range of ultraviolet (UV) radiation, of which UVA and UVB affect our skin. UVA rays have wavelengths of 320 to 400 nanometers; UVB rays have wavelengths of 290 to 320 nanometers. UVB radiation causes sunburn, while UVA radiation does not produce any visible short-term evidence of skin damage. Nonetheless, UVA radiation creates serious cumulative changes in skin that may be far greater than the sunburn caused by UVB radiation. Research has shown that unprotected exposure to UVA rays can, within one week, create distinct injury, such as inflammation, abnormal cell production, thickening of the stratum corneum (outer layer of skin), depletion of immune-stimulating cells, and evidence of the possibility of elastin deterioration (Sources: *Journal of the American Academy of Dermatology*, May 2001, pages 837–846; *Bulletin of the Academy of National Medicine*, 2001, volume 185, number 8, pages 1507–1525; *Photodermatology, Photoimmunology, and Photomedicine*, August 2000, page 147; and *Journal of the American Academy of Dermatology*, January 1995, pages 53–62).

To be truly effective and beneficial for skin, sunscreens must protect skin from both the sun's UVA and UVB radiation. In the United States, there are four ingredients approved by the FDA that protect across the full UVA range: titanium dioxide, zinc oxide, avobenzone (also called Parsol 1789 and butyl methoxydibenzoylmethane), and Mexoryl SX (ecamsule). Outside the United States, Tinosorb is another. Mexoryl SX is a L'Oreal-patented sunscreen ingredient that received FDA approval in July 2006 for use in a single sunscreen, Anthelios SX SPF 15, from the L'Oreal-owned line La Roche-Posay. This is the only sunscreen with Mexoryl SX that is approved for sale in the United States (Sources: *International Journal of Pharmaceutics*, June 2002, pages 85–94; *Photodermatology, Photoimmunology, Photomedicine*, August 2000, pages 147–155 and www.photodermatology.com/sunprotection.htm; *Skin Therapy Letter*, volume 2, number 5, 1997; and www.fda.gov/bbs/topics/NEWS/2006/NEW01417.html). However, L'Oreal has been adding Mexoryl SX to products in their namesake line as well as in other lines they own, including Lancome and Kiehl's.

***Uva ursi* extract**. *See* arbutin and bearberry extract.

UVB. Ultra-violet **B** radiation. *See* UVA.

VA/crotonates. Film-forming agent. *See* film-forming agent.

VA/crotonates copolymer. *See* VA/crotonates.

Vaccinium myrtillus. *See* bilberry extract.

valine. *See* amino acid.

***Vanilla planifolia* fruit extract**. Extract used primarily as a fragrance and flavoring agent. The vanilla plant is a source of catechins (also known as polyphenols), which exhibit antioxidant activity and serve as anti-inflammatory agents (Source: *Drugs Experimental Clinical Research*, 2004; 30(1):1–10).

vascular endothelial growth factor (VEGF). Stimulates the growth of blood vessels. *See* human growth factor.

verbena extract. Fragrant extract that can be a skin irritant.

vetiver oil or extract. Fragrant component in skin-care products that also has some antibacterial properties (Source: *Applied Microbiology*, June 1999, pages 985–990). It can also be a skin sensitizer.

***Viola tricolor* extract**. *See* pansy extract.

vitamin A. Considered a good antioxidant in some of its various forms, particularly as retinol and retinyl palmitate. *See* retinol and Paula's article, "Vitamin A: Retinol," at www.cosmeticscop.com.

vitamin B1. *See* thiamine HCL.

vitamin B12. May be effective in the treatment of psoriasis (Source: *Dermatology*, 2001, volume 203, number 2, pages 141–147). Overall there is limited research showing vitamin B12 has any benefit when applied topically on skin.

vitamin B2. There is no research showing this has any benefit when applied topically to skin. However, there is a small amount of research showing that riboflavin may be photosensitizing and thus cause the breakdown of skin (Sources: *Free Radical Biology and Medicine*, 1997, volume 22, number 7, pages 1139–1144; and *Toxicology Letters*, August 1985, pages 211–217).

vitamin B3. *See* niacinamide.

vitamin B5. Also known as pantothenic acid. *See* pantothenic acid.

vitamin B6. There is no research showing it to have benefit for skin.

vitamin C. Considered a potent antioxidant for skin (Sources: *Journal of Investigative Dermatology*, February 2002, pages 372–379, and June 2001, pages 853–859; and *Toxicology in Vitro*, August–October 2001, pages 357–362). Claims that vitamin C can prevent or eliminate wrinkling are not proven. An article in *Plastic and Reconstructive Surgery* (January 2000, pages 464–465) discussed the issue of vitamin C and concluded that "Vitamin C is a valuable antioxidant and protectant against photodamage that is created by sunlight in both the UVB and UVA bands.... Although oral supplementation may also be useful, topical preparations are able to deliver a higher dosage to the needed area. Topical vitamin C does not absorb or block harmful ultraviolet radiation like a sunscreen. Instead, it augments the skin's ability to neutralize reactive oxygen singlets [free-radical damage] that are created by the ultraviolet radiation, thereby preventing photodamage to the skin. It becomes an integral part of the skin and remains unaffected by bathing, exercise, clothing, or makeup. Used appropriately, topical vitamin C is an important adjunct to the use of sunscreens, an adjunctive treatment to lessen erythema [redness] in skin resurfacing, a helpful adjunct or an alternative to Retin-A in the treatment of fine wrinkles, and a stimulant to wound healing." *See* Paula's article, "Vitamin C," at www.cosmeticscop.com.

vitamin D. Provides no known benefit for skin when applied topically, though it may have antioxidant benefits. Vitamin D formed in the skin by sunlight, or in an oral supplement form, is essential for health. *See* Paula's article, "Vitamin D," at www.cosmeticscop.com.

vitamin E. Considered an antioxidant superstar. Vitamin E is a lipid-soluble vitamin (meaning it likes fat better than water) that has eight different forms, of which some are known for being excellent antioxidants when applied topically to skin, particularly alpha tocopherol and the tocotrienols (Sources: *Current Problems in Dermatology*, 2001, volume 29, pages 26–42; *Free Radical Biology and Medicine*, May 1997, pages 761–769; *Journal of Nutrition*, February 2001, pages 369S–373S; and *International Journal of Radiation Biology*, June 1999, pages 747–755). However, other studies have indicated the acetate form (tocopherol acetate) is also bioavailable and protective for skin (Source: *Journal of Cosmetic Science*, January–February 2001, pages 35–50), and still other research points to tocopherol sorbate as providing significant antioxidant protection against ultraviolet radiation–induced oxidative damage (Source: *Journal of Investigative Dermatology*, April 1995, pages 484–488). Pointing to the significance of vitamin E for skin is an article in the *Journal of Molecular Medicine* (January 1995, pages 7–17), which states: "More than other tissues, the skin is exposed to numerous environmental chemical and physical agents such as ultraviolet light causing oxidative stress [free-radical damage]. In the skin this results in several short- and long-term adverse effects such as erythema [redness], edema [swelling], skin thickening, wrinkling, and an increased incidence of skin cancer.... Vitamin E is the major naturally occurring lipid-soluble ... antioxidant protecting skin from the adverse effects of oxidative stress including photoaging [sun damage]. Many studies document that vitamin E occupies a central position as a highly efficient antioxidant, thereby providing possibilities to decrease the frequency and severity of pathological events in the skin." *See* Paula's article, "Vitamin E," at www.cosmeticscop.com.

vitamin F. Name sometimes used to represent essential fatty acids of linoleic acid and linolenic acid. These are considered essential fatty acids (EFA) because they cannot be produced by the body. There are many fatty acids that have benefit for skin, including arachidonic, eicosapentaenoic, docosahexaenoic, and oleic acids to name a few. These all have emollient, water-binding, and often antioxidant properties for skin. *See* gamma linolenic acid and linoleic acid.

vitamin H. *See* biotin.

vitamin K. Some cosmetics companies sell creams and lotions containing vitamin K, claiming it can reduce or eliminate surfaced spider veins (technically referred to as telangiectasias). These creams cannot change spider veins. The only research concerning vitamin K's effectiveness on skin or surfaced spider veins comes from the companies that sell these products. There are no published or peer-reviewed studies that add up to results you can even remotely count on (Source: *Archives of Dermatology*, December 1998, pages 1512–1514). *See* Paula's article "Vitamin K," at www.cosmeticscop.com.

***Vitis vinifera*.** Latin name for the vines that produce wine grapes. *See* grape seed oil and grape seed extract.

***Vitreoscilla* ferment.** Made from a bacterium that can help cells utilize oxygen better in vitro (Source: *Journal of Biotechnology*, January 2001, pages 57–66). Whether that effect can be translated to benefit skin cells via a cosmetic formulation is unknown.

volatile oil. Group of volatile fluids derived primarily from plants and used in cosmetics primarily as fragrant additives. These components most often include a mix of alcohols, ketones, phenols, linalool, borneol, terpenes, camphor, pinene, acids, ethers, aldehydes, and sulfur, all of which have extremely irritating and sensitizing effects on skin.

VP/hexadecene copolymer. Synthetic polymer. *See* film-forming agent.

walnut extract. Extract that can have antioxidant properties (Source: *Journal of Nutrition*, November 2001, pages 2837–2842). There is no research showing this has any benefit for skin.

walnut oil. Emollient, nonfragrant plant oil. *See* natural moisturizing factor (NMF).

walnut-shell powder. Abrasive used in scrub products; not preferred to polyethylene beads.

water. The most widely used cosmetic ingredient; water is almost always listed first on an ingredient label because it is usually the ingredient with the highest concentration. Yet, despite claims of the skin's need for hydration and the claims regarding special types of water used, it turns out that water may not be an important ingredient for skin. Only a 10% concentration of water in the outer layer of skin is necessary for softness and pliability in this part of the epidermis (Source: *Skin Pharmacology and Applied Skin Physiology*, November-December 1999, pages 344–351). Studies that have compared the water content of dry skin to that of normal or oily skin do not find a statistically significant difference in moisture levels between them (Source: *Journal of Cosmetic Chemistry*, September/October 1993, page 249). Further, too much water in the skin can be a problem because it can disrupt the skin's intercellular matrix, the substances that keep skin cells bonded to each other (Source: *Contact Dermatitis*, December 1999, pages 311–314). The most significant aspect of the skin's health is the structural organization of the intercellular lipids and the related materials that keep skin intact and prevent water loss (Sources: *Trends in Cell Biology*, August 2002, page 355; and *Journal of the American Academy of Dermatology*, August 2002, pages 198–208). *See* natural moisturizing factor (NMF).

water-binding agent. Wide range of ingredients that help skin retain water (moisture). Glycerin is one of the more typical and effective water-binding agents used in cosmetics. One group of water-binding agents can mimic the skin's actual structure and can be of benefit in a formulation; these include ceramide, lecithin, glycerin, polysaccharides, hyaluronic acid, sodium hyaluronate, mucopolysaccharides, sodium PCA, collagen, elastin, proteins, amino acids, cholesterol, glucose, sucrose, fructose, glycogen, phospholipids, glycosphingolipids, and glycosaminoglycans. No single one of these is preferred over another because even though they are all effective, none of them can permanently change the actual structure of skin. *See* natural moisturizing factor (NMF).

watercress extract. There is a small amount of research showing that dietary intake of watercress can inhibit the proliferation of breast and other cancer cells (Sources: *Journal of Applied Pharmacology*, December 2005, pages 105–113; and *Expert Opinion on Pharmacotherapy*, December 2004, pages 2485–2501). Research also indicates that watercress extracts can have antioxidant activity, but that information is limited (Source: *Applied Biochemistry and Microbiology*, July 2001, pages 392–399). However, it is important to note that this research was carried out either in vitro or as animal experiments, definitely not in skin-care products.

wheat germ glycerides. Used as emollient and thickening agents in cosmetics. *See* glyceryl ester and natural moisturizing factor (NMF).

wheat germ oil. Emollient plant oil similar to all nonfragrant plant oils. *See* natural moisturizing factor (NMF).

wheat protein. *See* natural moisturizing factor (NMF) and protein.

whey. Milk contains two primary proteins, casein and whey. When cheese is produced these more liquid components, whey and casein, are separated from the cheese. When eaten or taken in oral supplements, whey protein can have significant antioxidant properties (Source: *Journal of Dairy Science*, December 2001, pages 2577–2583) as well as anticancer properties (Source: *Anticancer Research*, November–December 2000, pages 4785–4792) because it generates the production of glutathione in the body, which is a significant antioxidant. Whether or not any of those benefits translate into benefit for skin is unknown. In skin-care products it is most likely a good water-binding agent.

white nettle. Contains components that can have both anti-irritant as well as inflammatory properties (Source: www.bastyr.org/academic/botmed/herbs.asp?Herbld=5).

white oak bark extract. *See* oak root extract.

white tea leaf extract. Extract from the minimally processed buds and leaves of green tea. There is research showing that white and green teas have the highest concentration of antioxidant properties (via their polyphenol and flavonoid content) of all teas, and several in vitro and animal studies have shown that green tea and white tea have anticancer and antimutagenic properties. However, even though tea flavonoids are effective antioxidants, it is unclear to what extent they increase the antioxidant capacity of humans, and there is no research showing what their activity means for skin. It appears that white and green teas have similar amounts of the polyphenol epigallocatechin-3-gallate (EGCG), which is the main antioxidant in tea. The conclusion to be drawn is that white and green tea have nearly identical antioxidant activity (Source: *Biochemical and Biophysical Research Communications*, volume 296, issue 3, August 23, 2002, pages 584–588.) *See* green tea.

white willow. *See* willow bark.

wild ginger. *See* ginger extract.

wild yam extract. The roots of wild yams were used in the first commercial production of oral contraceptives, topical hormones, androgens, estrogens, progesterones, and other sex hormones. Diosgenin, a component of wild yam, is promoted as a natural precursor to dehydroepiandrosterone (DHEA). Some wild yam products are promoted as "natural DHEA." Although diosgenin can be converted to steroidal compounds, including DHEA, in the laboratory, this chemical synthesis does not occur in the human body. So taking wild yam extracts orally will not increase DHEA levels in humans (Source: www.naturaldatabase.com). There is no research showing that wild yam has any effectiveness when applied topically on skin. If anything, the studies that do exist demonstrate that topical application of wild yam has little to no effect on menopausal symptoms (Source: *Climacteric*, June 2001, pages 144–150). *See* DHEA.

willow bark. Contains salicin, a substance that when taken orally is converted by the digestive process to salicylic acid (beta hydroxy acid). The process of converting the salicin in willow bark to salicylic acid requires the presence of enzymes, and is complex. Further, salicin, much like salicylic acid, is stable only under acidic conditions. The likelihood that willow bark in the tiny amount used in cosmetics can mimic the effectiveness of salicylic acid is at best questionable, and in all likelihood impossible. However, willow bark may indeed have some anti-inflammatory benefits for skin because, in this form, it appears to retain more of its aspirin-like composition.

willow herb. *See Epilobium angustifolium* extract.

wintergreen oil. Can be very irritating and sensitizing (Source: www.naturaldatabase.com). *See* counter-irritant.

witch hazel. Can have potent antioxidant properties (Sources: *Phytotherapy Research*, June 2002, pages 364–367; and *Journal of Dermatological Science*, July 1995, pages 25–34) and some anti-irritant properties (Source: *Skin Pharmacology and Applied Skin Physiology*, March-April 2002, pages 125–132). However, according to the *Consumer's Dictionary of Cosmetic Ingredients* (Sixth Edition, Ruth Winter, 2005, Three Rivers Press), "Witch hazel has an ethanol [alcohol] content of 70 to 80 percent and a tannin content of 2 to 9 percent. Witch hazel water … contains 15% ethanol." The alcohol can be an irritant. Witch hazel's high tannin content (and tannin is a potent antioxidant), can also be irritating when used repeatedly on skin, although when used for initial swelling from burns it can reduce inflammation. *See* tannin.

xanthan gum. Used as a thickening agent.

Xi xin. *See* ginger extract.

***Ximenia americana* oil**. Plum oil; it can have emollient properties.

xylitol. *See* sorbitol.

xylose. Form of sugar. Similar to other sugars, xylose has water-binding properties for skin.

xymenynic acid. Synthetic fatty acid that functions as a skin-conditioning agent.

yarrow extract. Extract for which there is little research showing it to have any benefit for skin. What studies do exist were performed in vitro, and indicate that it may have anti-inflammatory properties (Sources: *Planta Medica*, 1991, volume 57, pages 444–446, and 1994, volume 60, pages 37–40). However, yarrow also has properties that may cause skin irritation and photosensitivity (Source: *Healthnotes Review of Complementary and Integrative Medicine*, www.healthwell.com/healthnotes/herb).

yeast. Group of fungi that ferment sugars. Yeast is a source of beta-glucan, which is a good antioxidant. Yeasts are basically fungi that grow as single cells, producing new cells either by budding or fission (splitting). Because it reproduces well, *Saccharomyces cerevisiae* is the organism that is most widely used in biotechnology. Nevertheless, some forms of yeast are human pathogens, such as *Cryptococcus* and *Candida albicans*.

In relation to skin, there is limited information about how *Saccharomyces cerevisiae* may provide a benefit. Live yeast-cell derivatives have been shown to stimulate wound healing (Source: *Archives of Surgery*, May 1990, pages 641–646), but research about this is scant. Much of what is known about yeast's effects for skin is theoretical, and concerns yeast's tissue-repair and protective properties (Source: *Global Cosmetic Industry*, November 2001, pages 12–13) or yeast's antioxidant properties (Source: *Nature Genetics*, December 2001, pages 426–434). As a skin-care ingredient yeast has potential, but what its function may be or how it would affect skin is not fully understood.

yerba mate extract. Used for the preparation of the most popular tea-like beverage in South America. It has anti-inflammatory and antioxidant properties (Sources: *Fitoterapia*, November 2001, pages 774–778; and *Life Sciences*, June 2002, pages 693–705).

ylang ylang. Fragrant, volatile oil that can also be a skin irritant. *See* volatile oil.

yogurt. There is no research showing that yogurt is effective when applied topically on skin. Yogurt consumption may negatively impact those with atopic dermatitis (Source: *The Journal of Dermatology*, February 2003, pages 91-97).

yucca extract. Plant extract that can have anti-inflammatory benefits.

Zanthoxylum piperitum. *See* Szechuan pepper.

zeolite. Group of minerals used as an absorbent in cosmetics. Zeolites been shown to have anticancer properties (Source: *Journal of Cancer Research and Clinical Oncology*, January 2002, pages 37–44).

zinc. There is growing evidence that zinc can be a significant anti-irritant and antioxidant. It also can have anti-acne benefits when combined with a topical antibiotic such as erythromycin. Taken orally, zinc may have positive effects for wound healing and other health benefits (Sources: *Dermatologic Surgery*, July 2005, pages 837–847; *International Journal of Dermatology*, September 2002, pages 606–611; and *Journal of the European Academy of Dermatology and Venereology*, September 1998, pages 13–19).

zinc carbonate. *See* calamine.

zinc gluconate. Combination of zinc with a form of glucose (a sugar) that is commonly used in cold lozenges for its antiviral effects. A study reported in *Dermatology* (2001, volume 203, issue 2, page 40) evaluated "the place of zinc gluconate in relation to antibiotics in the treatment of *Acne vulgaris*. Zinc was compared to minocycline [an antibiotic] in a multicenter randomized double-blind trial. 332 patients received either 30 milligrams elemental zinc or 100 milligrams minocycline over 3 months. The primary endpoint was defined as the percentage of the clinical success rate on day 90...." The study concluded that "Minocycline and zinc gluconate are both effective in the treatment of inflammatory acne, but minocycline has a superior effect evaluated to be 17% in our study." Whether or not this relates to topical applications is unknown. Note, however, that high doses of zinc can be toxic, so avoid taking more than 100 mg of zinc per day from a supplement (Source: www.drweil.com).

zinc oxide. Inert earth mineral used as a thickening, whitening, lubricating, and sunscreen ingredient in cosmetics. Along with titanium dioxide, zinc oxide is considered to have no risk of skin irritation. It can also be an anti-irritant and potentially an antioxidant (Sources: *Journal of Postgraduate Medicine*, July 2004, pages 131–139; *International Journal of Dermatology*, July 2003, page 505; *Wound Repair and Regeneration*, May 2002, page 130; *Alternative Therapies in Health and Medicine*, May–June 2001, pages 49–56; and *Scandinavian Journal of Plastic and Reconstructive Surgery*, December 1994, pages 255–259.) *See* UVA and zinc.

zinc phenolsulfonate. Antimicrobial agent that can also be a skin irritant.

zinc sulfate. Chemical compound resulting from the interaction of zinc with sulfuric acid. There is little research showing this to be beneficial for skin. The little information that is available shows that it does not help skin healing (Source: *Acta Dermato-Venereologica*, 1990, volume 154, Supplemental, pages 1–36) and it can be a skin irritant. *See* zinc.

***Zingiber officinale* Roscoe**. *See* ginger extract.

Zingiber zerumbet. *See* ginger extract.

Zingiberaceae. *See* ginger extract.